Dele Oguns

KOENIG AND SCHULTZ'S DISASTER MEDICINE

Second Edition

As societies become more complex and interconnected, the global risk for catastrophic disasters is increasing. Demand for expertise to mitigate the human suffering and damage these events cause is also high. A new field of disaster medicine is emerging, offering innovative approaches intended to optimize disaster management. However, much of the information needed to create the foundation for this growing specialty is not objectively described or is scattered among multiple different sources.

This definitive work brings together a coherent and comprehensive collection of scientific observations and evidence-based recommendations with expert contributors from around the globe. This book identifies essential subject matter, clarifies nomenclature, and outlines necessary areas of proficiency for healthcare professionals handling mass casualty crises. It also describes in-depth strategies for the rapid diagnosis and treatment of victims suffering from blast injuries or exposure to chemical, biological, and radiological agents.

Dr. Kristi L. Koenig, Professor of Emergency Medicine and Public Health, Director of Public Health Preparedness, and Director of the Center for Disaster Medical Sciences at the University of California, Irvine, is an internationally recognized expert in the fields of homeland security, disaster and emergency medicine, emergency management, and emergency medical services. During the U.S. terrorist attacks of 9/11, she served as National Director of the Emergency Management Office for the Federal Department of Veterans Affairs. Professor Koenig is a Fulbright Scholar and fellow of the International Federation for Emergency Medicine. She holds multiple appointments including Visiting Professor at universities in Australia, Italy, and Belgium. With a strong health policy and academic background, including more than 100 peer-reviewed publications and nearly 500 invited lectures in about 35 countries, she is widely sought for presentations at regional, national, and international forums.

Dr. Carl H. Schultz is a Professor of Emergency Medicine and the Director of Research at the Center for Disaster Medical Sciences, University of California, Irvine, School of Medicine. He is an internationally recognized expert and researcher in the fields of disaster and emergency medicine. He has written more than 100 peer-reviewed publications, and his investigations have resulted in two first-author publications in the *New England Journal of Medicine*. He chaired the Disaster Preparedness and Response Committee of the American College of Emergency Physicians and received the College's Disaster Medical Sciences Award. He has served as a consultant for the U.S. Department of Defense, the Joint Commission, and the State of Israel. Dr. Schultz holds faculty appointments at universities in Belgium and Italy.

In loving memory of my mother, whose unwavering love, guidance, and support allowed me enormous life opportunities, including the ability to create this book
And with appreciation and admiration for my students, residents, EMS and Disaster Medical Sciences Fellows, International Fellows, and the European Master of Disaster Medicine family who will continue to move the science of disaster medicine forward into the future to mitigate loss of life and human suffering from disasters

Kristi L. Koenig, MD, FACEP, FIFEM

To all the organizations worldwide that support the emerging specialty of disaster medicine
To Noriaki Aoki, MD, PhD, whose premature death robbed our specialty of a truly gifted and visionary talent, and me of a great friend
To my father, Irwin M. Schultz, MD, and in memory of my mother, Ruth L. Schultz, BSN, whose love and encouragement have sustained me throughout my career

Carl H. Schultz, MD, FACEP

Koenig and Schultz's Disaster Medicine Comprehensive Principles and Practice

Second Edition

EDITED BY

Kristi L. Koenig

University of California, Irvine, Center for Disaster Medical Sciences

Carl H. Schultz

University of California, Irvine, Center for Disaster Medical Sciences

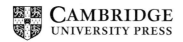
CAMBRIDGE
UNIVERSITY PRESS

CAMBRIDGE
UNIVERSITY PRESS

32 Avenue of the Americas, New York, NY 10013-2473, USA

Cambridge University Press is part of the University of Cambridge.

It furthers the University's mission by disseminating knowledge in the pursuit of education, learning, and research at the highest international levels of excellence.

www.cambridge.org
Information on this title: www.cambridge.org/9781107040755

© Kristi L. Koenig, Carl H. Schultz 2016

First published 2016

Printed in the United States of America

A catalog record for this publication is available from the British Library.

Library of Congress Cataloging in Publication Data

Names: Koenig, Kristi L., editor. | Schultz, Carl H. (Carl Herman), editor.
Title: Koenig and Schultz's disaster medicine : comprehensive principles and practice / edited by Kristi L. Koenig, Carl H. Schultz.
Other titles: Disaster medicine : comprehensive principles and practice
Description: Second edition. | Cambridge ; New York : Cambridge University Press, 2015. | Includes bibliographical references and index.
Identifiers: LCCN 2015041206 | ISBN 9781107040755
Subjects: | MESH: Disaster Medicine. | Disaster Planning. | Disasters.
Classification: LCC RA645.9 | NLM WA 295 | DDC 616 – dc23
LC record available at http://lccn.loc.gov/2015041206

Contents

CONTRIBUTORS

Ernest B. Abbott, JD, MPP practices emergency management law at Baker Donelson in Washington, DC, after 12 years at FEMA Law Associates, PLLC and four years' service as General Counsel of FEMA (from 1997 to 2001). He is a graduate of Harvard Law School and a frequent author, editor, and speaker on emergency management law. He is coeditor of *A Legal Guide to Homeland Security and Emergency Management* and adjunct professor of Disaster Law at the George Washington University Law School.

Carl Adrianopoli, PhD, MS is the Regional Administrator for the Office of Preparedness and Emergency Operations in the U.S. Department of Health and Human Services, Federal Region V. He represented the Department of Homeland Security in the multi–federal agency development of the *Excessive Heat Events Guidebook* (2006) and most recently was one of the co-authors on a Presidential Climate Change Work Group. He has presented and published numerous papers on extreme heat events and integrated response to disasters including the uses of Chemical, Biologic, Radiologic, Nuclear and Explosive Weapons of Mass Destruction. He deployed in response to the 1995 Chicago Heat Wave, the World Trade Center disaster in 2001, Hurricane Katrina in 2005, the Florida Hurricanes in 2004–2005, the BP Oil Spill in 2010 and the Unaccompanied, Migrant Children's Mission in Nogales, Arizona in 2014.

Jamie Agius, BA, MA is an environmental engineering teacher at a secondary charter school in Pacific Palisades, CA. She holds a BA in Urban Studies with a focus on Environmental Sustainability and an MA in Teaching from the University of California, Irvine. While attending UC Irvine, she conducted research with the Center for Unconventional Security Affairs in the areas of climate change mitigation and adaptation projects in peacebuilding, as well as on climate change and emergency medicine.

George J. Annas, JD, MPH is the Warren Distinguished Professor at Boston University, and Chair of the Department of Health Law, Bioethics & Human Rights at Boston University School of Public Health. He is the cofounder of Global Lawyers and Physicians, a transnational professional association of lawyers and physicians working together to promote human rights and health. He is the author or editor of 20 books on health law and bioethics, including *Worst Case Bioethics: Death, Disaster, and Public Health*.

Donna Barbisch, RN, MPH, DHA, a retired U.S. Army Major General, is President of Wicked Solutions and Senior Policy Advisor for the Center for Disaster Medical Sciences at UC Irvine. She is a visionary who drives senior leader decision-making to improve threat reduction and outcomes associated with catastrophic disasters. She is widely published and frequently an invited speaker at national and international meetings on building resilience and the process and policy underlying preparedness.

Peter J. Baxter, MD recently retired as consultant physician in occupational and environmental medicine at the University of Cambridge and Addenbrooke's University Hospital, Cambridge. He has researched the human impacts of volcanic eruptions and advised governments and the World Health Organization since his involvement with the eruption of Mount St. Helens in 1980, when he was a medical epidemiologist at the U.S. Centers for Disease Control and Prevention in Atlanta. He has also advised the U.K. government on the public health effects of air quality standards, major industrial incidents, climate change, and other disasters. He is honorary visiting research fellow in the Institute of Public Health at the University of Cambridge.

COL David M. Benedek, MD is Professor/Deputy Chair, Department of Psychiatry, Uniformed Services University School of Medicine and Associate Director/Senior Scientist at the University's Center for the Study of Traumatic Stress. He has authored over 100 publications and has presented extensively on military, disaster, and forensic psychiatry at regional, national, and international conferences. Dr. Benedek is a Distinguished Fellow of the American Psychiatric Association (APA) and past president of the APA's military district branch. He was principal consultant to the APA's Practice Guideline working group in their development of the Practice Guideline for the Treatment of Acute Stress Disorder and Posttraumatic Stress Disorder (PTSD), lead author of the APA's subsequent PTSD Guideline Watch and co-editor of the APA's Clinical Manual for Management of PTSD.

Ulf Björnstig, MD, PhD is Senior Professor of Surgery at Umeå University in Sweden. He is the Deputy Director of the Center for Disaster Medicine at Umeå University, as well as Director of Traffic Safety Center North. He has published 135 original scientific articles and approximately 75 book chapters, traffic safety plans, and other articles. Dr. Björnstig was Traffic Safety Director in the Swedish National Road Administration from 1998 to 2000. He holds several board positions in national and international scientific organizations.

Connie J. Boatright-Royster, MSN, RN, COL, USA (Ret.) is a Senior Crisis and Continuity Advisor with the MESH Coalition, a partner of the Indiana University Schools of Medicine and Nursing. She also serves as faculty for the Federal Emergency Management Agency (FEMA) national Center for Domestic Preparedness. An expert in emergency management in healthcare, COL Boatright-Royster served for over 20 years as a national leader in the Department of Veterans Affairs Emergency Management System, where she contributed significantly to national disaster medicine standards and guidelines.

Linda B. Bourque, PhD is Professor in the Department of Community Health Sciences in the Fielding School of Public Health at the University of California at Los Angeles, where she teaches research methodology with focus on the design, data processing and analysis of data collected with questionnaires in population-based surveys. Her professional interests include impacts of natural, technological and human-initiated disasters on communities and household preparedness for disasters, with an emphasis on preparedness for earthquakes in California, and ophthalmic clinical trials. Her publications are featured in several journals, including in *Environment and Behavior*, *Risk Analysis*, and *Earthquake Spectra*.

Peter W. Brewster, BS is the Program Manager, Strategic Planning/Quality for the Office of Emergency Management, Veterans Health Administration (VHA). He participates on several National Fire Protection Association technical committees and supports the Emergency Management Accreditation Program as an assessor and member of the Program Review Committee. In 2011–2012, Mr. Brewster was detailed to the Department of Health and Human Services, Assistant Secretary for Preparedness and Response as the Acting Director, National Disaster Medical System. His experience prior to joining VHA includes work as an Emergency Management Coordinator for the Consolidated City of Indianapolis/Marion County, and with the National Park Service at Grand Teton National Park and the U.S. Forest Service in Medicine Bow National Forest in Wyoming.

Sharon W. Bryson, MC is the Director of the Office of Transportation Disaster Assistance at the National Transportation Safety Board. Prior to serving on the Board, she worked as the Director of the Family Support Center at Dover Air Force Base. She served as adjunct faculty in psychology and sociology at Wilmington College, Wesley College, and the University of Delaware. She is certified by the National Board for Certified Counselors and is a Licensed Professional Counselor of Mental Health.

Frederick M. Burkle, Jr., MD, MPH, DTM, FAAP, FACEP has extensive global experience, research and publications relating to complex emergencies. He has worked for nongovernmental agencies, the World Health Organization, the Red Cross, the U.S. government, and the military. He is a Senior International Public Policy Scholar at the Woodrow Wilson International Center for Scholars, a Senior Fellow and Scientist at the Harvard Humanitarian Initiative, Harvard School of Public Health, a Senior Associate in the Departments of International Health and Emergency Medicine at Johns Hopkins, and an elected member of the Institute of Medicine, National Academy of Sciences.

Glenn Burns, MD, FACEP is an emergency physician and Associate Professor of Emergency Medicine and Military Medicine. Over his career, he has engaged with key international partners in developing military medical education curricula and training programs for point-of-injury care, medical disaster leadership, medical response to weapons of mass destruction and child/family reintegration in disaster response. He has published on medical leadership education, blast injury, tactical combat casualty care, mass casualty response and point-of-injury care.

Theodore J. Cieslak, MD, FAAP, FIDSA received his MD degree at the Ohio State University prior to completing a Pediatric Residency at Baylor and Infectious Disease fellowship at Walter Reed. Retired from the U.S. Army after a 30-year career, notable assignments included: Chairman of Pediatrics in San Antonio, Defense Department Liaison to CDC, and Chief of Operational Medicine at USAMRIID. He also served as Biodefense Consultant to the Army Surgeon General and as Head of delegation to NATO's Biomedical Advisory Council. He recently joined the faculty at the University of Nebraska's School of Public Health.

David C. Cone, MD is Professor of Emergency Medicine and EMS Section Chief at the Yale University School of Medicine in New Haven, Connecticut. A graduate of the European Master in Disaster Medicine, he has worked in emergency medical services for 30 years and as a firefighter for 15. Dr. Cone has served as Medical Team Manager for two urban search-and-rescue task forces. He is a past president of the National Association of EMS Physicians and editor-in-chief of the journal *Academic Emergency Medicine*.

Adam W. Darkins, MBChB, MPHM, MD, FRCS is Vice President for Medical Affairs and Enterprise Technology Development for Medtronic Plc. He formerly led the National Telehealth Program at the U.S. Department of Veterans Affairs. With a clinical background in Neurosurgery and in health services development in the U.S. and UK; his background as a clinician, healthcare executive, and director of enterprise technology programs gives him unique insights into developing virtual care services to increase access to healthcare. Dr. Darkins is internationally recognized as an expert in developing the clinical, technology and business processes necessary to create and sustain new models of healthcare delivery.

Zygmunt F. Dembek, COL (USAR, Ret), PhD, MS, MPH, LHD (Hon) is an internationally recognized bioterrorism preparedness and public health expert. He has authored over 80 publications, many directly relevant to civilian and military defense against bioterrorism and biological weapons; served as Senior Editor for the *Textbook of Military Medicine: Medical Aspects* *of Biological Warfare 2007;* and as the lead editor for USAM-RIID's *Medical Management of Biological Casualties Handbook (Blue Book) 7th Edition, 2011.*

William H. Dice, MD is Assistant Professor in the Department of Emergency Medicine at the State University of New York, Buffalo. He has more than 35 years of experience with disasters, humanitarian assistance, preparedness training, and response. He has served as Director for Emergency Planning in the Office of the Assistant Secretary of Defense for Health Affairs, and as Department of Defense Liaison to Emergency Support Function 8 for Hurricane Andrew. He is an alpine patroller for the National Ski Patrol and is an emergency preparedness consultant for county and state departments of health.

Rebecca Forsberg, RN, PhD holds a BA in peace and conflict management. She works as a researcher and project manager at the Center for Disaster Medicine at Umeå University, Umeå, Sweden. Dr. Forsberg has worked many years with research and development with a focus on passenger safety within the rail-bound transport system. The work is supported by the Swedish National Board for Health and Welfare.

Shantini D. Gamage, PhD, MPH is a Health Science Epidemiologist with the Department of Veterans Affairs (VA), National Infectious Diseases Service, where she focuses on translating science and epidemiologic data into infectious diseases policy in the healthcare setting. She has contributed to numerous national VA and interagency biopreparedness initiatives, including the National Biosurveillance Integration System and the National Biosurveillance Science and Technology Roadmap. She holds an adjunct affiliation with the University of Cincinnati College of Medicine where she lectures on infectious diseases and public health policy.

Ronald E. Goans, MD, PhD, MPH is an Associate Professor at the Tulane School of Public Health and Tropical Medicine and Senior Scientist at the Radiation Emergency Assistance Center/Training Site. He is also the senior medical adviser at MJW Corporation, a major health physics consulting firm. His current research activities include development of early radiation triage techniques and the mathematical modeling of local and systemic radiation damage.

Susan E. Gorman, BS, PharmD, MS, DABAT, FAACT is the Associate Director for Science, Division of Strategic National Stockpile, U.S. CDC. Her primary roles include oversight of the stockpile formulary and provision of technical and scientific advice on pharmacological and toxicological issues regarding the stockpile. She participates in numerous intergovernmental counterterrorism working groups involving radiological, chemical, and biological agents. She is a nationally and internationally recognized speaker on stockpiling for terrorist events and other large-scale public health emergencies.

James E. Gosney, MD, MPH, MS serves as the chair of the Committee on Rehabilitation Disaster Relief (CRDR) of the International Society of Physical and Rehabilitation Medicine (ISPRM) which advocates for the emerging disaster medicine specialization of disaster rehabilitation. He is a peer-reviewed author, journal reviewer, and speaker on this topic and has performed related research following large-scale disasters in China, Haiti, and the

Philippines. He is also coauthor of the chapter "Natural Disasters, Health-related Aspects" in *The International Encyclopedia of the Social & Behavioral Sciences, 2nd edition.*

Lawrence O. Gostin, JD is University Professor (Georgetown University's highest academic rank), O'Neill Chair in Global Health Law, and Director of the O'Neill Institute for National and Global Health Law. Professor Gostin holds international professorial appointments at Oxford University, University of Witwatersrand, and Melbourne University. He is Director of the WHO Collaborating Center on Public Health Law & Human Rights, and serves on expert WHO advisory committees on mental health, international health regulations, and pandemic influenza preparedness. Professor Gostin holds several editorial appointments, notably for the *Journal of the American Medical Association.*

Richard J. Hatchett, MD is Chief Medical Officer and Deputy Director of the U.S. Biomedical Advanced Research and Development Authority (BARDA), where he oversees programs to develop medical countermeasures against chemical, biological, radiological and nuclear threats, pandemic influenza, and emerging infectious diseases. Previously, he was Director for Medical Preparedness Policy on the White House National Security Staff and Associate Director for Radiation Medical Countermeasures and Emergency Preparedness at the National Institutes of Health. He completed a fellowship in medical oncology at Duke University Medical Center.

Josef Haik, MD, MPH is Professor of Plastic and Reconstructive Surgery, Director of the Division of Plastic and Reconstructive Surgery and Director of the National Burn Center at the Sheba Medical Center, affiliated with the University of Tel Aviv, Israel. He is a leader in burn management in Israel, a member of the Israeli Council of Trauma, chairman of the Israel Burn Prevention Committee, and serves as a civilian and military advanced trauma life support instructor. Professor Haik is an active reserve forces captain in the Israeli Defense Forces. He is an established author in the burn management literature and serves as a reviewer for the Journal of Burns. Dr. Haik is an awardee of the Talpiyot Medical Leadership Program.

James G. Hodge, Jr., JD is Associate Dean and Professor of Public Health Law and Ethics at the Sandra Day O'Connor College of Law, Arizona State University (ASU). Through scholarship, teaching, and varied applied and funded projects, Professor Hodge explores multiple areas of public health, law, and ethics. He is Director of ASU's Public Health Law and Policy Program and the Western Region Office of the Network for Public Health Law. He has published extensively on law, medicine, public health, and bioethics topics, notably including emergency legal and ethical preparedness.

John D. Hoyle, Sr., MHA, CHE, LFACHE has been active in disaster medical preparedness and response for 35 years. He was a hospital executive for 31 years, including 22 years as CEO of a three-hospital system. He served as National Disaster Medical System Hospital Coordinator in greater Cincinnati for 19 years and led a Disaster Medical Assistance Team for 15 years. He has responded to numerous hurricanes, airline crashes, the World Trade Center disaster, and medical preparedness operations for the Olympics in Atlanta and Salt Lake City. He also has served as commissioned officer in the U.S. Public Health Service.

Irving Jacoby, MD, FACP, FACEP, FAAEM is Emeritus Professor of Emergency Medicine at the UCSD School of Medicine. He is an attending physician in the ED, and served as Hospital Director for Emergency Preparedness and Response. As Commander of the San Diego Disaster Medical Assistance Team (DMAT CA-4), he has responded to more than 18 federally-declared disasters in the U.S. and its territories. He is Disaster Section Editor for the *Journal of Emergency Medicine*, co-developer of a healthcare facilities evacuation course, and has authored numerous articles and book chapters in disaster medicine.

Christopher A. Kahn, MD, MPH is Associate Professor of Emergency Medicine and Division Chief for Emergency Medical Services and Disaster Medicine at the University of California, San Diego (UCSD). He serves as Medical Co-Director for Emergency Preparedness and Response and Base Hospital Medical Director for the UCSD Health System. He is the "NHTSA Notes" section editor for *Annals of Emergency Medicine*, having formerly trained as the National Highway Traffic Safety Administration Medical Fellow during his EMS/Disaster Medical Sciences fellowship at UC Irvine. Dr. Kahn is a member of DMAT CA-4.

Megumi Kano, DrPH is Technical Officer for the World Health Organization, Center for Health Development in Kobe, Japan. Her areas of focus are urban health, health inequity and health metrics. Her previous work includes research in disaster public health as Senior Researcher at the Southern California Injury Prevention Research Center, University of California, Los Angeles, Fielding School of Public Health.

Mark E. Keim, MD, MBA is the founder of DisasterDoc, LLC, a consulting firm specializing in disaster risk reduction as applied to health. He is recently retired from CDC. His awards include: the U.S. Department of Health and Human Services Secretary's Award for Distinguished Service (twice) and the Special Service Award. In 2015, he was nominated for the prestigious United Nations Sasakawa Award for Disaster Risk Reduction.

Ian T. R. Kennedy, BSc (ClinMed), MB ChB, FFPH is Consultant in Public Health Medicine (Communicable Disease and Environmental Health) in the Public Health Protection Unit, NHS Greater Glasgow and Clyde since August 2015. His principle interests are communicable disease epidemiology, "natural" disasters and global health. During his training he worked with a variety of organizations including Public Health England's (PHE) Extreme Events and Health Protection team, PHE Centre for Infectious Disease Surveillance and Control, and WHO Patient Safety team.

Kelly R. Klein, MD, FACEP is Associate Professor of Emergency Medicine at UT Southwestern Medical Center in Dallas, Texas, and a supervising medical officer with the MI-1 Disaster Medical Assistance Team (DMAT). She received her fellowship training in weapons of mass destruction, disaster medicine, and emergency medical services at Wayne State University/Detroit Receiving Hospital in Detroit, Michigan. She has deployed for multiple DMAT missions, including the 2009 Presidential Inauguration and Hurricane Katrina. She is an invited lecturer both nationally and internationally and has published on disaster topics in textbooks and peer-reviewed journals.

Kristi L. Koenig, MD, FACEP, FIFEM, Professor of Emergency Medicine and Public Health and Director of Public Health Preparedness at the University of California, Irvine, is an internationally recognized expert in the fields of homeland security, disaster and emergency medicine, emergency management, and emergency medical services. During the U.S. terrorist attacks of 9/11, she served as National Director of the Emergency Management Office for the Federal Department of Veterans Affairs. Professor Koenig is a Fulbright Scholar and fellow of the International Federation for Emergency Medicine. She holds multiple appointments including visiting professor at universities in Australia, Italy and Belgium. With a strong health policy and academic background, including more than 100 peer-reviewed publications and nearly 500 invited lectures in about 35 countries, she is widely sought for presentations at regional, national, and international forums.

Stephen M. Kralovic, MD, MPH is Medical Epidemiologist with the National Infectious Diseases Service for the Department of Veterans Affairs. He is an Associate Professor of Medicine in the Division of Infectious Diseases at the University of Cincinnati College of Medicine. He holds a secondary faculty appointment in the Division of Epidemiology and Biostatistics within the Department of Environmental Health. His major expertise is in infectious diseases epidemiology within large patient populations, particularly within healthcare settings.

E. Brooke Lerner, PhD is Professor at the Medical College of Wisconsin in Milwaukee. She has authored more than 90 emergency medical services and disaster-related peer-reviewed publications. She is principal investigator on federally funded research projects examining trauma triage and led the U.S. CDC–sponsored workgroup that developed the Model Uniform Core Criteria, the national guideline for mass casualty triage. She also serves on the Board of Directors of the National Disaster Life Support Foundation.

Howard W. Levitin, MD, FACEP is a practicing emergency physician at Franciscan St. Francis Health and Clinical Assistant Professor of Medicine at the Indiana University School of Medicine. He has served as subject matter expert in the areas of victim decontamination, chemical and biological weapons, medical surge capacity planning, and emergency management for hospitals, national think tanks, and government agencies. He has several publications on decontamination and emergency preparedness and speaks nationally and internationally on these topics.

Hoon Chin Steven Lim, MBBS, MRCS, FCDMS is Chief and Senior Consultant at the Accident and Emergency Department, Changi General Hospital, Singapore. Dr. Lim is an Adjunct Assistant Professor at the Yong Loo Lin School of Medicine, National University of Singapore, and is also an advanced hazmat life support course instructor. He is the vice president of the Society for Emergency Medicine in Singapore and Program Director of the Diploma in Emergency Medicine Course. He is an International Fellow at the Center for Disaster Medical Sciences, University of California, Irvine.

Jeffrey H. Luk, MD, MS is Medical Director for Emergency Medical Services, Critical Care Transport, and UH MedEvac at University Hospitals Case Medical Center, the primary teaching affiliate for Case Western Reserve University School of Medicine, in Cleveland, Ohio. He is Assistant Professor of Emergency Medicine and is board-certified in emergency medicine and EMS. He is co-chair of the Emergency Management Subcommittee at UHCMC. He is an Associate Medical Physician for the Cleveland Browns and medical director for First Energy Stadium.

Richard A. Matthew, PhD is a Professor of Planning, Policy and Design and Political Science; Director of the Blum Center for Global Engagement (http://blumcenter.uci.edu); Director of the Center for Unconventional Security Affairs (www.cusa.uci.edu); and Co-Principal Investigator of the FloodRISE Project (http://floodrise.uci.edu), all at the University of California at Irvine. He is also a member of the United Nations Expert Group on Environment, Conflict and Peacebuilding, and has served on several UN peacebuilding missions, including two he led in Sierra Leone. He has over 170 publications, including 11 books.

Kenneth T. Miller, MD, PhD serves as the Medical Director of the Orange County Fire Authority, Assistant Medical Director of the Orange County Healthcare Agency/Emergency Medical Services, and Director of Operational Medicine for the Center for Disaster Medicine Sciences at the University of California at Irvine. He is the Medical Team Manager of Federal Emergency Management Agency (FEMA) Urban Search and Rescue Task Force 5 and Medical Officer of the FEMA Urban Search and Rescue Incident Support Team.

Michael S. Molloy, MB, BAO, BCh, EMDM, MCEM, MFSEM, MFSEM (U.K.) Grad Dip Medicine (NUI), Dip Sports Med (RCSI) is an emergency medicine specialist registrar in Ireland with expertise in disaster medicine and mass gathering medical care. He completed a fellowship in disaster medicine at Beth Israel and Harvard and was awarded a master degree in disaster medicine in Europe with research focusing on alert systems for major incidents. He served as past President of the Irish Medical Organization and has been part of the Mass Gathering Medical Care team for 10 years, acting as Chief Medical Officer in recent years.

Virginia Murray, FFPH, FRCP, FFOM, FRCPath is Public Health Consultant in Global Disaster Risk Reduction for Public Health England since April 2014. This appointment is builds on her work as vice-chair of the UN International Strategy for Disaster Reduction (ISDR) Scientific and Technical Advisory Group for the Post-2015 Framework for Disaster Risk Reduction. Prior to this she was appointed as Head of Extreme Events and Health Protection, Public Health England where she led the development of evidence-based information and advice on flooding, heat, cold, volcanic ash, and other extreme weather and natural hazards events.

Jonathan Newmark, MD, FAAN, COL (ret.), Medical Corps, US Army is Adjunct Professor of Neurology at the Uniformed Services University of the Health Sciences, Bethesda, Maryland, attending neurologist at the University of Cincinnati Medical Center, Cincinnati, Ohio, and Special Government Employee in the Chemical Preparedness Program, Office of Health Affairs,

U.S. Department of Homeland Security, Washington, DC. From 2002 to 2012 he served as Chemical Casualty Care Consultant to the U.S. Army Surgeon General.

Colleen M. O'Connell, MD FRCPC is Assistant Professor, Dalhousie University Faculty of Medicine, specializing in brain and spinal cord injury and upper limb amputation rehabilitation. She is past president of the Canadian Association of Physical Medicine and Rehabilitation, and member of the International Spinal Cord Society Disaster Committee. Through research and delivery of rehabilitative care and training in low resource and disaster environments, she has collaborated with Handicap International, Team Canada Healing Hands, and the International Committee of the Red Cross Special Fund for the Disabled.

Tina L. Palmieri, MD, FACS, FCCM, is Professor and Director of the Firefighters Burn Institute Burn Center at the University of California at Davis, Assistant Chief of Burns at Shriners Hospital for Children, Northern California, and past-president of the American Burn Association. She directs the U.C. Davis Burn Data Coordinating Center and has been active in the development and conduct of international burn multicenter outcome trials for more than 10 years. She is board certified in surgery and critical care and treats burned adults and children.

David Petley, PhD is Pro-Vice-Chancellor (Research and Enterprise) at the University of East Anglia in eastern England. A geologist by background, he has worked extensively on the mechanisms of landslides and the human costs that they inflict on society. His field areas have focused on high mountain areas, often in poor countries, including Nepal, Bhutan, China, Pakistan, Taiwan and New Zealand. He has worked extensively on landslides triggered by intense rainfall (for example from monsoons and typhoons) and by earthquakes.

Betty Pfefferbaum, MD, JD is George Lynn Cross Research Professor in the Department of Psychiatry at the University of Oklahoma College of Medicine in Oklahoma City, Oklahoma. She is the Co-Director of the Terrorism and Disaster Center of the National Child Traumatic Stress Network. Her expertise is in child trauma and disaster mental health. She is a general and child psychiatrist and holds a law degree.

Rose L. Pfefferbaum, PhD, MPH is a project director with the Terrorism and Disaster Center (TDC) of the National Child Traumatic Stress Network. She is responsible for TDC community resilience activities. A recently retired Professor of Economics and Director of Terrorism and Disaster Preparedness at Phoenix Community College in Phoenix, Arizona, she has had extensive experience in community-based programs including work with community disaster response groups. Her PhD is in economics.

Brenda Phillips, PhD is Associate Dean and Professor of Sociology at Ohio University in Chillicothe. She is an author of multiple books, including *Disaster Recovery, Introduction to Emergency Management, Qualitative Disaster Research* and *Mennonite Disaster Service: Building a Therapeutic Community after the Gulf Coast Storms*. She has co-edited *Social Vulnerability to Disasters* and *Women and Disasters*. Dr. Phillips earned the Blanchard Award for excellence in emergency management education and the Myers Award for work on the effects of disasters on women.

Jean Luc Poncelet, MD, a national of Belgium, physician, Master in Public Health and Specialist in Tropical Medicine, is the Pan American Health Organization (PAHO)/ World Health Organization (WHO) representative in Haiti. Until April 2013, he directed the Emergency Response and Disaster Risk Reduction Program in the PAHO/WHO regional office for Latin America and the Caribbean. He has actively participated in almost all major emergencies that have affected the Western Hemisphere since 1986 by either leading health field response, or in PAHO's regional capacity to coordinate international health assistance in support to member states. He has many technical publications in emergency and disaster medicine.

Richard Reed, MSW is Senior Vice President, Disaster Cycle Services, American Red Cross. He leads the development and execution of programs which help Americans prepare for, respond to, and recover from disasters. His 20 years of federal government service includes positions in the Department of Veterans Affairs, Federal Emergency Management Agency, and the General Services Administration. He served at the White House as Special Assistant to the President (2006–2012), Deputy Assistant to the President (2012–2013), and Deputy Ebola Coordinator (2014–2015).

Dori B. Reissman, MD, MPH (Captain, U.S. Public Health Service) leads the World Trade Center Health Program at the National Institute for Occupational Safety and Health, within the U.S. CDC. She has deployed to many disasters, serving in both emergency operations and field positions. Dr. Reissman is an expert in disaster mental and behavioral health. She integrates resilience into command and programmatic structures dealing with worker health and safety and consults with a variety of organizations.

Barbara J. Reynolds, PhD has been a Crisis Communication Specialist at the U.S. CDC since 1991. She currently serves as an Adjunct Assistant Professor at Tulane University. Dr. Reynolds's communication expertise has been used in the planning or response to pandemic influenza, vaccine safety, emerging infectious disease outbreaks, and bioterrorism. Internationally, she has acted as a crisis communication consultant on health issues for France, Hong Kong, Australia, Canada, former Soviet Union nations, the North Atlantic Treaty Organization, and the World Health Organization.

Gary A. Roselle, MD, FACP is Director of the National Infectious Diseases Service, Department of Veterans Affairs (VA) Central Office in Washington, DC. The scope of this national program includes infectious diseases, infection prevention and control, national bioterrorism surveillance, and VA's Emerging Pathogens Initiative. Recent emphasis has been placed on control of multidrug resistant organisms and implementation of antimicrobial stewardship. Dr. Roselle is a member of the Forum on Microbial Threats of the National Academy of Sciences, Institutes of Medicine. He is also a physician on staff at the Cincinnati VA Medical Center and Professor of Medicine, Department of Internal Medicine, Division of Infectious Diseases, University of Cincinnati College of Medicine.

Shira A. Schlesinger, MD, MPH is a practicing emergency physician in Los Angeles and Orange Counties, California. She completed her Fellowship in EMS and Disaster Medical Sciences at the University of California at Irvine. Dr. Schlesinger lectures on EMS topics for both prehospital and hospital providers. Her current research focuses on Community Paramedicine. Other research interests include hospital preparedness in disaster response, quality improvement in EMS, and public health integration in emergency medicine. Dr. Schlesinger is a member of the American College of Emergency Physicians EMS Committee and the California EMS for Children Technical Advisory Committee, and serves as the EMS Section Editor for the Western Journal of Emergency Medicine.

Merritt D. Schreiber, PhD is Associate Professor of Emergency Medicine at University of California Irvine School of Medicine in the Center for Disaster Medical Sciences. He is involved in the development of best practice models bridging public health and mental health for mass casualty events. He developed the PsySTART Rapid Mental Health Triage and Incident Management System for victims and responders; a psychological first aid program called Listen, Protect and Connect; and a responder resilience system known as Anticipate-Plan-Deter. He received a special commendation from the U.S. surgeon general for his response to Hurricane Katrina and a Joint Service Meritorious Service Medal from U.S. Northern Command/Department of Defense. He was a responder to the Sandy Hook School Tragedy and the Boston Marathon Bombing.

Carl H. Schultz, MD, FACEP is Professor of Emergency Medicine and Director of Research at the Center for Disaster Medical Sciences, University of California Irvine School of Medicine. He is an internationally recognized expert and researcher in the fields of disaster and emergency medicine. He has over 100 peer-reviewed publications and his investigations have resulted in two first-author publications in the *New England Journal of Medicine*. He chaired the Disaster Preparedness and Response Committee of the American College of Emergency Physicians and has served as a consultant for the U.S. Department of Defense, The Joint Commission, and the State of Israel. Dr. Schultz holds faculty appointments at universities in Belgium and Italy.

Gilead Shenhar, MBA is Senior Consultant on Homeland Security and an expert in risk communication. He is an instructor and the academic coordinator at Tel Aviv University's Master Program for Emergency and Disaster Management. He is also an investigator at the Israel Center for Trauma Research. During large-scale emergencies, he is a national spokesperson for the public. He is also a UN expert in UNDAC. He was previously Head of Doctrine and Development for the Israeli Defense Forces, Home Front Command and assisted with planning and executing risk communication for the civilian population.

Frank Fuh-Yuan Shih, MD, PhD is Assistant Professor of Emergency Medicine at National Taiwan University in Taipei. He is also the Chief Operating Officer for the Taipei Region Emergency Operations Center in the Taiwan Department of Health. He received disaster medical preparedness fellowship training at George Washington University. He was involved in the emergency response to the 1999 Taiwan Earthquake, the severe acute respiratory syndrome epidemic in 2003, and many other incidents. He was one of the founders of the Disaster Medical Assistance Team, Urban Search and Rescue, and hazmat and biohazard response systems in Taiwan.

Judith M. Siegel, PhD, MSHyg is Professor of Public Health in the Department of Community Health Sciences, University of California at Los Angeles, Fielding School of Public Health. She investigates the impact of disaster exposure on psychological distress. She has expertise in individual and community characteristics that may increase vulnerability to disaster-related distress, as well as the factors that may mediate this relationship.

Paul S. Sledzik, MS is director of the Transportation Disaster Assistance Division of the U.S. National Transportation Safety Board. Trained as a forensic anthropologist, he specializes in forensic issues related to mass fatality events. He has responded to numerous disasters of all types. He is a Fellow of the American Academy of Forensic Sciences and has consulted for the Joint Prisoner of War/Missing in Action Accounting Command and the National Center for Missing and Exploited Children.

Laura M. Stough, PhD is Associate Professor of Educational Psychology, Fellow at the Hazard Reduction and Recovery Center, and Faculty at the Center for Disability and Development at Texas A&M University. She coedited the book *Disaster and Disability: Exchanges and Explorations* and has authored over 40 publications that explore inequities in emergency management, social, and educational services provided to individuals with disabilities. She serves on the Office of Emergency Management Disability Task Force for the State of Texas.

Samuel J. Stratton, MD, MPH, FACEP is Professor at the University of California at Los Angeles, School of Public Health and a Deputy Health Officer for the Orange County California Health Care Agency. He is also the Medical Director for the Orange County, California Health Care Agency Health Disaster Management/Emergency Medical Services Division. Dr. Stratton serves as the Editor-in Chief for the journal, *Prehospital and Disaster Medicine* and is a senior reviewer for the *Annals of Emergency Medicine*.

Hock Heng Tan, MBBS, FAMS, FRCSEd (A&E), DABT is an emergency physician and clinical toxicologist with Changi General Hospital Emergency Department, Singapore. He was involved with the Ministry of Health Disaster Site Medical Command until 2011. He directs the Clinical Toxicology Consultation Service, Joint Environmental Occupational Toxicology Clinic and is Secretary for the Toxicology Society of Singapore. He is the chief editor of the local Hazmat Basic Provider Manual and lectures at hazmat medical life support courses locally and overseas.

Ariel Tessone, MD is a physician in the Department of Plastic and Reconstructive Surgery. He is a member of the Israeli Burn Center team and the microsurgical reconstruction team located at the Sheba Medical Center and affiliated with the University of Tel Aviv, Israel. Dr. Tessone is also a specialist in breast reconstruction and oncoplastic surgery, and is an awardee of the Talpiyot Medical Leadership Program.

Arthur G. Wallace, Jr., DO, MPH, FACEP is an emergency physician at Magnum Health St. Johns Healthcare System and MedNow urgent care in Tulsa, Oklahoma. He serves as Clinical Instructor at Oklahoma State University-College of Health Sciences. He is a former member of the Senior Medical Working Group, National Disaster Medical System, and former team commander for the Oklahoma-1 Disaster Medical Assistance Team. He has been involved with disaster medical responses for 22 years and has extensive experience treating tornado victims.

David Weinstock, MD is Associate Professor of Medicine at the Dana-Farber Cancer Institute and Harvard Medical School, Associate Member of the Broad Institute and Affiliated Scientist of the Harvard Stem Cell Institute. He currently serves as the Medical Advisor for the Radiation Injury Treatment Network and a member of the National Preparedness and Response Science Board in the Office of the Assistant Secretary for Preparedness and Response, Department of Health and Human Services. He is a frequent author and lecturer on hematologic radiation toxicity management.

James C. West, MD is Assistant Professor of Psychiatry at the Uniformed Services University of the Health Sciences and Scientist at the Center for the Study of Traumatic Stress. He is a graduate of University of Michigan Medical School. As a military psychiatrist he deployed to both Iraq and Afghanistan in support of Marine Expeditionary Forces and led behavioral health services at Walter Reed National Military Medical Center. He coauthored *Psychological Responses to Disaster* in Tasman's *Psychiatry*, 4th edition.

John M. Wightman, EMT-T/P, MA, MD, FACEP, FACFE is Director of the Human Research Protections Program and Biosurety at the 711th Human Performance Wing, Air Force Research Laboratory, Wright-Patterson Air Force Base, Ohio. He is also Professor and Assistant Director for Academics, Division of Tactical Emergency Medicine, Department of Emergency Medicine, Boonshoft School of Medicine, Wright State University, Dayton, Ohio. He published the definitive review on blast injuries and has been a highly sought consultant, author, and speaker on integration of mechanistic and clinical knowledge into disaster, emergency, military, and tactical planning and response for explosive incidents.

Michele Wood, MPH, PhD is Associate Professor in the California State University, Fullerton Department of Health Science. She teaches graduate and undergraduate courses in research methods, statistics, and program design and evaluation. She holds a master degree in Community Psychology and a doctoral degree in Public Health from the Department of Community Health Sciences in the School of Public Health at the University of California at Los Angeles. Her research focus is on risk communication for disasters, including preparedness and alerts and warnings.

Andreas Ziegler, MD, MSc EMDM, MBA serves within Vienna Emergency Medical Services as Teaching Physician of the EMS Academy and CBRN Advisor. He is responsible for NBC-Defence and involved in education and training. He is a member of numerous working groups and committees regarding radiation protection and CBRN management. He was also author of the Austrian *Federal Medical Emergency Plan for Diagnosis and Treatment after Radiation Accidents*. He graduated from Vienna Medical School and acquired degrees from the Universities of Leicester, Novara and Krems.

FOREWORD

Marvin L. Birnbaum, MD, PhD

Emeritus Professor of Medicine and Physiology, University of Wisconsin

Past-President, World Association for Disaster and Emergency Medicine (WADEM)

Editor-in-Chief Emeritus of Prehospital and Disaster Medicine

Co-Editor, Health Disaster Management: Guidelines for Evaluation and Research

Medical care and public health textbooks are published to document what we know about a particular subject and what to expect when an event occurs, and to define current evidence-based best practices. Textbooks are based on the latest evidence as distilled by the authors and synthesized with their experience and knowledge. This is particularly relevant given the current state of the science in the relatively new discipline of disaster medicine. The textbook, *Disaster Medicine: Comprehensive Principles and Practices*, Second Edition, edited by Koenig and Schultz, successfully identifies this body of knowledge and presents it in an objective and accurate manner.

Assembling textbooks addressing evolving disciplines can be difficult. While there are an abundance of epidemiological descriptions of the health aspects of disasters in the peer-reviewed disaster literature, for the most part, such reports have no standardized format. Without structure, it is difficult, at best, to compare findings with those of studies conducted in other similar or dissimilar settings. Failure to identify similarities and differences between descriptions makes it difficult to establish what to expect epidemiologically or evidence as to the impacts of interventions; these difficulties threaten the external validity of the findings. External validity for such evidence is based on the same or similar findings obtained in other studies and is essential for the design of interventions aimed at reducing the risks for future disasters.

Additional challenges faced in the development of disaster medicine textbooks involve capturing all the available evidence. This can be inspiring particularly when studying disaster-related interventions. These investigations are conducted to identify the *changes* in levels of function that resulted from the implementation of an intervention. The findings are used to determine best practices for management of the needs during an emergency or disaster or for reduction of the disaster risks in a given setting. To date, interventional studies of the health aspects of disasters (relief, recovery, and risk-reduction) rarely have been published in the peer-reviewed literature. The information that does exist has been published primarily in the grey literature, and is not only unstructured, but lacks information of what changes resulted from the intervention (such as outcomes and impacts). Much

of the information provided is limited to achievement indices (how many of something was accomplished). Such information does not provide evidence as to what worked and what did not. Unstructured information is difficult to compare. Without an ability to conduct randomized, controlled trials, comparisons with other studies have remained elusive, are replete with opinions, and often do not contribute to the establishment of both external and internal validity (cause-effect). Therefore, currently, there is little evidence available to define best practices to be used in a given setting.

These factors complicate the development of a textbook on disaster medicine. The assembly of accurate and valid information is a very difficult task. Building on the worldwide success of the first edition (including translations into Arabic and Mandarin Chinese), Koenig and Schultz have assembled a cadre of seventy-six noted authorities who have been at the forefront of disaster medicine and public health responses and risk-reduction for decades. For this second edition, additional chapters have been added: Climate Change; Community Resilience; Rehabilitation of Disaster Casualties; and Landslides. The text expands its international authors and global perspectives to include content discussions from academic, military, civilian, and intergovernmental perspectives. This integrated approach coupled with scientific rigor delivers both a conceptual framework for strategic decision making as well as practical information for use in disaster management.

The task for the assembled global team of national and international experts was to sift and winnow through the available information and synthesize their findings with their own knowledge and experience. Each chapter provides a systematic review of the existing peer-reviewed and grey literature related to the assigned topic, much as is done by the systematic reviews conducted by Evidence Aid and the Cochrane Collaboration. This very difficult and lengthy process synthesizes the best information currently available. The resultant second edition of *Koenig and Schultz's Disaster Medicine: Comprehensive Principles and Practices* captures the essence of disaster medicine as we know it today. As a definitive reference, it reflects the state of the science, codifies current practices in all aspects of the field of disaster medicine, and lays the foundation for the development of a research agenda for the study of the health aspects of future disasters.

DISCLAIMER FOR ACEP

The American College of Emergency Physicians (ACEP) makes every effort to ensure that contributors to its educational products are knowledgeable subject matter experts. Readers are nevertheless advised that the statements and opinions expressed in this work are provided as the contributors' recommendations at the time of publication and should not be construed as official College policy. ACEP recognizes the complexity of emergency medicine and makes no representation that this work serves as an authoritative resource for the prevention, diagnosis, treatment, or intervention for any medical condition, nor should it be the basis for the definition of or standard of care that should be practiced by all healthcare providers at any particular time or place. To the fullest extent permitted by law, and without limitation, ACEP expressly disclaims all liability for errors or omissions contained within this work, and for damages of any kind or nature, arising out of use, reference to, reliance on, or performance of such information.

PERSPECTIVE

Carl H. Schultz

The specialty of disaster medicine has witnessed significant progress in the last 20 years. New organizations and publications have arisen as governments and societies have become more determined to address the impact of disasters. However, a brief review of just one of history's previous catastrophes illustrates how much significant work remains ahead. Although the event in question occurred in the United States, its root cause and consequences apply to all countries.

This event is a disaster that many anticipated but were unable to prevent. Multiple clues and warnings existed but were ignored. Had even one entity or person of influence attended to these alarms and responded, the tragedy would have been averted. In the end, over 2,200 people died preventable deaths. In any real sense, this event represents the quintessential challenges faced by the disaster community.

Most reading this text will probably assume the event was the attack on the World Trade Center in New York on September 11, 2001. However, this disaster occurred 125 years ago in the city of Johnstown, in the state of Pennsylvania. An earthen dam, poorly managed and maintained by disinterested parties, collapsed in a rainstorm, flooding the town downriver. The text entitled *The Johnstown Flood* by David McCullough chronicles the missteps and arrogance leading up to the disaster. This work should be mandatory reading for anyone who commits to the study of and response to disasters.

The errors committed by those responsible in the Johnstown tragedy have been repeated multiple times in the ensuing years during different disasters throughout the world, resulting in similar outcomes. A reluctance persists to invest significant resources that bolster community resilience. Governments continue to assign low priority to rigorous disaster preparedness and mitigation. In the United States, the National Disaster Medical System, which is responsible for coordinating the acute medical response after a disaster from the national level, remains largely a volunteer organization without permanent funding from the federal government. The commitment is lacking to provide this entity with appropriate resources so it can properly protect the public's safety.

Such observations support the contention that we continuously learn the same lessons without making real progress. Unfortunately, this has been true until fairly recently. The term "lessons learned" has become part of the disaster medicine lexicon and disaster responders still refer to acquired knowledge using this phrase.

In truth, knowledge is not a lesson, learned or otherwise. It is an established fact that is identified and recorded for all to acquire. It represents scientific advancement and information that should be incorporated into a growing body of knowledge. One does not find physicists or biologists referring to newly identified discoveries as "lessons learned." The perpetuation of the term "lessons learned" has its origins in the creation and development of our specialty. When disaster medicine was in its infancy, no formal educational curriculum or scientific journal dedicated to the field existed. As individuals accepted appointments to disaster-related positions, they discovered a dearth of legitimate training opportunities. Given these limitations, they had no choice but to acquire knowledge by personal experience. Hence the term "lessons learned" crept into the disaster medicine taxonomy.

The problem with lessons, however, is that they are personal and cannot be generalized or systematically disseminated. A good example is the small child who learns not to touch a hot stove by experiencing a burn. The child has learned the lesson, but as an adult, will find it difficult to pass on that knowledge to his or her own child. Each child must learn the lesson as a personal unique event.

In a field where knowledge is acquired by personal experience, an individual may gain wisdom and understanding but will have difficulty distributing such information to others. When the knowledgeable person leaves the job, retires, or dies, the knowledge goes with that individual and others must begin all over again. As such, the system perpetuates itself with the new employee needing to "learn the lesson" anew. The bottom line is that no progress is made and the field of disaster medicine remains a cottage industry, devoid of new developments and science. At best, the term "lessons learned" provides tacit support for this suboptimal method of knowledge acquisition. At worst, it is disrespectful of those who pursue disaster medicine as a career and the field as a whole. The phrase incorrectly implies the specialty lacks a systematic body of literature that can be used to advance the field and better prepare for catastrophes.

Fortunately, this is beginning to change. There is an early but clear movement away from learning the field of disaster medicine through personal experience and an evolving emphasis on developing knowledge through formalized education and training. Although every disaster has unique and unanticipated features, underlying patterns exist. Employing a formal education and training approach can impart this growing body of information in the classroom by systematizing knowledge gained through objective investigation and observation. Many universities in the United States and Europe now offer master's degrees in disaster-related studies and several sponsor doctorate degree programs. Some medical schools offer fellowships in disaster medicine, emphasizing both clinical and research skills. Professional organizations are creating clinical competencies for those who would respond to disasters. There is an international movement to professionalize response teams and train them to essential skill levels prior to permitting deployment. The specialty is finally beginning the evolution to a science.

Publishing the second edition of *Koenig and Schultz's Disaster Medicine: Comprehensive Principles and Practice* marks a milestone of sorts. It attests to the establishment of an authoritative text with international input and support. While insufficient by itself, this definitive reference is a necessary achievement in a long process that will ultimately result in creation of a scientific specialty and cadre of true experts. This will significantly improve the care of populations impacted by disasters. Besides the emphasis on science, the text also focuses on the functional impact of disasters and strategies for effective management regardless of etiology. Less emphasis is placed on such issues as who is "in charge" of the response or whether the event is "natural or manmade." Such classifications do little to improve understanding or outcome. If successful, our journey toward science will render the term "lessons learned" obsolete. Someday, one will only find the term listed in Wikipedia under the disaster medicine heading as, "an archaic term of historical interest only."

PREFACE

Welcome to the second edition of *Koenig and Schultz's Disaster Medicine: Comprehensive Principles and Practices*. We are pleased to offer the next evolution of the book with timely updates by world-renowned contributors. This definitive reference on disaster medical sciences also contains new chapters that reflect the progression of the science of disaster medicine.

With more than 1,000 copies of the first edition sold, translation into Arabic completed, and translation into Mandarin Chinese ongoing, disaster medical sciences is moving forward. We include a new "Perspective" in the front matter to provide a solid framework as you digest this new knowledge.

Please enjoy this new edition. Use the knowledge for teaching and practical applications to improve all-hazard emergency management and provide the best possible outcomes for populations affected by disasters.

Part I

Conceptual Framework and Strategic Overview

1

DISASTER RESEARCH AND EPIDEMIOLOGY

Megumi Kano, Michele M. Wood, Judith M. Siegel,
and Linda B. Bourque

OVERVIEW

The effective application of research can deepen understanding of a disaster's impact on health and societies. Such systematic study can inform disaster management across the entire response spectrum: from preparedness and prevention, through the immediate aftermath, to coping and rebuilding. Research allows for the identification of best practices that are subsequently refined and updated through further study. Meaningful improvement in any field is based on sound research. Without this activity, a field becomes stagnant and eventually irrelevant. In addition, thoughtful analysis of research data may demonstrate where accepted practices are no longer appropriate or, in some cases, where assumptions that directed disaster responses are in error. A body of research that continually builds on previous studies is the best tool for guiding practitioners, policymakers, and program planners in their efforts to reduce the impact of disasters on individuals and communities.

This chapter provides an overview of the wide range of disaster research conducted to date across various disciplines and documents changes that have occurred in the last few years. The first section reviews definitions of disaster, provides a historical overview of disaster research, and summarizes the characteristics of recent articles published in major epidemiology journals and some social science journals. The second section reviews the current state of the art, including the methods used, objectives, and settings within which disaster research takes place, and the application of information technology to disaster research. Also included are sections on research ethics, disaster vulnerability, morbidity and mortality, and the consistency of estimation methods used. The chapter ends with recommendations for further research. While the methodology remains largely unchanged, numerous new studies have been conducted indicating sustained development in this field of research.

Defining Disaster

There is no single, agreed-upon definition of disaster either within or across disciplines. Definitions used in practice and research vary widely, reflecting different objectives and interests in regard to the causes, consequences, and processes involved in disasters. The following discussions touch on the broad spectrum of processes involved in disasters, including, but not limited to, the impact on the healthcare system; the short- and long-term effects on people's health and livelihood; and the behaviors of individuals, groups, and organizations in relation to disasters.

Accordingly, a disaster is "any community emergency that seriously affects people's lives and property and exceeds the capacity of the community to respond effectively to the emergency."[1] As an extreme example, the 2011 Tōhoku Earthquake and Tsunami (M9.0) that occurred on March 11, 2011, in the Pacific Ocean off the coast of Japan's northeastern region was the biggest earthquake ever recorded in Japan. It caused powerful tsunami waves 10 to 40 meters high, which reached up to 6 km inland, devastating the coastal areas and leaving over 18,000 people dead or missing. The disaster was further compounded by the loss of power and subsequent meltdown of reactors at a nuclear power station affected by the earthquake and tsunami. Large quantities of radioactive contaminants were released, which led to evacuations of surrounding areas. More than 2 years later, many of the victims of this disaster who lost their homes, neighborhoods, and livelihoods still lived in temporary housing settlements, depending on their savings, disaster compensation, and donations. National and local governments are struggling over reconstruction and redevelopment. This event clearly overwhelmed the response and recovery capacity of the community at the individual, household, and organizational levels. Studies of this disaster legitimately go beyond its impact on people's health and the healthcare system.

The term disaster is often used interchangeably with the terms "emergency" and "hazard," although there are formal distinctions. An emergency is a threatening situation that requires immediate action but may not necessarily result in loss or destruction. If an emergency is managed successfully, a disaster may be averted. A hazard is a possible source of danger that upon interacting with human settlements may create an emergency situation and may lead to a disaster. For the purposes of this chapter, all three terms will be used, and the distinctions in meaning will be maintained.

Historical Overview of Disaster Research

Historically, sociological disaster research has been dominated by exploratory research designs, whereas epidemiological research emphasizes the importance of explanatory designs.[2–8] Exploratory studies usually focus on examining new areas of research or the feasibility of conducting more structured research with an emphasis on developing hypotheses. Descriptive and explanatory studies, in contrast, start with hypotheses and emphasize minimizing bias and maximizing external validity, with explanatory studies also attempting to infer causality. The next section of this chapter (Current State of the Art) provides greater detail on study design.

The perceived need to enter the field immediately after a disaster encouraged disaster researchers to utilize exploratory study designs rather than more structured descriptive designs. Researchers thought they were dealing with perishable data that had a limited time frame for collection. Information was thought to be unavoidably fleeting, vanishing quickly after a disaster because of memory decay, removal of debris, and other activities. Furthermore, it was assumed that disaster-associated in- and out-migrations were rapidly changing the target population and their communities in ways that could not be captured by the research. Consequently, early research on disasters relied on data obtained through semi-structured interviews with selected informants after quick entry into a community immediately post-impact. Over time, this perceived need to enter the disaster area immediately has been referred to as the "window of opportunity" and has been adopted by practitioners and policymakers as well as other research disciplines including engineering, seismology, medicine, and public health.

Disaster researchers trained in the social sciences have been concerned with the applicability of social theory to the study of disasters and, in reverse, the contributions that disaster research can make to the development of theory. References to theory in the early disaster epidemiology literature are oblique, with the exception of concerns about biological plausibility. Contemporary social epidemiological research more frequently incorporates theory, a subject that is discussed more fully later in this chapter, under the heading of Disaster Vulnerability.

Early Disaster Research

Samuel Prince's Columbia University dissertation, which examined the impact of the collision and explosion of two ships in the inner harbor of Halifax, Nova Scotia, in 1917, is recognized as the first scholarly study of a disaster.[9,10] With few exceptions, other systematic studies of disaster were not undertaken until World War II. Table 1.1 organizes the milestones in disaster research linearly by date, initiating agency and funding sources, primary disciplines conducting the research, research strategies, contributions to the field, and key sources for accessing disaster research. In the United States, through 1959, all of the early research was initiated and funded by the federal government, often the military.

The United States Strategic Bombing Surveys (1944–1947) examined the effect of U.S. strategic bombing and the resultant physical destruction on industry, utilities, transportation, medical care, social life, morale, and the bombed population's will to fight in Germany and Japan. Fritz noted, "people living in heavily bombed cities had significantly higher morale than people in the lightly bombed cities," and that "neither organic neurologic diseases nor psychiatric disorders can be attributed to nor are they conditioned by the air attacks."[11] In other words, the problems that were anticipated did not emerge, including social disorganization, panicky evacuations, criminal behavior, or mental disorders. In fact, morale remained high and suicide rates declined. These findings were not widely disseminated and were at variance with prewar expectations and prevailing views on the behavior of people under extreme stress.[12,13]

With the advent of the Cold War, federal government agencies ignorant or unaware of these findings expressed concern about how people might react to new war-related threats. A second set of studies, funded by the U.S. Army Chemical Corps Medical Laboratories and conducted at the National Opinion Research Center (NORC) at the University of Chicago (1949–1954), hypothesized that disasters cause extreme stress, which in turn results in social disorganization, the breakdown of social institutions, and the manifestation of antisocial and psychotic behavior by individuals and groups. Field studies were conducted following disasters, with a major objective being to use these situations as surrogates for what might occur during an invasive war of the U.S. and the Americas. "Comparing the state of knowledge prior to the NORC studies with the new field research findings, it became clear that previous studies . . . were sorely deficient," and that "except for a few notable exceptions, the literature was loaded with gross stereotypes and distortions."[11] Researchers compiled the NORC disaster studies into a three-volume report.[14]

In 1952, the U.S. National Academy of Sciences–National Research Council established the Committee on Disaster Studies (later the Disaster Research Group) at the request of the Surgeons General of the Army, Navy, and Air Force to "conduct a survey and study in the fields of scientific research and development applicable to problems which might result from disasters caused by enemy action."[11] This third set of studies refined theories about human behavior in disasters and improved the methodologies. Exploratory field studies conducted in the immediate aftermath of a disaster focused on how individuals behaved in crisis.

The general theoretical structure brought to this research, although not always explicitly stated, was developed from the theories espoused by Mead and Cooley of symbolic interaction and theories of collective behavior, particularly those specific to crowd behavior and the development of emergent groups.[15,16] It was hypothesized that the norms which determined social interaction might be challenged as a result of a disaster. Different social norms might evolve either temporarily, while the environment stabilized, or permanently, leading to different forms of social organization. Disasters were seen as triggers that disrupted the social order. Of interest was the behavior of individuals, groups, and organizations during either a brief or prolonged period of normlessness.[17,18]

> Societies are composed of individuals interacting in accordance with an immense multitude of norms, i.e., ideas about how individuals *ought* to behave . . . . Our position is that activities of individuals . . . are guided by a normative structure in disaster just as in any other situation . . . . In disaster, these actions . . . are largely governed by *emergent* rather than established norms, but norms nevertheless.
>
> –Drabek as cited by Perry[19]

Consistent with the interests in emergent norms and in behavior during and immediately after a disaster, the research conducted

Table 1.1. Milestones in Disaster Research

Dates	Primary Research Agency/ Funding Source	Primary Disciplines Conducting Research	Research Strategies	Contributions to Disaster Research and Knowledge	Key Sources
1920	Doctoral dissertation	Sociology	Exploratory case/field study	Recognized as first scholarly study of a disaster[9,10]	
Nov. 1944–Oct. 1947	U.S. War Department, Army and Navy	Civilian and military experts headed by a civilian chair	Exploratory and descriptive research using field observations, archival data, and personal interviews	Countered prevailing views that extreme stress lowers morale, causes mental disorders and social disorganization[13]	U.S. National Archives and Records Administration, Records of the United States Bombing Survey [http://www.archives.gov/research/guide-fed-records/groups/243.html]
1949–1954	National Opinion Research Center at the University of Chicago; funded by the U.S. Army Chemical Corps and Medical Laboratories	Social science; Psychology	Exploratory field studies	Laid the groundwork for the study of human behavior in disasters[14]	
1952–1959	Committee on Disaster Studies (1952–1957), Disaster Research Group (1957–1959), National Academy of Sciences-National Research Council; requested by Surgeons General of Army, Navy, and Air Force; funded by the Armed Forces, Ford Foundation, National Institute of Mental Health, Federal Civil Defense Administration	Social science; Psychology; Medicine	Exploratory and descriptive research involving field studies, experiments, clinical, economic and demographic studies	Showed that routine crises are qualitatively different from large-scale disasters, although there are similarities in human responses across disaster types. Also shed light on the positive outcomes of disasters[11,14,65,129–131]	
1963–present	Disaster Research Center at Ohio State University and later at the University of Delaware; funded by Office of Civil Defense, FEMA and other federal agencies	Sociology	Exploratory field studies during immediate aftermath of a disaster, and descriptive surveys	Generated sociological disaster research over four decades. Remains one of the main academic centers for disaster research in the U.S.	Disaster Research Center [http://www.udel.edu/DRC/] International Journal of Mass Emergencies and Disasters [http://www.ijmed.org/] Mass Emergencies [http://www.massemergencies.org/]
1970–present	Center for Disease Control, and later, the Centers for Disease Control and Prevention (CDC)	Public health, especially epidemiology	Descriptive and some explanatory epidemiology	The first epidemiological study of a disaster is published.[23] *Morbidity and Mortality Weekly Report (MMWR)* becomes the main source for epidemiological disaster research in the U.S.	MMWR [http://www.cdc.gov/mmwr/]

(continued)

5

Table 1.1. *(continued)*

Dates	Primary Research Agency/ Funding Source	Primary Disciplines Conducting Research	Research Strategies	Contributions to Disaster Research and Knowledge	Key Sources
1973–present	Centre for Research on the Epidemiology of Disasters at the School of Public Health of the Université Catholique de Louvain in Brussels, Belgium	Epidemiology	Descriptive and explanatory epidemiology. Emphasis on applied research	Established an academic center for the study of disaster epidemiology. Maintains database on disasters worldwide and their human and economic impact by country and type of disaster	Bulletin of the World Health Organization [http://www.who.int/ bulletin/en/] Disasters [http://onlinelibrary.wiley .com/journal/10.1111/(ISSN)1467- 7717] Epidemiologic Reviews [http://epirev .oxfordjournals.org/] Lancet [http://www.thelancet.com/]
1976–present	Natural Hazards Center at the University of Colorado; funded by a consortium of federal agencies and the Public Entity Risk Institute	Geography; Sociology; Economics	Various research objectives and strategies. Promotion of interdisciplinary research	Brought together hazard researchers and disaster researchers. Increased interaction across disciplines, and between researchers, practitioners and policymakers both in the U.S. and internationally	Natural Hazards Center [http://www .colorado.edu/hazards/] Natural Hazards Review [http://www .colorado.edu/hazards/publications/ review.html]
1976–present	World Association for Disaster and Emergency Medicine	Emergency medicine	Exploratory and descriptive research utilizing case studies and surveys	Marked emergency medicine's entry into disaster research	Prehospital and Disaster Medicine [http://journals.cambridge.org/action/ displayJournal?jid=PDM/]
1977–present	Numerous grants awarded by the National Science Foundation, U.S. Geological Survey, National Institute of Science and Technology, FEMA, and the National Oceanic and Atmospheric Administration through the National Earthquake Hazards Reduction Program	Geography; Sociology; Political science; Psychology; Economics; Decision science; Regional science and planning; Public health; Anthropology	Various research objectives and strategies	Expanded the diversity in and quantity of disaster research[132]	

between 1949 and 1960 gradually identified an underlying time-line in the natural history of a disaster, starting with prepared-ness and proceeding through warning, evacuation, impact, and response and recovery periods. The early studies focused on the middle four stages, with little attention paid to preparedness or recovery. The stages enumerated have changed over time, but an underlying timeline is assumed, whether stated or not, in most contemporary disaster research.

The establishment of the Disaster Research Center (DRC) in 1963 – first at Ohio State University and later at the University of Delaware, by Russell Dynes and Enrico Quarantelli – was a natural extension of this early research. The DRC continued to conduct field studies immediately after disasters, focusing on the behavior of formal, informal, and emergent groups rather than the behavior of individuals. Although primarily studying disasters within the United States, field studies were also conducted in a number of other countries. Most studies were exploratory in design and many continue to be today, but some investigations were conducted using descriptive designs.[20,21] The Defense Civil Preparedness Agency (precursor to the Federal Emergency Management Agency, FEMA) funded most of the research, with the focus on major community organizations involved in disasters, such as police, fire departments, hospitals, and public utilities. Some funding was received from the National Institute of Mental Health and the Health Resources Administration to examine the delivery of medical care and mental health services.[22]

Gilbert White established the Natural Hazards Research and Applications Center (NHRAC) at the University of Colorado in 1976. With primary funding from the National Science Foundation as part of the National Earthquake Hazards Reduction Program agencies, the center served as a catalyst for bringing social scientists, physical scientists, academic researchers, practitioners, and policymakers together in multidisciplinary research projects, yearly workshops, and training programs. It encouraged the merger of disaster and hazard research. Interestingly, it was not until 1990 that the workshops drew participants from medicine, emergency medicine, epidemiology, and public health.

Epidemiology, Public Health, and Emergency Medicine

The first disaster research by investigators who identified themselves as epidemiologists was a study of the East Bengal cyclone of November 1970 by Sommer and Mosley.[23] They showed that death rates were highest for children and the elderly, and that women fared poorly relative to men. A decade later, in the first article published on disaster research in *Epidemiologic Reviews*, Logue and colleagues noted that, "research on the epidemiology of disasters has emerged as an area of special interest."[24] The authors observed that a few university groups in the United States (e.g., DRC and NHRAC) were conducting extensive research on disasters, and also made note of the work by the Center for Research on the Epidemiology of Disasters at the School of Public Health of Louvain University in Brussels, Belgium. They described the efforts as focusing on the immediate post-impact period with emphasis on surveillance for outbreaks of communicable diseases and on increased mortality directly attributable to the disaster. Importantly, they also recognized three "controlled long-term health studies" of the 1968 floods in Bristol, England; the floods in Brisbane, Australia, in 1974; and the 1972 Hurricane Agnes in Pennsylvania, respectively.

In 1990, a discussion of the epidemiology of disasters appeared as a brief update in *Epidemiologic Reviews*.[25] Many of the disasters discussed occurred outside the United States.

Notably, the public belief about the high prevalence of communicable diseases post-disaster was countered. Unlike the earlier review, however, there was no cross-referencing to studies conducted by social scientists or others traditionally associated with disaster research. In 2005, *Epidemiologic Reviews* devoted a full issue to the topic "Epidemiologic Approaches to Disasters." Included were original reviews of research conducted following cyclones, floods, earthquakes, and the Chernobyl reactor meltdown, and of the development of posttraumatic stress following disasters.

Disaster epidemiology concentrates on estimating the direct and indirect incidence and prevalence of morbidity or other adverse health outcomes over the short and long term, with the objective of developing surveillance systems, prevention strategies, and estimations of the public health burden caused by the disaster.[26] Ideally, studies would be population based and longitudinal in design. Case-series, cross-sectional, case-control, and cohort designs are all represented in the epidemiological studies of disasters, but where field studies are common in other disciplines, the case series predominates in the epidemiological disaster literature. The U.S. Centers for Disease Control and Prevention (CDC) and others have encouraged and sometimes funded the conduct of post-disaster, rapid-assessment surveys, using modified cluster sampling.[27] However, a substantial number of epidemiological studies are restricted to coroners' reports and the description of persons who present at emergency departments and other points of service. Many of these studies make no effort to describe the denominator population from which the dead, the injured, and the sick were drawn. A further complication is the lack of agreement on what constitutes a disaster-related death, injury, or disease.[28] With the exception of one article, none of the contributions to the aforementioned 2005 special issue of *Epidemiologic Reviews* makes any reference to theory, and most of the articles call for more rigorous methodology in epidemiological studies of disasters.

Epidemiology Publications, January 2007–April 2013

In the first edition of this chapter, the authors conducted systematic, although not exhaustive, searches for disaster-related research articles in the epidemiological literature published between 1987 and 2007. The review that follows covers the period of January 2007 through April 2013. We examine articles published in the *Morbidity and Mortality Weekly Report*, *Prehospital and Disaster Medicine*, and four epidemiologic journals (*American Journal of Epidemiology*, *Annals of Epidemiology*, *Epidemiology*, and *Epidemiologic Reviews*). We identify the location of the disaster, the research team, and the extent to which bibliographies include references to the broad social science literature, in addition to medical and epidemiologic journals. As a means of comparison, we provide a similar review of articles on disasters in two social science journals known for publishing disaster research (*Environment and Behavior* and *International Journal of Mass Emergencies and Disasters*) and determine the extent of cross-reference to the medical and epidemiologic literature (see Table 1.2).

A total of seventy-seven articles were identified with the following distribution: twenty-nine in the *Morbidity and Mortality Weekly Report* (*MMWR*), twenty in the *American Journal of Epidemiology*, fourteen in the *Annals of Epidemiology*, twelve in *Epidemiology*, and two in *Epidemiologic Reviews*. Although our review focuses on journals published in English,

Table 1.2. Number of Disaster-Related Articles Published in Six Selected Journals by Geographic Location of the Index Disaster Event, January 2007–April 2013

Journal	U.S. Disaster	Non-U.S. Disaster	Geographic Scope of Non-U.S. Disaster/Event (Number of articles)
Epidemiology Journals			
American Journal of Epidemiology	6	11	Australia (2), Britain, China, Europe, Iceland, Italy, Netherlands, Vietnam; International (2)
Annals of Epidemiology	10	4	China (2), UK; Asia
Epidemiology	5	7	Bangladesh, Canada, Chile, China, Liberia; 15 European cities; International
Morbidity and Mortality Weekly Report	18	12	Greece, Haiti (3), Kenya, Mexico, New Zealand, Pakistan, Sudan; International (3)
Social Science Journals			
International Journal of Mass Emergencies and Disasters	41	32[1]	Australia, Bangladesh, Cameroon, Canada (2), Haiti, India, Israel, Japan, Korea, Liberia, New Zealand (2), Sweden, Turkey, UK; Asia (3); International
Environment and Behavior	10	7	China, Japan, Netherlands, New Zealand, UK; International

[1] Includes twelve articles, of which six each were published in two special issues of the *International Journal of Mass Emergencies and Disasters* – one on Theory of Disaster Recovery (August 2012, Vol. 30, No. 2) and one on the National Evacuation Conference (March 2013, Vol. 31, No. 1).

thirty-four of the articles report on disasters that occurred outside the United States, and most of those articles were written by non-U.S. researchers. These articles examine the full range of disasters and disaster-associated morbidity, mortality, service delivery, and needs assessments. Topics of study included the 2009 H1N1 pandemic influenza (n = 23, of which 19 were in *MMWR*); other influenza outbreaks including historical events (n = 4); combat and war in both contemporary and historical settings (n = 15); weather events involving extremes of heat and cold (n = 5); the terrorist attacks of September 11, 2001 (n = 3); wildfires (n = 3); floods (n = 3); earthquakes (n = 2); preparedness for disasters (n = 2); a pub fire; a dioxin spill; dust storms; a power outage in the northeast United States; a typhoon; a hurricane; a coal mine disaster; a tornado; school mass homicides; two review articles on global surveillance and humanitarian relief workers; and two historical vignettes on the Halifax explosion and the Johnstown flood.

In contrast to the earlier 20-year period when the *American Journal of Epidemiology* published an average of one disaster article each year, an average of more than three articles was published each year between 2007 and 2013. Most of the studies are atheoretical (not designed to test a hypothesis or theory), and many combine existent cohort studies with a natural experiment. As before, the emphasis has been on mortality, morbidity, injuries, and psychological distress. Like the early field research conducted by social scientists and psychologists, many studies lack denominator data or information about the population they represent.

The journal *Epidemiology*, sponsored by the International Society for Environmental Epidemiology, publishes mostly conference abstracts, but also published twelve disaster-related articles between 2007 and 2013. Of these, five were conducted by U.S.-based researchers, five by research groups outside the U.S., and two by groups comprised of both U.S. and non-U.S. researchers. There were a total of eleven references to social science research. During this same time period, the *Annals of Epidemiology* published fourteen articles on disasters. Data were collected using surveys, registries, and other existent secondary sources of information. Eleven references were made to social science literature in the fourteen studies.

Prior to 2007, in addition to the literature noted previously, *Epidemiologic Reviews* published review articles on psychiatric distress from disasters, pandemic influenza, toxic oil syndrome, and heat-related mortality. Since 2007, two review articles, one on global public health surveillance and the other on trauma-related mental illness, have at least tangential relevance to the study of disaster epidemiology.[29,30]

Since January 2007, the CDC periodical *MMWR* has published twenty-nine articles about disasters throughout the world, with fifteen published in 2009. Most articles combined surveillance with a case series, but articles on school-associated homicides and coal mining included historical reviews of similar events with contemporary surveillance reports. A case-control study in Sudan evaluated an intervention designed to reduce the spread of cholera, and a population-based needs assessment following Hurricane Ike reported on injuries and other health-related needs. Two studies of household preparedness for emergencies and disasters were surveys. There are no references to social science research in any of the twenty-nine articles in *MMWR*. The lack of such references is particularly surprising in the two articles about household preparedness, given that household preparedness and evacuation behavior have been the focus of a substantial amount of social science research dating back to 1950.

Prehospital and Disaster Medicine, January 2007–April 2013

The establishment of the World Association for Disaster and Emergency Medicine by Peter Safar and other leading international experts in resuscitation/anesthesia in 1976 and that of the American Board of Emergency Medicine as a conjoint specialty board in 1979 mark emergency medicine's entry into disaster research.[31] Originally an invitation-only group called the Club of Mainz, membership was eventually broadened in 1997. In 1985, Safar founded the journal *Prehospital and Disaster Medicine* (*PDM*). Much of the disaster research conducted in emergency medicine is published in *PDM*, but in our original review we reported that very few articles contained references to disaster research conducted outside of medicine or to those published before 1985. More of the mainstream emergency medicine journals are now regularly featuring disaster medicine research but some of these same limitations remain.

Using a broad definition of "disaster research" and "nonmedical citations," twenty-three issues of *PDM* were reviewed for articles on disaster research in the first edition of this chapter. Seventy-one articles were identified, which included a total of ninety-two citations to nonmedical sources; these references were found in only a limited number of articles. Most references were to other emergency medicine or medical journals, including the *Annals of Emergency Medicine*.

This review was repeated for articles published between January 2007 and April 2013. Here we assumed that all articles published in *PDM* were directly or indirectly related to emergency medicine and disasters. During that period, 488 articles were published, with 175 about disasters and emergencies in the United States, 294 focused on non-U.S. disasters, and 19 having an international focus. A few authors of non-U.S.-based articles were from the United States, but the overwhelming majority was not.

PDM publishes a broad range of articles. Some focus on policy issues and editorial commentary. A substantial number of articles are based on case series or retrospective review of records. Some issues are largely devoted to publication of conference proceedings with, for example, Issue 5 in 2007 focused on the First Annual Humanitarian Health Conference convened by the Dartmouth Medical School and the Harvard Humanitarian Initiative. Occasionally case-control studies and evaluations of interventions are reported. Almost all research articles were atheoretical.

Over the period reviewed, there were 118 references to social science research in the 474 articles. When references appeared, they were concentrated in just a few articles, and the plurality of references was to Enrico Quarantelli's articles and chapters. When articles are focused on emergency medical interventions and treatment, such as triaging or crush injuries, lack of references to social science research is logical; however, when articles are focused on crowd behavior or evacuation, the lack of attention to historical social science research can be seen as a critical oversight. Earlier we noted that much of the theoretical interest in studying disasters evolved from theories of collective behavior, particularly those specific to crowd behavior and the development of emergent groups. At least four articles in *PDM* focus on mass gatherings and crowd control but only one editorial comment correctly identifies the origin of such research in social psychology over 100 years ago and its use as a context for studying disasters starting in 1950.[32]

In 2009, Smith et al. published a review of disaster-specific literature from 1977–2009.[33] The authors noted that the formal study of disasters dates to Samuel Henry Prince's dissertation on the 1917 ship explosion at Halifax, Nova Scotia, which was followed by "empirical and theoretical research throughout the 1930s, 40s and 50s," and that, "throughout the 1960s and 1970s, academics from a variety of disciplines began to examine the nature and concepts of disasters." Nonetheless, they make no attempt to include the social science literature in their review.

Social Science Publications, January 2007–April 2013

For a brief comparison, we also examined articles on disasters that were published in two social science journals to see whether authors cited research conducted in medicine or epidemiology. Because traditional disaster research primarily originated in soci-

ology, the number of articles published in traditional sociology journals between 2007 and 2013 was examined first. Over that period, only a total of five articles were published in the *American Sociological Review*, the *American Journal of Sociology*, and *Social Problems*, and a single special issue with seven articles was published in *Social Forces*. The absence of articles in these journals emphasize the extent to which the traditional disaster research paradigm in sociology has become restrictive and unproductive as suggested both by Tierney and in the special issue of *Social Forces*.[34,35] Tierney notes that:

> Disaster researchers must stop organizing their inquiries around problems that are meaningful primarily to the institutions charged with managing disasters and instead concentrate on problems that are meaningful to the discipline. They must integrate the study of disasters with core sociological concerns, such as social inequality, societal diversity, and social change. They must overcome their tendency to build up knowledge one disaster at a time and focus more on what disasters and environmental crises of all types have in common with respect to origins, dynamics, and outcomes. And they must locate the study of disasters within broader theoretical frameworks, including in particular those concerned with risk, organizations and institutions, and society-environment interactions.[34]

As a consequence, disaster researchers have become isolated from mainstream sociology and tend to publish in extreme event and multidisciplinary journals such as *Environment and Behavior*, the *International Journal of Mass Emergencies and Disasters*, *Disasters*, the *Natural Hazards Review*, the *Journal of Contingencies and Crisis Management*, *Risk Analysis*, and *Natural Hazards*. *Environment and Behavior* and the *International Journal of Mass Emergencies and Disasters* were selected as two examples of this broader social science literature.

Environment and Behavior published seventeen articles on disasters between January 2007 and April 2013. Nine articles focused on disasters in the United States and eight on non-U.S. disasters. All articles cited at least one theoretical context for the research being conducted, and data were collected through environmental observation, self-administered and internet questionnaires, in-person interviews, telephone surveys, panel studies, and the combination of multiple sources of data. Across the seventeen articles, there were twenty-one references to medical or epidemiology journals.

The *International Journal of Mass Emergencies and Disasters (IJMED)* – established in 1983 by the International Sociological Association's Research Committee on Disasters – focuses on theory, research, planning, and policy related to the social and behavioral aspects of disasters or mass emergencies. Papers concerned with medical, biological, physical engineering, or other technical matters are accepted if social and behavioral features of disasters are also discussed. Between January 2007 and April 2013, seventy-three articles were published in *IJMED* with forty-five focused on disasters in the United States and twenty-eight on disasters outside the United States. Articles in *IJMED* were less likely than those in *Environment and Behavior* to provide a theoretical context for the study, but all cite previous relevant research. Two special issues were published during this period on Gender and Disasters (August 2010), and the Theory of Disaster Recovery (August 2012). Across the 73 articles there were

119 references to medical journals and 11 to epidemiology journals. Interestingly, the articles focused on the identification of bodies after disasters had only a few references to relevant medical and epidemiologic literature.

Summary

The previous review demonstrates that roughly half of the disaster-related articles published between 2007 and early 2013 in some of the key English-language epidemiology journals, and a few social science journals, are about disasters occurring outside the United States. Articles published in epidemiology and emergency medical journals rarely cite a theoretical context for their analyses or provide cross-citations to the social science research on disasters. In contrast, articles published in the social science journals reviewed here are often placed within a theoretical structure but with limited references to relevant literature in medicine and epidemiology. These findings suggest that the many disciplines engaged in hazard and disaster research remain largely self-contained, with restricted knowledge of research conducted in other areas and disciplines, constraining the diversity of perspectives that could be brought to bear on critical issues.

CURRENT STATE OF THE ART

State of the art is described in regard to three aspects of disaster research: methodology, vulnerability, and estimates of morbidity and mortality. The first portion provides an overview of key methodological issues pertinent to disaster research, ranging from disaster research settings to ethical considerations. The second portion explores the concept of vulnerability, focusing on different approaches to determining who might be most vulnerable to the impact of a disaster. The last section is relevant to the impact and aftermath of a disaster. It reviews the factors that influence estimates of disaster-related morbidity and mortality.

Disaster Research Methods

There are multiple scientific perspectives involved in disaster research, and the methods used to study disasters are equally varied. The appropriateness of one methodological approach over another is determined by the specific question the researcher is trying to answer and the discipline in which the researcher was trained. A number of books provide expert guidance on disaster research methods.[36–38]

Disaster Research Objectives

The objective of disaster research can be exploratory, descriptive, or explanatory. Exploratory studies are the least structured type of research endeavor, often examining new areas of research or the feasibility of conducting more structured research. The emphasis is on developing hypotheses, frequently involving in-depth data collection from a relatively small group of purposively selected research subjects. It should not be assumed that exploratory studies are easier to conduct or less time consuming simply because they tend to be performed on a smaller scale or without the use of large sets of quantitative data.

Descriptive studies, in contrast, start with formal hypotheses or research questions and seek to accurately describe a situation by deriving estimates of important outcome distributions (e.g.,

disease occurrence by person, place, and time) or associations between variables and theoretical constructs in a population. Like descriptive studies, explanatory studies are driven by hypotheses. The aim, however, is to explain causal relationships. Explanatory research is also referred to as analytic research in epidemiology.[39] In both descriptive and explanatory studies, emphasis is placed on selecting samples that are representative of the population being studied and minimizing bias in data collection.

Disaster Research Settings

The study of disasters can occur in many different physical and temporal contexts. Among disaster health researchers and epidemiologists, data collection activities have been focused largely in high yield areas where disaster victims are likely to congregate, such as emergency departments. Research conducted in these settings captures the numerator, that is, the number of people with different health afflictions who present themselves in these settings. This approach provides no information on the larger community from which these individuals emerged (i.e., the denominator) or the extent to which they represent the range and severity of disaster-related morbidity in a population. It can even lead to misattribution of the cause for morbidity in the absence of a rigorous protocol. As a case in point, Peek-Asa and colleagues examined coroner and hospital records following the 1994 Northridge earthquake in California.[40] They found that, when compared with their systematic, individual medical record review, initial reports overestimated earthquake-related deaths and hospital admissions by misattributing deaths and injuries that presented for care shortly after the earthquake.

Population-based studies, in contrast, enable researchers to estimate the number of individuals in a community who were afflicted in some manner because they focus on the denominator, or the entire community at risk. A study conducted in Iceland after a volcanic eruption in 2010 utilized an existing population registry to identify and survey all adult residents in the municipalities closest to the volcano and an additional sample of demographically matched residents from a non-exposed area in the northern part of the country.[41] This population-based cross-sectional survey was able to estimate the proportion of the population afflicted by symptoms likely related to the volcano eruption and determine that residents living in the exposed area had markedly increased prevalence of respiratory and other physical symptoms compared to non-exposed residents. The dose–response pattern that emerged, with the highest symptom prevalence found in those living closest to the volcano, strengthened the evidence that the symptoms found in the study were caused by exposure to the eruption.

Disaster research may also occur in different temporal contexts. An organizational structure for disaster planning, response, and research conceptualizes disaster events as occurring in a cycle. There are slight variations in the way different researchers divide and label the critical periods, but three phases are common to all schemas.[42] These are the "pre-impact," "trans-impact," and "post-impact" periods, also described as the "disaster mitigation and preparedness," "emergency response," and "disaster recovery" periods. The U.S. National Research Council recommends that cycles typical of hazards on one hand, and disasters on the other, be integrated in recognition of the importance of collaborative cross-disciplinary research.[43]

The pre-impact period is the time frame leading up to a disaster event. This period involves two major activities, hazard mitigation and disaster preparedness, which help reduce vulnerability to disaster impact. Emergency preparedness planning and research may be conducted during this phase. Baseline information about disaster readiness and emergency planning may be collected as well. The trans-impact period focuses on warning, evacuation, immediate response, and disaster relief activities. The post-impact period revolves around disaster recovery. It is important to note that these divisions serve as an organizational scheme and are neither fixed nor absolute. In fact, they may blend together depending on the outcome of interest.

More recently, studies have been conducted during all phases of the disaster cycle, extending the window of post-impact data collection and using longitudinal designs (comparing data before and after a disaster) when appropriate baseline data are available. The notion that disaster-related memory is stable over time is supported by research conducted in three successive time periods following the 1994 Northridge earthquake in California.[44]

The stages of the "disaster cycle" can be related to the different levels of morbidity and mortality prevention. Within the field of epidemiology, the term "prevention" is broadly used to understand the spectrum of efforts to eliminate or reduce the negative consequences of disease and disability[45]. Traditionally the term has been defined in levels of primary, secondary, and tertiary prevention to help delineate different healthcare foci. Primary prevention involves individual and group efforts to protect health through activities such as improving nutrition and reducing environmental risks. These efforts are made before disease or disability occurs, and they are the main focus of public health. In terms of the health threats posed by disasters, primary prevention efforts represent individual and group disaster mitigation and preparedness activities.

Secondary prevention consists of measures that facilitate early detection and treatment, such as health screening, to control disease or disability and reduce the potential for harm. In terms of disasters and their health consequences, secondary prevention can be likened to early warning systems, evacuation efforts, and immediate disaster response and relief because these efforts are designed to reduce later harm in the face of a newly introduced disaster health threat.

Tertiary prevention strives to reduce the long-term impact of disease and disability by eliminating or reducing impairment and improving quality of life. These efforts are generally the focus of rehabilitation. Tertiary prevention of disaster-related health effects might be understood as disaster recovery efforts, in which the goal is to eliminate impairment caused by a disaster and to rebuild communities and infrastructures. Figure 1.1 integrates the temporal stages of a disaster, levels of prevention, and disaster-related activities.

Disaster Research Variables

Regardless of the phase of the disaster cycle that is being studied, the choice of research variables requires careful consideration. This selection is guided by the researcher's disciplinary or theoretical background as well as by the unit of analysis (i.e., individuals, groups, organizations, or communities). Variables that are expected to have an effect on the outcome of interest are the independent variables. A key independent variable in epidemiologic disaster research is the level or dose of exposure to a disaster. This exposure can be measured in various ways, such as the intensity of shaking experienced in an earthquake or the extent of personal loss due to a disaster. Alternatively, dose can

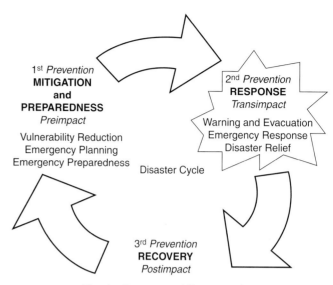

Figure 1.1. The Disaster Cycle.

be measured in terms of pre-disaster exposure to public information campaigns or other preparedness messages.[46] Demographic characteristics of the population at risk or those exposed to the disaster are also considered as independent variables or as effect modifiers that influence people's experiences in an event.

The range of possible outcomes or dependent variables in disaster research is extremely wide due to the multidimensionality of the disaster phenomenon and the corresponding multidisciplinary nature of disaster research. The major disciplines involved in disaster research today include geography, geology, engineering, economics, sociology, psychology, public policy, urban planning, anthropology, public health, and medicine.

Geographers and geologists study the relationship between human settlements and hazards (e.g., earthquake faults, hillsides, and floodplains), or the "hazardscape," and engineers examine the extent of structural damage that can be caused by a disaster. Economists assess the economic and financial impact of disasters, sociologists and psychologists study the behavioral responses to disasters and disaster risk, and health professionals are primarily interested in the effect of disasters on people's health and the healthcare infrastructure. Depending on when (i.e., during which part of the disaster cycle) the dependent variables are measured and how the study is designed, researchers can forecast the amount of loss and damage that might be done or prevented, measure the actual impact of a disaster, assess the effectiveness of interventions in reducing disaster impact, and predict the course of long-term recovery, each in terms of the dependent variables of interest to the researcher.

As the number of disasters increases worldwide, the field of disaster research grows, with new disciplines being added or previously minor disciplines becoming more prominent. These changes affect the dependent variables that are studied in disaster research. For example, subsequent to September 11, 2001, the study of terrorism has grown dramatically within this field. Studies have assessed different outcomes of terrorism, including the public's response to terrorism and the health impact of terrorism events.[47] Similarly, the occurrence of SARS and influenza pandemics and their repercussions on a global scale have given further impetus to public health emergency research in recent years.[48,49]

Disaster Research Study Designs

The appropriate study design depends on the research objective; whether it is exploratory, descriptive, or explanatory/analytic (as described earlier); and the feasibility of the study given available resources. The designs described here are frequently used in the social sciences and in epidemiology to study a wide range of phenomena, including those related to disasters.

Experimental studies involve comparing outcomes between those who receive a certain treatment and those who do not, holding all other known factors constant. A treatment can be any independent variable that is expected to have an effect on the dependent variable. In experiments, the researcher controls the level of the independent variable, or exposure, in an attempt to isolate its effect. Experiments involve random assignment of subjects to treatment groups (i.e., randomization) to increase the likelihood that the groups will be comparable in regard to characteristics other than the main independent variable that may affect the outcomes. Truly experimental designs can offer evidence with the highest internal validity (i.e., evidence of causality) and thus are suitable for explanatory research. As an example, researchers tested the effectiveness of a behavioral treatment for earthquake-related posttraumatic stress disorder by randomizing a group of survivors of the 1999 Turkey earthquake with a clinical diagnosis of posttraumatic stress disorder into treatment and non-treatment groups. This study identified significant effects of the behavioral intervention at weeks 6, 12, and 24, and 1–2 years post-treatment. Experiments might also be conducted in which human subjects are not involved, for example, to test whether certain structural designs mitigate damage in an earthquake. They are not used, however, to investigate how people are affected by or respond to disasters because it is unethical and, in most cases, impossible to manipulate exposure to a disaster.

There are many natural social settings in which the researcher can approximate an experimental design without fully controlling the stimuli (determining when and to whom exposure should be applied and randomizing the exposure) as in a true experiment. Collectively, such situations can be regarded as quasi-experimental.[50–52] Quasi-experiments are frequently used in the social sciences for explanatory research. This includes studies in which a group of individuals who were naturally exposed to a disaster is compared to a group of non-exposed individuals, or to those with varying degrees of exposure, to identify possible differences in the occurrence of key outcomes. In the absence of an actual disaster, level of exposure to disaster "risk" (e.g., distance from a hazard) instead of exposure to the disaster itself can be the exposure of interest in studying certain behavioral responses (e.g., emergency preparation). As will be discussed in a later section, people may also be indirectly exposed to a destructive event, for example, via media reports.

In epidemiology, study designs that are not experimental, including quasi-experimental designs, are called observational studies.[39] Here, subjects are studied under natural conditions without any intervention by the researcher. Only naturally occurring exposures and outcomes are examined in these types of studies. A cohort study is one of the typical designs used in epidemiology in which the researcher identifies a group of exposed individuals and a group of non-exposed individuals, or individuals with varying degrees of exposure, and follows the groups

to compare the occurrence of specific outcomes. In disaster research, for example, long-term health outcomes could be compared between groups of residents in the same disaster-affected community based on their level of exposure to the index disaster or between residents of a disaster-affected community and residents of a similar community not affected by a disaster.

Following the 1995 Kobe, Japan earthquake, a cohort of school children were assessed for posttraumatic stress reactions at four points in time over the 2 years after the disaster. Children who lived in areas directly affected by the earthquake were compared with children of the same age group who lived in distant areas that were not directly affected.[53] It was found that greater exposure to the earthquake was associated with more fear, anxiety, and depression or physical symptoms, with younger children exhibiting greater vulnerability. Exposure was defined as the extent of survivors' experiences related to home damage, injuries to oneself, fatalities or injuries among family members, and having to be rescued or to stay in shelters after the earthquake.

Another common study design in epidemiology applied to disaster research is the case-control study. As with cohort studies, this design is appropriate for explanatory research aimed at understanding the association between exposure and outcomes. In contrast with cohort studies, however, instead of determining exposure status first and then observing outcomes, a case-control study begins by identifying groups of people who naturally have or do not have the outcome of interest (i.e., cases and controls, respectively) and then retrospectively determining their exposure status. For example, a matched case-control study was conducted in a village of Southern China where a powerful typhoon struck in August 2006.[54] A census was conducted to determine residents who had died or been injured in the typhoon (i.e., the outcome of interest). A comparison with those residents who had survived without injury led to the identification of risk factors for typhoon-related injury and death. These included proximity of the house to the sea and behavioral factors such as failure to reinforce doors or windows and staying near a door or window during the typhoon.

Quasi-experimental, cohort, and case-control studies can all offer relatively high internal validity. They can also maximize external validity, or generalizability to a larger population, if population-based sampling is used. One of the major challenges to using these designs is defining disaster exposure. For example, one might posit that everyone in the United States was exposed to the September 11, 2001, attacks on the World Trade Center and Pentagon, even though most people were not proximal to the disaster sites. Nonetheless, they may have experienced it vicariously through the media, their friends, or family. A quasi-experimental study conducted in the United Kingdom (UK) compared the responses collected before and after the September 11 terrorist attacks in a longitudinal household panel survey. Investigators demonstrated that a terrorist attack in one country negatively impacted the wellbeing of residents in another country through vicarious exposure.[55] However, the amount of this exposure was not measured or validated in this study. As an example, researchers did not assess whether or how much the respondents had actually viewed or heard any media coverage of the event. Rather, given the extensive and prolonged worldwide media coverage of the disaster, it was assumed that all of the surveyed population had been exposed by the time of the post-9/11 survey. Epidemiologists are often interested in identifying dose–response relationships, that is, the relationship of observed outcomes to varying levels of exposure. A dose–response relationship strengthens the internal validity (i.e., causal claims) of the research findings.

Observational study designs are also appropriate for descriptive studies, in which the objective is to accurately describe the distribution of variables or associations between variables in a population. Non-experimental designs have low internal validity but can have a high degree of external validity if they are conducted with a probability sample of the population. The greatest challenge in conducting population-based studies in disaster research is identifying the population to which the study results can be generalized, or, in other words, establishing the denominator for population estimates. Catastrophic disasters further complicate this issue because the population from which data is collected may be unstable or different from what it had been before the event due to disaster-associated in- and out-migrations, deaths, and alterations in procedures used to compile administrative records.[56] A study of migration patterns in the wake of Hurricanes Katrina and Rita in the United States found that places characterized by greater proportions of disadvantaged populations, housing damage, and more densely built environments were significantly more likely to experience out-migration following the hurricanes.[57] In this case, surveying only the people who remained in the area will likely underestimate the full extent of physical and socioeconomic damages caused by the storms. Any population-based study conducted post-disaster will need to account for such nonrandom patterns of change in the base population.

A non-experimental observational study design that is suitable for in-depth, exploratory research is the case study (or a case series). In this type of study, cases are deliberately selected for examination without insuring they are statistically representative of a population, thus compromising external validity. Internal validity is also low because systematic comparisons between cases and non-cases are not performed. The main benefit of case studies is that they lead to a better understanding of rare or new phenomena and the development of hypotheses. Much of the early disaster research in the social sciences used case studies (see earlier section on Historical Overview of Disaster Research). Case studies are also used in disaster medicine and epidemiology to describe the unique characteristics of deaths, injuries, illnesses, and other health outcomes associated with disasters.[58]

In addition to the distinction between experimental and observational designs, there is also a difference between methodologies in terms of how frequently data are collected over a study period. When data are collected at only one point in time, it is called a cross-sectional or prevalence study. It is best used to describe the state of a population at a given time. Cross-sectional designs can also be used to identify causal associations between variables, where the evidence for causation is based on the application of theory and inferential logic rather than time sequence.[59] In other words, theoretical models are used to determine whether the hypothesized independent variable logically precedes the dependent variable. Therefore, cross-sectional designs can also be used in explanatory research, although they are most naturally used for descriptive research.

Cross-sectional studies conducted before a disaster occurs can provide valuable baseline data on health status, knowledge of risks, attitudes toward preparedness, and actual preparedness behavior at the individual, organizational, or community level. In reality, most disaster studies using a cross-sectional design are conducted after the event has occurred to assess its impact. Examples of these kinds of studies include the post-disaster, rapid

health surveys routinely conducted by the CDC as well as by local public health officials. Results of post-disaster, cross-sectional studies must be interpreted with care, especially when baseline data are not available. Although it is tempting to associate post-disaster observations with the index event, it must be recognized that findings from a post-disaster, cross-sectional study reflect conditions that existed before the event as well as conditions that arose during or afterward. Therefore, not all cases or conditions identified in a post-disaster, cross-sectional study are new (i.e., incident cases). The cases identified in a cross-sectional study, including both old and new, are referred to as prevalent cases.

Even new cases that occur after a disaster may have little or no causal association with the incident itself. Among the prevalent cases identified after an event, errors are frequently made in distinguishing between incident cases (or conditions) caused by the disaster, incident cases unrelated to the disaster, preexisting cases that were exacerbated by the disaster, and preexisting cases that were unaffected by the disaster. Chronic conditions are especially prone to such classification errors, although a carefully designed study can allow researchers to make causal attributions to the index event. As an example, following the magnitude 8.8 earthquake that struck Chile in 2010, the Chilean government re-interviewed a subsample of respondents to a national socioeconomic survey for a longitudinal study of posttraumatic stress symptoms, which had just been completed before the earthquake.[60] This enabled a clear distinction of pre- and post-exposure conditions. The study also employed new statistical methods to match the exposed and unexposed individuals on forty-six covariates to further strengthen internal validity. As a result, this study was able to produce strong evidence of elevated posttraumatic stress symptoms associated with earthquake exposure.

Longitudinal studies collect data more than once over a long period of time. This methodology is used less frequently than cross-sectional designs because it typically requires more resources and a longer-term commitment to the study. It has the advantage, however, of allowing researchers to examine trends and changes over time. It can also provide stronger evidence for causality because temporal ambiguity is reduced or eliminated. In disaster research, longitudinal designs are often used for documenting a community's course of recovery from a disaster, or for observing changes between periods interrupted by a disaster (i.e., pre- and post-disaster).

Examples of longitudinal designs include repeated cross-sectional studies (in which new samples of the population are studied each time) and cohort studies, also referred to as panel studies or repeated-measures studies (in which data are collected at multiple times from the same group of subjects). Repeated cross-sectional designs are especially useful when pre-disaster data are available for a population that was later affected by an incident. To illustrate, a study was conducted to estimate the impact of Hurricane Katrina on mental illness by comparing results of a post-hurricane survey with those of an earlier survey.[61] The populations from which the probability samples were drawn were comparable (although the post-hurricane population frame was limited to survivors) and the measures used to assess outcomes were identical. Results showed that the estimated prevalence of mental illness doubled after the hurricane.

Although repeated cross-sectional studies have the advantage of studying samples that are representative of the population at each time of data collection, cohort studies allow for the examination of change over time within a group. Cohort studies, however, often suffer from loss of follow-up (i.e., respondents intentionally or unintentionally stop participating in the study). For instance, respondents to a survey conducted after the 1994 Northridge, California earthquake were re-interviewed 4 years later to determine if their prior experience affected their response to another anticipated disaster, a slow-onset El Niño weather pattern.[62] Of the 1,849 households originally interviewed after the 1994 earthquake, 1,353 (73%) agreed to a follow-up interview, but less than half of them could be contacted at the time of the follow-up study. Ultimately, 414 were interviewed, yielding a 22.4% response rate of those interviewed at baseline. Loss of follow-up is expected to be high in areas where the population is very mobile, such as in large urban areas.

A further aspect of study designs is the timing of data collection in relation to the outcome of interest associated with the index disaster. In a concurrent design, both exposure and outcome data might be collected at the time the event occurs, or shortly afterward. In a prospective study, which is only possible using a longitudinal design, exposure data are collected from the target population before the event (in this case, the disaster) has occurred, and outcome data are collected subsequently. In these instances, the study may be initiated for other purposes but can be adapted to the disaster researchers' needs. Lastly, in a retrospective design, data are collected on events or conditions that occurred in the past by using archival or recalled information. An example here is a study based on a review of hospital records after a disaster. Case-control studies are retrospective by design because prior exposure data are collected after cases are identified. Although most observational studies can use any one of these designs, or a combination of them, experiments by definition can only be concurrent or prospective because it is impossible to go back in time to manipulate study variables.

Some study designs have been underutilized in disaster research. Case studies using laboratory simulations were used in early disaster research, but have not been used in recent times, perhaps because of the difficulty of simulating the complexities of a disaster.[63] Moreover, the external validity, or generalizability, of results from laboratory simulation studies might be compromised due to the highly artificial and decontextualized nature of a laboratory setting. It has been noted, however, that disaster simulation exercises in the field, which are routinely conducted to train emergency management personnel, are underutilized opportunities for disaster research.[7] A recent study has also noted that disaster exercises are an opportunity to test and evaluate research protocols.[64]

Retrospective designs are relatively underutilized compared to concurrent or prospective designs because they are not as suitable for research during the immediate post-disaster period, where researchers frequently focus. These include retrospective case studies (which involve the historical analysis and reconstruction of events that occurred in the past), historical cohort studies (which involve the analysis of data on cohorts that were followed up in the past), and case-control studies.[10] Case-control studies are appropriate for studying rare outcomes and thus would be suitable for studying disaster-associated phenomena.

Disaster Research Data Collection

As with most other types of investigations, disaster research utilizes both qualitative and quantitative data. Qualitative data are often collected through field observations, in-depth interviews, focus group discussions, and archival research. They offer very detailed information about a specific individual or group, place, time, and/or phenomenon that is of interest to the researcher. Qualitative data collection methods are frequently used in exploratory or descriptive studies in which the objective is to investigate an issue or describe a phenomenon about which there is little existing information. A historical example of qualitative disaster research is Form and Nosow's 1958 study of community responses to a tornado in Michigan.[65] A more recent study examined the dynamics of existing and emerging social networks among Latino survivors of Hurricane Katrina, which struck the Gulf Coast of the United States in 2005.[66] Data gathered from individual, in-depth interviews brought to light: 1) the role of social networks in gathering information, making decisions, and accessing resources; 2) broader structural constraints, including poverty, a lack of transportation, and marginalized status as immigrants; and 3) the emergence of new, if temporary, social networks based primarily on shared nationality, language, and a sense of collective commitment. These and other examples of well-performed qualitative disaster research demonstrate that despite a common misperception that qualitative studies are less scientifically rigorous than quantitative studies, they are indeed important and have been published in prominent journals.

Quantitative data complement qualitative data by expanding the breadth of knowledge about a particular issue. The most popular and efficient method for collecting quantitative data is the use of surveys based on representative sampling. Surveys can be of individuals, households, institutions, or communities, and data in surveys can be collected with questionnaires and record reviews. Surveys of individuals are typically conducted using questionnaires that are self-administered by the respondent or administered by interviewers over the telephone or in person. For surveys of households, organizations, or communities, a representative of the group can be designated to participate in the survey instead of all members of the group.

Survey topics that are common in social science research include: pre-disaster knowledge, attitudes, and behaviors; immediate emotional and behavioral responses to an event; and the course of post-disaster recovery. Commonly perceived limitations of survey use in disaster research include victims' reluctance to discuss their experiences with investigators and the inconsistent reliability of self-reports, although these concerns have been refuted by several researchers.[44,67,68] Another obstacle to using surveys for disaster research is the recent general decline in participation rates for household surveys.[69]

Surveys of individuals, healthcare providers, and healthcare organizations are heavily utilized in disaster epidemiology to obtain quantitative data about the health status of a population and possible associations between disaster exposure and health outcomes. These data are critical for assessing the immediate and ongoing healthcare needs in a population during and following a disaster. In addition to directly surveying members of the population, epidemiological disaster surveys often collect aggregated data from healthcare providers, emergency response agencies, coroners, and other relevant sources, either prospectively or retrospectively. Public health officials might survey emergency shelters on a weekly basis by reviewing medical records to enumerate shelter residents diagnosed with acute respiratory and gastrointestinal illnesses to detect possible outbreaks of infectious disease.

Standardization of the data collection method is especially important with quantitative data in order to allow comparisons across different events, populations, settings, and times.

In this respect, post-disaster rapid health surveys frequently suffer from inconsistencies in sampling methods, data reporting periods, criteria for establishing whether health outcomes are disaster-related, and completeness of data collection for identifying disaster-related injuries and medical conditions. Lack of standardized definitions and survey instruments is one of the major challenges to quantitative data collection in disaster research.

While qualitative and quantitative methodologies complement each other, use of both together in a single investigation (referred to as mixed methods) has yet to become an established approach in disaster research. Mixed methods is broadly defined as research in which the investigator collects and analyzes data, integrates the findings, and draws inferences by using both qualitative and quantitative approaches in a single study or program of inquiry.[70]

The Multihazard Mitigation Council of the National Institute of Building Sciences in the United States conducted a mixed method research study to determine the future savings gained from investments by FEMA in hazard mitigation activities.[71] FEMA funded hazard mitigation projects to reduce loses from earthquakes, high winds, and floods. Future savings from these endeavors were measured in two interrelated studies by using different methods to address the common question: What is the ratio of hazard mitigation benefit versus cost? The first study component used benefit/cost ratio analyses and a statistically representative sample of FEMA mitigation grants so that findings in the sample could be applied to the entire population of these FEMA grants. In the second study component, eight communities were selected using purposive sampling to examine if, why, and how mitigation activities percolate through communities. Field studies were conducted in each community by using semistructured telephone interviews with informants, field visits, and the review of documents. Findings suggest that natural hazard mitigation activities funded by the three FEMA grant programs between 1993 and 2003 were cost effective and reduced future losses from earthquakes, wind, and floods; yielded significant net benefits to society as a whole; and represented significant potential savings to the federal treasury. Specifically, the quantitative benefit/cost analysis found that on average, every dollar spent on natural hazard mitigation saves society approximately $4. The community studies suggest that the 1:4 cost/benefit ratio may be an underestimate because federally funded hazard mitigation often leads to an increase in non-federally funded mitigation programs.

Information Technology Applications in Disaster Research

The application of information technology (IT) in both disaster management and disaster research has remarkably advanced in recent years. The use of Geographic Information Systems (GIS) technology is a prime example. Dash, Thomas, and colleagues have written on the use of GIS technology in disaster management and research.[72,73] There have also been discussions on the utility of GIS-based spatial analysis in health research and epidemiology.[74,75] The main strength of GIS technology is its ability to integrate geographical data with other information, such as demographic data, extent of physical damage caused by a hazard, morbidity and mortality rates, and access to resources. It also has the capability to analyze data as well as to generate maps and other visual summaries of the data.

FEMA has developed a software program, HAZUS-MH, which uses GIS technology to map and display hazard data and also to produce estimates of potential losses (i.e., physical damage, economic loss, and social impact) from earthquakes, floods, and hurricane winds. GIS-based risk assessment tools such as these are extremely useful to disaster management officials and policymakers who are responsible for developing and implementing disaster mitigation, preparedness, and response strategies for geographically defined areas.

The most common application of GIS technology in disaster epidemiological research is to facilitate post-disaster rapid assessment surveys, which frequently use cluster–random sampling. The cluster–random sampling design, which was originally developed to estimate immunization coverage in a population, allows investigators to obtain expedient and accurate population-based information at relatively low cost.[76] GIS is used to aid the random selection of households, field navigation, data management and analysis, and presentation of results. For example, less than 3 weeks after Hurricane Katrina struck Hancock County, Mississippi, the CDC was asked to conduct a rapid assessment of public health needs. Using GIS, they cluster–random sampled 200 households. Using global positioning system technology to navigate to those locations, they physically surveyed 197 households and completed interviews with 77 of them in 2 days.[77] The results of the assessment, which indicated a need for water, trash/debris removal, and access to health services, were provided to the state health department and emergency management to guide relief and recovery operations.

There are other applications of GIS in disaster epidemiology that involve more extensive data collection and spatial referencing. Peek-Asa and others used GIS to link separate data elements derived from studying the 1994 Northridge, California earthquake. These included geophysical characteristics (i.e., shaking intensity, strong ground motion, and soil type), individual characteristics of people who were injured in the earthquake (i.e., physical address and demographics), and building data (i.e., damage state, year of construction, structure type), each obtained from a different source.[78] Their analyses indicated that a person's age and sex, intensity of ground motion, and multiunit building structures independently predict heightened risk for injuries in an earthquake.

GIS has the potential to facilitate data collection, analysis, and presentation for describing or predicting the geographical distribution of various disaster-relevant variables. The usefulness of GIS to disaster research, and especially disaster health research, depends on the quality and availability of spatial data. Health data generally lack spatial attributes (i.e., geocodes) unless they were collected specifically for use in GIS. In addition, there is a legitimate concern about preserving individual confidentiality within spatial information. Researchers have shown, for instance, that a map of Hurricane Katrina-related mortality locations in Orleans and St. Bernard Parishes published in a local newspaper could be reengineered to reveal the actual addresses associated with the points, even though the original map included very little secondary spatial data.[79]

Examples of relatively novel applications of IT include tracking population movements with mobile phone network data; real-time monitoring of calls made to a disaster communication hub (e.g., 211 calls for community information and referral services in the United States and Canada); crowd-sourced online mapping services; geo-targeted imminent threat alerts and warnings delivered to cell phones and other mobile devices; and use of social media for tracking events and distributing alert and warning messages.[80–85] While not without limitations, these applications may pave the way for further innovations in the use of IT to improve the efficiency of rapid assessments and the coverage of disaster relief services, as well as facilitate research-related activities.

Ethics in Disaster Research

As with any study, ethical considerations are integral to disaster research. The central concern is whether the investigational activity could, directly or indirectly, harm the research participants and the wider community. For example, field observations and interviews of evacuees and emergency responders during or immediately after the disaster might impede the progress of relief operations. Likewise, interviewing disaster victims about their experiences has the potential to cause emotional stress and pain, compounding that already caused by the event. Such an investigation might not be justified by the expected benefits of the study. Other ethical considerations include the ability of researchers to maintain a neutral stance. This situation might emerge when grave human suffering seemingly is attributable to social injustice and an incompetent response by the organizations responsible for protecting people's welfare. Despite a sense of urgency to deploy post-impact, disaster researchers must consider these and other ethical issues in designing their study and before having contact with research subjects. Readers are referred to Chapter 7 of this book, as well as to writings by Stallings, Fleischman et al., and Collogan et al. for further discussion about the ethical issues involved in disaster research.[4,86,87]

Disaster Vulnerability

There is a general consensus within the disaster community that vulnerability interacts with the physical hazard agent to produce disaster risk.[88–90] Vulnerability is conceptualized as, "the characteristics of a person or group and their situation that influence their capacity to anticipate, cope with, resist, and recover from the impact of natural hazards."[90] Thus, greater vulnerability of an individual or group is associated with increased risk from a given level of disaster exposure. In many instances, estimations of who might be most vulnerable to a disaster can be formulated before an event occurs, although disasters often function to bring attention to underserved segments of the population.

Health professionals may be most familiar with conceptualizing vulnerable populations as those that are physiologically susceptible because of age and/or physical and mental health conditions. Examples include children, the elderly, pregnant women, and people with disabilities. Physiological vulnerability can indeed affect people's ability to withstand external shock (such as the physical force of an earthquake, tornado, or hurricane) and survive trauma injuries. Also at risk is their capacity to cope with short- or long-term disruptions of access to basic resources, including food, shelter, and healthcare. It is widely recognized, however, that disaster vulnerability is multidimensional; there are many other factors that contribute to people's capacity to anticipate, cope, and recover from the impact of hazards.

The most commonly mentioned dimensions of vulnerability in disaster research are physical, economic, political, social, and psychological.[91–94] The social epidemiologic theory of fundamental cause is relevant to several of these dimensions, although the theory does not address disasters directly.[95] The central notion is that one's socioeconomic position shapes exposure to health risk factors and the individual's capacity to respond to those risk factors. The measured components of socioeconomic position are occupational prestige, educational attainment, and income, while the construct itself is thought to encompass political power and other forms of social stratification. The inverse relationship of social class with mortality and almost every measure of morbidity is consistent and strong. In fact, other predictors of health outcomes are often considered provisional until it can be shown that relationships exist independently of socioeconomic position, viewed as the fundamental cause.

Physical vulnerability refers to an individual's proximity and/or inadequate physical and structural resistance to a hazard.[94,96,97] Physical vulnerability is important for high physical force disasters, such as earthquakes and tornadoes, in which the potential for damage to physical structures is increased.

Economic vulnerability can be conceptualized at the macro level, in terms of international and national economic practices and conditions. However, it is more often conceptualized at the micro, or household level, in terms of employment conditions (e.g., income opportunities and job characteristics).[98] The nature of economic vulnerability is different for disasters with a rapid onset and short duration, such as earthquakes, than for those of a slow onset and/or long duration, such as droughts. In rapid-onset disasters, economic vulnerability is defined by the ability to withstand short-term social and economic disruption and the ability to finance reconstruction and repairs of structural damages. In contrast, economic vulnerability to slow-onset/chronic disasters depends on the flexibility of the economy to adjust to prolonged disaster situations (e.g., importing food stock, creating jobs for farmers), the availability of assets at the household level, and the diversity of income-producing opportunities.[99] Extended exposure to adverse conditions, including food scarcity, mass population movement, and psychological stress, can lower immunity levels and increase risk for infectious diseases, as well as exacerbate any preexisting health conditions. Although the risk for communicable diseases is actually quite low for any major disaster, these concerns are relevant in chronic disaster situations, like droughts and famines.[100]

Political vulnerability encompasses having little or no political power, representation, or autonomy.[91,93,101,102] Political values and priorities determine which hazards will be addressed, the degree of emphasis and support placed on hazard mitigation, and the willingness to meet the needs of divergent groups in the aftermath of a disaster. Political vulnerability, like psychological vulnerability described later, is relevant to any type of disaster. Political power affects the likelihood that an individual or a community will receive government support to ensure a safe environment or have the resources and resilience to take self-protective measures. Those who are marginalized in society tend to live in the least safe areas and have the greatest exposure to hazardous conditions. Political vulnerability is particularly relevant for disasters in conflict situations, where political or military motivations by warring parties determine who receives the most aid and protection.[103] The philosophy that increasing political influence is the key to reducing overall vulnerability, including vulnerability to disasters, underlies individual and community empowerment efforts.[102]

Social vulnerability includes the formal institutional structures that marginalize certain groups and individuals based on their socioeconomic characteristics, such as gender, race, or ethnicity.[94,97,104,105] Informal social relations with friends, family, and others are included here as well.[91] A community is socially vulnerable when people feel victimized, fatalistic, or dependent, often resulting in apathy and a low sense of personal responsibility.[92,93,101] This global sense of alienation can become immersed in a broader cultural system of beliefs and customs and may manifest itself in disaster-relevant behaviors, such as low levels of motivation and/or knowledge about implementing preparedness measures.

In an effort to quantify social vulnerability, the Social Vulnerability Index was developed, using factor analytic techniques to reduce thirty community-level variables (e.g., percent below poverty threshold) to a few factors that group similar data items together.[106] The index provides a score for each county in the United States and is envisioned as a tool for policymakers and practitioners. Consistent with predictions from fundamental cause theory, the variables of race (Black), class, poverty, and wealth contribute heavily to scores on the Social Vulnerability Index. The concept is a promising one and research on indices that attempt to quantify social vulnerability should be expanded.

Psychological vulnerability is studied at the level of the individual in terms of the psychological characteristics that influence coping skills with disaster stress and the likelihood of experiencing an emotional injury or distress.[107] In the extant literature, previous mental health problems are the most robust and consistent predictors of post-disaster distress.[108] Contrary to popular belief, psychological effects of non-terrorist disasters tend to be mild and transitory in the general population, rarely resulting in psychopathology.[109–111] Severe levels of psychological impairment are more likely to occur in disasters involving mass violence compared with other types of disasters.[112] Thus, psychological vulnerability is a more prominent factor in exposure to intentional disasters, with high exposure and loss of significant others as risk factors, in addition to previous mental health problems.[113]

The dimensions of vulnerability concept is a convenient schematic but it should be recognized that these dimensions mutually interact, and the distinctions among them are often blurred. For example, the 2010 earthquake in Haiti, which killed more than 220,000 people and injured another 300,000, occurred in a country where 80% of the population lived in poverty (economic and social vulnerability).[104] Lack of a clean water supply (physical vulnerability), both before and after the quake, contributed to a cholera epidemic that broke out later in 2010. Deforestation (physical vulnerability) and long-term political instability (political vulnerability) enhanced the impact of the quake and the government's ability to respond. In a country with a low priority on mental health, the earthquake magnified the inadequacy of mental health services (psychological vulnerability). Recovery continues to be slow, with some of the aid intended for rebuilding diverted to other projects (political vulnerability). The sharp reduction in foreign aid and focused attention may foster feelings of abandonment, futility, and hopelessness (psychological vulnerability). Focusing on the interplay among the dimensions of vulnerability is compatible with an ecological approach that emphasizes the mutuality of nature and human activity.[114–117] According to this approach, disasters occur when the social and cultural systems of a population fail to provide adequate adaptation to the environmental conditions that surround it or when these systems themselves produce a threat to the population.[116]

Disaster Morbidity and Mortality

The discussion of disaster morbidity and mortality describes how these estimates are derived, as well as the many factors that can influence their accuracy and introduce variability across studies.

Patterns of Morbidity and Mortality by Disaster Type

The health impact of a disaster varies by: 1) the physical characteristics of the hazard that triggers an abnormal event; 2) the physical, social, and political environment in which the hazard event occurs; and 3) the characteristics of the population that is affected. For instance, the number of people who die or suffer from physical or mental health problems as a result of an earthquake depends on multiple factors. These include: 1) the intensity of the ground shaking, the duration of shaking, the soil type, and the intensity and frequency of aftershocks (hazard characteristics); 2) the population density and proximity of human settlements to the areas where the greatest shaking occurs; 3) common types of building construction; 4) the emergency response and health-care infrastructure in place (physical environment); 5) cultural norms regarding earthquake awareness and preparedness, common human activity at the time of the earthquake occurrence, and political will and capacity to mitigate against and respond to earthquake disasters (social and political environment); and 6) the age, preexisting health conditions, and socioeconomic status of the population (population characteristics).

This is why earthquakes of a similar magnitude, as measured on the Richter scale, result in vastly different outcomes in regard to human casualties. To illustrate, official reports indicate that the 2001 Seattle/Nisqually, Washington earthquake (M6.8) resulted in one death and 407 injuries; the 1994 Northridge, California earthquake (M6.7) 57 deaths and 1,500 injuries (Note: A thorough county-wide screening of hospital admission records and a review of relevant medical records and coroner's reports in Los Angeles County verified 33 fatalities and 138 hospital admissions); the 1988 Armenian earthquake (M6.8) 25,000 deaths and 130,000 injuries; and the 2003 southeastern Iran earthquake (M6.6) 26,200 deaths and 30,000 injuries.[40,118]

Differences in reports of morbidity and mortality also reflect variability in the methods used to estimate the health impact. These methods are reflective of the infrastructure for systematic data collection that exists before the event, and the extent to which damage and disruption caused by the event interfere with post-disaster data collection. Thus, it is important to recognize this multifactorial nature of both the actual and reported morbidity and mortality in disasters. When possible, researchers should attempt to put the numbers into context by accounting for the various factors that could have influenced estimates of morbidity and mortality.

Hazard type is a common classification scheme for disaster-associated morbidity and mortality.[28,119] The CDC, through their publication *MMWR*, is the main source for disaster-attributable morbidity and mortality data in the United States. The amount of knowledge or research that is available about the health effects of a particular hazard depends on several factors. These include: 1) how frequently events involving that hazard occur; 2) whether there is a clear beginning and end point to the hazard event, thus making causal attributions less ambiguous; 3) whether the hazard tends to cause multiple human casualties; and 4) whether there have been especially devastating or dramatic events that surround the disaster.

As an example, there is an accumulation of literature and knowledge about the health impact of hurricanes (and floods associated with them) and tornadoes, especially in the United States. Both types of events are seasonal hazards that occur annually. Earthquakes also have been well studied internationally, even though they are irregular events, because there is little ambiguity about when an earthquake begins and ends, and because large earthquakes have caused numerous deaths. In comparison, relatively little research has been devoted to the health impact of volcanoes, wildfires, tsunamis, and droughts, due to one or more of the reasons noted. These limiting characteristics include infrequent event occurrence, ambiguous event thresholds, and low human impact. Concomitant with recent interest in the effects of global warming, there has been a recent rise in the number of heat-related health consequence studies, with a greater willingness to conceptualize extreme temperatures as a disaster.[120] The occurrence of a catastrophic event can re-energize or completely change the research activity in these areas. The Indian Ocean tsunami in December 2004 and the 2011 Tōhoku Earthquake and Tsunami in March 2011 have spawned an unprecedented amount of research on the physical and psychological morbidity and mortality associated with tsunamis.

Among the hazards that are not "environmental," unintentional releases of hazardous materials caused by industrial accidents have been studied the most. In regard to intentional events, the effects of terrorism, usually involving explosive devices, have also been well documented. This is especially true for the 1995 Oklahoma City and 2001 New York City bombings. In contrast, there have been very few studies on the intentional use of biological, radiological, or chemical agents. Nonetheless, the medical or physical health consequences of direct exposure to these hazards are perhaps better known than those resulting from exposure to other hazards, partly because exposure can be defined more clearly.

The psychological morbidity resulting from disasters is less differentiated by the type of hazard and more affected by whether a disaster was due to unintentional or intentional causes. The latter type causes greater psychological distress to victims who are aware it is intentional. Posttraumatic stress disorder is by far the most common malady studied, followed by depression, anxiety, and panic disorders.[121,122] Most studies reveal a significant drop in symptoms over time.[122,123]

Consistency of Estimation Methods

Lack of consensus on what constitutes a disaster, exposure to disaster, and a disaster-related death, injury, or disease complicates disaster research. One focus of disaster research is classifying types of disasters by types of health outcomes. Although a number of schemes for classifying health outcomes do exist, there is no standard method for classifying exposure to a disaster. Despite efforts to develop standardized procedures, disaster researchers continue to develop and use their own definitions and classification protocols, often with little regard for prior research. The sprawling disciplinary landscape of disaster research contributes to this tendency.

The definition of what constitutes a death or injury caused by a disaster varies not only within, but also across disaster types. The CDC has attempted to develop a protocol for classifying outcomes attributable to disasters based on the time the death or injury occurs relative to the event, and also based on whether the event is directly or indirectly related to the disaster. According to the authors, "disaster-attributed deaths [are] those caused by either the direct or indirect exposure to the disaster. Directly related deaths are those caused by the physical forces of the disaster. Indirectly related deaths are those caused by unsafe or unhealthy conditions that occur because of the anticipation, or actual occurrence, of the disaster."[124] Although strong in theory, the schema is difficult to apply in practice, especially when estimating indirect effects.

Estimates of morbidity are harder to ascertain than those of mortality. In many cases, assessments of U.S. disaster-related morbidity are based on the best guesses of a public health employee who contacted the Red Cross and local hospitals for their number estimates of the injured and ill individuals served in emergency departments. It has been established that most of the injured and sick do not utilize emergency departments, and persons staffing emergency departments are not necessarily aware of, or knowledgeable about, which injuries are attributable to a given disaster.[40] Thus, morbidity estimates often include a fairly substantial margin of error, including both under- and over-reporting. Careful review of emergency department logs and admission records is essential and will improve estimates but cannot eliminate ambiguity in every case.[28,108]

RECOMMENDATIONS FOR FURTHER RESEARCH

The key message that underlies this chapter is captured well in the following quote from Lurie et al.: "The knowledge that is generated through well-designed, effectively executed research . . . is critical to our future capacity to better achieve the overarching goals of preparedness and response: preventing injury, illness, disability, and death and supporting recovery."[125] Research is essential in generating the evidence base for policy development and decision-making to help ensure that fewer people and societies suffer from the devastating impact of disasters in the future. This final section offers some recommendations on the way forward for research on disasters.

In the first edition of this book, we had recommended the following: 1) facilitating closer collaborations between disciplines as well as between researchers and practitioners; 2) enhancing capacity in disaster research; 3) strengthening the validity of research findings through the use of population-based and longitudinal designs; 4) improving consistency of methods and measurements, with specific reference to the guidelines recommended by an international task force for the reporting of disaster medical research; and 5) improving access to disaster research strategies and findings.[126] These recommendations are still relevant today.

However, despite the fact that interdisciplinary and multi-sector collaborations have become common approaches in most research fields, it remains quite limited in practice when it comes to disaster research. Given how disasters are become increasingly complex within such contexts as climate change, urbanization, and population dynamics (e.g., ageing, racial/ethnic diversity, migration), multidisciplinary approaches to research are needed to understand the various factors and interactions that determine the causes and sequelae of disasters. Urban settings would be especially ideal for such research because these factors tend to converge in heavily populated areas. In addition, researchers, practitioners, and institutions from multiple disciplines and sectors can be found in urban centers. Research on urban disasters is also important because local city governments are frequently responsible for the first level of official preparedness, mitigation, and response to a disaster. In view of the fact that over half of the world's population lives in urban areas (a proportion which continues to grow) and that the most populous cities in the world are at risk of major disasters, we should expect more urban disaster research in the future.[127]

Access to reliable health and medical data remains a significant challenge. One approach to improving data collection is to classify injuries and illnesses that arise from officially declared disasters as reportable diseases. Identifying these outcomes as reportable will facilitate efforts by public health personnel to obtain critical information on disaster victims. The public health community has a long history of obtaining such information effectively while protecting the confidentiality of those exposed to the disaster. This approach will facilitate research across disciplines and make analyses more efficient, in that each group of researchers will not be repeating the process of independently collecting data. In addition, the recommended change will improve rapid access to data that may be lost over time or difficult to obtain, secondary to various governmental regulations.

With regard to enhancing training and capacity building in disaster research, increased efforts should be directed toward the developing regions of the world. Statistics show that 90% of all deaths caused by disasters over the past two decades have occurred in developing countries.[127] Even though the majority of the world's disaster-related human suffering occurs in these countries, much of the disaster research continues to be conducted in more developed regions. Disasters that affect developing countries are not limited to just rare, sudden-onset, catastrophic events. They also include recurrent, slow-onset events, such as floods and droughts. Improving the understanding of disasters in developing countries is in everyone's best interest in this increasingly interdependent, globalized world. Building capacity for research in these areas of the world can be realized through traditional cooperation between more resourced and less resourced countries, as well as through interactions between less developed countries which share common challenges and perspectives. Such initiatives have been shown to be successful in other fields of research, like mental health.[128] Funding initiatives are also important. In June 2013, a new collaboration between the UK government's Department of International Development and the Wellcome Trust was established to support world class research examining public health interventions during humanitarian disasters. The first *Call for Proposals for Research for Health in Humanitarian Crises Programme* was launched with a series of town hall meetings held in Delhi, Nairobi, London, and New York. Participants included those interested in applying for funding or seeking to build research partnerships. It is anticipated that initiatives like this can provide the impetus and funding necessary for building disaster research capacity in areas with limited resources.

The sustained frequency of disaster events should be utilized appropriately to improve the quality of disaster research. It is an unfortunate fact that disasters have continued to occur with such regularity around the globe. The year 2011 was one of the worst disaster years in history, with more than 300 disasters recorded, nearly 30,000 people killed, and over 350 billion U.S. dollars in losses.[127] Some of the same places are struck repeatedly, such as China by earthquakes, the Philippines by floods, and the United States by hurricanes and tornadoes. However, the frequency and predictability of these events should allow researchers to plan and conduct well-designed studies that could potentially yield strong evidence of causality with a high degree of generaliz-ability. Furthermore, it is important to generate greater knowledge about effective interventions that limit secondary effects over the course of recovery from a disaster.[26] While social science research has extensively studied pre-disaster preparedness and evacuation behavior, and health research has focused on immediate health consequences of disasters, societies could benefit from more multidisciplinary research analyzing longer-term impacts. Such topics include the indirect, medium- to long-term effects on individuals and communities, and how these impacts can be effectively addressed through interventions. Population-based, longitudinal designs would be ideal for capturing such effects.

We have previously advocated for improved consistency across studies and better access to completed research. The importance and relevance of these two recommendations has not changed. Some activities, if implemented and funded, have the potential to increase mechanisms that integrate disaster research at both the national and global level. For example, in 2011, an advisory committee to the U.S. Department of Health and Human Services (HHS) issued an endorsement to include scientific investigations as an integral component of disaster planning and response. It further recommended that the HHS develop infrastructure for strengthening the research response to emergencies.[125] At the same time, however, the CDC's funding and support for academic centers on public health preparedness and research has been inconsistent and, in fact, declining. How these contrasting approaches by the U.S. government to support health sciences research on disasters will evolve is open to speculation.

Finally, researchers are encouraged to explore new domains, such as the role of emerging technological and social innovations in the context of disasters. This may include research on entirely new topics, such as the efficacy of wireless emergency alerts, or on "old" topics with a new twist, such as disaster volunteerism through the use of social networking. It is through a continuous process of both learning from the past and staying abreast of new developments that the field of disaster research can further mature and generate critical knowledge toward building sound public policy and more resilient societies.

REFERENCES

1. Noji E. Public health consequences of disasters. *Prehosp Disaster Med* 2000; 15: 147–157.
2. Cisin IH, Clark WB. The methodological challenge of disaster research. In: Baker G, Chapman D, eds. *Man and Society in Disaster*. New York, Basic Books, 1962; 23–54.
3. Gordis L. *Epidemiology*. 3rd ed. Philadelphia, Elsevier Saunders, 2004.
4. Stallings RA. Methodological issues. In: Rodríguez H, Quarantelli EL, Dynes RR, eds. *Handbook of Disaster Research*. New York, Springer, 2006; 55–82.
5. Killian LM. An introduction to methodological problems of field studies in disasters. In: Stallings RA, ed. *Methods of Disaster Research*. International Research Committee on Disasters, Xlibris Corp., 2002; 49–93.
6. Quarantelli EL. The Disaster Research Center (DRC) field studies of organized behavior in the crisis time period of disasters. In: Stallings RA, ed. *Methods of Disaster Research*. International Research Committee on Disasters, Xlibris Corp., 2002; 94–126.

7. Drabek TE. Following some dreams: Recognizing opportunities, posing interesting questions, and implementing alternative methods. In: Stallings RA, ed. *Methods of Disaster Research*. International Research Committee on Disasters, Xlibris Corp., 2002; 127–153.

8. Guetzkow H. Joining field and laboratory work in disaster research. In: Baker GW, Chapman DW, eds. *Man and Society in Disaster*. New York, Basic Books, 1962; 337–355.

9. Prince SH. *Catastrophe and Social Change: based upon a Sociological Study of the Halifax Disaster*. ADD 1920. Proquest Dissertations and Theses, 1920.

10. Scanlon TJ. Rewriting a living legend: Researching the 1917 Halifax explosion. In: Stallings RA, ed. *Methods of Disaster Research*. International Research Committee on Disasters, Xlibris Corp., 2002; 266–301.

11. Fritz CE. Disasters and mental health: therapeutic principles drawn from disaster studies. 1996. http://dspace.udel.edu:8080/dspace/handle/19716/1325 (Accessed June 20, 2013).

12. Ikle F. The effects of war destruction upon the ecology of cities. *Soc Forces* 1951; 29: 283–291.

13. United States Strategic Bombing Survey. *Reports*. Washington, DC, Government Printing Office, 1947.

14. Marks ES, Fritz CE. *Human Reactions in Disaster Situations*. Vols. 1–3. Unpublished report, Chicago, IL, National Opinion Research Center, University of Chicago, 1954.

15. Morris CW, ed. *Mind Self and Society from the Standpoint of a Social Behaviorist*. Chicago, University of Chicago Press, 1932.

16. Cooley CH. *Social Organization*. New York, Charles Scribner's Sons, 1909.

17. Perry RW. What is a disaster? In: Rodríguez H, Quarantelli EL, Dynes RR, eds. *Handbook of Disaster Research*. New York, Springer, 2006; 1–15.

18. Turner RH, Killian LM. *Collective Behavior*. 1st ed. Englewood Cliffs, NJ, Prentice-Hall, 1957.

19. Perry RW. Evacuation decision-making in natural disasters. *Mass Emergencies* 1979; 4: 25–38.

20. Connell R. *Collective Behavior in the September 11, 2001 Evacuation of the World Trade Center*. Preliminary Paper #313. Newark, University of Delaware Disaster Research Center, 2007.

21. Taylor VA. *The Delivery of Mental Health Services in the Xenia Tornado: a Collective Behavior Analysis of an Emergent System Response*. DAI-A 37/02, Proquest Dissertations and Theses, 1976.

22. Quarantelli EL, Dynes RR. Editors' introduction. *Am Behavior Sci* 1973; 16: 305–311.

23. Sommer A, Mosley WH. East Bengal cyclone of November, 1970: epidemiological approach to disaster assessment. *Epidemiol Rev* 2005; 27: 13–20.

24. Logue JN, Melick ME, Hansen H. Research issues and directions in the epidemiology of health effects of disasters. *Epidemiol Rev* 1981; 3: 140–162.

25. LeChat MF. The epidemiology of health effects of disasters. *Epidemiol Rev* 1990; 12: 192–198.

26. Dominici J, Levy JI, Louis TA. Methodological challenges and contributions in disaster epidemiology. *Epidemiol Rev* 2005; 27: 9–12.

27. Noji EK. Disasters: introduction and state of the art. *Epidemiol Rev* 2005; 27: 3–8.

28. Bourque LB, Siegel JM, Kano M, et al. Morbidity and mortality associated with disasters. In: Rodríguez H, Quarantelli E, Dynes R, eds. *Handbook of Disaster Research*. New York, Springer, 2006; 97–112.

29. Castillo-Salgado C. Trends and directions of global public health surveillance. *Epidemiol Rev* 2010; 32: 93–109.

30. Connorton E, Perry JJ, Hemenway D, et al. Humanitarian relief workers and trauma-related mental illness. *Epidemiol Rev* 2012; 34: 145–155.

31. Srikameswaran A. Dr. Peter Safar Renowned Pitt physician called 'father of CPR.' Obituary. *Pittsburgh Post-Gazette*. August 5, 2003.

32. Ammar A. Role of leadership in disaster management and crowd control. *Prehosp Disaster Med* 2007; 22: 527–528.

33. Smith E, Wasiak J, Sen A, et al. Three decades of disasters: A review of disaster-specific literature from 1977–2009. *Prehosp Disaster Med* 2009; 24: 306–311.

34. Tierney K. From the margins to the mainstream? Disaster research at the crossroads. *Annu Rev Sociol* 2007; 33: 503–525.

35. Brunsma D, Picou JS. Disasters in the twenty-first century: modern destruction and future instruction. *Soc Forces* 2008; 87: 983–991.

36. Norris F, Galea S, Friedman MJ, Watson PJ. *Methods for Disaster Mental Health Research*. New York, Guilford Publications, 2006.

37. Rodríguez H, Quarantelli E, Dynes R, eds. *Handbook of Disaster Research*. New York, Springer, 2006.

38. Stallings RA, ed. *Methods of Disaster Research*. International Research Committee on Disasters, Xlibris Corp., 2002.

39. Kelsey JL, Whittemore AS, Evans AS, Thompson WD. *Methods in Observational Epidemiology*. 2nd ed. New York, Oxford University Press, 1996.

40. Peek-Asa C, Kraus JF, Bourque LB, Vimalachandra D, Yu J, Abrams J. Fatal and hospitalized injuries resulting from the 1994 Northridge earthquake. *Intl J Epidemiol* 1998; 27: 459–465.

41. Carlsen HK, Hauksdottir A, Valdimarsdottir UA, et al. Health effects following the Eyjafjallajökull volcanic eruption: a cohort study. *BMJ Open* 2012; 2: e001851.

42. Tierney KJ, Lindell MK, Perry RW. *Facing the Unexpected: Disaster Preparedness and Response in the United States*. Washington, DC, Joseph Henry Press, 2001.

43. National Research Council. *Facing Hazards and Disasters: Understanding Human Dimensions*. Washington, DC, The National Academies Press, 2006.

44. Bourque LB, Shoaf KI, Nguyen LH. Survey research. In: Stallings RA, ed. *Methods of Disaster Research*. International Research Committee on Disasters, Xlibris Corp., 2002; 157–193.

45. Last JM. *A Dictionary of Epidemiology*. 4th ed. Oxford, Oxford University Press, 2001.

46. Wood MM, Mileti DS, Kano M, Kelley MM, Regan R, Bourque LB. Communicating actionable risk for terrorism and other hazards. *Risk Anal* 2012; 32: 601–615.

47. Kano M, Wood MM, Bourque LB, Mileti DS. Terrorism preparedness and exposure reduction since 9/11: the status of public readiness in the United States. *Journal of Homeland Security and Emergency Management* 2011; 8.

48. Bensimon CM, Smith MJ, Pisartchik D, et al. The duty to care in an influenza pandemic: A qualitative study of Canadian public perspectives. *Soc Sci Med* 2012; 75: 2425–2430.

49. Fang LQ, Wang LP, de Vlas SJ, et al. Distribution and risk factors of 2009 pandemic influenza A (H1N1) in mainland China. *Am J Epidemiol* 2012; 175: 890–897.

50. Cook TD, Campbell DT. *Quasi-experimentation: Design and Analysis Issues for Field Settings*. Boston, Houghton Mifflin, 1979.

51. Campbell DT, Stanley JC. *Experimental and Quasi-experimental Designs for Research*. Boston, Houghton Mifflin, 1963.

52. Rothman KJ, Greenland S. *Modern Epidemiology*. 2nd ed. Philadelphia, Lippincott-Raven Publishers, 1998.

53. Uemoto M, Asakawa A, Takamiya S, et al. Kobe earthquake and post-traumatic stress in school-aged children. *Int J Behav Med* 2012; 19: 243–251.

54. Shen J, Feng Z, Zeng G, et al. Risk factors for injury during Typhoon Saomei. *Epidemiology* 2009; 20: 892–895.

55. Metcalfe R, Powdthavee N, Dolan P. Destruction and distress: using a quasi-experiment to show the effects of the September 11 attacks on mental well-being in the United Kingdom. *The Economic Journal,* 2011; 121: F81–F103.

56. Smith SK, McCarty C. Demographic effects of natural disasters: a case study of Hurricane Andrew. *Demography* 1996; 33: 265–275.

57. Myers CA, Slack T, Singelmann J. Social vulnerability and migration in the wake of disaster: the case of Hurricanes Katrina and Rita. *Popul Environ,* 2008; 29: 271–291.

58. U.S. Centers for Disease Control and Prevention. Deaths associated with Hurricane Sandy, October–November 2012. *MMWR* 2013; 62: 393–397.

59. Aneshensel CS. *Theory-based Data Analysis for the Social Sciences.* 2nd ed. Los Angeles, CA, Sage, 2013.

60. Zubizaretta JR, Cerdá M, Rosenbaum P. Effect of the 2010 Chilean earthquake on posttraumatic stress reducing sensitivity to unmeasured bias through study design. *Epidemiology* 2013; 24: 79–87.

61. Kessler RC. Mental illness and suicidality after Hurricane Katrina. *Bull World Health Organ* 2006; 84: 930–939.

62. Siegel JM, Shoaf KI, Afifi AA, Bourque LB. Surviving two disasters: does reaction to the first predict response to the second? *Environ Behavior* 2003; 35: 637–654.

63. Drabek TE, Haas JE. Laboratory simulation of organizational stress. *Am Sociol Rev* 1969; 34: 223–238.

64. Legemaate GAG, Burkle FM Jr., Bierens JJLM. The evaluation of research methods during disaster exercises: Applicability for improving disaster health management. *Prehosp Disaster Med* 2012; 27: 18–26.

65. Form WH, Nosow S. *Community in Disaster.* New York, Harper, 1958.

66. Hilfinger MDK, Barrington C, Lacy E. Latino social network dynamics and the Hurricane Katrina disaster. *Disasters* 2012; 36: 101–121.

67. Beckett M, Da Vanzo J, Sastry N, Panis C, Peterson C. The quality of retrospective data: an examination of long-term recall in a developing country. *J Hum Resources* 2001; 36: 593–625.

68. Norris FH, Kaniasty K. Reliability of delayed self-reports in disaster research. *J Trauma Stress* 1992; 5: 575–588.

69. Curtin R, Presser S, Singer E. Changes in telephone survey nonresponse over the past quarter century. *Public Opin Q* 2005; 69: 87–98.

70. Tashakkori A, Creswell JW. The new era of mixed methods [Editorial]. *J Mixed Meth Res* 2007; 1: 3–7.

71. Multihazard Mitigation Council. *Natural Hazard Mitigation Saves: An Independent Study to Assess the Future Savings from Mitigation Activities.* Washington, DC, National Institute of Building Sciences, 2005.

72. Dash N. The use of geographic information systems in disaster research. In: Stallings RA, ed. *Methods of Disaster Research.* International Research Committee on Disasters, Xlibris Corp., 2002; 320–333.

73. Thomas DSK, Kivanç E, Kemeç S. The role of geographic information systems/remote sensing in disaster management. In: Rodríguez H, Quarantelli E, Dynes R, eds. *Handbook of Disaster Research.* New York, Springer, 2006; 83–96.

74. Moore DA, Carpenter TE. Spatial analytical methods and geographic information systems: use in health research and epidemiology. *Epidemiol Rev* 1999; 21: 143–161.

75. Rushton G. Public health, GIS, and spatial analytic tools. *Ann Rev Public Health* 2003; 24: 43–56.

76. Malilay J, Flanders WD, Brogan D. A modified cluster-sampling method for post-disaster rapid assessment of needs. *Bull World Health Organ* 1996; 74: 399–405.

77. U.S. Centers for Disease Control and Prevention. Rapid community needs assessment after hurricane Katrina–Hancock County, Mississippi, September 14–15, 2005. *MMWR* 2006; 55: 234–236.

78. Peek-Asa C, Ramirez M, Seligson HA, Shoaf KI. Seismic, structural, and individual factors associated with earthquake-related injury. *Injury Prevent* 2003; 9: 62–66.

79. Curtis AJ, Mills JQ, Leitner M. Spatial confidentiality and GIS: Re-engineering mortality locations from published maps about Hurricane Katrina. *Intl J Health Geographics* 2006; 5: 44. http://www.ij-healthgeographics.com/content/5/1/44 (Accessed June 11, 2013).

80. Bengtsson L, Lu X, Thorson A, et al. Improved response to disasters and outbreaks by tracking population movements with mobile phone network data: a post-earthquake geospatial study in Haiti. *PLoS Med* 2011; 8: e1001083.

81. Bame SI, Parker K, Lee JY, et al. Monitoring unmet needs: using 2–1–1 during natural disasters. *Am J Prev Med* 2012; 43: S435–S442.

82. Zook M, Graham M, Shelton T. Volunteered geographic information and crowdsourcing disaster relief: a case study of the Haitian earthquake. *World Medical & Health Policy* 2010; 2: 7–33.

83. Nagele DE, Trainor JE. Geographic specificity, tornadoes, and protective action. *Weather, Climate, and Society* 2012; 4: 145–155.

84. National Research Council. *Public Response to Alerts and Warnings on Mobile Devices: Summary of a Workshop on Current Knowledge and Research Gaps.* Washington, DC, The National Academies Press, 2011.

85. National Research Council. *Public Response to Alerts and Warnings Using Social Media: Report of a Workshop on Current Knowledge and Research Gaps.* Washington, DC, The National Academies Press, 2013.

86. Fleischman AR, Collogan L, Tuma F. Ethical issues in disaster research. In: Norris FH, Galea S, Friedman MJ, Watson PJ, eds. *Methods for Disaster Mental Health Research.* New York, Guilford, 2006.

87. Collogan LK, Tuma F, Dolan-Sewell R, Borja S, Fleischman AR. Ethical issues pertaining to research in the aftermath of disaster. *J Trauma Stress* 2004; 17: 363–372.

88. Dilley M, Boudreau TE. Coming to terms with vulnerability: a critique of the food security definition. *Food Policy.* 2001; 26: 229–247.

89. Maskrey A. *Disaster Mitigation: A Community Based Approach.* Oxford, Oxfam, 1989.

90. Wisner B, Blaikie P, Cannon T, Davis I. *At Risk: Natural Hazards, People's Vulnerability, and Disasters.* 2nd ed. London, Routledge, 2004.

91. Morrow BH. Identifying and mapping community vulnerability. *Disasters* 1999; 23: 1–18.

92. Anderson MB, Woodrow PJ. *Rising from the Ashes: Development Strategies in Times of Disaster.* Boulder, CO, Lynne Rienner Publishers, 1998.

93. Aysan YF. Keynote paper: Vulnerability assessment. In: Merriman PA, Browitt CWA, eds. *Natural Disasters: Protecting Vulnerable Communities.* London, Thomas Telford, 1993; 1–14.

94. Cardona OD. The need for rethinking the concepts of vulnerability and risk from a holistic perspective: a necessary review and criticism for effective risk management. In: Bankoff G, Frerks G, Hilhorst D, eds. *Mapping Vulnerability: Disasters, Development and People.* London, Earthscan, 2004; 37–51.

95. Phelan JC, Link BG, Tehranifar P. Social conditions as fundamental causes of health inequalities: theory, evidence, and policy implications. *J Health Soc Behav* 2010; 51: S28–S40.

96. Horlick-Jones T, Jones DKC. Communicating risks to reduce vulnerability. In: Merriman PA, Browitt CWA, eds. *Natural Disasters: Protecting Vulnerable Communities.* London, Thomas Telford, 1993; 25–37.

97. McEntire DA. Tenets of vulnerability: An assessment of a fundamental disaster concept. *J Emerg Manage* 2004; 2: 23–29.

98. Cannon T. A hazard need not a disaster make: vulnerability and the causes of 'natural' disasters. In: Merriman PA, Browitt CWA, eds. *Natural Disasters: Protecting Vulnerable Communities.* London, Thomas Telford, 1993; 92–105.

99. Ezra M, Kiros G-E. Household vulnerability to food crisis and mortality in the drought-prone areas of northern Ethiopia. *J Biosoc Sci* 2000; 32: 395–409.

100. Morgan O. Infectious disease risks from dead bodies following natural disasters. *Pan Am J Public Health* 2004; 15: 307–312.

101. McEntire DA. Triggering agents, vulnerabilities and disaster reduction: towards a holistic paradigm. *Disaster Prevent Manage* 2001; 10: 189–196.

102. Heijmans A. From vulnerability to empowerment. In: Bankoff G, Frerks G, Hilhorst D, eds. *Mapping Vulnerability: Disasters, Development, and People.* London, Earthscan, 2004; 115–128.

103. Jaspars S, Shoham J. Targeting the vulnerable: a review of the necessity and feasibility of targeting vulnerable households. *Disasters* 1999; 23: 359–372.

104. Horton L. After the earthquake: gender inequality and transformation in post-disaster Haiti. *Gend Dev*, 2012; 20: 295–308.

105. Saito F. Women and the 2011 East Japan Disaster. *Gend Dev*, 2012; 20: 265–279.

106. Cutter SL, Boruff BJ, Shirley WL. Social vulnerability to environmental hazards. *Soc Sci Q* 2003; 84: 242–261.

107. Gerrity E, Flynn BW. Mental health consequences of disasters. In: Noji EK, ed. *The Public Health Consequences of Disasters.* New York, Oxford University Press, 1997; 101–121.

108. Bourque LB, Siegel JM, Kano M, Wood MM. Weathering the storm: the impact of hurricanes on physical and mental health. *Ann Am Acad Politic Soc Sci* 2006; 604: 129–151.

109. Bravo M, Rubio-Stipec M, Canino GJ, Woodbury MA, Ribera JC. The psychological sequelae of disaster stress prospectively and retrospectively evaluated. *Am J Community Psychol* 1990; 18: 661–680.

110. Lindell MK, Prater CS. Assessing community impacts of natural disasters. *Natural Hazards Rev* 2003; 4: 176–185.

111. Thompson MP, Norris FH, Hanacek B. Age differences in the psychological consequences of Hurricane Hugo. *Psychol Aging* 1993; 8: 606–616.

112. Norris FH, Friedman MJ, Watson PJ, Byrne CM, Diaz E, Kaniasty K. 60000 disaster victims speak, Part I: An empirical review of the empirical literature, 1981–2001. *Psychiatry* 2002; 65: 207–239.

113. Neria Y, DiGrande L, Adams BG. Posttraumatic stress disorder following the September 11, 2001, terrorist attacks: a review of the literature among highly exposed populations. *Am Psychol* 2011; 66: 429–446.

114. Hilhorst D. Complexity and diversity: Unlocking social domains of disaster. In: Bankoff G, Frerks G, Hilhorst D, eds. *Mapping Vulnerability: Disasters, Development, and People.* London, Earthscan, 2004; 52–66.

115. Oliver-Smith A. Global changes and the definition of disaster. In: Quarantelli EL, ed. *What is a Disaster? Perspectives on the Question.* New York, Routledge, 1998; 177–194.

116. Bates FL, Pelanda C. An ecological approach to disasters. In: Dynes RR, Tierney KJ, eds. *Disasters, Collective Behavior, and Social Organization.* Cranbury, NJ, Associated University Presses, 1994; 145–159.

117. Oliver-Smith A. Theorizing vulnerability in a globalized world: a political ecological perspective. In: Bankoff G, Frerks G, Hilhorst D, eds. *Mapping Vulnerability: Disasters, Development and People.* London, Earthscan, 2004; 10–24.

118. Kano M. Characteristics of earthquake-related injuries treated in emergency departments following the 2001 Nisqually earthquake in Washington. *J Emerg Manage* 2005; 3: 33–45.

119. Noji EK, ed. *The Public Health Consequences of Disasters.* New York, Oxford University Press, 1997.

120. Bey T, van Weizsaecker E, Koenig KL. Global warming: polar bears and people – implications for public health preparedness and disaster medicine: a call to action. *Prehosp Disaster Med* 2008; 23: 101–102.

121. Norris FH, Friedman MJ, Watson PJ. 60000 disaster victims speak, Part II: *Summary and implications of the disaster mental health literature.* Psychiatry 2002; 65: 240–260.

122. Vlahov D, Galea S, Resnick H, et al. Increased use of cigarettes, alcohol, and marijuana among Manhattan, New York, residents after the September 11th terrorist attacks. *Am J Epidemiol* 2002; 155: 988–996.

123. Briere J, Elliott D. Prevalence, characteristics, and long-term sequelae of natural disaster exposure in the general population. *J Trauma Stress* 2000; 13: 661–679.

124. Combs DL, Quenemoen LE, Parrish RG, Davis JH. Assessing disaster-attributed mortality: development and application of a definition and classification matrix. *Intl J Epidemiol* 1999; 28: 1124–1129.

125. Lurie N, Manolio T, Patterson AP, et al. Research as part of public health emergency response. *N Engl J Med* 2013; 368: 1251–1255.

126. Sundnes KO, Birnbaum ML, eds. Health disaster management: guidelines for evaluation and research in the Utstein style. *Prehosp Disaster Med* 2003; 17: Suppl. 3.

127. Maurice J. Mitigating disasters – a promising start. *Lancet* 2013; 381: 1611–1613.

128. Siriwardhana C, Sumathipala A, Siribaddana A, et al. Reducing the scarcity in mental health research from low and middle income countries: A success story from Sri Lanka. *Int Rev Psychiatry* 2011; 23: 77–83.

129. Chapman DW. Issue editor introduction. *Journal of Social Issues, Human Behavior in Disaster: A New Field of Social Research.* 1954; 10: 2–4.

130. Moore HE. *Tornadoes over Texas.* Austin, University of Texas Press, 1958.

131. Williams HB. Fewer disasters, better studied. *Journal of Social Issues, Human Behavior in Disaster: A New Field of Social Research.* 1954; 10: 5–11.

132. Committee on Disaster Research in the Social Sciences: Future Challenges and Opportunities, Division on Earth and Life Studies, National Research Council. *Facing Hazards and Disasters, Understanding Human Dimensions.* Washington, DC, The National Academies Press, 2006.

133. Basoglu M, Salcioglu E, Livanou M, Kalender D, Acar G. Single-session behavioral treatment of earthquake-related posttraumatic stress disorder: a randomized waiting list controlled trial. *J Trauma Stress* 2005; 18(1): 1–11.

2

DISASTER HEALTH EDUCATION AND TRAINING: LINKING INDIVIDUAL AND ORGANIZATIONAL LEARNING AND PERFORMANCE

Peter W. Brewster

OVERVIEW

What Is Disaster Health? Who Is Involved?

Disaster health is a term that refers to the disciplines and organizations involved with governmental public health, public and private medical care delivery including Emergency Medical Services (EMS), and governmental emergency management.[1] In 2004, the World Association for Disaster and Emergency Medicine led an effort to establish international standards for disaster health education and training.[2] A framework for "disaster health" was established that included: 1) primary disciplines; 2) support disciplines; 3) community response, resilience, and communication; and 4) a sociopolitical context. The framework functions as a scope of practice and suggests that educational standards should be developed first for undergraduates in various relevant professions and for practicing professionals (the "core of public health"). Subsequently, standards are developed for those academics, professionals, and policy experts seeking recognition as disaster health specialists (the "breadth of disaster health"). Other levels in the scope of practice could include community-level and doctoral-level specialists (see Table 2.1).[3]

What is Individual Learning and How Is It Linked to Organizational Learning?

Disaster health education and training is content delivered through various methods that prepare an individual to competently and proficiently perform their role in response to emergencies. A balance between theory (education) and practice (training) ensures an individual can retain and translate knowledge to a variety of situations in a dynamic environment.[4] Current perspectives assert that individual learning in disaster health occurs through formal (classroom), non-formal (workplace), and informal education and training (reading journals, experience with disasters).[5]

Experiential learning theorists suggest that learning occurs at two levels: conceptual and operational. These principles form an individual's mental model or view of the world. Conceptual learning is equated to education with content related to theory

or principles. Operational learning or training represents learning at the procedural level. One's mental model is composed of both frameworks of theory and principles, and of routines. Learning occurs through the process of having an experience, making observations on the experience, reflecting on and forming generalizations about the experience, testing these ideas in a new situation, and making changes to existing frameworks and routines. Thus, individual learning increases one's capacity to take effective action. The connection between individual learning and organizational learning is two-fold. Individuals can share their mental models in order to create a collective, organizational mental model.[6] In addition, they can create a process for analyzing the collective mental model and making changes to organizational structure, management processes, funding levels, policies, plans and procedures, training, facilities, equipment, and supplies to improve performance of the organization's core mission and objectives.[7]

Foundations for Disaster Health Education and Training

The 1994 Yokohama Strategy and Plan for a Safer World, part of the United Nations' International Decade for Natural Disaster Reduction, was based on the recognition that the impacts from disasters and societal vulnerability worldwide were increasing. It emphasized that: 1) prevention, mitigation, preparedness, and relief contribute to sustainable development policies; 2) disaster prevention, mitigation, and preparedness are more cost-effective than disaster response; and 3) the focus on disaster response should shift to an emphasis on prevention and mitigation.[8] The 2005 Hyogo Framework for Action assessed the progress of the Yokohama Strategy and articulated an International Strategy for Disaster Reduction (ISDR). ISDR's mission is to reduce "human, social, economic and environmental losses due to natural hazards and related technological and environmental disasters."[9] One of the major challenges or gaps was knowledge management and education in multiple areas. These included: 1) risk reduction; 2) building community resilience; 3) strengthening disaster response on community, regional, national, and international levels; and 4) involving citizens, private businesses, and government officials.[10]

Table 2.1. International Guidelines and Standards for Education and Training in Disaster Health

Category	Target	Description	Core & Electives	Delivery	Formal Assessment	Certificate Issued	Continuing Professional Development Required	Instructor Level
Level 1	Community	Civilian, community-based emergency preparedness and awareness	Common core for all, plus local needs	Short, didactic, competency-based, manageable	No	Certificate of Attainment (time limited)	No	Yes
Level 2	First responders; basic	First contact, primary care providers, all disciplines and responders. Categories: Bronze (provider); Silver (tactical); and Gold (strategic). Basic general emergency preparedness (USA model), MIMS (UK model), basic discipline, specific fundamentals	Common core for all, plus local needs	Short, didactic, competency-based, manageable	Yes	Certificate (time limited)	Yes	Yes
Level 3	First responders: Advanced or specific disciplines or specialty areas	First contact, primary care providers, all disciplines and responders. Categories: Bronze (provider); Silver (tactical); and Gold (strategic). Advanced general emergency preparedness (USA model), MIMS (UK model), specific discipline specialty areas, e.g. CBRN, communications	Common core for all, plus local needs	Short, didactic, competency-based, case-related, manageable	Yes	Advanced Certificate (time limited)	Yes	Yes
Level 4	First responders – curriculum enhancement units for course awards at diploma or Bachelor's degree	"Valued" content and process to enable Level 2/3 holders to receive academic credit for their prior studies and undertake additional related unit(s) in tertiary courses at an academic or professional organization to obtain diploma or Bachelor's degree	Yes	As determined by specific academic, professional organizations	Yes	Diploma or degree, issued by specific academic or professional organization	Yes	Academic or professional staff
Level 5	Professional – Master's degree	Formal education courses at professional level, i.e. Bachelor's or Master's for recognition as "Professional." Course curriculum to meet local, national, and international standards. Consider external accreditation by international body.	Core of each of the three disciplines in Paragraph 9.2.3, plus electives related to discipline and regional needs.	As determined by specific academic, professional organizations	Yes	Diploma or degree, issued by specific academic or professional organization	Yes	Academic or professional staff
Level 6	Specialist / Consultant – Master's plus specialized experience	For holders of formal education course award at Master's level to add formal, supervised, mentored professional experience in real-time "disaster medicine" situations. Course curriculum to meet local, national and international standards. Consider external accreditation by international body.	Core of each of the three disciplines in Paragraph 9.2.3, plus electives related to discipline and regional needs.	"In the field" specification of supervised, mentored, professional experience in "disaster medicine" situations.	Yes	Formal course award, e.g. fellowship or specialist endorsement as determined by specific academic or professional organization.	Yes	Academic or professional staff
Level 7	Researcher – National Leader – Doctoral	For holders of formal education course award at Master's level to add formal training in research and/or delivery and/or management and/or education at doctoral level, e.g., professional doctorate with course work and major thesis, or PhD by major thesis only. Could be PhD by major thesis only. Course curriculum to meet local, national, and international standards. Consider external accreditation by international body.	Core of each of the three disciplines in Paragraph 9.2.3, plus electives related to discipline of doctoral studies.	As determined by specific academic, professional organizations	Yes	Doctoral degree issued by specific academic organization.	No	Academic or professional staff

For the United States, the terrorist attacks in the fall of 2001 were critical to the development of many best practices in disaster health-related initiatives. But in 2002, when the U.S. Agency for Healthcare Research and Quality reviewed publications addressing effective ways to train clinicians for responses to a bioterrorist attack or other public health event, the report noted a lack of studies from which answers were available. At that time in history, the priorities lay in strengthening the public health system, enhancing surveillance systems, and building stockpiles of vaccines and drugs.[11]

In 2009, U.S. Homeland Security Presidential Directive (HSPD) 21, Public Health and Medical Services, was issued, calling for a National Health Security Strategy and a new approach to addressing the needs of disaster health.[12] Experience from the U.S. Health Resources and Services Administration, through the Bioterrorism Training and Curriculum Development Program (2003–2008), provided recommendations for the future of emergency preparedness education and training for health professionals. From these recommendations, a list of essential elements for health professional education and training were created and include: 1) personal and family preparedness; 2) an all-hazards and multidisciplinary approach; 3) partnerships across government and non-governmental organizations; 4) a standardized curriculum based on a set of core competencies; 5) recognizing the needs of diverse populations; 6) processes customized to the needs of learners; 7) use of various learning modalities; 8) providing incentives for participation; and 9) ensuring continuous evaluation and improvement.[13]

HSPD 21 created a joint program for disaster medicine and public health housed at the Uniformed Services University of the Health Sciences. This new entity would lead national efforts to develop and disseminate core curricula, training, and research related to disaster medicine and public health in disasters. Specifically, the program would consolidate education and research in the related specialties of domestic medical preparedness and response, international health, international disaster and humanitarian medical assistance, and military medicine.[12] The National Center for Disaster Medicine and Public Health (NCDMPH) was established in 2008 and has made many contributions to the development of disaster health education and training.

The Problem

Is the Workforce Prepared?

In the United States, a survey assessing five aspects of disaster readiness was administered in all fifty states. The five components included: 1) statewide disaster planning; 2) coordination; 3) training; 4) resource capacity; and 5) preparedness for biological/chemical terrorism. About half of the states offered disaster training to medical professionals, and only about 10% of those states required the training.[14] Estimates by public health leaders in 2004 placed the readiness of health professionals for public health emergencies around 20%.[15] In 2011, NCDMPH studied the question and cited the lack of a disaster health workforce development program within the various federal departments involved with disaster health, and across the intergovernmental system (federal, state, and local government as well as the private sector). They found that each agency develops and conducts its own training and education programs. In addition, exercises stop short of evaluating staff competencies, focusing

mainly on the review of plans and operational procedures.[16] As a result of these and other investigations, it appears three gaps exist in the current state and practice of disaster health education and training: 1) knowledge on the effectiveness of various education and training methods targeting different audiences; 2) linkage between disaster health core content and emergency plans and incident management systems; and 3) linkage to the requirements generated by disasters on population health and health service delivery.

EFFECTIVENESS OF DISASTER HEALTH EDUCATION AND TRAINING

The costs of education and training are significant at the organizational level and so effectiveness is a primary concern. Additional important considerations include efficiency, realism, and retaining trained personnel. However, a lack of knowledge exists regarding the effectiveness of education and training techniques for the various target audiences within the disaster health field. This is due to: 1) a lack of uniformity in evaluation when designing education and training methods; 2) the limited amount of research on disaster health education and training; 3) a lack of consensus on terms and definitions for research and evaluation; and 4) the incomplete development of the educational system supporting disaster health (core content, scope of practice, educational standards, accreditation, and certification). Competencies used in the design of disaster health education and training are the products of subject matter experts and have not been validated through performance testing, nor have they been aligned with the capability framework used in the disaster management systems descriptions.

LINKAGE BETWEEN DISASTER HEALTH AND DISASTER MANAGEMENT SYSTEMS

The development of an educational system supporting disaster health depends on the mission descriptions of the various organizations that comprise disaster health, public health, and medical services. Educational curricula must link to the disaster management system descriptions for prevention, protection, mitigation, preparedness, response and recovery. Once this is established, disaster health organizations can better focus the design of their emergency operations plans to fulfill their internal requirements and external support. Also, the incident management system should be refined to more adequately describe the roles and responsibilities for the various identified tasks/functions such as public health and medical services. Position descriptions and task books for public health and medical operational activities should serve as the basis for the design of role-specific education and training.

LINKAGE TO ACTUAL REQUIREMENTS GENERATED BY DISASTERS

A system that uses disaster-generated data to inform the design and refinement of education and training methods, systems descriptions, and organizational missions does not currently exist. The design of disaster prevention, protection, mitigation, preparedness, response, and recovery systems descriptions share a common capability framework. However, the incident management system used to implement these frameworks is not tied to the capabilities, and no uniform data reporting on the effects of disasters, the performance of capabilities, or the incident management system is in place. Without these data, quality management system approaches that support organizational learning, and thus the design and refinement of education and training, cannot perform optimally.

STATE OF THE ART

Establishing an Evidence Base

Compared to approaches used in medicine, questions in disaster medicine are not easily testable through controlled studies. Prospective investigations are difficult to perform due to issues of informed consent and inability to anticipate events in advance. Because situations are dynamic and concurrently evolving, valid information is difficult to obtain. As one author notes, disaster relief operations continue to rely heavily on "eminence-based" decisions by parties striving to broker goodwill and consensus. A more objective approach is limited due to a lack of expertise, a lack of effective coordination between responding agencies, and an imbalance between established minimum standards, health status indicators, and decision processes.[17] This lack of an evidence base reflecting response and recovery requirements and the impact from disasters limits the validation of core content. However, foundations for establishing an evidence base are being created both internationally and domestically.

One such development is the articulation of desired health outcomes and standards. The World Health Organization, an agency of the United Nations, is concerned with keeping health as a focus during disaster risk reduction discussions, and is the lead agency for providing health assistance during humanitarian crises worldwide. It does this through the Global Health Cluster (GHC) which is made up of thirty-eight international health organizations and four observers. The mission of the GHC is to build consensus on humanitarian health priorities and related best practices, and to strengthen system-wide capacities to ensure an effective and predictable response. In its 2012–2013 Strategic Framework, the GHC set an objective to demonstrate progress toward agreed health outcomes, impacts, and service availability to affected populations, and to use data for more effective health cluster advocacy. The GHC has established performance standards for health surveillance, coordination of health organizations, and the maintenance of health outcomes in the affected population.[18] Minimum standards were established for the health system and essential health services (control of communicable diseases, child health, sexual and reproductive health, injury, mental health, and non-communicable diseases). These standards for international humanitarian disaster health services – and tools for the assessment of health needs and the monitoring of interventions – serve as models that can be used for developing an evidence base on which the design of educational curricula and methodology could be based.[19]

In the United States, sustained efforts to enhance national preparedness focus on a "secure and resilient nation with the capabilities required across the whole community to prevent, protect against, mitigate, respond to, and recover from the threats and hazards that pose the greatest risk."[20,21] The National Health Security Strategy seeks to build community resilience by strengthening and sustaining health and emergency response systems through monitoring data on a unified public health and healthcare preparedness framework.[22–24] The U.S. Veterans Health Administration is establishing a quality management system to support its comprehensive emergency management program that will monitor value through the use of five outcomes: 1) continuity and access to care; 2) medical outcome and functional status; 3) patient satisfaction; 4) readiness and competence; and 5) cost.[25]

The World Association for Disaster and Emergency Medicine's (WADEM) Education and Standards committee continues its work establishing procedures to link the evidence base for disaster medicine to the development of educational standards. This will hopefully lead to developing a system for the accreditation of disaster health educational programs offered through academic centers and organizations.[26]

Another foundation is common terminology and a universal framework for research and evaluation. One challenge to developing disaster health educational standards was creating a common terminology between the fields of public health, EMS, healthcare, and emergency management. The 2003 Health Disaster Management Guidelines for Evaluation and Research in the Utstein Style emphasized the importance of common terms and definitions to the developing field of disaster health. The guidelines supported creation of standardized research methods for use by public health practitioners to produce sound information on the health impacts of disasters and the effectiveness of interventions.[27]

In addition, the capability to identify, collect, and analyze universal data indicators is evolving. Within the humanitarian assistance field, the World Health Organization is focused on monitoring progress toward certain health outcomes and service availability to affected populations, and using this data for improvement activities. It has developed three systems to support data collection and performance monitoring: initial health assessment, health resource availability mapping, and the health information record.[18] Domestically, web access to information on some existing health conditions improves responders' abilities to provide optimal care.[28] The U.S. National Disaster Medical System uses integrated medical records to document patient treatment and tracking, and for disaster medical assistance team quality improvement processes.[29] A template for reporting the acute medical response during disasters identified fifteen data elements with indicators for both research and quality improvement.[30] Efforts are underway to promote template use and the establishment of an international database to facilitate data collection and sharing. One important output from this process will be creation of evidence-based education and training programs.[31]

Use of Quality Management System Approaches

Continuous quality improvement processes have been at the center of the healthcare service design and delivery evolution for over a decade. Increasingly, standards for emergency management, business continuity, resiliency, and societal security incorporate a quality management system structure.[32–35] The U.S. National Preparedness System, released in 2011, uses an approach that resembles a quality management system (see Figure 2.1).[19]

This process begins with the identification of threats and hazards. These include: 1) a risk assessment (vulnerability and likelihood of occurrence); 2) determining the desired levels of each core capability (desired outcomes); and 3) an impact estimation of those threats/hazards on the various core capabilities. When taken together with the desired outcome, these assessments establish the capability target.[36,37] For example, one desired outcome might be, *during the first 72 hours of an incident, conduct operations to recover fatalities.* The estimated impact of a theoretical earthquake is 375 fatalities. Therefore, the capability

Figure 2.1. National Preparedness System Process

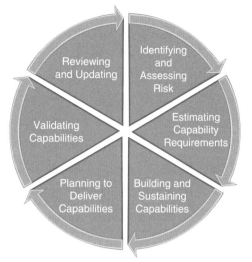

Mission Area Components of the National Preparedness System (U.S. Federal Emergency Management Agency).

target for fatality management services is, "during the first 72 hours of an incident, conduct operations to recover 375 fatalities." Estimating the resource requirements for capability targets is based on the existing resource baseline compared to the required levels for the desired outcomes.[38] Delivery of such capabilities involves the development of Emergency Operations Plans (EOPs) that are implemented through the Incident Command System (ICS).

Planning Frameworks and Core Capabilities

National and international response frameworks describe the concept of operations for the response to disaster events.[39,40] These frameworks have been traditionally organized around functional areas, for example, communications, transportation, public health, and medical services. However, there has been a recent trend in the United States to organize plans/frameworks around "mission areas" (protection, prevention, mitigation, response and recovery), and for each mission area, to identify the capabilities that will be needed. Note that in this conceptual model, preparedness is a component of each mission area and not a separate one. While both the functional and the mission area concepts support an all-hazards approach, capability-based planning enables a closer connection to competency-based education and training.[41] Capabilities for emergency management, public health, and healthcare have been designed to address the full spectrum of requirements needed to manage disasters (see Table 2.2).[21,23,24,42]

Capability development is a process involving hazards identification, gap analysis, resource management, education and training, and exercises.[43]

In 2007, the president of the United States issued a national preparedness directive that called for the establishment of a national preparedness goals and guidelines. The guidelines were designed to: 1) unify federal, state, local, tribal, and territorial preparedness efforts; 2) describe the capability-based and risk-based planning process; 3) establish metrics to measure progress; and 4) create a system to assess the nation's overall preparedness capability for response to major emergencies.[44] Key to the devel-

opment of national preparedness was the Target Capability List (TCL). These thirty-seven target capabilities were derived from the tasks planners and responders must perform to prevent, protect against, respond to, and recover from the fifteen National Planning Scenarios. These scenarios represent the range, scope, magnitude, and complexity of major incidents that could affect the United States, including terrorism, natural disasters, and other hazards (see Table 2.3).[45]

Other countries using the same approach might develop a slightly different set of national planning scenarios based on the threats they face.

The national preparedness directive was reaffirmed in March 2011 as a presidential policy directive, with the purpose to strengthen the security and resilience of the United States through an integrated, nationwide capability-based approach.[46] The TCL was revised to a set of "core capabilities" that address the five mission areas that define homeland security and emergency management program activity: prevention, protection, mitigation, response, and recovery (see Table 2.4).[21]

While the five mission areas may seem to be a departure from the classic "mitigation, preparedness, response and recovery" orientation, they represent greater unity in the United States between emergency management, law enforcement, public health, business continuity, and social services communities.

Planning frameworks were developed for each of these five mission areas. The purpose of the frameworks is to clarify roles, responsibilities, and a coordinating structure between federal, state, local, tribal and private sector organizations. Disaster health (public health and medical services) is one of fifteen functional areas included in the National Response Framework and is identified as the eighth Emergency Support Function (ESF 8) (see Table 2.5).[40]

Within this framework, ESF 8 coordinates the assistance to an actual or potential public health and medical disaster or incident. It provides the core capabilities of public health and medical services, fatality management services, mass care services, critical transportation, public information and warning, environmental response/health and safety, and public and private services and resources.[40]

NATIONAL INCIDENT MANAGEMENT SYSTEM

The National Incident Management System (NIMS), the subject of HSPD 5 (2003), is a comprehensive structure used to organize the response to emergencies in the United States and as such is the principal vehicle for implementing the capabilities developed through the preparedness process described in the previous section.[47] The current system has its roots in the National Inter-agency Incident Management System, created by the National Wildland Fire Coordinating Group in the early 1980s due to the need to better coordinate the efforts of federal, state, and local wildland firefighting agencies in Southern California.[48] NIMS consists of the three main components: command and management (ICS); communications and information management; and resource management. The ICS organizational structure consists of command and general staff positions with additional units filling out the structure. The particular organizational structure needed to manage any particular incident at any point in time is driven by a management-by-objectives process called incident action planning. Inter-agency involvement is achieved through structures for unified command and multi-agency coordination. Efforts to prepare individuals to serve in ICS positions has been led by the wildland firefighting

Table 2.2. Capabilities for Emergency Management (EM), Public Health (PH), and Healthcare

EM Capabilities	PH Capabilities	Healthcare Capabilities
Planning	Community Preparedness	Healthcare Preparedness
Public Info/Warning	Community Recovery	Healthcare Recovery
Operational Coordination	Emergency Operations Coord.	Emergency Operations Coordination
Forensics and Attribution	Public Information/Warning	Fatality Management
Intel/Info Sharing	Fatality Management	Medical Surge
Interdiction/Disruption	Information Sharing	Responder Safety and Health
Screening/Detection	Mass Care Services	Volunteer Management
Access Control	Medical Countermeasure Dispensing	
Cybersecurity	Medical Materiel Management/Distribution	
Physical Protection	Medical Surge	
Risk Management	Non-Pharmaceutical Interventions	
Supply Chain Integrity	Public Health Laboratory Testing	
Vulnerability Reduction	Public Health Epidemiological Surveillance	
Resilience Assessment	Responder Safety and Health	
Hazard Identification	Volunteer Management	
Critical Transportation		
Environmental Response		
Fatality Management		
Infrastructure Systems		
Mass Care Services		
Mass Search and Rescue		
Security and Protection		
Operational Communications		
Public and Private Services		
Public Health and Medical		
Situational Assessment		
Economic Recovery		
Health and Social Services		
Housing		
Natural/Cultural Resources		

community and include the development of a position quali-fications system; position-specific procedures or task books; a standardized, competency-based curriculum; and a certification system.[49,50] The Department of Homeland Security (DHS) and FEMA are working to replicate the system structure in support of NIMS.

NIMS resource typing includes efforts to organize resources using consistent terminology and organizational structures, and an overarching management process that helps ensure accountability and safety. Resource typing is a process of defining and categorizing, by capability, the various resources that are requested, deployed and used in incidents. Resource typing definitions are used to establish a common language and define the minimum capabilities of equipment and teams of personnel.[51] The Emergency Management Assistance Compact (http://www.emacweb.org/index.php/mutualaidresources/

mission-ready-packages/get-started), an organization serving the interests of state emergency management agencies, has developed several public health and medical mission-ready packages created under the NIMS principles.

Incident Management Systems for Public Health and Medical Services

While the use of ICS had been part of firefighting efforts since the 1980s, the use of ICS in the emergency management, public health, and medical communities was slower to evolve. In 2002, a key document was developed that introduced both the ICS structure and management process. It did so in the form of a planning tool for communities to use in developing a compre-hensive approach to address the various requirements created by mass casualty incidents.[52] It was the foundation for the current system description and concept of operations for the delivery

Table 2.3. National Planning Scenarios (2006)

Nuclear Detonation – 10-Kiloton Improvised Nuclear Device

Biological Attack – Aerosol Anthrax

Biological Disease Outbreak – Pandemic Influenza

Biological Attack – Plague

Chemical Attack – Blister Agent

Chemical Attack – Toxic Industrial Chemicals

Chemical Attack – Nerve Agent

Chemical Attack – Chlorine Tank Explosion

Natural Disaster – Major Earthquake

Natural Disaster – Major Hurricane

Radiological Attack – Radiological Dispersal Devices

Explosives Attack – Bombing Using Improvised Explosive Devices

Biological Attack – Food Contamination

Biological Attack – Foreign Animal Disease (Foot and Mouth Disease)

Cyber Attack

Table 2.5. Emergency Support Functions

Transportation

Communications

Public Works and Engineering

Firefighting

Information and Planning

Mass Care Services

Logistics

Public Health and Medical Services

Urban Search and Rescue

Oil and Hazardous Materials

Agriculture and Natural Resources

Energy

Public Safety and Security

Long-term Community Recovery

External Affairs

of disaster public health and medical services used by the U.S. Department of Health and Human Services. This current tool organizes the department's preparedness and response activities and grant funding opportunities for states (see Table 2.6).[53]

The Hospital Incident Command System expands on the Tier 1 level shown in this table.[54]

Key to successful implementation of an incident management system during an event is the strength of the linkages between the various professional disciplines and organizations that would work together in that response. These participants include: hospital personnel; representatives from the healthcare coalition; public health officials; EMS personnel; fire service personnel; law enforcement officers; emergency management personnel; state-level emergency managers; and other organizations that may become involved such as the American Red Cross, Salvation Army, and the local medical society.

Table 2.4. Core Capabilities for the Five Mission Areas

Prevention	Protection	Mitigation	Response	Recovery
Planning Public Information and Warning Operational Coordination				
Forensics and Attribution	Access Control and Identity Verification	Community Resilience	Critical Transportation	Economic Recovery
Intelligence and Information Sharing	Cybersecurity Intelligence and Information Sharing	Long-term Vulnerability Reduction	Environmental Response/ Health and Safety	Health and Social Services
Interdiction and Disruption	Interdiction and Disruption	Risk and Disaster Resilience Assessment	Fatality Management Services	Housing
Screening, Search, and Detection	Physical Protective Measures	Threats and Hazard Identification	Infrastructure Systems	Infrastructure Systems
	Risk Management for Protection Programs and Activities		Mass Care Services	Natural and Cultural Resources
	Screening, Search, and Detection		Mass Search and Rescue Operations	
	Supply Chain Integrity and Security		On-scene Security and Protection	
			Operational Communications	
			Public and Private Services and Resources	
			Public Health and Medical Services	
			Situational Assessment	

Table 2.6. Operational System Structure for Public Health and Medical Services

Tier 1	Individual Healthcare Asset
Tier 2	Healthcare Coalition
Tier 3	Jurisdiction
Tier 4	State/Intra-State
Tier 5	Inter-State/Regional
Tier 6	Federal Support to State, Tribal, and Jurisdiction

HOMELAND SECURITY EXERCISE AND EVALUATION PROGRAM

Validating the baseline capability performance levels would occur through exercises developed using a process similar to the Homeland Security Exercise Evaluation Program (HSEEP). This program provides a structured exercise design and evaluation process that leads to an After Action Report and Improvement Plan (IP). Capability performance is evaluated utilizing standardized Exercise Evaluation Guides (see Table 2.7) that are used by subject matter expert observers to identify strengths and weaknesses. In producing the IP, weaknesses are analyzed to determine what changes are needed to organizational structures, plans and procedures, management processes, equipment and supplies, resources and funding, and training that sustain existing performance and build additional capability. This information is organized into a multi-year work plan that would include review and revision to the various components of the preparedness system.[55,56]

Conceptual Basis for Linking Disaster Requirements, Organizational Capabilities, and Individual Competencies

A series of workshops in the United States conducted for the Federal Education and Training Interagency Group (FETIG) in 2010–2011 sought to establish a conceptual basis for the relationship between disaster requirements, national policy, strategy, and planning frameworks (see Figure 2.2).[57]

In this diagram, competencies are related to capabilities through the term "domains." The domain is the overall category

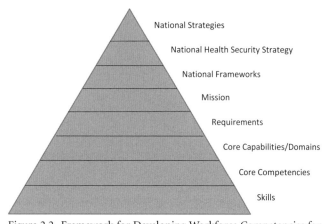

Figure 2.2. Framework for Developing Workforce Competencies for Public Health and Medical Disciplines.

Table 2.7. DHS, Target Capability List, Exercise Evaluation Guide, Medical Surge

Capability – Medical Surge
Activity 1: Pre-event Mitigation and Preparedness
Tasks:
Conduct Hazard Vulnerability Analysis.
Define incident management structure and methodology.
Establish a bed tracking system.
Develop protocols for increasing internal surge capacity.
Determine medical surge assistance requirements.
Develop plans for providing external surge capacity.

Activity 2: Incident Management
Tasks:
Activate the healthcare organization's EOP.
Conduct incident action planning.
Disseminate key components of incident action plan.
Provide emergency operations support to incident management.

Activity 3: Increase Bed Surge Capacity
Tasks:
Implement bed surge capacity plans, procedures, and protocols.
Maximize utilization of available beds.
Forward transport less acutely ill patients.
Provide medical surge capacity in alternate care facilities.

Activity 4: Medical Surge Staffing Procedure
Tasks:
Recall clinical staff in support of medical surge capacity.
Augment clinical staffing.
Augment non-clinical staffing.

Activity 5: Decontamination
Task:
Provide mass decontamination capabilities, if necessary.

Activity 6: Receive, Evaluate and Treat Surge Casualties
Tasks:
Establish initial reception and triage site.
Provide medical equipment and supplies.
Initiate patient tracking.
Execute medical mutual aid agreements.
Activate procedures for altered nursing and medical care standards.

Activity 7: Provide Surge Capacity for Behavioral Health Issues
Tasks:
Institute strategy to address behavioral health issues.
Provide behavioral health support.
Provide family support services.

Activity 8: Demobilize
Tasks:
Coordinate decision to demobilize with incident management.
Provide a staff debriefing.
Reconstitute medical supply equipment inventory.

Source: see note 89.

from which the competency is derived. For example, if the competency domain is surge management, then it includes four capabilities: fatality management, mass care, medical surge, and volunteer management. By definition, competencies describe employee behavior that supports effective and efficient organizational performance.[58]

Table 2.8. Disaster Health Core Competencies

1.0	Maintain personal and family preparedness for disasters and public health emergencies.
2.0	Demonstrate knowledge of one's expected role(s) in organizational and community response plans activated during a disaster or public health emergency.
3.0	Maintain situational awareness of actual/potential health hazards during a disaster or public health emergency.
4.0	Communicate effectively with others in a disaster or public health emergency.
5.0	Use personal safety measures in a disaster or public health emergency.
6.0	Demonstrate knowledge of surge capacity assets, consistent with one's role in organizational, agency, and/or community response plans.
7.0	Demonstrate knowledge of principles and practices for the clinical management of all ages and populations affected by disasters and public health emergencies, in accordance with professional scope of practice.
8.0	Demonstrate knowledge of public health principles and practices for the management of all ages and populations affected by disasters and public health emergencies.
9.0	Demonstrate knowledge of ethical principles to protect the health and safety of all ages, populations, and communities affected by a disaster or public health emergency.
10.0	Demonstrate knowledge of legal principles to protect the health and safety of all ages, populations, and communities affected by a disaster or public health emergency.
11.0	Demonstrate knowledge of considerations for recovery of all ages, populations, and communities affected by a disaster or public health emergency.

Source: see note 68.

Establishing Core Content

Competency Development

Course development has moved from traditional, content-focused training, such as training clinicians on smallpox, anthrax, and radiation illness to role-specific, outcome-based courses that teach individual students what is expected of them in preparedness and in response.[58] This is the basis for competency-based education and training models. Most definitions of the term "competency" include reference to the grouping of knowledge, skills, abilities, and behaviors demonstrated by employees that support the successful attainment of the organization's mission, vision, and values.[15,59] Calhoun et al. identified progressive levels of development for the affective and cognitive domains ("domain" as used here refers to the affective, cognitive, and psychomotor areas defined in Blooms's *Taxonomy of Educational Objectives*) to produce a common framework on which to base curriculum development. Proficiencies (novice to expert) are examples of development stages of the psychomotor domain.[58]

Competency development in disaster health over the past decade includes notable works by: 1) the American College of Emergency Physicians; 2) the University of Michigan; 3) the Johns Hopkins University; 4) the Council on Linkages between

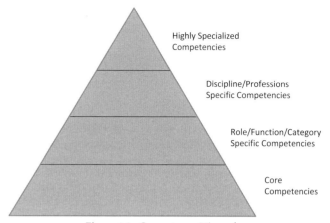

Figure 2.3. Competency Hierarchy.
Source: see note 67.

Academia and Public Health Practice; 5) the Federal Emergency Management Agency and the National Wildland Fire Coordinating Group; 6) Schultz and Koenig; 7) the George Washington University; and 8) the American Medical Association.[49,58,60–68] Currently, there is a consensus-based set of core competencies for disaster health (see Table 2.8). There are now many examples of disaster-related competencies that have been developed for healthcare workers.[69] A hierarchy was created to provide a method for aligning and stratifying the many models (see Figure 2.3).

Other alignment proposals have focused on standardizing the content, structure, and process of disaster health competency models using the research, development, test, and evaluation construct. Here, initial research is conducted to identify all the possible competency model components. Then individuals review this information and develop a proposal that could potentially identify the correct components. Next, a model is created using this list of identified components and tested on a population of disaster responders. Finally, their performance in actual disasters is evaluated to determine if the training based on the new model was effective. Additional work is needed to validate existing competency models against actual disaster-derived benchmarks.[70] The long-term expectations of competencies include their use as the basis for educational standards in curriculum design and certification, their application to accreditation processes across undergraduate, graduate, and continuing education programs, and their influence on the evolution of current position-specific job aids and emergency procedures.[71,72]

Existing Courses

As part of its role to coordinate national efforts to develop and propagate core curricula, education, training, and research in disaster health, NCDMPH inventoried no cost, online training courses available from the following groups: 1) the Bioterrorism Training and Curriculum Development Program Resource Center; 2) the Public Health Foundation's Training Finder Real-time Affiliate Integrated Network; 3) the CDC Preparedness and Emergency Response Learning Centers; and 4) the Training Repository for Assessing Integrated Learning Standards. The courses were organized by the topical areas relating to the learning needs of disaster responders and include: Health System Preparedness and Planning, Cultural Awareness and Community Preparedness, Baseline Disaster Response Education, Leading

Teams/Building Teams, Disaster-Specific Education, Risk Communication, and Mental/Behavioral Health.[73]

Education and Training Methods

The Agency for Healthcare Research and Quality in the United States has studied the effectiveness of various clinician training methods for responding to bioterrorism and other public health events. It found that the use of standardized patient descriptions was an effective way to train physicians in detection and management of infectious disease outbreaks. Additional findings include: 1) presentations delivered over satellite broadcasts was an effective way to train large numbers of clinicians and served to standardize training across geographically separated groups; 2) tabletop exercises had some use in training healthcare professionals; 3) exercises can improve clinicians' knowledge of emergency operations plans and identify potential problems; and 4) didactic programs had been shown to help train infection control nurses to identify and report certain infectious diseases to a central agency.[11]

Providing education to adults requires instructors to engage the student as an active, self-directed participant in his or her own learning. Course developers need to recognize and incorporate motivational factors into the educational process and utilize work-relevant situations. By implementing situational learning, instructors acknowledge the various professional experiences of the students and create a collaborative environment.[74]

Target Groups and Sources of Education and Training

Broadly speaking, there are three target groups for disaster health education and training: 1) those who are employed locally in various healthcare, public health, EMS, and emergency management positions; 2) citizens; and 3) those who are part of organizations that respond to requests for staff augmentation during an emergency. In the United States, sources of education and training for citizens, aside from those available online, include the American Red Cross for first aid and CPR and the local emergency management agency for participation in Community Emergency Response Teams or Medical Reserve Corps/Citizen Corps.[75–78] Sources of training for local disaster health professionals include continuing education offered by: 1) their employer; 2) the healthcare coalition; 3) the local National Disaster Medical System program; and 4) the state public health, emergency management, or EMS agencies. The National Disaster Life Support Foundation offers regional deliveries of its Basic Disaster Life Support and Advanced Disaster Life Support courses.[79] Response to disasters has recently been added to the Residency Review Committee Program Requirements in Community Medicine.[80] Curricula that involve live actors and human simulators is being used increasingly to train clinicians.[81–83] For disaster health professionals involved with faith-based organizations and groups affiliated with the Emergency Management Assistance Compact or Disaster Medical Assistance Teams, just-in-time training courses offer an orientation to their deployment with opportunities for discussing mission-specific issues, field living skills, and provision of field medical care in distant emergencies.[84–88]

Evaluation

Evaluation science as applied to disaster health education and training is at an early stage of development. Most training evaluations occur at the individual course or student level. Accomplishments cannot be aggregated to demonstrate achievement of national preparedness goals because standard indicators are lacking. While the TCL and core capabilities provide examples of these standardized indicators, these have been principally used to guide the development of national preparedness and are not linked to competency models.[89] If designed correctly, the evaluations of training would serve as a proxy measure of the learner's abilities to realize the desired outcomes for patients and populations in an actual disaster.[13]

Experts believe that evaluating the impact of training on disaster health professionals requires a new and unique framework. Such an evaluation would include processes and outcomes of the actual training program itself, and public health and patient care processes and outcomes. Each of these categories (public health, patient care, and the training program itself) has different performance measures and very different outcome measures (see Table 2.9).[13]

Exercises

U.S. hospitals use exercises as tools for training and rehearsal of their emergency operations plans, and such activities are required for accreditation.[35] Experience shows that training provided prior to the exercise will increase proficiency. However, many emergency management drills are conducted at great expense and disruption to the hospital, with a minority of people acquiring some benefit in terms of skills.[15] Nonetheless, exercises do enable staff to test emergency procedures, reinforce coordination and collaboration, provide a baseline level of understanding for new employees, and give the organization an opportunity to reaffirm partnerships with community organizations.[13] The most effective exercises involve criteria that will enable the performance evaluation of staff using the actual emergency operations plan.[90,91]

Using the EMS Education Agenda for the Future as a Template Plan of Action

It is acknowledged that a nationally recognized education and training standard is needed for disaster health in the United States. The National Highway Traffic Safety Administration confronted a similar problem regarding EMS in 2000. The agency observed that there was no established national EMS education system or master plan and proposed a systems approach to develop such standards: the Emergency Medical Services Education Agenda for the Future. The components of this framework included: core content, a scope of practice model, education standards, educational program accreditation, and individual provider certification.[5]

In 2004, influenced by the EMS Education Agenda for the Future, WADEM produced an issues paper that provides leadership and direction toward the development of standards and guidelines for education and training in the multidisciplinary disaster health field. WADEM's work was intended to: 1) develop consensus around concepts and attributes of disaster medicine; 2) develop a scientific foundation for disaster medicine education and training; 3) identify barriers to effective education and training; and 4) articulate the general principles and a conceptual framework needed to establish the standards and guidelines.[3]

As previous sections of this chapter have discussed, the current status of core content educational standards development for disaster health education and training is the identification of

Table 2.9. Evaluation Framework for All-Hazards Preparedness Training for Health Professionals

Preparedness Entity	Professional and Pre-Professional Education/Training	Public Health Systems	Patient Care Delivery Systems
What is the goal?	Certify/credential trainees	Ensure healthy populations	Ensure healthy individuals
Who is responsible?	Schools/universities	Local, state, federal government	Hospitals, clinics, private practitioners, et al.
Examples of outcome measures?	Didactic knowledge; performance-based competencies and skills	Mass casualties; population-based measures of morbidity and mortality	Death, disability, illness, disease, psychosocial morbidity at individual and aggregate service levels
Examples of intermediate process or performance measures?	Pre- and post-tests of knowledge; individual/group performance in exercises or drills; self-report; training "rate" where numerator = number trained at basic, intermediate, advanced levels, denominator = all eligible health professionals by self-selected expertise preference	Delivery of mass drug prophylaxis or mass immunizations; isolation and quarantine; evacuation or shelter-in-place; post-disaster evaluation	Patient triage; ventilation; resuscitation; surgery; medication; clinical indicators; post-disaster evaluation
Examples of the "ultimate" test of the system?	Placement and performance of trainees	Widespread disaster	Surge
What is a success?	Measured in the roles the trainees assume in Public Health or Health Care Delivery sectors	Averting morbidity and mortality	Treating morbidity and averting mortality
Sources of funding?	Student tuition; state or federal grants; private grants	Public tax revenues; state or federal grants	Health insurance companies; state or federal programs; patient payments

core competencies on which curricula can be based.[61,62,68,70,92] Currently, the WADEM Education and Standards committee continues its work to: 1) establish a science base for disaster medicine; 2) develop educational standards; and 3) create a system for accreditation of disaster health educational programs offered through academic centers and organizations.[26,93]

RECOMMENDATIONS FOR FURTHER RESEARCH

The disaster health and disaster management communities need to collaboratively develop processes that will capture and analyze data on the impacts and requirements generated by emergencies and disasters, and on the performance of the responding organizations. These data, applied within a quality management system structure, could then be used to effectively refine current plans and procedures, and the education and training provided to response officials. Through the end of 2014, the core capabilities used in generating planning frameworks were not effectively connected to the incident management system used for implementing those frameworks, nor were these capabilities derived from actual data and observations resulting from disaster analysis. The current evaluation and improvement framework is limited in its impact due to these reasons and because competencies used in courses to train personnel are not aligned with the core capabilities. As such, training for personnel is not based on the requirements for effective disaster management. Finally, the evaluations of exercises and real events do not include assessments of role performance by officials and key staff − an important design component of future disaster health education and training. Further research and development are needed to correct these deficiencies.

Core content for disaster health should be based on data derived from existing health conditions and impacts caused by disasters on population health and health service delivery. Standards for international humanitarian disaster health services, tools for the assessment of health needs, and the monitoring of interventions serve as models that can be used for developing the processes that will yield an evidence base on which the refinement of existing models can be used to design improved educational standards.[33,94] Additional investigations in these areas are warranted.

Over a decade ago, the EMS community provided an example for building a comprehensive education and training system. A similar approach could be used by the disaster health community but this will require unified action on the part of national and international organizations involved with disaster health and disaster management.

REFERENCES

1. Fowkes V, Ablah E, Oberle M, et al. *Emergency Preparedness Education and Training for Health Professionals: A Blueprint for Future Action.* Whitepaper for the Assistant Secretary for Preparedness and Response, 2010.
2. Saynaeve G, et al. International Standards and Guidelines on Education and Training for the Mutli-disciplinary Health Response to Major Events that Threaten the Health Status of a Community, Education Committee Working Group, World Association for Disaster and Emergency Medicine. *Australasian Journal of Paramedicine*, April–May 2004. http://ro.ecu.edu.au/jephc/vol2/iss1/4 (Accessed August 29, 2014).
3. Archer F, Seynaeve G. International guidelines and standards for education and training to reduce the consequences of events

that may threaten the health status of a community. A Report of an Open International WADEM Meeting, Brussels, Belgium, October 29–31, 2004. http://www.ncbi.nlm.nih.gov/pubmed/17591184 (Accessed August 29, 2014).

4. Margolis G, Mercer S. EMS Education Agenda for the Future: A Systems Approach. National Highway Traffic Safety Administration, 2000. http://www.nhtsa.gov/people/injury/ems/EdAgenda/final/index.html (Accessed August 29, 2014).

5. Altman BA, Strauss-Riggs K, Schor KW. Capturing the Range of Learning: Implications for Disaster Health in a Resource Constrained Future. National Center for Disaster Medicine and Public Health, December 2012. http://ncdmph.usuhs.edu/Documents/201212-Range-of-Learning.pdf (Accessed August 29, 2014).

6. Kim D. The Link Between Organizational and Individual Learning. Sloan Management Review, 1993. Article: http://www.iwp.jku.at/born/mpwfst/03/0312_IVkim.pdf and diagrams: http://www.iwp.jku.at/born/mpwfst/03/0312_IVkimbilder.pdf (Accessed August 29, 2014).

7. ICDRM/GWU Emergency Management Glossary of Terms. The Institute for Crisis, Disaster, and Risk Management (ICDRM) at the George Washington University (GWU), Washington, DC, June 30, 2009. www.gwu.edu/~icdrm (Accessed August 29, 2014).

8. Yokohama Strategy and Plan for a Safer World, Guidelines for Natural Disaster Prevention, Preparedness and Mitigation, 1994. http://unpan1.un.org/intradoc/groups/public/documents/APCITY/UNPAN009632.pdf (Accessed August 29, 2014).

9. International Strategy for Disaster Reduction: Latin America and the Caribbean. Web page for the United Nations International Strategy for Disaster Reduction. http://www.eird.org/herramientas/eng/partners/isdr/Mission.pdf (Accessed July 31, 2015).

10. Hyogo Framework for Action 2005–2015: Building the Resilience of Nations and Communities to Disasters, International Strategy for Disaster Reduction. United Nations, 2005. http://www.unisdr.org/we/coordinate/hfa (Accessed August 29, 2014).

11. Catlett C, et al. Training of Clinicians for Public Health Events Relevant to Bioterrorism. Agency for Healthcare Research and Quality, Department of Health and Human Services, January 2002. http://www.ncbi.nlm.nih.gov/books/NBK36521 (Accessed August 29, 2014).

12. Homeland Security Presidential Directive 21, Public Health and Medical Services. Office of the President, 2009. http://www.fas.org/irp/offdocs/nspd/hspd-21.htm (Accessed August 29, 2014).

13. Fowkes V, et al. *Emergency Preparedness Education and Training for Health Professionals: A Blueprint for Future Action.* Whitepaper for the Assistant Secretary for Preparedness and Response, 2009.

14. Mann NC, MacKenzie E, Anderson C. Public Health Preparedness for Mass Casualty Events: A 2002 State-by-State Assessment, 2002. http://www.ncbi.nlm.nih.gov/pubmed/15571201 (Accessed August 29, 2014).

15. Spear T. Education and Training for a Qualified Workforce. Agency for Healthcare Research and Quality Archives, 2004. http://archive.ahrq.gov/news/ulp/btsurgeau/surgetrans.htm (Accessed August 29, 2014).

16. Report on the Natural Disaster Health Workforce. National Center for Disaster Medicine and Public Health, November 2011. http://ncdmph.usuhs.edu/Documents/Workforce2011/WorkforceProject2011-B.pdf (Accessed August 29, 2014).

17. Bradt DA, Aitken P. Disaster Medicine Reporting: The Need for New Guidelines and the CONFIDE Statement. Emergency Medicine Australia, December 2010. http://onlinelibrary.wiley.com/doi/10.1111/j.1742-6723.2010.01342.x/full (Accessed August 29, 2014).

18. Strategic Framework 2012–2013. Interagency Standing Committee, Global Health Cluster, World Health Organization, 2012–2013. http://www.preventionweb.net/english/professional/contacts/profile.php?id=2747 (Accessed August 29, 2014).

19. Minimum Standards in Health Action, Humanitarian Charter and Minimum Standards in Humanitarian Response. The Sphere Project, 2011. www.sphereproject.org (Accessed August 29, 2014).

20. National Preparedness Goal. FEMA, Department of Homeland Security, 2012. https://www.fema.gov/national-preparedness-goal (Accessed August 29, 2014).

21. Core Capabilities. FEMA, Department of Homeland Security, 2012. https://www.fema.gov/core-capabilities (Accessed August 29, 2014).

22. National Health Security Strategy. Assistant Secretary for Preparedness and Response, Department of Health and Human Services, 2009. http://www.phe.gov/Preparedness/planning/authority/nhss/Pages/default.aspx (Accessed August 29, 2014).

23. Public Health Preparedness Capabilities: National Standards for State and Local Planning. Centers for Disease Control and Prevention, March 2011. http://www.cdc.gov/phpr/capabilities (Accessed August 29, 2014).

24. Healthcare Preparedness Capabilities: National Guidance for Healthcare System Preparedness. HHS Office of the Assistant Secretary for Preparedness and Response, January 2012. http://www.phe.gov/preparedness/planning/hpp/pages/default.aspx (Accessed August 29, 2014).

25. Performance Improvement Management System. Veterans Health Administration, Office of Emergency Management, 2010. http://www.va.gov/vhaemergencymanagement (Accessed August 29, 2014).

26. Education and Standards Committee. World Association for Disaster and Emergency Medicine. April 2013. http://www.wadem.org/ed_and_standards.html (Accessed August 29, 2014).

27. Sundnes KO, Birnbaum ML. Health Disaster Management Guidelines for Evaluation and Research in the Utstein Style. Task Force on Quality Control of Disaster Management, 2009. http://www.laerdalfoundation.org/dok/Health_Disaste_%20Management.pdf (Accessed August 29, 2014).

28. Health Indicator Sortable Statistics. Centers for Disease Control and Prevention, 2013. http://wwwn.cdc.gov/sortablestats (Accessed August 29, 2014).

29. System of Records, National Disaster Medical System. Assistant Secretary for Preparedness and Response, Department of Health and Human Services, 2009. http://www.hhs.gov/foia/privacy/recordsnotices/09-90-0040.html (Accessed August 29, 2014).

30. Research Group on Emergency and Disaster Medicine. Utstein Template Project, 2012. http://currents.plos.org/disasters/article/utstein-style-template-for-uniform-data-reporting-of-acute-medical-response-in-disasters (Accessed August 29, 2014).

31. Debacker M. Data Reporting Disasters. Emergency Management and Disaster Medicine Academy, 2012. http://www.cochrane.org/sites/default/files/uploads/Evidence_aid/DEBACKER%20-%20Data%20reporting%20in%20disasters.pdf (Accessed August 29, 2014).

32. National Fire Protection Association 1600, Standard for Disaster/Emergency Management and Business Continuity Programs. National Fire Protection Association, 2013. http://www.nfpa.org/codes-and-standards/document-information-pages?mode=code&code=1600&DocNum=1600 (Accessed August 29, 2014).

33. International Organization for Standardization 22301, Societal Security Business Continuity Management, 2012. http://www.iso.org/iso/catalogue_detail?csnumber=50038 (Accessed August 29, 2014).

34. ASIS SPC-1, Organizational Resilience, Security, Preparedness and Continuity Management Systems, 2009. http://www.amazon.com/dp/B008MNFWN2 (Accessed August 29, 2014).

35. Emergency Management Standards. The Joint Commission 2014. http://www.jointcommission.org/standards_information/standards.aspx (Accessed August 29, 2014).

36. Strategic National Risk Assessment. Department of Homeland Security, December 2011. http://www.dhs.gov/xlibrary/assets/rma-strategic-national-risk-assessment-ppd8.pdf (Accessed August 29, 2014).

37. Threat and Hazard Identification and Risk Assessment Guide, Comprehensive Preparedness Guide 201. Department of Homeland Security, April 2012. http://www.fema.gov/library/viewRecord.do?id=5823 (Accessed August 29, 2014).

38. Comprehensive Preparedness Guide 201, Second Edition. Department of Homeland Security, August 2013. https://www.fema.gov/media-library/assets/documents/26335 (Accessed August 6, 2015).

39. Emergency Response Framework. World Health Organization, 2013. http://www.who.int/hac/about/erf_.pdf (Accessed August 29, 2014).

40. National Response Framework. FEMA, 2010. http://www.fema.gov/national-preparedness-resource-library (Accessed August 29, 2014).

41. Marcozzi DE, Lurie N. Measuring Healthcare Preparedness. October 2012. http://www.ncbi.nlm.nih.gov/pubmed/23098101 (Accessed August 29, 2014).

42. Capability Assessment Program. Veterans Health Administration Office of Emergency Management, 2015. Electronic planning document on system server. Copy available from author upon request.

43. Integrated Emergency Management System, FEMA, 1983. http://link.springer.com/referenceworkentry/10.1007/978-1-4020-4399-4˙197 (Accessed August 6, 2015).

44. National Preparedness Guidelines. Department of Homeland Security, 2007. http://www.dhs.gov/national-preparedness-guidelines (Accessed August 29, 2014).

45. National Planning Scenarios. Department of Homeland Security, 2006. http://info.publicintelligence.net/national_planning_scenarios.pdf (Accessed August 29, 2014).

46. Presidential Policy Directive 8, National Preparedness. Executive Office of the President, March 2011. http://www.dhs.gov/presidential-policy-directive-8-national-preparedness (Accessed August 29, 2014).

47. National Incident Management System Overview. Department of Homeland Security, 2013. http://www.fema.gov/library/viewRecord.do?id=6449 (Accessed August 29, 2014).

48. National Interagency Incident Management System. Oklahoma State University, Fire Protection Publications, Stillwater, Oklahoma, 1984.

49. Incident Command System Core Competencies. FEMA, 2007. http://training.fema.gov/EMIWeb/IS/ICSResource/index.htm (Accessed August 29, 2014).

50. Product Management System. National Wildland Fire Coordinating Group, June 2013. http://www.nwcg.gov/pms/docs/docs.htm (Accessed August 29, 2014).

51. NIMS Resource Types. Department of Homeland Security, January 2013. http://www.fema.gov/national-incident-management-system/resource-management-mutual-aid (Accessed August 29, 2014).

52. Barbera JA, Macintyre AG. Medical and Health Incident Management (MaHIM) System: A Comprehensive Functional System Description for Mass Casualty Medical and Health Incident Management. Institute for Crisis, Disaster, and Risk Management, GWU, Washington, DC, October 2002. http://www.gwu.edu/~icdrm/publications/MaHIM%20V2%20final%20report%20sec%202.pdf (Accessed August 29, 2014).

53. Medical Surge Capacity and Capability, A Management System for Integrating Medical and Health Resources During a Large-Scale Incident. 2nd ed. Department of Health and Human Services, 2007. http://www.phe.gov/Preparedness/planning/mscc/Pages/default.aspx (Accessed August 29, 2014).

54. Hospital Incident Command System. California Emergency Medical Services Authority, 2014. http://www.emsa.ca.gov/disaster_medical_services_division_hospital_incident_command_system_resources (Accessed August 29, 2014).

55. Homeland Security Exercise Evaluation Program. Department of Homeland Security, April 2013. https://hseep.dhs.gov/support/HSEEP_Revision_Apr13_Final.pdf (Accessed August 29, 2014).

56. Lessons Learned Information Sharing. FEMA, May 2008. https://beta.fema.gov/about-lessons-learned-information-sharing (Accessed August 29, 2014).

57. Smith SD. From Process to Practice: Coordinating Core Competencies for Medical Disaster Preparedness and Response. Presentation to the Federal Education and Training Interagency Group, 2011.

58. Calhoun JG, et al. Competency Mapping for Public Health Preparedness Training Initiatives. Michigan Center for Public Health Preparedness, University of Michigan School of Public Health, 2005. http://www.ncbi.nlm.nih.gov/pmc/articles/PMC2569994 (Accessed August 29, 2014).

59. Newsome S, Catano VM, Day AL. Leader Competencies: Proposing a Research Framework. Sponsored Research Report: Canadian Forces Leadership Institute, 2003. http://www.arladay.com/2009/technical-consulting-reports (Accessed August 29, 2014).

60. Waeckerle JF, et al. *Competencies for the Response to Weapons of Mass Destruction Incidents*. American College of Emergency Physicians, 2000.

61. Hsu EB, et al. Healthcare Worker Competencies for Disaster Training. BMC Medical Education, 2006. http://www.ncbi.nlm.nih.gov/pmc/articles/PMC1471784 (Accessed August 29, 2014).

62. Core Competencies for Public Health Professionals. The Council on Linkages Between Academia and Public Health Practice, 2010. http://www.phf.org/resourcestools/Documents/Core_Competencies_for_Public_Health_Professionals_2010May.pdf (Accessed August 29, 2014).

63. Emergency Management Core Competencies. FEMA, 2011. https://training.fema.gov/EMIWeb/edu/localEM1.asp (Accessed August 29, 2014).

64. Schultz CH, Koenig KL, Whiteside M, Murray R. Development of National Standardized All-Hazard Disaster Core Competencies for Acute Care Physicians, Nurses, and EMS Professionals. *Ann Emerg Med* 2012; 59: 196–208.

65. Barbera JA, MacIntyre AG, Shaw G, et al. Healthcare Emergency Management Competencies: Competency Framework Final Report. Institute for Crisis, Risk and Disaster Management, GWU developed under contract with the U.S. Veterans Health Administration, 2007. http://www.va.gov/VHAEMER GENCYMANAGEMENT/Documents/Education_Training/ Healthcare_System_Emergency_Management_Competency_ Framework_2007.pdf (Accessed August 30, 2014).

66. Subbarao I, Lyznicki JM, Hsu EB, et al. A consensus-based educational framework and competency set for the discipline of disaster medicine and public health preparedness. *Disaster Medicine and Public Health Preparedness* March 2008. http://www .ncbi.nlm.nih.gov/pubmed/18388659 (Accessed August 30, 2014).

67. Building Core Competencies in Disaster Medicine and Public Health Preparedness. American Medical Association, 2011. http://journals.cambridge.org/action/displayAbstract? aid=8849122 (Accessed August 30, 2014).

68. Walsh L, et al. Core Competencies for Disaster Medicine and Public Health. *Disaster Medicine and Public Health Preparedness* March 2012; 6(1). http://journals.cambridge. org/action/displayFulltext?type=6&fid=8849123&jid=DMP &volumeId=6&issueId=01&aid=8849122&bodyId= &membershipNumber=&societyETOCSession=&fulltextType= RA&fileId=S1935789300004122#fig1 (Accessed August 30, 2014).

69. Disaster-related Competencies for Health Care Providers. Disaster Information Management Research Center, National Library of Medicine, October 2010. http://disasterinfo.nlm.nih .gov/dimrc/professionalcompetencies.html (Accessed August 30, 2014).

70. Schor KW, Altman BA. Proposals for Aligning Disaster Health Competency Models. *Disaster Medicine and Public Health Preparedness* 2013; 7(1). https://journals.cambridge. org/action/displayAbstract?fromPage=online&aid= 8901679&fulltextType=RV&fileId=S1935789313000190 (Accessed August 30, 2014).

71. Daily E, Williams J. White Paper on Identifying and Assessing Competencies in Disaster Health. World Association for Disaster and Emergency Medicine, April 2013. http://www .wadem.org/documents/competencies_in_disaster_health.pdf (Accessed August 30, 2014).

72. Study to Determine the Current State of Disaster Medicine and Public Health Education and Training and Determine Long-term Expectations of Competencies. Yale New Haven Center for Emergency Preparedness and Disaster Response, 2011. http://ncdmph.usuhs.edu/KnowledgeLearning/KL_ Workshops.htm (Accessed August 30, 2014).

73. Compendium of Disaster Health Courses. National Center for Disaster Medicine and Public Health, May 2011. http:// ncdmph.usuhs.edu/Documents/NCDMPH_Compendium_V1 .pdf (Accessed August 30, 2014).

74. National Incident Management System Training Program. Department of Homeland Security, 2011. http://www.fema.gov/ pdf/emergency/nims/nims_training_program.pdf (Accessed August 30, 2014).

75. Training and Certification.American Red Cross, June 2012. http://www.redcross.org/take-a-class (Accessed September 30, 2014).

76. Community Emergency Response Teams. FEMA, May 2010. http://www.fema.gov/community-emergency-response-teams (Accessed August 30, 2014).

77. CERT Training Program. FEMA, May 2010. http:// www.fema.gov/community-emergency-response-teams/ training-materials (Accessed August 30, 2014).

78. Citizens Corps. FEMA, April 2013. http://www.ready.gov/ citizen-corps (Accessed August 30, 2014).

79. National Disaster Life Support Foundation, September 2013. http://register.ndlsf.org/mod/page/view.php?id=2056 (Accessed August 30, 2014).

80. Huntington MK, Gavagon TF. Disaster Medicine Training in Family Medicine: A Review of the Evidence. *Family Medicine* January 2011. http://www.ncbi.nlm.nih.gov/pubmed/21213132 (Accessed August 30, 2014).

81. Scott LA, Maddux PT, Schnellmann J, et al. High-fidelity multiactor emergency preparedness training for patient care providers. *American Journal of Disaster Medicine* 2012. http:// www.ncbi.nlm.nih.gov/pubmed/23140061 (Accessed August 30, 2014).

82. Emergency Preparedness Simulation Scenarios Developed for Disaster Training. Laerdal, September 2009. http://www.laerdal.com/us/docid/42057682/Emergency-Preparedness-Simulation-Scenarios-Developed-for-Disaster-Training-utilizing (Accessed August 30, 2014).

83. Healthcare Leadership Course. Noble Training Center, Center for Domestic Preparedness, Department of Homeland Security, December 2012. https://cdp.dhs.gov (Accessed August 30, 2014).

84. Mission Ready Packages. Emergency Management Assistance Compact, National Emergency Management Association, May 2013. http://www.emacweb.org/index.php?option=com_ content&view=article&id=88&Itemid=310 (Accessed August 30, 2014).

85. Disaster Medical Assistance Team. National Disaster Medical System, Department of Health and Human Services, April 2013. http://www.phe.gov/Preparedness/responders/ndms/teams/ Pages/dmat.aspx (Accessed August 30, 2014).

86. Disaster Resistant Communities Group, June 2013. http:// www.drc-group.com/project/jitt.html (Accessed August 30, 2014).

87. Urban Search and Rescue Just in Time Training Course. FEMA, November 2012. http://www.fema.gov/library/viewRecord.do? id=5398 (Accessed August 30, 2014).

88. U.S. Agency for International Development, Global Health Cluster Training Materials. American College of Emergency Physicians, August 2013. http://www.acep.org/_InternationalSection/ Training-Material (Accessed August 30, 2014).

89. Exercise Evaluation Guide Library. Department of Homeland Security, April 2013. https://hseep.dhs.gov/pages/1002_EEGLi .aspx (Accessed August 30, 2014).

90. Gebbe KM, Valas J, Merrill J, et al. Role of Exercises and Drills in the Evaluation of Public Health in Emergency Response. *Pre-Hospital and Disaster Medicine* May–June 2006. http:// www.researchgate.net/publication/6893957_Role_of_exercises_ and_drills_in_the_evaluation_of_public_health_in_emergency_ response (Accessed August 30, 2014).

91. Sarpy SA, Warren CR, Kaplan S, et al. Simulating public health response to a severe acute respiratory syndrome (SARS) event: a comprehensive and systematic approach to designing, implementing, and evaluating a tabletop exercise. *Journal of Public Health Management and Practice* November 2005. http:// www.ncbi.nlm.nih.gov/pubmed/16205548 (Accessed August 30, 2014).

92. Public Health Preparedness and Response Competency Map. American Society of Public Health, 2010. http://www.phf.org/programs/preparednessresponse/Pages/Public_Health_Preparedness_and_Response_Core_Competencies.aspx (Accessed August 30, 2014).

93. Shultz JM, Loretti A. White Paper on Setting Standards for Selecting a Curriculum in Disaster Health. World Association for Disaster and Emergency Medicine, April 2013. http://www.wadem.org/documents/curriculum_in_disaster_health.pdf (Accessed August 30, 2014).

94. Risk Reduction and Emergency Preparedness, WHO's Six-Year Strategy for the Health Sector and Community Capacity Development. World Health Organization, 2007. http://www.who.int/hac/techguidance/preparedness/emergency_preparedness_eng.pdf (Accessed August 30, 2014).

3

Surge Capacity and Scarce Resource Allocation

Donna F. Barbisch

OVERVIEW

A fundamental issue in disaster response is the need to provide appropriate patient care and public health support as demands for medical and health resources exceed existing supply. Developing the capacity and capability to handle a rapid increase in demand for medical care and public health services is known as medical surge. The mismatch or gap between needs and the capability and/or capacity to fill those needs is the focus of building surge capacity. The gap varies depending on the type and magnitude of the event. In addressing the gaps, perspectives differ across health and medical communities (hospitals, public health, and other health-related communities) as well as across different levels of response (local, regional, national, international). Planning for and managing an event requires an in-depth review of the changing demand for health-related services created by an event, an assessment of existing capability and capacity, a realistic assessment of where excess capacity exists or might exist, and finally a realistic timeline for when resources will be available. The ultimate goal in creating surge capacity and scarce resource allocation protocols is to manage and balance available resources to optimize outcomes. These outcomes will shift from focusing on individual care to maximizing outcomes for the greatest number of people (overall population health).

Defining the Gap in Medical Surge

Health and medical capability to meet an overwhelming demand for care is not uncommon. Overcrowding in emergency departments is a regular occurrence. This "daily surge" to meet routine healthcare requirements exacerbates the challenge in managing large-scale events. This is true regardless of whether the surge results from a sudden large increase in patient numbers for a brief period, a sustained increase in patient volume, or a rise in demand for complex care in a specialized field, such as burn care. Daily surge is characterized as predictable and manageable.[1] Disaster medical surge is more challenging. As surge needs grow, it is imperative to balance capability and capacity. A structured approach, referred to as the "3-S System," can address this need by balancing the triad of personnel (Staff), supplies and equip-

ment (Stuff), and facilities (Structure) to meet needs in a timely fashion as shown in Figure 3.1.

It is not beds or ventilators alone that provide patient care. Effective management requires integration of all healthcare system components. A 3-S System's approach addresses this challenge by integrating policies, procedures, and the Stuff, Staff, and Structure to provide realistic planning and response, creating the capability to adequately manage the crisis.[2]

The proliferation of large-scale events over the course of the past two decades highlights the need for planning to surge in a resource constrained environment. Increasingly, the delivery of healthcare to large numbers of victims has been a central feature of the response. Events caused by natural disasters, as well as those related to terrorist actions, contribute to a fundamental focus on integrating the provision of healthcare into overall response efforts.

In general, events fall into two distinct categories based on how the incident evolves. One event type is characterized by a slow, steady, and progressive rise in patient demand for healthcare services, such as might be seen in an emerging infectious disease or biological event. These events may be obscure and are often characterized by unusual and unclear etiologies. They develop gradually over time, plateau at some point, and then slowly recede, allowing a return toward the baseline delivery of healthcare services. The other type of medical surge event is defined by the suddenness in which its impact occurs. These events may be anticipated, as in a hurricane or cyclone, or unexpected as in an explosion or earthquake. They generate a rapid, but not usually sustained, demand for healthcare services. The need for medical services peaks much faster in these incidents than in the slow-onset event.

Most commonly, the need for medical surge is associated with a sudden-onset event, such as a blast, earthquake, or tsunami. In a sudden impact event, there is usually an awareness of the incident and the immediate need for increased medical response capacity and capability. The medical community surges to respond but resources often become exhausted within a relatively short time period. The timeline for flow and integration of external support and resources is variable and should be factored into plans. A distinct strategy for shortening the timeline includes

Modular Systems Approach

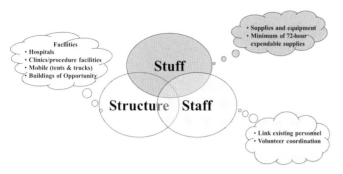

3-S: Coordinate and Balance across ALL Domains

Figure 3.1. 3-S System.

Sudden Onset Event

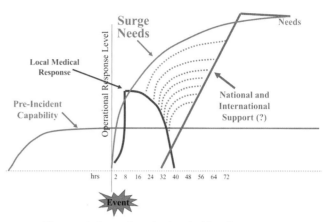

Figure 3.2. Surge Capacity in a Sudden-Onset Event.

efforts focused on pre-event planning and selective positioning of resources. While the sudden impact event is relatively finite in nature, the secondary impact of improper management can have a profound effect on the total number of casualties. An example of such an occurrence is the cholera outbreak in Haiti, resulting from the arrival of United Nations (UN) troops from Nepal that carried cholera into the country. This unfortunate consequence resulted in 657,117 cases and 8,096 deaths as of May 22, 2013.[3] The return to baseline demand for medical services is dependent on the magnitude of the event and the capability of the community to restore services.[4] Figure 3.2 depicts a timeline for a sudden onset event.

The 1918 pandemic is an extreme example of a slow-onset event requiring a surge in medical services. Individuals begin presenting to the medical community with generalized complaints, an unknown etiology, and symptoms that developed over hours and days. A slow-onset event can continue for weeks to months. It may also affect multiple geographic regions, which can limit deployment of external resources from these areas to the location where the disease first appeared. Public health may be overwhelmed with demands to monitor or restrict travel (see Chapter 17) or report symptoms.

Figure 3.3 depicts a slow-onset timeline reflecting the escalation of casualties presenting to the medical community, the follow-up response of local medical resources, the point at which the local resources are exhausted, and the gap between exhaustion and when external resources may become available. The system may not return to baseline for months to years. The 2014 Ebola outbreak also illustrates these concepts, although to a lesser degree.

STATE OF THE ART

Definitions and Perspectives

In its broadest context, surge is defined as representing a sudden rise in some measurable entity to excessive or abnormal values. However, detailed approaches to interpreting this definition differ based on geographical/political areas of responsibility (local, regional, national, or international) and on the specific mission of the healthcare entity (hospital, prehospital, pharmacy, mental health, special populations, and public health). In addition, medical surge can be further defined as requiring both a

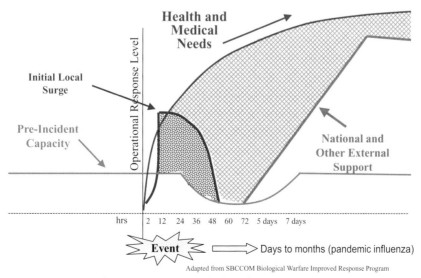

Adapted from SBCCOM Biological Warfare Improved Response Program

Figure 3.3. Surge Capacity in a Slow-Onset Event.

2.2.1 | WHO has the following grade definitions:

Ungraded: an event that is being assessed, tracked or monitored by WHO but that requires no WHO response at the time.

Grade 1: a single or multiple country event with minimal public health consequences that requires a minimal WCO response or a minimal international WHO response. Organizational and/or external support required by the WCO is minimal. The provision of support to the WCO is coordinated by a focal point in the regional office.

Grade 2: a single or multiple country event with moderate public health consequences that requires a moderate WCO response and/or moderate international WHO response. Organizational and/or external support required by the WCO is moderate. An Emergency Support Team, run out of the regional office,[6] coordinates the provision of support to the WCO.

Grade 3: a single or multiple country event with substantial public health consequences that requires a substantial WCO response and/or substantial international WHO response. Organizational and/or external support required by the WCO is substantial. An Emergency Support Team, run out of the regional office, coordinates the provision of support to the WCO.

Figure 3.4. WHO International Grading System.

medical surge "capacity" and surge "capability." Medical surge capacity is the provision of services that are normally available from an entity to a greater percent of the population. Development of medical surge capacity recognizes that the response to a sustained or sudden increase in demand for healthcare services requires a certain concomitant rise in available surge resources including hospital beds, hospital staff, equipment, supplies, and pharmaceuticals needed to support such care. Medical surge capability is the provision of new or expanded services that an entity does not normally offer, such as burn or trauma care. This concept recognizes the need to expand capabilities to manage patient care needs, particularly those that may require unique services not generally available in locations other than specialty centers.

At the global level, the World Health Organization (WHO) approaches medical surge from a broad perspective and with regard to international laws and independent jurisdictions. Their guiding document is the International Health Regulations of 2005.[5] The WHO Emergency Response Framework uses a grading system designed to: 1) inform and identify the extent, complexity, and duration of operations; 2) initiate action to re-purpose support resources; and 3) support implementation of disaster policies and procedures. Should an event occur, local WHO Country Office (WCO) staff will respond immediately, forming an initial Emergency Response Team (ERT) within the country. However the process of identifying the scale and urgency of an event, as well as the appropriate international response and authority of member nations, can take hours to days. Once the public health consequences are determined, WHO follows a two-phase surge process over 3 months to grade and manage an international response to the emergency. Phase 1 deployments occur within 72 hours to supplement the WCO; phase 2 occurs within 2 weeks of grading the emergency. Grading occurs within 24 hours of completing a risk assessment for a sudden-onset event, and within 5 days of performing a risk assessment for a slow-onset event. Figure 3.4 depicts the WHO international grading system.

An overview of the U.S. framework for medical surge is contained in the Department of Health and Human Services Medical Surge Capacity and Capability Handbook.[6] This guidance provides organizational clarity to develop surge planning across multiple jurisdictions. It classifies groups into six tiers that range from an individual operating unit through local, regional, state, and federal efforts. Other countries and states have their respective guidance on medical surge, proposing how the jurisdictional and overlapping needs and resources can be coordinated.

When considering medical surge guidelines within specialties or practice areas, interdependencies between different healthcare groups can create cascading untoward effects in other parts of the surge system. One group's surge strategy may conflict with that of another. Consider a hospital plan that redirects home health staff to the hospital in an effort to increase the hospital's capacity to manage individual care. This shift in personnel may initially increase the in-hospital care capacity. However, as the need for in-patient care continues to rise, patients will require discharge to home healthcare. However, due to insufficient numbers of personnel working in the home health environment, the overall system's patient care capacity is actually reduced. Planning for one area without consideration of the impact in another area creates critical points of failure that reduce overall medical system surge capacity. Resources such as qualified healthcare

Pandemic Influenza
Planning Assumptions

Based on U. S. Population 2010:　Aprox 300,000,000*

- **50% of ill persons will seek medical care****
- **Hospitalization and deaths will depend on the virulence of the virus**

	Moderate (1957-like)	Severe (1918-like)
Illness	90 million (30%)	90 million (30%)
Outpatient medical care	45 million (50%)	45 million (50%)
Hospitalization	865,000	9, 900,000
ICU care	128,750	1,485,000
Mechanical ventilation	64,875	745,500
Deaths	209,000	1,903,000

Source: * Census data
** Projections using CDC FluAid planning tool

Figure 3.5. Pandemic Influenza Planning Assumptions Using CDC Planning Tool *FluAid.*

staff are mostly a fixed asset, even if one includes those who come from outside the affected disaster area in support of the response. Hospitals, public health agencies, and specific elements within communities (emergency departments, intensive care settings, home health services, and hospice facilities) must consider each other as they optimize their planning priorities. Other surge concepts have been developed to address specific types or causes of injury and illness. Examples include trauma, burns, and infectious diseases. If uncoordinated, multiple entities can be competing for the same resources rather than complementing each other.

Consider the assumptions used to decide where to manage a critical care patient when both the emergency department and the intensive care unit of a hospital are filled to capacity. Members in both environments understand that the patient will not get optimal care if the appropriate 3-S resources (Staff, Stuff, and Structure) are unavailable and if the system is not coordinated to provide all necessary services. In some cases, patients are placed in hallways without provision of all essential services while awaiting appropriate care environments. The practice raises several questions: Which environment will create the best outcomes for the patient, for the other patients, for the staff, and for the hospital? Depending on the goal, the answers may change. In a true scarce resource environment, the goal will be to optimize outcomes for the entire population of patients, rather than for each individual.

Detailed surge plans are complex and challenging to implement. Specific elements of the plan can be incomplete or ill defined, particularly as it relates to the availability of actionable information that warrants a surge response effort. For example, deciding when a given healthcare organization or health system is truly overwhelmed can be difficult to ascertain. The importance of situational awareness is critical to supporting the administrative decisions needed to move toward implementing surge response plans. Yet, the communication of information that results in actions is often subject to the effects of the ensuing disaster event, and therefore may be impeded. The disrupted communication capability that frequently occurs after a disaster

leads to incomplete information, and time-sensitive critical decisions must be made in a vacuum. Understanding that a health system has reached appropriate trigger points for action poses a vexing challenge, particularly when the event is unfolding and information is limited or inaccurate.

Such challenges that occur in planning for and managing medical surge are categorized as "wicked problems," that is, those associated with complex issues that have incomplete, contradictory, and changing requirements.[7] Defining best outcomes in wicked problems requires: 1) understanding the environment and assumptions of all stakeholders; 2) acceptance of differing perspectives; and 3) comparing the impact of actions that may not be optimal for each individual stakeholder, but deliver best outcomes for the community at large. Using the wicked problems approach, enduring processes can be developed to link the seemingly disparate influences in the health and medical environment with the desired outcome.

With these challenges in mind, identifying the underlying issues can be accomplished by measuring capacity and capability across the continuum of healthcare. A simple view of this approach is to consider the throughput of patients from the time they enter the healthcare system until they return to health. Using this strategy, it is clear that simply having the current level of hospital capacity (or current number of hospital beds) does not ensure the healthcare system is prepared. As an example, based on the U.S. Center for Disease Control and Prevention (CDC) influenza planning tools, projections for pandemic influenza suggest: 1) 30% of the U.S. population will become ill; 2) 50% of those will need outpatient services; 3) more than 10% will require hospitalization; 4) 1.6% will require intensive care; 5) 0.8% will require mechanical ventilation; and 6) 2% will die.[8]

Figure 3.5 provides the numbers for a 1918 and a 1957-like pandemic. Comparing this information with historical data from 1918 suggests the majority of illnesses will occur in a 1-month period. Data on the influenza pandemic of 1918 within the United States show that the death rate escalated from 14 per 1,000 to 44 per 1,000 in October. It then immediately declined

U.S. Crude Death Rates
1917–1919
per 1,000 population*

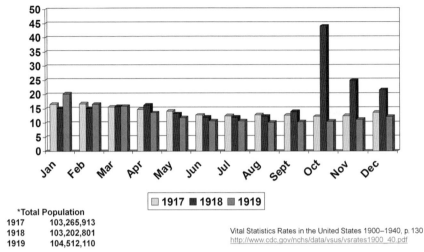

*Total Population
1917   103,265,913
1918   103,202,801
1919   104,512,110

Vital Statistics Rates in the United States 1900–1940, p. 130
http://www.cdc.gov/nchs/data/vsus/vsrates1900_40.pdf

Figure 3.6. United States Crude Death Rates, 1917–1919.

to 24.9 per 1,000 in the following month, returning to nearly baseline in less than 2 months as shown in Figure 3.6.

If this surge event occurred in the United States during 2014, the projected supply of healthcare resources would not be sufficient to meet the population's medical needs in the peak month. This raises several questions. What is "hospitalization" if hospitals are not available? How many victims will actually receive hospital care? If not managed in a hospital, where will care take place? Who will provide the care? Will appropriate triage occur to dedicate scarce resources to those who are expected to live? If not, will more suffer and die?

It is critical to use assumptions that not only project the level of demand for care, but also correlate such demand with what will realistically be available. With a surge in requirements for medical resources similar to the magnitude seen in the 1918 pandemic, traditional healthcare will be unavailable. Therefore, planning should address methods to optimize patient outcomes using nontraditional approaches. One model, the Seamless Emergency Medical Logistics Expansion System (SEMLES) originally designed for the Washington, DC, Department of Health in 2003, demonstrates a cost-effective and integrated approach to surge planning. The concept synchronizes parallel systems to create critical surge capacity for a rapid and sustained response. The process requires extensive inter-organizational collaboration in assessing existing medical emergency capability, projecting needs in a variety of disasters and catastrophic events, and analyzing capability gaps. The program establishes a hub within the health department that links resources into a modular system that can expand capability as needs grow. Components of this modular system include prehospital EMS, hospitals, outpatient medical care providers, and infrastructure support agencies. Regardless of the resource, SEMLES enables connectivity to optimize capability. Despite inevitable organizational, financial, and political obstacles, SEMLES coordinates and synchronizes programs to provide a template to optimize surge capacity. (See Figure 3.7).[9]

Healthcare Facility Surge Capacity

The implementation of surge capacity strategies in healthcare facilities requires a graded approach using a variety of strategies. There are a number of steps that healthcare facilities can take to expand capacity over discrete timeframes and augment the delivery of care for an increased volume of high acuity patients. Space to deliver care, clinical staffing availability, and the critical use of supplies must all be considered. Examples of methods to support conventional care that are outside the normal operations of daily patient care delivery include doubling of beds in single patient rooms and canceling elective surgical procedures. At the other end of this spectrum, the delivery of crisis care might involve the placement of patients in non-conventional treatment settings, referred to as alternate care sites. In addition, some experts recommend that hospitals with intensive care units should prepare to deliver such care for a daily critical care census that is three times their usual capacity, for up to 10 days of care delivery. Further research is necessary to validate this recommendation.

The identification and utilization of alternate care sites can support overall surge capacity. While many potential facilities exist, several offer clear advantages. The U.S.-based Joint Commission identified the following examples as options for consideration.

Hospitals that have been closed (shuttered hospitals) may offer an option for surge capacity. The process of opening a facility that has been closed requires considerable attention to environmental safety. Planning is critical as the cost of improving the facility may be more than the cost of replacement. Recently closed facilities offer the most viable expansion solutions.

A second option, "facilities of opportunity," are nonmedical buildings that can serve to enhance healthcare facility surge. Examples include veterinary hospitals, convention centers, exhibition halls, empty warehouses, airport hangars, schools, sports arenas, or hotels. Considerations such as staffing, ease of patient care, sanitary facilities, and food service should be considered.

Modular / Phased Planning
Immediate and Sustained Capability

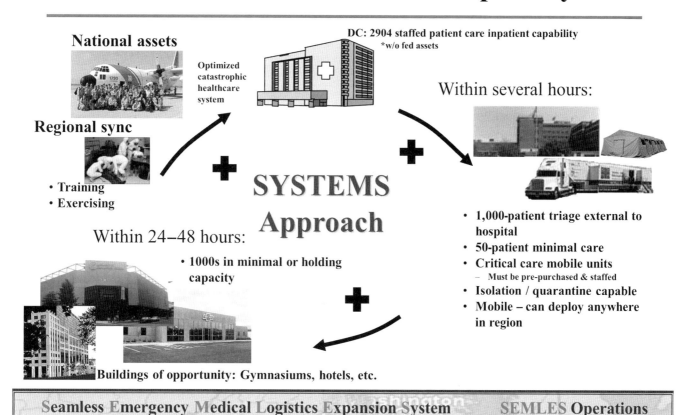

Figure 3.7. Seamless Emergency Medical Logistics Expansion System (SEMLES).

Facilities such as day surgery centers and other existing healthcare facilities may provide options for expansion with minimal cost and effort.

Lastly, mobile and portable facilities build on the military model of independent hospital facilities. Many models exist commercially that may offer expansion capability. As with other options, a cost benefit analysis along with assessment of the ability to deliver care in a timely manner is critical in developing the capability. A major problem with such facilities is not just acquisition costs, but the ongoing expense generated by maintenance. These facilities may remain unused for decades and the cost for maintaining them in a continuous state of readiness is substantial.

Staff Support Options

Staffing for surge capacity presents many challenges. Uninvited but well-meaning volunteers may converge on the disaster region. Often there is no plan to integrate these spontaneous volunteers into the local command and control structure and their management consumes resources that were programmed for the response. In addition to anticipating this group of volunteers, a better approach is to establish systems to coordinate volunteer resources prior to rather than during an event. Even with pre-event initiatives, there are difficulties related to confirming current qualifications, identifying sufficient providers who are not already committed to other responsibilities, and compliance with existing country-specific regulations. For example, in the United States, multiple entities may have requirements for credentialing personnel including states and local healthcare facilities. These initiatives are focused on identifying health personnel who may be mobilized to help support the surge in demand for patient care service delivery.

In the United States, state-based registry systems have been established under the Emergency System for Advance Registration of Volunteer Health Professionals (ESAR-VHP) program. Additional federal resources are being developed within the Medical Reserve Corps (MRC) program to identify local volunteers in the medical and public health arenas who can contribute their skills during times of disaster response. Nevertheless, significant controversy surrounds credentialing and management of volunteers. For example, Schultz and Stratton argue that all of the currently available credentialing options have serious limitations that would make it difficult for hospitals to use the healthcare workers provided by such entities. Most of these systems require significant time to activate and implement. In addition, they don't all provide volunteers with skill levels that hospitals can utilize. Hospitals require highly trained professionals within hours of a disaster. These two authors suggest a hospital-based credentialing system that is shared among local facilities within one jurisdiction. All credentialed healthcare providers at each hospital are listed in a database and this information is distributed to all facilities. Immediately after a disaster, hospitals can consult the database to verify the credentials of volunteers in the area. This system would permit rapid credentialing of qualified volunteers in the first hours and help to maintain hospital function.[10]

In addition to utilization of local responders, many countries have organized deployable medical teams. In the United States, the National Disaster Medical System (NDMS) is a nationally driven, top-down program designed to provide resources to local jurisdictions upon their request, in the event of a disaster. NDMS constitutes the primary federal response mechanism for management of mass casualty events in the United States, with focus placed on three discrete areas of response. The first is the provision of deployable teams designed to provide basic emergency healthcare support in the disaster-affected area. The teams mobilize under federal authority to provide support as requested.

Disaster Medical Assistance Teams (DMATs) are the basic unit of NDMS and have demonstrated the ability to deploy between 6 and 12 hours after activation. They are expected to arrive on site within 48 hours and maintain operations for 72 hours without resupply. Teams consist of thirty-five people who are capable of providing primary and acute care, triage, initial resuscitation and stabilization, advanced life support, and preparation of sick or injured for evacuation. DMAT members are capable of providing ambulatory care for up to 250 patients per 24-hour mission cycle, with limited laboratory point of care testing and bedside radiology services. They have the means to stabilize and hold six patients for extended treatment for up to 12 hours, and can support an additional two critical care patients for up to 24 hours. Other teams with different missions also exist, such as Disaster Mortuary Operational Response Teams and Veterinary Medical Assistance Teams. Additional

groups support the care of burn, pediatric, and mental health patients.

Medical Supply Surge

Options for managing increased demand for medical supplies and equipment exist and include optimizing utilization for the population instead of the individual. But scarce resource allocation protocols are only effective for a limited time. At some point, resupply is necessary. Strategies for eventually providing increased supply usually involve stockpiles.

An example of this approach is the Strategic National Stockpile (SNS), a program created by the U.S. federal government designed to supplement and resupply state and local governments with medical materiel supplies. It contains antibiotics, medical supplies, antidotes, antitoxins, antiviral medications, vaccines, and other pharmaceuticals. The SNS program coordinates governmental and nongovernmental capabilities including the National Veterinary Stockpile, commercial business vendor managed inventory process, and commercial carriers. The purpose is to integrate critical medical supplies for distribution in emergencies. The program also coordinates with the research and development community to acquire medical countermeasures for Chemical, Biological, Radiological, and Nuclear (CBRN) threats and to expedite access to drugs that are not commercially available for non-research purposes. The SNS maintains 12-hour push packs that are strategically located across the United States near major transportation hubs as well as forward-placed caches of chempacks that are integrated into local hazardous material response programs. A Technical Advisory Response Unit (TARU) is also available to support local authorities in receipt and coordination of distribution of the SNS.

In addition to the 12-hour push packages, ventilators and vaccines are stored and managed under a managed inventory program. This consists of either vendor managed inventory

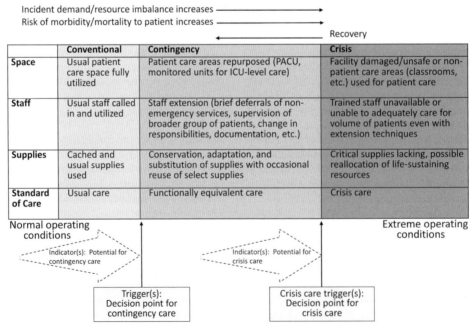

Figure 3.8. Continuum of Surge Response and Implications for Provision of Medical Care under Increasingly Austere Conditions (Courtesy of the Institute of Medicine, *Crisis Standards of Care: A Toolkit for Indicators and Triggers*. National Academies Press, 2013).

(VMI) or strategic stockpile managed inventory (SMI). When specific supplies are required to support the medium- to long-term objectives of a disaster surge response, VMI or SMI will be used to supplement the initial shipments. VMI is maintained by the primary corporate vendor under contract with the federal government. VMI and SMI supplies are designed to arrive 24 to 36 hours following the initial receipt of the push packages.

Considerations in Development of Surge Capacity

Another framework to organize and conceptualize surge suggests categorizing surge into conventional capacity, contingency capacity, and crisis capacity.[11] In crisis capacity, the degraded resources force the practice environment into provision of crisis care using previously determined scarce resource allocation protocols. A key goal of the framework was to aid in phased implementation of surge capacity plans (see Figure 3.8).

At the individual level, a review of patient care requirements from the moment an event begins through recovery is useful in determining how to build system resiliency and sustainable surge capacity. Barbisch and Koenig describe an outcomes-based, scalable, time-sensitive system applicable across the continuum of care that will provide appropriate capacity or capability. It takes into consideration the 3-S System as previously mentioned to support the full spectrum of needs for patient care.[12] The 3-S system terminology was further endorsed by Hick et al. in 2009. However, in doing so, they changed the terminology to Staff, Space, and Supplies.[13] Early surge models often focused on critical supplies (Stuff) like ventilators or hospital beds while overlooking the critical need for Staff and Structure. In addition, surge planning that emphasizes the needs of only one group, such as trauma or burn patients, would overlook the secondary impact on other practice areas. As an example, the cross-training of hospital staff caring for patients in non-acute areas to also provide burn care in support of burn center personnel may seem reasonable. However, it is highly likely that during a large-scale surge, these same staff would also be overwhelmed with an increase in volume of non-acute patients and so be unavailable.

Patient care delivery requiring integrated surge planning can be divided into five basic elements: 1) emergency medical services (initial triage and treatment); 2) hospital care; 3) out-of-hospital healthcare (clinics, physician offices, nursing homes, home health, hospice, and rehabilitation facilities); 4) out-of-hospital health and medical assets (public health assets, laboratory, pharmacy, radiology, occupational health, and medical supply); and 5) assets that are not health or medical, but provide operational support (communications, power, water, security, and transportation). Catastrophic events require increased capacity across all elements. Depending on the scenario, surge capacity may only be needed for a portion of these elements at any given time. Critical issues arise when any one of the elements is mismanaged or managed in a vacuum.

Appropriate triage at the onset of the event is critical. Mismanagement of fragile populations (populations with functional or access needs) increases the risk for poor outcomes secondary to the primary event. This designation applies to those victims of disaster that are extraordinarily vulnerable members of society due to socioeconomic standing, chronic disease state, age, and other characteristics. Triage is critical to ensure that these unique populations have access to support services such as pharmacy, dialysis, and oxygen therapy. Without appropriate support, populations with functional or access needs can easily become secondary casualties.[14] Development of robust community-based surge strategies that address the delivery of care to the medically fragile is an important component of developing a community's approach to surge capacity and capability planning. A key component that contributes to this community-based approach includes the utilization of home healthcare services. Assuring the delivery of home healthcare will be an important strategy to prevent patients who might otherwise not need hospital-level care from using these critical resources. With a clear understanding of patient care requirements and the ability to develop a cohesive plan for patient throughput, implementation of surge policies and procedures will likely improve outcomes in a timely and cost-effective manner under catastrophic disaster conditions.

Evolution and Historical Context of Surge Capacity

The early 1980s witnessed an emerging international emphasis on coordinating efforts to bridge the gap between medical needs and available care during disasters. The 1983 *Health Services Organization in the Event of Disaster*, published by the Pan American Health Organization (PAHO), stressed the importance of preventive planning for disaster management.[15] The publication outlined a process for disaster management to involve every organization and sector that directly or indirectly performs health activities in the country. It suggested comprehensive national planning and set forth clear and precise objectives and targets to parallel national planning efforts. The document called for the delivery of medical services to victims using a tiered system of care. Personnel provide initial first aid followed by coordinated and more focused efforts in cooperation with every institution in the health sector. The system emphasizes the importance of institutional organization requirements to meet disaster care needs outside of hospital facilities. Special emphasis is placed on middle- and low-income countries where government resources are not always sufficient.

U.S. efforts to close operational gaps in medical surge can be traced to the 1982 legislation mandating the development of the Department of Veterans Affairs (VA) and Department of Defense (DOD) Contingency Hospital System. The VA/DOD Contingency Hospital System required the VA to serve as the primary contingency backup to DOD medical services if a surge in combat casualties requiring hospitalization could not be accommodated by military treatment facilities. At the time, DOD facilities were experiencing a reduction in both medical capacity and capability. Given this situation, the VA/DOD Contingency Hospital System had to expand its capability to meet potential wartime needs. In 1984, the program was incorporated into the federally mandated NDMS, transferring the lead to the Department of Health and Human Services and adding civilian hospitals as partners. Planning for disaster management at the federal level was coordinated under the Federal Emergency Management Agency (FEMA). FEMA developed a Federal Response Plan (FRP), which was later refined to the National Response Framework (NRF). NDMS, an early public-private partnership, has evolved over the years from its initial focus on supporting care of military casualties that overwhelmed the military medical care system to its initial secondary mission of supporting civilian disasters.[16] With increased emphasis on the need for medical surge to support the care of disaster victims, NDMS began developing the concept of deployable civilian response teams to increase their operational reach. The DMATs were designed to mobilize at a local level and deploy to disaster stricken areas to augment medical response.[17] Specialty teams were added to support specific shortfalls in medical surge needs such as Disaster Mortuary Operational Response Teams and National Veterinary Response Teams.[18] With an increasing awareness of the evolving terrorist threat, additional critical medical specialty needs drove the development of pharmacy, burn, pediatric, and management teams. The concept expanded in 1999 to include International Medical Surgical Response Teams.

In the mid-1990s, WHO increased its emphasis on managing emergencies as it developed a strategy and organization to support countries' needs during emergencies and humanitarian relief operations.[19] In 2013, WHO published the previously mentioned Emergency Response Framework.

Numerous efforts to build surge capacity evolved from models used to provide for medical surge in times of war. Many models are hospital-based and include numerous underground medical facilities across Europe and Australia.[20,21] The facilities were designed to add capacity and provide for security. In 2013, Rambam Medical Center in Haifa built a Fortified Underground Emergency Hospital. Its design allowed conversion of a 1,500-vehicle parking lot into a 2,000-bed acute care emergency hospital protected against conventional and non-conventional warfare.[22]

Recent Developments

While much has been done in disaster management, medical surge remains a challenge. Efforts to develop a common framework for time-phased implementation of medical surge are not uniformly adopted. Professional organizations continue to recognize medical surge as a critical need, but publish only limited guidance recommending goals of surging to 200% of current hospital based capacity and alignment of policies with other organizations. Although more must be done, these organizations recognize that support from the government, improved communication systems, advanced planning, and realistic exercises are critical.[23] Research is still considered in its infancy, especially in middle- and low-income countries given the fragmentation of emergency health service systems and inconsistent application of policy.[24]

Much of the work presented at the 2006 Society for Academic Emergency Medicine Consensus Conference on the Science of Surge, and the recommendations contained within the Department of Health and Human Services Medical Surge Capacity and Capability Handbook continue as foundational guidance in developing medical surge.[25,26] In the United States, the State of California developed comprehensive surge capacity standards and guidelines in 2008 with the input of a broad group of stakeholders from both government and private sectors. These activities provided organizational clarity to develop surge planning across multiple jurisdictions that ranged from the individual operating unit level all the way through local, regional, state, and national efforts. In 2010, the National Academies of Sciences Institute of Medicine (IOM) examined the approach to provision of care when demand overwhelms capacity. It found that current surge capacity plans would not allow providers to adhere to normal treatment protocols and that even basic life sustaining interventions might not be possible.[27]

The State of California's and the IOM's efforts both emphasized concerns related to scarce resource allocation decision-making. Their findings reflected the top priorities for health planners and medical responders regarding the complex issues related to the provision of medical care in a disaster. Long before either of these efforts came to fruition, there were a few focused efforts involving a multidisciplinary group of legal scholars, operational medical experts, and public health professionals that were already beginning to examine this issue in greater detail. Peer reviewed journals began publishing a small but growing body of literature focusing on the threats of an impending pandemic crisis or the experiences of managing the SARS outbreak a few years earlier.[28,29]

The evolution of thought and scholarly effort on this topic has resulted in three independent reports completed by the Institute of Medicine entitled Crisis Standards of Care.[46,47] Rather than focusing on actual standards of care, the IOM committee elected to use the framework for surge capacity elucidated by Hick et al. This concept recognized that the development of surge capacity is not an all or none phenomenon, but is implemented across a spectrum of increasingly austere environments. Surge capacity is best considered as occurring over a continuum that ranges from conventional surge to contingency surge to crisis surge responses. Within each of these categories, it is expected that there will be an increase in demand for health and medical service delivery, and a concomitant decrease in the availability of resources required to deliver and sustain such services. The IOM committee adopted the position that under conventional surge response, the probable strategy for resource allocation that most would view as rational and achievable would largely follow "conventional" processes. These are allocation policies that traditionally govern day to day delivery of healthcare, and that are very much focused on individual patient care outcomes. Under contingency response conditions, healthcare providers would implement contingency allocation protocols, which begin to value improved population outcomes over individual care. In the event that a crisis surge response was necessary, the delivery of care would be governed by crisis resource allocation guidelines.

The publication of this report was surrounded by a significant degree of uncertainty, specifically regarding the impending second wave of the H1N1 pandemic. The published Letter Report was intended as basic guidance that health officials could use, should the need arise, to establish and implement response plans allocating resources based on pervasive shortages or insufficiencies. One of the most concerning issues involved the availability of mechanical ventilators and the difficult decisions facing medical personnel determining which patients would receive them. Challenging issues might arise should such resources be taken from one cohort of patients who were not improving, and shifting them to provide life-sustaining treatment to another group more likely to survive. Such actions would almost certainly result in a transition to palliative care, comfort measures, and death for those patients removed from the ventilators. This was recognized as both medically and legally unprecedented territory, and the ensuing guidance was intended to persuade medical surge planners to confront such unlikely but extremely problematic scenarios. With respect to the H1N1 pandemic, the envisioned worst-case scenario never arose. The second wave of H1N1 cases resulted in relatively few critically ill patients succumbing to the influenza strain and related respiratory infections.

What the committee emphasized in its approach was the importance of developing a cohesive systems framework for catastrophic disaster response planning. It should be based on the description of ethical and legal principles as the foundation for all such planning. Key steps required to establish such plans include an emphasis on the importance of provider and community engagement and the development of indicators and triggers that highlight the transitions of care along the surge continuum.

The 2012 Report emphasized that the planning process must be inclusive of all emergency response system elements including hospitals and healthcare facilities, outpatient healthcare services, public health agencies, EMS, and the emergency management and public safety agencies. The committee emphasized that such efforts must occur under the auspices of a performance improvement model. Health systems should evaluate and monitor their own efforts at delivering care under the worst-case scenarios, and be prepared to make mid-event corrections when warranted. Rather than focus on a specific resource allocation guideline, which conditions generated by the disaster could alter, the IOM Committee felt strongly that their work detailed a process to improve existing discussions that focus on surge capacity and capability development.

Clinical Development and Tools to Support Medical Surge Plans

Planning and response tools have been developed to support the full spectrum of local, regional, national, and global medical surge. Globally, the UN Office for the Coordination of Humanitarian Affairs addresses surge coordination through the Surge Capacity and Logistics Section in its Emergency Services Branch. WHO, in its 2013 Emergency Response Framework, identifies performance standards relative to event coordination and timeline of deployment. However, the actual implementation of such global planning may be encumbered by international policy and treaties and can be obscure when viewed by local responders. As mentioned earlier in the chapter, global response timelines can be prolonged. Local planners may have access to some international support in a Grade 2 event, given its moderate public health consequences. However, significant international support will likely be critical in a Grade 3 event, as these disasters are associated with substantial public health consequences.

One of the most detailed clinically focused surge planning efforts has been undertaken by the critical care community.[30,31,32] Threshold targets for critical care surge planning have been described, and include suggested approaches to managing a surge of critically ill or injured patients. Key recommendations related to basic equipment, supplies, pharmaceuticals, staffing, and the adjustment of facility operations were described, and are summarized in Table 3.1.

Response to the Haitian Earthquake of 2010 demonstrated that augmented staffing models such as DMATs supported by NDMS, international response teams, and mobile field hospitals (when coordinated appropriately) have a significant impact on disasters. In addition, just-in-time training and cross training models were demonstrated as viable templates for increasing critical staffing shortages.[33] The use of field hospitals (military and civilian) and deployable medical teams in response to complex disasters has increased over the past decade, as evidenced by deployments to Iran, Haiti, Indonesia, and Pakistan. Analyses of field hospital efficacy have demonstrated mixed results, depending on when the evaluations were performed. Prior to the Haitian Earthquake of 2010, after-action reports indicated that field hospitals arrived too late to have a significant impact on the need for emergency medical and trauma care. They were, however, found to have some value in substituting for existing hospitals that were damaged or destroyed.[34] A 2003 PAHO study found field hospitals to be costly, late in arriving, and not effective in improving patient outcomes. Additionally, field hospitals apparently undermined efforts to restore services to baseline because they diverted staff, supplies, and patients away from regular services in the aftermath of the disaster.[35] More recently, PAHO/WHO convened a working group to create recommendations that ensure deployable teams and field hospitals meet basic standards when caring for disaster victims, and that these response assets are coordinated so they support national efforts.[36] This working group is currently addressing issues related to accreditation, medical standards and qualifications, level of service provided, quality of care, logistics, quality of insurance, and coordination. This detailed assessment was initiated as a direct result of the experience of deployed foreign medical teams (FMT) to Haiti in 2010, and resulting concerns related to the delivery of quality healthcare services as part of the international surge response.[37] The review recommends developing a process of global accreditation, identifying minimum standards for foreign medical teams in case of disaster, and identifying a process to ensure the deployable assets support and do not replace the work of national governments.

In the United States, medical surge is designated as one of fifteen critical capabilities in the continuum of healthcare system preparedness under the National Guidance for Healthcare System Preparedness published in 2012.[38] The guidance provides an operational approach to planning, equipping, training, and implementing integrated surge capacity. It addresses integrating multi-agency planning, prehospital emergency services, hospital and healthcare organizations, standard of care assessment, and evacuation. The Hospital Surge Model, updated in 2013, further supports planners in estimating hospital resources needed to treat casualties arising from biological (anthrax, smallpox, pandemic influenza), chemical (chlorine, sulfur mustard, or sarin), nuclear (1 KT or 10 KT explosion), or radiological (dispersion device or point source) attacks.[39]

Additional interest developed in creating and implementing fundamentally important interventions addressing behavioral and mental health needs in the context of surge planning. Surge planners have recognized that a disproportionate number of individuals consider themselves victims of a disaster even if not suffering from any physical impairments. This may be driven by the need for reassurance, the fear that something wrong has befallen them that they can't detect, or the development of an acute psychological or psychiatric condition. A variety of psychological first aid tools exist, many focused on increasing mental health surge capacity. Given the likelihood that many more patients without physical ailments will present for care in comparison to those with acute medical conditions, these efforts are extremely important to support ongoing medical surge planning. Most recently, innovative efforts have explored creation of a triage tool to assess the risk for psychological harm, including a project referred to as PsySTART (see Figure 3.9).[40] This is a simple effort focused on the basic principles of self-triage, and has been adopted by the American Red Cross as a tool for field utilization. It is an evidence-based approach to the triage of mental health needs in the disaster setting.

RECOMMENDATIONS FOR FURTHER RESEARCH

Numerous areas of research and investigation can add to the evidence-based data supporting local, national, and international operational planning, education of providers, and

Table 3.1. Equipment, Supplies, Pharmaceuticals, Staffing, Facility Operations and Other Key Recommendations for Critical Care Surge Capacity (created with the assistance of Melinda Byrns, Inova Health System)

Equipment	Supplies	Pharmaceuticals	Staffing	Facilities/Operations	Other Considerations
▪ Basic modes of mechanical ventilation ▪ Elevate head of bed ▪ Ventilator recommendations ▪ 1 ventilator/patient; used for patient with significant airflow obstruction or ARDS; able to function with low-flow O2 & with high pressure medical gas; accurately deliver prescribed minute ventilation; sufficient alarms to note apnea, disconnect, low gas source, low battery, high peak airway pressure ▪ Reducing cold stress ▪ Pediatric critical care teams may need to bring their own equipment & supplies ▪ Plan for surge in need of Pediatric Intensive care Unit (PICU) beds whose age & size distribution is similar to the ordinary PICU (6 age categories) ▪ 1.5 endotracheal tube/patient ▪ 10 IV catheters/patient ▪ 1 central line/2 patients ▪ 1 chest tube/4 patients	▪ IV fluid resuscitation (48-hour stockpile) ▪ Stockpile personal protective equipment (PPE) – 48-hour supply ▪ Pulse oximeters, thermometers, blood pressure cuffs ▪ Maintain additional 30% of disposable supplies ▪ Pediatric critical care teams may need to bring their own equipment & supplies ▪ Plan for surge in need of PICU beds whose age & size distribution is similar to the ordinary PICU (6 age categories) ▪ 1.5 ETT/patient ▪ 10 IV catheters/patient ▪ 1 central line/2 patients ▪ 1 chest tube/4 patients	▪ Vasopressors ▪ Antibiotics (48-hour stockpile) ▪ Thromboembolism prophylaxis ▪ Drugs for sedation & analgesia ▪ Optimal therapeutics & interventions (renal replacement therapy; nutrition) ▪ Rules/guidelines for drug administration (such as substitution, conservation, etc.)	▪ Modify staff to include non-ICU physicians/nurses (2-tiered staffing model) ▪ Non-ICU physicians manage 6 critically ill patients; intensivists coordinate efforts of up to 4 non-intensivists ▪ Non-critical care nurse assignments ▪ Non-ICU nurses assigned to 2 critically ill patients; 1 ICU nurse works with 3 non-ICU nurses ▪ Staff training on use of PPE; bioterrorism response training for non-critical care practitioners on basic principles of critical care management ▪ Principles for staffing models include pharmacists & respiratory therapists in 2-tiered staffing models ▪ Assign critical care lead physician ▪ Transfer skilled pediatric critical care teams to non-pediatric hospitals ▪ Identify staff with experience in care of pediatric patients pre-event	▪ Augment isolation capacity ▪ Concentrate ICU surge in non-ICU hospital rooms that are on specific wards/floors ▪ IT capabilities for analyzing clinical data ▪ Approximately 20% of total hospital rooms would need to provide Emergency Mass Critical Care (EMCC) ▪ Achieve 300% of usual ICU capacity ▪ Deliver EMCC for 10 days with sufficient external assistance ▪ EMCC should occur in hospitals or equivalent structures; designated areas for treatment of critically ill patients assigned ▪ Consider phased expansion to double ICU capacity ▪ Prioritization of support services; instruction of utilization of diagnostics (lab, x-ray) ▪ Duplicate liquid oxygen systems; allow interface with trailer-based system ▪ Ensure generator power sufficient to supply maximal load required for critical care delivery ▪ Plan for water needs (including support for hemodialysis)	▪ Modify usual care delivery; how to identify trigger shift to EMCC ▪ Define essential elements of care ▪ Regional hospital coordination should be the goal ▪ Provision of adequate palliative care ▪ Establish regional triage process ▪ EMCC definition; communities should develop graded response plans ▪ Crisis care: adoption of conventional/contingency/crisis approach to ICU surge ▪ Hospital remodel or building projects incorporate O2 ports ▪ Continuity of operations planned ▪ Mass fatality planning ▪ Must be prepared to deliver pediatric EMCC in non-pediatric hospitals (all hospitals must plan to care for children) ▪ Establish referral network

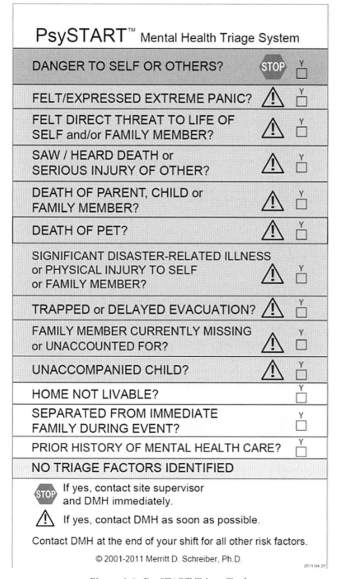

Figure 3.9. PsySTART Triage Tool.

nontraditional methods of providing medical surge. Fundamental to evidence-based planning is the validation of assumptions. Commonly held assumptions are often incorrect, including consideration by some that the number of hospital beds is a reflection of capability, or that stockpiling of ventilators is a measure of readiness. While beds and ventilators may be critical components of a plan, acquisition of these resources alone will not create surge capacity. To be effective, deployment of supplies and equipment must be augmented by arrival of trained personnel and identification of appropriate facilities and management strategies to deliver such care. Additionally, assumptions that the creation of deployable teams and the purchasing of costly field hospitals will enhance the care of disaster victims must be reviewed to identify if the acquisition of these resources actually improves outcomes.

The efficacy of proposed interventions is generally designed and assessed by experts within the specific focus area. An independent review is required to assess second- and third-order impact to interdependent healthcare environments. For example, the practice of shifting personnel from traditional care envi-

ronments to alternate care areas may have unintended consequences and deserves further study. Modeling and simulation with an attempt to establish metrics for surge response may offer insight into the process of addressing realistic timelines for delivery of resources during crisis. Modeling and simulation have the potential to train responders to better manage their own ability to function. Using virtual reality can support the emersion into situations often described as extremely stressful and outside the experience of most healthcare personnel. In 2009, the CDC initiated a virtual reality program to prepare responders for the stress of deployment. The program was expanded in 2013 to better prepare CDC emergency workers to handle the sights, sounds, and smells of a real disaster.[41] "Serious gaming," a term referring to the use of video game environments for education rather than for entertainment, offers the potential to imagine the unimaginable and reinforce best outcomes behavior.[42]

A process known as reverse triage rapidly assesses the need for continuing inpatient care and expedites patient discharge to create surge capacity for disaster victims.[43] The process was analyzed during the Royal Darwin Hospital's response to the Ashmore Reef disaster. Investigators demonstrated that surge capacity was created to accommodate victims through a process of cancelling all scheduled admissions, discharging patients at least 1 day earlier than planned, and discharging all patients earlier in the day. While the process of reverse triage resulted in no increase in clinical risk, further study could determine the sustainability of such action.

Another area of current investigation involves the use of telemedicine to serve as a force multiplier. Although not a new concept for use in disaster events, telemedicine solutions can help extend the delivery of surge capability to patients who may be geographically isolated from specialty centers, yet can still benefit from their expertise.[44,45] This modality for medical surge support was utilized with some success during the Haiti Earthquake response and has continued to play a role in the long-term recovery efforts.[46] This modality remains under-utilized in disaster responses. Additional investigations of effect methods to deploy this technology during disasters could make a significant contribution to the care of victims in developing countries and in isolated regions.

An additional innovative use of available technologies to support medical surge response is the creation of Internet-based triage methods. This was first implemented in an adult population during the H1N1 outbreak in 2009 in the United States.[47] The same strategy was also replicated in pediatric aged patients.[48] The ability to utilize web-based tools may make an important contribution to ameliorating the effects of a surge in demand for healthcare services, particularly during the onset of an infectious disease outbreak. Making a decision regarding the need to seek care, whether by utilizing web-based tools or relying on more traditional methods of information exchange (telephone advice lines), will likely impact the balance of the demand–supply equation.[49] If patients can safely rely on advisory information to make an informed decision regarding the need to seek care, this may lessen the impact of such events on the need for outpatient services. This includes emergency services provided in hospital emergency departments and urgent care settings. Reducing the demand for care can have a beneficial impact on delivering medical services to those who are most in need. However, these efforts require additional study, to ensure that decisions regarding care prioritization can be safely made using such algorithms.

Progress has been made in promulgation of recommendations for improving medical surge capacity. These include the creation of: 1) scarce resource allocation protocols; 2) transition strategies for adjusting the medical response to increasing surge needs; and 3) identifying triggers for implementing and withdrawing surge protocols. One example of this is the series of publications by the IOM on surge capacity. However, much of the data to date supporting these guidelines are derived from consensus groups using the Delphi method, studies using hospitalized patients and not disaster victims, and expert opinion based on individual disaster experiences. While this is a reasonable start, more robust data supporting or refuting these recommendations are necessary using information collected from disaster victims in multiple events.

Finally, the business of healthcare reimbursement for services rendered requires further study. Because surge planning proposes use of alternate care environments, existing reimbursement codes may not apply. In the United States, the publication of *Standards and Guidelines for Healthcare Surge during Emergencies* by the California Department of Public Health provides a review of reimbursement and a starting point for further research. As reimbursements are tied to practice environments, no latitude currently exists in reimbursement coding practices that would permit the use of alternate care environments or providers whose credentials are extended in resource constrained situations.[50]

REFERENCES

1. Jenkins JL, O'Connor RE, Cone DC. Differentiating Large-scale Surge versus Daily Surge. *Acad Emerg Med* 2006, 13: 1169–1172.
2. Barbisch DF, Koenig K. Understanding Surge Capacity: Essential Elements. *Acad Emerg Med* 2006; 13(11): 1098–1102.
3. CDC Cholera in Haiti watch level. http://wwwnc.cdc.gov/travel/notices/watch/haiti-cholera (Accessed November 2014).
4. CDC Cholera in Haiti watch level.
5. *International Health Regulations* (2005). 2nd ed. World Health Organization, 2007. http://www.who.int/ihr/9789241596664/en (Accessed November 12, 2014).
6. Barbera JA, MacIntyre AC. *Medical Surge Capacity and Capability: A Management System for Integrating Medical and Health Resources During Large-Scale Emergencies.* 2nd ed. Washington, DC, US Department of Health and Human Services, 2004. http://www.phe.gov/Preparedness/planning/mscc/handbook/Pages/default.aspx (Accessed November 12, 2014).
7. Rittel H, Webber M. Dilemmas in a General Theory of Planning. In: *Policy Sciences.* Vol. 4. Amsterdam, Elsevier, 1973; 155–169. http://www.uctc.net/mwebber/Rittel+Webber+Dilemmas+General_Theory_of_Planning.pdf (Accessed November 12, 2014).
8. FluAid 2.0. Pandemic Influenza Resources, Centers for Disease Control and Prevention. http://www.cdc.gov/flu/tools/fluaid/index.htm (Accessed November 12, 2014).
9. Barbisch D. Developing Sustainable Surge Capacity for a Regional Public Health Response to Terrorism and Other Medical Disasters. American Public Health Association: Public Health and the Environment. Washington, DC, November 6–10, 2004. https://apha.confex.com/apha/132am/techprogram/paper_83055.htm (Accessed November 12, 2014).
10. Schultz CH, Stratton SJ. Improving hospital surge capacity: a new concept for emergency credentialing of volunteers. *Ann Emerg Med* 2007; 49: 602–609.
11. Hick JL, et al. Refining surge capacity: conventional, contingency, and crisis capacity. *Disaster Med Public Health Prep* June 2009; 3(2 Suppl.): S59–S67. http://www.ncbi.nlm.nih.gov/pubmed/19349869 (Accessed November 12, 2014).
12. Hick JL, et al. Refining surge capacity: conventional, contingency, and crisis capacity. *Disaster Med Public Health Prep* June 2009; 3(2 Suppl.): S59–S67.
13. Hick JL, et al. Refining surge capacity: conventional, contingency and crisis capacity. Disaster Med Public Health Prep June 2009; 3(2 Suppl.): S59–S67.
14. Bethel JW, Foreman AN, et al. Disaster preparedness among medically vulnerable populations. *Am J Prev Med* 2011; 40(2): 139–143. http://www.ncbi.nlm.nih.gov/pubmed/21238861.
15. PAHO. *Health Services Organization in the Event of Disaster.* PAHO/WHO, 1983.
16. Franco C, et al. The National Disaster Medical System: Past, Present, and Suggestions for the Future. *Biosecur Bioterror* 2007; 5(4). http://www.upmchealthsecurity.org/our-work/pubs_archive/pubs-pdfs/2007/2007–12–04-natldisastermedsystempastpresfut.pdf (Accessed November 12, 2014).
17. Couig MP. Annual Review of Nursing Research: Disasters and Humanitarian Assistance. 2012; 30: 29.
18. Barbisch DF. *Identification of barriers to the use of Department of Defense Medical Assets in Support of Federal, State, and Local Authorities to Mitigate the Consequences of Domestic Bioterrorism.* Doctoral Dissertation, Medical University of South Carolina, 2000.
19. Menu J-P. A New Role for WHO in Emergencies. December 1996. www.who.int/disasters/repo/6608.doc (Accessed November 12, 2014).
20. Underground hospital systems at Ft Bribie, Bribie Island, Queensland, Australia. http://indicatorloops.com/fb_hospital.htm (Accessed November 12, 2014).
21. Swedish military hospitals. http://www.militaryphotos.net/forums/showthread.php?65025-Musk%F6-underground-navalbase/page3 (Accessed November 12, 2014).
22. http://www.timesofisrael.com/worlds-most-advanced-underground-hospital-opens-in-haifa
23. Dichter JR, et al. System-level planning, coordination, and communication: care of the critically ill and injured during pandemics and disasters: CHEST consensus statement. *Chest* 2014; 146(4 Suppl.): E87S–E102S. http://journal.publications.chestnet.org/article.aspx?articleid=1899978 (Accessed November 12, 2014).
24. Zhong S, et al. Progress and challenges of disaster health management in China: a scoping review. *Global Health Action* 2014; 7: 24986. http://dx.doi.org/10.3402/gha.v7.24986 (Accessed November 12, 2014).
25. Koenig KL, Kelen G. Executive Summary: The Science of Surge Conference. *Academic Emergency Medicine* 2006; 13: 1087–1088. http://onlinelibrary.wiley.com/doi/10.1197/acem.2006.13.issue-11/issuetoc (Accessed November 12, 2014).
26. Barbera JA, MacIntyre AC. *Medical Surge Capacity and Capability: A Management System for Integrating Medical and Health Resources During Large-Scale Emergencies.* 2nd ed. Washington, DC, U.S. Dept. of Health and Human Services, 2004.
27. Stroud C, Altevogt BM, Nadig L, et al, *Crisis standards of care: Summary of a workshop series.* Washington, DC, The National Academies Press, 2010.
28. Hick JL, O'Laughlin DT. Concept of Operations for Triage of Mechanical Ventilation in an Epidemic. *Acad Emerg Med* 2006; 13: 223–229.
29. Christian MD, Hawryluck L, Wax RS, et al. Development of a triage protocol for critical care during an influenza pandemic *CMAJ* November 21, 2006; 175(11): 1377–1381.

30. Rubinson L, Nuzzo J, Talmor D, et.al. Augmentation of hospital critical care capacity after bioterrorist attacks or epidemics: Recommendations of the Working Group on Emergency Mass Critical Care. *Crit Care Med* October 2005; 33(10): 2393–2403.

31. Rubinson L, Hick JL, Hanfling D, et. al., Definitive care for the critically ill during a disaster: A framework for optimizing critical care surge capacity. *Chest* 2008; 133; 18–31.

32. Kissoon N, et. al, Deliberations and recommendations of the Pediatric Emergency Mass Critical Care Task Force: executive summary. *Pediatr Crit Care Med* November 2011; 12(6 Suppl.): S103–S108.

33. Registration and coordination of Foreign Medical Teams responding to sudden onset disasters, the way forward. Foreign Medical Team Working Group, WHO, May 5, 2013. http://www.who.int/hac/global_health_cluster/fmt_way_forward_5may13.pdf (Accessed November 12, 2014).

34. von Schreeb J, Riddez L, Samnegård H, Rosling H. Foreign field hospitals in the recent sudden-onset disasters in Iran, Haiti, Indonesia, and Pakistan. *Prehosp Disaster Med* March–April 2008; 23(2): 144–151, discussions 152–153.

35. *Guidelines for Use of Foreign Field Hospitals in the Aftermath of Sudden-Impact Disasters.* WHO-PAHO, 2003. http://www.who.int/hac/techguidance/pht/FieldHospitalsFolleto.pdf (Accessed November 12, 2014).

36. FMT Concept Paper. WHO. http://www.who.int/hac/global_health_cluster/about/ghc_annex9_field_medical_team_concept_note_18march2011.pdf (Accessed November 12, 2014).

37. de Ville de Goyet C, Sarmiento JP, Grunewald F. *Health response to the earthquake in Haiti January 2010: lessons to be learned for the next massive sudden-onset disaster.* PAHO, Washington, DC, 2011.

38. National Guidance for Healthcare System Preparedness. DHHS, Office of the Assistant Secretary for Preparedness and Response, Hospital Preparedness Program, January 2012. http://www.phe.gov/preparedness/planning/hpp/reports/documents/capabilities.pdf (Accessed November 12, 2014).

39. Bayram JD, et al. Critical Resources for Hospital Surge Capacity: An Expert Consensus Panel. Version 2. *PLoS Curr* October 7, 2013 [revised]; 5. http://www.ncbi.nlm.nih.gov/pmc/articles/PMC3805833 (Accessed November 12, 2014).

40. Schreiber M. Overview. The PsySTART Rapid Mental Health Triage and Incident Management System. http://www.cdms.uci.edu/pdf/psystart-cdms02142012.pdf (Accessed November 12, 2014).

41. Bayram JD, Zuabi S, Subbarao I. Disaster Metrics: Quantitative Benchmarking of Hospital Surge Capacity in Trauma-Related Multiple Casualty Events. *Disaster Med Public Health Prep* 2011; 5: 117–124.

42. The Problem with Serious Games: Solved. MIT Technology Review, Emerging Technology From the arXiv, February 24, 2014. http://www.technologyreview.com/view/525061/the-problem-with-serious-games-solved (Accessed May 20, 2014).

43. Kelen GD, Kraus CK, McCarthy ML, et al. Inpatient Disposition Classification for the Creation of Hospital Surge Capacity: A Multiphase Study. *Lancet* 2006; 368: 1984–1990.

44. Llewellyn CH, The role of telemedicine in disaster medicine. *J Med Syst* February 1995; 19(1): 29–34.

45. Nicogossian AE, Doarn CR. Armenia 1988 earthquake and telemedicine: lessons learned and forgotten. *Telemedicine and e-Health* 2011; 17(9): 741–745.

46. Freudenheim M. In Haiti, Practicing Medicine from Afar. *New York Times.* February 8, 2010. http://www.nytimes.com/2010/02/09/health/09tele.html?_r=0 (Accessed November 12, 2014).

47. Kellermann AL, Isakov AP, Parker R, et al. Web-based selftriage of influenza-like illness during the 2009 H1N1 influenza pandemic. *Ann Emerg Med* 2010; 56(3): 288–294, e6.

48. Price RA, Fagyubi D, Harris R, et al. Feasability of Web Based Self-Triage by Parents of Children with Influenza-Like Illness. *JAMA Pediatrics* 2012; 166(12): 1–7.

49. Koonin L, Hanfling D. Broadening access to medical care during a severe influenza pandemic: the CDC nurse triage line project. *Biosecur Bioterror* March 2013; 11(1): 75–80.

50. *Standards and Guidelines for Healthcare Surge During Emergencies.* California Department of Public Health, May 2005. http://www.beprepparedcalifornia.ca.gov/CDPHPrograms/PublicHealthPrograms/EmergencyPreparednessOffice/EPO ProgramsandServices/Surge/SurgeStandardsandGuidelines/Documents/FoundationalKnowledge_FINAL.pdf (Accessed November 12, 2014).

4

CLIMATE CHANGE

Richard A. Matthew and Jamie L. Agius

OVERVIEW

The scientific basis for climate change has strengthened considerably since 1896, when the Swedish physicist and chemist Svante Arrhenius first hypothesized that emissions of carbon dioxide could accumulate in the atmosphere to create a greenhouse gas effect resulting in global warming.[1] In the past two decades, the Intergovernmental Panel on Climate Change (IPCC), a planetary network of climate scientists established by the United Nations, has released four assessment reports as well as more than a dozen special publications and methodology reports. The principal conclusion of IPCC is that human activities, and especially those involved in generating carbon emissions and reducing carbon storage, are almost certainly forcing global climate change.[2,3]

This growing body of research links changes in the composition of the earth's atmosphere (that is, a net increase in CO2 and other greenhouse gases) to the retention of solar energy on the surface of the planet, in the atmospheric boundary layer which touches the surface, and in the troposphere which extends to about 2.6 km (1.6 miles) above the surface. Such a high level of trapped solar energy has not been experienced for at least several thousand years. This, researchers contend, warms the planet's surface, disrupting its hydrological cycle and weather patterns. As a result of this warming, different regions of the world, depending on elevation, latitude, and related factors, may be experiencing more severe drought, severe flooding, and severe storms than in the past several millennia. Climate change science assesses the impacts of the alteration in atmospheric composition by investigating variations in the statistical characteristics of weather aggregated over time and space.

Scientists are well aware that climate change has been a regular feature of planet earth since it took shape from space debris some 4.5 billion years ago. In fact, in geological time, much larger climate transformations took place in the pre-Anthropocene era (earth history before the age of transformative human impact on the planet). Today's transformations may appear rather small compared to some of the climate change periods that occurred in the past, such as the oxidation of the atmosphere. However, they are unique in that they are being forced by human activ-

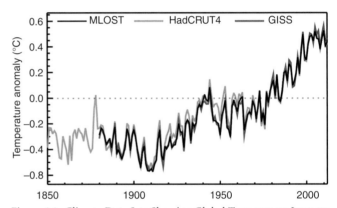

Figure 4.1. Climate Data Sets Showing Global Temperature Increase since 1850 (MLOST is the Merged Land-Ocean Surface Temperature Analysis produced by the National Climatic Center of the National Oceanic and Atmospheric Administration; HadCRUT4 is produced by the Hadley Centre of the UK Met Office and the Climatic Research Unit of the University of East Anglia; and GISS is produced by the Goddard Institute of Space Studies at the National Aeronautics and Space Administration). Adapted from: IPCC Fifth Assessment Report (AR5), 2013. https://www.ipcc.ch.

ities such as: 1) the consumption of cheap and plentiful fossil fuels; and 2) the conversion of forest into farmland, firewood, and framing for construction. These routine activities increase the concentration of carbon dioxide and other greenhouse gases in the atmosphere and reduce carbon storage on the earth's surface. The measurable outcome from this activity is that the earth's average surface temperature has increased by 1 degree centigrade since the mid-nineteenth century (see Figure 4.1).[4]

This measurable outcome is grounded in considerable research and has enabled a high level of scientific agreement.[5] This research began with information from ice cores, tree rings, and weather data that have been collected since the 1600s. The International Meteorological Organization, founded in 1873, developed protocols and standards for collecting weather data which made possible longitudinal analysis. Approximately 50 years later, scientists such as G. S. Callendar began to collect

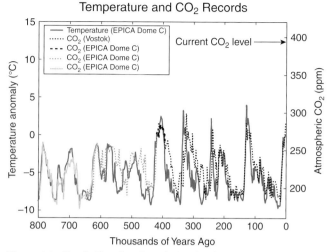

Figure 4.2. Graph Showing the Relationship between CO_2 Levels and Global Temperature over the Past 400,000 Years (EPICA is the European Partnership for Ice Coring in Antarctica; Dome C is the site of the Concordia Research Station, which is jointly run by France and Italy. Vostok data are collected by Russia at its Vostok Station in Antarctica).[6]

time series data on temperature. In addition, "The high-accuracy measurements of atmospheric CO_2 concentration, initiated by Charles David Keeling in 1958, constitute the master time series documenting the changing composition of the atmosphere."[6] These changes are depicted in Figure 4.2.

The universal narrative that has emerged today from this research is familiar to everyone worldwide. Contemporary global warming is being driven by human behavior. No matter what our response, this process will continue for decades and perhaps centuries because changes in the composition of the atmosphere and land cover have triggered transformative processes that have not yet played themselves out and established new equilibria. However, action today could have an important mitigating effect. The best models suggest that the distinguishing impact of climate change is an accentuation of familiar phenomena such as drought, flooding and extreme weather. Arid areas will tend to receive less precipitation, whereas coastal areas and flood plains will tend to receive more, and storms will tend to worsen. How intense and how frequent these amplifications are may depend on how much more greenhouse gas we continue to add to the atmosphere.

Social and ecological systems are currently being affected in multiple ways, and this impact will continue into the future. However, these patterns will not be uniform across the planet and will display considerable variability by region. Some changes will not be foreseen at all. This is partly because climate change is affected by phenomena that have proven impossible to model, at least so far. Examples include changes in cloud cover and unpredictable feedback responses from both natural and human systems. This unpredictability is in part because complex adaptive systems, such as forests, display non-linear behavior and generate new properties. In short, while much is known about anthropogenic climate change, and broad patterns of future climate change are being predicted, there remain important areas of uncertainty.

Based on these current research findings, it is widely assumed that disasters will increase in the decades ahead. IPCC concludes

that climate change "leads to changes in the frequency, intensity, spatial extent, duration, and timing of extreme weather and climate events, and can result in unprecedented extreme weather and climate events."[7] In addition, a 2012 report by the Joint United Nations Environment Programme/Office for the Coordination of Humanitarian Affairs (UNEP/OCHA) Environment Unit states that

> The lack of precise data about future emissions levels and climate change impacts translates into a growing degree of uncertainty concerning the frequency and intensity of extreme weather events, as historical trends and risks no longer apply. As such, communities living in areas exposed to storm surges, flooding, and landslides face greater exposure to climate risks, even while it is unclear just how much greater those risks will be.[8]

In short, disasters are expected to increase dramatically but what, where, and when are uncertain.

The broad contours of future disasters related to climate change can be summarized in terms of:

▪ an expected increase in the frequency and intensity of extreme events such as fires, cyclones and floods; and
▪ an expected increase in the intensity and duration of longer term events such as heat waves and droughts.

These will be experienced by human populations that, in many cases, are likely to be more vulnerable to such future weather events than they have been in the past. This vulnerability results from the likelihood of:

▪ demographic changes including an increase in the number of elderly and in the number of urban dwellers;
▪ the displacement of large numbers of people into high risk areas such as flood plains due mainly to poverty;
▪ public health setbacks in many regions due to water scarcity, food scarcity, and the spread of pathogens, which are themselves challenges intensified by climate change;
▪ the degradation of infrastructure, such as waste management and drainage systems, in many regions of the world;
▪ the erosion of ecosystems such as forests that provide a natural buffer against many forms of natural disaster;
▪ difficult local conditions under which aid is delivered, especially when the provision of emergency assistance occurs in places where access, sanitation, mobility, and resource allocation are problematic; and
▪ heightened competition for scarce emergency assistance resources.

Patterns of vulnerability are expected to reflect demographic and socioeconomic indicators, with risk closely associated to age, gender, and income. But the actual rate and scale of disasters related to climate change also will likely be affected by:

▪ whether climate change leads to unforeseen feedbacks and new equilibria that change its current trajectory; and
▪ whether human ingenuity leads to better levels and forms of communication, preparedness, and resilience.

In other words, the evidence in support of global climate change is compelling and the processes through which this is occurring are well-understood. From a contemporary data-based perspective, it is reasonable to predict an increase in weather-related disasters such as floods, storms, tornados, droughts, fires, and heat waves. This increase will tend to amplify familiar conditions – that is, areas prone to floods, droughts, or heat waves are likely to experience more of the same. Much analysis suggests that the vulnerability of people throughout the world is increasing because of demographic changes, public health setbacks, and the erosion of infrastructure and natural ecosystems that have the capacity to buffer against disaster. At the same time, climate is a complex system that can transform and stabilize in unexpected ways, and humans are a resourceful species that can adapt to new environments. Hence, the passage of time could find the world's population better or worse off than current global climate models predict.

The IPCC argues that

Projected changes in climate extremes under different emissions scenarios generally do not strongly diverge in the coming two to three decades, but these signals are relatively small compared to natural climate variability over this time frame. Even the sign of projected changes in some climate extremes over this time frame is uncertain. For projected changes by the end of the 21st century, either model uncertainty or uncertainties associated with emissions scenarios used becomes dominant, depending on the extreme. Low-probability, high-impact changes associated with the crossing of poorly understood climate thresholds cannot be excluded, given the transient and complex nature of the climate system. Assigning "low confidence" for projections of a specific extreme neither implies nor excludes the possibility of changes in this extreme. The following assessments of the likelihood and/or confidence of projections are generally for the end of the 21st century and relative to the climate at the end of the 20th century.[9]

The final conclusion is that the more extreme weather expected over the next three decades will still likely fall within the stable natural variability parameters of the past several millennia. After that, the parameters themselves could change but there is less confidence in predicting this.

Given the previous information, it is easy to understand why efforts to link climate change and disaster tend to aggregate into one of two quite different scenarios. The first scenario has received most of the attention in scientific communities, political arenas, and popular media, Here, the negative impacts of climate change increase steeply throughout the next several decades, damaging natural and social systems and displacing, killing, and injuring hundreds of millions and possibly billions of people. Severe weather events like Hurricanes Katrina and Sandy ravage coastal communities around the world. Heat waves devastate cities like London, Los Angeles, and Shanghai – perhaps as often as thirty or forty times a year. Stagnant air traps ozone and particulates in urban space and respiratory ailments like asthma increase sharply. The warming of the planet allows tropical insects to migrate into upper and lower latitudes, leading to malaria and other epidemics in places where people have no experience with them. Droughts transform much of sub-Saharan Africa and large areas of the United States and China into dust bowls. Much of the world faces chronic food and water insecurity. Wildfires burn out of control around the world and some places

experience a new disaster – the fire tornado. Meanwhile, the melting of the Greenland ice sheet and the sudden release of vast quantities of methane gas trapped in permafrost lead to a reversal of the ocean conveyer. This results in the loss of ocean flow that today warms much of the United Kingdom and Europe and disruption of the monsoon upon which the livelihoods of billions of people in Asia depend. Much of humankind must confront a struggle to survive against a turbulent, erratic, and inhospitable climate. In fact, by as soon as 2025 a state shift could occur – a situation in which the global climate experiences a sudden and dramatic shift to a new regime, and extremely inhospitable weather (the extremes of the past millennia) becomes the new global norm. Efforts to survive often become violent, and as a result, disasters and wars tend to occur together.[10–19]

Given the areas of uncertainty noted previously, however, a second scenario has also been developed in which the social effects of climate change are imagined to be rather small. Milder impacts would result because phenomena arise that have not been captured in global climate models. Increases in cloud cover could blunt global warming and establish new equilibria that maintain a fairly stable and congenial global climate regime. Moreover, climate change could prove to have benefits for large parts of the world such as longer growing seasons and easy access to natural resources previously hidden by ice. Humans would play a major role in this scenario, because wherever climate change effects create significant damage, human ingenuity might discover effective coping and adaptation responses.[20]

While these two scenarios both have thoughtful and well-informed advocates, the first is clearly dominant.[21] Ironically, this has not translated into the aggressive mitigation and adaptation responses that such a scenario would seem to authorize. As such, the world has gravitated toward accepting the worst-case scenario in words but not in actions.[22] Hence, a future of unprecedented disasters affecting much of the world's population is fully plausible.

CURRENT STATE OF THE ART

While many studies exist on the real and potential social impacts of climate change, the issue that receives the greatest attention from the disaster perspective is hydrological intensification, and especially flooding. This is because flooding causes approximately 50% of all of the damage from natural disasters. Floods have directly affected almost half of the world's population in the past four decades, and there is a clear trend toward more flooding. A considerable amount of infrastructure is situated in flood plains, and major reinsurance companies like Swiss Re and Munich Re have suggested that much of this will soon be uninsurable by the private sector.

A recent overview of flood activity from 1980 to 2009 reports that an average of 131 floods occur each year. Eighty-one percent of all floods identified in the study occurred in the last two-thirds of the survey time period. During this period, flooding caused about 540,000 deaths and affected over 2.8 billion people. No other natural disaster comes close to this level of devastation on an annual basis.[23]

However, trends in the broader set of disasters that could be associated with climate change are also alarming. According to a 2012 UNEP/OCHA report that examines the interaction between climate change and urbanization, "The period between 2002 and 2011 included over 4000 disasters linked to natural hazards, resulting in over one million deaths and greater than $1 billion in losses."[24] In 2010, the International Federation of the Red Cross and Red Crescent (IFRC) reported that 7,184 disasters took place in the first decade of the new millennium causing 1,105,352 deaths, affecting over 2.5 billion people, and costing some $986,691,000,000 USD. A total of 4,014 of these were natural disasters, and in turn 91% of these were climate-related disasters.[25] This larger set of climate-related disasters includes:

■ cyclones
■ drought
■ flooding
■ heat waves
■ hurricanes
■ pandemic disease outbreaks
■ tornado fires
■ tornados
■ wildfires

From the perspective of IPCC, UNEP, OCHA, and many other organizations, humankind is likely to experience more devastating disasters in the next few decades than it has in the past several millennia. This is due to two interrelated phenomenon: climate change is pushing weather toward and even beyond historical extremes and, at the same time, human exposure and vulnerability are increasing due to multiple factors, including climate change itself.

The widespread perception that the world's inhabitants are becoming more vulnerable is based partly on the increasing occurrence rates for many forms of natural disasters as well as on the net impact assessments of several global trends. In particular, world population is growing at the rate of about 90 million people per year. Even though fertility rates in the vast majority of countries are at or below replacement levels, this growth is not expected to reach a plateau until at least mid-century due to the large proportion of women who are fertile.

This growth is largely taking place in the urban areas of the developing world. These urban areas are often situated along coastlines and in flood plains, and typically do not have infrastructure, such as drainage systems, that is likely to be effective under most climate change scenarios. In other words, large numbers of people are living in areas vulnerable to natural hazards. In addition, both the number of people and the number of hazards are increasing even as the infrastructure is aging and often of low quality. Developed countries generally are not experiencing population growth, but their citizens are undergoing an unprecedented aging. Soon, these nations will have substantial populations at heightened risk for extreme weather events such as heat waves. It is an alarming prospect that more people in developing countries, and more elderly people in developed countries, are all living in brittle cities that are potentially exposed to the most severe weather events in human history.

Other global trends may add layers of complication to this situation. For example, recent analyses of Gravity Recovery and Climate Experiment (GRACE) satellite data, which record fluctuations in gravitational force on the surface of the earth, show that large groundwater systems worldwide are shrinking. This is mainly due to unsustainable pumping for irrigation. Of particular concern is the groundwater depletion being experienced by both the Indian subcontinent and the Tibetan Plateau, home to some 2 billion people. Climate change could accelerate the decline of some ground water reserves through contamination

from saltwater intrusion due to sea level rise and reduction of replenishing surface waters. However, the major threat is that certain forms of hydrological intensification induced by climate change, such as extreme drought, will be an even greater burden in areas where the alternate source of water is diminishing. In the case of Asia, such changes are taking place in the region that already is the most vulnerable to natural disasters on the planet. Maplecroft's Natural Disaster Risk Ranking, for example, identifies South Asia as the highest risk region of the world, including Bangladesh (ranked 1), Pakistan (ranked 4), and India (ranked 11).

The expansion of the built environment could add another source of stress to this volatile situation. For example, many of Asia's major rivers such as the Brahmaputra, Ganges, Indus, Irrawaddy, Mekong, Salween, Yangzi, and Yellow Rivers originate in Tibet. They have enormous hydroelectric power potential, and there are plans in China and India to build hundreds of new dams to harness this power and to store water for emergencies. However, little is known about the resilience of contemporary dam designs under conditions of extreme weather. They might fail. In addition, serious concerns exist that such plans will also weaken the resilience of downstream countries by amplifying water insecurity. The dams will also reduce the flow of silt, which aggregates into barriers that provide natural protection against flooding in countries such as Bangladesh.

The list of global trends that could increase vulnerability to the impact of climate change could be expanded for pages. For example, the 2007 recession underscored the potential magnitude of any economic crisis today. Such events are an almost inevitable outcome of a globalized economy in which there are powerful incentives to diffuse and shift risk. Economic crisis reduces the surge capacity of a country, curtails investment into resilience, and makes emergency response more difficult. Similarly, medical researchers are concerned that the misuse of large quantities of powerful drugs has created conditions amenable to a growing array of multiple drug resistant (MDR) and extremely drug resistant (XDR) pathogens that could seriously weaken public health around the world. The main point is that there are many reasons for concern that vulnerability to climate-related disasters is growing, and will continue to grow for decades.

The combination of more extreme weather events, a growing population of people vulnerable to these events, fragile infrastructure, weak governments, public health setbacks, and economic crises aligns nicely with the scenario described previously that focuses on the likelihood of escalating catastrophe. What, then, can disaster response mean in a world in which the lives, livelihoods, and property of tens and perhaps hundreds of millions of people are put at considerable and escalating risk each year? The answer to this question depends on three types of social investment.

The first area of investment involves mitigation and associated technologies, institutions, and practices. In the disaster literature, mitigation refers to "the effort to reduce loss of life and property by lessening the impact of disasters. Mitigation is taking action *now* – before the next disaster – to reduce human and financial consequences later (analyzing risk, reducing risk, insuring against risk)."[26] In the realm of climate change, mitigation

refers to efforts to reduce or prevent emission of greenhouse gases. Mitigation can mean using new technologies and renewable energies, making older equipment more energy efficient, or changing management practices or consumer behavior. It can be as complex as a plan for a new city, or as a simple as improvements to a cook stove design. Efforts underway around the world range from high-tech subway systems to bicycling paths and walkways. Protecting natural carbon sinks like forests and oceans, or creating new sinks through silviculture (forest management) or green agriculture are also elements of mitigation.[27]

IPCC describes the second area of investment as adaptation. It is widely believed that mitigation efforts have had limited impact to date. Human-generated climate change has taken place and will continue to unfold for decades and possibly centuries. Therefore, humans and many other species will need to adapt to new, extreme weather patterns and to the intensification of the planet's hydrological system. IPCC defines adaptation as follows: "In human systems, [adaptation is] the process of adjustment to actual or expected climate and its effects, in order to moderate harm or exploit beneficial opportunities. In natural systems, [adaptation is] the process of adjustment to actual climate and its effects; human intervention may facilitate adjustment to expected climate."[28]

Insofar as disasters are concerned, adaptation tends to cluster around three areas:

1) Preparedness: improving early warning systems and community resilience through measures such as training programs, stockpiling emergency supplies, and encouraging self-reliance at the household level.
2) Response: ensuring response capacity remains consistent with the likely magnitude of disasters.
3) Recovery: Rebuilding after an event in ways that maximize adaptive capacity and resilience.

In 2013, IPCC introduced the concern that mitigation and adaptation might be insufficient to manage the impact of climate change. The panel proposed a third area of investment, the implementation of geoengineering. This concept is described as "the deliberate large-scale intervention in the Earth's natural systems to counteract climate change."[29] Geoengineering can be organized into two broad areas. The first, solar geoengineering, focuses on how to: 1) reflect significant amounts of solar energy back into space; or 2) prevent it from reaching the earth's surface. An example of the former would be albedo-enhancing technologies (interventions that increase reflection of solar energy from Earth back into space) such as painting large areas of the land surface white. An example of the latter would be dispersing reflective materials in space to deflect energy away from the earth.

The second form of geoengineering, carbon geoengineering, focuses on affecting the growth of the planet's carbon economy by removing large amounts of carbon from the atmosphere. This might be achieved simply by covering large areas of land with new forest, or through accelerating natural processes such as the rate at which biological activity in the oceans uses atmospheric carbon dioxide. Other strategies include developing technologies that could clean carbon dioxide from the air or capture it before it is released into the atmosphere.

Few observers contend that social investments into mitigation, adaptation, and geoengineering have been adequate to date. In fact, current available evidence suggests that these efforts remain insufficient. For example, in 1997, the developed countries of the world negotiated the Kyoto Protocol, which had the modest objective of reducing key greenhouse gas emissions by 5% below 1990 levels. When the protocol expired in 2012, this goal had not been met; to the contrary, emissions had increased by 58% during this period.[30] A publication called *Germanwatch* reports annually on what countries are doing in response to climate change. It wrote in its 2012 report: "As in the years before, we still cannot reward any country with the rankings 1–3, as no country is doing enough to prevent dangerous climate change."[31] Capturing the sense that too little is being accomplished, journalist Fred Pearce has written that climate change "scares me, just as it scares many of the scientists I have talked to – sober scientists, with careers and reputations to defend, but also with hopes for their own futures and those of their children, and fears that we are the last generation to live with any kind of climatic stability."[32]

An apparent gap exists between the future credible scenarios that climate scientists have developed and the human response to these scenarios that occurred over the past two decades. This gap may be explained by construal level theory, which developed in the field of social and behavioral psychology. This theory links information to human behavior through the lenses of proximity and certainty. The core insight is that as distance and uncertainty decrease, the impact of information on behavior increases. The converse is also true. Therefore, people are less likely to act in response to the narrative of climate science as it suggests problems that seem far away spatially and temporally, appear to have a low probability of occurrence in the near term, and may be more likely experienced through a third party.[33] Discussions of climate change are so fraught with conditionality that they simply may be too abstract and vague to catalyze much action. In other words, the delivery of climate science information to citizens may be ineffective, making it easier for individuals to focus on other, more concrete and pressing priorities that do require immediate attention and resources.

RECOMMENDATIONS FOR FURTHER RESEARCH

From a global perspective, human activity creating climate change is continuing more or less unchecked. Carbon is being added to the atmosphere and carbon storage is being reduced on the surface of the planet. No one knows exactly how this will affect weather over the next few decades. However, the dominant concern is that weather considered to be extreme during the past several millennia is becoming the normal weather pattern for the years ahead. This new normal weather is likely to impose extremely high costs on societies around the world as well as introduce enormous instability. The sort of severe flooding and drought that a society might have previously experienced once a century or even less frequently, could in the future be experienced by a single generation many times. Additionally, such future weather extremes could be of an intensity that the human species has not experienced for thousands of years.

Given the scale of this challenge, important research is emerging around geoengineering solutions – from technologies that might deflect solar radiation back into space away from the atmosphere, to new ways of capturing and storing carbon. Another promising line of research, referred to as biomimicry, focuses on finding solutions to challenges such as storing carbon, managing heat waves, or cultivating food under arid conditions by observing nature and identifying the efficient responses to these problems generated through millennia of evolution. Sophisticated systems models are maturing that seek to capture the complexity of climate change, and better understand how feedback generates new equilibria, or what triggers systems collapse or change.

The drama of climate change is poised to unfold just as billions of people are moving into urban areas, doubling the size of urban space in a matter of decades. This expanding population will be dependent on aging and ineffective infrastructure. This, too, is unprecedented. Yet, the image of highly vulnerable populations impacted by a cascade of extreme floods, storms, droughts, and heat waves currently seems too distant and uncertain to warrant action. Politicians, policymakers, business leaders, and the general public seem unwilling to make the level of investment that climate science experts believe is needed to mitigate climate change and adapt to its inescapable effects. In short, there is a reasonable chance that the world is headed toward a period of truly unprecedented environmental disaster. Climate change could ultimately have the same consequences as a large asteroid hitting the planet.

Of course, there has been some behavioral response to climate science. Indeed, across the planet, many communities and countries are developing and implementing climate action plans; however, this vibrant and important activity is not yet having a discernible impact on global climate trends. Moreover, it is not clear that these investments are being made in the right places, or that they will aggregate into an adequate global response. The promise of the ingenuity, experimentation, and policy innovation that are evident around the world in mainly very local contexts has yet to be assessed. It would be of great value to develop a framework for cataloguing and assessing this activity, and for measuring the significance of the myriad measurable responses to physical and informational stimuli that now exist.

Another important step concerns communication. What is the most effective way to communicate climate science? In this regard, two interesting research agendas have emerged in recent years. One focuses on how climate change is framed. For example, would linking it to health raise awareness and catalyze action? Would people respond to an evidence-based narrative depicting how often significant medical conditions such as severe respiratory distress experienced by an asthmatic child, a skin disorder seen in a 30-year-old, or a senior citizen having a myocardial infarction are caused by climate change? Would it be useful to present climate change as an obstacle to poverty alleviation, as a cause of war, or as a platform for famine? Investigators should examine what works insofar as behavioral response is concerned, and what does not. In other words, which frames of reference inspire people to act, and which ones leave people feeling overwhelmed or helpless?

A related strand of research is exploring techniques for downsizing climate science so that people can understand how it is likely to impact their communities. The goal of this research is to communicate at a local level the damage scientists believe climate change-related flooding is likely to impose on individual neighborhoods in Los Angeles, Beijing, or Paris. There is, of course, a risk that some communities will learn that climate change impacts are expected to be mild or even positive for their region, thereby potentially reducing their willingness to support aggressive response strategies.

Another important consideration for future research would be improving analysis of the social effects of climate change by including things like human ingenuity in scenario building. Without this, the linear move from extreme weather event to human tragedy is not very compelling after the first few instances.

However, the most important next step is perhaps to imagine with greater sophistication what it would be like to experience a world of unprecedented disasters. This would motivate identification of measures that will be critical to addressing the associated consequences. Implementation of such measures would prevent climate-related changes that are morally unacceptable, economically devastating, and seriously threaten population health. Emphasis could be placed on problems that could be prevented at low cost.

It is possible future research will ultimately conclude that the worst-case scenarios of climate science will not materialize. In this eventuality, many nations will have invested significantly into mitigation, adaptation, and geoengineering on a false premise. The resources invested in preventing or mitigating climate change will be lost, in much the same way as the individual who purchases homeowner's insurance but never makes a claim has lost opportunities to invest the insurance premiums in other endeavors. On the other hand, if we fail to make these investments and the worst-case scenarios do unfold, populations will suffer egregiously and unnecessarily, like the individual whose uninsured home is completely destroyed by fire. The prudent course of action under these uncertain circumstances would be to continue investing in forms of preparedness, mitigation, and resilience while simultaneously pursuing research efforts to improve our understanding of this challenge.

REFERENCES

1. Weart S. *The Discovery of Global Warming*, Revised and Expanded Edition, Cambridge, MA, Harvard University Press, 2008.

2. Intergovernmental Panel on Climate Change (IPCC). *Climate Change 2013: The Physical Science Basis*. 2013. http://www.ipcc.ch/report/ar5/wg1/#.UksGlxbWTFI (Accessed October 1, 2013).

3. Solomon S. et al., eds. *The Physical Science Basis: Contribution of Working Group I to the Fourth Assessment Report of the Intergovernmental Panel on Climate Change.* Cambridge, Cambridge University Press, 2007.

4. Intergovernmental Panel on Climate Change (IPCC). *Climate Change 2013: The Physical Science Basis*. 2013. http://www.ipcc.ch/report/ar5/wg1/#.UksGlxbWTFI (Accessed October 1, 2013)

5. Weart S. *The Discovery of Global Warming*, Revised and Expanded Edition, Cambridge, MA, Harvard University Press, 2008.

6. Le Treut H., Somerville R, Cubasch U, et al. Historical overview of climate change. In: Solomon S, Qin D, Manning M, et al., eds. *Climate Change 2007: The Physical Science Basis. Contribution of Working Group I to the Fourth Assessment Report of the Intergovernmental Panel on Climate Change*, Cambridge, Cambridge University Press, 2007; 98.

7. Intergovernmental Panel on Climate Change (IPCC). *Climate Change 2013: The Physical Science Basis*. 2013. http://www.ipcc.ch/report/ar5/wg1/#.UksGlxbWTFI (Accessed October 1, 2013)

8. Joint UNEP/OCHA Environment Unit. Keeping up with Megatrends: The Implications of Climate Change and Urbanization for Environmental Emergency Preparedness and Response. Joint UNEP/OCHA Environment Unit, Switzerland, 2012; 6. https://docs.unocha.org/sites/dms/Documents/Keeping%20up%20with%20Megatrends.pdf (Accessed September 1, 2013).

9. Intergovernmental Panel on Climate Change (IPCC). Summary for Policymakers. In: Field CB et al., eds. *Managing the Risks of Extreme Events and Disasters to Advance Climate Change Adaptation. A Special Report of Working Groups I and II of the Intergovernmental Panel on Climate Change.* Cambridge, Cambridge University Press, 2012; 11–12.

10. National Security and the Threat of Climate Change. CNA, 2007. http://securityandclimate.cna.org (Accessed March 6, 2013).

11. German Advisory Council on Global Change. *World in Transition: Climate Change as a Security Risk.* London, Earthscan, 2008.

12. Gleick PH, Climate change, exponential curves, water resources, and unprecedented threats to humanity. *Climatic Change* 2012; 100: 125–129.

13. Gleick PH, Heberger M. The coming mega drought. *Scientific American* 2012; 306: 1–14.

14. McElroy M, Baker DJ. Climate extremes: recent trends with implications for national security. 2012. http://environment.harvard.edu/sites/default/files/climate_extremes_report_2012-12-04.pdf (Accessed February 15, 2013).

15. National Research Council. *Himalayan Glaciers: Climate Change, Water Resources, and Water Security.* Washington, DC, The National Academies Press, 2012.

16. Pearce F. *With Speed and Violence: Why Scientists Fear Tipping Points in Climate Change.* Boston, Beacon Press, 2007.

17. Stern N. *The Economics of Climate Change.* Cambridge, Cambridge University Press, 2007.

18. Welzer H. *Climate Wars: Why People Will Be Killed in the 21st Century.* Cambridge, Polity Press, 2012.

19. Pearce F. *With Speed and Violence: Why Scientists Fear Tipping Points in Climate Change.* Boston, Beacon Press, 2007.

20. Lomborg B. *The Skeptical Environmentalist: Measuring the Real State of the World.* Cambridge, Cambridge University Press, 2001.

21. Hulme M. *Why We Disagree about Climate Change: Understanding, Controversy, Inaction and Opportunity.* Cambridge, Cambridge University Press, 2009.

22. The Climate Change Performance Index: Results 2012. Germanwatch, 2011. http://germanwatch.org/klima/ccpi.pdf (Accessed April 30, 2012).

23. Doocy S, Daniels A, Murray S, Kirsch T. The Human Impact of Floods: A Historical; Review of Events 1980–2009 and Systematic Literature Review. *PLOS Currents Disasters* April 16, 2013; 1.

24. United Nations Environment Programme (UNEP)/Office for the Coordination of Humanitarian Affairs (OCHA). *Keeping Up With Megatrends: The Implications of Climate Change and Urbanization for Environmental Emergency Preparedness and Response.* Geneva, Joint UNEP/OCHA Environment Unit, 2012; 3.

25. World Disasters Report 2010: Focus on Urban Risk. International Federation of the Red Cross and Red Crescent (IFRC), 2010. http://www.ifrc.org/Global/Publications/disasters/WDR/wdr2010/WDR2010-full.pdf (Accessed on October 1, 2013).

26. FEMA Website. http://www.fema.gov/what-mitigation (Accessed October 1, 2013).

27. UNEP Website. http://www.unep.org/climatechange/mitigation (Accessed October 1, 2013).

28. Intergovernmental Panel on Climate Change (IPCC). Summary for Policymakers. In: Field CB et al., eds. *Managing the Risks of Extreme Events and Disasters to Advance Climate Change Adaptation. A Special Report of Working Groups I and II of the Intergovernmental Panel on Climate Change.* Cambridge, Cambridge University Press, 2012; 9.

29. Oxford University Website. http://www.geoengineering.ox.ac.uk/what-is-geoengineering/what-is-geoengineering/? (Accessed October 1, 2013).

30. Paris M. CBC News: Kyoto Climate Treaty Sputters to a Sorry End, December 31, 2012. http://www.cbc.ca/news/politics/story/2012/12/20/pol-kyoto-protocol-part-one-ends.html (Accessed September 1, 2013).

31. The Climate Change Performance Index: Results 2012. Germanwatch, 2011; 4. http://germanwatch.org/klima/ccpi.pdf (Accessed September 30, 2013).

32. Pearce F. *With Speed and Violence: Why Scientists Fear Tipping Points in Climate Change.* Boston, Beacon Press, 2007; xxx.

33. Eyal T, Liberman L, Trope Y. Judging near and distant virtue and vice. *Journal of Experimental Social Psychology* 2008; 44: 1204–1209; Fujita K, Henderson M, Eng, J, et al., Spatial distance and mental construal of social events. Psychological Science 2005; 17: 278–282; Liberman N, Sagristano M, Trope Y. The effect of temporal distance on level of construal. Journal of Experimental Psychology 2002; 38: 523–535; Todorov A, Goren A, Trope Y. Probability as a psychological distance: construal and preferences. Journal of Experimental Social Psychology 2007; 43: 473–482.

5

INTERNATIONAL PERSPECTIVES ON DISASTER MANAGEMENT

Jean Luc Poncelet

OVERVIEW

For many years, disasters were perceived as unavoidable and only attributable to "natural" events. Over the last forty years, however, professionals in the health field have begun studying the subject, realizing that there is potential to avoid the many negative consequences linked to such hazards. Public health, sociology, and emergency medicine specialists were among the first groups to investigate these issues scientifically, examining ways to protect lives from the impact of disasters.

Pioneers in this new area of research included Professor Michel Lechat from the University of Louvain in Belgium, Professor Peter Safar from the University of Pittsburgh in the United States, and Professor Rudolph Frey from the University of Mainz in Germany. Professor Lechat established the Center for Research on the Epidemiology of Disasters in 1973, which hosts the only comprehensive worldwide hazard database. Professors Safar and Frey founded the Club of Mainz in 1976, which would become the World Association for Disaster and Emergency Medicine. Its focus was improvement in the worldwide delivery of pre-hospital and emergency care during everyday events and mass casualty disasters.[1] More recently, the approval of the International Health Regulations in 2005 by the World Health Assembly empowered public health officers, infectious disease specialists, and epidemiologists to manage evolving epidemics with the potential to reach catastrophic levels such as seen in the 1918 "Spanish flu." The disciplines of public health and emergency medicine have both made substantial contributions to the field and are now intimately linked. Subsequently, a growing number of professionals have systematically investigated disasters from a multidisciplinary and multihazard perspective.

This chapter will provide an international perspective that focuses on the evolution of the approach health specialists have used to reduce the health consequences linked to disasters. It will highlight some of the main aspects of humanitarian disaster response training and disaster risk reduction. The first section explores how disaster management has evolved to its present status, whereas the latter section explores avenues for future growth. Examples of developments in emergency medicine education and research will also be discussed.

STATE OF THE ART

40 Years of Steady Improvement in the Approach to Preparedness

In 1976, a major shift took place in the field of humanitarian disaster response. Several disasters occurred in a relatively short period of time in a same geographical region. The most significant of these were earthquakes impacting Peru in 1970, Nicaragua in 1972, and Guatemala in 1976. These caused significant devastation and loss of life, and the ministers of health in Latin America and the Caribbean subsequently called for changes in the international humanitarian response mechanism. Until that point, disaster response was mostly reactive both at the national and international levels.

Recognizing the shortcomings of an improvised disaster response, these ministers of health requested assistance from the Pan American Health Organization (PAHO) to propose ways to reduce disaster health consequences. PAHO is the regional office for the World Health Organization (WHO) in the Americas. In response, PAHO created a disaster preparedness program that improved the national capacity for responding to catastrophes. The resulting plan, passed as Resolution X at the PAHO 24th Directing Council, called on member states to, "develop plans, and, as necessary, enact legislation, set standards, and take preventive or palliative measures against natural disasters and disseminate these measures throughout the sectors concerned [with] coordinating their action with that taken by the corresponding services of the Pan American Health Organization."[2] Passage of this resolution represented a turning point in disaster response strategy, switching from an ad hoc response to a systematic preparedness approach. What was considered by many as an act of God or nature became viewed as an event with consequences that could be significantly reduced by improving governmental and institutional preparedness.

In the field of public health, disasters are defined as situations in which the local health response capacity is overwhelmed to the point that external (often international) assistance is required. Typically, in these events, the number of injuries and deaths exceeds the level the emergency services can absorb. At the same time, the health system loses capacity because its infrastructure

Table 5.1. Topics Frequently Included in Disaster Health and Medicine Curricula

Acute medical response	Prehospital emergency plans
Long-term medical support	Epidemiology
Surveillance	Hazard vulnerability analysis
Reconstruction of the medical and health system	Refugees
Disaster impact on public health	Sanitation
Transportation and communication	Water supply
Mental health	Nutrition and food supply
Hospital emergency plans	Shelter
Management of donations	Reconstruction of infrastructure
Mass casualty management	Disaster legislation

Table 5.2. Recommendations for International Donations

1. Donations of cash or credit provided to health authorities or international agencies should be used whenever possible.

2. Donations should be aimed at restoring the quality of healthcare to pre-disaster levels.

3. Perishables or short-life donations should only be made on request from, and with prior approval by, the National Health Disaster Coordinator or other Ministry of Health authority.

4. The World Health Organization's list of essential drugs and supplies should be used as a guideline by those wishing to donate.

5. Recipient countries should improve their distribution systems to ensure the best utilization of donated resources.

is seriously affected or completely overwhelmed and healthcare personnel have suffered injuries and deaths or are unable to work.

Hence, disasters are situations in which a system can no longer meet the demands for health and medical services. The science of disaster response integrates all existing resources to increase capacity and address the needs that could not be met using standard operating procedures. The central objective of a disaster program is to prepare entities for coordination of necessary resources to reduce the disaster's negative impact on health. The funding needed for preparedness activities can be relatively small; what is most needed is the political support empowering the disaster management entity to assume the necessary leadership role to conduct the coordination function. It is very difficult for politicians to invest resources in the management of disasters as such events are rare and unlikely to occur during the tenure of any one individual. In addition, efforts invested in disaster preparedness are much less likely to attract the interest of voters.

More recently, the concepts reflected in Resolution X have been applied not only to "natural" disasters but to all hazards. This preparedness methodology is now widely accepted and used to address any public health event of international interest, such as a possible influenza pandemic, as described in the International Health Regulations (IHR).[3] Professionals in the field of chemical and radiological disasters have also adopted similar preparedness approaches.[4–6]

The first pillars of health preparedness began in the late 1970s with simulations or tabletop exercises, and drills or live exercises that included the participation of several institutions through a multidisciplinary approach. Following suit, a number of countries started preparedness planning in their hospitals and later expanded activities to other institutions such as water systems.[7] Presently, a wealth of guidelines exist on the web covering a variety of topics, from establishing an Emergency Operations Center to describing the amount of water in liters that should be distributed to displaced populations or those in shelters.[8–10] This and other information can now be found at virtual knowledge centers such as the Knowledge Center on Public Health and Disasters.[11]

Training in disaster preparedness has expanded over these last few decades. According to a survey performed in 2003, 70%

of the faculties of medicine in Latin America and the Caribbean were teaching at least a few hours of disaster management.[12] A sample of the most frequent topics included in such trainings is listed in Table 5.1.

Health and disaster legislation has also greatly improved.[13,14] In many countries, the progressive expansion of health and disaster-related standards and legislation resulted largely in response to the occurrence of disasters. These events helped governments identify problems and propose solutions. Based on these experiences, research activities, and field work, new standards and legislation were eventually created.[14] Some examples of these are found in countries where they form the basis of establishing hospital emergency committees and defining hospital construction standards. On a broader scale, subregional institutions – such as the Ministries of Health for Central America, South American Andean Countries, and South East Asia – also pass resolutions providing standards and defining the scope of regulations that form and implement a National Disaster Relief and Prevention System.

Although great progress has been made in preparedness, issues first identified in the 1980s remain as significant challenges. For example, nongovernmental organizations (NGOs), representatives from governments, and United Nations (UN) agencies met in Costa Rica in 1986 and established a series of specific recommendations to guide direct international donations (see Table 5.2).[15]

Although these approved policy guidelines have been updated over time, relief agencies remain far from being compliant with the recommendations. Examples of such noncompliance are reflected in the continually perpetuated disaster myths and misconceptions of disaster management realities, which contradict these recommended standard procedures (see Table 5.3).

In the 2010 Haitian earthquake, more than 400 health and medical groups provided services. While several were excellent, many of them were of questionable skill and efficiency, and some may have actually inflicted harm.[16]

From Preparing the Response to Mitigating the Impact

In a perfectly designed health disaster preparedness plan, all existing resources, including those at the local, national, and international levels, are used in the most efficient way to minimize the number of lives lost, contain diseases, and limit disabilities. However, preparedness has it limits as reality has shown. The Mexico City earthquake of 1985 illustrated the limits of preparedness,

Table 5.3. Disaster Myths and Realities

Myth	Reality
Foreign medical volunteers with any kind of medical background are needed.	The local population almost always covers immediate life-saving needs. Only medical personnel with skills that are not available in the affected country may be needed.
Any kind of international assistance is needed, and it is needed now!	A hasty response that is not based on an impartial evaluation only contributes to the chaos. It is better to wait until genuine needs have been assessed.
Epidemics and plagues are inevitable after every disaster.	Epidemics do not spontaneously occur after a disaster and dead bodies will not lead to catastrophic outbreaks of exotic diseases. The key to preventing disease is to improve sanitary conditions and educate the public.
The affected population is too shocked and helpless to take responsibility for their own survival.	On the contrary, many find new strength during an emergency, as evidenced by the thousands of volunteers who spontaneously united to sift through the rubble in search of victims after the 1985 Mexico City earthquake.
Disasters are random killers.	Disasters strike hardest at the most vulnerable group, the poor, and especially women, children, and the elderly.
Locating disaster victims in temporary settlements is the best alternate.	Temporary settlements should be the last alternate. Many agencies use funds normally spent for tents to purchase building materials, tools, and other construction-related support in the affected country.
Conditions are back to baseline within a few weeks.	The effects of a disaster last a long time. Disaster-affected countries deplete much of their financial and material resources in the immediate post-impact phase. Successful relief programs gear their operations to the fact that international interest wanes as needs and shortages become more pressing.

Source: PAHO/WHO.[17]

when one of the best-prepared medical response teams in the city was killed in a hospital collapse. Almost 20 years later, Hurricane Ivan struck Grenada in 2004 (a Caribbean island of 90,000 inhabitants). The country suffered such a level of destruction that no response could be generated from the island's resources, regardless of its previous preparedness level. The 2010 earthquake in Haiti destroyed most public buildings and homes in the capital. The 2011 Tōhoku earthquake and tsunami in Japan that caused a nuclear reactor breech and released radiation surprised authorities who did not plan for a combination mega-disaster with all three events taking place nearly simultaneously.

These extreme situations illustrate the limits that preparedness can achieve. If destruction is complete and only victims remain after a major disaster, such as in the Philippines after Typhoon Haiyan in 2013, there is little that a preparedness approach can offer, no matter how well developed it is. These types of situations require a different perspective and new approach. The new approach developed after the 1985 earth-

quake in Mexico is based on the concept of mitigation, emphasizing protection of infrastructure and the health system.

In 1987, the UN Assembly adopted a resolution launching the International Decade for Natural Disaster Reduction.[17] Its goal was to reduce loss of life, property damage, and social and economic disruption caused by disasters, especially in developing countries. The resolution establishing the International Decade for Natural Disaster Reduction was implemented in 1990.[18] The concept of mitigation was born.

Later, the mitigation approach helped produce the concept of risk reduction, which recognizes the importance of moving beyond preparedness. Risk can be defined as a function of the hazard and vulnerability in which the hazard is an environmental (e.g., earthquake or hurricane), technological (e.g., chemical or radiological accident), or political (e.g., war or civil strife) event. The essential idea of mitigation focuses on separating the hazard (an earthquake or biological agent) from the vulnerability of the institution or the system. If a building collapses, it is not attributed to the earthquake; rather, it was a consequence of poor building design or failure to use appropriate shake-resistant construction techniques.

Since the late 1980s, an ongoing effort has existed in the health sector, especially in Latin America and the Caribbean, to protect health facilities so that life-saving functions can continue after a disaster. In the beginning, efforts centered on mitigating and refurbishing health facilities. Currently, the approach includes a more comprehensive vision, not just focusing on the construction aspects (structural and nonstructural dimensions), but also considering the functional aspects of a hospital.[19,20] In this context, "functional" refers to all organizational components needed to provide service.

Enormous progress has been achieved in the field of mitigation. For example, methodologies now exist that can produce a vulnerability analysis for buildings. This is the detailed study on how a building would perform if a maximum magnitude event (such as an earthquake or hurricane) occurs. The information generated by these analyses provides guidance on how to improve construction and revise existing building codes.

Mitigation can be a very efficient strategy. For example, some structures have been protected from collapse through targeted adjustments, such as retrofitting. The cost of the additional construction requires a relatively small financial investment compared with the overall value of the building. However, mitigation can be expensive when applied to existing facilities in poor condition and it frequently reaches the point at which it is too expensive to be considered. Hence, a lower cost approach is needed to reduce vulnerability.

From Mitigation to Resilience

In the late 1990s and early 2000s, the increasing engagement of financial institutions in risk reduction opened the door to considering new incentives and justifications for such activities in addition to typical health-centered metrics such as lives saved. Participating institutions included the World Bank through its Global Facility for Disaster Reduction and Recovery and regional banks in Asia and Latin America.[21,22]

Increasingly, studies demonstrate that the perception commonly accepted 40 years ago, that it is too costly to make a society resilient to disasters, does not hold true. Contrary to earlier thoughts, if mitigation is part of the development process, it is not too costly to make a society disaster resistant. For example, when hazards are taken into account before construction begins, the increase in expenditures represents less than 4% of the total construction cost.[23]

Although cost is an essential factor in justifying risk reduction, it is not the only element. It would be unacceptable to construct a critical facility, such as one providing an emergency service, in so suboptimal a manner that it collapses during an earthquake simply due to financial considerations.

The integration of these financial and other technical considerations is an extremely positive step, as it allows development professionals to include "risk reduction" in their projects. The end result is an improvement in society without increasing the risk from disasters. For example, development professionals have begun to take into consideration locating critical services on higher ground, instead of flood prone areas. With these advances, it is possible to design technical tools and to train experts to conceive new development projects in such a way that they will remain functional even after a major event occurs.[24] The objective is no longer simple mitigation, but to build resiliency by considering vulnerability in a more comprehensive way through the risk reduction approach.

Although at the time of this writing the risk reduction approach is still in the initial stages of development, it has already generated some results. The World Bank established an online tutorial for "Strengthening essential public health functions," and one of these essential functions refers to disasters.[25]

This tool allows the user to estimate a country's level of preparedness and some aspects of risk reduction. Another example is the WHO/PAHO Hospital Safety Index.[26] This instrument allows trained local professionals to assess the safety level of health facilities. By applying this tool, government authorities can determine the likelihood that health and medical facilities will remain functional during and after exposure to known hazards.

Additional medical tools have also been developed to improve the quality of patient care. These instruments provide guidance on how to ensure quality care in disaster situations. For example, the U.S. Institute of Medicine within the National Academies has proposed a series of protocols referred to as "Crisis Standards of Care: A Systems Framework for Catastrophic Disaster Response."[27] Many organizations have succeeded at improving the quality of care under catastrophic conditions. In 2012 and 2013, groups such as the ICRC (the International Committee of the Red Cross), MSF (Médecins Sans Frontières), and AusAID (Australian Agency for International Development) have developed their own guidelines, especially for the delivery of care during armed conflicts.

The UN launched a 2-year campaign in 2008 called "Hospitals Safe from Disasters" to ensure that these institutions are prioritized in reducing their vulnerability to hazards. Spearheaded by WHO and the UN International Strategy for Disaster Reduction (UNISDR), "the campaign will focus on structural safety of hospitals and health facilities, on keeping health facilities functioning during and after disasters, and on making sure health workers are prepared when natural hazards strike."[28]

However, simply having safe structures and processes may not be comprehensive enough or may not apply to a given situation. For example, countries with very weak economies could not expect to have a state of the art safe society in a decade. However, these countries could improve their overall disaster readiness by increasing their resilience. UNISDR defines resilience as the ability of a system, community, or society exposed to hazards to resist, absorb, accommodate to, and recover from the effects of the hazard in a timely and efficient manner, including through the preservation and restoration of its essential basic structures and functions. The principle is to permit a community to experience the disaster with the capacity to absorb the impact without sustaining significant permanent damage. The first practical definition and documentation of resilience was achieved by the United Kingdom's Department for International Development in 2011.[29] Hundreds of such projects now exist, created by this British agency in support of community resilience.

Although this topic has been proposed previously in other forms, the concept of resilience goes far beyond what has been done to date by the humanitarian community. It requires that all development activities fully embrace disaster risk and ensure that all tools are used in an integrated manner.

Shift in the Institutional Approach

Both governmental and regional institutions have significantly improved their disaster management efforts over the last 40 years. In a recent WHO survey report, 85% of the Ministries of Health globally have policies or programs related to disaster preparedness.[30] In Latin America and the Caribbean region, all countries with more than 20 million inhabitants have a formal multidisciplinary disaster agency and a staffed national disaster coordination office within the Ministry of Health.[31,32] The goals of these groups are civil protection and disaster risk reduction at the national level. These departments within the Ministries of Health are the designated entities for protecting the public's health from the consequences of disasters. The national disaster coordination office's mission is to ensure the synchronization of all governmental disaster reduction efforts. These agencies promote preparedness and risk reduction responsibilities across all sectors, such as a federal emergency management agency or other organizations that provide civil protection. Over the last few years, especially since the adoption of the international health regulation renewed mandate, Ministries of Health have developed centers that catalogue information and coordinate responses for events with international consequences.[33] Such events include epidemics and any event occurring at a border, such as a volcanic eruption. In some countries, like the United States, the offices responsible for IHR and disaster management are integrated into the same department within the government.

Although these achievements represent a major step forward in national preparedness, the sustained improvement in quality and institutional continuity of these offices still relies on the frequent occurrence of disasters. In fact, the rate at which disasters occur has a substantial impact on institutional development of these agencies. Just as these national disaster programs and offices were established or have been significantly strengthened as the consequence of a catastrophe, they have also experienced reductions in their capacity or disappeared entirely when such events do not occur for prolonged periods. This tendency has been noted in both wealthy and developing countries. In the latter, a change of government is another common reason for reducing the disaster preparedness investment or for assigning new personnel with no experience to these offices. In countries where the percentage of career disaster employees is small (staff that earned their position rather than being politically appointed), it is difficult to maintain a capable disaster management program. The absence of a disaster in such countries is a threat to institutionalizing preparedness and changes the nature of the roles and functions within these offices. With time, these agencies focus increasing attention on smaller events. When a government institution attends only to smaller emergencies, it loses its perspective and hence its capacity for cross-cutting coordination – its main function. Over time, the institution will isolate itself from other administrative entities and it will lose its close relationship with the top authority.[34]

On the international scene, similar progress and challenges exist. In 1974, the international community made a significant commitment with the creation of the UN Disaster Relief Organization (the precursor entity to the Office for the Coordination of Humanitarian Affairs, OCHA) as a way to improve the international response to disasters. The reaction to the 2004 tsunami in Southeast Asia clearly showed that OCHA and many other agencies could successfully deliver aid, but also suggested that a stronger mechanism is needed to make the international response more efficient. Establishing a mechanism that attracts and coordinates more UN agencies (as is intended by UN humanitarian reform efforts) is an important step, but remains insufficient on its own.

Even in an ideal situation, in which all UN agencies and major NGOs agree to coordination using a single unified command structure, planners could not guarantee the most effective response. Instead, the efficiency of international assistance is mostly dependent on the recipient country's capacity to absorb, coordinate, and distribute the deluge of resources that could reach the affected population. Any international response effort that is not strictly and exclusively complementary with the national response will result in competition with, and disruption of, the country's relief activities. In other words, the best international humanitarian response is the one that complements the local response. The only exception to this is when no local organization exists or when the local authority is the reason for the chaos, such as in some complex public health emergencies (see Chapter 27). Even in those rare situations when the local population relies primarily on an international response, the objective must remain to rebuild the local response capacity that existed before the disaster. International assistance cannot be considered successful if the recipient country is left with minimal institutional capacity when support is withdrawn.

Institutionalization of Knowledge

Four decades ago, disaster-related issues were viewed simplistically, primarily guided by the lack of resources and the limited number of professionals in the field. The decision-making process was also less complex, because those issues that could be addressed were solved quickly and efficiently because few people were involved. Today, with the availability of more human and financial resources, institutions are compelled to both raise and respond to more complex issues. As a consequence, this expansion of the field requires a lengthy and more sophisticated consultation process, through networks of various professionals and professional associations.

The knowledge base for the field of international humanitarian assistance increases every day. This explosion of information is reflected not only in the number of experts in the field, but also in the number of related scientific and technical publications. A few examples are listed in Table 5.4.

The U.S. National Library of Medicine has inventoried more than 30,000 publications related to disasters.[35] Disaster management, however, is still a relatively new field, and the majority of the technical "knowledge" is derived from anecdotes and personal experiences, rather than from scientifically rigorous studies published in peer-reviewed journals, although this is chang-

Table 5.4. Sample List of International Disaster Medicine Journals

Publication	Sponsoring Institution or Society
Japanese Journal of Disaster Medicine	Japanese Association for Disaster Medicine (first published in 1996)
Prehospital and Disaster Medicine	World Association for Disaster and Emergency Medicine, editorial offices in the United States (first published in 1985)
Disaster Medicine and Public Health Preparedness	Society for Disaster Medicine and Public Health (first published in 2007)
International Journal of Disaster Medicine	Published by Taylor & Francis, editorial offices in Sweden (first published in 2004)
American Journal of Disaster Medicine	American Society of Disaster Medicine (first published in 2006)
Annals of Disaster Medicine (web-based journal)	Taiwan Society of Disaster Medicine (first published in 2002)

ing. The number of sophisticated investigations published to date is limited by a lack of research funding for such projects and the fact that disasters occur relatively infrequently. Therefore, the best training centers today must still rely significantly on post facto documentation of individual and group experiences. On the other hand, the number of institutions invested in disaster-related education, training, and research are growing. In the United States alone there are approximately 180 institutions sponsoring emergency management–related programs. Several websites document available courses.[36]

Some information centers such as the Regional Disaster Information Center have been compiling an inventory of gray (non-peer reviewed) literature.[37] More than 15,000 publications are now accessible on the web without cost through this resource.

Within emergency medicine, formal education and certification in disaster-related fields is also developing. The Department of Emergency Medicine at the University of Paris, France, in collaboration with the Paris Fire Brigade, introduced a "Capacité de Médecine de Catastrophe" in 1981. The name of the certificate (capacité), although a postgraduate diploma, clearly indicated it was not meant to be a specialty.[38] This capacité was later organized in other French-speaking countries, such as Morocco. The European Center for Disaster Medicine was founded by the Council of Europe in the aftermath of earthquakes in southern Italy that occurred during the early 1980s. Since 1989, the Center has organized courses on emergency and disaster medical response, targeting mostly an Italian audience, but also countries from the Mediterranean basin. In the United States, Johns Hopkins University in Baltimore, Maryland, and the U.S. Center for Disease Control (CDC) organized international workshops on earthquake injury epidemiology that mainly focused on mitigation and response.[39] Several other U.S.-based universities have developed postgraduate programs for trained emergency physicians. For example, in 2006, the University of California at Irvine founded its Emergency Medical Services and Disaster Medical Sciences Fellowship, a 2-year program that includes completion of a master's degree.[40] Another example of postgraduate training is at the University of Linkoping in Sweden where they collaborated with the regional health authorities and founded a Center for Teaching and Research in Disaster Medicine and Traumatology. The center introduced a certificate in disaster management, which subsequently was offered to international students. The university continued to expand its educational portfolio and in 2006 granted its first Doctor of Philosophy in disaster medicine.

In addition to individual institutions offering advanced degrees, international consortia of universities now exist, creating a global educational effort. One example is a program initially developed in Europe called the European Master in Disaster Medicine (EMDM). In 1998, at the European Society for Emergency Medicine's first European Congress, organizers discussed the idea of an education platform for disaster medicine. The European Center for Disaster Medicine had offered training in emergency and disaster medicine since 1989. Similarly, the Department of Emergency Medicine at the Catholic University of Leuven, Belgium, had taught a postgraduate course on disaster medicine and management since 1988, in collaboration with the Medical Service of the Belgian Armed Forces. Integration of these two courses led to the establishment in 2001 of an educational program in which students could obtain EMDM certification. All partners agreed that this certificate was meant to acquire the status of a university diploma, as soon as requirements listed in the European Directives on Higher Education were satisfied. In 2004, the diploma designated as the European Master in Disaster Medicine was established as a second-level master's degree, (a master's degree obtained by an individual already holding a master's degree or equivalent), according to the Directives of the European Union. The two sponsoring organizations are the University of Eastern Piedmont, Vercelli, Italy, and the Free University of Brussels, Belgium. The diploma is issued by the University of Eastern Piedmont on behalf of both universities. Subsequently, several institutions in the United States have formally affiliated with the EMDM and supply faculty; these include Harvard, Yale, and the University of California at Irvine.

The EMDM program emphasizes concept development and strategic thinking, with less weight placed on operational training. The basic content is offered in a modular format and the modules address all subjects commonly classified under the terms "disaster medicine" and "public health." The design of the EMDM consists of an electronic textbook with problem-based interactive simulation exercises, delivered via the Internet. This distance-learning component is combined with a residential session, a master's thesis, and a final examination also administered over the Internet. Student evaluation is continuous.[41] Due to the format chosen (Internet), the student population (between twenty-five and thirty-five per year) is international in scope. Total enrollment to date represents all five continents and more than fifty countries. Although the EMDM is European, as it is based on European Directives and the title is issued by European Universities, it is global as far as the faculty and the students are concerned.

Broadening the Approach to Include Multiple Institutions

The central premise of disaster health response and risk reduction is management of resources for a *population's* health, as opposed to therapeutic measures applied to large numbers of individual patients in an emergency medical situation. Not surprisingly, disaster response, preparedness, and vulnerability reduction rely not only on a multiplicity of institutions within the health sector (e.g., the Ministry of Health, the Red Cross and Red Crescent societies), but also require resources administered by organizations outside of the healthcare field. Involvement of other sectors including national disaster coordination entities, financial institutions, military, fire brigade, and meteorological centers is essential. In theory, determining the entity that can and should coordinate these multiple organizations is straightforward. In practice, however, it remains a challenge.

Some countries that have marginalized the Ministry of Health's role in disaster response have met with catastrophic results. Such poor outcomes have occurred when the health response is assigned to agencies outside the ministry. It eliminates the health institution's ownership of the process and creates an unproductive competition with entities outside the health sector. Experience has shown that the Ministry of Health should lead the health sector as a complement to the national disaster coordination system. The Ministry of Health is recognized by sovereign states as being the highest decision level entity dealing with health issues. A Ministry of Health without a functional disaster program will leave a country's population vulnerable to disasters and reduce effective management of health resources.

The humanitarian reform movement has generated the concept of dividing humanitarian assistance into several topic-specific groups called clusters. Under this approach, one UN agency has been assigned to lead each cluster, as described in Table 5.5.[42] Although this approach has great advantages from a management perspective, it also raises new challenges as health-related topics such as nutrition, water quality, or sanitation are split among different clusters. Continued improvement in multiagency coordination at the international level is necessary. This issue was discussed at the PAHO/WHO 2012 assembly, where the ministers of health of Latin America and the Caribbean clarified responsibilities.[43]

Table 5.5. Global Cluster Leads

Sector or Area of Activity	Global Cluster Lead Agency
Food Security	Food and Agriculture Organization/World Food Program
Camp Management & Coordination	UN High Commissioner for Refugees/International Organization for Migration
Early Recovery	UN Development Program
Education	UN Children's Fund/Save the Children
Emergency Shelter	UN High Commissioner for Refugees/International Federation of Red Cross and Red Crescent Societies
Emergency Telecommunications	World Food Program
Health	World Health Organization
Logistics	World Food Program
Nutrition	UN Children's Fund
Protection	UN High Commissioner for Refugees
Sanitation, Water, and Hygiene	UN Children's Fund

Source: http://www.unocha.org/what-we-do/coordination-tools/cluster-coordination.

RECOMMENDATIONS FOR FURTHER RESEARCH

Striking the Appropriate Balance between International Response and National Preparedness

International institutions continue to improve their disaster response capabilities. However, further improvement is needed, especially for mega-disasters such as the Southeast Asian tsunami of December 2004, the Haitian earthquake in 2010, and Hurricane Ivan that completely destroyed the Island of Grenada in 2004. New mechanisms resulting from the humanitarian reform movement, such as the cluster approach, and new sources of funding like the UN Central Emergency Response Fund, are signs of progress.[44] These and other developments are likely to stimulate further advances in international disaster response programs. However, coordination in situations where an overwhelming number of international response entities arrive in just a few days remains a challenge. Another area of concern is that improving international institutional response capability will only be successful if the level of individual countries' national preparedness improves simultaneously.

The difference in the preparedness levels between low-income countries and the international community is increasing. As a consequence, national authorities, especially in fragile states, increasingly see this gap as a threat to their authority. Countries that are more dependent on external assistance due to lack of wealth are less able to control those providing international assistance. This loss of autonomy and authority in developing countries is considered by some as a minor inconvenience, as it is outweighed by the immediate benefit from international assistance. However, there is some evidence that this gap in preparedness results in long-term political instability and negative impacts on the population after international aid arrives. The struggle for control between the national government and the international community has the potential to negatively impact the effective delivery of assistance.

In contrast to response efforts, national disaster preparedness receives much less international attention. The perceived failures in response coordination have been more visible than the contributing effects of inadequate national preparedness. As a consequence, analysts focus more on response issues when discussing deficiencies in disaster management. The conclusions that misattribute all the problems with disaster relief activities to failed response efforts frequently result from a lack of proper analysis. Although many failures in disaster response coordination exist, the root cause is primarily due to the lack of support for preparedness activities prior to the event.

This situation is of particular concern because disaster preparedness is the most efficient way to improve disaster response. Effective preparedness, especially in the least developed countries, is also the only way to ensure cost-effective mobilization of national resources and cost-effective international assistance. Focusing on preparedness is a more challenging approach because the international community has no control over planning efforts of individual countries, and these nations must juggle the competing priorities of daily emergencies with planning for the "what if." In the long run, however, it is the only possible solution for true improvement in disaster management.

Although this topic has been discussed for twenty years, the scientific evidence supporting the impact of preparedness is limited. For example, no rigorous comprehensive study exists analyzing the cost effectiveness of providing a region with needed infrastructure, supplies, and equipment to manage a disaster prior to its occurrence in order to avoid the response deficiencies that result from the absence of these resources in the aftermath. This would provide low-income states a better idea of how much and on what preparedness activities to invest. Having just 1% of the operations budget dedicated to such research could make a difference.

Strengthening Emergency Medicine

Progress is possible, as is exemplified by a WHO document produced during the 60th World Health Assembly on May 23, 2007, which emphasizes improvements in national disaster preparedness. The document, entitled "Health systems: emergency-care systems," recognizes that "improved organization and planning for provision of trauma and emergency care is an essential part of integrated health-care delivery, plays an important role in preparedness for and response to mass-casualty incidents, and can lower mortality, reduce disability, and prevent other adverse health outcomes arising from the burden of everyday injuries." In addition, the document urges member states to assess comprehensively their prehospital and emergency care systems with regard to identifying unmet needs; ensuring involvement by Ministries of Health; establishing integrated emergency care systems; monitoring performance as a solid basis for ensuring minimum standards for training, equipment, infrastructure, and communication; ensuring that appropriate core competencies are part of relevant health curricula; and promoting continuing education.[45]

However, additional issues remain. Large disasters with high casualty numbers, such as earthquakes, create ethical challenges for medical response teams. Can a team deployed by a country with high medical standards provide substantially lower quality medical services if these lower standards are the norm for the region in which they are working? Should a medical team be dispatched from a country that is not recognized for high healthcare standards to provide service to other countries? The WHO is now developing guidelines for Foreign Medical Teams, which have been implemented at least partially in the Philippines after hurricane Haiyan.[46] More operational research is required to identify the qualifications, selection criteria, and post-disaster evaluation metrics for these teams.

Improving Donations and Countering Disaster Myths

Appropriate handling of international donations remains an unresolved issue. At a conference in 1986, the main NGOs, government representatives, and UN agencies agreed on a set of recommendations for appropriate international humanitarian assistance.[15] Although these recommendations have been widely published and subsequently implemented by a small number of agencies (those with the most experience and largest donor support), they are still not commonly practiced.[47] Presently, there are still large quantities of mostly useless supplies, sent at a high cost, that arrive too late to be beneficial following a disaster.

The types and quantities of humanitarian assistance donations are largely determined by the needs of the donors rather than by those requesting aid. Donations are still motivated by the horror of images on a television screen, rather than the sudden pressing needs of the affected population. To move toward resolving the problem, an international information campaign to educate the public and the media on ways to make appropriate donations is urgently needed. Improving the quality of donations will require further research investigating ways to change the public's behavior and perceptions and will need to align incentives with institutional donors.

Instruments exist that provide more transparency in the management of humanitarian supplies. In the early 1990s, the Humanitarian Supply Management System was developed as a joint effort of Latin American and Caribbean countries, with the technical cooperation of PAHO. In 2004, the inter-agency Logistic Support System (LSS) was created to expand the experience of the Humanitarian Supply Management System in the Americas while building a global interface that serves agencies, NGOs, and donors, as well as countries. LSS was developed jointly with OCHA, the World Food Program, the UN Children's Fund, WHO, PAHO and the UN High Commissioner for Refugees, and is the most advanced example in the field.[48] This free instrument enables all users, both agencies and governments, to capture information on all humanitarian supplies received for the same disaster. This software enables the coordinating entity to collect and track the quantity of pledged and received donations. It complements existing tracking systems (systems designed to track supplies managed by one institution from the point of reception to the point of distribution). A large number of domestic disaster agencies have used the LSS software; however, this management tool and others similar to it are still rarely utilized proactively by international relief agencies. This challenge of managing donations is likely to remain unresolved until public opinion demands that the international community be held as accountable as national governments. For example, groups that constitute themselves as NGOs at the moment a disaster occurs, collect money, and then provide ineffective aid have not yet suffered consequences as a result of this dysfunction.

The issue of appropriate donations is only one of the recurring concerns identified more than twenty years ago as disaster myths and realities.[17] Each of these seven notorious myths requires further study to analyze why they persist and suggest new potential solutions to counter them.

Improving Knowledge Discovery

A systematic analysis of large disasters would be an effective technique to gain knowledge from previous experiences and many organizations have attempted to adopt this methodology. One problem is that only a few large-scale disasters (events that overwhelm national capacity) occur. Therefore, a systematic analysis at the institutional or even at the country level is problematic because the limited number of events makes it difficult to draw meaningful conclusions.

A second challenge is the difficulty in obtaining an impartial analysis. Some improvement has occurred in this area, as exemplified by the 2004 South-East Asia Tsunami review coordinated by WHO.[49] However, many post-disaster analysis exercises are still limited to providing success stories, and few address the issues that require change. Many such documents are not even peer-reviewed. No real progress can be expected without a scientific and objective evaluation of a disaster's management.

Finally, a method is needed to incorporate this information permanently into the growing body of knowledge in the science of disaster public health and medicine. One example is that the National Library of Medicine is now creating web sites compiling the best of the grey and peer-reviewed literature. However, until this is done in a more systematic fashion, information will be lost as those who "learn" it retire or change jobs. The fact that the same issues are identified again and again demonstrates that these recommendations have not been incorporated by institutions and universities into the growing body of science. The commonly used term "lessons learned" is problematic as it implies that this information is gained on a personal level (as when a child discovers that touching a hot object hurts) and not incorporated into an expanding permanent record. More appropriate terms for the results of these exercises would be "issues for action," "outcomes identified," or "new knowledge discovered." Research centers have a responsibility to collect these identified outcomes, retain them, and make them accessible to professionals in the field and to the public at large. Endeavors by universities such as those sponsoring the EMDM – or institutions offering postgraduate degrees in health disaster–related topics such as John Hopkins, the Hawaii Pacific Disaster Research Centers, and Cayetano Herredia University in Peru – are changing this pattern but more work must be done. This methodology offers the only real long-term solution for disaster coordination entities and international humanitarian agencies to absorb this knowledge into their operations and policies.

Strengthening the All-Hazard Approach

Previously unrecognized hazards, events, and threats are becoming national or international concerns. For example, chemical intoxication from dumping sites in Cote D'Ivoire, hemorrhagic dengue in Paraguay or Africa, severe acute respiratory syndrome in Asia, and the threat of bioterrorism are among the types of challenges that have recently justified declaring a national emergency. This trend is likely to increase and become more complex in the future. Experts from various specialties would have responded to these same disasters 10 years ago, but such events would not have attracted a great deal of political attention. Now, even incidents with smaller numbers of deaths or with the mere potential to threaten neighboring countries have become events of international interest. The disclosure of threats is expected to further increase because countries must now report all public health events with international implications under the International Health Regulations procedures.[3]

With the recognition of each emerging threat, the tendency has been to create a new mechanism at the national or international level to address it. Bioterrorism and pandemic influenza are among the recent examples. Addressing each hazard with a separate and unique mechanism, project, or agency is not sustainable. Such an approach weakens the existing coordination mechanisms by establishing parallel systems. One solution is implementation of a comprehensive all-hazard approach to managing threats. This would stimulate countries to revisit and strengthen their existing national disaster coordination system each time a new threat is perceived, rather than creating another separate strategy. This approach would initiate responses from both national and international systems during major crises, increasing inter-agency contact and enhancing mutual trust between all organizations. This all-hazard approach is logical but not yet widely recognized. The United States and several other countries have officially embraced an all-hazard strategy. However, rigid administrative procedures, departmental culture, and existing compartmentalization among professions and institutions are restrictive obstacles that require significant energy to overcome. Further identification and refinement of the essential disaster components associated with these events is required to promote a better understanding of this methodology.

Toward Stronger Inter-Agency Cooperation

Due to the increasing number of specialized disaster-related topics and the diversification of players in the humanitarian assistance field, it will be increasingly difficult for one entity to address sufficiently the multifaceted needs of disaster response and risk reduction – even in a specific sector. To be relevant, institutions will need to further specialize while simultaneously striving for stronger inter-agency cooperation. This also applies to national governments. These bodies will need to develop human resources in their respective Ministries of Health to specifically know what is available internationally, how to access such resources, and how to incorporate them as part of the national response.

Entities representing intergovernmental regional organizations, such as the Asian Development Bank or African Union, and subregional intergovernmental agencies, such as the Andean Committee for Disaster Prevention and Assistance, will become increasingly relevant and dually supported by national governments and donor countries. These groups, however, should maintain a limited scope and address the challenges of interconnectedness with a mosaic of partners. To be efficient, each entity must identify its unique valued-added specialty within the global village environment. In contrast, entities involved in improving global response processes must better recognize regional or subregional processes, and most importantly, include national systems in all of their considerations.

The International Federation of Red Cross and Red Crescent Societies have analyzed many multinational laws and regulations and created international protocols based on these evaluations.[50] More such efforts are needed. Subregional protocols, multinational agreements, and national legal frameworks are some additional examples of tools to improve inter-agency and intergovernmental cooperation that have been poorly documented and studied to date.

Addressing Climate Change and Security

Significant progress has occurred in risk identification, stemming mostly from the analysis of previous disasters. UNISDR is now regularly publishing the Global Assessment Report on Disaster Risk Reduction.[51] These reports are developed based on a large body of original research by a wide range of institutions including UN agencies, governments, NGOs, and businesses. Material incorporated into these reports includes original data, case studies, analysis, and survey results. It enables the identification of a number of socioeconomic and environmental variables that may point to causal processes of disaster risk. In addition to this publication, specific risk vulnerability assessments have been developed by WHO to protect health from climate change.[52]

New threats, such as the advent of climate change and its implications for disaster medicine, oblige relief organizations to revisit the concept of risk analysis. The 2003 heat wave, which is estimated to have killed approximately 15,000 persons in France, took Europe largely by surprise. In comparison, the threat of pandemic influenza has been much better anticipated. It is clear that efficient disaster management programs must guide their actions not only based on past experiences but also on future projections.

The concept of security is currently limited to discussions between northern hemisphere specialists. Developing countries remain more preoccupied by historically prevalent conditions rather than by lower probability "potential" threats. Bioterrorism and pandemic influenza are mostly overlooked in countries where they are not present today. This may change in the not too distant future.

Security threats and climate change are examples of recently emerging challenges. In the near term, disaster agencies will require tools that can assist them in recognizing and anticipating such potential risks. The methodology for identifying the risks a country is likely to face (mostly perceptions, based on probability analysis assessing rate of occurrence and magnitude of impact) is incomplete and must await future investigations. Once established, however, this methodology will allow disaster entities to switch from a reactive attitude (based on probability of past events) to a proactive stance (based on perceived risks in the future). This would be a much more scientifically valid method to focus disaster mitigation and preparedness efforts.

A Stronger Scientific and Professional Approach

Historically, disaster preparedness and risk reduction have been based on a nonscientific common sense analysis of past events. As new resources become available, a more scientific approach is required to address important issues such as a country's degree of preparedness. At present, there are no internationally recognized standards for estimating either a country's or an institution's level of readiness. Research focused on establishing benchmarks for the assessment of preparedness is necessary. The WHO Office for Southeast Asia has developed a framework of twelve national disaster preparedness benchmarks. These are associated with a corresponding set of standards and indicators that elaborate the best practices to facilitate political commitments through a uniform framework for planning and evaluating emergency preparedness actions for the countries of Southeast Asia.[53] Baseline surveys measuring progress in a region are necessary to provide a gauge for further growth and compliance with such benchmarks.[54] Other areas that would benefit from scientific inquiry include identification of where disaster preparedness and risk reduction programs are needed and the essential elements that comprise a national disaster management policy.

Scientific and professional organizations must be involved not only in the investigation of the aforementioned topics, but also in lending expertise in response to issues raised by disaster management personnel. WADEM is proposing some criteria to identify minimum standards that define a disaster professional. However, future progress requires that research centers and academic entities propose scientifically rigorous methods to study, analyze, and respond to present challenges. Therefore, universities and professional associations must be included as partners in the disaster preparedness field. Some of these professional societies exist; however, thus far most are in emergency medicine. These include the World Association for Disaster and Emergency Medicine, the European Society for Emergency Medicine, the American Public Health Association, the Australasian College of Emergency Medicine, and the American College of Emergency Physicians. Still, more professional associations should be encouraged to participate.

Determining precise definitions remains a problem due to the multiplicity of expertise involved in this field. More deliberation will be required to move beyond the current multitude of existing classifications and reach agreement on internationally accepted definitions. For example, the International Strategy for Disaster Reduction has proposed some excellent definitions of disaster risk reduction terminology; however, too few entities regularly accept and utilize these definitions.[55] Instead, they promulgate their own systems. Standardizing terminology would improve communication among sectors.

Research techniques will develop in new and innovative ways. The challenge imposed by difficulties in performing prospective investigations can be partially overcome through sophisticated simulation of disaster events. Simulation template models allowing experimental changes of environment, preparedness level, and response capabilities may serve as platforms for research and produce performance and outcome indicators. They may allow comparison of different scenarios and quantify the results of environmental manipulation, vulnerability reduction, and preparedness modification without creating risk to populations and care providers.

In this field, the tradition of using simulation exercises has continued to evolve and now has the ability to address massive public health problems. One such example is the U.S. "Top Officials" simulation exercise, referred to as "Top Off." This full-scale simulation was the largest and most comprehensive terrorism-response exercise ever conducted in the United States, involving multiple sectors and multistate participants.[56] The ConvEx simulation exercises, coordinated by the Inter-Agency Committee for the Response to Nuclear Accidents, test and evaluate the international emergency management system. They identify best practices, deficiencies, and areas requiring improvement that could not be detected in national exercises.[57] Sometimes these simulations precede real events (mass gatherings where there is a risk of disaster), such as the simulations conducted for the Cricket World Cup in the Caribbean in 2007. These types of simulations are considered one-time events and frequently do not include evaluation or continuity parameters to build cumulatively on previous exercises.

Another example of using simulations to improve disaster preparedness is the I SEE (Inter-active Simulation Exercise for Emergencies) project, financed by the Leonardo da Vinci Agency of the European Union. The goal of this endeavor was to develop an electronic platform and a pilot exercise for the team training of all the participants involved in disaster response management. The project involved a collaborative effort of universities and educational institutions from five European countries (Belgium, Italy, Romania, Spain, and Sweden) and started with a survey on the educational needs of 206 teaching institutions, providing different levels of education, from these five countries.[58] Project design was based on the survey results and followed by system development, formative evaluations, refining and retuning of the product, and development of a policy for implementation.

The I SEE project ran from October 2004 through September 2007. It was developed primarily as a research project to evaluate training methodologies in disaster medicine.[59] In the future, however, it may evolve into a tool for studying decision making, preparedness, and logistics, as the template allows customization of the exercise environment and scenario.

Improvements in disaster management will continue at a greater rate and more publications on disaster health management will appear. Subsequently, this expansion of information will require more intense participation of information centers. In the near term, the gray literature will remain among the best sources of information. New initiatives must be encouraged, especially in lower-income countries, which do not have ready access to or appropriately consider peer review as part of their daily operations.

Many governments have created positions within various agencies to manage disasters. These positions are mostly occupied by professionals with a variety of backgrounds and training. A consensus does not yet exist on what constitutes the minimum qualifications for a specialist in disaster management. Creating such criteria would encourage further development of the specialty and improve professionalization of those involved. Ultimately, acceptance of such standards would increase the quality in all components of disaster management. Further work is needed to define these qualifications.

Reconstruction

Increasingly, reconstruction following disasters has been included as part of humanitarian assistance and mostly funded by emergency budget lines. The issues that arise during reconstruction, although similar to the acute aspects of risk reduction, are not lifesaving time-related decisions, but rather must be approached using a more deliberate and orderly process. Expertise is needed from developers and planners that is unrelated to the required knowledge for those making immediate disaster risk reduction decisions. As such, it may not be optimal to have humanitarian assistance personnel involved in reconstruction.

Similar to the long-term aspects of risk reduction, humanitarian specialists should remain in the advocacy role and permit development specialists to supervise reconstruction. If the initial response and rehabilitation phase must be under the leadership of humanitarian specialists, the long-term reconstruction efforts should be the responsibility of development professionals.

Some financial institutions such as the World Bank are developing tools for reconstruction based on post-disaster assessment. More such instruments should be developed. For example, very few individuals tasked with providing infrastructure expertise within Ministries of Health have developed a reconstruction plan or strategy that anticipates the approach to rebuilding damaged hospitals that account for known vulnerabilities of these institutions.

Resilience

Many disaster management specialists have recently adopted the concept of resilience (see UNISDR definition earlier in this chapter). This concept now requires authorities to develop a more comprehensive view of disaster management. A non-resilient community will lack redundancies or viable response and recovery alternatives, rendering it more vulnerable to the initial and long-term consequences of a disaster's impact. The challenge is in identifying which components of a community's assets are the most crucial in maximizing resilience. It is recognized that many aspects of a community can fail during a disaster, however relatively few will significantly compromise response and recovery. It is easy to identify such critical community resources after an event has occurred, but more difficult to quantify beforehand, when it really matters. More work is need in the field of resilience to identify and implement effective strategies.

Conclusions

Disaster management has been a thriving global field for the last 40 years and remains a very promising area of specialization. In a short period of time, the discipline has evolved from using an ad hoc emergency response approach to a more comprehensive preparedness, mitigation, risk reduction, and resilience approach. It is now becoming intimately involved with emergency medicine and epidemiology. Presently, disaster management is at a critical point; it must move from utilizing a "common sense perspective" in analyzing disasters to one involving more systematic, scientific, and professional methodologies. Initial progress was possible utilizing accumulated individual experience. However, the topic is now so vast and complex that its evolution will depend on substantive investment of additional resources in the support of future research. One proposed funding strategy is to designate a percentage of the disaster response budget for research.

Disaster myths identified almost thirty years ago still persist, such as the ineffective manner in which donations are appropriated. These myths represent important areas for growth as they involve fundamental principles of disaster management. Although these issues have been identified and described over the years, they remain an ongoing concern.

The main risk for the future is that the importance of national preparedness will be minimized. Although there is still the need for a global response to disasters, it must be based on national coordination to be successful. Strong national coordination capacity is the best investment the international humanitarian community can make because it is the most effective way to ensure that international assistance is efficiently used. In addition, it preserves the function of local organizations and leaves behind a positive image among the assisted population.

Witnessing the significant negative impact of disasters on human life provokes a great deal of public sympathy. Often, the need to respond to such events seems overwhelmingly important. As such, the disaster response component of the overall disaster management strategy seems most significant. Hence investment in improving disaster response capabilities has seemed to be the appropriate answer. The last 30 years of disaster management indicate that preparedness and risk reduction play even more important roles than the response phase. A real improvement in response to disasters will only be possible when additional resources are invested prior to the event, rather than when it is already too late to make a real difference – when victims already exist.

Acknowledgment

The author and editors would like to thank Center for Disaster Medical Sciences International Fellow Wajdan Alassaf, MD for her assistance with obtaining and verifying the web-based references for this chapter.

REFERENCES

1. Mission and History. World Association for Disaster and Emergency Medicine. http://www.wadem.org/mission.html (Accessed June 20, 2014).
2. Resolution X of 1976 of Pan American Health Organization (PAHO) Directing Council.
3. International Health Regulations (IHR). World Health Organization. http://www.who.int/csr/ihr/finalversion9Nov07.pdf (Accessed June 20, 2014).
4. International Atomic Energy Agency (IAEA). Arrangements for Preparedness for a Nuclear or Radiological Emergency. http://www-pub.iaea.org/MTCD/Publications/PDF/Pub1265web.pdf (Accessed December 12, 2014).
5. WHO International Programme on Chemical Safety. http://whqlibdoc.who.int/publications/2004/9241546158.pdf?ua=1 (Accessed December 12, 2014).
6. International Programme on Chemical Safety (IPCS). IPCS Guidelines for the Monitoring of Genotoxic Effects of Carcinogens in Humans. http://www.who.int/ipcs/en/ (Accessed June 20, 2014).
7. Humanitarian Assistance Training Inventory. http://www.reliefweb.int/Training/orgs.html or Aid Workers Network. http://www.aidworkers.net/personal/AATG.doc (Accessed June 20, 2014).
8. Australian Government Emergency Management. Education and Training Bulletin No. 6, Summer 2007.
9. Medecins Sans Frontieres. Refugee Health: An Approach to Emergency Situations, 1997. http://refbooks.msf.org/msf_docs/en/refugee_health/rh.pdf (Accessed December 12, 2014).
10. UNHCR Handbook for Emergencies. http://www.unhcr.org/partners/PARTNERS/472af2972.html (Accessed June 20, 2014).
11. Knowledge Center on Public Health and Disasters. PAHO and WHO. http://saludydesastres.info/index.php?lang=en (Accessed May 3, 2014).
12. Florez Trujillo J. Estudio sobre el estado de la enseñanza de la administración sanitaria de emergencia en casos de desastres, en las facultades de Medicina y Enfermería – Mayo 2003
13. On November 30, 2007, the 30th International Conference of the Red Cross and Red Crescent unanimously adopted the Guidelines for the domestic facilitation and regulation of international disaster relief and initial recovery assistance.
14. International Federation of Red Cross and Red Crescent Societies (IFRC). International Disaster Response Laws, Rules and Principles (IDRL) Project. http://www.ifrc.org/en/publications-and-reports/idrl-database/ (Accessed June 20, 2014).
15. International Health Relief Assistance – Recommendations Approved at the Meeting of International Health Relief Assistance in Latin America Pan American Health Organization (PAHO), San Jose, Costa Rica, March 1986.
16. de Ville de GC, Sarmiento JP, Grünewald F. *Health response to the earthquake in Haiti: January 2010.* Pan American Health Organization, Washington, DC, 2011. http://new.paho.org/disasters/dmdocuments/HealthResponseHaitiEarthq.pdf (Accessed April 21, 2014).
17. United Nations Resolution 42/169 of December 11, 1987, designating 1990–1999 as the International Decade for Natural Disaster Reduction. Proposed by Frank Press.
18. United Nations Resolution A/RES/44/236. 85th Plenary Meeting of December 22, 1989.
19. Boroschek KR, Retamales SR. *Guidelines for Vulnerability Reduction in the Design of New Health Facilities.* Washington, DC, Pan American Health Organization, 2004.
20. Concheso TG. *Protecting New Health Facilities from Natural Disasters: Guidelines for the Promotion of Disaster Mitigation.* Pan American Health Organization/World Bank, Washington, DC, 2003. http://www.mona.uwi.edu/cardin/virtual_library/docs/1228/1228.pdf (Accessed on August 16, 2015).
21. World Bank Global Facility for Disaster Reduction and Recovery. http://www.gfdrr.org. (Accessed December 12, 2008).
22. Natural and Unexpected Disasters Policy (OP-704). Inter-American Development Bank (IADB). http://www.iadb.org/en/topics/topics-in-latin-america-and-the-caribbean,1125.html (Accessed June 20, 2014).
23. Boroschek KR, Retamales SR. *Guidelines for Vulnerability Reduction in the Design of New Health Facilities.* Washington, DC, Pan American Health Organization, 2004.
24. Gibbs T, et al. *Mitigation: Disaster Mitigation Guidelines for Hospitals and Other Health Care Facilities in the Caribbean,* Washington, DC, Pan American Health Organization, 1992.

25. World Bank. Strengthening Essential Public Health Functions. http://wbi.worldbank.org/wbi/event/strengthening-essential-public-health-functions-web-based-course (Accessed December 12, 2014).

26. Pan American Health Organization. Hospital Safety Index. http://www.paho.org/english/dd/ped/Safe%20Hospital%20Checklist.pdf (Accessed June 20, 2014).

27. *Crisis Standards of Care: A Systems Framework for Catastrophic Disaster Response.* Institute of Medicine, The National Academies Press, Washington, DC, 2012. http://www.iom.edu/reports/2012/crisis-standards-of-care-a-systems-framework-for-catastrophic-disaster-response.aspx (Accessed April 21, 2014).

28. UN International Strategy for Disaster Reduction. Hospitals Safe from Disasters Campaign. http://www.unisdr.org/2009/campaign/wdrc-2008–2009.html (Accessed June 20, 2014).

29. Defining Disaster Resilience: A DFID Approach Paper. Department for International Development, United Kingdom. https://www.gov.uk/government/uploads/system/uploads/attachment_data/file/186874/defining-disaster-resilience-approach-paper.pdf (Accessed June 18, 2014).

30. World Health Organization. *Global Assessment of National Health Sector Emergency Preparedness and Response: Phase 1 Report.* Geneva, WHO, 2006.

31. CD47/34 Pan American Health Organization 47th Directing Council. July 31, 2006.

32. CD47/INF4 Pan American Health Organization 47th Directing Council. July 31, 2006.

33. *International Health Regulations.* 2nd ed. Geneva, World Health Organization, 2005. http://www.who.int/ihr/9789241596664/en/index.html (Accessed April 24, 2014).

34. Drury CA, Olson R. Disasters and political unrest: an empirical investigation. *J Continge Crisis Manage.* 1998; 6: 153–161. http://onlinelibrary.wiley.com/doi/10.1111/1468–5973.00084/pdf (Accessed December 12, 2014).

35. Selected National Library of Medicine Resources for Disaster Preparedness and Response. National Library of Medicine, Specialized Information Services. http://sis.nlm.nih.gov/pdf/nlmdisasterresources.pdf (Accessed June 20, 2014).

36. Knowledge Center on Public Health and Disasters. Pan American Health Organization and World Health Organization. http://www.saludydesastres.info/index.php?option=com_content&view=article&id=351:diplomado-gestion-para-la-reduccion-del-riesgo-a-desastres&catid=203:oferta-educativa&Itemid=776&lang=en. (Accessed April 30, 2014).

37. Regional Disaster Information Center. http://www.cridlac.org/ing_index.shtml (Accessed December 12, 2014).

38. Landstinget I Östergötland KMC. Personal communication; Huguenard P. Médecine de catastrophe: Commerce des Idées et Enseignement. *Médecine de Catastrophe Urgences Collectives* 1998; 1(2–3): 67–70.

39. Noji EK. Advances in Disaster Medicine. *Eur J Emerg Med.* 2002; 9: 185–191.

40. Fellowship in Emergency Medical Services/Disaster Medical Sciences. Department of Emergency Medicine, University of California Irvine School of Medicine. http://www.emergencymed.uci.edu/fellowships.asp (Accessed June 20, 2014).

41. Debacker M, Delooz H, Della Corte F. The European Master Program in Disaster Medicine. *Intl J Disaster Med.* 2003; 1: 35–41.

42. United Nations Cluster Approach. www.unocha.org/what-we-do/coordination/leadership/overview (Accessed December 12, 2014).

43. Resolution CSP28.R18 – Bioethics: Towards the Integration of Ethics in Health. The 28th Pan American Sanitary Conference, Pan American Health Organization and World Health Organization, Washington, DC, 2012. http://www.paho.org/hq/index.php?option=com_content&view=article&id=7022&Itemid=39541&lang=en (Accessed April 30, 2014).

44. UN Central Emergency Response Fund (CERF). http://ochaonline.un.org/Default.aspx?alias=ochaonline.un.org/cerf (Accessed November 3, 2008).

45. 60th World Health Assembly, WHA60.22, A60/VR/11, 2007.

46. Classification and Minimum Standards for Foreign Medical Teams in Sudden Onset Disasters. World Health Organization, 2013. http://www.who.int/hac/global_health_cluster/fmt_guidelines_september2013.pdf (Accessed June 20, 2013).

47. *Humanitarian Assistance in Disaster Situations: A Guide for Effective Aid.* Washington, DC, Pan American Health Organization, 2000. http://www1.paho.org/English/DD/PED/pedhum.htm (Accessed June 20, 2014).

48. Logistics Support System. http://www.lssweb.net/ (Accessed June 20, 2014).

49. Tsunami 2004: A Comprehensive Analysis (Volume I & II). World Health Organization, Regional Office for South-East Asia, 2013. http://www.searo.who.int/entity/emergencies/documents/tsunami_2009/en/ (Accessed June 19, 2014).

50. Disaster Law. International Federation of Red Cross and Red Crescent Societies. http://www.ifrc.org/what-we-do/idrl (Accessed May 2, 2014).

51. Global Assessment Report on Disaster Risk Reduction. United Nations International Strategy for Disaster Reduction, 2013. http://www.preventionweb.net/english/hyogo/gar/2013/en/home/index.html (Assessed June 19, 2014).

52. Protecting Health from Climate Change: Vulnerability and Adaptation Assessment. World Health Organization, 2013. http://www.who.int/globalchange/publications/vulnerability-adaptation/en/ (Assessed June 19, 2014).

53. Benchmarks, Standards, and Indicators for Emergency Preparedness and Response. World Health Organization, Regional Office for South East Asia, 2007. http://www.searo.who.int/entity/emergencies/topics/EHA_Benchmarks_Standards11_July_07.pdf?ua=1 (Accessed December 12, 2014).

54. Progress Report on National and Regional Health Disaster Preparedness and Response. CD47/34 Pan American Health Organization 47th Directing Council. Washington, DC, Pan American Health Organization, September 2006.

55. Terminology: Basic Terms of Disaster Risk Reduction. International Strategy for Disaster Reduction (ISDR). http://www.unisdr.org/we/inform/terminology (Accessed June 20, 2014).

56. Top Officials (TOPOFF). U.S. Department of State Archives. http://2001–2009.state.gov/s/ct/about/c16661.htm (Accessed December 12, 2014).

57. Inter-Agency Committee on Response to Nuclear Accidents: Exercise Report on International Emergency Response Exercise ConvEx-3. International Atomic Energy Agency, 2005. http://www-ns.iaea.org/downloads/iec/convex-3.pdf (Accessed June 20, 2014).

58. Delooz H, Debacker M, Moens G, Johannik K. European Survey on Training Objectives in Disaster Medicine. *Eur J Emerg Med.* 2007; 14: 25–31.

59. ISEE Interactive Simulation for Emergencies. Inovaria. https://www.inovaria.com/inovaria/?products=isee-interactive-simulation-for-emergencies&lang=en (Accessed December 12, 2014).

6

COMMUNITY RESILIENCE

Rose L. Pfefferbaum, Richard Reed, and Betty Pfefferbaum

OVERVIEW

Disaster managers embrace the concept of community resilience, sometimes as a strategy and sometimes as a vision. Community resilience both requires and supports effective disaster management. To promote community resilience and to improve its application in disaster medicine, this chapter explores the concept, then describes principles for building community resilience and currently available resources and programs, and finally offers recommendations for future research.

DEFINITION OF RESILIENCE

Multiple disciplines (e.g., computer science, ecology, economics, engineering, geography, health, physical science, psychology, sociology) define and use "resilience" in application to their specific, and sometimes unique, contexts and purposes. The term is used to describe individuals, materials, networks, ecosystems, and/or communities, all of which have relevance to disasters. For the purposes of this chapter, resilience is defined as "the process of successfully adapting to, and recovering from, adversity." While this definition has the advantage of being straightforward, it conceals some complexities that may be of importance to practitioners, policymakers, and researchers interested in assessing resilience and in generating and implementing evidence-based strategies to enhance it.

RESILIENCE AS AN EMERGENT PROCESS

Resilience is a process of adaptation and recovery that emerges in response to adversity. While some definitions characterize community resilience as an attribute or outcome, a process definition is used here. This distinguishes it from the attributes (e.g., ability, capacity) that characterize a resilient system, and from the outcome of adaptation and recovery. Norris et al. define resilience as "a process linking a set of adaptive capacities to a positive trajectory of functioning and adaptation after a disturbance"

(p. 130).[1] Thus, resilience emanates from adaptive capacities, which are resources with dynamic attributes, as described later in this chapter. Resilience leads to adaptation, an outcome characterized by wellness.

Resilience is not the absence of adversity, but successful progress in spite of, in the midst of, and in response to it.[2] A system may be resilient with respect to some adversities and not others, and it may respond differently to a given stressor at different times and differently to different stressors. Definitions of resilience as an attribute are likely to recognize that it can be affected by circumstances over time, thereby lending a dynamic quality to it.[3] Such descriptions, along with process definitions, realize that resilience can be influenced by a variety of determinants, an appreciation of which is important for those who seek to understand and build resilience.

DIFFERENCES BETWEEN PERSONAL RESILIENCE AND COMMUNITY RESILIENCE

Although similar definitions may apply, community resilience is not merely a collection of personally resilient individuals. The distinction, which is substantive, may be understood, in part, by recognizing that the whole is more than the sum of its parts.[4] Rather than a group of individuals acting independently on their own behalf, community resilience involves collective activity in which individuals work together in ways that support response and recovery for the whole. Brown and Kulig describe a community as requiring dynamic, interactive relations between members so that individuals "in communities are resilient together, not merely in similar ways" (p. 43).[5] Hence, a community of personally resilient individuals is not necessarily resilient.

In addition to inter-relational aspects in which individuals join together in support of the aggregate, community resilience requires physical and social conditions and structures that buttress individual and collective activity and facilitate the resilience process.[5–7] Medical, public health, and disaster medicine infrastructures are examples of systems that help create resilient communities by their attention to identifying, studying, preventing, and resolving threats and potential threats to individual and communal health. These infrastructures, as examples of systems that help create resilient communities, must also be resilient so that they continue to function during and after an event.

Just as personal resilience does not guarantee community resilience, community resilience does not guarantee personal resilience. Community resilience can strengthen the personal resilience of some, perhaps many, community members through systems that attend to behavioral and functional problems at the individual level.[6] This does not mean, however, that all members will adapt well to particular adversities. Indeed, in the case of disasters, it is unlikely that all members of a community will adapt well. Thus, communities may recover successfully even though some members do not. Communities may be resilient even when some members are not.

Resilient communities care for and support their members. Moreover, for many adversities in which survivors and other community members contribute to response and recovery efforts, the presence of personally resilient individuals benefits others in the community. Such contributions are less likely to be realized during a disaster that affects many members of the community since individuals may be forced by circumstances to focus primarily on themselves and their families, thereby leaving them with little to offer others. This scenario illustrates one way in which disasters can overwhelm a community. In such circumstances, a resilient community is aided by established linkages with external public and private sources of assistance.

THE ROLE OF HUMAN AGENCY

Community resilience reflects an ability to change and adapt[1,3,8] and, in the definition of some researchers, the potential to grow from a crisis.[5-7] Brown and Kulig[5] base the concept of community resilience in human agency, that is, in the capacity for people to take deliberate, meaningful actions. Community members must communicate effectively to interpret their environment and act together to heal in the aftermath of a crisis. Recovery results from individual and collective decisions and activities that potentially transform the environment to mitigate future adversities. Community resilience thus requires both proactive and reactive efforts.

PROPERTIES OF COMMUNITY RESILIENCE

Bruneau, Chang, et al.[9] describe four properties of resilience for physical and social systems: robustness, redundancy, resourcefulness, and rapidity. Robustness refers to strength or the ability of elements, resources, and systems to withstand stress without degradation or loss of function. Redundancy is the extent to which essential components are substitutable so that critical functional requirements can be met in the event of a crisis. Resourcefulness is the ability to identify problems, determine priorities, and mobilize resources in response to threats and disruptions. Resourcefulness also refers to the ability to use human and material resources to meet priorities and accomplish goals. Rapidity is the ability to meet priorities and reach goals in a timely manner to limit losses and prevent future disruption (Table 6.1).

Table 6.1. Community Resilience Properties, Attributes, and Adaptive Capacities

Properties[9]	Attributes[7]	Adaptive Capacities[1]
Robustness	Connectedness, Commitment, and Shared Values	Economic Development
Redundancy	Participation	Social Capital
Resourcefulness	Support and Nurturance	Information and Communication
Rapidity	Structure, Roles, and Responsibilities	Community Competence
	Resources	
	Critical Reflection and Skill Building	
	Communication	
	Disaster Management	

ATTRIBUTES OF RESILIENT COMMUNITIES

Pfefferbaum et al.[7] drew on community competence and capacity literatures[10-15] to describe eight attributes of community resilience. The eight attributes, which are described subsequently, are: 1) Connectedness, Commitment, and Shared Values; 2) Participation; 3) Support and Nurturance; 4) Structure, Roles, and Responsibilities; 5) Resources; 6) Critical Reflection and Skill Building; 7) Communication; and 8) Disaster Management (Table 6.1).

Connectedness, Commitment, and Shared Values. Connection to a group or a place characterized by shared history, laws, values, interests, and customs is the cornerstone of community. One's commitment and sense of belonging to a community are likely to be enhanced by the perception that personal well-being is improved by membership in the community and that members are treated fairly. Relationships of mutual concern and benefit can encourage cooperation and consensus building. Communities that support diverse members may be better able to address the plethora of needs that arise during and in the aftermath of disasters.

Participation. Participation in community organizations and activities can strengthen feelings of ownership and a sense of belonging, resulting in increased personal contribution and a commitment to safeguarding community well-being. When participation is valued and fostered, communities are likely to find their members more actively invested and engaged in civic roles. Communities that extend opportunities for involvement to diverse members in ways that are respectful and sensitive to their interests and demographics may be better able to identify and address concerns that arise during and after disasters.

Support and Nurturance. Supportive and nurturing communities attend to the needs of their members regardless of socioeconomic status, ethnicity, experience, education, and background. Such communities listen to and help members to overcome challenges and accomplish goals. They promote member well-being, empower individuals and groups, and instill hope. Communities that are adept at mobilizing and equitably allocating resources may be better able to provide support and nurturance. In resilient communities, support includes early and ongoing assessment of, and assistance to, potentially vulnerable members before, during, and in the aftermath of disasters. Support must be sustained if it is to buffer the personal, social, and economic losses that accompany crises.

Structure, Roles, and Responsibilities. Community structure, roles, and responsibilities must help create and support the capacity for mitigation of, as well as decisive and timely response to crises. Resilient communities reflect an appreciation for equity in establishing and applying community standards, rules, and procedures. Members must learn, and can teach each other, to navigate the complex reciprocal links and overlapping networks of individuals, groups, organizations, and agencies that exist within their community. In resilient communities, interactions are relatively frequent and supportive, with individuals and groups identifying and addressing common concerns. Associations that arise, formally or informally, to establish priorities and resolve issues give rise to solutions. Responsive and effective leadership; teamwork; clear organizational structures; and well-defined roles, responsibilities, and lines of authority advance adaptation and recovery. In a highly uncertain, all-hazard environment, structural elements (e.g., emergency management and medical systems) must permit sufficient flexibility to address unforeseen threats and vulnerabilities. Communities also must manage relations with the larger society.

Resources. A community's resources include natural, physical, financial, human, and social assets belonging to individual members as well as those attached to the community itself. In addition to land and other raw materials, resources include existing infrastructure and machinery and tools for production. Money and credit are financial resources that facilitate the acquisition of other resources, the production and distribution of goods and services, and exchange within and across communities. Human resources include a workforce, skills and expertise, and leadership, along with member qualities such as hope, work ethic, and the will to improve personal and community well-being. Relationships and support systems within a community and characteristics such as cohesion and collaboration constitute social resources. Community resources may be augmented after a disaster by an infusion of resources from other communities (through, e.g., mutual aid agreements in which emergency assistance is made available across jurisdictional boundaries) and from the larger society, domestically and internationally. Resilient communities acquire, mobilize, allocate, invest in, and utilize resources effectively to serve members and meet community goals. Resources can substitute for and complement each other. Redundancy in critical resources can help maintain essential functions. Ongoing investment in physical, human, and social capital – such as improvements in health facilities, job training, and neighborhood development – may be necessary to create infrastructures and systems that can endure and respond to a wide variety of potential disasters and threats.

Critical Reflection and Skill Building. Resilient communities identify and address local issues, needs, and problems; establish structures to collect, analyze, and use information; recognize and frame collective experiences; and plan, manage, and evaluate programs. Critical reflection about values, community history and experiences, and the experiences of others can help informal and formal community leaders to reason, problem solve, set goals and objectives, and develop and implement strategies for the benefit of the community and its members. Resilient communities evaluate their performance, study their successes and failures, and learn from adversity. They also support skill building at individual and systemic levels. Learning, accommodation, and growth can lead to enhanced capacity and improved disaster resilience.

Communication. Clear, timely, accurate, and effective communication among community members, between authorities and community residents, and with other communities and the larger society is essential for community resilience. To be productive, communication must be based on common meanings and must be perceived to be honest and transparent. All community members and groups should have opportunities to identify and express their views and their needs, and they should be encouraged to participate in community problem-solving, especially so that diversity is embraced. Effective communication fosters trust in leadership, promotes preparedness, increases the likelihood of compliance with disaster directives, facilitates effective response, and simplifies the resolution of existing and emerging unmet needs as well as those arising from disasters. Disaster resilience depends on sufficient redundancy in communication channels to ensure timely resource mobilization and deployment.

Disaster Management. Measures to mitigate, prepare for, and respond to disasters, which limit adverse consequences and set the stage for reconstruction and recovery, are necessary for community resilience. Prevention and mitigation include activities to avoid or control an incident, to reduce risks to people and property, and to lessen actual or potential adverse effects of an incident. Implemented prior to, during, or after an incident, mitigation measures focus on decreasing the likelihood of hazardous incidents and reducing exposure to, or potential loss from, such events. Preparedness is a continuous process that assesses threats, identifies vulnerabilities, determines resource requirements, and amasses resources for response and recovery. Disaster response relates to activities that occur as soon as feasible after an incident. Along with emergency assistance, response includes efforts to limit further damage during and immediately after a disaster; support basic human needs; and maintain the social, economic, and political structure of the affected community. The relatively short-term response phase transitions to a longer period of recovery and reconstruction during which survivors begin to rebuild their lives and their community.

ADAPTIVE CAPACITIES

Norris and colleagues[1] describe a set of four primary adaptive capacities (resilience resources) from which community resilience emerges: Economic Development, Social Capital, Information and Communication, and Community Competence (Table 6.1). Resilience depends on these four resources and their dynamic attributes, which are described by three of the properties identified by Bruneau and colleagues:[9] robustness, redundancy, and rapidity. Resilience can fail when adaptive capacities are damaged or disrupted by a stressor. Public health and disaster medicine systems contribute to the adaptive capacities of communities to the extent that they establish conditions necessary for the health and wellness of community members through personal and community mitigation, preparedness, response, and recovery programs and services.

Economic Development. As an adaptive capacity, economic development involves the volume and diversity of economic resources (e.g., raw materials; machinery, tools, and equipment; physical infrastructure; service systems; labor force) and equity in resource distribution. Poor and developing communities are not only at greater risk for destruction, they often are less successful in mobilizing support during and in the aftermath of a disaster. Community resilience is directly influenced by the ability to distribute resources to those most in need post disaster.[1]

Social Capital. Social capital can be defined as the collection of resources, both actual and potential, that are needed for a durable network of relationships.[1,16] As an adaptive capacity, social capital involves network structures and linkages; social support; and community roots, bonds, and commitments. Network structures and linkages include overlapping, inter-organizational systems with reciprocal links, frequent supportive interactions, and processes for cooperative decision making.[1,13] Social support includes social interactions that provide assistance (received or delivered social support) and those that are expected to provide assistance when the need for it arises (perceived or expected social support). Community roots, bonds, and commitment involve place attachment (i.e., an emotional connection to one's community), a sense of community involving feelings of trust and belonging, and citizen participation in formal organizations and grassroots leadership.[1]

Information and Communication. A communication infrastructure, including the media, is an important element of this adaptive capacity since information and communication are necessary for effective emergency management. Longstaff[8] argues that a trusted source of accurate information is an individual's or group's most important resilience asset. Communal narratives, which give shared meaning to a disaster, also are a beneficial element of the information and communication resource.[1]

Community Competence. Community competence involves collective action and decision making, which may stem from collective efficacy and empowerment. Collective efficacy depends on mutual trust and willingness to work toward the common good.[1] Cottrell[10] describes a competent community as one in which various community components collaborate effectively to identify community problems and needs; reach a working consensus on goals and priorities; agree about how to implement these goals; and take effective, collaborative action.

CHARACTERISTICS OF SAFE AND RESILIENT COMMUNITIES

An International Federation of Red Cross and Red Crescent Societies (IFRC)[17] study of its community-based disaster risk reduction programs[18] identifies community perceptions of characteristics required of safe and resilient communities. The six characteristics embody many of the attributes and adaptive capacities described in the previous section. Safe and resilient communities:

1) are knowledgeable and healthy. Safe and resilient communities are able to assess, manage, and monitor their risks. They can learn from past experiences and develop new skills.
2) are organized. Safe and resilient communities have the capacity to identify problems, set priorities, and take action.
3) are connected. Safe and resilient communities have relationships with external sources of support that can supply goods, services, and technical assistance when needed.

4) have infrastructure and services. Safe and resilient communities have strong housing, transportation, power, water, and sanitation systems and the ability to maintain, repair, and renovate them.
5) offer economic opportunities. Safe and resilient communities offer a diverse range of employment opportunities and have diverse income and financial services. These communities are flexible, resourceful, and able to accept uncertainty and respond proactively to change.
6) are able to manage their natural resources and other environmental assets. Safe and resilient communities recognize the value of these assets, and they can protect, enhance, and maintain them.

STATE OF THE ART

As both a vision and a strategy for disaster management, community resilience has captured the attention of community leaders, emergency managers, policymakers, and researchers. This has resulted in the availability of resources and programs to assess and promote community resilience. Principles for enhancing community resilience and examples of current resources and programs are described.

PRINCIPLES

Ultimately, community resilience emanates from the engagement and collective action of the units (e.g., individuals, families, groups, organizations) comprising a community. Ideally, the development and application of resources, strategies, and programs to build community resilience are guided by underlying principles drawn from research and practice. Fundamental among these principles is an all-hazard approach with attention to the local context that is necessitated by the inherent variation among communities across many dimensions. Other supporting principles involve community engagement, bioethical duties, assessment, asset-based approaches, and attention to skill development and personal resilience.

Community engagement. Community resilience requires the participation of individuals and organizations that reflect the diversity of the community. Public engagement efforts should identify and enlist traditionally underrepresented and underserved populations as well as those in the mainstream. Marginalized individuals or groups may have unexpected perceptions of the relevant roles and responsibilities that support a community's structure and operations, they may ask fresh questions, and they may bring new insight and energy to the process.[19] Resilience-building efforts should seek to create and bolster connections among constituents. Insofar as feasible, community members and organizations should be empowered to act in the interest of the community.

Bioethical duties. Bioethical principles derive from a system of values regarding relations among individuals. These principles establish obligations for professional and organizational behavior and for research with human subjects. While these principles sometimes give conflicting guidance in a disaster setting, as with all aspects of emergency management, they should be upheld to the extent possible in the development and implementation of activities that build community resilience. The principle of autonomy (respect for persons) requires that individuals be respected, that they be treated as autonomous agents, and that those with diminished autonomy be protected. The principle of beneficence requires contributions to the welfare of others and that interventions be designed to protect people from harm and promote their well-being. When that is not possible, the principle of non-maleficence demands that no harm be done. The principle of justice establishes a duty to be fair, particularly when imposing burdens and allocating benefits. Distributive justice requires an equitable allocation of scarce resources. Other ethical principles (e.g., the principle of fidelity, which requires faithfulness and that one keep promises) establish additional duties for professionals and organizations involved in community resilience work.[20]

Community assessment. Efforts to enhance community resilience should be based on an assessment that identifies the community's assets and challenges and its specific vulnerabilities and threats related to disasters and other potential crises. Information from community members and organizations with knowledge of their locality, relationships, and networks can be particularly useful in understanding the local context and dynamics that support or limit disaster resilience. This information should be augmented with risk assessment data, often available through official emergency management agencies. Other sources of information include studies conducted by foundations, newspapers, universities, and other agencies and organizations in the public and private sectors.

Asset-based approaches. Asset-based community development contributes to community resilience. Kretzmann and McKnight[19] recommend asset-based approaches as an alternate to traditional needs-driven approaches to community development. They maintain that needs-based approaches teach people about their problems, encourage reliance on services and resources that may need to be imported from outside the community, and foster a perception of oneself as a consumer rather than a producer. Used in conjunction with needs-based approaches or as an alternate to them, asset-based development identifies, links, and capitalizes on the capacities, skills, and strengths of individuals and their neighborhoods. A community is enriched and becomes more self-reliant when residents work with each other to address problems and when organizations collaborate to take collective action.

Skill development. In the process of community development, community resilience activities should help cultivate and exercise local skills and personal resilience among community members. Leadership, team building, and risk management skills can be important ingredients, as well as potential byproducts, of community resilience efforts. Creating a consciousness of community resilience (e.g., as part of processes that define and develop community resilience such as those described later in the chapter) also can be beneficial by galvanizing community members and organizations, highlighting shared values, focusing on critical reflection and skill development, and reinforcing the belief that resilience must be sustained over time and across adversities.[7]

PROCESSES

A number of processes (such as those described in handbooks and toolkits[21-25]) are available to assist communities in assessing and building disaster resilience. Three of these[23-25] described here can be implemented in communities of any size and level of economic development and have the potential for global application. Two additional processes[21,22] described here are designed for rural communities but have broader applicability.

Making Cities Resilient Campaign. The United Nations International Strategy for Disaster Reduction (UNISDR)[26] launched its Making Cities Resilient: My City is Getting Ready! Campaign in May 2010 to help local governments (subnational administrations of various sizes and hierarchical levels such as cities, municipalities, townships, and villages) to address disaster risk reduction.[27] As of August 2012, 1,050 local governments worldwide had enrolled in the campaign and pledged to take steps to improve disaster resilience. Twenty-nine of these governments, recognized as role models in disaster risk management and reduction, share best practices in the UNISDR *Making Cities Resilient Report 2012.*[28] The UNISDR *Handbook for Local Government Leaders*[25] provides an overview of key strategies and actions needed to build disaster resilience as part of a broader strategy to achieve sustainable development. It presents a checklist of ten essential requirements for making cities resilient and identifies steps for implementing them. The UNISDR Handbook also includes a Local Government Self-Assessment Tool to assist local governments in establishing baselines, identifying gaps, undertaking action planning, and measuring advancements over time. The UNISDR assessment is implemented by local government and involves multiple stakeholders (e.g., citizen groups, nongovernmental and community-based organizations, businesses, local academia). Governing authorities can use their findings when setting priorities and making budgetary decisions. The results can be recorded in a UNISDR web-based system, thus enriching the Making Cities Resilient Campaign's online profile of local governments.

The Community Resilience Strategy (CRS). CRS[23] is an approach developed by the American Red Cross[29] that empowers societies to build disaster resilience by becoming connected, problem-solving, prepared communities. These communities are characterized by strengthened relationships and linkages between and across sectors, the ability of stakeholders to work together, and the capacity to manage all phases of the disaster cycle. The CRS process, which is cyclical, flexible, and participatory, makes community preparedness a community-led responsibility that uses existing local capabilities and resources and identifies external resources as necessary. The CRS process consists of four phases: Understanding the Community, Crafting Solutions and Taking Action Together, Monitoring Progress, and Reassessing Goals and Moving Forward. A lead agency (e.g., a local Red Cross Chapter) guides networks of community stakeholders through the process to identify, prioritize, and act on preparedness issues. The lead agency also provides expertise, resources, and support as needed. A guidebook[23] details the four phases, explains how to implement them, provides tools, and shares case studies and best practices. Results of five CRS pilot studies, conducted from July 2011 through October 2012, indicate success of the strategy in developing active community networks capable of implementing resilience-enhancing activities.

The Communities Advancing Resilience Toolkit (CART). Created by the TDC[30] of the NCTSN[31] in the United States, CART[24,32,33] is a community-driven, publicly available, theory-based, and evidence-informed community intervention. Designed for use by community-based organizations and/or affiliated volunteer responder teams, the CART process engages community stakeholders in collecting and using assessment data to develop and implement strategies for building community resilience. The online version of CART[24] includes the rationale, instructions, templates, and a discussion of special considerations for using a variety of CART instruments. Instruments include a field-tested assessment survey questionnaire, key informant interviews, community conversations, neighborhood infrastructure maps, community ecological maps, stakeholder analysis, and capacity and vulnerability assessments. Research conducted in the development of CART[32] identified four interrelated, overlapping domains that both reflect and contribute to community resilience: 1) Connection and Caring (including relatedness, participation, shared values, support and nurturance, equity, justice, hope, and diversity); 2) Resources (including natural, physical, information, human, social, and financial resources); 3) Transformative Potential (deriving from the ability of communities to frame collective experiences, collect and analyze relevant data, assess community performance, and build skills); and 4) Disaster Management (including prevention and mitigation, preparedness, response, and recovery). The primary value of CART lies in its ability to stimulate analysis, collaboration, skill building, resource sharing, and purposeful action and to advance community participation, communication, self-awareness, cooperation, and critical reflection.

The Community Resilience Project. The Community Resilience Project of the Canadian Centre for Community Renewal[34] was the impetus for the development of a model of community resilience, a process to guide application of the model, and manuals to facilitate implementation of the process. Although specifically designed for small, economically-distressed towns, these resources also are appropriate for other communities seeking to assess and build their resilience. The community resilience model used in this project addresses four interrelated dimensions (people, organizations, resources, and community process, which consists of approaches and structures for organizing and using resources) detailed in terms of twenty-three characteristics that form the basis for assessment. The process involves four steps to be undertaken locally: 1) presenting the model and creating an organizational structure for implementation; 2) assessing community resilience; 3) setting community priorities; and 4) planning to strengthen selected priorities. *The Community Resilience Manual: A Resource for Rural Recovery & Renewal*[21] describes the community resilience model, explains the field-tested process for implementing it, and provides worksheets (with tools, forms, and other resources) to support execution of the process. A companion manual, *Tools & Techniques for Community Recovery & Renewal*,[35] is a catalog of methods for community economic development organized around five topics: planning, research, and advocacy; human resources; jobs; financial gaps; and special sectors. Each catalog entry includes a description of the method, its benefits and challenges, practical steps for implementation, and useful resource organizations and publications.

Building Resilience in Rural Communities: Toolkit. An outcome of a three-year research project to develop, implement, and evaluate a model for enhancing psychological wellness in rural people and communities,[36] the *Building Resilience in Rural Communities: Toolkit*[22] provides information and ideas for enhancing personal, group, and community resilience. The toolkit can be used by program coordinators (e.g., social workers, health professionals) and community leaders to introduce resilience into existing social programs, to develop new programs, and

as part of workshops. The toolkit is organized around eleven resilience factors (referred to as resilience concepts): Social Networks and Support, Positive Outlook, Learning, Early Experience, Environment and Lifestyle, Infrastructure and Support Services, Sense of Purpose, Diverse and Innovative Economy, Embracing Differences, Beliefs, and Leadership. Information sheets for each factor explain the concept, pose basic questions for consideration, offer constructive ideas for enhancing resilience, describe case studies, present a community perspective, and provide a brief literature review. While developed with and for a rural Australian community, the toolkit is applicable in many settings.

COMMUNITY-BASED ACTIVITIES

In addition to efforts designed specifically to address community resilience, programs developed for other purposes may enhance community resilience. Many community development activities, by their very nature, contribute to community health and capacity and, thus, resilience. Local disaster management and relief programs also contribute to community resilience. Among these are programs that support local affiliated volunteer responder teams such as Community Emergency Teams in Israel[37] and Community Emergency Response Teams in the United States.[38]

Local affiliated volunteer responder teams are neighborhood (or business) based with membership trained in personal and community preparedness and response. Teams learn about a variety of hazards that may affect their local area, and they acquire and practice disaster response skills (e.g., light search and rescue, basic disaster medical operations, psychological first aid, teamwork). Teams help organize their neighborhoods in advance of disasters and, after a community crisis, they respond before official responders arrive and assist official responders once they arrive on the scene. Ideally, team members continue to learn and work together over time. Affiliation, organizational structure, and specific functions vary across programs. To be most effective, team membership should reflect the diversity of the neighborhood, roles should be established in conjunction with official responders and respected by community members, and teams should be supported to help prevent burnout.[37,38]

INTERNATIONAL ORGANIZATIONAL SUPPORT FOR COMMUNITY RESILIENCE

A number of organizations support the development of disaster resilient communities on a global basis. These include IFRC[17] through many community-based disaster risk reduction programs worldwide, UNISDR[26] through its Making Cities Resilient Campaign,[27] and the World Resources Institute[39] through research and action related to the environment and socioeconomic development. The Global Platform for Disaster Reduction,[40] organized by UNISDR[26] and first convened in 2007, is a major international, biennial forum that seeks to advance disaster risk reduction and community resilience through improved stakeholder communication and coordination. The Chair's Summary of the Fourth Session of the Global Platform,[41] held in Geneva, Switzerland, in May 2013, recognizes the importance of culturally sensitive approaches, inclusiveness, participation, and empowerment in building resilience.

RECOMMENDATIONS FOR FURTHER RESEARCH

Research on community resilience to disasters is in its infancy. Thus, the potential research agenda is substantial and complex. Some of the issues that demand attention parallel those of research in personal resilience, which has a much longer history. At the most basic level, there remain questions regarding the definition of resilience as a process, an attribute, an outcome, or some combination of these. Other challenges relate to assessment and measurement of community resilience; the context from which it emanates; its attributes and capacities; sustainment; and the development, implementation, and evaluation of interventions. Community-based research is one appropriate methodology for studying community resilience to disasters.

ASSESSMENT AND MEASUREMENT

There is much interest in measuring community resilience as a way of determining the status of communities. It is difficult to assign scores to communities that objectively describe their level of resilience in a dynamic, all-hazard environment. Nonetheless, quantification and measurement of aspects of community resilience are increasingly important for an understanding of the construct, for the creation of tools to build disaster resilience, and for the development and implementation of public policy directives. Thus, efforts to operationalize the concept of community resilience must progress even in the absence of a consensus regarding the definition and measurement of resilience. These efforts can proceed in tandem with, and will help guide, further analysis and the development of interventions.

Assessment and measurement can be facilitated by addressing relevant aspects of community resilience. For example, in discussing performance measures for community resilience with respect to earthquakes, Bruneau and colleagues[9] identify and suggest indicators for measuring four interrelated dimensions: 1) technical (concerning the ability of physical systems to meet acceptable performance standards when subjected to stress); 2) organizational (relating to the ability of organizations responsible for managing critical facilities and performing essential disaster-related functions to make decisions and act in ways that improve the four properties of robustness, redundancy, resourcefulness, and rapidity); 3) social (entailing measures designed to reduce adverse consequences due to the loss of critical services resulting from a disaster); and 4) economic (referring to the ability to limit direct and indirect economic losses associated with a disaster). Longstaff, Armstrong, Perrin, Parker, and Hidek[42] describe, and provide a framework for assessing, five subsystems: 1) ecological (the combined biological and physical elements of the environment); 2) economic (associated with the production, distribution, and consumption of goods and services); 3) physical infrastructure (including basic installations and facilities related to production); 4) civil society (referring to nongovernmental channels for social organization and action); and 5) governance (including public organizations and the processes and mandates of government). Sherrieb et al.[43] use survey results in an effort to measure adaptive capacities (Economic Development, Social Capital, Information and Communication, and Community Competence) in a sample of U.S. school principals. In assessing relevant aspects of community resilience (using a framework based on, e.g., interrelated dimensions,[9] subsystems,[42] or adaptive capacities[43] as described pre-viously), research should consider the relative importance of identified components within any specific framework, potential threshold levels, the consequences of limitations or failures in one or more of the components, and how to enhance the components.

CONTEXT

Community resilience can only be fully understood in context. Elements to consider include: the nature and scale of hazards, characteristics of the affected community, and the availability of aid and assistance. Future research is needed to address the many issues associated with context.

Nature and scale of hazards. While efforts to build community resilience typically take an all-hazard approach, it would be imprudent to assume that a community can be resilient to all of the great variety of adversities to which it is potentially exposed. Rather, a community's disaster resilience varies with respect to the nature and severity of events and the extent of disruption and destruction. As the severity of events and the associated disruption increase, the need for resilient responses increases and the ability to enact resilient responses becomes increasingly compromised.[44] Future research should address the importance of disaster type, scale, and duration in community resilience.

Community resource base and economic development. Given similar threats, poor communities that lack individual and communal resources, a solid economic base, and capable transitional leadership generally will be less able than better endowed communities to mount effective disaster management programs.[7] The problem is exacerbated for communities in countries struggling to develop economically. The World Resources Institute,[45] with its concern for socioeconomic development in the midst of climate change and other environmental challenges, argues that three essential elements are precursors to resourceful and resilient communities: 1) ownership (resulting from a foundation of governance that grants to the poor real authority over local resources and elicits efficient management of those resources); 2) capacity (the capacity to manage and leverage ecosystems competently and to equitably distribute the income from resulting ecosystem enterprises); and 3) connection (establishing adaptive networks that connect and support ecosystem enterprises so that they can learn, adapt, attach to markets, and become self-sustaining businesses). Case studies by the World Resources Institute provide insight into the "scaling up" of ecosystem enterprises, and they support recommended actions that government at all levels can take to address poverty and build resilience. Research is needed to more fully understand the difficulties of developing resilience in resource-poor communities.

Income and wealth inequalities. Communities characterized by significant inequalities in income and wealth may be at increased risk for adverse disaster effects. Cutter describes the "social vulnerability of communities" borne of inequalities (p. 3).[3] Impoverished segments of the population that live with danger and insecurity on a daily basis are particularly vulnerable to the destruction that accompanies disasters. Morrow[46] maintains that it is unreasonable to expect these population groups to anticipate and respond effectively to external threats without assistance. Norris and colleagues[1] recommend that economic and social resources, which are essential to disaster readiness and response, be acquired and shared to reduce risk and address the social vulnerability associated with disasters. Public policies and programs that address resource inequities within and across communities must be a feature of comprehensive local and national approaches for disaster-resilient communities within a disaster-resilient country. Such policies and programs are both practical and moral.[46] Future research should address the implications of inequality of income and wealth and effective ways to improve equity.

Availability of external assistance. The influence of aid and assistance in disaster response and recovery deserves attention. By definition, disasters overwhelm communities, creating the need for aid and assistance from the larger society. While some amount of aid and assistance may be essential, Aldrich maintains that "little systematic evidence connects greater levels of aid and assistance to better long-term recoveries" (p. 10).[47] Sizeable amounts of aid may, for example, complicate existing social relationships and undermine traditional social practices. Future research should investigate the importance of external assistance, including the influence of various forms of assistance (both positive and negative), in disaster response and recovery.

ATTRIBUTES AND CAPACITIES

Future research should examine the nature and function of various attributes, capacities, and domains associated with community resilience. This research should consider, for example, social capital; communication; roles, responsibilities, and accountability; leadership; and diversity.

Social capital. Aldrich[47] focuses on the role of social capital (the networks and resources available to people through their interpersonal connections) to explain the variation in disaster recovery across communities. Aldrich addresses three dimensions of social capital: bonding (which involves the bonds among community members), bridging (which connects community members to networks outside the local area extending beyond local identities), and linking (involving interactions across formal power centers). Social capital and its dimensions deserve further exploration. Bonding social capital, for example, potentially creates unintended negative consequences when identification and bonding of members within a group result in detrimental treatment of those outside the group such as might arise in the presence of racism, sexism, or ageism.[47]

Communication. Communication is an important ingredient in disaster resilience. It can foster connections among community members and organizations, and it is essential for effective disaster management and for the transmission of information that contributes to critical reflection, skill building, and transformation.[24] Considerable attention has been given to crisis and emergency risk communication. More research is needed to address issues associated with the role of communication in community resilience including, but not limited to, the influence, cost, and effectiveness of traditional and social media in resilience and resilience building.

Roles, responsibilities, and accountability. Individuals, families, organizations, businesses, and governments all play important roles that contribute to community resilience. Roles and responsibilities, which may vary across communities, provide a foundation for accountability. Future research should seek to better clarify and understand appropriate roles and responsibilities and how to improve responsibility and accountability among private and public stakeholders.

Leadership. Community resilience is inherently community-based. While there are benefits associated with community-driven developmental processes, there are also important roles for leadership. Research should explore multiple issues associated with leadership including informal versus formal leadership, public and private responsibilities, and leadership approaches for engaging and empowering community members.

Diversity. The role of diversity in community resilience deserves scrutiny. Resource diversity is generally considered to be beneficial, especially when it contributes to redundancy of critical functions.[42] The benefits of demographic diversity are less obvious. Whether demographically homogeneous communities recover more or less quickly and thoroughly than do diverse communities likely depends, in part, on community-specific demographics. Future research should consider benefits and costs of various types of diversity as well as how to support diverse community members.

SUSTAINING RESILIENCE

Resilience is not an endpoint but a process. Over time, existing problems evolve and new ones emerge, stakeholders change, and the resource base varies. While many communities have become involved in preparedness and resilience building, their efforts may be thwarted, in part, by a lack of attention to sustainability. Future research should address the complexities associated with sustaining disaster resilience.

DEVELOPMENT, IMPLEMENTATION, AND EVALUATION OF INTERVENTIONS

Further research is necessary to inform the development, implementation, and evaluation of interventions to enhance community resilience and to establish an evidence base for their use. An in-depth study by IFRC[18] of its response and recovery operation in the aftermath of the 2004 Indian Ocean tsunami supports the benefit of such research. Based on a review of programs implemented in 600 communities, the study identifies characteristics of safe and resilient communities and detects essential determinants of successful community-based disaster risk reduction programs. These key determinants relate to: 1) an enabling environment (motivation and capacity of the community and its leaders; motivation and capacity of stakeholders and the strength of partnerships between them; and the capacity of external contributors and the strength of partnerships with them); 2) program design (the level of community participation and ownership of the program; the level of program integration within other sectors; and an appropriate balance between flexibility and standardization in design); and 3) program management (sufficient time and funding to implement the program and adequate assessment, monitoring, and evaluation procedures).

COMMUNITY-BASED RESEARCH

In an otherwise complicated selection of research methodologies, community-based research is one appropriate approach for studying community resilience. As described by Israel, Schulz, Parker, and Becker,[48] community-based research: 1) acknowledges the community as a unit of identity; 2) identifies and builds on community assets including resources and relationships; 3) facilitates collaboration; 4) informs community action; 5) fosters individual and community empowerment; 6) involves a process that advances policy, action, and sustainability; 7) emphasizes physical, mental, and social well-being; and 8) provides feedback to the community.

CONCLUSION

Future research and practice in the development and assessment of community resilience will help elucidate the important properties, attributes, and capacities that characterize disaster resilience. Underlying principles (associated with a myriad of issues including an all-hazard approach, community engagement, bioethics, community assessment, asset-based approaches, and skill development) can guide research and the creation of programs and processes that contribute to effective disaster management and community resilience. Ultimately, the goal of both research and practice should be to encourage and support the ongoing work that communities must undertake in the process of becoming more resilient. An emphasis on *becoming* resilient highlights that community resilience is not an endpoint but an ongoing, dynamic process of adaptation and recovery in managing an ever-changing environment.

ACKNOWLEDGMENTS

This work was supported in part by the Terrorism and Disaster Center (TDC) located at the University of Oklahoma Health Sciences Center (OUHSC) in Oklahoma City, Oklahoma, a partner in the National Child Traumatic Stress Network (NCTSN), which is funded by the Substance Abuse and Mental Health Services Administration (SAMHSA), U.S. Department of Health and Human Services (HHS); by the National Consortium for the Study of Terrorism and Responses to Terrorism (START), located at the University of Maryland in College Park, Maryland, which is funded by the U.S. Department of Homeland Security (DHS); and by the U.S. Centers for Disease Control and Prevention (CDC), HHS.

The findings, conclusions, opinions, and contents of this chapter are those of the authors and do not represent the official position of NCTSN, SAMHSA, HHS, START, USDHS, CDC, or the American Red Cross.

REFERENCES

1. Norris FH, Stevens SP, Pfefferbaum B, Wyche KF, Pfefferbaum RL. Community resilience as a metaphor, theory, set of capacities, and strategy for disaster readiness. *Am J Community Psychol* 2008; 41: 127–150.
2. Pfefferbaum B, Pfefferbaum RL, Norris F. Community resilience and wellness for children exposed to Hurricane Katrina. In: Kilmer RP, Gil-Rivas V, Tedeschi RG, Calhoun LG, eds. *Helping Families and Communities Recover from Disaster: Lessons Learned from Hurricane Katrina and Its Aftermath*. Washington, DC, American Psychological Association. 2010; 265–288.
3. Cutter SL, Barnes L, Berry M, Burton C, Evans E, Tate E, Webb J. Community and Regional Resilience: Perspectives from Hazards, Disasters, and Emergency Management. Oak Ridge,

TN, Community and Regional Resilience Initiative (CARRI), National Security Directorate, Oak Ridge National Laboratory. CARRI Research Report 1. September 2008. http://www.resilientus.org/publications/research-reports (Accessed June 16, 2013).
4. Ross WD, trans. *Metaphysics by Aristotle*. Adelaide, University of Adelaide Library, 2007. http://ebooks.adelaide.edu.au/a/aristotle/metaphysics/index.html (Accessed June 21, 2013).
5. Brown DD, Kulig JC. The concept of resiliency: Theoretical lessons from community research. *Health Can Soc* 1996–1997; 4(1): 29–50.
6. Pfefferbaum B, Reissman DB, Pfefferbaum RL, Klomp RW, Gurwitch RH. Building resilience to mass trauma events. In: Doll LS, Bonzo SE, Mercy JA, Sleet DA, Haas EN, eds. *Handbook of Injury and Violence Prevention*. New York, Springer, 2007; 347–358.
7. Pfefferbaum RL, Reissman DB, Pfefferbaum B, Wyche KF, Norris FH, Klomp RW. Factors in the development of community resilience to disasters. In: Blumenfield M, Ursano RJ, eds. *Intervention and Resilience after Mass Trauma*. Cambridge, Cambridge University Press, 2008; 49–68.
8. Longstaff PH. Security, Resilience, and Communication in Unpredictable Environments Such as Terrorism, Natural Disasters, and Complex Technology. Cambridge, MA, Program on Information Resources Policy. November 2005. http://www.pirp.harvard.edu/pubs'pdf/longsta/longsta-p05-3.pdf (Accessed August 7, 2015).
9. Bruneau M, Chang SE, Eguchi RT, et al. A framework to quantitatively assess and enhance the seismic resilience of communities. *Earthquake Spectra* 2003; 19(4): 733–752.
10. Cottrell LS, Jr. The competent community. In: Kaplan BH, Wilson RN, Leighton AH, eds. *Further Explorations in Social Psychiatry*. New York, Basic Books, Inc, 1976; 195–209.
11. Gibbon M, Labonte R, Laverack G. Evaluating community capacity. *Health Soc Care Community* 2002; 10(6): 485–491.
12. Goeppinger J, Baglioni AJ, Jr. Community competence: A positive approach to needs assessment. *Am J Community Psychol* 1985; 13(5): 507–523.
13. Goodman RM, Speers MA, McLeroy K, et al. Identifying and defining the dimensions of community capacity to provide a basis for measurement. *Health Educ Behav* 1998; 25(3): 258–278.
14. Labonte R, Laverack G. Capacity building in health promotion, Part 1: for whom? And for what purpose? *Crit Public Health* 2001; 11(2): 111–127.
15. Labonte R, Laverack G. Capacity building in health promotion, Part 2: whose use? And with what measurement? *Crit Public Health* 2001; 11(2): 129–138.
16. Bourdieu P. The forms of capital. In: Richardson J, ed. *Handbook of Theory and Research for the Sociology of Education*. New York, Greenwood, 1986; 241–258. http://www.marxists.org/reference/subject/philosophy/works/fr/bourdieu-forms-capital.htm (Accessed June 16, 2013).
17. International Federation of Red Cross and Red Crescent Societies. Geneva, Switzerland, International Federation of Red Cross and Red Crescent Societies, c2013. http://www.ifrc.org (Accessed June 22, 2013).
18. International Federation of Red Cross and Red Crescent Societies. Understanding Community Resilience and Program Factors that Strengthen Them: A Comprehensive Study of Red Cross and Red Crescent Societies Tsunami Operation. Geneva, Switzerland, International Federation of Red Cross and Red Crescent Societies, June 2012. http://www.ifrc.org/PageFiles/96984/Final_Synthesis_Characteristics_Lessons_Tsunami.pdf (Accessed June 22, 2013).

19. Kretzmann JP, McKnight JL. *Building Communities from the Inside Out: A Path Toward Finding and Mobilizing a Community's Assets.* Chicago, ACTA Publications, 1993.

20. Beauchamp TL, Childress JF. *Principles of Biomedical Ethics.* 7th ed. New York, Oxford University Press, 2012.

21. Colussi MM. The Community Resilience Manual: A Resource for Rural Recovery & Renewal. Port Alberni, BC, Canada, Canadian Centre for Community Renewal, 2000. http://communityrenewal.ca/community-resilience-manual (Accessed July 26, 2013).

22. Hegney D, Ross H, Baker P, et al. Building Resilience in Rural Communities: Toolkit. Toowoomba, Australia, University of Southern Queensland, Centre for Rural and Remote Area Health, 2008. http://www.usq.edu.au/bluecare/docs/toolkit_v5.pdf (Accessed August 7, 2015).

23. Herbst K, Yannacci J. *Guidebook on Creating Resilience Networks.* Washington, DC, The American National Red Cross, 2013.

24. Pfefferbaum RL, Pfefferbaum B, Van Horn RL. Communities Advancing Resilience Toolkit (CART)©. Oklahoma City, Terrorism and Disaster Center, University of Oklahoma Health Sciences Center, 2011; May 2013 (revised). http://www.oumedicine.com/psychiatry/research/terrorism-and-disaster-center/interventions/community-resilience-(cr) (Accessed July 26, 2013).

25. United Nations International Strategy for Disaster Reduction (UNISDR). How to Make Cities More Resilient: A Handbook for Local Government Leaders. Geneva, Switzerland, United Nations International Strategy for Disaster Reduction, March 2012. http://www.unisdr.org/campaign/resilientcities/toolkit/handbook (Accessed June 22, 2013).

26. UNISDR. Geneva, Switzerland, United Nations Office for Disaster Risk Reduction. http://www.unisdr.org (Accessed July 22, 2013).

27. UNISDR. Making Cities Resilient: My City is Getting Ready. Geneva, United Nations International Strategy for Disaster Reduction, c2012. http://www.unisdr.org/campaign/resilientcities (Accessed June 22, 2013).

28. UNISDR. Making Cities Resilient Report 2012. My City is Getting Ready. A Global Snapshot of How Local Governments Reduce Disaster Risk. 2nd ed. Geneva, United Nations International Strategy for Disaster Reduction, October 2012. http://www.unisdr.org/campaign/resilientcities/toolkit/report2012 (Accessed June 22, 2013).

29. American Red Cross. Washington, DC, The American Red Cross, c2013. http://www.redcross.org (Accessed June 22, 2013).

30. Terrorism and Disaster Center. Oklahoma City, OK, Terrorism and Disaster Center, University of Oklahoma Health Sciences Center, c2013. www.oumedicine.com/tdc (Accessed June 22, 2013).

31. National Child Traumatic Stress Network. Los Angeles, CA, National Center for Child Traumatic Stress. http://www.nctsn.org (Accessed June 22, 2013).

32. Pfefferbaum RL, Pfefferbaum B, Van Horn RL, Klomp RW, Norris FH, Reissman DB. The Communities Advancing Resilience Toolkit (CART): An intervention to build community resilience to disasters. *J Public Health Manag Pract* 2013; 19(3): 250–258.

33. Pfefferbaum RL, Pfefferbaum B, Van Horn RL, Neas BR, Houston JB. Building community resilience to disasters through a community-based intervention: CART© applications. *J Emerg Manag* 2013; 11(2): 151–159.

34. Canadian Centre for Community Renewal (CCCR). Port Alberni, BC, Canada, c2011. http://communityrenewal.ca (Accessed July 22, 2013).

35. Perry SE. Tools & Techniques for Community Recovery and Renewal. Port Alberni, BC, Canada, The Centre for Community Enterprise, 2000. http://communityrenewal.ca/tools-and-techniques (Accessed July 21, 2013).

36. Hegney D, Ross H, Baker P, et al. Identification of personal and community resilience that enhance psychological wellness: A Stanthorpe study. Toowoomba, Australia, University of Southern Queensland, Centre for Rural and Remote Area Health, 2008. http://www.uq.edu.au/bluecare/identifying-models-of-personal-and-community-resilience-that-enhance-psychological-wellness-a-stanthorpe-study (Accessed August 7, 2015).

37. Lahad M, Nesher UB. Community coping: Resilience models for preparation, intervention and rehabilitation in manmade and natural disasters. In: Gow K, Paton D, eds. *Phoenix of Natural Disasters: Community Resilience.* New York, Nova Science Publishers, Inc, 2008; 195–208.

38. Federal Emergency Management Agency (FEMA). Community Emergency Response Teams. Washington, DC, USA, FEMA, DHS. http://www.fema.gov/community-emergency-response-teams (Accessed June 22, 2013).

39. World Resources Institute (WRI). Working at the Intersection of Environment and Human Need. Washington, DC, USA, World Resources Institute. http://www.wri.org (Accessed June 22, 2013).

40. Global Platform for Disaster Reduction. Geneva, Switzerland, UNISDR. http://www.preventionweb.net/globalplatform/2013 (Accessed July 22, 2013).

41. Dahinden M. Chair's Summary. Presented at: Global Platform for Disaster Risk Reduction, Fourth Session. Geneva, Switzerland, May 19–23, 2013. http://www.preventionweb.net/files/33306_finalchairssummaryoffourthsessionof.pdf (Accessed July 20, 2013).

42. Longstaff PH, Armstrong NJ, Perrin K, Parker WM, Hidek MA. Building resilient communities: Preliminary framework for assessment. *Homeland Security Affairs* September 2010; VI(3): 1–23. http://www.hsaj.org/?article=6.3.6 (Accessed June 24, 2013).

43. Sherrieb K, Louis CA, Pfefferbaum RL, Pfefferbaum B, Diab E, Norris FH. Assessing community resilience on the US coast using school principals as key informants. *Int J Disaster Risk Reduction* 2012; 2: 6–15.

44. Tierney K. Disaster Response: Research Findings and Their Implications for Resilience Measurement. Oak Ridge, TN, CARRI, National Security Directorate, Oak Ridge National Laboratory. CARRI Research Report 6. March 2009. http://www.resilientus.org/publications/research-reports (Accessed June 25, 2013).

45. WRI, in collaboration with United Nations Development Programme, United Nations Environment Programme, and World Bank. World Resources 2008: Roots of Resilience–Growing the Wealth of the Poor. Washington, DC, WRI, 2008. http://pdf.wri.org/world_resources_2008_roots_of_resilience.pdf (Accessed June 22, 2013).

46. Morrow BH. Community Resilience: A Social Justice Perspective. Oak Ridge, TN, CARRI, National Security Directorate, Oak Ridge National Laboratory. CARRI Research Report 4. September 2008. http://www.resilientus.org/publications/research-reports (Accessed June 22, 2013).

47. Aldrich DP. *Building Resilience: Social Capital in Post-Disaster Recovery.* Chicago, University of Chicago Press, 2012.

48. Israel BA, Schulz AJ, Parker EA, Becker AB. Review of community-based research: Assessing partnership approaches to improve public health. *Annu Rev Public Health* 1998; 19: 173–202.

7

ETHICAL ISSUES IN DISASTER MEDICINE

George J. Annas

OVERVIEW

Disasters are exceptional occurrences. Responders are frequently required to make decisions in extreme circumstances with limited resources and information. Such situations are very different from the usual, day-to-day practice of medicine and healthcare, and it often seems that ethics has little applicability to such catastrophes. As will be explored in this chapter, however, ethics is at the core of all healthcare decisions in disasters. This should not be surprising, and is explained by two primary propositions. The first is that while any particular disaster and its response may be unique, it follows the experiences of previous disasters, and the knowledge gained from them. The second is that the victims of disasters are all human beings, and basic ethical principles apply to healthcare decision making for all people, including equality and fairness. How these principles are applied may vary from one disaster to another, but the ethical and human rights principles remain constant.[1]

War and plagues have historically produced the largest number of human fatalities and provided the greatest challenges to human survival. It is within these contexts that the bulk of applied ethics in disaster medicine has been developed. More recently, the tactic of terrorism has taken center stage, as have a variety of environmental disasters including earthquakes, hurricanes, and floods. This chapter will draw on all of these examples to help illustrate basic ethical and human rights principles that should help guide physicians when responding to disasters. Principles spelled out in humanitarian law and international human rights law provide a solid foundation on which to build an ethical framework for medical response to disasters.

STATE OF THE ART

Theories of Medical Ethics

Theories of medical ethics have been constructed almost exclusively around the physician-patient relationship in the context of a normal peacetime setting, in which resources are not severely constrained.[2] That is why the focus has generally been on patient autonomy and the doctrine of informed consent. Physicians, at

least since Hippocrates, were enjoined to "do no harm," and also to act in a manner consistent with the best interests of the patient. Only later did the patient's role expand to that of a co-equal decision-maker. Under the doctrine of informed consent, physicians are required to provide the patient with information not just regarding the recommended treatment, but also available alternatives, and their associated risks and benefits. In all circumstances, patients retain the right to refuse any medical treatment.[3] These basic principles apply to disaster medicine, although the circumstances will change the manner in which they are applied. In routine medical practice, for example, it has become common to use consent forms to summarize information presented to patients in the informed consent process, and have the patient sign this form. This will be impossible in many disasters, and even the oral presentation of alternatives (sometimes as stark as amputation or death) will likely be truncated. The ethical obligation of the physician remains constant, however: to do the best one can under the circumstances, with the patient's consent. Some disasters, like those involving contagious diseases, may require extraordinary interventions, such as quarantine, to protect others. This is an exception to the rule of informed consent, but should be implemented only when necessary to protect the lives of others, and only for as long as necessary to preserve the public's health.[4]

The most difficult medical decisions in disasters are those generated by a lack of resources. This circumstance necessitates that treatment of some patients occurs before others, and that some patients may receive no treatment at all. It is sometimes asserted that decisions under scarcity should be based strictly on utilitarianism: saving the most patients possible, or the most years of life possible. This is a reasonable place to start the decision-making process, but it is only a beginning. Ethics requires that fairness and equality are given weight as well. All disaster victims must be treated fairly. This requires application of the Justice Principle. In this context, justice can be defined as the fair and equitable (not necessarily equal) distribution of resources, taking into account the patient's medical condition and prognosis. For example, rich and poor patients should be treated equally, without providing special consideration based on wealth. In addition, discrimination based on race or ethnicity is never ethically permissible. Conversely, it will often be ethically reasonable and responsible to deny medical resources to patients who will likely die even if treated heroically. The same denial could also apply to patients who have some chance of survival, but only at the expense of depriving other patients of adequate medical care who would almost certainly survive. The point is that decisions based on objective medical criteria regarding prognosis can be ethically acceptable in a disaster setting, whereas decisions based on race or income can never be ethically acceptable.[1,2,4]

In large-scale disasters involving responses by government, modern human rights law will be directly applicable as well, and it is completely consistent with medical ethics doctrine. In war, international humanitarian law will also be applicable, as interpreted most definitively by the International Committee of the Red Cross.

War and Humanitarian Law

Humanitarian law is the unlikely term for the law of war (although it is often used simply for relief efforts after a mass disaster). It most prominently includes the pre-World War I Hague Convention, and the post-World War II Geneva Conventions. Many ethical principles that apply to disaster medical care are derived from these treaties that aim to protect civilians from the ravages of war by, among other things, protecting their access to food, shelter, and medical care. The law of war is divided into two parts: primary prevention, that is, preventing war in the first place (*jus ad bellum*); and secondary prevention, that is, rules designed to contain the destructiveness of war, especially by protecting civilians (*jus in bello*). More specifically, *jus as bellum* is defined as agreements limiting the justifiable reasons for one country to declare war against another. *Jus in bello* refers to a body of independent and objective rules applying to all belligerents and governing the conduct of war to protect all persons. Examples of this second principle include the Geneva Conventions, which attempt to protect civilians caught in a war.[5]

War requires justification, usually by application of a version of the "just war" doctrine that states war be waged by a public authority, be started only for self-defense or grievous injury, and be conducted to achieve only just ends. The United Nations (UN) was founded not only to promote human rights, but primarily to keep the peace. The killing of at least 40 million civilians during World War II, as well as millions of prisoners of war deaths, led directly to the expansion of the Geneva Conventions of 1949 and to two additional protocols written in 1977, which have direct application to civil wars. The conventions are designed to ensure that the general population is provided with food, medical supplies, clothing, bedding, shelter, and "other supplies essential to the survival of the civilian population." Prisoners of war are also specifically protected by the Geneva Conventions.[6]

The International Committee of the Red Cross (ICRC) has promulgated a definitive interpretation of humanitarian law in its three volumes on *Customary International Humanitarian Law*.[7] Rules most directly applicable to war-related disaster responses by physicians include guidance designed primarily to protect civilians and physicians. These include: Rule 1: Attacks must not be directed against civilians; Rule 3: All members of the armed forces of a party to the conflict are combatants, except medical and religious personnel; Rule 25: Medical personnel exclusively assigned to medical duties must be respected and protected in all circumstances; Rule 26: Punishing a person for performing medical duties compatible with medical ethics or compelling a person engaged in medical activities to perform acts contrary to medical ethics is prohibited; Rule 29: Medical vehicles designated exclusively for the purpose of medical transportation must be respected and protected in all circumstances; Rule 30: Attacks directed against medical and religious personnel and objects displaying the distinctive emblems of the Geneva Conventions in conformity with international law are prohibited; and Rule 31: Humanitarian relief personnel must be respected and protected.[7]

Human Rights Law

Like modern humanitarian law, modern human rights law is primarily a product of World War II. The three most important sources are the Charter of the United Nations, the Nuremberg Trials, and the Universal Declaration of Human Rights (UDHR). All share a common basic premise that all individuals are equal in rights and dignity. The first two goals of the UN, as spelled out in its charter, are "to save succeeding generations from the scourge of war . . . and to reaffirm faith in fundamental human rights, in the dignity and worth of the human person, [and] in the equal rights of men and women." In what has come to be known as the Nuremberg Principles, the International Military Tribunal affirmed the existence of war crimes and crimes against humanity (including murder, torture, and slavery). Individuals can be held criminally responsible for committing such acts, and the response that one was simply "obeying orders" is not a valid defense.[5,6]

The UDHR was adopted by the UN General Assembly in 1948 without dissent as "a common standard of achievement for all peoples and all nations." Its precepts apply in both war and peace, and articulate several important principles. These include: 1) "Everyone has the right to life, liberty and security of person"; 2) "Everyone has the right to freedom of thought, conscience and religion"; and 3) "No one shall be subjected to torture or to cruel, inhuman or degrading treatment or punishment." This last phrase also appears in Common Article 3 of the Geneva Conventions. Of particular interest to physicians is Article 25 of the UDHR, often referred to as the "right to health":

1) Everyone has the right to a standard of living adequate for the health and well-being of himself and his family, including food, clothing, housing and medical care and necessary social services . . .
2) Motherhood and childhood are entitled to special care and assistance.

The UDHR was meant to articulate a set of principles, which can reasonably be seen as aspirational and even ethical. To make these concepts part of international human rights law, two separate treaties were developed: the International Covenant on Civil and Political Rights (ICCPR) and the International Covenant on Economic, Social, and Cultural Rights (ICESCR). Both were opened for signatures in 1966 and currently each has been adopted by approximately 150 nations. The division of rights listed in the UDHR into these two treaty categories was necessitated by the Cold War, with the United States championing the first document and the former Soviet Union the second.[6]

Human rights law is applicable to both war and peace. Regardless of the emergency, some human rights cannot be compromised by the state. These include: the right to life; the right not to be tortured or subjected to cruel, inhuman, or degrading

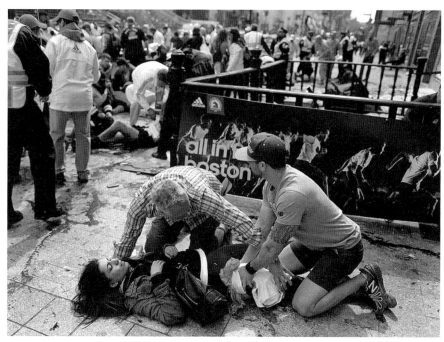

Figure 7.1. Front page of the *Boston Globe* describing the attack at the Boston Marathon.

treatment or punishment; the right not to be held in slavery; and the right not to be subject to arbitrary arrest or imprisonment. Article 4 of the ICCPR provides that, "In a time of public emergency which threatens the life of the nation . . . , a state may derogate from its obligations under the treaty if contrary measures are strictly required for its survival and are not inconsistent with their other obligations under international law and do not involve discrimination solely on the ground of race, color, sex, language, religion or social origin." Rights to freedom of thought, conscience, and religion are also protected absolutely.

Standards known as the Siracusa Principles explain how to apply the emergency derogation provision just identified in Article 4 in the previous paragraph. They require that when a derogation of the other rights in the ICCPR is made for an emergency, including a public health emergency, the aim must be legitimate and the measure "proportionate to that aim," and "a state shall use no more restrictive means than are required for the achievement of the purpose of the limitation."[5,6]

Case-Based Examples of Applying Ethical and Human Rights Principles

The Boston Marathon Bombing

The medical response to the Boston Marathon bombing in the United States is a useful initial example of the medical ethics issues in disaster medicine. On April 15, 2013, two bombs exploded near the finish line of the Boston marathon (see Figure 7.1).

The bombs were designed to inflict the most damage to the runners' legs. Because the bombing took place near the end of the marathon, the medical aid station (designed to help dehydrated runners with intravenous fluids among other things) was available to receive casualties, and ambulances were already on scene. Nonetheless, as with virtually all disasters, the first responders were the bystanders. It was somewhat unusual that at least several responders were also physicians. One such individual, a pediatric resident who was participating in the race, heard the

explosions and ran toward those injured to provide assistance. She administered CPR to a severely injured woman and helped others apply pressure to the victim's bleeding leg wounds. In addition, she treated two others who had severely injured lower extremities. In the meantime, a radiologist was tending to other runners.[8] Also on scene, and only 10 yards from the blast, was an emergency physician from Georgia. He immediately began applying tourniquets to the victims to prevent massive blood loss, and eventually transported them to the medical aid tent (which had at least eight physician volunteers and as many as two dozen nurses) where he continued to assist others. Victims arriving at the tent were triaged, primarily to decide who should be treated immediately and who could wait. Despite the surrounding chaos, one of those present described the medical tent as "a pretty controlled environment."[9]

The scene quickly shifted from the finish line to Boston's level 1 trauma centers as ambulances and other vehicles delivered victims to the hospitals. The medical personnel also changed roles from volunteers to physicians working in their natural environments. These individuals included emergency physicians, trauma surgeons, and other specialists commonly found in hospitals.[10] The results were remarkable. Of the 267 injured victims, only three died and all before reaching the hospital. Every patient who reached a hospital alive survived, including the twenty who sustained critical injuries. Medical skill is widely credited for this outcome, but luck also played a part. Several of these fortuitous factors included: 1) the bomb's location – it detonated near the end of the race and thus near the medical aid station and waiting ambulances: 2) the time of day the explosion occurred – the area hospitals' day shift personnel were leaving and the evening shift staff were arriving so that double staffing was present; and 3) the marathon occurred on a holiday when few surgeries were scheduled so operating rooms were mostly unoccupied and immediately available.[10,11,12]

The planning and training of Boston EMS personnel also played a significant role. They initiated triage, rapid treatment, and the loading of patients onto ambulances. Paramedics applied tourniquets to victims based on data obtained from the military's experiences in Iraq and Afghanistan showing that early tourniquet use dramatically reduces deaths from limb exsanguination associated with blast injuries.[10,11] At the Boston EMS dispatch center, a physician assisted the loading officer with the distribution of the most critically ill patients triaged as immediate (red-tagged). The initial thirty red-tagged patients were triaged, treated, and transported within 18 minutes after the explosions.[10]

Attacks similar to the marathon bombing are weekly, if not daily, occurrences in Syria, Afghanistan, Iraq, and Pakistan. While not as frequent in the United States, the impact of such bombings on all populations is the same. Pakistani artist Imran Qureshi created an art installation on the roof garden at the Metropolitan Museum of Art reflecting the effects of violence. His work, titled "And How Many Rains Must Fall Before the Stains are Washed Clean," suggests a blood-soaked street after the bodies of a bombing have been removed, but also includes images depicting the possibility of hope and new life.[13] The work also suggests not only our common humanity, which is often emphasized in mass tragedies, but also that there are patterns in disasters that can help us prepare to better deal with them. These patterns include not just the types of injuries inflicted, but also the necessity for quick and coordinated action in response.

The context in which medical decisions are made can vary radically, but the principles of medical ethics do not vary with the situation. Religious beliefs vary from country to country, but principles of medical ethics do not. That is why such organizations as the World Medical Association can set ethical standards for physicians, and why the United Nations Educational, Scientific, and Cultural Organization could promulgate an international declaration on medical ethics and human rights. No respected authority argues for the existence of special ethics or special standards of care for hospital emergency departments, intensive care units, or operating rooms. In the same context, how can one propose that evidence exists for "special ethics" or even a special "crisis standard of care" for disasters with limited medical resources? Physicians, for example, always have an ethical obligation to their patients – to act in the patients' best interests and with their consent. How individual patients actually define "best interests" may vary depending on the nature of their condition, especially whether their malady is likely to be fatal or cause permanent and severe disability. Ethical decisions regarding amputations call for informed consent protocols whether the decision is being made in a major Boston hospital after a terrorist attack, or with a patient trapped in the rubble left after an earthquake in Haiti.[14] However, consent is sometimes impossible to obtain, as when the patient is unconscious and next of kin or prior directive are not available to help guide the physician. Such practical issues can be difficult enough in day-to-day practice, but extreme situations can make them appear overwhelming. Unless decision-making criteria are considered before a disaster strikes, ethics is unlikely to play the role it should when physicians respond.[4]

Medical Ethics and Response to Haiti Earthquake

The basic mission of the military relates to armed conflict. However, it is not unusual for governments to request that their military forces respond to natural disasters. In extreme circumstances, governments may send troops to other countries to provide assistance in disaster situations. This happened not only in response to the Asian tsunami but also to the massive Haitian earthquake in January 2010. For example, within 48 hours after the earthquake, the Israeli government dispatched a military task force of 230 people to run a field hospital. The Israelis maintain two such mobile field hospitals on constant alert to respond to attacks on Israel. However, they also will deploy one of them to other countries if the need arises. The mobile hospital contains sixty inpatient beds, four intensive care unit beds, and two operating rooms. Once established, the field hospital in Haiti treated more than 1,100 patients.[15]

The situation they encountered was extremely challenging. Many said they were practicing medicine in a manner more reminiscent of the 1930s or the 1950s.[14] At some hospitals, conditions were primitive, with vodka being used to sterilize instruments and hacksaws to perform amputations. A *Boston Globe* reporter commenting on conditions about a week after the earthquake stated, "This is catastrophe medicine, where resources are scarce, time short, options few. It is a world apart from the exacting standards of the high temples of modern medicine in Boston."[14] Five physicians reflected on the ethics of their actions after returning home.[15] They worried most about their triage decisions involving which patients they elected to treat and which ones were denied care at the field hospital. Their triage protocol evaluated three criteria: 1) How urgent was the patient's condition? 2) Did they have adequate resources to meet the patient's needs? 3) Assuming the patient was admitted and provided appropriate care, could the patient's life be saved? The physicians acknowledged that the more time that passed since a patient's open fracture occurred, the more likely infection and death would follow. Therefore, they considered implementing a time limit for treatment eligibility. However, they ultimately decided that "each case had to be evaluated individually."[15] Other considerations also played a role:

> The potential for rehabilitation was an additional consideration in the triage process. Patients who arrived with brain injuries, paraplegia secondary to spinal injuries, or a low score on the Glasgow Coma Scale were referred to other facilities. Since we had neither a neurosurgical service nor computed tomography, we believed it would be incorrect to use our limited resources to treat patients with such a minimal chance of ultimate rehabilitation at the expense of others whom we could help.[15]

Those decisions were difficult, but ethically justifiable under the circumstances. More difficult to objectively evaluate, but equally understandable, was the dilemma of dealing with patients trapped for a week or more under the rubble who were finally being rescued. Even though their chances of survival were remote, the physicians "believed it would be [ethically] inappropriate to deny treatment to a patient who had survived days under the rubble before a heroic rescue, even though this policy meant potentially diverting resources from other patients with a better chance of a positive outcome."[15] This action cannot be ethically justified on the basis of a strict utilitarian principle, "the greatest good for the greatest number," or even a more focused ethical interpretation of "save the most lives possible." It must instead be justified by an ethics that requires individual patient evaluation, and considers the mechanism of injury and the method of rescue in deciding whether it is appropriate to deny the patient treatment.[16]

Such decisions could appear arbitrary. To avoid this, and to share the ethical responsibility of these judgments, the group created a system of ad hoc ethics committees. The treating physicians would present cases to a panel of three senior physicians who would then decide how to proceed. This system relieved individual doctors of the burden of determining a given person's outcome.[15] The concept of diffusing responsibility for life and death decisions has been previously described as one of the positive attributes of an ethics committee.[17] Nonetheless, it should be emphasized that there is nothing "ethical" about such a committee. The Israeli committee was composed entirely of physicians and was not required to either construct an ethical algorithm or use ethical principles to make decisions. Instead, they acted much more like a prognosis committee, making decisions about appropriate medical intervention based on the likely prognosis of the patient, and the resources required to continue patient treatment.[18]

The Standard of Care

It is in the context of medical decision making that many commentators have become confused regarding how the standard of care applies to disasters. As both the Israeli field hospital physicians and the *Boston Globe* reporter make clear, the standard of care as practiced in major hospitals of developed countries cannot be directly transported and applied in the wake of a massive earthquake. Beds and medical equipment are severely limited, and some resources that are routinely available in modern hospitals, such as CT scanners and dialysis machines, simply do not exist. This has raised the question, should the law be changed to protect volunteer physicians from potential legal liability for injuries to patients that would have been prevented had they followed the standard of care under typical conditions? This question is evidence of confusion, rather than a reflection of reality. This is because all proposals to change the medical standard of care for disasters are based on a misunderstanding of the "standard of care," both in the field and in the courtroom.[19]

The legal standard of care for physicians represents a formal description of a physician's duty to provide care. It states they are required to act as a "reasonably prudent physician [with the same medical qualifications] would act in the same or similar circumstances" taking into account the resources available.[20] *By its own terms*, the standard varies with the conditions under which the physician is providing treatment, including emergency and disaster conditions.[14,20,21] Given this language, there is no difference between the medical standard of care and the legal standard (or duty) of care. As previously summarized, "The [legal] standard of care is flexible and fact-dependent."[22] Nor can the standard of care in any situation be seen as encompassing only one rigid method, as is illustrated by the Israeli field hospital experience. As observed by others, "at any given moment, doctors employing a wide variety of treatments and skills for identical conditions may be practicing non-negligently in the eyes of the law."[23] Although wide variations exist in everyday medical practice patterns, no one suggests that physicians who practice in cities or regions at the extremes of these variations are guilty of medical malpractice. As such, there is no legal necessity to change or alter the standard of care in emergencies, as it changes on its own to reflect reality. The American Bar Association officially endorsed this position in a resolution adopted in August 2011 by its House of Delegates (which includes members representing both physician groups

and preparedness organizations).[24] A report accompanying the resolution states:

> It is unnecessary and unwise to remove or alter the legal duty of care owed to disaster victims by relief organizations and health care professionals. That duty is the duty to exercise the same degree of knowledge and skill that a competent practitioner would exercise in the same or similar circumstances, a time-honored principle that should not be altered, especially on the basis of confusion and speculation. Disaster victims are entitled to expect that their health care practitioners will provide them with reasonable care as the circumstances permit.[24]

Two other issues are involved in the altered standards of care discussion: diffusing fear of liability that might inhibit physician volunteers, and resource allocation. The first is a belief that physicians will not volunteer to offer medical assistance in disasters unless they are guaranteed virtually absolute legal immunity from malpractice claims. There is some suggestion from physician surveys in the United States that they would prefer such immunity. However, examining the actual experiences of physician volunteers in disasters, "There is no evidence that immunity is needed to encourage altruistic physicians to volunteer in an emergency, nor any evidence that granting malpractice immunity would be sufficient to get unwilling physicians to volunteer."[21] Every new disaster simply provides additional support for this conclusion. In addition, no evidence exists that immunity was a major concern for physicians responding either to out-of-country catastrophes, like the Haiti earthquake, or to U.S. emergencies, such as the marathon bombings.[8,9,16]

Resource Allocation

What the Israeli physicians in Haiti were actually dealing with was not a modified standard of care. Rather, they were struggling with the second issue, the distinct question of resource allocation; specifically, who gets access to the limited available resources and who does not.[15] Put more succinctly, how are decisions made to offer treatment to some and withhold it from others (often life and death decisions), and on what basis, when the resources are insufficient to treat everyone?

The answer offered to this question is often based on utilitarian ethics (i.e. do the greatest good for the greatest number). This proposition seems simple, but in reality, it raises as many questions as it answers. For example, what is meant by "good," and are these short-term or long-term considerations? Does it matter if the lives saved are children or the elderly? Although many assume triage involves the application of utilitarian ethics only, in fact the history of triage also highlights its emphasis on equality and fairness.[16] Born in the military of Napoleon and the French Revolution, the concept was to abandon the previous practice of treating officers first and ordinary soldiers second, by adopting new sorting or "triage" ethics that treated all wounded the same without regard to rank.[25]

Likewise, utilitarianism was not used to resolve the primary rationing problem impacting medicine in developed countries: Who gets the next organ for transplant? When kidney dialysis machines were first used in Seattle, Washington, an anonymous screening committee was established to select who among competing candidates would receive the life-saving technology. One lay member of the committee is quoted as saying:

The choices were hard . . . . I remember voting against a young woman who was a known prostitute. I found I couldn't vote for her, rather than another candidate, a young wife and mother. I also voted against a young man who, until he learned he had renal failure, had been a ne'er do well, a real playboy. He promised he would reform his character, go back to school, and so on, if only he were selected for treatment. But I felt I'd lived long enough to know that a person like that won't really do what he was promising at the time.[26]

Unsurprisingly, when the biases and selection criteria used by this group were exposed in a *Life Magazine* cover story, the committee method for patient selection was abandoned. Shortly thereafter, Congress passed a statute providing federal funding to support dialysis for everyone in renal failure. This measure served simply to postpone the difficult selection decisions among candidates for organ transplantation. The limiting resource was no longer money, but organs available for transplantation. Having abandoned the committee selection process, three other models for identifying organ recipients were examined: the market approach, the lottery approach, and what may be called the customary medical approach.[26]

In the market approach, the next organ goes to the person who is willing to pay the most for it. While very simple to implement, it utterly fails on the criteria of fairness and equality. The lottery approach, which has been endorsed by courts in extreme cases – such as deciding who should be killed in a lifeboat so that some may live by eating the deceased – assumes fairness is the ultimate and only value. Applying this to transplant recipients, everyone has an equal chance to get the organ. On the other hand, it offends our values of efficiency and fairness. It makes no distinctions among such things as the candidates' capacity to comply with medical care, their potential for survival with treatment, or their quality of life. Finally, the customary medical approach would permit physicians to choose their patients on the basis of medical criteria or clinical suitability. The major problem with this method is that it hides selection criteria based on social worth. It allows physicians to discriminate against individuals on the basis of poor family support, poverty, low intelligence, mental illness, criminal records, drug and alcohol addiction, age, or even geographical location, by terming these social status contraindications "medical."[26,27]

In organ transplantation, society has ultimately decided to use a combination of approaches to solve its rationing problem. This is because no one approach can meet all the reasonable criteria of being fair, efficient, reflective of societal values of equality, and life-affirming. To promote efficiency, for example, it is important that no one receive a transplant unless they truly desire one and are likely to obtain significant benefits measured in years of life at a reasonable level of functioning. This makes an initial evaluation based exclusively on medical criteria a reasonable screen. It determines the probability of a transplant being successful in extending years of life that are high quality. Once it is determined that the person is a good candidate to benefit from the transplant, the next screen could be a lottery – made more palatable by using a first-come first-served rationing approach.[23] This avoids making arbitrary and capricious decisions about individual social characteristics. On the other hand, there is some flexibility to allow individuals near death to advance on the list, at least as long as they are not so near death that their ability to survive the transplant with a reasonable quality of life is compromised.

Triage strategies, like organ transplant allocations, are not ultimately based solely on utilitarian ethics, but rather are tempered with ideals of equality and fairness.[16] These goals are achieved in a disaster or emergency situation by making treatment priority decisions based primarily on objective medical prognosis criteria. This is why it has been argued that experienced providers are likely to be the best triage officers.[28] Several experts have also persuasively argued that no single or even multiple principles can adequately account for ethical allocation decisions in life and death situations. These authors suggest combining four morally relevant principles to assist with decision making: youngest-first, prognosis, lottery, and saving the most lives. The proper ethical strategy, they argue, is to "embrace the challenge of implementing a coherent multi-principle framework rather than relying on simple principles or retreating to the status quo."[29] Other experts have also tried to use a more complex scheme to determine which groups should get priority for the flu vaccine at the outset of a pandemic.[30]

Triage decisions can be seen from two points of view: deciding who gets treatment first, and deciding who will not receive care. Using a nautical analogy, when a ship is sinking and not everyone can be saved, the customary rule has been to allocate women and children first to the lifeboats, leaving the men and sailors "untreated."[31] Although this rule was applied by the captain of the Titanic, recent scholarship has documented that it is more of a guideline than a rule, and that more recently "every man for himself" more accurately describes what happens when a ship sinks.[32] For the medical community, abandoning a hospital or nursing home in the middle of a disaster is a more commonly faced problem. In this regard, Hurricane Katrina provides a useful example.

Hurricane Katrina

In the immediate aftermath of Hurricane Katrina in the United States, decisions were made about how to evacuate the patients from one of New Orleans's impacted hospitals, Memorial Medical Center (see Figure 7.2). This was a privately owned institution that experienced flooding in its lower floors and subsequently lost electrical power. The decision made was thought to be medical, but was based on a profound misunderstanding of a particular medical order, the do not resuscitate (DNR) order. About two dozen physicians and a few nurse managers met to decide how to evacuate the hospital's 180 patients and an additional 55 patients on the seventh floor. The patients on the seventh floor were actually under the care of a separate company called LifeCare that leased this space. These LifeCare patients required long-term intensive nursing care.[33,34] The medical team quickly agreed that those who would suffer most from the heat should receive first priority for evacuation on rescue helicopters. These included infants in the neonatal intensive care unit, pregnant women, and critically ill adults in the ICU. Then a leading physician at the hospital suggested that all patients with DNR orders should go last.

Other physicians agreed, and the plan was adopted, even though it is now clear that many of the physicians did not understand the meaning of a DNR order.[33,35] The intent of this medical order is to prevent aggressive resuscitative interventions if a patient suffers a cardiac or respiratory arrest. It does not imply, as many physicians believed, that a patient with a DNR order

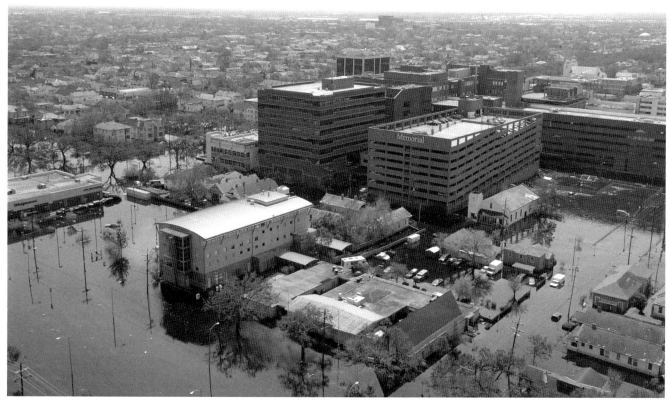

Figure 7.2. Memorial Medical Center in New Orleans during the flooding caused by Hurricane Katrina.

has an extremely poor prognosis and is likely to die in the near future.[3] It is also worth noting that for competent patients, a DNR order requires informed consent, and a competent patient can withdraw that consent at any time. A significant number of patients with DNR orders were competent and likely would have rescinded the order if it meant he or she could advance on the evacuation priority list.[34] It is acknowledged that using medical prognostic judgments to determine the order of patient evacuation is a reasonable strategy for physicians to adopt in extreme situations. However, creating patient evacuation priorities based on a misunderstanding of their code status is not.[34]

Many family members objected to assigning patients with DNR orders to the lowest evacuation priority. Some patients in this category were not ultimately evacuated at all, even after resources to transport them became available.[34] This suggests the need to emphasize situational awareness and for frequent reassessment of patients being evaluated by triage protocols.[36] In this case, revisions of the triage rules seemed to suggest that at least some of the patients should not be evacuated at all. Specifically, at least two other triage rules were later adopted. One revision stated:

> The standard of rescue [had] changed from Tuesday to Thursday; initially the sickest patients were evacuated first. When we realized that help was not imminent . . . the standard of rescue changed to that of reverse triage. It was recognized that some patients might not survive, and priority was given to those who had the best chance of survival. On Thursday morning, only category 3 patients [the most gravely ill] remained on the LifeCare unit.[37]

About a week after the evacuation, an unnamed physician described a still later triage revision for the remaining patients to a British newspaper:

> We divided patients into three categories: those who were traumatized but medically fit enough to survive, those who needed urgent care, and the dying. People would find it impossible to understand the situation. I had to make life-or-death decisions in a split second. It came down to giving people the basic right to die with dignity.[35]

In July 2006, Dr. Anna Pou and two nurses were arrested and charged with second-degree murder for allegedly injecting four patients from the LifeCare floor with morphine and midazolam to cause their deaths. Autopsies were conducted on more than twenty of the patients who had died, including the nine LifeCare patients who expired just prior to the hospital evacuation. In September, Dr. Pou offered this explanation for her actions: "I do not believe in euthanasia. I don't think that it's anyone's decision to make when a patient dies. However, what I do believe in is comfort care. And that means that we ensure that they do not suffer pain."[38]

The grand jury did not begin work until May 2007, and in July it decided not to indict Dr. Pou. New Orleans residents generally applauded the decision. The general feeling was that no one person should have been singled out for blame. Forensic experts, who thought there should have been a trial in this case, said the main reason was determining responsibility.[34] On the other hand, the case illustrates that after a major disaster, even though criminal law is not suspended, the likelihood of conviction for medical personnel is vanishingly small. It is worth noting that although the Pou case continues to be used as the rationale for granting physicians immunity in responding to disasters, no one has seriously argued that such immunity should cover criminal acts, or that physicians, no matter how accomplished or distinguished, should be above the law, even in extreme circumstances. After Hurricane Katrina, the attorney general's office for the State of Louisiana investigated at least 140 deaths in hospitals and nursing homes. However, when the cases were turned over to local district attorneys for possible prosecution, there were no convictions.[38]

Plagues

Albert Camus closes his narrative of *The Plague* by observing that those who "fought against its terror and relentless onslaughts," although they were "unable to be saints," refused to "bow down to pestilences [and strove] their utmost to be healers." Camus's novel is used as an introduction to an essay published in 1988 about physician obligations at the beginning of the AIDS epidemic.[39] At least some physicians were refusing to treat patients with AIDS, arguing that they did not possess the expertise needed. Resolution of the problem rested almost completely within the ethical sphere, since the law was of limited applicability in dealing with this dilemma, addressing only a restricted area of medical practice. The U.S. common law, for example, requires physicians in emergency departments to treat any patient regardless of illness who requests care for an emergency medical condition.[3] There is no exception for HIV/AIDS. Of course, emergency department personnel have the right to take reasonable precautions to protect themselves from harm, and hospitals have an obligation to provide their staff with protective clothing and to follow protective procedures.[39] Failure to implement such precautions helped facilitate the spread of SARS to physicians and nurses in ICUs, and to greatly amplify the 2014 Ebola outbreak in Western Africa. But protecting does not include acts that would amount to refusal of treatment or that would compromise good patient care.

Outside of the emergency department, however, physician obligations were much more limited. In the absence of some contractual rights (such as membership in a health insurance plan), or statutory rights (such as admission to a United States Government Department of Veterans Affairs hospital or clinic), the general rule is that physicians can choose which patients they wish to treat. There are additional statutes that prohibit rejection of patients for certain discriminatory reasons such as race and disability, and arguably the latter applied to HIV/AIDS.[39]

In general, however, medical ethics proved a more important stimulus to influence physician behavior than law. In 1986, for example, the American Colleges of Physicians urged "all physicians, surgeons, nurses, and other medical professionals and hospitals to provide competent and humane care to all patients, including patients with AIDS and AIDS-related conditions." In addition, they stated that, "Denying appropriate care to sick and dying patients for any reason is unethical."[39] A statement by the American Medical Association was similar: "Neither those who have the disease [AIDS] nor those who

have been infected with the virus[HIV] should be subjected to discrimination based on fear or prejudice, least of all by members of the health care community."[39] As medical societies have no enforcement mechanism, the statements by state licensing boards likely had more weight. In 1987, for example, the New Jersey State Medical Board adopted the following "AIDS Policy": "A licensee of this Board may not categorically refuse to treat a patient who has AIDS or AIDS-related complex, or an HIV positive blood test, when he or she possesses the skill and experience to treat the condition presented."[39] Perhaps most impressive, however, was the powerful policy statement adopted by the State of New York's thirteen medical schools, which decreed that physicians had a "most fundamental responsibility to treat AIDS patients" and that any faculty member, hospital resident or medical student who refused to treat an AIDS patient would be dismissed.[39]

All of these ethics policies could be directly applied to pandemic flu, SARS, and other infectious diseases.[4] The conclusion is that physicians do have special legal and ethical obligations because they have been granted special privileges by society. "Their continued practice is voluntary; and their conduct is properly judged by standards higher than those we hold others to, even higher than those to which we hold fire and police personnel."[39]

Ethics and Ethical Codes

Everyone is familiar with the Hippocratic injunction, "first, do no harm." If this in fact was the primary rule of medical ethics, physicians could meet it in disasters simply by refusing to provide any help at all.[2,40] However, that is not a useful prospect, and the real ethical rule for physicians responding to a disaster is to perform to the best of one's ability in providing medical care to victims without intentionally causing harm. Attempts have been made to articulate medical ethics standards in disasters, including efforts in Canada after the SARS epidemic.[41] Perhaps the most successful statement on disaster medical ethics has been written by the World Medical Association (WMA), but it should nonetheless still be considered a work in progress. At its 2006 meeting, the WMA adopted the code set forth in Table 7.1 (a revision of a code first adopted in 1994).

This is a credible summary of the issues in disaster medicine, but, like all codes of ethics, leaves much to interpretation and suggests future revisions. Two points regarding the triage section stand out. The first is the notion of "beyond emergency care," which could imply a fair degree of subjectivity rather than a decision based on objective criteria. While the concept itself is sound, the section's descriptive language contains comments that could be better quantified by currently available data. The second point, also related to this concept, is the seeming acceptance of applying just one measure (rather than multiple principles) to determining the ethical underpinnings of triage. The WMA accepts as the primary triage goal to save the maximum number of individuals/lives. While an appropriate metric, its sole use as a principle to guide triage may simply be too narrow. It disregards other factors that deserve consideration such as age, prognosis, and even first-come, first-served prioritization under certain circumstances.[29,42]

A related issue that deserves mention is the role of nongovernmental organizations (NGOs) in responding to disasters in resource-poor countries such as Haiti. In 1995, the International Federation of Red Cross and Red Crescent Societies (IFRC)

Table 7.1. The World Medical Association Statement on Disaster Medical Ethics

WMA Statement on Medical Ethics in the Event of Disasters

1. The definition of a disaster for the purpose of this document focuses particularly on the medical aspects.

   A disaster is the sudden occurrence of a calamitous, usually violent, event resulting in substantial material damage, considerable displacement of people, a large number of victims, and/or significant social disruption. This definition excludes situations arising from conflicts and wars, whether international or internal, which give rise to other problems in addition to those considered in this paper. From the medical standpoint, disaster situations are characterized by an acute and unforeseen imbalance between the capacity and resources of the medical profession and the needs of survivors who are injured whose health is threatened, over a given period of time.

2. Disasters, irrespective of cause, share several features:
   a. their sudden and unexpected occurrence, demanding prompt action;
   b. material or natural damage making access to the survivors difficult and/or dangerous;
   c. adverse effects on health due to pollution, and the risks of epidemics, and emotional and psychological factors;
   d. a context of insecurity requiring police or military measures to maintain order;
   e. media coverage.

   Disasters require multifaceted responses involving many different types of relief ranging from transportation and food supplies to medical services. Physicians are likely to be part of coordinated operations involving other responders such as law enforcement personnel. These operations require an effective and centralized authority to coordinate public and private efforts. Rescue workers and physicians are confronted with an exceptional situation in which their normal professional ethics must be brought to the situation to ensure that the treatment of disaster survivors conforms to basic ethical tenets and is not influenced by other motivations. Ethical rules defined and taught beforehand should complement the individual ethics of physicians.

   Inadequate and/or disrupted medical resources on site and the large number of people injured in a short time present specific ethical challenges.

   The World Medical Association therefore recommends the following ethical principles and procedures with regard to the physician's role in disaster situations.

3. Triage
   a. Triage is a medical action of prioritizing treatment and management based on a rapid diagnosis and prognosis for each patient. Triage must be carried out systematically, taking into account the medical needs, medical intervention capabilities, and available resources. Vital acts of reanimation may have to be carried out at the same time as triage. Triage may pose an ethical problem owing to the limited treatment resources immediately available in relation to the large number of injured persons in varying states of health.
   b. Ideally, triage should be entrusted to authorized, experienced physicians or to physician teams, assisted by a competent staff.
   c. The physician should separate patients into categories and then treat them in the following order, subject to national guidelines:
      1. patients who can be saved but whose lives are in immediate danger should be given treatment straight away or as a matter of priority within the next few hours;
      2. patients whose lives are not in immediate danger and who are in need of urgent but not immediate medical care should be treated next;
      3. injured persons requiring only minor treatment can be treated later or by relief workers;
      4. psychologically traumatized individuals who do not require treatment for bodily harm but might need reassurance or sedation if acutely disturbed;
      5. patients whose condition exceeds the available therapeutic resources, who suffer from extremely severe injuries such as irradiation or burns to such an extent and degree that they cannot be saved in the specific circumstances of time and place, or complex surgical cases requiring a particularly delicate operation which would take too long, thereby obliging the physician to make a choice between them and other patients. Such patients may be classified as "beyond emergency care."
      6. Since cases may evolve and thus change category, it is essential that the situation be regularly reassessed by the official in charge of the triage.
   d. The following statements apply to treatment beyond emergency care:
      1. It is ethical for a physician not to persist, at all costs, in treating individuals "beyond emergency care," thereby wasting scarce resources needed elsewhere. The decision not to treat an injured person on account of priorities dictated by the disaster situation cannot be considered a failure to come to the assistance of a person in mortal danger. It is justified when it is intended to save the maximum number of individuals. However, the physician must show such patients compassion and respect for their dignity, for example by separating them from others and administering appropriate pain relief and sedatives.
      2. The physician must act according to the needs of patients and the resources available. He/she should attempt to set an order of priorities for treatment that will save the greatest number of lives and restrict morbidity to a minimum.

4. RELATIONS WITH THE PATIENTS
   a. In selecting the patients who may be saved, the physician should consider only their medical status, and should exclude any other consideration based on non-medical criteria.
   b. Survivors of a disaster are entitled to the same respect as other patients, and the most appropriate treatment available should be administered with the patient's consent. However, it should be recognized that in a disaster response there may not be enough time for informed consent to be a realistic possibility.

5. AFTERMATH OF DISASTER
   a. In the post-disaster period the needs of survivors must be considered.
   b. Many may have lost family members and may be suffering psychological distress. The dignity of survivors and their families must be respected.
   c. The physician must respect the customs, rites and religions of the patients and act in all impartiality.
   d. If possible, the difficulties encountered and the identification of the patients should be reported for medical follow-up.

6. MEDIA AND OTHER THIRD PARTIES
   The physician has a duty to each patient to exercise discretion and ensure confidentiality when dealing with third parties, and to exercise caution and objectivity and act with dignity with respect to the emotional and political atmosphere surrounding disaster situations. This implies that physicians are empowered to restrict the entrance of reporters to the medical premises. Media relations should always be handled by appropriately trained personnel.

(continued)

Table 7.1. (*continued*)

7. DUTIES OF PARAMEDICAL PERSONNEL
The ethical principles that apply to physicians also apply to personnel under the physician's direction.
8. TRAINING
The World Medical Association recommends that disaster medicine training be included in the curricula of university and post-graduate courses in medicine.
9. RESPONSIBILITY
The World Medical Association calls upon governments and insurance companies to cover both civil liability and any personal damages to which physicians might be subject when working in disaster or emergency situations.
  The WMA requests that governments:
  a. accept the presence of foreign physicians and, where demonstrably qualified, their participation, without discrimination on the basis of factors such as affiliation (e.g. Red Cross, Red Crescent, ICRC, and other qualified organizations), race, or religion.
  b. give priority to the rendering of medical services over visits of dignitaries.

and the ICRC adopted a basic code of conduct for NGOs in disasters which states:

1) The humanitarian imperative comes first.
2) Aid is given regardless of the race, creed, or nationality of the recipients and without adverse distinction of any kind. Aid priorities are calculated on the basis of need alone.
3) Aid will not be used to further a particular political or religious standpoint.
4) We shall endeavor not to act as instruments of government foreign policy.
5) We shall respect culture and custom.
6) We shall attempt to build disaster response on local capacities.
7) Ways shall be found to involve program beneficiaries in the management of relief aid.
8) Relief aid must strive to reduce future vulnerabilities to disaster as well as meeting basic needs.
9) We hold ourselves accountable to both those we seek to assist and those from whom we accept resources
10) In our information, publicity, and advertising activities, we shall recognize disaster victims as dignified humans, not hopeless objects.

Two things are especially important in this code. The first is that the welfare of the victims should always be the priority, and, consistent with international human rights law, all must be treated equally. Second is the assertion that NGOs should be apolitical and accountable to those they seek to assist. This has not always been the case, and number 10 responds to NGOs that use pictures of victims in their own fundraising – suggesting that the primary goal of NGOs is not relief, but financing themselves. Accountability and coordination among NGOs has been a major problem in international disaster relief efforts, perhaps nowhere as well-illustrated as in Haiti.

As Subbarao, Wynia, and Burkle have persuasively argued, much has been published on "the challenges such as triage and crisis standards of care" but very little has been written on the social justice aspects of responding to disasters.[43] They suggest that much more attention should be focused on the ethics of relief organizations themselves during disasters, especially what they term "high-profile disasters." This is because many NGOs actively seek publicity which they need for fundraising. This can lead to competition among NGOs rather than cooperation. This competition both distracts from their mission and can endanger

the lives of the very people these organizations were designed to help. The authors further state:

High-profile disasters... bring an influx of newly arriving NGOs from around the world... [which] are driven to get the highest possible visibility for their good works.... There arises a frenzied attempt by individual NGOs to outmaneuver one another for prime locations and media attention.... [E]very NGO would like to plant its flag in the most photogenic areas – the ones trafficked by more journalists and media – in order to solicit prime donations.[43]

They make specific suggestions, the most important of which are: 1) for all NGOs to adopt the Sphere Standards for humanitarian assistance, and 2) for all disaster workers to be educated and trained not just for emergency response, but also for the stages of transition and recovery that follow the event. Other leaders from international humanitarian groups have also called for increasing the oversight of aid workers and aid organizations that respond to large-scale disasters.[20,44] The ethical concern is that humanitarian responders, including physicians, have no accountability even if their interventions make a difficult situation worse.

Summary

There are no special medical ethics for disaster relief. However, there are principles from humanitarian law, international human rights law, and medical ethics that have direct application to disaster response. Humanitarian law (the law of war) is designed both to prevent war, and also to mitigate its worse effects by protecting civilians and the physicians who tend to them during the conflict. Human rights law operates both during war and peace, and is founded on the principle that all humans are equal in dignity, and must be treated equally. Governments, nonetheless, have special obligations toward children and the mothers who care for them. Certain human rights obligations apply everywhere and always, including the right not to be killed or tortured, not to be enslaved, and not to be arbitrarily arrested. These rights can be termed civil and political, or even "negative" rights. Additional state obligations include the "right to health." In disasters, this is similar to the state's obligations to civilians in war. Governments must provide the basic necessities of life: food, shelter, clean water and sanitation, and medical care.

Treatment decisions made under disaster conditions must take into account available resources. The legal standard of care (or duty of a physician) is to act in the way a reasonably prudent physician (with the same training) would act in the same or similar circumstances. Calls to modify this standard or to grant physicians prospective immunity are misguided and dangerous to disaster victims. Triage decisions can be difficult, and need to include more than the ethical rationale based on utilitarianism. They should acknowledge an ethics that takes three or more ethical principles into account. No perfect medical ethics code exists, but the WMA's declaration is an excellent work in progress that provides a useful summary of the major issues. Perhaps the major ethical issue in disaster response is accountability, and reasonable voices have recently been raised to encourage NGOs and professional organizations to enforce standards for disaster care delivery, recovery, and coordination.

RECOMMENDATIONS FOR FURTHER RESEARCH

Future work should focus on more explicit and transparent policies that can be developed both locally and globally, incorporating ethical and human rights principles into more concrete operational guidelines. When the functioning and viability of civil society is at stake, human rights remain but humanitarian law comes to the forefront. Disaster triage protocols must be both fair and tested to show that they improve outcomes. Furthermore, studies are needed to determine fair and equitable allocation of scarce resources during a catastrophic disaster. The provision of an untested drug, ZMapp, to two American health workers during the Ebola epidemic, for example, may have been done in an ad hoc manner without ethical analysis. Leaders must inform the public of the need to embrace the difficult issues of social worth and prioritization within disease and illness strata; a policy of first come, first served without consideration of the overall circumstances is insufficient as a moral rule. Specific endeavors might focus on examining classic dilemmas from previous disasters, identifying those that were managed effectively and those that were managed poorly. Such new knowledge could be incorporated into better training for managers and responders.

Several examples illustrate this approach. Documenting the post-Haiti earthquake experience could yield important information. The investigation could include interviews with the Israeli responders on the effect of their "ethics committee" triage system, how well they believe it worked in retrospect, and what system they currently use. A follow-up study of the cholera epidemic spread by the UN Nepalese peacekeepers could identify what responsibility the UN is taking for the epidemic and whether the UN (or any NGO) has ever been found liable for harms they have may have caused during a disaster response. Another option is surveying as many physician-responders to disasters as can be identified to ask about their ethics training for disaster response, if any. Queries could include the ethical principles they used in the field, whether they ever worried about legal liability for their actions (why or why not), and listing as many examples as they can provide of specific ethical dilemmas and how they resolved them. It has been suggested that research protocols, including those for experimental drugs potentially deployable in a pandemic, could be "pre-approved" by review committees.[45,46] It remains unclear how many times this has been attempted, and if it has ever succeeded.

Beyond the application of public health ethics, disaster situations create a parallel need for a host of virtues not commonly required in daily medical practice, including vigilance, courage, stewardship, prudence, resilience, justice, and self-effacing charity. Ongoing research suggests that such traits form a cadre of core competencies, "the right stuff," from which the ideal disaster worker is made. Future work should evaluate the ability of such virtues to act as a polyvalent counterpoint to the vices of apathy, cowardice, profligacy, recklessness, inflexibility, and narcissism. Outcome data may validate virtues that empower providers in all positions to integrate vertically principles of safety, public health, utility, and medical ethics at all organizational levels. Longitudinal and prospective studies should explore if, over time, virtuous behavior can be modeled, mentored, practiced, and institutionalized to become a useful vaccine against the vast array of moral threats inherent in disaster preparedness and response.

Insufficient data exist identifying effective methods for: 1) communicating to the general public the ethical challenges faced by responders during disasters; and 2) obtaining their cooperation for implementation of policies addressing these problems. The population at large must not only understand these problems, but agree to or at least cooperate with proposed solutions (mass casualty triage protocols, scarce resource allocation policies, etc.).

Future empiric research in the field should help discern the feasibility of screening for, selecting, teaching, and modeling the cardinal virtues among provider candidates in advance of a disaster or multiple casualty incidents. Multisite studies must also be conducted that validate the ability to measure and imbue core values of fairness, utility, and virtue in a multicultural context. Future codes of conduct must also incorporate practical aspects of provider discretion, the importance of good intent, and the challenge of dynamic decision making amid changing disaster circumstances.

REFERENCES

1. Dworkin R. *Justice for Hedgehogs.* Cambridge, MA, Harvard University Press, 2013.
2. Veatch RM. *A Theory of Medical Ethics.* New York, Basic Books, 1981.
3. Annas GJ. *The Rights of Patients.* 3d ed. New York, New York University Press, 2004.
4. Annas, GJ. *Worst Case Bioethics: Death, Destruction and Public Health.* New York, Oxford University Press, 2010.
5. Annas GJ, Geiger HJ. War and Human Rights. In Levy BS, Sidel VW, eds. *War and Public Health.* New York, Oxford University Press, 2008; 37–50.
6. Alston P, Goodman R. *International Human Rights.* New York, Oxford University Press, 2013.
7. ICRC. *Customary International Humanitarian Law.* 3 vols. Cambridge, Cambridge University Press, 2005.
8. Abel D. Runners and spectators raced to save lives. *Boston Globe.* April 17, 2013.
9. Kolata G, Longman J, Pilon M. Saving lives, if not legs, with no time to fret. *New York Times.* April 17, 2013; A1.
10. Biddinger PD, Baggish A, Harrington L, et al. Be prepared – The Boston Marathon and mass-casualty events. *N Engl J Med* 2013; 368: 1958–1961.
11. Walls RM, Zinner MJ. The Boston Marathon response: why did it work so well? *JAMA* 2013; 309: 2441–2443.

12. Kellerman AL, Peleg K. Lessons from Boston. *N Engl J Med* 2013; 368: 1956–1957.

13. Johnson K. Savagery, mulled in airy precincts. *New York Times.* May 16, 2013; C1.

14. Annas GJ. Standard of care: In sickness and in health and in emergencies. *N Engl J Med* 2010; 362: 2126–2131.

15. Merin O, Ash N, Levy G, Schwaber MJ, Kreiss Y. The Israeli field hospital in Haiti: Ethical dilemmas in early disaster response. *N Engl J Med* 2010; 362: e38.

16. Baker R, Strosberg M. Triage and Equality: An historical reassessment of utilitarian analysis of triage. *Kennedy Institute of Ethics Journal* 1992; 2: 103–123.

17. In re Quinlan, 70 N.J.10, 335 A.2d 647 (1976). Describes the case of Karen Ann Quinlan on the right to refuse treatment.

18. Teel K. The physician's dilemma: a doctor's view. *Baylor Law Rev* 1975; 27: 6–12.

19. E.g., Institute of Medicine. *Guidance for Establishing Crisis Standards of Care for Use in Disaster Situations: A Letter Report.* Washington DC, National Academies Press, 2009.

20. Schultz CH, Annas GJ. Altering the standard of care in disasters: Unnecessary and dangerous. *Annals of Emergency Medicine* 2012; 59: 191–195.

21. Rothstein MA. Malpractice immunity for volunteer physicians in public health emergencies: adding insult to injury. *Journal of Law, Medicine & Ethics* 2010; 149–153.

22. Hoffman S. Responders' responsibility: Liability and immunity in public health emergencies. *Georgetown Law Journal* 2008; 96: 1913–1969.

23. Annas GJ, Miller FH. The empire of death: how culture and economics affect informed consent in the U.S., the U.K., and Japan. *American Journal of Law & Medicine* 1994; 20: 357–394.

24. American Bar Association Resolution 125, Opposes Regulation of Disaster Relief Care, adopted by the House of Delegates August 8, 2011.

25. Larrey DJ. *Surgical Memoirs of the Campaign in Russia.* trans. Mercer J. Philadelphia, Cowey & Lea, [1863], 1971.

26. Annas GJ. The prostitute, the playboy, and the poet: rationing schemes for organ transplantation. *American Journal of Public Health* 1985; 75: 187–189.

27. Calabresi G, Bobbitt P. *Tragic Choices.* New York, Norton, 1978.

28. Hick JL, Hanfling D, Cantrill SV. Allocating scarce resources in disasters: emergency department principles. *Annals of Emergency Medicine* 2012; 59: 177–187.

29. Persad G, Wertheimer A, Emanuel EJ. Principles for allocation of scarce medical interventions. *Lancet* 2009; 373: 423–431.

30. Emanuel EJ, Wertheimer A. Who should get influenza vaccine when not all can? *Science* 2006; 312: 854–855.

31. Hanson N. *The Custom of the Sea.* New York, John Wiley, 1999.

32. Elinder M, Erixson O. Every man for himself: gender, norms and survival in maritime disasters. Working paper. Department of Economics, Uppsala University, Uppsala, Sweden,. 2012; 8. http://www.nek.uu.se (Accessed August 9, 2015).

33. Fink S. The deadly choices at Memorial. *New York Times Magazine.* August 30, 2009; 28–46.

34. Fink, S. *Five Days at memorial.* New York, Crown, 2013.

35. Deichmann RE. *Code Blue: A Katrina Physician's Memoir.* Bloomington , IN, Rooftop Publishing, 2007.

36. Fink S. Worst case: rethinking tertiary triage protocols in pandemics and other health emergencies. *Critical Care* 2010; 14: 103–105.

37. Okie S. Dr. Pou and the hurricane: implications for patient care during disasters. *N Engl J Med* 2008; 358: 1–5.

38. Wecht CH, Kaufmann D. *A Question of Murder.* Amherst, NY, Prometheus Books, 2008.

39. Annas GJ. Not saints, but healers: the legal duties of health care professionals in the AIDS epidemic. *American Journal of Public Health* 1988; 78: 844–849.

40. Beauchamp TL, Childress JF. *Principles of Biomedical Ethics.* 6th ed. New York, Oxford University Press, 2009.

41. Singer PA, Benatar SR, Bernstein M, et al. Ethics and SARS: lessons from Toronto. *BMJ* 2003; 327: 1342–1345.

42. McCullough LB. Taking seriously the 'what then?' question: an ethical framework for the responsible management of medical disasters. *Journal of Clinical Ethics* 2010; 21: 321–327.

43. Subbarao I, Wynia MK, Burkle FM. The elephant in the room: collaboration and competition among relief organizations during high-profile disasters, *Journal of Clinical Ethics* 2010; 21: 328–334.

44. Walker P, Hein K, Russ C, et al. A blueprint for professionalizing humanitarian assistance. *Health Affairs (Millwood).* 2010; 29: 2223–2230.

45. Schopper D, Upshur R, Matthys F, et al. Research ethics review in humanitarian contexts: the experience of the independent ethics review board of Médecins Sans Frontières. *PloSMed* 2009; 6(7): e1000115.

46. Rid A, Emanuel EJ. Ethical considerations of experimental interventions in the Ebola outbreak. *Lancet* 2014; 384: 1896–1899.

8

EMERGING INFECTIOUS DISEASES: CONCEPTS IN PREPARING FOR AND RESPONDING TO THE NEXT MICROBIAL THREAT

Shantini D. Gamage, Stephen M. Kralovic, and Gary A. Roselle

OVERVIEW*

Former U.S. Surgeon General William H. Stewart has been attributed with stating in the late 1960s that the time had come to "close the book" on infectious diseases as major threats to public health. Even though this statement's authenticity has been questioned,[1] it is often used to convey the optimism expressed at the time by health experts and world leaders.[2] At the time, it did appear that the age of infectious diseases that had plagued humans for millennia was coming to an end. Vaccines and antibiotics had substantially reduced the incidence and mortality of many diseases. The smallpox eradication campaign was on its way and it was thought that eradication of other diseases (for example tuberculosis and polio) would not be too far behind. Improved food and water safety resulted in less exposure to disease-causing microbes, and the use of pesticides to control arthropod populations had reduced vector-borne diseases. It seemed the battle with the microbial world had been won, and it was time to focus efforts and funding on the looming threat of chronic diseases.

This confidence, however, largely ignored the burden of infectious diseases in the developing world. Five decades later, although great strides have been made to control infectious diseases, microbial pathogens are still major threats to public health throughout the world. The last few decades have unveiled new challenges: "old" pathogens once thought to be controlled by antibiotics have developed multidrug resistance, new pathogens have emerged, and traditional pathogens have appeared in new locations. Furthermore, factors such as increased global commerce and travel and the threat of the intentional release of pathogens have set the stage for infectious disease disasters with large numbers of casualties. In this chapter, "casualties" includes all persons with symptoms of the infectious disease, not just fatalities.

There is a wide body of knowledge on the emergence and reemergence of pathogens of public health importance. Humans are in a delicate balance with microbial cohabitants of the earth;

circumstances can tip that balance in favor of microbes with new or renewed pathogenic vigor. There will always be emerging pathogens, and consequently there is always the chance that a virulent microbe will cause extensive human disease and death. Exactly what the causative agent of the next big infectious disease disaster will be and when it will happen is not known. Using examples from past events, this chapter addresses the concepts and tools necessary to prepare better for and respond to infectious disease disasters in general.

OVERVIEW

The Threat of Emerging Infectious Diseases

Infectious diseases are caused by microorganisms such as bacteria, viruses, fungi, and protozoa, and by proteinaceous particles called prions. The majority of microbes on earth are benign to humans; many are necessary for ecological stability, and even human and animal health. Microbes that do cause disease are collectively referred to as pathogens. There are more than 1,400 pathogens known to cause disease in humans.[3]

Some pathogens are prevalent at a constant and stable rate in a given population and are considered "endemic." Other infectious diseases are not common to a given population but, at times, a number of cases occur that is higher than expected. This situation is considered an "outbreak" (for a more localized increase in disease incidence) or an "epidemic" (for a larger regional increase in disease incidence). The concept of the epidemiological triangle (Figure 8.1) is used to understand the factors involved in promoting such an outbreak or epidemic. This model highlights the interactions among an agent (e.g., *Salmonella*), a host (e.g., elderly patients at a nursing home), and an environment (e.g., undercooked chicken left at room temperature) that cause disease (e.g., acute gastroenteritis). Table 8.1 provides a comprehensive list of terms related to infectious disease biology.

Many pathogenic microbes have been associated with human disease for hundreds or thousands of years. Examples of infectious diseases with long human histories include smallpox, plague, cholera, malaria, tuberculosis, and syphilis. These diseases, and others, resulted in millions of deaths over the

---

* The views expressed in this chapter are those of the authors and not necessarily those of the University of Cincinnati or U.S. Department of Veterans Affairs.

Table 8.1. Infectious Diseases Biology Terminology

	Description	*Example*
Airborne Transmission	The process whereby agents are spread by small-particle (≤ 5 μm) droplet nuclei that can suspend in the air and travel by air currents or through ventilation systems; respiratory PPE (N95 respirator) is often required to prevent infection in responders.	*Mycobacterium tuberculosis*
Biological Incident	The presence of a pathogen in a population from a natural, accidental, or intentional exposure that has the potential to cause extensive public harm and/or fear.	2012 MERS emergence in the Middle East (natural); 2010 return of epidemic cholera to Haiti (accidental); 2001 dissemination of anthrax spores in U.S. mail (intentional)
Communicable	The ability of an infectious agent to be transmitted from one host to another; contagious.	Influenza, smallpox
Contact Transmission	The process whereby agents are spread by direct contact with a person or indirect contact with contaminated objects.	Direct contact: skin (MRSA); mucous membrane (HIV) Indirect contact: fecal-oral (norovirus)
Droplet Transmission	The process whereby agents are spread by large-particle (> 5μm) droplet nuclei produced by, for example, coughing and sneezing; agent does not remain suspended in the air for a long time and infection usually occurs when susceptible person is within 1 m of infected person. A surgical mask may offer protection.	Influenza Meningococcal disease
Endemic	A disease that is consistently present in a population at a certain level or rate without requiring introduction from another area.	Malaria in India and Africa
Epidemic	A level of disease that is higher than the expected level at a time or location. Similar to an "outbreak" but usually refers to disease incidence that spans a large region, country, or multiple countries for a prolonged period of time.	Cases of measles in Wales in 2012–2013 Chikungunya fever on La Réunion Island in 2005–2006
Host – Resistant	The state in which a person is immune to infection by a specific pathogen.	In general, a person who has had hepatitis A is resistant to subsequent infection with the hepatitis A virus.
Host – Susceptible	The state in which a person can be infected by a specific pathogen. May be due to lack of immunity and/or to host factors that promote infection (e.g., a specific receptor).	A person who has not had the Measles/Mumps/Rubella (MMR) vaccine is susceptible to the agents that cause these diseases.
Isolation	The separation of infectious disease cases from the general population to prevent transmission of the agent to susceptible people; instead of physical separation, may use barriers such as masks on cases to "isolate" the infection and prevent transmission (this may be necessary in disasters with many casualties).	In 2003, SARS cases were sequestered on specific hospital wards.
Mode of Transmission	The mechanism a pathogen uses to spread from one host to another.	Airborne transmission by small particles in the air
Outbreak	An increased incidence of a disease in a region. Usually on a smaller scale (regionally and temporally) than an epidemic. A food-borne outbreak typically refers to disease caused by food(s) contaminated with a specific pathogenic microorganism.	*Neisseria meningitidis* outbreak on a college campus Norovirus outbreak on a cruise ship
Pandemic	The global spread of an epidemic.	1918 influenza pandemic 2009 H1N1 pandemic
Quarantine	A form of isolation that restricts the movements of *healthy people who were exposed* to a contagious agent to prevent contact with the general public. The duration of the quarantine period is usually the longest time for symptoms to appear after exposure (incubation time). Home quarantine refers to isolation of exposed persons in the home, provided that basic needs can be met and contact with other household members can be avoided. Work quarantine refers to permitting exposed healthcare workers and emergency responders to go to work using appropriate PPE so that disaster operations can remain intact; this modification does not apply to workers in the general public.	In Ontario, Canada in 2003, people who were exposed to SARS were quarantined for 10 days. At times during the epidemic, over half of the paramedics in the Toronto area were operating under work quarantine conditions.
Reproductive Rate (R_0)	For an infectious agent, the number of people to whom an infected person spreads the disease in the absence of control measures (such as vaccination, isolation of cases).	According to historical data, a person with pandemic influenza will transmit the disease to three other people

Table 8.1. (*continued*)

	Description	*Example*
Reservoir	The environmental niche of a pathogenic organism, usually another organism unaffected by the infectious agent.	Specific rodent species are the reservoirs for particular hantavirus strains.
		Human-made water sources for *Legionella* species infections
Vector	An organism (e.g., insects or other arthropods) that harbors and transfers agents that are pathogenic to another organism (e.g., humans).	*Ixodes* ticks transfer *Borrelia burgdorferi*, the causative agent of Lyme disease, to humans; *Anopheles* mosquitoes transfer *Plasmodium* sp, the causative agents of malaria, to humans
Zoonoses	Infectious diseases in which the pathogenic agent is transmitted to humans from animals.	West Nile virus encephalitis is transmitted to humans from birds (via the mosquito vector)

centuries and were the focus of targeted efforts of varying degrees around the world to reduce the burden of infectious diseases on human populations. Improvements to public health systems, such as sanitation, drinking water treatment, and education, reduced human contact with pathogens. Scientific advances, such as antibiotics and vaccines to treat and prevent infectious diseases, revolutionized the medical arsenal against microbes. As a result, by the middle of the twentieth century, the incidence of many infectious diseases plummeted, particularly in the developed world. It was widely thought that science had conquered the threat that infectious diseases posed to human health.

What is appreciated now is that microbes are constantly interacting with their environment and evolving. As they do, circumstances may allow for the emergence of new infectious agents/diseases, or the reemergence of previously controlled contagions. These emergences fall into many categories:[4]

▦ Microorganisms that have not been known previously and that cause new diseases (e.g., severe acute respiratory syn-

drome coronavirus [SARS-CoV] and Middle East respiratory syndrome coronavirus [MERS-CoV]; human immunodeficiency virus [HIV] that causes acquired immunodeficiency syndrome [AIDS]);

▦ Agents that have been known previously and that cause new diseases (hantavirus in the United States in 1993 that caused respiratory distress instead of kidney disease);

▦ Microbes that have been known previously to cause disease, but the incidence of disease is noticeably increasing in a region (e.g., whooping cough caused by *Bordetella pertussis* in the United States; diphtheria caused by *Corynebacterium diphtheriae* in Russia);

▦ New, and often more virulent, strains of a known pathogen that cause disease (e.g., *Vibrio cholerae* O139 and epidemic diarrheal disease; highly virulent *Clostridium difficile* NAP1/027 and increased incidence of *C. difficile*-associated disease in North America and Europe). Increased virulence often occurs when a pathogen acquires a genetic element that allows for the production of a new virulence factor such as a toxin (e.g., *Staphylococcus aureus* that produces TSST-1 and causes toxic shock syndrome);

▦ Microbial pathogens that cause disease in a new geographical location (e.g., West Nile virus encephalitis in North America; reintroduction of epidemic cholera in Haiti; Chikungunya virus in the Caribbean; Ebola virus in West Africa);

▦ Microbes of animal origin that infect humans (zoonoses). This includes animal-associated microorganisms to which humans are newly exposed (e.g., hantavirus pulmonary syndrome due to Sin Nombre virus from the rodent population in the United States), or animal-associated microbes that are newly able to infect humans (e.g., influenza virus from birds or swine);

▦ Microbial pathogens that have acquired the ability to resist the effects of antimicrobial agents (e.g., multidrug-resistant tuberculosis [MDR-TB]; methicillin-resistant and vancomycin-resistant *S. aureus*; amantadine-resistant influenza A virus; carbapenem-resistant Enterobacteriaceae [CREs]).

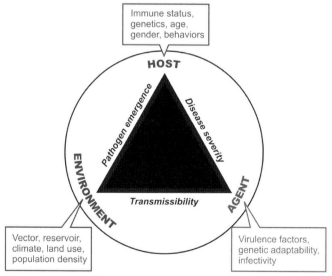

Figure 8.1. The epidemiological triangle. This type of diagram is widely used to represent the interconnectedness of the three major components involved in the emergence of infectious diseases. The "Host" is the organism that is affected by the pathogen or toxin and can develop disease. The "Agent" is the infectious microorganism (pathogen) or toxin. The "Environment" refers to the circumstances that influence the interaction between the Host and the Agent. Examples of influencing factors are given for each component.

The occurrence of emerging infectious diseases (EIDs) or reemerging infectious diseases in human history is not new. The great plague and influenza pandemics are well-known historical examples. The last few decades have witnessed a recrudescence of EIDs. Furthermore, as global surveillance of diseases has developed, the awareness that new EIDs are occurring has increased. Although exact numbers of EIDs are debatable due to differences

Table 8.2. Factors that Drive the Emergence or Reemergence of Infectious Diseases

Factor in Emergence	Description	Example
Microbial Adaptation	Microbes are under constant selective pressure from the environment to adapt genetically for survival. Evidence of adaptation includes: the evolution or acquisition of antibiotic resistance genes that allow bacteria to survive exposure to antibiotics, the mutation of genetic material, and the horizontal transfer of virulence genes from one microbe to another.	The emergence of MDR-TB, which is resistant to at least two of the primary antibiotics used to treat the disease. Even more alarming is the appearance of extensively drug-resistant tuberculosis (XDR-TB), resistant to many first-line *and* second-line antibiotics.

The emergence of CRE, for example by transfer of the New Delhi metallo-beta-lactamase-1 (NDM-1) gene, which confers resistance to a range of antibiotics to bacteria that carry it.

The strain of Shiga-toxin-producing *E. coli* that caused an outbreak of food-related illness in 2011 in Germany and other countries was a rarely seen strain that had virulence factors from two different types of pathogenic *E. coli* and resulted in severe disease in a higher proportion of cases than usual. |
Human Susceptibility	The ability to stave off a pathogenic infection is predominantly due to host immunity, a multi-organ system involving physical barriers, complex cell–cell signaling, recognition, and memory to fight invading pathogens. A healthy immune system is a function of many factors. The extremes of age, poor nutrition, and presence of chronic and/or infectious diseases could result in an immunocompromised state.	The increased incidence of *Pneumocystis jiroveci* (formerly known as *Pneumocystis carinii*) pneumonia in the United States as the HIV/AIDS population increased.
Climate and Weather	Changes in climate and weather affect every organism in a region. As plant and animal life is affected, so too is the interaction between humans and these organisms, and the microorganisms they may harbor. Climatic changes can also affect human activities. For example, a negative effect on crop production can increase malnutrition and render a population more susceptible to disease. Furthermore, agricultural practices may be altered, exposing populations to different vectors and microbial agents.	Certain species of zooplankton are associated with the presence of pathogenic *Vibrio cholerae*. In South America, the El Niño southern oscillation of 1991–1992 increased coastal water temperatures, zooplankton density, and, consequently, exposure of people to *V. cholerae*. The ensuing cholera epidemic was the first in the region in a century.
Changing Ecosystem	The environment can have a profound impact on the emergence of pathogens, predominantly through wildlife ecology and the interaction of humans with the vectors and animals that carry potential pathogens. Environmental changes in forestation, humidity, and predator density due to natural or anthropogenic causes can all affect vector and pathogen biology.	Dam building in Ethiopia to improve agricultural productivity had the undesired side effect of increasing mosquito breeding grounds, an outcome implicated in increases in malaria cases in children.
Human Demographics and Behavior	At over 7 billion people, the world population is four times as large as it was at the beginning of the twentieth century when advances in science, medicine, and public health first allowed for the widespread control of infectious diseases. The increasing population has resulted in crowded living conditions and habitation of previously undeveloped areas, exposing more individuals to new diseases. Human behaviors, often for economic gain, can also influence disease emergence.	Live-animal markets that put humans and pathogens in close contact (e.g., SARS-CoV and influenza viruses).

Commercial sex workers who engage in unprotected sexual intercourse (e.g., HIV emergence in Asia). |
| Economic Development and Land Use | Globalization of national economies has resulted in an unprecedented interdependence in trade and commerce, and an increase in the volume of goods produced. Land use for industry and agriculture, and for population expansion, can influence emerging diseases. | Widespread deforestation in Malaysia for the expansion of plantations encroached on the natural habitat of fruit bats, the reservoir for the previously unknown Nipah virus. The fruit bats found food in the orchards that were adjacent to swine farms and infected the swine with Nipah virus. In 1988, human disease emerged. |
| Technology and Industry | Medical technology has improved lives, but also has led to an increase in immunocompromised persons (e.g., transplant recipients).

Technology has allowed for mass production in the food industry. Larger animal feedlots and processing plants facilitate the transmission of infectious agents from one animal to another. Refrigeration, packaging, and transportation networks allow foods from different regions and countries to be distributed throughout a nation.

Advanced water distribution systems for consumption, hygiene, recreation, and indoor temperature regulation are comforts particularly associated with and expected in the developed world. With this technology comes the risk of mass distribution of pathogens. | Hemophiliacs who were infected with HIV from infected blood products

Spinach contaminated with *E. coli* O157:H7 affected people in over twenty-five U.S. states in 2006.

Viral gastroenteritis outbreaks associated with swimming pools

Growth of *Legionella* bacteria in building water distribution systems and transmission to occupants resulting in Legionnaires' disease |

Table 8.2. (*continued*)

Factor in Emergence	Description	Example
International Travel and Commerce	The movement of people across regions means the movement of microbes and vectors as well. In addition to traveling for pleasure or for business, people move across borders for temporary employment, as military personnel, as immigrants, as refugees, as undocumented persons, or in situations of forced labor. Commerce is highly dependent on international production and trade of goods. For example, foods once considered exotic or seasonal are available in the United States year round due to importation from other countries.	One infected person spread the SARS-CoV from Guangdong Province, China to twelve guests at a Hong Kong hotel. The twelve people spread the virus to five other countries. In 6 months, the SARS-CoV spread from China to over thirty countries on six continents.
Breakdown of Public Health Infrastructure	Public health measures, such as sanitation, health education, vaccinations, and access to care, are critical for preventing infectious diseases. These measures must be consistently upheld, or microbial pathogens will return to the niche they once inhabited. Reasons for public health inadequacies or collapse include economic hardship, political instability, war, complacency, disasters, and lack of priority standing.	In the early 1990s, diphtheria reemerged in the former Soviet Union amidst a turbulent political, economic, and social environment. In 2000, approximately 2,300 people in Walkerton, Ontario, Canada became ill after consuming inadequately treated and monitored drinking water contaminated with *E. coli* O157:H7 and *Campylobacter jejuni*.
Poverty and Social Inequality	Increased populations, political unrest, and/or inadequate food production in some areas have resulted in increased numbers of persons who are malnourished and without access to medical care. Infectious disease outbreaks in these areas tax already overburdened healthcare systems. Inadequate resources spread disease by failing to reach the sick, transmitting the pathogen in the healthcare setting due to crowding and reusing supplies, and neglecting to educate the population on safe practices. In addition, the lack of adequate courses of medication leads to incomplete treatment of disease and the emergence of antibiotic-resistant pathogens.	The incidence of AIDS, malaria, and tuberculosis has reached alarming rates in developing countries where resources are scarce.
War and Famine	War often unsettles populations and increases the reliance on public health infrastructures to provide medicines, food, and emotional support to affected persons. These health systems are often inadequate during peacetime and cannot undertake additional responsibilities during unrest. Furthermore, poor health status in a population may result from: 1) substandard housing in refugee camps; 2) guerilla-controlled access to food and medicines; 3) elevated pollution; and 4) interrupted power and water distribution. Infectious diseases can spread from contaminated food or water, from persons with contagious respiratory diseases, or from sexual assaults. Famine, like poverty, deteriorates the health of populations and renders them more susceptible to old and new infectious diseases.	Cholera outbreaks in the 1990s among Rwandan refugees in the Democratic Republic of Congo resulted in thousands of deaths in weeks.
Lack of Will	Four segments of the global society that must commit to combating emerging infectious diseases are monetary donors, health professionals, governments, and patients and civil society. Donors, both private and public, are necessary to provide funding for research and for health programs. Health professionals must be available to design and implement intervention and prevention programs. Governments must prioritize infectious disease science, surveillance, and reporting; build public health infrastructures; and collaborate with other nations and global partners. And the community needs to motivate the other segments to act by voicing concerns and participating in intervention and prevention programs.	In the West, early efforts to understand HIV and determine intervention strategies were stalled by political and societal discomfort that the disease was spreading in the male homosexual population. Inadequate education on the myths and facts of sexually transmitted infection prevention led to widespread transmission of HIV throughout Africa and Asia.
Intent to Harm	There is heightened awareness of the threat of an intentional attack with a bioweapon. In addition to the unpredictability of when and where such an attack will occur, the type of microbe that will be used is largely unknown. There is concern that the agent used will be one not regularly encountered in the afflicted area. In effect, a bioterrorist attack could result in the emergence or reemergence of infectious diseases in an area, with the potential to cause many casualties. In addition, the social, political, and economic disruption could be far reaching.	2001 release of anthrax spores via the U.S. postal system.

Adapted from: IOM. *Microbial Threats to Health: Emergence, Detection and Response.* Washington, DC, National Academies Press, 2003.

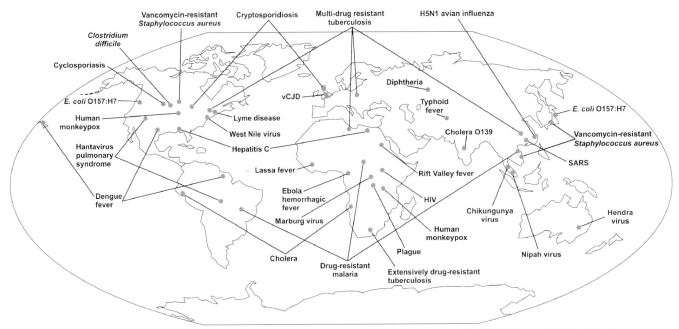

Figure 8.2. Emerging and reemerging infectious diseases/agents, 1990–2013. The diseases/agents in the black boxes with the white dots represent select emergences that have occurred since the first edition of this textbook was published in 2010. *E. coli, Escherichia coli*; vCJD, variant Creutzfeldt–Jakob disease; HIV, human immunodeficiency virus; SARS, severe acute respiratory syndrome; MERS, Middle East respiratory syndrome; NDM-1, New Delhi metallo-beta-lactamase-1.Adapted from the National Institutes of Health website (www3.niaid.gov/about/overview/planningpriorities/strategicplan/emerge.htm).

in criteria used, Taylor and colleagues suggest that 175 of the 1,400-plus known human pathogens are EIDs (approximately 12%).[3]

Figure 8.2 shows recent EIDs and reemerging infectious diseases in both the developed and developing world.

The question then is: Why are EIDs occurring so frequently despite the optimism of past generations? In 2003, the Institute of Medicine (IOM) published *Microbial Threats to Health: Emergence, Detection and Response*,[5] which outlined thirteen factors that contribute to the emergence or reemergence of new pathogens.

Although now more than a decade old, the IOM report remains a seminal work in framing the understanding of why infectious diseases emerge. The factors reflect a very different world from previous decades. "Globalization," often characterized by changes in global movement, economic development, and environmental and agricultural practices, has unwittingly exposed the world's populations to microbial threats. Not all of the categories are necessary for every emerging pathogen; however, neither are they mutually exclusive. The emergence or reemergence of a pathogen is usually a function of many factors. An understanding of all the factors is necessary to prevent or quickly detect future EIDs and to determine how to effectively mitigate an EID disaster.

Table 8.3 uses pandemic influenza, dengue hemorrhagic fever, MDR-TB, HIV/AIDS, and cholera to demonstrate how these factors interplay in the emergence or reemergence of diseases.

Another example of the convergence of factors resulting in disease emergence and transmission is the Ebola virus disease (EVD) outbreak in West Africa,[6] the first such outbreak in that region and a situation still evolving at the time of this writing

in August 2014. With 3,069 cases and 1,552 deaths reported as of August 26, 2014 in Guinea, Liberia, Sierra Leone, and Nigeria, it is the largest EVD outbreak to date. The outbreak started in Guinea; phylogenetic analysis suggests evolution of the virus in the area as opposed to importation of the outbreak strain from other countries.[7] The initial EVD cases and transmission were unrecognized, likely a result of local clinicians' unfamiliarity with the disease and its symptoms, and also due to inadequate healthcare availability and resources. Human behaviors in the area may have also played a role in the emergence and persistence of the disease, including: funeral practices that involve touching the deceased; food habits such as consumption of bats, a likely vector; mistrust of government officials, aid organizations, and healthcare workers resulting in delayed or avoided care; and fear, resulting in actions such as airplane flight limitations that affect resources and response capabilities. Indication that residents attacked and looted an EVD clinic in a poor neighborhood of Monrovia, Liberia suggests instability in the area is resulting in unconventional risks for further transmission of this disease. Likely the most critical factors related to the scope of this EVD outbreak compared to previous outbreaks are modernization and urbanization. Cases have occurred in larger cities with more mobile populations, and travel by land and air has transmitted disease between countries, hindering the comprehensive contact tracing necessary to prevent continued transmission.

Many of the thirteen factors outlined by IOM drive disease emergence by influencing the interaction of humans with animal reservoirs of potential pathogens. In fact, approximately 75% of recently emerged pathogens are zoonotic. The abundance, location, and behaviors of putative animal reservoirs, and human influences on them, are important factors in

Table 8.3. Examples of How Multiple Factors Influence the Emergence or Reemergence of Infectious Diseases

Infectious Disease (Agent)	Pandemic Influenza* (highly pathogenic avian influenza [HPAI] virus)	Dengue Hemorrhagic Fever (dengue virus; transmitted to humans by mosquito vector)	Multidrug-resistant Tuberculosis (Mycobacterium tuberculosis)	AIDS (HIV)	Epidemic cholera in Haiti (Vibrio cholerae)
Emergence Factor					
Microbial Adaptation	Reassortment of, or mutations in, influenza virus genes that allow for human–human transmission of HPAI virus	Adaptation of viral strains to urban mosquitoes facilitated emergence	Improper use of antibiotics allowed M. tuberculosis to develop resistances	Mutation of simian immunodeficiency virus to infect humans; emergence of drug-resistant HIV; high mutation rate complicates vaccine development	Mutations in toxin genes have resulted in an altered El Tor strain of V. cholerae with increased virulence
Human Susceptibility	Extensive viral adaptations means no inherent immunity in humans; no vaccine-enhanced immunity in the initial months of the pandemic	No cross-immunity to the four different viral strains; heterologous infection increases chance of severe disease	Increased tuberculosis in HIV-endemic areas	Lack of host immunity when virus emerged; no vaccine-enhanced immunity	Immunologically naive population on Hispaniola (Haiti and Dominican Republic) where cholera had not been seen for a century
Climate and Weather	Cold weather in some countries during flu season encourages social clustering and, consequently, viral transmission	Rainy seasons increase mosquito population			
Changing Ecosystems	Changing marshland habitats and waterfowl distribution	Repopulation of New World by mosquito species after mid-twentieth century mosquito eradication programs ended			
Human Demographics and Behavior	Increased worldwide poultry production to feed increased human population; cohabitation with potential zoonotic sources	Disease centers in overpopulated urban areas with poor housing and utility management that promote mosquito breeding grounds	Failure to adhere to medication regimens; people in remote areas hard to treat consistently; immigration of infected persons	Unprotected sexual activity; illicit intravenous drug use; prostitution	Disaster relief being provided in response to the 2010 earthquake
Economic Development and Land Use	Live markets put humans and infected birds in close contact	Dam building promotes mosquito breeding grounds			
Technology and Industry	Crowded poultry feedlots favor viral transmission between birds	Possible disease transmission through blood products		Disease transmission through blood products	
International Travel and Commerce	Global travel can rapidly spread disease; illegal exotic bird trade can transfer infectious birds	Travelers can spread strains between endemic areas; outbreaks in nonendemic areas with appropriate mosquito species (e.g., southern United States)	Dissemination of M. tuberculosis on airplanes via recirculation of air	Global travel spreads disease	Travel of international relief workers to Haiti to aid in the earthquake disaster response; relief workers from Asia, where cholera is endemic/epidemic, may have been incubating cholera at the time of deployment
Breakdown of Public Health Infrastructure	Prolonged nature of the pandemic strains resources	Lack of effective mosquito control; poor water and sewage systems in developing areas	Inability to monitor tuberculosis population; high treatment interruption rates in developing countries; HIV epidemic areas overwhelmed	Lack of education and intervention programs, overwhelmed workforce in developing countries	Disruption of already-poor sanitation, water treatment, and healthcare infrastructures by the earthquake disaster

99

(continued)

Table 8.3. (continued)

Infectious Disease (Agent)	Pandemic Influenza* (highly pathogenic avian influenza [HPAI] virus)	Dengue Hemorrhagic Fever (dengue virus; transmitted to humans by mosquito vector)	Multidrug-resistant Tuberculosis (Mycobacterium tuberculosis)	AIDS (HIV)	Epidemic cholera in Haiti (Vibrio cholerae)
Poverty and Social Inequality	Rapid spread of the virus in the developing world	Developing countries that lack vector control programs risk high incidence	Expense of directly observed therapy inhibits consistent use in poorer nations	Expense of antiretroviral therapy; stigmatization of men who have sex with men, especially in early days of the emergence; marginalized women's rights in some societies	Occurrence in a developing nation with few resources for public health infrastructure and response; waning aid and funding
War and Famine	Increased global travel during World War I facilitated propagation of the 1918 influenza pandemic		Tuberculosis spreads quickly through refugee camps (e.g., in Somalia)	Treatment programs are difficult to administer in areas of conflict	Malnutrition in the population resulting in increased disease severity and poor outcomes
Lack of Will	Pharmaceutical industry and vaccine/therapeutic development	Poor surveillance in endemic countries	Inadequate infection control policies or practices	Initial low research and intervention priorities for an agent primarily spreading in men who have sex with men; refusal of officials in some developing countries to acknowledge HIV in the population	Low priority for vaccine development; initial reluctance of international relief force to acknowledge that response efforts may have contributed to the reemergence, leading to mistrust of the nation
Intent to Harm	Theoretical potential of genetically reconstructed 1918 pandemic influenza virus to be used in a terrorist attack				

* At the time of this writing, pandemic HPAI has not reemerged. Based on knowledge from prior influenza pandemics and extensive studies on influenza virus epidemiology and genetics, experts have uncharacteristically broad insight into factors that affect how these zoonotic pathogens emerge.

disease emergence. Microbes often live in harmony with animal hosts and the pathogenic infection of humans is inadvertent.

Infectious Diseases and Disaster Medicine

History has shown that infectious disease outbreaks, epidemics, and pandemics have the potential to afflict large numbers of people. Estimates for the next severe influenza pandemic suggest millions of cases in the United States alone with hundreds of thousands of flu-related fatalities. The 2001 deliberate release of anthrax spores in the United States through the postal system and the 2003 SARS pandemic are reminders that the scope of the disaster is not just a function of actual case numbers, but of the ability to manage the outbreak and to the public reaction during the event. Both situations taxed the available resources of some of the most sophisticated public health systems in the world despite relatively low numbers of cases.[6,7]

Disasters are commonly considered to be acute, often regional, events. Even in the realm of infectious diseases, the anthrax letters incident in the United States is often cited as an example of the type of response required for an infectious disease disaster. More likely, however, biological situations (of either intentional or unintentional origin) that strain response efforts will unfold in a more gradual manner. Furthermore, if disasters are defined as situations that require external resource assistance, then the global AIDS pandemic (now decades long) can be considered a disaster. Disasters due to EIDs are of particular concern given the paucity of information on the biology of the agent, the course of disease, and mechanisms of treatment. Even a local outbreak of a known infectious agent can strain a response effort.

Management of infectious disease disasters shares many general aspects of the management of other disasters. The basic principles of leadership and collaboration, resource management, surge capacity, triage, and public relations are all important; however, the specifics of response activities can have special considerations when an infectious agent is the cause of the disaster.

Table 8.4 provides a description of unique features of infectious disease disasters that are not usually encountered in many other disaster response efforts.

The Infectious Agent

Infectious disease disasters, unlike physical and chemical incidents, are caused by biological entities that are diverse and under constant selective pressures to change. It may be clear that an outbreak has occurred due to the contagiousness and nature of the illness that characterize cases presenting to healthcare facilities; however, the identity of the agent that is sickening patients may be elusive, and any effort to mitigate the disease and spread

Table 8.4. Challenges of Infectious Disease Disasters that May Differentiate Them from Other Types of Disasters

Category*	Challenge
Infectious Agent	Novel agent or one not previously associated with disease
	No known treatment or cure
	Unknown reservoir
	May not initially be recognized as the causative agent of the disaster
Disease	Not characterized previously
	Medical community lacks experience identifying and treating
	Symptoms are similar to other infectious diseases
	People who are concerned about exposure but not truly exposed
Transmission	Contagious agent – large numbers infected over time
	Global response may be necessary to contain agent
	Multiple cities affected
	Disaster could last weeks, months, years or decades
	How to decide when the disaster is over
Personnel	Exposure of response personnel to agent
	Healthcare workers' absenteeism due to concern of contracting agent
Resources	Isolation of cases in the healthcare facility
	Decontamination of hospital equipment
	Capacity of laboratory to process samples
	Distribution of limited supplies (drugs, equipment)
	May be other infectious disease outbreaks concurrently
The Public	Quarantine and Isolation
	Screening for symptoms (at hospitals, airports)
	Controlling movement (closed borders)
	Closing services (schools, churches, public transportation)
	Psychological fears
	Media relations
Ethics and Law	Mass vaccinations
	Quarantine/restriction of movement
	Allocation of resources
	Demands on healthcare workers, first responders
Terrorism	Balancing epidemiological and criminal investigations

* The first three categories (agent, disease, transmission) are unique to infectious disease disasters. The remaining categories (personnel, resources, the public, ethics and law, and terrorism) may apply to other types of disasters, but the challenges listed are unique or particularly applicable to infectious disease disasters.

of the agent will be compromised. Cases of severe atypical pneumonia perplexed physicians in Guangdong province, China in 2002. Chinese officials maintained the causative agent to be a bacterium called *Chlamydia*.[8] It was not until months later, after global spread occurred requiring a then-unprecedented international response effort, that a new coronavirus was publicly identified as the cause of a heretofore-uncharacterized disease, SARS.

For a number of infectious agents, previously known or unknown, there is no specific treatment or cure. Medical management is limited to supportive care, which may require long hospital stays. Depending on the number of afflicted persons, this could affect resource availability (discussed later). The unknown nature of some pathogens also limits detection and diagnostic capabilities.

Infectious agents are often zoonoses. Human infection from the animal reservoir occurs when environmental and behavioral factors coincide to allow for transmission of the agent. In the case of EIDs, the identity of the animal reservoir may be unknown. Successful mitigation of disease spread is contingent on discovering the reservoir. The 1993 emergence of hantavirus pulmonary disease in different locations in the United States occurred due to increased contact between rodent and human populations; disease eradication followed reduction of human contact with rodent excreta.

The Disease

In some situations, the medical literature may not have previously described the disease (e.g., the various viral hemorrhagic fevers that have emerged over the years), or a particular disease was not previously associated with a type of infectious agent (e.g., acute respiratory disease and hantaviruses). In either case, understanding the mechanism of disease is important to provide effective care and prevent future cases. Incomplete or incorrect disease classification hampers an effective response effort. Alternatively, a disease may be classically associated with an infectious agent; however, outbreaks are rare (e.g., SARS) or historical (e.g., smallpox) and the medical community lacks experience in identifying and treating the disease. This scenario can also affect the timeliness with which a disaster is controlled.

In many instances, an EID has similar symptoms to other diseases that are endemic to a region. SARS patients had general symptoms of fever, headache, and malaise that typically progressed to pneumonia. Healthcare workers had the daunting task of differentiating patients with respiratory ailments to properly isolate and treat the SARS cases.[9] Likewise, a 1995 *Neisseria meningitidis* outbreak in Minnesota occurred during flu season, overwhelming a hospital emergency department and complicating triage.[10] Additionally, some cases of EVD in West Africa in 2013 and 2014 may initially have been diagnosed as malaria[6] – a disease that requires different clinical and infection control practices to prevent illness and transmission.

Particularly during epidemics with common symptoms such as headache and fever, healthcare facilities may be inundated with the so-called worried well. Although psychology experts have advocated for abandoning this phrase and replacing it with more appropriate terminology such as "medically unexplained symptoms," it is still often used to refer to persons who think they may have symptoms although they do not actually have the disease, or to well persons who present to healthcare facilities in the hopes of receiving prophylaxis "just in case." These situations are understandable given the fear of contracting the infectious disease and the desire to protect oneself and one's family. Communication with the public is an important component of the response. It provides information on the disease and actions to take if people think they have been exposed. Crowd control, screening, and triage may be necessary actions to separate infected and uninfected persons.

Transmission of the Infectious Agent

An infectious disease may be contagious. This occurs when the reproductive rate (R_0) – the average number of secondary cases to which an infected person spreads the disease when no control measures are used – is greater than 1. Some agents, such as *Bacillus anthracis* (the causative agent of anthrax) are not contagious ($R_0 < 1$) and containment of the disaster is dependent on prevention of human contact with *B. anthracis* spores in the environment. Many other infectious agents are contagious ($R_0 > 1$). Pandemic influenza R_0 estimations vary, but most are approximately 2–3.[11] This means that one person with influenza will likely infect two other people. Interestingly, in the case of SARS-CoV, the R_0 was usually approximately 2–4, yet some people appeared to be super spreaders, passing the virus to at least ten people.[12] This variance in R_0 among different hosts complicates predictions of the magnitude of the epidemic.

There are many implications of a communicable disease agent for disaster relief. Large numbers of afflicted persons could result from a single "emergence" of an agent or from one bioterrorist attack because more and more people are exposed to the agent. Due to travel of infected persons (e.g., SARS in 2003, MERS in 2013), or environmental factors that influence animal ecology (e.g., hantavirus pulmonary syndrome in 1995), the infectious disease may affect many cities, straining the ability of national and regional agencies to assist in local response efforts. Furthermore, as multiple neighboring public health jurisdictions are affected, communication and collaboration becomes important. If the infectious agent crosses international borders, a global effort may be required to end the spread of disease. This could include travel restrictions, surveillance, and the sharing of resources (e.g., vaccines and antibiotics) and technology (e.g., diagnostics).

The communicability of an infectious agent can also affect the duration of the disaster. Rather than resulting in an acute incident, an infectious disease disaster could last weeks, months, or even years as waves of people are affected in a region or across the globe. Pandemic influenza is predicted to last 18–24 months. The AIDS disaster has lasted for decades. Sustaining disaster relief for years will be challenging – resource utilization, a fatigued healthcare workforce, even changing political administrations, can all affect response and recovery efforts. As mentioned previously, other infectious disease outbreaks will surely occur, requiring an even greater effort from an already overwhelmed system.

Transmissibility of infectious agents in the context of disaster medicine and infectious disease emergence is poignantly exemplified by the cholera epidemic in Haiti that followed the devastating January 2010 earthquake. The country, already burdened with suboptimal public health, medical, and sanitation infrastructures, was critically in need of assistance to respond to victims of the earthquake. The world reacted, and thousands of aid workers descended on Haiti in the days, weeks, and months after. In October 2010, a new issue began to emerge – increasing cases of severe, acute gastrointestinal illness in areas along the Artibonite River that spread to all parts of the country. Surprisingly, the disease was cholera, which had not been seen in Haiti in over 100 years. It was possible that a local strain of the bacteria had reemerged after the earthquake. However, extensive analysis revealed an unexpected source – molecular characterization of the strain and epidemiological evidence strongly indicate that the epidemic strain of *Vibrio cholerae* was introduced to the region by a vessel of United Nations relief workers from Asia. It appears that sewage disposal practices on the ship introduced a particularly virulent South Asian strain of *V. cholerae* to the Artibonite River and eventually exposed millions of immunologically naive people to the agent, largely due to insufficient sanitation and healthcare systems. By the fall of 2013, hundreds of thousands of people had become ill and over 8,000 people had died in Haiti,[13] and the bacteria had spread to neighboring Dominican Republic and Cuba. This is the first widely documented case of the international disaster response resulting in a second large-scale disaster of an infectious nature. This occurrence has not only led to mass casualties, but also to the reemergence of an infectious disease in a region.[14]

Implementation of the incident command system for disaster relief of an acute event such as a fire is relatively straightforward, with a clear start and end point. The beginning and end of an infectious disease disaster can be much less clear. Often, a period of days occurs when no new cases are diagnosed, the outbreak is determined to be over, and public health response activities return to normal; then, the community experiences a second wave of cases and public health and healthcare entities must work quickly to reinstate outbreak procedures. This concept is illustrated by the 2003 SARS epidemics in Ontario, Canada and in Taiwan, with a focus on infectious disease transmission in the healthcare setting. The 2003 SARS epidemic curve for Ontario, Canada demonstrates two phases of increased disease incidence (Figure 8.3).

Provincial public health officials had assumed that the outbreak in Ontario was contained at the end of April 2003 because no new cases of SARS were diagnosed after April 20. World Health Organization (WHO) officials concurred; the travel advisory to Toronto was lifted on April 30 and Toronto was removed from the WHO list of locations with disseminated SARS on May 14, 2003. Ontario health officials relaxed the strict hospital infection control directives for SARS. Days later, the second phase of the epidemic in Ontario began. Apparently, patient-to-patient and patient-to-visitor spread of the virus was still occurring unnoticed at one hospital. When SARS control measures were lifted, viral exposure of hospital workers led to a resurgence of cases.

Once again, infection control directives were issued, the hospital ceased admitting new patients, and hospital workers faced restrictions and quarantine.[15] Taiwan also had transmission of SARS among healthcare workers.[16] In contrast to the Toronto experience, some patients and staff were quarantined in the affected healthcare facility, infection control practices were enhanced at all facilities, and extensive community

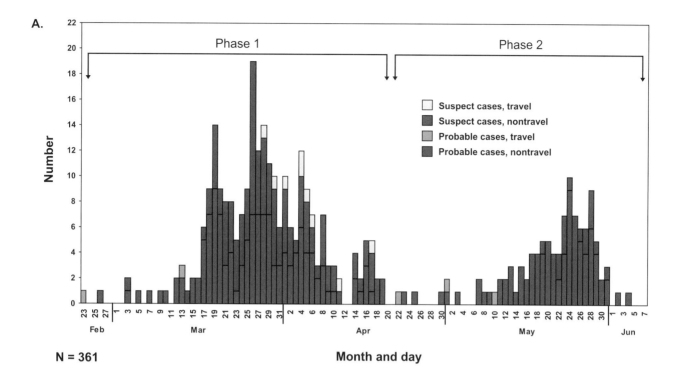

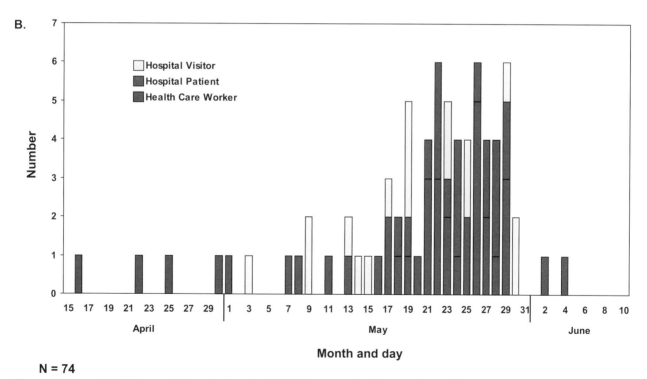

Figure 8.3. Reported SARS cases in Ontario, Canada in 2003 demonstrating the two phases of the epidemic. A) Number of reported cases of SARS by classification and date of illness onset – Ontario, Canada, February 23–June 7, 2003. B) Number of reported cases of SARS in the second phase of the epidemic by source of infection and date of illness onset – Toronto, Canada, April 15–June 9, 2003. Adapted from U.S. Centers for Disease Control and Prevention. 2003. Update: Severe acute respiratory syndrome – Toronto, Canada. *MMWR*; 52(23): 547–550.

screening, outreach, and infection control practices were instituted. Although the total case count was higher in Taiwan, the outbreak curve was not bimodal. The experiences of these two cities stress a number of points: 1) Surveillance is critical to limiting the spread of an infectious agent in the healthcare setting. All patients and healthcare workers should be monitored for development of symptoms. 2) Decision-makers must be wary of relaxing strict infection control measures too soon. Although officials in Ontario and at WHO waited at least 20 days (two incubation periods) before lifting the SARS directives, this action was complicated by the difficulty in differentiating SARS patients from patients with other respiratory ailments. 3) The psychological toll on affected citizens, and especially healthcare workers who may have witnessed their colleagues become sick and die, was immense in both cities and must be factored into the situational awareness for the event for determination of response actions. The very nature of infectious agents is often unpredictable, especially when the agent is newly emerging. This reality needs to be balanced with the desire to return an overwhelmed staff and system to normal operations.

Food-borne transmission of infectious agent adds other facets to the epidemiological investigation. Identification of the contaminated product(s) can involve: obtaining food histories from cases and controls, sometimes weeks after the initial cases surface; extensive laboratory analysis of food and environmental samples; consideration of food distribution networks and trace-backs to food sources; implications on the food industry and consumer perceptions; differences in local, regional, and national food outbreak surveillance protocols; and ramifications of/to the economy and international trade. The 2008 *Salmonella* serotype Saint Paul outbreak, associated with over 1,400 cases in the United States and Canada – initially attributed to tomatoes and then to Mexican hot peppers – has been the subject of numerous hearings and analyses to elucidate shortcomings in food safety and outbreak response in North America.[17] Likewise, the 2011 outbreak of *E. coli* O104:H4 in Germany and other parts of Europe, which resulted in about 4,000 illnesses and 53 deaths, was misattributed to Spanish cucumbers before Egyptian sprouts were identified as the likely transmission vehicle. International response included the banning of Spanish and/or European Union produce by some countries (e.g., Russia), a UN epidemiological investigation of Egyptian fenugreek seed suppliers, and the Egyptian government refuting claims that seeds from their growers were the source of the outbreak.[18]

Response Personnel

The communicability of infectious diseases poses a unique threat to first responders, hospital emergency departments, and primary care providers. Although a radiological attack can result in exposure of healthcare workers, the mechanism and nature of the injuries is well-defined and the threat, once identified, can be relatively easily contained and avoided. In contrast, containing an infectious agent in the healthcare setting can be far more insidious – some people may be asymptomatic carriers of the agent, surfaces may be contaminated, and appropriate personal protective equipment (PPE) may not be in use. The infectious nature itself of a newly emerging pathogen, including whether it is contagious prior to symptom onset, may not even be recognized. All of these factors can result in exposure of healthcare workers to the agent. In the 1957 influenza pandemic, healthcare workers constituted a large proportion of the infected. The emergence of Ebola-Zaire virus in 1976 devastated the region, including the

clinic run by Belgian missionary Sisters. Almost 20 years later, 30% of physicians and 10% of nurses were infected with Ebola-Zaire during an outbreak in the Democratic Republic of the Congo (formerly known as Zaire).[19] SARS in Toronto primarily spread in the healthcare setting (72% of cases were healthcare related), and 44% of cases were healthcare workers.[20] MERS transmission in 2013 was also documented in the healthcare setting.[21,22]

It may be necessary to restrict the movement of individuals in a community to prevent spread of the infectious agent. This is particularly true in the healthcare setting where infectious people congregate and where immunocompromised patients can be exposed. During the SARS pandemic, many healthcare workers were directed to function under work quarantine. These workers were instructed to go to work or stay home, with minimal contact outside these areas. Many healthcare workers are stationed at different facilities or have more than one healthcare-related job. The movement of workers between facilities could expose many more patients to the infectious agent, yet prohibiting this movement would leave facilities understaffed.

Health professionals are a dedicated group of individuals who adhere to a code of ethics to provide care for the ill and injured (often referred to as "duty to care"); however, the management of infectious disease outbreaks is stressful. The long hours often due to understaffing, high volume of patients, duration of the outbreak, and publicity can have adverse psychological impacts on responders and primary care providers. If the infectious agent is emerging and unknown, highly communicable and/or highly lethal, it is possible that healthcare workers will be unwilling or unable to perform their duties. Various studies have been conducted to assess healthcare worker willingness to provide care during infectious disease disasters (notably SARS[23] and influenza pandemics[24]) and the contributing factors for refusing the duty to care. An analysis of published, peer-reviewed articles found that personal obligations and protection of self and loved ones from disease via availability of antiviral medication and/or vaccine were important determinants in willingness to report to work.[25]

The personnel "on call" during an infectious disease disaster are not just the direct patient care staff. Public health staff (nurses, epidemiologists, sanitarians, and laboratory technologists) will be involved from the beginning to determine the extent of the disaster and how to stop the spread of the infectious agent, and to identify the infectious agent source. These efforts necessitate long work hours for days and often weeks. A second unrelated infectious disease outbreak or disaster could occur during or shortly after the first disaster, requiring the same personnel to act without respite. This protracted demand on the workforce may require recruitment of additional personnel not specifically trained for a particular task to maintain the increased level of service (surge capacity). For example, in the 1995 *N. meningitidis* outbreak in Minnesota, extra people were needed to dispense antibiotics, a job that legally could only be performed by a registered pharmacist until the licensing board provided emergency authorization for others to do so. Understanding surge capacity needs is critical to timely, consistent, and effective remediation of the event.

Resources

The availability of resources in public health is a concern even in the absence of a disaster situation. The 2004 shortage of seasonal influenza vaccine in the United States resulted in long lines, distribution issues, and public attention – the shortage itself became a disaster of sorts. This scenario of limited vaccine availability was heightened in the 2009 H1N1 influenza pandemic,[26] even though disease severity was not high. During an outbreak or epidemic, mobilization of potentially large volumes of preventive and/or prophylactic medicines to the affected area(s) is necessary in a short period of time. Approximately 10,000 courses of ciprofloxacin were required to treat the people *possibly exposed* to anthrax spores in the United States in October 2001.[27] The 1995 *N. meningitidis* outbreak in Minnesota resulted in the vaccination of 30,000 people, more than half the population of the town. The vaccine stock was not available locally and it took 2 days to deliver the medication to the impacted area. In the 2010 emergence of cholera in Haiti, oral cholera vaccine was not used based on a number of factors including unavailability of enough doses for the population and logistical issues with implementing a vaccination campaign in the aftermath of the earthquake.[28]

Healthcare workers and other response personnel at risk of exposure must use appropriate PPE to prevent exposure to the infectious agent. U.S. hospitals use national guidelines for the types of PPE required based on the mode of pathogen transmission (e.g., contact, droplet, or airborne). Details on the types of PPE required for the different modes of transmission are available at the U.S. Centers for Disease Control and Prevention (CDC) website.[29] The World Health Organization also espouses use of PPE for response to infectious conditions.[30] Public health experts may recommend extra precautions when the agent initially emerges and there is incomplete information on the mode(s) of transmission. For example, evidence suggested that SARS-CoV was not spread by airborne transmission (characterized by dissemination through the air on small particles); however, healthcare workers were often directed to wear airborne PPE (N95 respirators). Consideration should be given to ensuring that PPE can be used properly in an emergency situation (e.g., some respirators need to be fit-tested for optimal functioning) and to contingency plans if PPE availability is insufficient.

The healthcare workforce is a resource itself. As workers become ill, stressed, or quarantined, fewer people will be available to care for patients (in fact, the number of patients may increase as workers become patients). Some of the most qualified people to treat disease will be on the front lines at the beginning of the disaster and at increased risk of contracting disease. This may require less experienced individuals from other departments to fill the void. Many healthcare workers died from SARS in 2002 and 2003, including Dr. Carlo Urbani, the WHO infectious diseases specialist in Vietnam who is credited with discovering the outbreak and taking steps to prevent its spread.

Even with the proper use of PPE, a contagious microbe can spread in the healthcare setting. Examples include patient-to-patient or patient-to-visitor transmission. Therefore, the isolation of infectious patients to one area of the facility is recommended. This may necessitate extra equipment and supplies dedicated for use in the isolation area. Patients infectious with pathogens spread by airborne transmission (or with emerging pathogens for which airborne transmission is suspected) should be sequestered in negative pressure rooms from which air is released directly outside or filtered before recirculation throughout the facility. There are, however, limited numbers of these units and a large infectious disease disaster may require cohorting multiple patients in the same room or even the establishment of facilities committed to treating only infectious patients. During other types of large disasters, patients are often transferred to various hospitals in the region. Although this has been successfully accomplished in some infectious disease disasters (e.g., in Singapore during the SARS epidemic), any patient transfer risks further spreading of the disease and should be undertaken within the context of overall containment strategies. Furthermore, in systems that allow it, neighboring hospitals may be unwilling to accept patients from hospitals with confirmed cases due to concern of the disease spreading to their own patients and staff. If the original hospital is designated as an infectious disease facility, these other hospitals may be willing to accept nonexposed patients in transfer, thereby increasing capacity for contagious patients within the original facility.

Equipment that is used to treat multiple patients, ranging from stethoscopes to ventilators, must be properly managed between patients using disposal or decontamination processes as appropriate. This may be particularly difficult for new infectious agents for which effective decontamination protocols are not known. Furthermore, taking equipment out of circulation, even temporarily, may delay treatment of patients.

There are usually two general aspects to mitigating an infectious disease outbreak: the care of individual patients (to alleviate disease and suffering) and the population epidemiological investigation and response (to prevent further transmission). In both cases, laboratory testing of human and/or environmental samples for evidence of the pathogen is important to ensure the correct intervention strategies are directed to the right people and areas. Although an increase in the number of patient samples during an outbreak is often expected, the number of environmental samples can be quite large. At times, the magnitude of testing required is overwhelming to even the larger regional, national, and international laboratories, whose services are required for sizeable incidents and/or for the testing of certain pathogens. For example, thousands of analytical assays were performed on environmental samples in the 1993 U.S. hantavirus pulmonary disease epidemic, in the 1999 West Nile virus emergence in the United States, in the 2001 U.S. anthrax attacks, and in the 2012 *E. coli* O104:H4 outbreak in Germany. The response to an EID outbreak may be largely dependent on the local public health workforce, but this response may be directly reliant on the capacity of other health departments and agencies.

The Public

The 2003 SARS epidemic in Toronto provides numerous examples of unique considerations for interacting with the public during an infectious disease disaster. The etiology of SARS was initially unknown, but it was apparent that person-to-person transmission was occurring. Therefore, voluntary quarantine measures were implemented, representing the first time in 50 years that such measures were used in North America to control disease transmission in a community. Approximately 23,000 people were asked to adhere to home quarantine (remain at home, wear a mask, have limited contact with family members, and measure their temperatures twice a day) and/or work quarantine. Studies after the epidemic ended suggest that complete compliance to home quarantine requirements was low.[31] Respondents to a web-based survey indicated confusion over the quarantine instructions and inability to contact public health officials for clarification. Furthermore, the quarantine period was necessarily 10 days, a relatively long time for most people to be away from work and community activities.

For this pandemic, it was not necessary to close borders (within and/or between nations) to general travel. Diseases with higher transmission rates, such as smallpox from a bioterrorist attack (estimated $R_0 = 10$),[32] may require such stringent measures. Issues to consider are enforcement, the effect on businesses, and the effect on the supply chain for disaster management. Institutions within a community where people congregate may require closure, including schools and places of worship.

Whether or not movement or quarantine measures are implemented, public concern and psychological trauma will likely be high for both contagious and noncontagious diseases. This concern will be a function of exposure risk to the agent and subsequent infection, the severity of illness, and the availability of treatment for oneself and one's dependents. Media coverage during the disaster influences community resilience and either exacerbates or alleviates fears, depending on perceptions of the mitigation effort and truthfulness and accuracy of the messages.

Ethics and Law

There are many ethical and legal considerations in the management of an infectious disease disaster. The following issues are illustrative:[33]

- The process of making population-based decisions for infection control during a disaster (e.g., mass vaccinations, quarantine, and movement restrictions) will raise concerns about the legality and necessity of infringements of individuals' rights.
- A scarcity of resources such as vaccines, therapeutics, or hospital equipment will require difficult decisions about who receives the resources and who does not.
- In the event of a disaster caused by a highly contagious, highly virulent, uncharacterized, and/or genetically engineered agent, to what extent should first responders and other healthcare workers be expected to comply with "duty to care" orders for the public good?

Terrorism

This chapter will not elaborate on preparedness and response for infectious disease events caused by bioterrorism because their presentation and management is similar to that for other microbial threats. Criteria include most of those already described, albeit some may be particularly relevant (e.g., public fear, the number of areas affected, and laboratory capacity). The U.S. Department of Health and Human Services (HHS), specifically CDC, and the U.S. Department of Agriculture, Animal and Plant Health Inspection Service jointly administer the Federal Select Agent Program, which maintains and oversees use of a list of select agents and toxins that "have the potential to pose a severe threat to public, animal or plant health or to animal or plant products."[34] Diseases caused by many of the agents on this list, including anthrax, smallpox, and the viral hemorrhagic fevers, are not commonly encountered by the medical community in the Western hemisphere. A bioterrorist may use an agent that has been genetically engineered to be highly virulent, resistant to therapeutics, and/or to cause a novel disease. In these cases, health professionals will be at a further disadvantage to prevent disease and death.

As with every terrorist attack, a criminal investigation should ensue after a bioweapon is used. In other types of attacks, this investigation begins immediately after the actual incident has occurred (e.g., an explosion), during the aftermath and rescue efforts. When a bioweapon is used, it may be days or longer before exposed people develop symptoms. Depending on the agent used, it may be an even longer time before a crime is

Table 8.5. Indications that an Infectious Disease Outbreak May Be Due to a Bioterrorist Attack

Category	Indication of Bioterror Attack*
Agent	The disease or agent is not usually seen in the region (e.g., smallpox anywhere in the world; plague caused by *Yersinia pestis* on the East Coast of the United States).
	Multiple geographically distant areas have disease outbreaks occurring at the same time due to a genetically identical strain of an agent. (e.g., identical *Francisella tularensis* strain causes outbreaks in Washington, DC, St. Louis, MO, and Las Vegas, NV). Note: unintentional food-borne outbreaks may display this incidence pattern if the contaminated product is widely distributed.
	Genetically engineered to be resistant to multiple antibiotics, particularly those commonly used to treat disease (e.g., ciprofloxacin-resistant *B. anthracis*).
	Genetically engineered to cause a novel disease for that agent (e.g., incorporation of genes that cause symptoms of a chronic disease).
	Genetically engineered to be more virulent than usual (e.g., incorporation of genes for toxin production; reconstructed 1918 influenza virus).
Host/ Environment	Larger number of casualties in a region in a short period of time compared to expected incidence.
	Cases do not have risk factors for exposure (e.g., brucellosis cases without known exposure to contaminated foods or infected animals). This may indicate an unconventional infection route, such as aerosolization of the *Brucella* pathogen.
	Cases may have risk factors for exposure, but no common exposures (e.g., all salmonellosis cases ate from restaurant salad bars, but they ate different foods at different restaurants).
Environment	Case distribution and/or environmental distribution of the agent follow wind trajectories (e.g., accidental release of anthrax spores in Sverdlovsk, USSR in 1979).
	Other types of attacks (e.g., chemical, radiological) occur at the same time.
	More than one outbreak (with potentially larger numbers than usual) in a region caused by different agents, especially if one or more agents is uncommon.
	An outbreak of disease in an unexpected season, or that does not follow usual global incidence trends. Unnatural distribution mechanism of the agent (e.g., anthrax spores in letters).

* More than one indication may be present after an attack. Indications listed do not necessarily mean a bioterror attack has occurred, and should be substantiated with epidemiological and/or criminal investigations.

suspected. The site or mechanism of the actual agent release may never be known. If the agent used in the attack occurs naturally in the region, foul play may not even be suspected.

Table 8.5 lists some clues that suggest an outbreak could be due to criminal activity. Although the criminal investigation will focus on finding the perpetrators of the attack, a second investigation – an epidemiological investigation – will be progressing as well to determine the cause and spread of disease. Both public health and law enforcement investigations will require sample analysis and interviews with the public and must progress in a collaborative manner despite each entity having different goals.

The amount of microbiological sampling after an act of bioterrorism will likely be extensive. Contaminated areas could have very high concentrations of the bioweapon, risking cross-contamination of PPE and transfer of the agent to other surfaces in the area, or other regions. The criminal investigators must take precautions to avoid contracting disease. In the 2001 U.S. anthrax attacks, investigators had to develop microbiological methods specifically for dried spores. Despite these precautions, handling the most contaminated samples, including both the attack letters and cross-contaminated letters, created aerosolized spores and a very hazardous situation.[35]

STATE OF THE ART

As with other types of events, the response to an infectious disease incident of any origin is only as effective as the monitoring and relief infrastructure in place. In the United States, heightened awareness of infectious disease threats followed the 2001 anthrax attacks. An era of preparedness ensued, with the U.S. Congress allocating unprecedented sums of money to enhance the public health response to bioterrorism. Internationally, a significant driver for public health preparedness has been the International Health Regulations (2005) which entered into force in 2007. The immediacy for response action plans was amplified by the 2003 emergence of SARS,[36] and has been reinforced by other international biological incidents such as the 2009 H1N1 influenza pandemic, the 2012 emergence of MERS-CoV, human cases of H7N9 avian influenza in China in 2013, and Ebola virus disease in 2014.

Preparedness is the state of being ready to act. In the infectious disease disaster context, it broadly refers to the ability to detect a pathogen, act to prevent its spread, and mitigate disease in humans (or animals or plants). Related components include an ability to forecast emerging incidents and to provide reliable situational awareness as a biological incident progresses. Accomplishing this is challenging, given the large number and variability of pathogenic microbes, the potentially rapid global spread of disease, and the extent of communication required between individuals, agencies, governments, and nations. Furthermore, the working definition of "infectious diseases disaster preparedness" and the mechanisms and priorities to achieve it can vary widely between jurisdictions and nations. Because the exact nature of the infectious disease in a disaster situation cannot be known in advance, planning procedures are largely dependent on assessment and subsequent remediation of response vulnerabilities (often identified from previous events and training exercises).

Figure 8.4 shows a general schematic of selected response stakeholders and the activities that occur before, during, and after a biological incident. While not all-inclusive, the diagram serves to illustrate: 1) the ongoing nature of EID preparedness, surveillance, and response; 2) the complexity of the response; 3) the overlapping responsibilities of stakeholders; and 4) the current "feedback" approach to EID preparedness. The light grey

circle just outside the heavy black line (designated "Biological Incident Occurs") is the "incident threshold." This circle represents the time it takes for detection of the biological incident (during which time agent transmission progresses essentially unchecked), and can determine the extent of response measures necessary. This section of the chapter discusses the components of infectious disease preparedness that aim to facilitate response activities and minimize the duration, disruptiveness, and impact of the incident. The discussion uses the U.S. perspective to illustrate one approach to EID preparedness. Other countries may address these issues differently. Nonetheless, the section highlights conceptual considerations for infectious disease disaster preparedness.

Disaster Response Plans

As illustrated by Hurricane Katrina in 2005 and Super Storm Sandy in 2012 in the United States, the earthquake in Haiti in 2010, and the Tōhoku Earthquake and Tsunami in 2011, a large-scale event can overwhelm a response system in both developed and developing nations. The predicted characteristics of infectious disease disasters outlined in the previous section, coupled with evidence from past incidents, serve as tools for understanding the challenges of the next EID disaster. Questions such as "Who is in charge?" and "How well do different jurisdictions or nations interact?" have been the subject of many workshops, symposia, and planning meetings that have occurred at local, regional, national, and international levels.

An important distinction between typical infectious disease disasters and many other disasters is the lack of a specific and immediately recognized incident initiation point (rather, there is an "incident threshold" period). By the time a biological incident is detected and response plans are initiated, many people in diverse areas may already be affected. Biological incidents also have the potential to spread internationally, meaning that response capabilities, plans, and actions in one country can potentially affect many others.

International Plans – the International Health Regulations (2005)

WHO has had international regulations for preventing the spread of disease since 1951, although narrow in scope to select infectious diseases. In May 2005, the World Health Assembly adopted the International Health Regulations (IHR)[37] – this edition is extensively revised and expands the scope beyond a few diseases to any potential "public health emergency of international concern." In this way, the IHR will remain relevant as infectious diseases emerge or reemerge. The overarching purpose of the IHR is "to prevent, protect against, control and provide a public health response to the international spread of disease in ways that are commensurate with and restricted to public health risks" while limiting unnecessary interruption of global traffic and trade. In general, State Parties to the IHR became bound by the agreement on June 15, 2007. State Party obligations for compliance with the IHR include, among others, reporting of biologic events that are potential public health emergencies of international concern to WHO, and developing minimum core public health capabilities (e.g., surveillance, laboratory capabilities, reporting, implementation of control measures, workforce training) for effective and prompt response to biologic events. The core capabilities were to be achieved within 5 years of the IHR entering into force; evidence suggests, however, that less

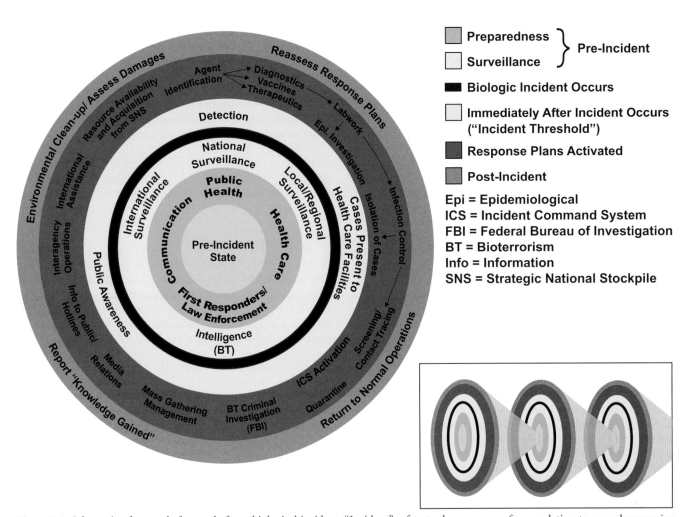

Figure 8.4. Schematic of events before and after a biological incident. "Incident" refers to the exposure of a population to a newly emerging disease (e.g., SARS), to an infectious disease with the potential for extensive casualties and/or public concern (e.g., *Neisseria meningitidis*), or to an act of bioterrorism. Represented are examples of the factors that need to be considered before, during, and after an incident. Increased size of the concentric circles generally corresponds with the progression of time; however, events in larger circles may "feed back" on smaller circles. The use of circles symbolizes the interconnectedness of entities and events within each ring.

The center of the diagram ("Pre-Incident State") represents the situation prior to a biological incident; during this phase, the various response stakeholders (e.g., Public Health, Healthcare, First Responders/Law Enforcement and Communications) enhance preparedness by, for example, improving response plans and participating in practice exercises. This aims to fortify comprehensive preparedness plans (second ring labeled "Preparedness") and surveillance activities (third ring labeled "Surveillance"). The heavy black line represents the occurrence of an actual biological incident. After this happens, a period of time ensues when response stakeholders should become aware of the incident (fourth ring labeled "Incident Threshold"), either by active detection through surveillance efforts or passively by presentation of cases to healthcare personnel. Depending on the agent, the incident may not be initially apparent. The border between the occurrence of the incident and the incident threshold is blurred, representing the often unknown occurrence and/or nature of the emergence when it happens. Response plans are activated (fifth ring labeled "Response Plans Activated") when the incident is recognized. Some elements of the response are shown to illustrate the types of actions the preparedness stakeholders may need to take. This includes agent identification and development of diagnostics/vaccines/therapeutics, activities that will not be timely for an EID unless solid scientific programs are in place in the Pre-Incident State. The events in the final circle (sixth ring labeled "Post-Incident") largely occur in the post-incident phase when disease transmission has been controlled and no new cases are detected. Some actions such as the clean-up of environmental contamination may initiate sooner to prevent disease transmission. Disaster mitigation efforts are analyzed in the post-incident phase. "Knowledge Gained" is used to optimize preparedness plans for the next potential biological incident (this flow of information is symbolized in the inset). Effective planning and surveillance in the circles before an incident occurs can reduce the incident threshold time and make the events of the subsequent circles easier to manage.

than 20% of the 194 parties to the IHR had met this obligation by the June 2012 deadline.[15] A number of challenges have been described, for example, gaps in resources, insufficient laboratory infrastructure, difficulty in capacity building at the local level, and lack of priority due to the need to address other endemic health and healthcare issues.[38] These challenges highlight that compliance capabilities are not globally uniform but a reflec-

tion, at least in part, of disparities between the developed and developing world.

U.S. Local, State, and National Systems

Management of an infectious disease outbreak usually begins with local authorities as the first cases of disease are reported. Therefore, local preparedness plans can be essential for preventing dissemination of the infectious agents to other regions. This is particularly important when more than one locality is affected concurrently, straining national and international assistance mechanisms. In the years after the terrorist events of 2001, the U.S. government appropriated over a billion dollars to states to augment disaster preparedness. The CDC Public Health Emergency Response Guide, version 2.0 (April 2011) provides guidance and information to U.S. local, state, and tribal health departments for initiating public health response activities in the first 24 hours of an emergency or disaster. The guide includes the following preparedness assumptions that health departments must develop prior to an incident in order to effectively respond to an emergency or disaster:

- establishment of working relationships between local public health partners (e.g., neighboring health jurisdictions, emergency management agencies and services, fire and law enforcement, volunteer/aid organizations, emergency planning committees and response coordinators, academic institutions, and private businesses)
- risk and hazard assessments for the area
- a risk communication plan
- resource capacity assessment and surge capacity plan
- operational plans consistent with those used by other response agencies in the community
- procedures that are consistent with the U.S. Department of Homeland Security (DHS), National Response Framework (NRF), and the National Incident Management System (NIMS)
- surveillance systems to monitor public health
- a trained public health workforce (e.g., on proper use of PPE, emergency operations procedures, incident command system)
- exercises to evaluate and review response plans[39]

Specific plans for biological incidents should address operations in the event that the agent spreads to or from neighboring jurisdictions.

Within the U.S. system, the NRF (second edition, published in 2013) emphasizes involvement of the whole community for "implementing nationwide response policy and operational coordination for all types of domestic incidents." The NRF is structured in alignment with the NIMS framework, a unified command approach to disaster response that directs different organizational branches as required and is scalable, flexible, and adaptable as incidents change in size, scope, and complexity. When the scope of an incident is expected to surpass the response capabilities of the local and state governments, federal assistance can be requested by the state under the Stafford Act. The all-hazard approach of the NRF necessarily gives broad guidelines for the organization of the response so that procedures apply to many situations. The NRF also outlines more specific considerations for certain types of incidents; for example, depending on the nature of the incident, certain Emergency Support Functions (ESFs) can be implemented. The Biologic Incident Annex outlines "the actions, roles, and responsibilities associated with response to a human disease outbreak of known or unknown origin requiring Federal assistance."[40] This annex, coordinated by HHS, evokes primarily ESF 8 – Public Health and Medical Services. This ESF defines the core functions for supplemental federal aid to be the assessment of public health and medical needs, public health surveillance, medical care personnel, and

medical equipment and supplies. The Biologic Incident Annex also delineates special considerations (e.g., surreptitious nature of a bioterrorist attack, the importance of surveillance systems), policies (e.g., collaboration with the Environmental Protection Agency in the case of environmental contamination, involvement of the Federal Bureau of Investigation during a bioterrorist attack), concepts of operations (e.g., effective response elements such as detection and containment), and planning assumptions (e.g., multiple jurisdictions may be affected, disease transmission mode is important) that are unique and/or fundamental to a biological incident response.

Hospital Emergency Management Systems

Hospitals should be aware of the unique aspects of large infectious disease outbreaks that could compromise the usual functioning of a disaster management system. These include the transmissibility of the infectious agent to persons not involved in the initial outbreak, the protracted nature of the incident as the agent spreads through the community, and the possibility of infection and absenteeism in hospital staff. Contagious agents necessarily confer an environment of population-based decisions to prevent widespread transmission to the community, which differs from the individual-based care customary of critical care and emergency medicine.

Hospitals should be prepared to operate using an Incident Command System (ICS) during an infectious disease disaster situation. Functioning within an ICS has the advantages of pre-event assignment of roles, ease of coordination of multiple facility responses, and scalability of the response as the disaster progresses or is resolved. Within the United States, hospitals and healthcare facilities (i.e., those that receive medical and trauma patients on a daily basis) that receive federal preparedness funding are required to be NIMS compliant, which allows for the coordination of response efforts on a national level. Compliance includes the implementation of a number of elements in the areas of command and management systems, preparedness planning, workforce training, preparedness exercises, resource management, and communication and information management.[41] Within these areas, hospitals and healthcare facilities must plan for possible bioterrorism or large-scale infectious disease events. For these types of disasters, infectious disease specialists and infection control experts should be included in the incident command organizational chart to provide guidance on the management of potentially infectious patients with respect to triage, medical care, further assessment, and the handling of infectious decedents.[42]

An important component of the hospital response to a communicable disease is infection control policy to prevent the spread of the agent within healthcare settings. This concept was exemplified by the transmission of MERS-CoV in hospitals in Saudi Arabia, where a WHO mission to the country in May 2014 cited lapses in implementation of WHO-recommended hospital infection prevention and control measures as contributing to a surge in cases.[43] Hospital ICS plans for communicable disease disasters must account for prevention of transmission within the facility, and must also assume that a proportion of the people in the command structure will be unavailable for duty due to illness or personal obligations such as the need to care for ill family members. Preparedness includes a mechanism for real-time alternate assignments for each role in the command structure. Hospital infection control may also result in the temporary discontinuation of elective procedures. With adequate prior training, personnel from these areas can be diverted to critical response areas that are overwhelmed.

In an infectious disease disaster, potentially exposed persons present to many hospitals in a region. A coordinated incident command Emergency Operations Center for all hospitals in a region is a particularly relevant system given the issue of resource limitations; however, cooperation between facilities may be challenging. Hospitals not yet affected by the disaster must balance the responsibility to assist in the emergency and accept patients with the need to prevent spread of a contagious agent. Transfer of resources such as ventilators and prophylactic medications to overwhelmed facilities may also be hindered because hospitals not yet involved anticipate future casualties. Therefore, hospital preparedness plans for mass casualty bioevents should also include response actions in the situation of limited outside assistance. Additional recommendations have been published on infection control, the types of interventions to use, deciding who should be treated, and who should administer care.[44] These recommendations, although developed for an intentional attack, can guide planning for all types of infectious disease disasters.

The need for extensive infectious disease disaster management plans is controversial. Some experts argue that the threat of an infectious disease disaster with a high human toll, such as pandemic influenza, is greatly exaggerated. Supporting this viewpoint, the 2009 H1N1 influenza pandemic – the first global influenza emergence since the focus on preparedness plans in the new millennium – did not result in the disease incidence or severity expected. Furthermore, modern day medicines and technologies have provided an arsenal against microbes not available during historical epidemics. Yet preparedness needs are difficult to gauge for novel pathogens, including new pandemic influenza strains. Nonetheless, some assert that the constant barrage of reports on the lack of preparedness only serves to either reduce public confidence or foster an atmosphere of complacency.[45] SARS is often used as an example: public concern and economic losses were extensive, but there were only approximately 8,000 cases and 750 deaths worldwide. It would seem that the world overreacted. Recall, however, that the causative agent, reproductive rate, transmission mode(s), treatment, and mortality of this new respiratory infection were not known at the beginning of the pandemic. During this time of uncertainty, global spread occurred only weeks after international awareness of a new disease. Fortuitously, the SARS-CoV was not as infectious as initially thought. This pandemic serves as a warning that preparedness plans are necessary, especially in the event of an EID with high transmissibility.

Mechanisms to Prevent Disease Transmission in the Community

Specific actions taken by responders during an infectious disease disaster will depend on the nature of the agent. In general, the reproductive rate will determine the extent of the measures necessary for containment. There may be uncertainties at the beginning of an EID outbreak. Epidemiological data on the initial cases will guide predictions. In the event that the agent is transmissible from person to person, mechanisms of varying degrees of restriction can be implemented. The concepts of isolation, quarantine, evacuation, shelter-in-place, and social distancing are important containment strategies. Whether these measures are implemented on a voluntary or mandatory basis will depend on characteristics of the agent, and on legal and ethical considerations. Control of a contagious disease may also require contact tracing, which involves identifying and locating the people with whom an infectious person has come in contact, and the mass distribution of prophylactic medication or vaccination, if available. Implementing controls at national borders to prevent inbound travelers from importing the infectious agent are an option but may be very difficult in some countries and may not be highly effective. Models of pandemic influenza in the United States, for example, suggest that even if incoming infections were reduced by as much as 99%, this would only delay peak disease incidence by approximately 3 weeks.

Some infectious disease outbreaks may require rodent or arthropod control programs to eliminate reservoirs or vectors that carry the agent. This can be challenging for EIDs of unknown (or mistaken) etiology. An outbreak of suspected St. Louis virus encephalitis in New York in 1999 prompted mosquito control and public education activities. Experts soon realized that the encephalitis cases were actually caused by West Nile virus, a closely related virus not previously associated with disease in North America that is transmitted by a broader range of mosquitoes. Initial intervention strategies were sufficiently expansive to be constructive but were optimized with the new diagnosis to the different habitat and activity patterns of West Nile virus–carrying mosquitoes.[46]

Control of zoonotic diseases may require extensive elimination of animals of agricultural importance. The emergence of Nipah virus in Malaysia and avian influenza in Asia in the early 2000s resulted in the slaughter of millions of pigs and fowl, respectively.[47,48] Although arguably necessary to prevent disease transmission to humans, this type of activity can have negative consequences. Economically, segments of the agricultural industry may be devastated due to decreased production, costs of disease containment and clean-up, trade embargoes, and reduced consumer confidence. Associated industries such as transportation, suppliers, and food service would also be negatively affected.

Science and Technology

Scientific advances in molecular biology over the last half century, and particularly in the last 25 years, have greatly benefited infectious disease public health. The successes of the core goals of public health in any infectious disease disaster, namely detection of an outbreak, prevention of its transmission, and mitigation of disease, are all functions of the body of scientific knowledge on the pathogen and the technological capabilities to translate that knowledge into action. In the case of an EID, this specific kind of knowledge may initially be sparse. This highlights the need for solid work in basic infectious disease biology, because EIDs will often (but not always) be novel strains/species of known infectious agents.

Basic scientific research on the bioterrorism potential of select agents has increased dramatically in the last decade, providing insight into their pathogenic mechanisms. These advances can lead to the discovery of targets for novel countermeasures and/or to new diagnostic tools. Some critics have suggested that extensive funding for specific select agents is detrimental to preparedness goals. Biodefense research needs to be translatable to infectious diseases in general, and to public health policy.

Identification and Characterization of the Agent

Standardized techniques, such as microscopy and culture, are useful in determining the nature of the agent (e.g., the type of bacteria) and whether any known therapeutics are active against it. Further genetic and molecular analyses, including polymerase chain reaction and immunofluorescence techniques, can differentiate the agent from other similar microorganisms. Along with these types of assays, genome sequencing (the identification of the nucleic acid composition of the organism's entire DNA) can determine whether the etiological agent is a known or a novel pathogen. For example, the SARS coronavirus is only distantly related to other known human coronaviruses (an etiological agent of the common cold) and produces a very different disease, so it is considered to be a newly emerged variety of this type of virus.[49] Similarly, the epidemic of respiratory illness in 2012 and 2013, primarily in the Middle East, is caused by a coronavirus genetically distinct from SARS and therefore represents a new viral emergence – the MERS coronavirus.[22]

There are many obstacles to rapid and definitive identification and characterization of a novel agent. Known animal models may not exist, precluding the ability to link the isolated agent with disease or establish transmission modes. Culturing techniques to grow microbes in the laboratory are very specific for different types of agents, even within the same genus. Due to the unknown nature of transmission and disease severity, specialized containment labs with specifically trained staff may be required. Many regional testing laboratories do not have the equipment or experience to conduct molecular testing.

Diagnostic Assays

Diagnostic assays are important to quickly identify new cases of disease, to differentiate between cases and noncases with similar symptoms, and to determine environmental sources of the pathogen. Genetic tests are often developed due to the rapidity and relatively high analytic sensitivity (ability to detect small amounts of the agent) and analytic specificity (ability to differentiate the agent from other organisms) of the results compared with conventional laboratory techniques. Time is often required to create these assays. During an EID situation, significant pressure exists for rapid development of diagnostics so that clinicians and epidemiologists have tools to identify new cases. These first-line diagnostics are useful, but an understanding of the sensitivity (i.e., true positive rate), specificity (i.e., true negative rate) and accuracy of the diagnostics is important for assessing the interpretation and limitations of any results.

Therapeutics

Antimicrobial drug discovery waned in the 1960s when pharmaceutical companies turned their attention from the supposedly declining threat of infectious diseases to the more pressing and lucrative concerns of chronic illnesses. In modern times, in the face of increasing antimicrobial resistance and emerging agents, new therapies are needed. Scientists are using molecular and structural biology techniques to understand microbial pathogenesis. This information can enhance approaches to discovering novel classes of drugs that block pathogenic processes. Despite an increasingly alarming understanding of the emergence and burden of antimicrobial-resistant pathogens, the drive for the discovery of new drugs effective against bacteria and viruses has not been an industry priority. From 1998 to 2003, only nine new antibacterial drugs were approved, the same number as those approved for just one virus alone, HIV, in the same period. Importantly, only two of the nine antibacterial drugs had novel mechanisms of action.[50] A review published in 2013 indicates that the "innovation gap" of novel antimicrobial agents

continues, with only three new classes of antibiotics approved for use since 2000.[51]

Emerging agents provide a unique challenge for therapeutic design. As noted previously, treatment options for EIDs may be limited, with even broad-spectrum antimicrobial drugs having little or no effect. Information is learned about the causative agent and the disease as the outbreak or epidemic progresses; however, using conventional therapies that work for similar diseases, or emergency use of pre-event approved therapeutics, is risky without efficacy and/or safety studies. In a systematic review of more than fifty published studies that assessed treatment efficacy during the 2003 SARS pandemic, no therapy (including antivirals, corticosteroids, intravenous immunoglobulin, convalescent sera, and type I interferon) conclusively improved patient outcomes. In fact, some studies reported possible harmful effects of treatment with ribavirin or corticosteroids.[52] The development of novel drugs for an EID is challenging. Even if a molecular target is discovered, the design, development, and approval of a therapeutic agent would not be rapid. For example, in the United States it takes approximately 8 years for a new drug to complete clinical trial phases, gain approval, and be marketed. Furthermore, factoring in 1) the high cost of drug development, 2) the relatively low numbers of cases of an EID initially, and 3) the chance that the epidemic will end with no further cases, pharmaceutical companies would be unlikely to even initiate the discovery process without government intervention and/or incentives.

Vaccines

Vaccines are one of the most successful public health tools to improve the health of populations. By preventing infectious diseases, vaccines limit human suffering and the spread of contagious agents. There are many infectious diseases that are endemic in parts of the world for which no vaccines are available. Finding mechanisms to produce effective vaccines is the subject of extensive basic research. Molecular and genetic advances have vastly improved the understanding of immune system regulation and of vaccine delivery methods. Translating this knowledge into approved vaccine products has been slow for numerous reasons. In some cases, the knowledge base on the infectious agent is simply not advanced enough to make a vaccine. For example, some viruses have high mutation rates; consistent vaccine efficacy is difficult because mutated forms of the viruses arise that are not affected by vaccine-enhanced immune functions. As with therapeutic development, pharmaceutical companies are hesitant to engage in vaccine design. The return on investment is relatively low, demand for vaccines that target sporadically occurring agents is unpredictable, some vaccines for endemic diseases are not extensively used (e.g., yellow fever in Africa and South America), and safety and liability issues abound.

Government Incentives

After the terrorist attacks of 2001, the U.S. federal government passed the Project BioShield Act in 2004 (and reauthorized portions in 2013) to "accelerate the research, development, purchase, and availability of effective medical countermeasures against biological, chemical, radiological, and nuclear (CBRN) agents."[53] The three main goals of Project BioShield are to 1) provide funding for the procurement of critical medical countermeasures (MCMs); 2) give authority to the National Institutes of Health of HHS to prioritize the granting procedure for research and development of critical MCMs; and 3) assist in the use of MCMs during an emergency. BioShield lays the groundwork for increased vaccine and drug development for bioterrorist agents. Major pharmaceutical companies have not widely used this funding system primarily due to concerns about liability protection for expedited MCMs. Funding smaller biotechnology companies can help fuel an industry, but there are risks for both parties involved. Some companies may be unable to produce the contracted pharmaceutical after receiving federal funding, or the government may opt to purchase less of the product than projected.

The U.S. pharmaceutical industry needs motivation beyond Project BioShield to expand antimicrobial therapeutic and vaccine development. In this regard, the Pandemic and All-Hazards Preparedness Act was approved in December 2006. This act directed the formulation of the Biomedical Advanced Research and Development Authority (BARDA) within HHS. BARDA is charged with promoting the translation of scientific research into antimicrobial products, including provisions to induce participation by the pharmaceutical industry. The creation of BARDA was criticized. Consumer advocacy groups questioned the safety of using expedited drugs, even in emergency situations. Scientific associations were concerned about the lack of transparency of BARDA activities and decisions, the potential for gaps in or duplication of research efforts, and funding sources and amounts.[54] In 2013, the U.S. government passed the Pandemic and All-hazards Preparedness Reauthorization Act. This legislation clarifies and expands on U.S. Food and Drug Administration authority for supporting preparedness and rapid response capabilities, including components that address refinement of, or additional authorities for, emergency use of MCMs, pre-event positioning of MCMs, shelf-life extension of MCMs, and regulatory/review processes for MCM development.

Dual-Use Risk

The 2001 U.S. anthrax attacks heightened public awareness about bioterrorism. To increase preparedness against future strikes, the American government allocated billions of dollars for biodefense research on certain pathogens and toxins, termed "select agents." The select agents are categorized as those that affect humans, those that affect agriculture (animals and plants), and those that can affect both humans and agriculture. Policymakers realized that increased research on select agents could increase the risk that the agents, or scientific information learned about them, would fall into the hands of terrorists. As a result, measures have been taken through the Biopreparedness Act to limit access to the select agents, regulate genetic manipulations of these agents, and restrict publication of information that could lead to enhanced virulence of the select agents. The Biopreparedness Act also mandates FBI clearance rules for scientists working with select agents. The National Science Advisory Board for Biosecurity (NSABB) was formed to oversee the balance between increasing scientific research to prepare better for a bioterrorist attack and preventing potential adversaries from accessing scientific reagents and information.

Since the first adoption of the act, changes to "dual use" legislation and implementation have occurred. Revisions in 2012 to the select agents list removed a number of them to focus regulatory efforts on the agents of most concern to public or agricultural health. In addition, some agents, such as Ebola virus, botulinum neurotoxin and *Bacillus anthracis*, were designated as "Tier 1" to indicate the subset most at risk for deliberate misuse and with greatest potential for mass casualties, economic or infrastructure devastation, or erosion of public confidence. Additionally, rules for publication of research on pathogens with pandemic/bioterrorism potential that are engineered to increase pathogenicity or transmissibility came into question in 2011 after two research groups, one in the United States and one in the Netherlands, independently submitted manuscripts to scientific journals describing such work. NSABB initially recommended that the work not be published in full; the journals delayed publication, the research community halted work on related research until the issue could be resolved, and eventually NSABB reversed its recommendation to withhold publication of each paper after the manuscripts were revised to remove methodological details.[55]

Surveillance

Broadly speaking, public health surveillance refers to "the collection, analysis, and use of data to target public health prevention."[56] There are four basic components to surveillance: monitoring for disease, detection of disease, analysis of data, and dissemination of findings. A relatively newer term is "biosurveillance," which is often used to denote the assessment of health-related and other data for rapid recognition (i.e., "early warning") of a biologic incident or "real-time" situational awareness as an incident progresses. The sooner the detection of an infectious disease outbreak or emergence occurs, the faster the response can be to prevent spread of the agent and human disease. In addition, early detection can prevent the dissemination of the pathogen to other regions or countries and potentially prevent an epidemic or pandemic. The Surveillance Resource Center on the CDC website is an online clearinghouse of guidance and practice tools for surveillance capabilities.

Surveillance is also an assessment tool for the general functioning of a public health system. Monitoring disease incidence, morbidity, and mortality can indicate regions that must boost existing public health infrastructure. These regions are at increased risk for large numbers of casualties during an infectious disease disaster compared to regions with more robust infrastructures.

International Surveillance Efforts

Globalization has conversely made international infectious disease surveillance both increasingly necessary and possible. Emerging infectious agents can arise in any country and potentially spread globally due to travel and commerce. Quick determination of the emergence of an outbreak will give public health officials, clinicians, and researchers throughout the world an opportunity to prevent dissemination and to develop diagnostics and therapeutics. Increased global interactions, which can promote spread of a disease agent, can also encourage cooperation in surveillance efforts. The IHR obligates Member Parties to develop a minimum core surveillance capability for the detection of biologic events that may constitute a public health emergency of international concern.

Disparities exist in the capabilities of different countries with respect to workforce, tools, and effort. In Europe, where resources for surveillance were prioritized as in North America, sophisticated systems have been developed to collect, analyze, and disseminate information for public health action (e.g., the European Surveillance System). Many developing countries have a strained public health infrastructure that cannot expand to support intensive surveillance efforts. Therefore, global partnerships that link networks from many regions and countries, such as those supported by WHO Member States, serve to share expertise and information. For example, the WHO Integrated Disease Surveillance Programme is a strategy adopted by most countries in the WHO African Region for strengthening core surveillance capabilities at the district level.

Reporting is a critical component of effective global surveillance. The IHR includes reporting of potential public health emergencies of international concern to WHO as a core capability so that global response activities can be initiated if necessary. The obligation to report such events is intended to prevent countries from delaying reporting to avoid stigmatization and negative impacts on travel and trade, or assumptions that an outbreak is under control and of little threat for further spread. The situation of the emergence of SARS reinforced the need to include reporting in the IHR: although cases of SARS first appeared in Guangdong Province in November 2002, Chinese officials only confirmed the outbreak to WHO in February 2003 after international surveillance networks were alerted through media and Internet reports.[57] Chinese public health officials worked with WHO to control the outbreak, but international dissemination had already occurred. In response to the SARS pandemic, the Chinese government has overhauled its infectious disease surveillance and reporting systems.

The public health infrastructure problems that delayed the Chinese response are not unique to that country. This substantiates the need for international collaborations to detect EIDs and support mitigation efforts. Implementation of the IHR for reporting has not been uniform across nations, but the regulations provide a framework of expectations. In China, transparency in reporting cases of H7N9 influenza in 2012 and 2013 has been lauded by WHO as exemplary adherence to the IHR,[58] and is distinct from the experience with the lack of early reporting of cases of SARS a decade earlier. In contrast, Saudi Arabia has been accused of being less than forthcoming with information on the emergence of MERS, even in light of the IHR.[59]

National Surveillance Efforts – U.S. Model

Healthcare practitioners play a central role in the surveillance process by notifying public health authorities regarding patients with reportable diseases or atypical symptomatology. For example, U.S. physicians in the early 1980s noticed that young men were contracting *Pneumocystis carinii* pneumonia (now known as Pneumocystis jiroveci pneumonia) and/or certain malignancies not normally associated with that demographic group. This was one of the first indications that a new immunocompromising infectious disease (now known as AIDS) was circulating in the population.

This classic method of outbreak identification is a key component of disease control in a population, but relying on it solely is problematic. Recognition of cases that should be reported and subsequent data submission are not always timely. There is heavy reliance on subjective determination of what should be communicated to public health and not all infectious diseases are reportable. Furthermore, early surveillance opportunities that could potentially prevent human disease and death may be missed. In the first North American outbreak of West Nile virus in 1999, unexplained bird deaths had been noticed 2 months prior to the human outbreak investigation, but no extrapolation was made to possible human consequences.

Recognizing the value of time, many health departments, health agencies, academic institutions, and governments have developed a number of surveillance systems and networks to more rapidly and consistently detect disease events. Examples of the types of systems include those that 1) monitor the environment for the presence of bioterrorism agents (e.g., BioWatch in the United States); 2) use health and other data for early detection of outbreaks (i.e., syndromic surveillance; Chapter 13); and 3) aim to foster collaboration and information sharing among biosurveillance stakeholders (e.g., the U.S. National Biosurveillance Integration System).

The U.S. government executive leadership published a National Strategy for Biosurveillance in 2012 to emphasize that early detection of biological threats, and accurate and timely information for situational awareness, is important for decision making at all levels to save lives and protect national security.[60] This strategy aims to strengthen U.S. government national biosurveillance by leveraging and integrating existing national capabilities, building capacity, fostering innovation, and strengthening partnerships. These activities are in the context of maintaining a global health perspective by promoting reinforcement of international partnerships and encouraging surveillance development and integration across countries.

Workforce Preparedness

Workforce preparedness is the state of readiness of public health, public safety, and healthcare employees to act in an infectious disease emergency. Workforce readiness is primarily related to workforce capacity and education/training. The concept is often used to describe readiness at the community and state level, but EID or large biological incidents will likely require participation on a national level as well. The jobs performed by these employees are critical to the proper and sustainable functioning of the other preparedness requirements such as surveillance and resource management. Furthermore, training exercises and past disasters have demonstrated that mitigation and response are improved by good working relationships between public health, public safety, and healthcare workers.

Public Health Workforce

Inadequate public health workforce numbers and expertise are not limited to developing nations. For example, it is well established that decades of budget cuts and neglect have resulted in an understaffed public health infrastructure in the United States. This has compromised the ability to respond effectively during an infectious disease disaster. In some jurisdictions and facilities, especially smaller ones, the roles of public health nurses, laboratory technologists, epidemiologists, and infection control practitioners are accomplished by staff with multiple duties. Furthermore, these positions are often characterized by staff who are reassigned when needed, by employees working overtime, and/or by the use of temporary workers. These options will be limited during an infectious disease disaster as demand for these employees will increase and movement between facilities will be restricted.

Formal education of public health workers in the United States for epidemic situations is accomplished mainly by the CDC. The Epidemic Intelligence Service (EIS) is a well-known program. For more than 60 years, the EIS has trained public health professionals with hands-on field experiences in epidemiology. CDC Environmental Public Health Leadership Institutes prepare environmental public health workers for leadership positions at the state and local levels and promote networking between jurisdictions. CDC also funds Preparedness and Emergency Response Learning Centers at university schools of public health across the United States to train the public health workforce on core public health competencies.

Laboratory technologists are a fundamental part of infectious disease disaster management teams. Timely surveillance, detection, and diagnosis are all dependent on laboratory services and can reduce transmission and disease severity during an infectious disease disaster. Chronic underfunding has left many public health laboratories understaffed. As demonstrated by the 1999 West Nile virus emergence, 2001 anthrax attacks, and 2003 SARS pandemic, the laboratory workforce can quickly become overwhelmed with samples. The U.S. CDC implemented the Laboratory Response Network in 1999 to act as a networking platform for laboratories (local, state, federal, international, military, veterinary, and agricultural) in response to terrorism. This role has since been expanded to include EIDs and other public health emergencies.

The general public expects the public health workforce to provide accurate information. Such timely and reliable data are a vital resource for control of an epidemic. However, knowledge of the characteristics of an emerging biologic incident may change frequently as the incident unfolds, and messaging and resource planning may need continual assessment and updating. Public health telephone hotlines are a common mechanism to disseminate information and to answer specific questions. Disaster plans do not, however, always consider the volume of calls that an information hotline receives. Over 316,000 calls were placed to the Toronto SARS hotline, which was established the day after the first Toronto SARS case was announced at a press conference. Almost 60% of the callers selected the "listen to recorded information" option. Of the calls in which the "speak to a staff person" option was selected, almost 80% (104,852 calls) were *not* answered by a staff member.[61] This number illustrates the overwhelming service requirements that can be associated with infectious disease disasters. Case numbers alone do not always correlate with workload. The prevalence of use of social media will likely reduce the importance of telephone hotlines.

Public Safety Workforce

First responders such as law enforcement, firefighters, and emergency medical services personnel are important segments of the public workforce for management of an infectious disease disaster. These workers will be involved in the distribution of resources, crowd control at mass gatherings, the transfer of patients, and any criminal investigations resulting from a bioterrorist attack. In some countries, first responders have the advantage of extensive ICS training and experience; however, as outlined previously, biological incidents are unique in many facets. As one of the primary interfaces with the general public, first responders are at risk for exposure to infectious agents. Jurisdictions must determine in advance how best to protect first responders in the event of a contagious infectious disease disaster. The U.S. CDC website provides information for state, local, and tribal public health directors, and for first responders with respect to emergency response after a biological incident. These recommendations include use of PPE by first responders and suggestions for the handling of contaminated mail or containers. Preparedness also includes an understanding of public health law with respect to quarantine orders and other public movement restrictions, and plans for enforcing these orders.

Healthcare Facility Workforce

A component of NIMS hospital compliance in the United States is workforce training in core competencies so that hospital personnel will be able to function in a coordinated fashion during a disaster. The U.S. CDC found that the ICS format for disaster response was critical for providing stability and continuity to response efforts after Hurricane Katrina. As a result, the CDC pandemic preparedness plan uses the ICS to structure response efforts during a prolonged disaster with high staff turnover. Hospital ICS plans for an infectious disease disaster should account for reduced workforce capacity as the disaster progresses due to illness, absence to care for ill family members, refusal to work, and psychological stress. In that regard, healthcare workers should be trained in advance to understand possible implications of a contagious infectious disease disaster and methods to contain the disease. This training should include proper use of PPE, duty-to-care expectations, and infection control practices. Workforce preparedness must also address psychological consequences of a prolonged disaster. The toll on those expected to respond to disasters is significant and this stress has usually received inadequate attention. This is especially important when the workforce is already understaffed.

International Workforce

Infectious diseases affect more people in developing nations than in other areas of the world. An underdeveloped and understaffed public health workforce contributes to this poor outcome. For example, early management of the 2014 EVD outbreak in West Africa was hindered by insufficient numbers and training of local healthcare and public health staff. Response to the outbreak was largely reliant on clinical volunteers from international aid organizations, with little assistance from local or international governments until the threat of international dissemination of the virus increased.

Augmenting fields such as epidemiology and infection control in developing nations can reduce human suffering and increase detection of emerging pathogens and impending pandemics. International partnerships among aid organizations, government agencies, and industries have resulted in programs to develop global information networks and workforce alliances that train public health workers in developing countries. WHO's Global Health Workforce Alliance and Integrated Disease Surveillance programs are examples of international efforts to improve workforce capacity and training in developing nations.

Response Communications

Many aspects of successful management of an infectious disease disaster are dependent on timely and accurate communications between different stakeholders. Examples of such aspects include surveillance, implementation of scientific advances, resource allocation, and delivery of assistance.

International Communication

As previously outlined, infectious disease disasters and emerging new pathogens can rapidly become global in nature. Communication among governments and agencies is fundamental to limiting the extent of an infectious disease disaster. The initial delay in disclosure of a new severe respiratory disease to the world was a likely factor in the global spread of SARS. Once it was clear a new disease had emerged, the international response demonstrated unprecedented cooperation and communication. WHO, facilitated by the Global Outbreak Alert and Response Network, established secure communication networks and websites for the daily exchanges of information on surveillance, epidemiology, and disease characteristics. The utility of this networking system was nowhere more evident than in the discovery of the etiological agent. The Laboratory Network, which consisted of eleven laboratories in nine countries, shared data and information. Together, they identified the causative agent of SARS, sequenced its genome, and developed diagnostic tests, all in a matter of weeks. These laboratories were already in communication prior to the SARS pandemic via the well-established WHO Influenza Surveillance Network, substantiating the value of ongoing partnerships.

National Response Communication

One of the primary ways that new, cleared information is shared in the United States regarding urgent public health incidents is the CDC's Health Alert Network (HAN), which publishes CDC advisories and updates on clinical and epidemiological information, often as an incident is unfolding. For example, numerous HAN communications were published in 2012 regarding the multi-state outbreak of fungal meningitis resulting from injection of people with fungus-contaminated medications.[62] Communication between jurisdictions and between levels of government is vital during an infectious disease disaster due to the transmissibility of the agent. It can be the difference between a contained localized outbreak and a national epidemic. Unlike many other disasters, communications interoperability will likely remain intact during an infectious disease disaster. This is in contrast to the situation during Hurricane Katrina, where widespread physical disruption of communication systems made information exchange between response teams difficult. Without a distinct starting point for the biological incident, however, extensive and formal interagency and intergovernmental communication through the NRF may be delayed. This could undermine unified command and result in multiple and disparate efforts toward similar goals. Even in non-disaster situations, past experiences suggest that poor communication results in conflicting actions. For example, during the 2004 U.S. influenza vaccine shortage, agencies at different governmental levels gave inconsistent messages, recommending vaccination of different age groups.[63]

Communication with the Public

Communication of disease and containment information to the community by the public health system can determine, to a large degree, the extent of an epidemic. WHO held the first Expert Consultation on Outbreak Communication symposium in Singapore in 2004 to discuss risk communication to the public. It is widely agreed that providing the public with accurate and timely information is necessary to prevent spread of the infectious agent. Yet, these tasks are usually very difficult because the information may change as the epidemic unfolds. Inconsistent messages may be viewed as untrustworthy. Furthermore, while response plans should include general requirements for crisis and emergency risk communication to the public, the messages need to be tailored for each biological incident or circumstance. For example, although the Ministry of Health in Saudi Arabia recommended that people at high risk for contracting MERS cancel their participation in the 2013 Hajj pilgrimage, a French study found that all 179 survey-takers with conditions that put

them at high risk for contracting MERS still planned to participate even after pre-travel educational consultations.[64] Most, however, were receptive to prevention practices such as wearing masks. The authors suggest that risk perception may be influenced by cultural and religious beliefs, and risk messaging should account for that context.

The media is a powerful tool for disseminating information. In a survey of people quarantined in Toronto during the SARS epidemic, more people claimed that they got helpful information on the quarantine orders from the media than from public health officials or from their healthcare providers. Good working relationships between health department public relations liaisons and local news stations before an incident occurs can encourage cooperation during an outbreak. In a large disaster, it may be necessary to establish an information center to coordinate messages for the public. In addition to the disaster itself, the media also report on the management of the emergency.[65] Some decisions will need to be explained or justified. As defined by the ICS structure, a credible spokesperson should be selected as the point of contact with the media to ensure delivery of consistent and accurate messages to the public.

Resource Management

In a biological incident, critical resources are needed for detection of the pathogen in the community and for appropriate patient care. Yet, real outbreaks from the past and tabletop preparedness exercises have ascertained that resources will be limited.

National Resources

Within the United States, HHS and CDC maintain the Strategic National Stockpile (SNS).[66] The SNS is a supply of critical resources that includes antibiotics, antitoxins, ventilators, N95 respirators, and medical equipment for use in the event of a public health emergency. CDC distributes SNS resources to supplement local capabilities on request from the governors of affected states and on assessment of need. Aid is in the form of 12-hour Push Packages and Vendor Managed Inventory. The 12-hour Push Packages are designed for distribution of nonspecific critical resources from regional warehouses within 12 hours of federal approval of allocation. The Vendor Managed Inventory supplies additional and more specific resources within 24–36 hours directly from pharmaceutical companies; CDC may choose to supply Vendor Managed Inventory instead of a Push Package. CDC deploys Stockpile Service Advance Group staff to assist in receiving, organizing, and distributing the supplies.

The SNS is an extensive cache, but insufficient for a catastrophic disaster effecting multiple jurisdictions. A large infectious disease disaster, such as a bioterrorist attack, is an example of an event that will affect many areas at one time. CDC may have to prioritize which states receive aid from the SNS based on severity of the outbreak. Some SNS resources may even be reserved in the event of a second attack. Furthermore, the 12-hour response time refers to distribution from federal stocks to state authorities; it is up to the states to then determine which localities will receive the supplemental aid. Given all of these circumstances, hospitals should stockpile *at least* a 48-hour supply of PPE and drugs likely to be used during a mass casualty infectious disease event. A 3–7-day supply may be necessary in the event of a large or widespread disaster.

Hospital Resources

A large biological attack or epidemic could result in hundreds of people a day presenting to hospital emergency departments during peak disease incidence. As the number of ill patients increases, hospital critical care providers will have to assess resource capacity and may need to determine allocation procedures to save the most lives instead of focusing the majority of resources on a few critically ill patients. This is a difficult task because intensive critical care for the very ill in non-disaster situations may result in improved outcomes.

As discussed previously, hospital plans must include provisions for isolating infectious patients. These should include requirements for beds, equipment, and staff dedicated for that purpose. The availability of mechanical ventilators is a particular concern during an infectious disease emergency. Many microbial pathogens cause respiratory complications that require mechanical ventilation. Yet preparedness assessments have demonstrated that hospitals cannot accommodate ventilation for all patients, even operating under surge capacity guidelines. For example, during a Minnesota drill, regional vendors could only provide sixteen extra ventilators.[67] Proper allocation of resources is also a function of knowing what resources are available. An up-to-date list of available staffed beds, ventilators, and other limited resources can help with the triage process.

The hospital infectious disease triage system is an important process to quickly determine patient health and susceptibility status. People efficiently and accurately categorized as "susceptible," "exposed and/or infectious," or "immune" (due to vaccination or prior recovery from the disease) can receive the appropriate management with minimal suboptimal use of resources.[68] In the midst of a disaster, the tendency is to either over-classify people as "exposed" or to protect individuals who are at minimal risk. Both of these situations can result in increased numbers of people unnecessarily using limited hospital resources.

Allocation of Resources

Preparedness plans need to include guidelines for resource allocation in the event that supplies are limited. In other words, algorithms are needed to help identify which patients may not qualify for treatment. Making these decisions at the time of an infectious disease disaster without prior consideration can lead to heightened confusion among providers, contention among policymakers, and anger among the public. Legal, social, and political factors will be as much a part of the decision-making process as patient care.

Most agree that to save the most lives, the patients most likely to survive (that is, the least critically ill) should be treated with limited resources first. Whatever system is adopted, administration must be equitable and transparent to all patients and to the public. One mechanism to promote the just allocation of limited resources is to numerically code the survivability of patients based on clinical assessment. Resource distribution is then based on patient scores.

A Specific Case: 2009 H1N1 Pandemic Influenza and Resource Availability

For many years prior to the emergence of the novel H1N1 influenza A virus in April 2009, the threat of pandemic influenza was often used to examine resource availability in public health. The 2009 novel H1N1 event (declared a pandemic by WHO on June 11) highlighted that disease emergence characteristics can be unpredictable despite well-informed "best guesses." Viral emergence and disease were first detected in North America, not Asia; the pandemic virus was a novel H1N1 quadruple reassortant of swine, human, and avian genes, not (yet) a highly pathogenic H5N1 avian virus with increased transmissibility in humans; transmission and disease continued during the summer months in the United States; and worldwide disease severity was mild or moderate with low mortality rates. Unlike disease transmission and global spread, disease severity was not officially factored into the WHO decision to elevate the pandemic alert phase, but this pandemic demonstrated that concern for public overreaction and for response activities tied to elevation of alerts necessitated a carefully worded declaration statement addressing that disease was moderate. In 2013, based on knowledge gained from this pandemic, WHO issued interim guidance that proposed a revised influenza pandemic alert system. This system has four phases instead of six, with the pandemic phase accounting for "a period of global spread of human influenza caused by a new subtype. Movement between . . . phases may occur quickly or gradually as indicated by the global risk assessment, principally based on virological, epidemiological and clinical data."[69]

In the United States, the initial wave of the 2009 H1N1 influenza pandemic illustrated some of the suspected resource challenges of a novel disease outbreak, including increased volumes of patients in emergency departments, management of changing recommendations and information overload, scarcity of PPE (e.g., requirements for and availability of surgical masks and N95 respirators), viral resistance to existing therapeutics, hospital employee issues (e.g., absence due to influenza-like illness, wage compensation for absence after exposure, fatigue), availability of diagnostics, and lack of a vaccine at the onset. The anticipation of a second wave of H1N1 disease in the fall of 2009 coupled with the arrival of seasonal influenza led response stakeholders, such as the American College of Emergency Physicians, to issue guidance on the necessary resource and surge capabilities for management of novel H1N1 outbreaks.[70]

The 2009 H1N1 influenza pandemic marked the highly unusual situation where two viruses coexisted in elevated phases in the WHO pandemic alert system (novel H1N1 at pandemic level and avian H5N1 at phase 3). Viral unpredictability precludes definitive expectations of a "double influenza pandemic." Nonetheless, such a situation has serious consequences for response capabilities; robust pandemic preparedness is especially important for resource management, continuity of operations, and patient care.

Preparedness Training Exercises

Infectious disease disasters are rare events, yet a state of complacency or underpreparedness by response stakeholders can result in increased casualties when one does occur. Preparedness is more than just having meetings and written plans. Exercises are the current state of the art in testing the readiness of response systems and in identifying areas that need improvement. The time and resource commitments for this practical training must be balanced with those for normal operations, and an avoidance of "preparedness fatigue."

Some exercises are supplements to didactic lessons at institutions of higher learning, such as nursing and medical schools. Nurses and physicians may be the first to recognize that an infectious disease disaster is looming and/or they will be on the frontline of the response. It follows then that nursing and medical students should receive dedicated education and training in the mechanics of the response. The exercises are usually in the form of case scenario discussions that address the clinical, operational, and ethical issues of infectious disease disaster management.

Policymakers, resource managers, public health departments, first responders, and healthcare facilities often use tabletop exercises and drills to assess preparedness. These types of activities are useful for practicing coordination of efforts within and between different parties. The exercises usually involve the mock release of a biological agent such as the smallpox virus, with informational updates given by the exercise administrators to participants as the disaster unfolds. Factors such as resource availability and allocation, protection of healthcare workers, and public unrest are usually components of the exercise. Table 8.6 lists criteria typically considered for the development of a training exercise.

Since the anthrax attacks of 2001 and the 2003 SARS outbreak, regional preparedness drills are now commonplace throughout the world. In the United States, there have been large-scale national disaster exercises such as Dark Winter and TOPOFF (for "top officials") exercises starting even prior to 2001. These congressionally mandated exercises were designed to examine national preparedness. They involved officials and responders from all levels of government. All of these exercises substantiated the validity and importance of the preparedness factors that are outlined in this section. For example, TOPOFF 4, which occurred in October 2007, had over 15,000 participants and included the U.S. territory of Guam. It was designed to assess the response to multiple coordinated attacks with a Radiological Dispersal Device. TOPOFF 3, which took place in April 2005, included a bioterrorism component and participation from Canada and the United Kingdom. It was the first national practice of a response based on implementation of the NRF (then known as the National Response Plan) and NIMS in the capacity of the Homeland Security Operations Center. Concerns raised by the DHS Office of Inspector General[71] after completion of the exercise included: 1) insufficient understanding and training of participants on NRF and NIMS procedures, which resulted in "bureaucrat confusion" and operations under multiple different protocols; 2) confusion over the declaration of an Incident of National Significance and the consequences of such an action; 3) challenges with information collection and reporting; 4) inadequate collaborations between government and the private sector; 5) the high cost of TOPOFF 3 to participating states; and, importantly, 6) repeated weaknesses from TOPOFF 2.

Although not really "drills," recent outbreaks, epidemics, and events are arguably the most appropriate tools for assessing disaster responses. Public reaction, media relations, and interagency communication in a high-pressure situation are components not easily reproduced in an exercise. Response limitations in recent events such as the 2001 anthrax attacks (e.g., laboratory capacity), the 2003 SARS pandemic (e.g., contact tracing, implementation of quarantine, and healthcare worker safety), Hurricane Katrina in 2005 (e.g., interagency communication), and the 2009 H1N1 influenza pandemic (e.g., vaccine production and allocation) serve as reminders that certain aspects of preparedness plans are consistently deficient. Even local outbreaks of foodborne illnesses can inform health departments on areas in need of improvement. For exercises to be useful to a jurisdiction, government, or institution, they need to occur at regular intervals. Policies will change over time due to data from previous exercises, new legislation, and funding constraints. In addition, personnel

Table 8.6. Considerations for Exercise Development

Participants
- Health departments/Public health
- Government officials (local, state, federal)
- Hospital workers
  - Management
  - Patient care providers
  - Laboratory technologists
  - Epidemiologists/Infection control
  - Pharmacists
  - Health information management
  - Support personnel (e.g., housekeeping, security)
- Law enforcement
- First responders
  - Emergency medical services
  - Fire
- Media representatives
- U.S. Federal Bureau of Investigation and equivalent in other countries (bioterrorism exercises)

Areas for response assessment
- Resource availability
  - Hospital patient care areas and supplies
  - Therapeutics and vaccines
  - Personal protective equipment
  - Personnel
- Resource allocation
- Response coordination/Incident Command
- Infection Control
  - Spread of the agent through the community
  - Protection of healthcare workers and responders
- Communication
  - Interagency
    - Among jurisdictions or regions
    - Among levels of government
    - Media relations/Information to public
- Triage
- Information management
- Personnel management
  - Within facilities and agencies
  - Mobilized for large-scale action (vaccine distribution, epidemiology)
- Management of public reaction
  - Public fear
  - Civil unrest
  - Mass gatherings for resources
- Psychological ramifications
  - Response personnel
  - Public
- Understanding of legal implications of decisions
- Cost of implementing decisions

Exercise Evaluation
- Assessment of whether processes and outcomes of the response met goals
- Comparison of evaluation to previous exercises
- Cost of the exercise

Adapted from Bardi J. Aftermath of a hypothetical smallpox disaster. *Emerg Infect Dis* 1999; 5(4): 547–551.

turnover necessitates repeated training so that new employees can function within the system. The utility of the exercises is also contingent on proper evaluation after they are completed. An exercise with flawed design and/or execution can lead to a false sense of preparedness. For example, participants in the TOPOFF 3 exercise noted that federal assistance was provided in an unrealistically fast manner and may not correspond to the timing in an actual disaster.

Modeling

Given the rarity of infectious disease disasters, mathematical models are used as prediction and forecasting tools. These models use existing data from previous outbreaks, epidemics, or pandemics to provide insight into putative future transmissions of infectious diseases and/or ramifications of preparedness decisions. This is important because the process of designing and interpreting models can serve as a guide for discussions on the variables and assumptions involved in controlling disease. The uncertainty regarding use of various inclusion and exclusion parameters and the potential errors in selection of data values brings into question the significance of the models.

Epidemic emergence models using climatic data have been developed with success for *V. cholerae* O139, a pathogen endemic to certain regions of the world.[72] Modeling of novel or rare pathogens, such as pandemic influenza or intentionally released smallpox, is more problematic. Here, specific characteristics of the agent (transmissibility or drug resistance) and the host (susceptibility, super spreaders, public reaction and compliance) are unknown and must be assumed.

Modeling is also used for preparedness plans to determine how decisions will affect the progression of the epidemic. Models related to resource allocation, antimicrobial use, vaccination strategies, health economic implications, and public control (quarantine, isolation, social distancing) have all been published.[73–77] How to best validate these models (and the decisions they support) and incorporate their recommendations into the formulation or optimization of preparedness plans remains a challenge.

Evaluation

Since 2001, many countries have spent large amounts of money on public health preparedness for a biological event. For example, the United States has spent billions of dollars on surveillance, workforce preparedness, response strategies, and exercises and drills to prepare for an attack using biological weapons. Formal evaluation of these activities is crucial to ensuring that outcomes are properly reviewed and that funding is being used effectively. This mandates more than the simple creation and publication of after-action reports. Preparedness programs should be designed with the inclusion of specific evaluation components to empirically determine whether goals are being met and provide data for improvements. This type of evaluation is critical because some assessment questions may give a skewed sense of readiness. For example, in assessing a workforce readiness training program, asking whether or not people are trained (a structural measure) is different from asking how well employees perform their duties after training (a process measure) or even whether the training was successful in reducing the morbidity and mortality of an infectious disease disaster (an outcome measure). This last type of assessment is challenging given the rarity of infectious disease disasters and the difficulty of defining "success."[78]

The complexity of preparing for infectious disease disasters lies in the unknown nature of future threats. Because of this, individuals involved in their management may disagree on the necessity and requirements for effective preparedness plans. This is particularly true for bioterrorism preparedness, because the perceptions of the necessity for such specific plans vary widely.[79,80] For example, the campaign in the United States in 2003 to vaccinate 500,000 healthcare workers against smallpox had very low compliance. This was due, at least in part, to perceptions that the threat of a smallpox bioterrorist attack was low and concerns over the unknown safety of the vaccine.[81] Evidence-based assessments of the needs and priorities of response preparedness efforts and the probability of success (from sociological and scientific perspectives) are critical to preventing this type of program collapse. This is particularly important because the failure of these large programs causes the public to question the utility and funding of any EID preparedness initiative.

RECOMMENDATIONS FOR FURTHER RESEARCH

The traditional paradigm regarded pathogens as enemies to be battled as they emerged. As a better understanding of the relationship between humans and the microbial world is gained, the war analogy in approaching EID management has become insufficient.[82] It has become clear that relying on the current antimicrobial arsenal to react to EIDs is inadequate. With the exception of post-exposure prophylaxis, this is predominantly a treatment strategy for those who have already developed disease. Preventing acquisition of infection or disease is preferable to treatment to avert potential disaster situations. There have been successes with preventive mechanisms, such as vaccines to specific infectious disease agents; however, the diversity of EIDs and the potential for microbial adaptation and change precludes using current strategies against all known pathogens, and especially for still undiscovered or yet-to-emerge agents.

The emergence of infectious diseases, largely fueled by human practices, poses worldwide disaster threats. Immediate needs to expand the local and global public health infrastructure and workforce are obvious. The ultimate future of infectious disease disaster management rests on improving two broad but interrelated areas:

1. Preparedness strategies that surpass the usual unresolved obstacles by promoting multidisciplinary program design, and by substantiating early surveillance/detection and prevention of disease;
2. Research into novel countermeasure development, host–microbe relationships, host–immune responses, surveillance tools, and analysis of how behaviors of the human host and perturbations of the environment (whether at the macro- or micro-molecular level) affect infectious disease emergence. These essentially encompass a fresh perspective reevaluation of the approach regarding the understanding of the epidemiology of infectious diseases.

Preparedness

Preparedness Strategies

Repeated drills are used to determine areas for preparedness plan improvements; however, the usefulness of drills diminishes when identified obstacles are not addressed. Areas consistently identified for further improvement include resource allocation, communication between response stakeholders, and understanding of governmental roles. Current templates for planning need modification to first address why these "lessons learned" are not, or cannot be, actually implemented. This necessitates the study of the barriers to implementation of findings from previous drills and disasters by multidisciplinary teams that include social scientists, communications experts, and human factors specialists. Ultimately, drills should be used as a rehearsal tool for workforce training (i.e., to identify improvement goals on an individual basis), not as a mechanism for developing preparedness plans.

EID Surveillance

Although improved response preparedness is reassuring, preventing disease transmission will do much to reduce the dependence on limited resources and other preparedness obstacles. EID management needs to be changed beyond the state of relying on disease treatment when cases appear at the hospital doors. In essence, it must move from the conventional reactionary EID response to a more proactive approach.[83] Improving early EID detection can reduce the "incident threshold" and expedite agent characterization, assessment of response needs, and education of the public. This must be a global effort. Although new agents can emerge from any area, developing countries bear the burden of global infectious disease incidence and the likelihood of witnessing the development of new pathogens. The developed world has a responsibility to provide assistance in surveillance for both humanitarian reasons and the need for self-protection. Great strides have been made in global surveillance of human infectious diseases, especially after the infectious disease events of the new millennium and efforts to comply with IHR, but there are still political, social, and economic obstacles to further advancement.

As discussed, non-human sources of microbes can lead to emergence of human infectious diseases. A research need exists to broaden and strengthen surveillance beyond human symptom and disease reports. Past evidence shows that understanding animal infectious disease trends can benefit human health. Linking animal disease surveillance (including zoological, agricultural, and wild and companion animals) with human disease surveillance clearinghouses can potentially alert public health officials sooner to possible human infectious disease disasters, whether global in nature or constrained to a small location. The specificities of such tactics are complicated, given the current inconsistencies in animal disease surveillance and reporting and the unproven value of many human disease surveillance systems.

Research

Basic Research

The understanding of pathogens has been transformed by genomics and proteomics, fields of molecular biology that study the overall functions and regulation of the genes and proteins of an organism in an environment. These technologies allow scientists to identify disease-causing agents and comprehensively characterize microbial pathogenic mechanisms in a fraction of the time needed in previous decades. Future efforts must include the development of technologies to translate this knowledge into functional applications such as rapid screening of people and/or animals during an EID disaster, the development of sensitive handheld devices for remote screening applications, and more rapid determination of antimicrobial resistances and application of therapies.

For effective EID management, other areas of basic research must be enhanced to complement the more common agent-specific programs. Namely, there is a need to expand research on diverse biological disciplines associated with zoonotic and vector-borne diseases, such as reservoir ecology and entomology. Ideally, these specialties would be housed in interdisciplinary academic EID departments that include infectious diseases, molecular biology, and veterinary and conservation medicine experts to foster a collaborative atmosphere that has been increasingly referred to as a "One Health" approach to understanding disease emergence.

Drug and Vaccine Development

Improved pharmaceuticals alone will not be adequate to change the burden of EIDs on society, but they have an important role in mitigating disease severity, human suffering, and infectious agent transmission. The need and incentives for antimicrobial drug development has already been outlined. The future lies in the discovery of novel targets and mechanisms active against a broad spectrum of agents. This requires a more comprehensive understanding of host–pathogen relationships: how the host recognizes an invading pathogen, how pathogens evade host defenses, how hosts and microbes interact in nonpathogenic relationships (symbiosis), and how host–immune responses to pathogens can be modulated by drugs or by beneficial bacteria.

Revolutionary advances in understanding cellular immunology, structural biology, nanotechnology, diagnostics and monitoring, and bioinformatics have all contributed to the field of vaccine development. Scientists are on the brink of unlocking the secrets of improving vaccine efficacy by targeting both the innate and adaptive immune response.[84] DNA vaccines hold promise as future EID countermeasures because they can be designed and manufactured relatively rapidly, they can induce cross-strain immunity, and they can be administered by different routes.[85] As the basic sciences continue to inform the understanding of human and microbial biological processes, progress must be made in moving these advances to novel vaccine design and product development that result in effective vaccines. Thus far, such progress has been slow and effective vaccines against some long-studied, and globally-relevant, pathogens (e.g., HIV, *Plasmodium falciparum*) remain elusive. Further understanding of vaccine-induced protective immune responses in humans and immune evasion mechanisms in microbes is needed to accelerate next-generation vaccine development.[86]

The international community must take a more collaborative approach to drug and vaccine design for EIDs. Nowhere is this more evident than in the case of pandemic influenza vaccine. Current production capabilities may limit the number of courses available during an infectious disease disaster. Scientific research is necessary to: 1) develop rapid in vitro methods for vaccine component production; 2) increase vaccine efficacy at lower doses; 3) investigate less-specific vaccines that can be made and stockpiled prior to a pandemic; and 4) increase the shelf-life of vaccines. Advances in all four of these areas can benefit both influenza pandemic preparedness and vaccinology in general. WHO has convened meetings with international stakeholders to formulate plans for increasing the international production capacity of influenza vaccine. Such plans will need to address international differences in complicated issues such as production regulations, acceptable clinical safety data, and intellectual property.

In 2010, the Infectious Diseases Society of America (IDSA) called for a global commitment to antibiotic development; the "10 x '20 Initiative" challenges the development of ten new antibiotics by 2020.[87] Essential to the success of the initiative is a global approach that builds on international capabilities to foster an ongoing research and development infrastructure. In the European Union, the Innovative Medicine Initiative launched its New Drugs for Bad Bugs (ND4BB) core element in the sixth call for proposals in May 2012, and subsequent calls for proposals have also included topics that address antimicrobial development.[88] Despite the heightened attention given to antimicrobial research and development by key groups, it is not yet clear whether this high-level attention has yielded results. An update report from IDSA in 2013[89] deemed progress to be "alarmingly elusive," suggesting that efforts thus far to spur global innovation, funding, and regulatory progress have been largely unsuccessful. What more, then, is necessary? So and colleagues[90] suggest that the public-private dynamic important for fostering innovative antimicrobial development would be advanced by mechanisms and priorities that promote the sharing of the "3Rs": Resources (e.g., sharing of data from pharmaceutical companies that would not provide a competitive advantage), Risks (e.g., public funding for research that would share the risks with private companies), and Rewards (e.g., product development partnerships).

EID Surveillance Research

A more expansive approach to surveillance that encompasses monitoring beyond human and animal health is under investigation. Sometimes termed "conservation medicine," it utilizes interdisciplinary networks that examine the ecology of microbial interactions with animals, plants, and humans in the context of the drivers of disease emergence.[91] These networks should include the expertise of health workers, veterinarians, plant biologists, epidemiologists, ecologists, climatologists, and conservation biologists. Environmental specialists and global geologists must be involved in such endeavors to ensure inclusion of environmental aspects that may affect EIDs. Computational and theoretical biologists, and epidemiologists with expertise in transmission, host–agent interaction, host–environment interaction, and agent–environment interaction, need to develop cooperative research programs among themselves and with other specialists. The goal of such collaboration is to produce, and more importantly, validate, predictive models of disease occurrence. This holistic approach to surveillance is exemplified by geographical information systems that integrate infectious disease incidence, prevalence, and distribution data with satellite environmental data to predict disease emergence in other locations with similar conditions.[92]

The ultimate goal is the capability to predict human EIDs before they occur, or at least to detect an emergence earlier. These types of broad surveillance tools that include environmental components have been used for years by plant biologists to predict disease emergence in agricultural crops. The basic epidemiological triangle of host, agent, and environmental interactions described earlier in this chapter was officially conceptualized decades ago by plant biologists.[93] The link between environmental factors and plant diseases may be obvious, but the time is overdue to integrate this same approach into understanding human infectious diseases.

That said, in addition to improving methods for achieving better surveillance, *what* is monitored needs further assessment. The perceived pressing need for surveillance systems, especially in the United States after the 2001 terrorist attacks, has resulted in much research, development, and implementation of such systems using a variety of data and information, often incorporated due to availability. The general, albeit likely unintentional, assumption has been that such systematic analysis of "any" data and information will be useful and an improvement over a surveillance system vacuum. Now, over a decade later, it becomes clear that the field would benefit from the comprehensive study and development of mechanisms to assess whether or not data sources are relevant for the purposes of biosurveillance systems (early detection and situational awareness of outbreaks). Research is also needed to assess and advance the often-cited but heretofore largely unrealized capability to integrate information from different surveillance systems and efforts to provide a more comprehensive picture. Significant obstacles include lack of common architecture among systems, inability or unwillingness for entities to share systems or data, sustainment of efforts and collaborations, and lack of priority.

Finally, the EID surveillance field needs further research on analysis and interpretation of results. Ultimately, the goal of using surveillance tools is to provide information in "near real-time" to decision-makers regarding a disease emergence or progression of an outbreak. However, the expectation of timely information may not allow for the rigorous assessment that information providers would like to conduct before conveying results that may be used for actions. The ability to quantify, with some reliability, the confidence in the information will provide decision-makers valuable data when determining response activities.

Infectious disease disaster medicine is itself a growing field and has been the focus of extensive preparedness efforts. Further research on the impact of politics, international relations, social behavior, and public health policies on EID disaster management is warranted to develop sound and realistic action plans. As noted throughout the chapter, this multidisciplinary focus of effort toward the fields of infectious disease biology and epidemiology is a nascent application that holds promise for the future of both infectious diseases and disaster medicine.

REFERENCES

1. Spelling B, Taylor-Blake B. On the exoneration of Dr. William H. Stewart: debunking an urban legend. *Infectious Diseases of Poverty* 2013; 2: 3.

2. Pier GB. On the greatly exaggerated reports of the death of infectious diseases. *Clin Infect Dis* 2008; 47: 1113–1114.

3. Taylor LH, Latham SM, Woolhouse ME. Risk factors for human disease emergence. *Phil Trans R Soc Lond B Biol Sci* 2001; 356(1411): 983–989.

4. Lashley FR. Factors contributing to the occurrence of emerging infectious diseases. *Biol Res Nurs* 2004; 4(4): 258–267.

5. Institute of Medicine. *Microbial Threats to Health: Emergence, Detection and Response.* Washington, DC, National Academies Press, 2003.

6. Koenig KL, Majestic C, Burns MJ. Ebola Virus Disease: Essential Public Health Principles for Clinicians, WestJEM, 2014. http://www.escholarship.org/uc/item/1bh1352j#page-1 (Accessed August 8, 2015).

7. Fauci AS. Ebola – Underscoring the Global Disparities in Health Care Resources. *N Engl J Med* August 13, 2014. http://www.nejm.org/doi/pdf/10.1056/NEJMp1409494 (Accessed August 21, 2014).

8. Baize SB, et al. Emergence of Zaire Ebola Virus Disease in Guinea – Preliminary Report. *N Engl J Med* April 16, 2014. http://www.nejm.org/doi/full/10.1056/NEJMoa1404505 (Accessed August 11, 2014).

9. Institute of Medicine. *Biological Threats and Terrorism: Assessing the Science and Response Capabilities.* Washington, DC, National Academies Press, 2002.

10. Naylor CD, Chantler C, Griffiths S. Learning from SARS in Hong Kong and Toronto. *JAMA* 2004; 291(20): 2483–2487.

11. Enserink M. SARS in China. China's missed dance. *Science* 2003; 301(5631): 294–296.

12. U.S. Centers for Disease Control and Prevention (CDC). Update: severe acute respiratory syndrome – Toronto, Canada. *MMWR* 2003; 52(23): 547–550.

13. Osterholm MT. How to vaccinate 30000 people in three days: realities of outbreak management. *Pub Health Report* 2001; 116 (Suppl. 2): 74–78.

14. Ferguson NM, Cummings DAT, Fraser C, Cajka JC, Cooley PC, Burke DS. Strategies for mitigating an influenza pandemic. *Nature* 2006; 442(7101): 448–452.

15. Barbisch D, Koenig KL, Shih F-Y. Is There a Case for Quarantine? Perspectives from SARS to Ebola. *Disaster Medicine and Public Health Preparedness*, 2015. DOI: 10.1017/dmp.2015.38.

16. CDC. Severe acute respiratory syndrome – Singapore, 2003. *MMWR* 2003; 52(18): 405–411.

17. Bliss KE, Fisher M. Water and sanitation in the time of cholera: sustaining progress on water, sanitation, and health in Haiti. *Center for Strategic and International Studies.* September 2013. https://csis.org/publication/water-and-sanitation-time-cholera (Accessed September 20, 2013).

18. Stratton SJ. Cholera in Haiti: redefining emergency public health philosophy. *Prehosp and Disaster Med* 2013; 28(3): 195–196.

19. Braden CR, Dowell SF, Jernigan DB, Hughes JM. Progress in global surveillance and response capacity 10 years after severe acute respiratory syndrome. *Emerg Infect Dis* 2013; 19(6): 864–869.

20. Berg R. Salmonella Saint Paul: what went wrong? *J Environ Health* 2008; 71(5): 50–52.

21. Spanish farmers paid a price for Europe's E. coli O104 outbreak. *Food Safety News.* July 9, 2012.

22. Koenig KL. Identify-Isolate-Inform: A modified tool for initial detection and management of Middle East Respiratory Syndrome patients in the emergency department. *West JEM* 2015. http://escholarship.org/uc/item/3k27v8g1 (Accessed August 8, 2015).

23. Peters CJ, LeDuc JW. An introduction to Ebola: the virus and the disease. *J Infect Dis* 1999; 179(Suppl 1): ix–xvi.

24. McDonald LC, Simor AE, Su I-J, et al. SARS in healthcare facilities, Toronto and Taiwan. *Emerg Infect Dis* 2004; 10(5): 777–781.

25. Assiri A, McGeer A, Perl TM, et al. Hospital outbreak of Middle East respiratory syndrome coronavirus. *N Engl J Med* 2013; 369(5): 407–416.

26. Qureshi K, Gershon RRM, Sherman MF, et al. Health care workers' ability and willingness to report to duty during catastrophic disasters. *J Urban Health Bull NY Acad Med* 2005; 82(3): 378–388.

27. Balicer RD, Barnett DJ, Thompson CB, et al. Characterizing hospital workers' willingness to report to duty in an influenza pandemic through threat- and efficacy-based assessment. *BMC Public Health* 2010; 10: 436.

28. Devnani M. Factors associated with the willingness of health care personnel to work during an influenza public health emergency: an integrative review. *Prehosp Disaster Med* 2012; 27(6): 551–566.

29. Roos R. CDC says vaccine shortage likely to outlast current H1N1 wave. *CIDRAP News* November 4, 2009. http://www.cidrap.umn.edu/news-perspective/2009/11/cdc-says-vaccine-shortage-likely-outlast-current-h1n1-wave (Accessed September 20, 2013).

30. Shepard CW, Soriano-Gabarro M, Zell ER, et al. Antimicrobial postexposure for anthrax: adverse events and adherence. *Emerg Infect Dis* 2002; 8(10): 1124–1132.

31. Date KA, Vicari A, Hyde TB, et al. Considerations for oral cholera vaccine use during outbreak after earthquake in Haiti, 2010–2011. *Emerg Infect Dis* 12011; 7(11): 2105–2112.

32. Centers for Disease Control and Prevention. Healthcare Infection Control Practices Advisory Committee (HICPAC). 2007 Guideline for Isolation Precautions: Preventing Transmission of Infectious Agents in Healthcare Settings. http://www.cdc.gov/hicpac/2007ip/2007isolationprecautions.html (Accessed August 10, 2015).

33. World Health Organization. World Health Day. How to Safeguard Health Facilities. http://www.who.int/world-health-day/2009/safeguard_health_facilities/en (Accessed August 10, 2015).

34. Hawryluck L, Gold WL, Robinson S, Pogorski S, Galea S, Styra R. SARS control and psychological effects of quarantine, Toronto, Canada. *Emerg Infect Dis* 2004; 10(7): 1206–1212.

35. O'Toole T, Mair M, Inglesby TV. Shining light on "Dark Winter." *Clin Infect Dis* 2002; 34(7): 972–983.

36. Wynia MK, Gostin LO. Ethical challenges in preparing for bioterrorism: barriers within the healthcare system. *Am J Pub Health* 2004; 94(7): 1096–1102.

37. National Select Agent Registry. August 12, 2013. http://www.selectagents.gov (Accessed September 20, 2013).

38. Beecher DJ. Forensic application of microbiological culture analysis to identify mail intentionally contaminated with Bacillus anthracis spores. *Appl Environ Microbiol* 2006; 72(8): 5304–5310.

39. CDC Public Health Emergency Response Guide for State, Local, and Tribal Public Health Directors - Version 2.0. http://emergency.cdc.gov/planning/responseguide.asp (Accessed August 8, 2015).

40. LeDuc JW, Barry MA. SARS, the first pandemic of the 21st century. *Emerg Infect Dis* November 2004. http://www.cdc.gov/ncidod/EID/vol10no11/04–0797_02.htm (Accessed January 13, 2009).

41. International Health Regulations. 2005. http://www.who.int/ihr/en (Accessed September 24, 2013).

42. Katz RL, Fernandez JA, McNabb SJN. Disease surveillance, capacity building and implementation of the International Health Regulations (IHR[2005]). *BMC Public Health* 2010; 10(Suppl): S1.

43. U.S. Department of Homeland Security, Federal Emergency Management Agency. Biological Incident Annex. August 2008. http://www.fema.gov/media-library/assets/documents/25550 (Accessed October 10, 2013).

44. Federal Emergency Management Agency. NIMS Alert. NIMS implementation activities for hospitals and healthcare systems. September 12, 2006. http://www.fema.gov/pdf/emergency/nims/imp_act_hos_hlth.pdf (Accessed November 12, 2008).

45. Arnold JL, Dembry L-M, Tsai M-C, et al. Recommended modifications and applications of the hospital emergency incident command system for hospital emergency management. *Preshosp Disaster Med* 2005; 20(5): 290–300.

46. World Health Organization. WHO concludes MERS-CoV mission in Saudi Arabia. Press release. May 7, 2014. http://www.emro.who.int/media/news/mers-cov-mission-saudi-arabia.html (Accessed August 26, 2014).

47. Rubinson L, Nuzzo JB, Talmor DS, O'Toole T, Kramer BR, Inglesby TV, for the Working Group on Emergency Mass Critical Care. Augmentation of hospital critical care capacity after bioterrorist attacks or epidemics: recommendations of the Working Group on Emergency Mass Critical Care. *Crit Care Med* 2005; 33(10): 2393–2403.

48. Fumento MJ. The threat of an avian flu pandemic is over-hyped. *Virtual Mentor* 2006; 8(4): 265–270.

49. U.S. General Accounting Office. West Nile virus outbreak. *Lessons for public health preparedness.* GAO/HEHS-00–180. Washington, DC, General Accounting Office, 2000.

50. Chan PKS. Outbreak of avian influenza (H5N1) virus infection in Hong Kong in 1997. *Clin Infect Dis* 2002; 34(Suppl 2): S58–S64.

51. Chua KB. Nipah virus outbreak in Malaysia. *J Clin Virol* 2003; 26(3): 265–275.

52. Ksiazek TG, Erdman D, Goldsmith CS, et al. A novel coronavirus associated with severe acute respiratory syndrome. *N Engl J Med* 2003; 348(20): 1953–1966.

53. Spellberg B, Powers JH, Brass EP, Miller LG, Edwards JE, Jr. Trends in antimicrobial drug development: implications for the future. *Clin Infect Dis* 2004; 38(9): 1279–1286.

54. Bassetti M, Merelli M, Temperoni C, Astilean A. New antibiotics for bad bugs: where are we? *Annals Clin Microbiol Antimicrobials* 2013; 12: 22.

55. Stockman LJ, Bellamy R, Garner P. SARS: systematic review of treatment effects. *PLoS Med* 2006; 3(9): e343.

56. U.S. Department of Health & Human Services, Medical Countermeasures.gov, https://www.medicalcountermeasures.gov/barda/cbrn/project-bioshield-overview.aspx (Accessed August 10, 2015).

57. American Society for Microbiology. ASM comments on the Biodefense and Pandemic Vaccine and Drug Development Act of 2005. November 4, 2005. www.asm.org/Policy/index.asp?bid=38723 (Accessed November 12, 2008).

58. Malakoff D. U.S. accepts NSABB recommendation to publish H5N1 flu papers. *Science/AAAS News.* April 20, 2012. http://news.sciencemag.org/2012/04/breaking-u.s.-accepts-nsabb-recommendation-publish-h5n1-flu-papers (Accessed October 11, 2013).

59. Centers for Disease Control and Prevention Surveillance Resource Center. http://www.cdc.gov/surveillancepractice, Accessed Aug 10, 2015.

60. Institute of Medicine. *Learning from SARS: Preparing for the Next Disease Outbreak.* Washington, DC, National Academies Press, 2004.

61. Schnirring L. Medical conferences spotlight H7N9 threat. *CIDRAP News.* May 21, 2013. http://www.cidrap.umn.edu/news-perspective/2013/05/medical-conferences-spotlight-h7n9-threat (Accessed September 20, 2013).

62. Branswell H. Saudi silence on deadly MERS virus outbreak frustrates world health experts. *Scientific American* June 7, 2013. http://www.scientificamerican.com/article.cfm?id=saudi-silence-on-deadly-mers-virus-outbreak-frustrates-world-health-experts (Accessed September 20, 2013).

63. Executive Office of the President. National Strategy for Biosurveillance. July 2012. http://www.whitehouse.gov/sites/default/files/National_Strategy_for_Biosurveillance_July_2012.pdf (Accessed on October 11, 2013).

64. Svoboda T, Henry B, Shulman L, et al. Public health measures to control the spread of the severe acute respiratory syndrome during the outbreak in Toronto. *N Engl J Med.* 2004; 350(23): 2351–2361.

65. CDC. Health Alert Network Update: Multistate outbreak of fungal infections among persons who received injections with contaminated medication. December 12, 2012. http://emergency.cdc.gov/HAN/han00338.asp (Accessed September 20, 2013).

66. U.S. General Accounting Office. Influenza pandemic. *Challenges in preparedness and response.* GAO-05–863T. Washington, DC, General Accounting Office, 2005.

67. Gautret P, Benkouiten S, Salaheddine I, et al. Hajj pilgrims' knowledge about Middle East respiratory syndrome coronavirus, August to September 2013. *Eurosurveillance* October 10, 2013;18(41).

68. Bardi J. Aftermath of a hypothetical smallpox disaster. *Emerg Infect Dis* 1999; 5(4): 547–551.

69. CDC. Strategic National Stockpile (SNS). http://www.cdc.gov/phpr/stockpile/stockpile.htm (Accessed September 20, 2013).

70. Hick JL, O'Laughlin DT. Concept of operations for triage of mechanical ventilation in an epidemic. *Acad Emerg Med* 2006; 13(2): 223–229.

71. Burkle FM. Population-based triage management in response to surge-capacity requirements during a large-scale bioevent disaster. *Acad Emerg Med* 2006; 13(11): 1118–1129.

72. World Health Organization (WHO). Pandemic Influenza Risk Management; WHO Interim Guidance. June 10, 2013. http://www.who.int/influenza/preparedness/pandemic/influenza_risk_management/en (Accessed October 10, 2011).

73. American College of Emergency Physicians. National Strategic Plan for Emergency Department Management of Outbreaks of Novel H1N1 Influenza. http://acep.org/WorkArea/DownloadAsset.aspx?id=45781 (Accessed on July 12, 2009).

74. DHS Office of Inspector General. A review of the Top Officials 3 exercise. November 2005. https://www.dhs.gov/xoig/assets/mgmtrpts/OIG_06–07_Nov05.pdf (Accessed December 5, 2006).

75. Lobitz B, Beck L, Huq A, et al. Climate and infectious disease: use of remote sensing for detection of Vibrio cholerae by indirect measurement. *Proc Natl Acad Sci USA* 2000; 97(4): 1438–1443.

76. Stein ML, Rudge JW, Coker R, et al. Development of a resource modeling tool to support decision makers in pandemic influenza preparedness: The AsiaFluCap Simulator. *BMC Public Health* 2012; 12: 870.

77. Becker NG, Wang D. Can antiviral drugs contain pandemic influenza transmission? *PLoS One* 2011; 6(3): e17764.

78. Araz OM, Galvani A, Meyers LA. Geographic prioritization of distributing pandemic influenza vaccines. *Health Care Manag Sci* 2012; 15(3): 175–87.

79. Smith, RD, Keogh-Brown MR. Macroeconomic impact of pandemic influenza and associated policies in Thailand, South Africa and Uganda. *Influenza Other Respi Viruses* 2013; 7 (Suppl. 2): 64–71.

80. Maharaj S, Kleczkowski A. Controlling epidemic spread by social distancing: do it well or not at all. *BMC Public Health* 2012; 12: 679.

81. Asch SM, Stoto, M, Mendes M, et al. A review of instruments assessing public health preparedness. *Pub Health Report* 2005; 120(5): 532–542.

82. Amadio JB. Bioterrorism preparedness funds well used at the local level. *Am J Pub Health* 2004; 95(3): 373–374.

83. Cohen HW, Gould RM, Sidel VW. The pitfalls of bioterrorism preparedness: the anthrax and smallpox experiences. *Am J Pub Health* 2004; 94(10): 1667–1671.

84. Wortley PM, Schwartz B, Levy PS, Quick LM, Evans B, Burke B. Healthcare workers who elected not to receive smallpox vaccination. *Am J Prevent Med* 2006; 30(3): 258–265.

85. Institute of Medicine. *Ending the War Metaphor: The Changing Agenda for Unraveling the Host-Microbe Relationship.* Washington, DC, National Academies Press, 2006.

86. King DA, Peckham C, Waage JK, Brownlie J, Woolhouse ME. Epidemiology. Infectious diseases: preparing for the future. *Science.* 2006; 313(5792): 1392–1393.

87. Pulendran B, Ahmed R. Translating innate immunity into immunological memory: implications for vaccine development. *Cell* 2006; 124(4): 849–863.

88. Liu MA, Wahren B, Karlsson Hedestam GB. DNA vaccines: recent developments and future possibilities. *Hum Gene Ther* 2006; 17(11): 1051–1061.

89. Koff WC, Burton DR, Johnson PR, Walker BD, et al. Accelerating next-generation vaccine development for global disease prevention. *Science* 2013; 340(6136): 1232910.

90. Infectious Diseases Society of America. The 10 x '20 initiative: pursuing a global commitment to develop 10 new antibacterial drugs by 2020. *Clin Infect Dis* 2010; 50(8): 1081–1083.

91. Scott A. Europe invests $550 million into drug discovery and antibiotic development. *Chemical & Engineering News* 2013; 91(7): 8.

92. Boucher HW, Talbot GH, Benjamin DK, Jr., et al. 10 x '20 progress – development of new drugs active against Gram-negative bacilli: an update from the Infectious Diseases Society of America. *Clin Infect Dis* 2013: 56(12): 1685–1694.

93. So AD, Ruiz-Esparza Q, Gupta N, Cars O. 3Rs for innovating novel antibiotics: sharing resources, risks, and rewards. *BMJ* 2012; 344: e1782.

9

DISASTER BEHAVIORAL HEALTH

James C. West, Merritt D. Schreiber, David Benedek, and Dori B. Reissman

OVERVIEW

Communities exposed to disasters experience multiple traumatic events including threats to life, loss of property, exposure to death, and often economic devastation. Disasters by definition overwhelm institutions, healthcare, and social resources and require from months to years for both individuals and communities to recover.[1]

In the aftermath of disasters, a range of behaviors and symptoms emerge with profound individual and population-level public health implications. A number of terms have been used to describe the social, psychological, and emotional health of affected populations in the aftermath of disasters including those resulting from acts of terrorism. The term "behaviors" captures the actions people take to reduce perceived threats to safety, health, and well-being. Coping behaviors have social and emotional effects that may mitigate or aggravate the sense of loss and change triggered by the disaster or its aftermath. The term "symptoms" refers to more severe or pathological emotional and behavioral responses, which may be transient or persistent.

Characteristics of the disaster event may greatly increase the stress experienced, such as lack of familiarity with the hazard (e.g., radiation exposure following the Fukushima reactor accident), use of terror as a weapon, intensity of impact (e.g., degree of direct exposure to harm, loss, and change), predictability of the event (e.g., no warning, inability to avoid, unclear targets, protracted or stuttering course), or caused by intentional human action (purposeful intent to harm vs. accidental). This chapter describes the 1) range and timeline of typical reactions; 2) state of the art with respect to clinical and public health considerations for disaster mental health; and 3) recommendations for further study.

Range and Timeline of Typical Reactions

Disasters, including those resulting from acts of terrorism, produce a spectrum of common physiological, psychological, social, behavioral, emotional, cognitive, and spiritual reactions (Tables 9.1 and 9.2). Broadly speaking, these involve anxiety, mood, cognitive, and somatic symptoms.[2,3] An Institute of Medicine (IOM) Committee on Psychological Aspects of Terrorism report provides a useful framework to assist disaster and emergency planners in preparing for and managing anticipated clinical and population-level effects of disasters[4]. Their product captures a range of social and emotional impacts across the life cycle of the event (including pre-event, response, and recovery phases).[4] In their report, the IOM committee illustrates three overarching, time-phased, and interrelated aspects of population-level impact: 1) distress responses; 2) changes in behavior; and 3) clinically significant psychiatric disorders and impairment. Direct disaster exposure includes the following potential stressors: 1) serious injury; 2) traumatic bereavement; 3) loss of home or other critical resources; 4) witnessing severe or mutilating injury or death of others; 5) perceiving an immediate threat to one's own life or the life of a significant other; and 6) managing prolonged uncertainties about threats to health and safety.[1,2,5] Although disasters are associated with varied clinical outcomes, including complex comorbidity, post-traumatic stress disorder (PTSD) is the most widely investigated clinical outcome. PTSD is a disorder of characteristic symptoms of re-experiencing, hyperarousal, and avoidance following exposure to a traumatic event. Posttraumatic stress (PTS) is a commonly used term to describe any collection of PTSD symptoms insufficient to meet full diagnostic criteria. A review of the epidemiology of PTSD following disasters concludes the following:

> [The] prevalence of PTSD among direct victims of disasters ranges between 30% and 40%; the range of PTSD prevalence among rescue workers is lower, ranging between 10% and 20%, while the range of PTSD rates in the general population is the lowest and expected to be between 5% and 10%. The most consistently documented determinants of the risk of PTSD across studies are measures of the magnitude of exposure to the event. Particularly, degree of physical injury, immediate risk of life, severity of property destruction, and frequency of fatalities are strong predictors for high rates of PTSD.[6]

Population-level statistics can be misleading due to considerable heterogeneity in individual risk for development of PTSD

Table 9.1. Common Adult Responses to Disasters and Traumatic Events

Physiological Responses	Behavioral and Emotional Responses	Cognitive Responses
Fatigue	Anxiety, fear	Memory problems
Nausea, vomiting	Grief, guilt, self-doubt, sadness	Calculation difficulties
Insomnia, sleep disruption	Irritability, anger (sometimes displaced), resentment, increased conflicts with friends/family	Confusion in general and/or confusing trivial with major issues
Chest pain, choking, or smothering sensation	Feeling overwhelmed, hopeless, despair, depressed	Concentration problems, distractibility
Fine motor tremors, tics, paresthesias	Crisis of faith, anger at God, questioning basic religious beliefs	Recurring dreams or nightmares
Profuse sweating	Anticipation of harm to self or others; isolation or withdrawal	Decision-making difficulties, easily confused
Dizziness	Changes in usual eating, sleeping patterns	Preoccupation with disaster events
Gastrointestinal upset (diarrhea or constipation, abdominal pain)	Hypervigilance, startle reactions	Lessened ability to handle complexities
Racing pulse, heart palpitations	Crying easily, mood swings	Fear of crowds, strangers, or being left alone
Nonspecific joint or body aches or pain, headaches	Gallows humor	Anomia
Environmental intolerance (temperature, sound, smell)	Poor performance of usual roles (home, work, social)	Slowed rate of thinking, speech difficulties
	Regression to less mature or risky behaviors	
	Ritualistic behavior	

Table 9.2. Common Pediatric Responses to Disasters and Traumatic Events by Age

Children of All Ages	Preschool Age(1–5 y)	Early Childhood(5–11 y)	Adolescence(12–14 y)
Anxiety and irritability	Changes in eating habits	Increased aggressiveness	Abandonment of chores, schoolwork, and other prior responsibilities
Clinging, fear of strangers	Changes in sleeping habits	Changes in eating/sleeping	Disruptiveness at home or in the classroom
Fear of separation, being alone	Clinging to parent	Difficulty concentrating	Experimentation with high-risk behaviors such as drinking or drug use
Headache, abdominal pain, or other aches and pains	Disobedience	Regression to earlier behavior	Vigorous competition for attention from parents and teachers
Increased shyness or aggressiveness	Fear of animals, the dark, "monsters"	Competing more for the attention of parents	Resisting authority
Nervousness about the future	Hyperactivity	Fear of going to school, the dark, "monsters"	
Regression to immature behavior	Speech difficulties	Drop in school performance	
Reluctance to go to school	Regression to earlier behavior (thumbsucking, bedwetting)	Desire to sleep with parents	
Sadness and crying			
Withdrawal			
Worry, nightmares			

dependent on the unique features of each disaster. However, recent efforts to model population-level effects suggest common "trajectories" of outcome over time including: a resilience trajectory, an early emerging and chronic disorder course, an acute disorder with recovery, and a delayed disorder trajectory.[7] In a study of ongoing political violence, a resilience trajectory was not observed at all.[8] Following Hurricane Katrina in the United States, the majority of adults who developed presumptive PTSD did not recover within 18–27 months.[9] Serious psychiatric disorders, including suicidal ideation and plans increased over time.[10]

In a review of 60,000 disaster victims, Norris et al., found children (defined as age < 16 years) to be the single highest risk group by age.[11] A recent meta-analysis of ninety-six studies on children following a disaster also reported significant effects of disasters on youth. It further found that the existing needs of the child, the context of the disaster itself, and the child's exposure to the disaster all influenced risk for development of PTS symptoms.[12] Etiology of the disaster was inconsequential, however specific aspects of the incident, namely the mass casualty death toll, the child's perceived threat to self, peri-traumatic symptoms at the time of the disaster, and proximity to the event (i.e., extent of exposure) all correlated positively with risk for development of PTS and PTSD. Finally, traumatic loss of a loved one was also shown to increase risk of PTSD in children following a disaster.

Distress Reactions

Reflective of the multiple trajectories pathway models, for people who are directly exposed to a disaster, acute posttraumatic reactions such as hypervigilance, difficulty sleeping, and feelings of anxiety, event-specific fears, anger or rage, and vulnerability are prominent and tend to emerge early. Recovery is rapid for most, but occurs more slowly or not at all for some. Performance problems may develop at work, school (children), home (family roles), or socially. In addition to those directly exposed to the disaster, many other individuals may be traumatized by the event either through close ties with directly affected persons, intrusive and high-intensity media coverage,[13] or cascading changes (e.g., business closures, destruction of local facilities, parks, or neighborhoods) evoked by the disaster. Days after the September 11, 2001 terrorist attacks in the United States, a national survey found that 44% of adult respondents had one or more PTS symptoms, and one-third of responding parents reported their children to have at least one PTS symptom.[14] Intense media coverage or use of social media is associated with widespread psychological distress.[13,15] Children's distress reactions are tied to many factors, including developmental status, media exposure,[16] and, particularly for younger ages (i.e., preschool), parental coping abilities.[17–19] These reactions may include regression from previously achieved developmental milestones and the emergence of problems with separation, nighttime behavior, or learning. Older children and adolescents may develop new schemas of danger in their worlds and engage in variable types of risk-taking or resilience behaviors.[17] There is no single pattern of symptoms that account for the observed variety in traumatic stress reactions and behaviors. As such, PTSD and PTS are inadequate explanatory mechanisms for the population-level impact of disasters, including terrorism events and other public health emergencies. For example, many observational disaster research studies describe nonspecific indicators of distress[20] or perceived stress,[21] demoralization,[22] changes in world view,[23] physical health concerns,[3,24–26] health-

care utilization, and changes in perceived safety and security.[27] Recent studies suggest that most distress responses, including illness, are transient, with many of the affected population showing a long-term trend toward resilience.[28,29] There are numerous individual, community, and incident specific features associated with expression of risk and resilience (see Chapter 6).

Changes in Behavior/Health Risk Behaviors

A significant change in behavior, including engaging in health-risk activities, manifests in a proportion of people exposed to disasters.[4,30] In the immediate aftermath of a disaster or mass violence, individuals forced to cope with overwhelming psychological stress may respond in adaptive ways, or they may instead make fear-based decisions, resulting in maladaptive behaviors. Individuals exposed to terrorism and other disasters have been found to increase their use of alcohol, tobacco, and other substances. This tendency is more pronounced in those with existing alcohol use or other psychiatric illnesses.[31,32] Evidence suggests that this transient increase in substance use does not consistently result in persisting substance use disorders.[33] Additionally, prior studies report a surge in demands for medical evaluation induced by a significantly sized outbreak of infectious disease, or complicated by fear evoked by a mysterious or potentially toxic exposure. This surge in help-seeking behavior may merely be a consequence of the stress involved in managing uncertainty; however, the increased requirements for medical evaluation can easily overwhelm local healthcare systems. This substantial extra demand can trigger additional requests for assistance if perceptions of the adequacy of the response weaken.[34–36] Other risk behaviors may emerge with significant impact on health, safety, and well-being. Such behaviors include: aggressive or careless driving without a seatbelt or under the influence of drugs and alcohol; poor lifestyle choices such as eliminating exercise, poor nutrition, and promiscuity; provocative or assaultive behavior; work absenteeism or decline in performance; and increased conflict or violence within the home.[37,38] Suicidal behavior, from ideation to completed suicides, shows an inconsistent pattern, with some studies suggesting a delayed increase several years after a disaster.[39] Based on the experience of Hurricane Katrina, the risk for behaviors such as suicide can be aggravated and sustained if services and social support remain compromised for an extended period.[10]

Psychiatric Disorders

Disasters have the potential to both create and aggravate mental illness. Major disasters have historically devastated social services and medical infrastructure, placing additional stress on those with chronic mental illness. The additional stress of destruction of homes or death or injury of family members can destabilize previously stable mental illness. New-onset PTSD and major depressive disorder are predictable sequelae of disaster events in up to 30% of the population.[10] Other disorders commonly observed following disasters include insomnia, panic disorder, and generalized anxiety disorder. Risk of persisting mental illness increases in vulnerable populations. Those most directly exposed to death or serious injury, injured survivors, first responders, and those with existing mental illness are at increased risk for developing persisting illness following disaster trauma. Cukor et. al., identified an increased incidence of PTSD in World Trade Center disaster workers with prior trauma history and prior psychiatric history.[40] Significant peritraumatic reactions, such as dissociation or panic attacks, may predict persisting illness following trauma.[41] Overall, studies indicate the prevalence of post-disaster PTSD tends to decline rapidly in the years after disaster,[29,42,43] accompanied by the emergence of a smaller subset of delayed-onset disorders.[44] In addition to psychiatric illnesses, data suggest that overall population health declines years after a significant terrorist event.[45] As noted above, children and adolescents are among those at highest risk of adverse mental health outcomes, including PTSD, depression, disruptive behavioral disorders, impairments in learning, and disaster-specific fears.[17,19,46] Consideration of the community-wide magnitude of mental and behavioral health needs enables emergency managers and mental health workers to appropriately plan and allocate resources for both adults and children who are at risk for developing acute and long-term disorders.

STATE OF THE ART

Adherence to Public Health Measures

The involvement of the public as a key strategic partner has only recently been described and needs additional attention.[47] There is a large gap between recommended protective actions for the public and the population's actual behavior. This highlights a critical need for emergency planning, including scenario development, to include behavioral aspects.[34,48,49] The degree to which adequate proportions of the population comply with or adhere to public health directives (e.g., quarantine, movement restrictions, mass prophylaxis, school closures, appropriate healthcare seeking) can directly determine whether public health and emergency medical response efforts are successful. Numerous individual, group, and population-level behavioral changes occur in to the face of all types of hazards. These, in turn, have profound impacts on the success of public health emergency response efforts, economic trends, and the resilience of entire nations.

Disaster "myths" are embedded within response plan assumptions across many levels of government.[50] One such myth is that the public will "panic" (albeit, not defined) in response to emergencies. Another is that the public will adhere to directions if messages are crafted in a certain content style. There has been significant concern and confusion about the term "mass panic," aggravated by a lack of basic science to inform policy. In reality, it is uncommon for individuals to act without an underlying concern for others (i.e., totally self-focused or violent). In fact, neighbors or coworkers are most likely to be the "first responders," willing and able to help constructively and collectively.[51] Although panic-like behavioral phenomena are rare, they can and do occur within certain situations. Incident-specific features that might lead to panic include:

■ Belief that there is little chance of escape (e.g., engulfing fire in a crowded room)
■ Perceived high risk from event (e.g., running from a collapsing building)
■ Available, but limited, treatment resources
■ No perceived effective response
■ Significant loss of faith in authorities

Another, more recent view suggests that the public need only be clearly "instructed" by credible sources and people will comply. This prevailing perspective discounts the impact of a plethora of mediating factors and "tipping points" such as culture, special

needs, or the impact of hazard-specific perceptions of risk, and ability to take protective actions.[30,49,52] Government planning scenarios describe events with massive effects. Involved planners must anticipate and mitigate predictable triggers of panic-like behavior at the population level. For example, evacuation orders in response to the Three Mile Island nuclear accident resulted in gridlock from actions in surrounding areas where people were not instructed to leave. Following the Scud attacks in Israel, approximately 70% of hospital emergency department visits were related to psychological factors, including 230 (27%) individuals who self-injected themselves with nerve agent antidote – even though they had not actually been exposed to a nerve agent, and 544 (44%) with an admitting diagnosis of "acute stress reaction."[53] Although the evidence base is limited, prior experience, personal beliefs, and actions or beliefs shared by loved ones or local thought leaders are believed to greatly influence obedience behaviors.[54] Additionally, the content of crisis and emergency risk communication, trust or faith in social institutions, and a host of event- or risk-specific contextual features influence population adherence to governmental directives for protective actions.[55]

Some governmental efforts directed at planning for pandemic influenza address the potential for societal disruption and dysfunction, with attention directed at business and government operational continuity. Collective reactions may involve behaviors to demand, hoard or otherwise procure (in competition with public health channels) antiviral prophylaxis or other perceived life-saving treatments. In a modeling study of community measures to contain the spread of pandemic influenza, prompt closure of schools (requiring the active collaboration of public health, school districts and, notably, parents) resulted in a case rate reduction of approximately 14%. This represented the largest single reduction in rates of influenza; this action led to a "decompression of the peak burden."[56] Together with other strategies such as social distancing, a 40% reduction in peak disease burden was achieved. Clearly, strategies to enhance behavioral compliance with community mitigation strategies may significantly reduce the impact of the next influenza pandemic.

Understanding the impact of population compliance or adherence to instruction in controlling the spread of infectious diseases is informed by studies of those quarantined due to the Severe Acute Respiratory Syndrome (SARS) outbreak. Approximately 30% of people placed in even a relatively brief quarantine (up to 10 days) had symptoms of PTSD and depression.[57] Key risk factors for developing these psychological symptoms included the duration of quarantine and knowing someone, or direct exposure to a person, with a diagnosis of SARS. Compliance with quarantine in Toronto was associated with:

■ Fear of loss of income while quarantined
■ Inconsistencies in local application of quarantine from area to area
■ Inconsistencies in monitoring of compliance
■ Logistical support (e.g., access to groceries, transportation of family members)

Approximately 57% of Canadians neither in quarantine nor directly exposed to SARS in Toronto had fears about acquiring the illness, but did not report clinical manifestations. Taken collectively, the findings suggest that social distancing strategies used to contain disease resulted in pronounced behavioral health effects in the form of fears, isolation, stigma, and boredom. All of these negatively impacted compliance with quarantine and may be considerations in other scenarios. A practical implication for public health emergency response planning is that public acceptance and adherence is greater in voluntary as opposed to mandatory strategies, and where income protections are provided for those in quarantine.[54] These data are from the United States however, and effective strategies may vary in different countries with other cultural norms.

Management of Demand Surge

Acute demand surges for medical evaluation have been observed in reaction to disasters, mass violence, and traumatic events. The nature of health complaints is related to: 1) toxic exposure, 2) specific symptoms related to the current health threat, 3) exacerbations of underlying chronic disease (in part due to lack of access to regular medications including psychiatric drugs), or 4) troubling and nonspecific symptoms that may be related to distress or fear. This last issue often leads to dissatisfying provider–patient relations.[46] The proper triage and management of this demand surge has critical bearing on the following: 1) systemic ability to provide timely life-saving interventions for those with acute medical/surgical needs; 2) prevention of chronic psychiatric disorders and life dysfunction; 3) organizational chaos and cascading inefficiencies; 4) healthcare staff stress and burnout; and 5) customer (community) satisfaction. Nonspecific health complaints associated with disasters and mass violence have been called "multiple unexplained physical symptoms" or "disaster somatization reactions."[3,19] People with multiple unexplained physical symptoms or disaster somatization reactions sometimes markedly outnumber direct medical casualties. Ratios as high as 1,700:1 have been reported.[3] Following a nonionizing radiation event in Brazil with limited exposure and only 4 deaths, approximately 130,000 unexposed individuals presented acutely to be screened for radiation illness and approximately 5,000 displayed symptoms of acute radiation sickness. Other collective demand surges may emerge in attempts to obtain protective equipment (masks, gloves) or medical prophylaxis (e.g., distribution of pharmaceutical stockpiles), especially if there is high mortality, limited availability of effective treatment, or little warning and a short window of opportunity for prophylaxis. This highlights a need to better understand, integrate, and prepare for the emotional, behavioral, and social factors involved in demand surge and adherence to public health measures.

Understanding Community and Social Support Factors

Empirical observations by various disaster experts describe time-phased patterns of community-based responses after sudden-impact disasters such as hurricanes, fires, floods, or earthquakes.[58] Although oversimplifying the underlying social tensions before a disaster strikes, this phased approach helps planners, response and recovery workers, and healthcare providers anticipate common collective reactions based on elapsed time since the event. Inadequate disaster planning, preparedness, and response or faulty warning systems exert lasting effects on the population's overall psychosocial and behavioral health. Early in the aftermath of disasters people are mobilized to work together, with collective action and prosocial behavior. Heroic acts and bridging social divides help with search and rescue and early recovery activities. A period of disillusionment then emerges as barriers to rebuilding and economic and social recovery exacerbate underlying social discord. Such barriers include inadequate insurance payouts, business relocations, loss of "neighborhood," and perceived or real disparities in the distribution of public goods and services. The process of reconstruction or coming to terms with multiple layers and cycles of loss and change may take years, marked by anniversary reactions and other reminders of the traumatic events. The time-phased model captures useful phases for disasters within prescribed time periods and geography, but not all communities progress in the same fashion; phases may be skipped, prolonged, or revisited given the prevailing sociopolitical context. This model may not be useful for other types of disaster events, such as those caused by human action or inaction, or those involving biological or radiologic hazards.

Kaniasty and Norris analyzed social relationships as a critical element in communities impacted by disasters.[59] These disaster researchers contend "disasters exert their adverse impact on emotional distress both directly and indirectly, through disruptions of social relationships and loss of perceived social support (p. 207)." Initial social support mobilization is followed by a prolonged resource drain and a mismatch of expectations with postdisaster realities. There is a subsequent disruption of social support networks and loss of social resources. The investigators further observed fragmented, polarized, mistrustful, and antagonistic community social patterns after "human-caused" (technological) disasters. They highlighted the conflicting and insufficient information surrounding such events. Psychosocial impacts are even more pronounced when human actions produce intentional harm. Terrorism occurring in the U.S. in 2001 resulted in: 1) anger, stigma, and violence, sometimes under the guise of patriotism; 2) a historical reorganization of federal assets for homeland security;[60] and 3) a multitude of alterations in travel, banking, and business practices. The next section addresses the continuum of screening, triage, and referral for mental health treatment.

Approaches for Screening, Triage, and Referral

Many responses to trauma and disasters are expected and time limited. However, secondary assessment by professional mental health professionals is necessary for patients with certain risk factors for more prolonged or maladaptive responses. Results of several meta-analytic studies of PTS symptoms and disorders suggest that, while several classes of variables predict outcome, the potential predictors that occur closest in time to the event are the most highly correlated with acute and chronic disorders. These factors include peri-traumatic reactions (reactions occurring in the immediate post-impact phase), the extent of direct event exposures (e.g., life threat), and levels of social support.[61,62]

Although distress is common and exposure-based risk factors convey better estimation of risk, the following symptoms, when present, require evaluation by a mental health professional:

- ■ Significant disorientation (dazed, memory loss, unable to give date/time or recall recent events)
- ■ Suicidal or homicidal thoughts, plans, actions
- ■ Domestic violence, child or elder abuse/neglect
- ■ Acute psychosis (hearing voices, seeing visions, delusional thinking)
- ■ Inability to care for self (not eating, bathing, changing clothing, or otherwise managing activities of daily living)

- Severe anxiety (constantly on edge, restless, obsessive fear of another disaster)
- Inappropriate use of alcohol or drugs
- Clinical symptoms of depression (pervasive feeling of hopelessness and despair, withdrawal from others)

Longitudinal Incident Management: Toward a Disaster Mental Health Concept of Operations

From a population health perspective, time-limited distress is common, while behavioral changes can influence health and safety outcomes over much longer periods of time.[1,4,17] A smaller, yet significant, proportion of the affected population is at risk for clinically relevant psychiatric disorders and dysfunction in various life roles. To meet diagnostic criteria, symptoms of psychiatric disorders and dysfunction must persist for varying durations of time. Evidence-informed risk factors for severe reactions and degrees of impairment have been combined to develop a novel disaster mental health triage system called "PsySTART." The following are the risk markers[63–65]:

- "Dose of exposure," based on individual experience (e.g., injury or illness, fearing death, and separation from family)
- Death of loved ones (traumatic loss)
- "Secondary stress," such as impact of, or worry about, long-term health risks, loss or difficulty with access to key services related to housing, employment, insurance, stigma, reduced social support, and not being able to engage in valued pre-event activities (e.g., school, faith-based, and sports)
- History of mental illness or traumatic stress
- Ensuing life stressors (job change, marriage/divorce, relocation, loss of loved ones, children moving away)

Relatively small increases in prevalence rates of psychiatric disorders within affected populations can result in a significant surge of absolute numbers of individuals requiring definitive mental healthcare. This increases long-term demands on an already overtaxed and dysfunctional public mental healthcare system. This longitudinal model of impact suggests the need to align the delivery of disaster mental health services along a more appropriate timeline of need. The prospect of a mass casualty event, with unparalleled behavioral health impacts over an extended period, would tax traditional behavioral health approaches and unleash population-level psychological morbidity for many years to come. To mitigate the community-based behavioral health effects of an emerging global health threat such as pandemic influenza,[5,49] crisis and emergency risk communication should be combined with other public health measures. These include: education and information campaigns; skill building for sustainable resilience; rapid behavioral health triage; and incident management. The PsySTART model has been operationalized in the U.S. state of Washington (Seattle and King County) into a Mass Casualty Disaster Mental Health Incident Management Concept of Operations (CONOPS) and at the national level in a version specific to the needs of children and families.[65]

The American Red Cross Disaster Mental Health System adopted a PsySTART model with elements of the disaster mental health response (Figure 9.1). These elements form a continuum of services from identifying mental health needs (individual triage and mental health surveillance, element 1) to providing clinical interventions appropriate to clients and workers in the disaster setting (promoting resilience and coping, and providing targeted interventions, elements 2 and 3, respectively).[66]

In the absence of rapid triage and coordination between systems, those with the greatest needs may not be located until clinical levels of distress and impairment have become entrenched.[5,59] As large numbers of children move across different systems of care, inconsistent approaches to the definition and assessment of "acute need" may further hamper critical provision of psychological assistance and definitive care. For example, following the 1994 Northridge earthquake in California, many children at high risk due to intense event exposures remained undetected until months and, sometimes years later.[67] These included children injured and/or trapped inside structures. Evidence from New York City also found that only 27% of children with severe or very severe posttraumatic reactions received any mental health care 4–5 months after the U.S. terrorist attacks of September 11, 2001.[68] Acute-phase triage and incident management are critical because there is meta-analytic evidence that certain types of acute-phase interventions, applied early after the traumatic event, might afford a unique window of opportunity to interrupt the trajectory of risk, disorder, and impairment for those at high risk who are already symptomatic.[69,70] There are also limited data for the efficacy of an evidence-based acute intervention for children.[71]

Disaster mental health workers and other responders should apply timely, evidence-based care to individuals at risk. Optimally, there should be a seamless system of triage, needs assessment, clinical care, and long-term surveillance for disaster-related mental and behavioral health[5] matching acute and long-term evidence-based interventions for the subset of persons that require them. One approach involves partnerships among many entities including public health authorities, public information officers, emergency medical services, primary and advanced medical and behavioral healthcare facilities, medical examiner and mortuary services, faith-based communities, schools, businesses, and nongovernmental relief organizations. These "disaster systems of care" are positioned to significantly mitigate adverse outcomes and move populations toward improved mental health preparedness, response, and recovery[19] if appropriate preparedness and coordination has begun pre-event.[5] This requires dynamic and continuous coordination, communication, and resource (goods and services) delivery targeted to those at highest risk of adverse outcomes. A paradigm shift in disaster recovery planning is needed to manage the continuum of risk and adverse outcomes over the extended course of recovery. The emerging incident management model PsySTART for disaster mental and behavioral health is composed of three major components. This enables a common operational picture and real-time situational awareness for participating entities and jurisdictions.[5] The components are: 1) community-based "disaster systems of care"; 2) a common system for incident-specific rapid triage; and 3) a mobile-optimized web application for real-time triage linkage across diverse disasters and systems of care. In the PsySTART model, each participating system of care uses the same triage risk factors, which are based on objective evidence-informed exposure risks (not symptoms) for adverse post-disaster mental health outcomes. In field applications, the triage information were found to positively predict PTSD and depression among exposed children in the Indian Ocean tsunami[63] and the Laguna Beach, California wildfires.[72] PsySTART was also used in the federal response to the American Samoa Catastrophic Earthquake and Tsunami[64] and by the American Red Cross in 18,000 triaged

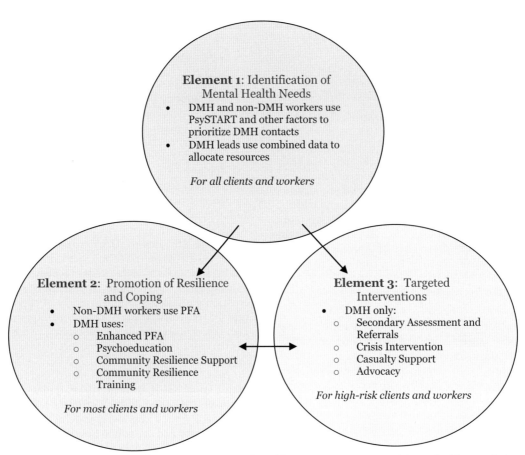

Figure 9.1. The American Red Cross Disaster Mental Health System PsySTART Model. Used with permission from the American Red Cross.

disaster mental health contacts within the first three weeks after Superstorm Sandy.[73] This rapid mental health triage system flexibly incorporates event- and hazard-specific exposure factors such as decontamination, mass prophylaxis or vaccination, shelter in place, quarantine, and/or evacuation in more complex public health emergencies. The triage data are used to inform incident managers of resources needs, match high-risk adults and children to available screening and clinical resources, and provide estimates of burden. In this way, stratified rapid triage data correspond to the concept of disaster medical triage and connect level of need with appropriate level of evidence-informed intervention throughout an extensive period of community recovery.[5,30]

Preventing and Managing Psychological Injuries

Estimates of Disaster-Related Behavioral Health Casualties

In catastrophic events, rates of disorder in the vulnerable child population are extremely high. For example, in a large earthquake in Armenia in villages with nearly 50% pediatric mortality, the surviving children exhibited comorbid psychiatric disorders approaching 90%.[74] Adults are also at risk. In a study published in 2006, 64% of the 5,383 survivors who were in collapsed and damaged buildings during the September 11, 2001, terrorist attacks reported new-onset depression, anxiety, or emotional problems after the event.[75] Estimates of mental health disorders within months post-event revealed an incidence of approximately 100,000 new cases in school-aged children alone.[76] As another example, approximately half of those

most severely impacted by Hurricane Katrina in the United States had clinically significant levels of distress, leading to federal funding requests for "specialized/enhanced services" beyond typically funded crisis counseling programs.

Psychological impact and resulting levels of psychiatric disorders vary as a function of event characteristics, such as terrorism (biological, explosive, chemical, nuclear, or radiation), which can cause mass casualties and societal disruption.[1] Weapons that involve sustained health risk over time can induce particularly pernicious mental and behavioral health morbidity on a population scale. Planning for mental and behavioral healthcare needs must anticipate demand surges during acute-phase distress and the behavioral reactive phase. This is followed by an extended trajectory of needs continuing and emerging throughout the duration of recovery, especially after mass casualty events.[5,30] A unique approach to modeling a continuum of population-level mental health effects was performed for an exercise in Southern California termed the "Shakeout Scenario." In this scenario, a mock 7.8 magnitude earthquake strikes eight counties and a population of 21 million in Southern California. Using the PsySTART triage model based on incident-specific features such as death, injuries, and home loss, investigators estimated the number of distressed, but resilient persons to be approximately 8 million, and a new incidence of mental health disorders requiring professional assessment and care for approximately 200,000 persons.[77]

In the United States, the approach of using incident-specific features to estimate the continuum of mental health impacts based on PsySTART triage has been further developed into a national model for planning for the mental health response at the local or state level focused on the needs of children and families.[65] In this model, PsySTART triage is used to estimate impacts for children and then convert them into estimates of service delivery requirements. This metric reveals a "gap" which then becomes the focus of local preparedness efforts. It is also used for triggers for "crisis standards of care," which are operationalized into a floating triage algorithm[78] such that those at higher risk are prioritized for care in a rational and ethical alignment of resources. In 2012, the National Children's Disaster Mental Health Concept of Operations model was extended to include a novel triage-driven disaster mental health incident action plan for coordination of response-phase operations.[65]

Basic Disaster Mental and Behavioral Health Intervention

Much of the initial on-site disaster mental health response focuses on 1) dampening anxiety and arousal by providing safety, comfort, and consolation; 2) assisting those directly affected to function effectively (reality testing and concrete problem solving); and 3) providing clear guidance and information to meet basic individual and family needs (e.g., safety, medical attention, water, food, shelter, clothing, essential medication, supervision of children and other dependents, and reunification of families).[58,79] An extensive literature review, including the findings of two consensus development workshops, defined key components of early intervention for survivors of mass violence.[79–81] Key components of this early intervention include: assess needs; monitor the recovery environment; and provide outreach, screening, triage, and treatment services for survivors. The goal is to foster resilience, effective coping, and recovery.[82]

Early Intervention

From a population health perspective, the following groups stand to benefit from early intervention: 1) persons with direct disaster exposure; 2) persons demonstrating extreme acute stress reactions, extreme cognitive impairment, or prolonged and intense distressful emotions; and 3) persons having a prolonged inability to sleep.[1,4,19,79,80] Risk factors in the early disaster aftermath include loss of personal and financial resources, loss of social support, displacement, loss of home, and proliferation of secondary stressors. Also at increased risk for psychiatric outcomes following disasters are persons living in poverty; low visibility groups (homeless, migrant, impaired mobility, institutionalized); and persons with trauma, psychiatric, or illicit substance use history. The goal is to deliver a compendium of pragmatically oriented interventions as soon as possible for individuals experiencing acute stress reactions or who appear unable to regain function.[80,82] At-risk persons should be connected early with evidence-based interventions such as acute prolonged exposure cognitive-behavioral therapy (CBT) for adults, or trauma-focused CBT for children. There is evidence of benefit to both adults and children when these interventions are provided early (~30 days). In addition to decreasing morbidity in high-risk and symptomatic individuals, overall cost of care is reduced.[69–71] In general, interventions are designed to aid adaptive coping and restore problem-solving capabilities as quickly as possible. During the 1980s and early 1990s, critical incident stress debriefing surged in popularity and was widely adopted by disaster response personnel. During this period, critical incident stress debriefing was applied indiscriminately to disaster survivors; however, the technique was found to have equivocal effects and in some appli-

Table 9.3. Core Actions of Psychological First Aid[84]

Contact and Engagement

Safety and Comfort

Stabilization

Information Gathering: Needs and Current Concerns

Practical Assistance

Connection with Social Supports

Information on Coping

Linkage with Collaborative Service

cations, to have the potential to cause harm. This led to consensus recommendations to abandon this approach.[80–82]

Psychological First Aid

Psychological First Aid (PFA) is currently the most widely accepted intervention for populations following disaster. PFA is based on a core set of principles: 1) promote a sense of safety; 2) promote calming; 3) promote self and community efficacy; 4) promote social connectedness; and 5) instill hope.[83] The core principles of PFA have been operationalized into a set of core actions summarized in Table 9.3.[84] PFA is intended to restore and maintain individual and community function, reduce health-risk behaviors in the population, and prevent or minimize psychiatric illness following disaster. While users must undergo a brief training, use of PFA does not require a licensed mental health provider or formal mental health training. National and international organizations endorse either PFA, or interventions based on its principles.[85,86] The American Red Cross also includes a version of PFA for use by all of its disaster relief workers as a key element of its disaster response strategy.[66] In Los Angeles and New York, "Listen, Protect and Connect," a "Neighbor-to-Neighbor" simplified version of PFA designed for family members (including parents with children), schools, the faith-based community, neighbors, and coworkers to use with each other, has been implemented as part of a broader all-hazard, community resilience initiative.[87,88] Both the American Red Cross and "Listen, Protect and Connect" PFA include PsySTART rapid mental health triage as a core competency. Application of this model to non–mental health medical reserve corps members revealed improvements in their awareness about the psychological impact of disasters and in their comfort level in providing PFA.[89]

Promoting a sense of safety and promoting calm (PFA principles 1 and 2) mitigate the physiological and psychological reactions to life-threatening events. Recommendations include reducing exposure to further trauma by discouraging repeated retelling or witnessing media coverage of events. Promoting calm facilitates the transition out of intense emotions experienced immediately after a disaster and reduces the development of avoidant behaviors. Techniques such as therapeutic grounding, breathing retraining, or deep-muscle relaxation are appropriate.[83] Promotion of self- and community efficacy (PFA principle 3) involves restoring a sense of control over outcomes in both individuals and communities. Individuals and communities can manage uncomfortable post-disaster emotions by successfully solving problems, facilitating the transition from "victim" to "survivor."[83] Promoting social connectedness (PFA principle 4) enhances and sustains attachments between affected individuals and within affected communities. This provides survivors with better access to the knowledge necessary for recovery and allows for collaborative problem solving. It also offers emotional understanding and acceptance.[83] Instilling hope (PFA principle 5) is the process of restoring a positive outlook against a worldview shattered by overwhelming events. At the individual level it requires countering catastrophic thoughts while promoting realistic benefit-finding.[83] Affected individuals gain the most when they identify a realistic outcome, even if the situation is worse than their pre-disaster circumstances. At the population level, psychological benefits accrue in a systemic manner by bridging together primary care and mental health systems (i.e., "disaster systems of care") and improving access to the broad range of human service needs (e.g., housing, employment, schooling, and child care). Such approaches, although not mental health interventions by mental health providers, may be the most effective for providing PFA and improving coping at the population level.

PFA research reports positive provider perceptions of efficacy,[90] but, at the time of this writing, controlled trials of interventions in a real-world disaster setting are lacking. Mental health practitioners cite providing safety and comfort, making contact and engaging with survivors, and providing practical assistance as the most beneficial interventions.[91]

World Health Organization Guidelines

In 2013, the World Health Organization (WHO) published guidelines for the management of acute stress in adults and children resulting from traumatic exposure.[92] Among the specific recommendations, WHO emphasizes basic principles such as communication and social support, and recommends that PFA be available to anyone recently exposed to a potentially traumatic event. For adults experiencing acute symptoms, WHO recommends acute trauma-focused CBT and avoidance of medications such as benzodiazepines and antidepressants in the first month. For those experiencing insomnia, relaxation and sleep hygiene techniques are advised for both children and adults. For children experiencing enuresis, WHO endorses non-punitive psychoeducation for children and parenting skills enhancement for adults. For those children and adults who develop PTSD more than a month after exposure, WHO advocates individual or group CBT with a trauma focus, eye movement desensitization and reprocessing, and stress management. Antidepressant medication should be considered for those who develop moderate to severe depression.

Behavioral Preparedness for Disaster Responders

Responder Resilience

Disaster responders represent a diverse collection of professional and volunteer workers that bring unique strengths and vulnerabilities. Resilience is common, even in the face of severe adversity.[93] Resilience is not a fixed attribute; instead, resilience is a process that evolves with changing disaster circumstances and experiences (see Chapter 6). Responders as a population may be self-selected for resilient psychological traits, but are vulnerable due to the duration and intensity of their exposure to disaster stressors. The disaster experience may be transformative, enabling more constructive ways of managing adversity and stress.[94] Responder resilience refers to the capacity of emergency personnel to rapidly adjust to the stresses of deployment, successfully respond to adverse cultural and situational challenges, and reintegrate into routine work in a healthy and adaptive fashion.

Responding optimally to mass trauma and mass casualty incidents requires an organizational culture that prioritizes both physical health and psychological well-being. Psychological preparedness improves disaster response for those who respond to incidents of all magnitudes. Enhancing resilience skills in the workforce will diminish the likelihood 1) that critical infrastructure personnel refuse to work during a disaster;[49] 2) that workers resign, requiring massive retraining and rehabilitation; and 3) of lost productivity, thus dampening the economy in a potentially cascading fashion. In the face of all-hazard planning and the need to maintain critical infrastructure and key resources, responder health, safety, and resilience must be integrated into organizational culture for public safety, health, and security. Emergency response personnel are often required to work extended hours in high-risk environments, where alertness and attention to detail are an absolute requirement for safe work practices. Hazards and risks to responders can be directly related to the reason for the deployment (e.g., infectious disease outbreak) or incidental to the deployment (endemic diseases, lack of medical facilities, and physical security hazards). Risk of psychological effects from exposure to these hazards must be assessed and appropriate control measures taken to reduce them.

Promoting Resiliency in Emergency Responders

Organizational policy can prevent or mitigate injuries and illnesses from environmental, occupational, and operational threats including psychological and traumatic stress. Disaster events in the United States over the last decade led to the creation of the National Planning Frameworks, promoting interagency coordination.[95] As part of this coordination, the National Institute for Occupational Safety and Health (NIOSH) created a recommended framework for health surveillance of emergency responders, to include psychological health.[96,97] This comprehensive plan identifies actions to be taken before, during, and after deployment. Before deployment, organizations should ensure personnel complete multiple requirements to foster a state of readiness. These include rostering and credentials verification to perform work assigned and health screening for both medical and behavioral fitness for deployment. In addition, pre-deployment training on safe work practices, use of appropriate personal protective equipment, and self-care (psychological, social, and behavioral), and other specialized training are needed to fulfill job-related responsibilities. During deployment, just-in-time briefings should be used to provide information about anticipated hazard exposure, including psychological and emotional hazards from response activities. Health monitoring of individual exposures and population surveillance for patterns of injury and disability, and communication of this information back to disaster workers are vital activities to maintain a resilient and ready workforce. At the conclusion of deployment, organizations should again screen responders for physical and psychological health during their outprocessing, and establish mechanisms to continue to follow workers post-event. This screening should include particular attention to those workers with the most hazardous exposures and those showing signs of adverse reactions at outprocessing.[98]

A similar approach, specifically designed and operationalized for disaster health workers, called "Anticipate, Plan and Deter" has been deployed in California for Los Angeles and Alameda County Emergency Medical Services providers as part of an overall evidence-based platform for community-wide disaster mental health for citizens and responders.[99] The "Anticipate, Plan and Deter" responder resilience model entails pre-event stress inoculation, basic PFA training for all responders using the "Listen, Protect and Connect" model and acute phase response, including responder self-triage and use of the novel, Internet-based intervention "Bounce Back Now."[100] Optimally, the individual responder has existing emergency plans and systems to manage concerns about the safety and welfare of loved ones. This avoids fractured attention on the job and decreases the likelihood of accidents, improper work practices, and poor decision making. Training and maintenance programs can be instituted for peer support, team building, and crisis leadership, with skill building to improve stress, anger, and grief management.[48]

RECOMMENDATIONS FOR FURTHER RESEARCH

Despite continued progress, several areas of disaster behavioral health require research attention. Quantifying the psychological, behavioral, and social consequences and management strategies for disasters and mass violence is critical. Continued efforts are needed to:

- further refine and test emerging rapid mental and behavioral health triage and assessment tools for population-based, facility-based, and clinical contact surveys, including assessment for mass casualty settings;
- integrate psychological and behavioral elements into population-based surveillance systems; and
- leverage modifiable risk factors to help design effective prevention and intervention programs.

Despite the knowledge that early intervention mitigates risk for extended traumatic stress syndromes, the field has been hampered by misapplication and misrepresentation of early intervention strategies. Prospective research to quantify the outcomes of PFA is essentially nonexistent and urgently needed.[88] Applied research is needed to test promising early interventions for those directly impacted by disasters and mass violence. Such studies should include:

- quantitative study and comparison among the various models of Psychological First Aid;
- further development and validation of acute phase, evidence-based interventions, including interventions for young children; and
- determination of optimal timing of strategies to implement interventions.

Research is also needed to evaluate the effectiveness of efforts to increase preparedness and adherence to behavioral aspects of public health emergency response strategies. These include compliance with incident-specific disaster response strategies, such as sheltering and evacuation. More research and program evaluation efforts are needed to understand the key ingredients of resilience of professionals performing emergency response, disaster recovery, and remediation work. Finally, research is needed to evaluate the value of organizational approaches such as Emergency Responder Health Monitoring and Surveillance

and "Anticipate, Plan and Deter" in enhancing resilience among disaster response professionals.

Conclusion

Planning for the behavioral and mental health needs of disaster-exposed individuals, families, communities, and responders is an essential public health and medical activity. Without it, available resources, monitoring efforts, and healthcare services may be overwhelmed. Although "panic" is ill-defined, anxiety, fear for one's children, and the absence of feeling safe can create personal and community confusion and disillusionment with leadership that has substantial real world consequences. Planning must address the range and trajectory of responses from distress to persisting illness, as well as numerous behavioral impacts (e.g., changes in travel, reverse quarantine). Communities receiving disaster victims must anticipate the need for additional mental health services, both for displaced persons with existing psychiatric conditions and for those with new disorders. Disaster mental health Concepts of Operations (such as the National Children's Disaster Mental Health CONOPS project) include triage, protection from secondary stressors, restoration of families and social networks, and a continuum of care from PFA acute and long-term evidence-based interventions. Novel Internet-based interventions are the primary cutting-edge, population-level interventions for codifying the behavioral and mental health consequences of disaster. Public messaging and leadership presence are critical to convey and implement the principles of mental health interventions. At appropriate times, grief counseling – an important task in advancing communities to recovery – becomes the focus of all community leaders. First responders represent a high-risk group and benefit from planned behavioral health support and surveillance to promote their resilience and readiness. Addressing knowledge gaps in disaster mental health, applying scientifically supported interventions, and tracking the trajectory of unresolved needs are important objectives.

REFERENCES

1. Fullerton CS, Ursano RJ, Norwood AE, Holloway HH. Trauma, terrorism, and disaster. In: Ursano RJ, Fullerton CS, Norwood AE, eds. *Terrorism and Disaster: Individual and Community Mental Health Interventions*. Cambridge, Cambridge University Press, 2003; 1–20. [see p. 1]
2. Norris FH, Elrod CL. Psychosocial consequences of disaster: a review of past research. In: Norris FH, Galea S, Friedman MJ, Watson PJ, eds. *Methods of Disaster Mental Health Research*. New York, Guildford Press, 2006; 20–42.
3. Engel CC. Somatization and multiple idiopathic physical symptoms: relationship to traumatic events and posttraumatic stress disorder. In: Schnurr PP, Green BL, eds. *Trauma and Health: Physical Consequences of Exposure to Extreme Stress*. Washington, DC, American Psychological Association, 2003; 191–216.
4. Butler AS, Panzer AM, Goldfrank LR, and Institute of Medicine Committee on Responding to the Psychological Consequences of Terrorism: Board of Neuroscience and Behavioral Health. *Preparing for the Psychological Consequences of Terrorism: A Public Health Approach*. Washington, DC, National Academies Press, 2003.
5. Schreiber M. Learning from 9/11: Toward a national model for children and families in mass casualty terrorism. In: Danieli Y, Dingman R, eds. *On the Ground after September 11: Mental*

Health Responses and Practical Knowledge Gained. New York, Haworth Press, 2005; 605–609.

6. Neria Y, Nandi A, Galea S. Post-traumatic stress disorder following disasters: a systematic review. *Psychological Medicine* 2008; 38(4): 467–480.

7. Pietrzak RH, Van Ness PH, Fried TR, Galea S, Norris FH. Trajectories of posttraumatic stress symptomatology in older persons affected by a large-magnitude disaster. *J Psychiatr Res* 2013; 47(4): 520–526.

8. Hobfoll SE, Mancini AD, Hall BJ, Canetti D, Bonanno GA. The limits of resilience: distress following chronic political violence among Palestinians. *Soc Sci Med* 2011; 72(8): 1400–1408.

9. McLaughlin KA, Berglund P, Gruber MJ, Kessler RC, Sampson NA, Zaslavsky AM. Recovery from PTSD following Hurricane Katrina. *Depress Anxiety* 2011; 28(6): 439–446.

10. Kessler RC, Galea S, Gruber MJ, Sampson NA, Ursano RJ, Wessely S. Trends in mental illness and suicidality after Hurricane Katrina. *Mol Psychiatry* 2008; 13(4): 374–384.

11. Norris FH, Friedman MJ, Watson PJ, Byrne CM, Diaz E, Kaniasty K. 60000 disaster victims speak: Part I. An empirical review of the empirical literature, 1981–2001. *Psychiatry* 2002; 65(3): 207–239.

12. Furr JM, Comer JS, Edmunds JM, Kendall PC. Disasters and youth: a meta-analytic examination of posttraumatic stress. *J Consult Clin Psychol* 2010; 78(6): 765–780.

13. Otto MW, Henin A, Hirshfeld-Becker DR, Pollack MH, Biederman J, Rosenbaum JF. Posttraumatic stress disorder symptoms following media exposure to tragic events: impact of 9/11 on children at risk for anxiety disorders. *Journal of Anxiety Disorders* 2007; 21(7): 888–902.

14. Schuster MA, Stein BD, Jaycox LH, et al. A national survey of stress reactions after the September 11, 2001, terrorist attacks. *N Engl J Med* 2001; 345(20): 1507–1512.

15. Goodwin R, Palgi Y, Hamama-Raz Y, Ben-Ezra M. In the eye of the storm or the bullseye of the media: Social media use during Hurricane Sandy as a predictor of post-traumatic stress. *J Psychiatr Res* 2013; 47(8): 1099–1100.

16. Pfefferbaum B, Seale TW, Brandt EN, Jr, Pfefferbaum RL, Doughty DE, Rainwater SM. Media exposure in children one hundred miles from a terrorist bombing. *Ann Clin Psychiatry* 2003; 15(1): 1–8.

17. Pynoos RS, Steinberg AM, Wraith R. A developmental model of child traumatic stress. In: Cicchetti D, Cohen DJ, eds. *Manual of Developmental Psychopathology.* New York, John Wiley and Sons, 1995; 72–83.

18. Laor N, Wolmer L, Cohen DJ. Mothers' functioning and children's symptoms 5 years after a SCUD missile attack. *Am J Psychiatry* 2001; 158(7): 1020–1026.

19. Gurwitch RH, Kees M, Becker SM, Schreiber M, Pfefferbaum B, Diamond D. When disaster strikes: responding to the needs of children. *Prehosp Disaster Med* 2004; 19(1): 21–28. Review.

20. Carr V, Lewin T, Webster R, Kenardy J, Hazell, P, Carter G. Psychosocial sequelae of the 1989 Newcastle earthquake: exposure and morbidity profiles during the first 2 years post-disaster. *Psychol Med* 1997; 27: 167–178.

21. Thompson M, Norris F, Hanacek B. Age differences in the psychological consequences of Hurricane Hugo. *Psychol Aging* 1993; 8: 606–616.

22. Dohrenwend B. Psychological implications of nuclear accidents: The Three Mile Island. *Bull NY Acad Med* 1983; 59: 1060–1076.

23. Smith B. Coping as a predictor of outcomes following the 1993 Midwest flood. *J Soc Behav Personality* 1996; 11: 225–239.

24. Baum A, Gatchel R, Schaeffer M. Emotional, behavioral and physiological effects at Three Mile Island. *J Consult Clin Psychol* 1983; 51: 565–572.

25. Krakow B, Haynes PL, Warner TD, et al. Nightmares, insomnia, and sleep-disordered breathing in fire evacuees seeking treatment for posttraumatic sleep disturbance. *J Trauma Stress* 2004; 17(3): 257–268.

26. Clayer J, Bookless-Pratz C, Harris R. Some health consequences of a natural disaster. *Med J Aust* 1985; 43: 182–184.

27. Grieger TA, Fullerton CS, Ursano RJ. Posttraumatic stress disorder, depression, and perception of safety 13 months after September 11. *Psychiatric Serv* 2004; 55(9): 1061–1063.

28. Zhang G, North CS, Narayana P, Kim Y, Thielman S, Pfefferbaum B. The course of postdisaster psychiatric disorders in directly exposed civilians after the US Embassy bombing in Nairobi, Kenya: a follow-up study. *Soc Psychiatry Psychiatr Epidemiol* 2013; 48(2): 195–203.

29. Pietrzak RH, Tray M, Galea S, et al. Resilience in the face of disaster: prevalence and longitudinal course of mental disorders following hurricane Ike. *PLoS One* 2012; 7(6): e38964.

30. Reissman DB, Spencer S, Tanielian TL, Stein BD. Integrating behavioral aspects into community preparedness and response systems. In: Danieli Y, Brom D, Sills J, eds. *The Trauma of Terrorism: Sharing Knowledge and Shared Care, an International Handbook.* New York, Haworth Maltreatment and Trauma Press, 2005. Co-published simultaneously in *J Aggress Maltreat Trauma* 2005; 10(3/4): 707–720.

31. Galea S, Ahern J, Resnick H, et al. Psychological sequelae of the September 11 terrorist attacks in New York City. *N Engl J Med* 2002; 346(13): 982–987.

32. Pfefferbaum B, Doughty DE. Increased alcohol use in a treatment sample of Oklahoma City bombing victims. *Psychiatry* 2001; 64(4): 296–303.

33. North CS, et al. Postdisaster course of alcohol use disorders in systematically studied survivors of 10 disasters. *Arch Gen Psychiatry* 2011; 68(2): 173–180.

34. Engel CC, Locke SL, Reissman DB, et al. Terrorism, trauma, and mass casualty triage: how might we solve the latest mind-body problem? *J Biosecur Bioterrorism* 2007; 5(2): 155–163.

35. Barbera JA, McIntyre AG. Hospital emergency preparedness and response. In: *Jane's Mass Casualty Handbook.* Surrey, Jane's Information Group, Ltd, 2003.

36. Auf der Heide E. The importance of evidence-based disaster planning. *Ann Emerg Med* 2006; 47: 34–49.

37. Harville EW, et al. Experience of Hurricane Katrina and reported intimate partner violence. *J Interpers Violence* 2011; 26(4): 833–845.

38. Schumacher JA, et al. Intimate partner violence and Hurricane Katrina: predictors and associated mental health outcomes. *Violence Vict* 2010; 25(5): 588–603.

39. Kolves K, Kolves KE, DeLeo D. Natural disasters and suicidal behaviours: a systematic literature review. *J Affect Disord* 2013; 146(1): 1–14.

40. Cukor JC, Wyka K, Jayasinghe N, et al. (2011). Prevalence and predictors of posttraumatic stress symptoms in utility workers deployed to the World Trade Center following the attacks of September 11, 2001. *Depress Anxiety* 2011; 28(3): 210–217.

41. Wood CM, Salguero JM, Cano-Vindel A, Galea S. Perievent panic attacks and panic disorder after mass trauma: a 12-month longitudinal study. *J Trauma Stress* 2013; 26(3): 338–344.

42. van der Velden PG, Wong A, Boshuizen HC, Grievink L. Persistent mental health disturbances during the 10 years after a disaster: four-wave longitudinal comparative study. *Psychiatry Clin Neurosci* 2013: 67(2): 110–118.

43. Cukor J, Wyka K, Mello B, et al. The longitudinal course of PTSD among disaster workers deployed to the World Trade Center following the attacks of September 11th. *J Trauma Stress* 2011; 24(5): 506–514.

44. Meewisse ML, Olff M, Kleber R, Kitchiner NJ, Gersons BPR. The course of mental health disorders after a disaster: predictors and comorbidity. *J Trauma Stress* 2011; 24(4): 405–413.

45. Neria Y, Wickramaratne P, Olfson M, et al. Mental and physical health consequences of the September 11, 2001 (9/11) attacks in primary care: a longitudinal study. *J Trauma Stress* 2013; 26(1): 45–55.

46. North CS, Nixon SJ, Shariat S, et al. Psychiatric disorders among survivors of the Oklahoma City bombing. *JAMA* 1999; 282(8): 755–762.

47. Glass TA, Schoch-Spana M. Bioterrorism and the people: how to vaccinate a city against panic. *Clin Infect Dis* 2002; 34(2): 217–223. Review.

48. Kaji A, Koenig KL, Bey T. Surge capacity for healthcare systems: A conceptual framework. *Acad Emerg Med* 2006; 13(11): 1157–1159.

49. Reissman DB, Watson PJ, Klomp RW, Tanielian TL, Prior SD. Pandemic influenza preparedness: adaptive responses to an evolving challenge. *J Homeland Secur Emerg Manage* June 2006; 3(2): 1–27.

50. Wenger DE, Dykes JD, Sebok TD, Neff JL. It's a matter of myths: An empirical examination of individual insight into disaster response. *Mass Emerg* 1975; 1: 33–46.

51. Mawson AR. Understanding mass panic and other collective responses to threat and disaster. *Psychiatry* 2005; 68(2): 95–113.

52. Covello VT. Best practices in public health risk and crisis communication. *J Health Commun* 2003; 8(Suppl. 1): 5–8, discussion 148–151.

53. Bleich A, Gelkopf M, Soloman Z. Exposure to terrorism, stress-related mental health symptoms, and coping behaviors among a nationally representative sample in Israel. *JAMA* 2003; 290(5): 612–620.

54. DiGiovanni C, Jr, Reynolds B, Harwell R, Stonecipher EB, Burkle FM, Jr. Community reaction to bioterrorism: prospective study of simulated outbreak. *Emerg Infect Dis* 2003; 9(6): 708–712.

55. Lerner JS, Gonzalez RM, Small DA, Fischhoff B. Effects of fear and anger on perceived risks of terrorism: a national field experiment. *Psychol Sci* 2003; 14(2): 144–150.

56. Germann T, Kadau K, Longini I, Macken C. Mitigation strategies for pandemic influenza in the United States. *Proc Natl Acad Sci USA* 2006; 11: 5935–5940.

57. Hawryluck L, Gold WL, Robinson S, Pogorski S, Galea S, Styra R. SARS control and psychological effects of quarantine, Toronto, Canada. *Emerg Infect Dis* 2004; 10(7): 1206–1212.

58. DeWolfe DJ. *Training Manual for Mental Health and Human Service Workers in Major Disasters.* 2nd ed. DHHS Publication No. ADM 90–538. Washington, DC: Substance Abuse and Mental Health Services Administration, 2000.

59. Kaniasty K, Norris FH. Social support in the aftermath of disasters, catastrophes, and acts of terrorism: altruistic, overwhelmed, uncertain, antagonistic, and patriotic communities. In: Ursano RJ, Norwood AE, Fullerton CS, eds. *Bioterrorism: Psychological and Public Health Interventions.* New York, Cambridge University Press, 2004; 200–231.

60. Koenig KL. Homeland Security and Public Health: role of the Department of Veterans Affairs, the U.S. Department of Homeland Security, and implications for the public health community. *Prehosp Disast Med* 2003; 19(4): 327–333.

61. Ozer EJ, Best SR, Lipsey TL, Weiss DS. Predictors of posttraumatic stress disorder and symptoms in adults: a meta-analysis. *Psychol Bull* 2003; 129(1): 52–73.

62. Brewin CR, Andrews B, Valentine JD. Meta-analysis of risk factors for posttraumatic stress disorder in trauma-exposed adults. *J Consult Clin Psychol* 2000; 68(5): 748–766.

63. Thienkrua W, Cardozo BL, Chakkraband ML, et al. Symptoms of posttraumatic stress disorder and depression among children in tsunami-affected areas in southern Thailand. *JAMA* 2006; 296(5): 549–559.

64. King ME, Schreiber MD, Formanski SE, Fleming S, Bayleyegn TM, Lemusu SS. A Brief Report of Surveillance of Traumatic Experiences and Exposures After the Earthquake-Tsunami in American Samoa, 2009. *Disaster Med Public Health Prep* 2012; 7(3): 327–331.

65. Schreiber M, Pfefferbaum B, Sayegh L. The Way Forward: the National Children's Disaster Mental Health Concept of Operations. *Disaster Med Public Health Prep* 2012; 6: 174–181.

66. American Red Cross Disaster Mental Health Handbook. *American Red Cross Disaster Services.* Washington, DC, American Red Cross, 2012.

67. Asarnow J, Glynn S, Pynoos RS, et al. When the earth stops shaking: earthquake sequelae among children diagnosed for pre-earthquake psychopathology. *J Am Acad Child Adolesc Psychiatry* 1999; 38(8): 1016–1023.

68. Fairbrother G, Stuber J, Galea S, Pfefferbaum B, Flieschman AR. Unmet need for counseling services by children in New York City after the September 11th attacks on the World Trade Center: implications for pediatricians. *Pediatrics* 2004; 113(5): 1267–1274.

69. Roberts NP, Kitchiner NJ, Kenardy J, Bisson JI. Systematic review and meta-analysis of multiple-session early interventions following traumatic events. *Am J Psychiatry* 2009; 166(3): 293–301.

70. Shalev AY, Ankri Y, Israeli-Shalev Y, Peleg T, Adessky R, Freedman S. Prevention of posttraumatic stress disorder by early treatment: results from the Jerusalem Trauma Outreach And Prevention study. *Arch Gen Psychiatry* 2012; 69(2): 166–176.

71. Berkowitz SJ, Stover CS, Marans SR. The Child and Family Traumatic Stress Intervention: secondary prevention for youth at risk of developing PTSD. *J Child Psychol Psychiatry* 2011; 52(6): 676–85.

72. Pynoos R, Schreiber M. The impact of Laguna Beach wildfire on children and parents. Presentation at the 42nd Annual Meeting of the American Academy of Child and Adolescent Psychiatry. New Orleans, LA, 1995.

73. Schreiber M, Yin R, Omaish M, Broderick J. Snapshot from Super Storm Sandy: American Red Cross Mental Health Risk Surveillance in New York. (Submitted).

74. Goenjian AK, Pynoos RS, Steinberg AM, et al. Psychiatric comorbidity in children after the 1988 earthquake in Armenia. *J Am Acad Child Adolesc Psychiatry* 1995; 34: 1174–1184.

75. Brackbill RM, Thorpe LE, DiGrande L, et al. Surveillance for World Trade Center disaster health effects among survivors of collapsed and damaged buildings. *MMWR* 2006; 55(SS-2): 1–11.

76. Hoven CW, Duarte CS, Lucas CP, et al. Psychopathology among New York City public school children 6 months after September 11. *Arch Gen Psychiatry* 2005; 62(5): 545–552.

77. Schreiber M. In Jones LM, Bernknopf R, Cox D, Goltz J, Hudnut K, Mileti D, Perry S, Ponti D, Porter K, Reichle M, Seligson H, Shoaf K, Treiman J, Wein A. The ShakeOut Scenario: U.S. Geological Survey Open-File Report 2008–1150. Prepared in cooperation with the California Geological Survey, U.S. Geological Survey Open File Report 2008-1150, California Geological Survey Preliminary Report 25 version 1.0. http://pubs.usgs.gov/of/2008/1150 (Accessed August 10, 2015).

78. Institute of Medicine. *Crisis Standards of Care: A Systems Framework for Catastrophic Disaster Response.* Washington, DC, The National Academies Press, 2012.

79. Gerrity ET, Flynn BW. Mental health consequences of disasters. In: EK Noji, ed. *The Public Health Consequences of Disasters.* New York, Oxford University Press, 1997; 101–121.

80. National Institute of Mental Health. *Mental health and mass violence: evidence-based early psychological intervention for victims/survivors of mass violence; A workshop to reach consensus on best practices (NIH Publication No. 02–5138).* Rockville, MD, National Institute of Mental Health, 2002.

81. Orner RJ, Kent AT, Pfefferbaum BJ, Raphael B, Watson PJ. The context of providing immediate postevent intervention. In: Ritchie EC, Watson PJ, Friedman MJ, eds. *Interventions Following Mass Violence and Disasters.* New York, Guilford Press, 2006; 121–133.

82. Watson PJ, Friedman MJ, Gibson LE, Ruzek JI, Norris FH, Ritchie EC. Early intervention for trauma-related problems. In: Ursano RJ, Norwood JE, eds. *Trauma and Disaster Responses and Management.* Washington, DC, American Psychiatric Publishing, 2003; 118–129.

83. Hobfoll SE, Watson P, Bell CC, et al. Five essential elements of immediate and mid-term mass trauma intervention: empirical evidence. *Psychiatry* 2007; 70(4): 283–315, discussion 316–269.

84. National Center for PTSD, National Center for Child Traumatic Stress. *Psychological First Aid: Operations Guide.* 2nd ed. Los Angeles, National Center for Child Traumatic Stress, 2006.

85. Department of Health and Human Services (HHS). Fact Sheet: Disaster Behavioral Health. 2012. http://www.phe.gov/Preparedness/planning/abc/Documents/disaster-behvioral-health.pdf (Accessed July 18, 2013).

86. Interagency Standing Committee (IASC). IASC Guidelines on Mental Health and Psychosocial Support in Emergency Settings (English). June 2007. http://www.who.int/hac/network/interagency/news/mental_health_guidelines/en (Accessed August 10, 2015).

87. Schreiber M, Gurwitch RH. Listen, protect, and connect model. Sponsored by the U.S. Department of Homeland Security. http://www.ready.gov/sites/default/files/documents/files/LPC_Booklet.pdf (Accessed July 30, 2013).

88. Plough A, Fielding JE, Chandra A, et al. Building community disaster resilience: perspectives from a large urban county department of public health. *Am J Public Health* 2013; 103(7): 1190–1197.

89. Chandra A, Kim G, Pieters H, Tang J, McCreary M, Schreiber M, Wells, K. Implementing Psychological First Aid Training for Medical Reserve Corps Volunteers. (in press).

90. Allen B. Perceptions of psychological first aid among providers responding to Hurricanes Gustav and Ike. *J Trauma Stress* 2010: 23(4): 509–513.

91. Fox JH, Burkle FM, Jr, Bass J, Pia FA, Epstein JL, Markenson D. The effectiveness of psychological first aid as a disaster intervention tool: research analysis of peer-reviewed literature from 1990–2010. *Disaster Med Public Health Prep* 2012: 6(3): 247–252.

92. World Health Organization. *Guidelines for the management of conditions specifically related to stress.* Geneva, WHO, 2013.

93. Foa EB, Meadows EA. Psychosocial treatments for posttraumatic stress disorder: a critical review. *Ann Rev Psychol* 1997–1938.

94. Reissman DB, Klomp RW, Kent AT, Pfefferbaum B. Exploring psychological resilience in the face of terrorism. *Psychiatr Ann* 2004; 34(8): 627–632. Review.

95. Federal Emergency Management Agency (FEMA). National Planning Frameworks Overview. 2013. http://www.fema.gov/national-planning-frameworks (Accessed July 30, 2013).

96. Centers for Disease Control and Prevention, NIOSH. Emergency Responder Health Monitoring And Surveillance (ERHMS). 2013. http://www.cdc.gov/niosh/topics/erhms (Accessed July 30, 2013).

97. National Response Team (NRT). Emergency Responder Health Monitoring And Surveillance (ERHMS). 2012. http://nrt.sraprod.com/ERHMS (Accessed July 30, 2013).

98. Reissman DB, Kowalski-Trakofler KM, Katz CL. Public health practice and disaster resilience: a framework integrating resilience as a worker protection strategy. In: Southwick SM, Litz BT, Charney D, Friedman MJ, eds. *Resilience and Mental Health.* Cambridge, Cambridge University Press, 2011.

99. Schreiber M, Shields S, Hanfling D. Behavioral Health Issues. In: Farmer CJ, Wax R, Baldisseri MR, eds. *Preparing Your ICU for Disaster Response.* Mount Prospect, IL: Society for Critical Care Medicine, 2012.

100. Amstadter AB, Broman-Fulks J, Zinzow H, Ruggiero KJ, Cercone J. Internet-based interventions for traumatic stress-related mental health problems: a review and suggestion for future research. *Clin Psychol Rev* 2009; 29(5): 410–420.

10

POPULATIONS WITH FUNCTIONAL OR ACCESS NEEDS

Brenda D. Phillips and Laura M. Stough

OVERVIEW

Some populations experience a greater vulnerability to injury, death, and/or property loss.[1] Populations particularly vulnerable to disaster may include people with disabilities, senior citizens, pregnant women, infants and children, children in school and day care settings, single parents, women, low-income families, rural and isolated populations, and racial and ethnic minorities. Examples of unique interventions that may support these individuals are targeted warnings (in various languages and literacy levels), evacuation and transportation assistance, priority rescue, medical treatment, accessible sheltering, and assistance with rebuilding. However, it is equally true that vulnerable populations also have access to resources and can demonstrate considerable resilience. The twin notions of vulnerability and resilience must be considered in order to construct a holistic picture of how individuals are affected by and respond to disaster. This chapter examines vulnerability and then discusses strategies for medical providers to support populations at risk, including fostering resilience and autonomy.

The terms "functional and access needs," as well as "vulnerable populations" and "populations at risk," have been applied to people who may need additional assistance in emergencies and disasters. Functional and access needs are often identified by the acronym C-MIST[2] which emphasizes the communication, medical conditions, independence, supervision, and transportation supports needed during disasters. However, this term does not encompass broader concerns that emerge in disaster settings, such as women's access to safe and sanitary facilities or to reproductive care.

To capture the most complete information about those potentially at risk, this chapter takes a broad-brush approach to vulnerability. Emergency managers can select relevant information by performing a needs assessment to determine which populations are of concern within a given jurisdiction, organization, or community. In some locations, it may be that the most vulnerable population includes senior citizens. In another location, it could be recent immigrants. This analysis allows emergency managers to understand the complexities of people's lives and circumstances. Gender, for example, can greatly increase

risk in some contexts including exposure to interpersonal violence and human trafficking.[3–5] Pregnancy may further complicate personal abilities to escape danger or can, itself, endanger both mother and fetus. Low-income households may lack the resources to afford protective action. If such households include seniors on fixed incomes, additional complications may include transportation assistance and nutritional or medical support. Because the prevalence of disability increases with age, seniors in these fixed-income households could also have mobility or cognitive disorders and require additional support.

The use of broad, inclusive terminology can also generate misclassification. People do not necessarily have functional or access needs simply because they fall into a given population. For example, a person with a disability can also live independently in the community, hold a job, and prepare adequately for a disaster event. Women, for example, may experience differential vulnerability that is tied to lower income levels or their status in society rather than simply because they are female. In addition, belonging to a vulnerable population is a dynamic process. People move into and out of poverty, experience temporary or adult-onset disabilities, and move from rural to urban areas. Local demographics can shift and change. For example, in the United States, the Census Bureau has found that minority populations will become the majority within 30 years and that important demographic shifts are occurring within various populations.

In addition, disasters generate new risks. For example, individuals with asthma may manage their condition well on a daily basis and not need special medical or functional supports. However, in a high-rise fire and evacuation, such as occurred on September 11, 2001 in the United States, an asthmatic condition may cause significant challenges. Consider the situation of a Muslim diabetic seeking refuge in a public shelter after Hurricane Katrina. With the only food available being ham and white bread, the evacuee would face a choice of either violating religious customs or going hungry. Physical deterioration could result without proper nutrition. Similar problems result when disasters disrupt access to medications, medical care, or other health-related services. Losing access to dialysis, cancer treatment, or to social services such as home healthcare can lead to life-threatening circumstances. When a disaster strikes at the

Demographic Shifts Changing the United States (U.S. Census Bureau, 2012, Verbatim)

Hispanics

■ California had the largest Hispanic population of any state on July 1, 2012 (14.5 million), as well as the largest numeric increase within the Hispanic population since July 1, 2011 (232,000). New Mexico had the highest percentage of Hispanics at 47.0%.

■ Los Angeles County had the largest Hispanic population of any county (4.8 million) in 2012 and the largest numeric increase since 2011 (55,000). Starr County – on the Mexican border in Texas – had the highest share of Hispanics (95.6%).

Blacks

■ New York had the largest Black or African-American population of any state or equivalent as of July 1, 2012 (3.7 million); Texas had the largest numeric increase since 2011 (87,000). The District of Columbia had the highest percentage of blacks (51.6%), followed by Mississippi (38.0%).

■ Cook, Illinois (Chicago) had the largest Black or African-American population of any county in 2012 (1.3 million), and Harris, Texas (Houston) had the largest numeric increase since 2011 (20,000). Holmes, Mississippi, was the county with the highest percentage of blacks or African-Americans in the nation (83.1%).

Asians

■ California had both the largest Asian population of any state (6.0 million) in July 2012 and the largest numeric increase of Asians since July 1, 2011 (136,000). Hawaii is the nation's only majority-Asian state, with people of this group comprising 56.9% of the total population.

■ Los Angeles had the largest Asian population of any county (1.6 million) in 2012 and the largest numeric increase (25,000) since 2011. At 60.9%, Honolulu County had the highest percentage of Asians in the nation.

American Indians and Alaska Natives

■ California had the largest American Indian and Alaska Native population of any state in 2012 (1,057,000) and the largest numeric increase since 2011 (13,000). Alaska had the highest percentage (19.5%).

■ Los Angeles County had the largest American Indian and Alaska Native population of any county in 2012 (232,000), and Maricopa, Arizona had the largest numeric increase (4,000) since 2011. Shannon County, South Dakota – on the Nebraska border and located entirely within the Pine Ridge Indian Reservation – had the highest percentage (93.5%).

Native Hawaiians and Other Pacific Islanders

■ Hawaii had the largest population of Native Hawaiians and other Pacific Islanders of any state (364,000) in 2012. California had the largest numeric increase since 2011 (6,000). Hawaii had the highest percentage (26.2%).

■ Honolulu had the largest population of Native Hawaiians and other Pacific Islanders of any county (238,000) in 2012. Los Angeles County had the largest numeric increase since 2011 (1,100). Hawaii County had the highest percentage (34.3%).

Non-Hispanic White Alone

■ California had the largest non-Hispanic white alone population of any state in 2012 (15.0 million). Texas had the largest numeric increase in this population group since 2011 (78,000). Maine had the highest percentage of the non-Hispanic white population (94.1%).

■ Los Angeles had the largest non-Hispanic white alone population of any county (2.7 million) in 2012. Maricopa County, Arizona, had the largest numeric increase in this population since 2011 (24,000). Leslie County, Kentucky, comprised the highest percentage (98.4%) of non-Hispanic whites.

Minorities

■ Five states or equivalents were "majority-minority" in 2012: Hawaii (77.2% minority), the District of Columbia (64.5%), California (60.6%), New Mexico (60.2%) and Texas (55.5%).

■ Maverick, Texas, had the largest share (96.8%) of its population in minority groups of any county, followed by Webb, Texas (96.4%) and Starr, Texas (96.1%).

Age Groups

■ Two groups of children saw their population decline between 2011 and 2012: those under age 5, from 20.1 million to just under 20 million, and high school-age children (ages 14–17), from 16.9 million to 16.7 million. In contrast, the number of elementary school-age children (ages 5–13) rose from 36.9 million to just over 37 million.

■ Nationally, the 65-and-older population grew 4.3% between 2011 and 2012, to 43.1 million, or 13.7% of the total population.

■ Florida had the highest percentage of its total population age 65 and older in 2012 (18.2%), followed by Maine (17.0%) and West Virginia (16.8%). Alaska had the lowest percentage (8.5%), followed by Utah (9.5%) and Texas (10.9%).

■ Among the nation's counties, Sumter, Florida, had the highest proportion of its population age 65 and older (49.3%), followed by Charlotte, Florida (36.0%) and La Paz, Arizona (34.9%). Chattahoochee, Georgia (3.6%) was at the other extreme.

■ The 85-and-older population grew by about 3% from 2011 to 2012, to almost 5.9 million. The number of centenarians grew to almost 62,000.

■ Utah had the highest percentage of its total population under age 5 at 9.0%, and Vermont (4.9%) the lowest. Among counties, the respective extremes were claimed by Shannon, South Dakota (11.6%) and Sumter, Florida (2.2%).

■ In 2012, there were 197 million working-age adults (ages 18–64), representing 61.6% of the total population, an increase of about 736,000 people from 2011.

■ New Hampshire experienced the largest increase in median age among states from 2011 to 2012, from 41.6 to 42.0. Among counties, the greatest upsurge belonged to Lake, South Dakota, whose median age rose 1.4 years to 42.8.

Gender

■ There were only ten states where males made up the majority of the population on July 1, 2012. Alaska had the highest percentage of men at 52.1%, followed by Wyoming (51.1%), North Dakota (50.8%), Nevada (50.4%) and Hawaii (50.4%).

■ The District of Columbia had the highest percentage of females of any state or equivalent at 52.3%, followed by Rhode Island (51.6%), Maryland (51.6%), Delaware (51.5%) and Massachusetts (51.5%).

end of the month, those reliant on social security or disability-related incomes may have to make hard choices between staying at home and being able to purchase needed medications and food or using their funds to evacuate. People can also sustain major, permanently disabling injuries in disasters. After the 2013 tornado outbreak in Oklahoma, a number of victims survived but experienced permanent injuries. Some experienced impalement while others required rehabilitation for mobility impairments. The same was true for the U.S. terrorist attacks on September 11, 2001, particularly for victims sustaining burn injuries. Other terrorist-generated injuries included first responders who faced a lifetime of respiratory conditions.[6] Such conditions meant job loss, health expenses, and even death.

Finally, many conditions remain invisible. It may be difficult to identify "people with hidden disabilities, people with serious mental illness, people with intellectual and cognitive disabilities, and people with a variety of visual, hearing, mobility, emotional and mental disabilities and activity limitations."[7]

Recent disasters in the United States have revealed the challenges for populations at risk. In 2005, Hurricane Katrina claimed over 1,300 lives and 50% of those who died in Louisiana were older than the age of 75.[8] A disproportionate percentage of these individuals were racial and ethnic minorities.[9] Horrific images linger of people who were exposed to heat exhaustion, lack of food or water, power losses, poor evacuation planning, transportation failures, and unavailable medications. These problems were not unexpected.[10] Hurricane Katrina revealed deeply embedded problems within the practice of emergency management, particularly the understanding of how to reduce risks for vulnerable populations. While improvements occurred, Superstorm Sandy that struck hard at New Jersey and New York in 2011 demonstrated the challenges of people living in high-rise buildings particularly seniors, women in labor, and people with disabilities and medical conditions. Loss of power to such facilities necessitated difficult evacuations and assistance for those with mobility impairments. Another example of the challenges with management of vulnerable populations is illustrated by deaths in elderly patients who were evacuated after the Fukushima accident in Japan in March 2011. People died not because of radiation exposure, but due to lack of attention to basic health and medical needs.[11]

Lack of preparedness or insight into what people truly require to survive can also produce new unmet needs. To illustrate, consider the following examples.

Recognizing and addressing a group's increased vulnerability to disasters can lead to significant reductions in risk.

- In Victoria, Australia, firefighters sought a reduction in the number of fires and subsequent burns among senior citizens. Recognizing a pattern in the fires, five firefighters learned Turkish, formed a partnership with the local Migrant Resource Center and Islamic schools, and provided information for Turkish senior citizens and the Turkish media. Fewer fires and injuries resulted.[12]
- As Hurricane Gustav neared the U.S. coast in 2008, the U.S. Postal Service released social security and other entitlement checks early to enable evacuation among low-income households and senior citizens across the Gulf Coast. This was especially important for people waiting on checks to refill medications.
- When a shortage of influenza vaccinations occurred in the United States, public health officials prioritized who should

Populations at Risk

- A low-income hotel burns to the ground and the local Red Cross opens a shelter. A woman, 8 months pregnant, arrives but no one realizes that she is pregnant because she has chronic malnutrition.
- A massive tornado nears an elementary school. Adults present must make a choice about how to save lives without any underground safe room to use.
- A teenager who is deaf and home alone does not get warning information about an impending hurricane and must wade through water contaminated with feces, chemicals, and petroleum to get to a safe location. Over the coming weeks, many that waded out through the water develop serious, persistent skin and wound infections.
- A paraplegic is airlifted to a safe shelter in another state but his wheelchair, which cost nearly $30,000, remains behind. When he arrives at the general population shelter where he could have been independent, he is sent to a medical needs facility that is already crowded and understaffed. His medical records are destroyed by the disaster and his medications have been lost during the storm.
- A Vietnamese-American family arrives at a shelter that is serving unfamiliar foods. The children, already upset by the events, refuse to eat. When they do begin to eat, several experience intestinal distress.
- Immigrant workers help to clean dust and debris from homes and offices damaged by a terrorist attack. They are not given protective clothing or equipment. They do not speak much English. Over the next year, they develop a persistent condition that comes to be known as the "World Trade Center cough."
- An individual becomes separated from his service animal. In addition to the individual's service-related needs, he experiences emotional trauma from the potential loss of a social relationship with the animal.
- Insufficient numbers of accessible, Americans with Disabilities Act–compliant Federal Emergency Management Agency (FEMA) trailers are available after a major disaster. A local disability organization sues FEMA to establish a hotline and case management procedures to move people out of hotels and shelters and closer to their healthcare and social service providers.

receive immunizations first including the elderly, people living in congregate facilities, children, and people with chronic health conditions and their partners.

- When a wildfire broke out in September 2011 in the urban-wildlife interface of Bastrop County, Texas, over 5,000 rural residents living across more than 34,000 acres of pine forest were successfully evacuated by local first responders and volunteer firefighters. Rural neighbors were instrumental in notifying each other about the spreading fire and posting evacuation notices via social media as the fire continued to burn for a full month.

▪ An EF5 tornado destroyed elementary schools in Moore, Oklahoma, in 2013. Teachers and staff moved rapidly to protect children at risk. The powerful storm collapsed school walls, injured adults, and claimed the lives of seven children at Plaza Towers Elementary. A similarly destructive storm in Joplin, Missouri, the previous year resulted in FEMA funds to rebuild Irving Elementary School. Two EF5-rated safe rooms will shelter 550 adults and children.

Understanding risk through an examination of the local population serves as a starting point for identifying who might need additional assistance during a disaster. The remainder of the chapter examines how the medical community can actively participate in reducing risk and empowering those who might be affected by disaster.

STATE OF THE ART

A Social Vulnerability Perspective

Social vulnerability theory examines how economic, social, cultural, and political conditions foster disproportionate impacts resulting from disaster.[13,14] Vulnerability theory suggests risk develops as a consequence of failure to collectively address social conditions such as affordable housing and healthcare, prejudice, or interpersonal violence. For example, low-income housing structures usually sustain more serious damage following a disaster, leading to more injuries and deaths. Most vulnerability theorists suggest that altering these conditions requires broad systemic change. Since this change tends to occur slowly, vulnerability theorists advocate for empowering those at risk to participate in their own risk reduction. The insights, experiences, and recommendations of those at risk can be used as the basis to increase the rate of positive change. People at risk should be encouraged to seek solutions in partnership with emergency management and disaster medicine professionals.

In an effort to understand and reduce vulnerability, researchers have focused attention on specific demographic groups.[1] The following sections examine a number of the populations historically considered vulnerable.

Age

Age clearly relates to vulnerability. In disasters, the very young and older persons tend to bear disproportionate impacts. This section first examines the elderly, and then addresses children.

The Elderly

Terms for people who are aging include "seniors," "elderly," and "aged" – all terms that reference age. On the other hand, descriptions such as "frail elderly" or "fragile elderly" are used to denote a health, mobility, or health impairment in addition to advanced age. There is sizable overlap between the category of "seniors" and those with disabilities. As people age, there are natural declines in physical and cognitive ability. Approximately 80% of all U.S. seniors have one chronic condition and 50% have at least two.[15] These additive consequences of normal aging and disease combine with other social factors to make older adults particularly vulnerable to disasters.[16,17]

Two general divergent points of view have emerged regarding seniors. The first is that disasters disproportionately deprive the elderly of social and economic resources relative to their younger counterparts, causing them to sustain greater losses.[18] The second perspective is that they demonstrate psychological resilience gained through prior life experiences.[19,20] Evidence supports both perspectives to varying degrees. Hurricane Katrina, for example, resulted in a significantly higher rate of mortality among the elderly, with almost 50% of the fatalities being older than 75.[21] The relative deprivation hypothesis emphasizes the lack of resources for transportation, evacuation, and recovery available to this population. It is also true, however, that the elderly can and will respond when they receive information from trusted sources. For example, warning and evacuation compliance is high when seniors receive messages and have the abilities to act.[22] Furthermore, researchers have found that "the significance of the event becomes relative to a lifetime of circumstances experienced by the individual,"[23] suggesting that the elderly consider the relativeness of their loss. The inoculation hypothesis thus holds some merit.

The recovery period also presents challenges for the elderly. Seniors appear to be reluctant to access relief and other recovery programs.[24] This may result from fear of institutionalization in residential care if it is assumed they cannot meet their own needs. Resistance may also result from pride, self-reliance, and an unwillingness to accept charity. Burdensome paperwork that challenges and fatigues some seniors has also been blamed. Elders who are socially isolated are at particular risk for not accessing disaster resources.[25] In addition, the digital divide (Internet, text messaging, pagers used for warning messages, and online aid applications) may increasingly segregate elders. In the United States, the online FEMA application times out for security purposes, a problem for those with slower responses or who are unfamiliar with the Internet, cannot type, and have eyesight or cognitive impairments. Outreach teams, with community relations personnel, have reduced these problems. Vulnerability theory suggests building capacity and establishing partnerships to increase resilience in the face of disaster. These solutions were embraced by the Baylor College of Medicine and the American Medical Association. Together, they produced a set of recommendations for assisting elderly disaster victims:[26]

▪ Involve gerontologists, geriatricians, geriatric nurse practitioners, and others in emergency operations planning.

▪ Conduct pre-disaster planning with local social services, public health services, and other key organizations, especially aging organizations, senior centers, and faith-based organizations.

▪ Offer specific training to those who interact with elderly disaster victims, including transportation personnel, shelter staff, and case managers.

▪ Protect seniors from abuse and fraud. Adult Protective Services can be a partner in this activity.

▪ Plan carefully for the frail elderly, the homebound, and those in nursing homes.

Children

Children are more vulnerable to disasters by virtue of their reliance on caregivers for assistance with protective behaviors, their greater physical vulnerability to impact, and the added risk that is created when they are separated from their families. Children's reactions to disasters vary by age. Younger children usually react well to being physically comforted after a frightening experience and by a quick return to a normal routine. Reactions of older children often depend on how the adults around them behave.[19,20,26] Because children lack a referential framework for behavior, they tend to look to trusted parents, childcare workers, or significant others for behavioral cues. If parents react poorly, children are likely to respond similarly. Children home alone at the time of a disaster can experience greater challenges than those accompanied by adults, unless they have been trained for the anticipated hazard.[5] Children with disabilities may require additional assistance in order to evacuate and may have their health compromised if needed supports are not quickly reconstituted following an event.[27]

Behavioral responses typical for younger children that usually diminish with time include being upset over losses (blankets, toys, and pets), aggression, fear of sleeping alone, nightmares, fear of similar events (wind, rain, and storms), crying, enuresis, thumb sucking, and psychosomatic responses, which can include headaches, gastrointestinal distress, and even fevers.[19,20,26] Younger children may not understand why they cannot go home after their houses have been destroyed. Older children and adolescents may have more difficulty coping with the disaster given their capacity to grasp the meaning of the event. Psychological responses are also affected by direct exposure to the disaster impact, particularly personal injuries or harm to others around them, loss of loved ones, and the ways in which parents or guardians handle the event.

Extreme events, such as the attacks on September 11, 2001, or the Newtown school shootings in December 2012 in the United States, are likely to create a more complex range of problems that include school disruption, displacement, and separation from family during evacuation or living in temporary locations. In addition, there can be loss of medical records, medications, and familiar healthcare providers.[28,29] Children in congregate settings such as schools or day care centers may experience more severe trauma due to exposure effects.[19,20] For example, the shootings in Newtown occurred in a populated setting where children personally witnessed the violence. Assessment of some of the psychological effects of a disaster progresses over time, as a diagnosable condition such as post-traumatic stress disorder (PTSD) is not confirmed until 6 months or more after the inciting event.

Recommendations typically include reintegrating children into school, reestablishing routines, and providing mental health support at shelters and other temporary locations.[30] By reentering children into their school routine, a "ripple effect" is believed to occur that moves through families, households, and into the broader community to accelerate recovery.[30]

Support from trusted adults, including parents, teachers, childcare workers, disaster volunteers, and shelter workers, is key to helping children.[31] Calm and competent adults serve not only as positive role models for children unfamiliar with disasters but also help them to feel safer. When an EF5 tornado destroyed Moore, Oklahoma, on May 20, 2013, two elementary schools and a day care facility were in its path (Figure 10.1). Teachers and day care employees moved the children to the safest locations they could find, laid their bodies over the children to protect them, and sang and prayed with them as the winds increased. Although seven people, including six children, died at the Plaza Towers Elementary School, hundreds survived.

Psychological treatment, school programs, and volunteer work are recommended as intervention strategies for older children. Mental health providers may need to offer a range of services to children. After the bombing in Oklahoma City, for example, trauma counselors created "Project Heartland," which trained teachers and others to recognize and manage signs of long-term trauma. More than 60,000 students received interventions.[32] Services to teachers and students included counseling and training for stressor identification and coping mechanisms. Researchers examining the attacks of September 11, 2001, found that approximately 10% of all children in New York City received counseling.[33] Schools served as the most common setting (44%) followed by professional treatment (36%) or spiritual care/other (20%). Children were more likely to receive counseling if parents also experienced traumatic reactions.[20] Structured environments, play and therapeutic activities, and

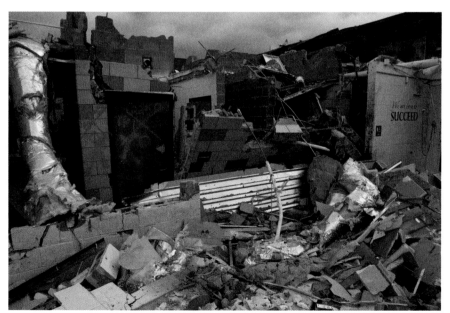

Figure 10.1. The Plaza Towers Elementary School in Moore, Oklahoma Shows Tornado Damage That Resulted in Loss of the Lives of Seven Children. Photo by Andrea Booher, FEMA.

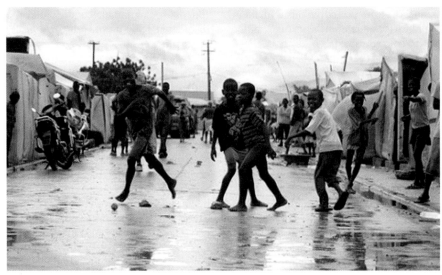

Figure 10.2. Haitian Children Still Living in Temporary Tent Cities 3 Years after the Massive Earthquake that Claimed over 200,000 Lives. Photo by USAID.

effective role modeling appear valuable in helping children cope with disasters.

Health concerns for children depend on the type of event. Concern about spread of severe illnesses is common in refugee camps and mass evacuation locations, particularly in developing nations. In the Philippines, for example, mothers express worry over the potential for epidemics in unsanitary evacuation centers, where "children are exposed to . . . lack of food and clean drinking water, unsanitary shelter, closed schools and poor health services. . . . [T]hey face hunger and epidemics, perhaps even death."[34] In Hurricane Katrina in the United States, concerns arose over toxic contamination of schools, homes, and playgrounds.[30] The dust from the World Trade Center prompted apprehension about the long-term effects of exposure on all populations including pregnant women, newborns, and people with existing respiratory conditions.[6] The 2010 earthquake in Haiti caused families with children to linger in tent encampments for years (Figure 10.2). At the end of the first year, an outbreak of cholera presumed to be imported by responders claimed over 1,000 lives.[34] Anxiety lingers over the potential radiological exposure of children from the 2011 Tōhoku Earthquake and Tsunami.

Disasters also impact the education of children, who spend much of their developmental period at school. Disasters often destroy school buildings, especially in locations where engineering standards and building codes are not enforced or where buildings have suboptimal structural integrity.[27] When instruction is disrupted, children lose not only educational skills but also opportunities for social growth through interaction with their classmates. Schools serve as community gathering places and a place for supervised and safe care for children. They are often the largest single employer in rural areas, so their loss also disrupts the lives of parents and other adults. For families of children with disabilities, teachers can be valuable supports. For example, after Hurricane Ike in the United States, teachers on Galveston Island provided information on the storm, contacted families during the evacuation from the island, and supported students with disabilities in returning to their instructional routines after the storm.[37]

Recovery can prove especially challenging for families with children. FEMA disbursements in the United States, for example, have been criticized for their "one size fits all" approach in which a single mother with several children receives the same funds as an adult man without any children.[30] Living in cramped, temporary housing is difficult for any family. For larger families or for single parents, the situation may create additional stress. Families in disaster trailer parks often lack access to amenities such as playgrounds or after school programs. Recovery among those displaced by disaster means rebounding from losing teachers, neighbors, and nearby kin, as well as learning new schools, making new friends, finding new places to play, and understanding new cultural contexts.[29] Nevertheless, as is the case with the elderly, children can prove to be resilient. Children developed coping skills after Hurricane Katrina while living in shelters and formed strong bonds with shelter workers.[31] Children in the Philippines are considered "indispensable helpers . . . . [T]he potential of elder children could . . . be developed and maximized through community daycare and other collective activities."[34]

Income

Income level affects all aspects of disasters. Lower-income households may be unable to afford emergency preparedness kits. Single mothers, of whom approximately 33% fall below the poverty line in the United States, may have trouble buying mitigation measures such as hurricane shutters to protect the contents of their homes.[38] Those living on fixed incomes have particular difficulties. For example, Hurricane Katrina occurred at the end of August, which meant that social security and disability checks had not yet arrived. Many people were waiting for checks to refill prescriptions. Furthermore, they could not afford gasoline or food to evacuate. Buses that should have been dispatched to evacuate people needing transportation did not arrive. Reluctant to leave a familiar environment and family on which they could depend, a disproportionate number of low-income households remained behind. Extensive damage occurred to many low-income homes located in floodplain areas. For hundreds of families, this meant the loss of a home that had been in their possession for generations and could no longer be replaced due to financial hardship. In a post-disaster context, low-income households face hard choices between recovery and ongoing needs. To survive, they may pawn remaining possessions, relocate to more affordable areas away from familiar healthcare providers, move in with other families, skip meals or eat poorly, delay healthcare, cut medications in half, or not follow through on expensive medical regimens.

Low-income homeowners often face serious rebuilding challenges. Because many are underinsured or cannot afford hazard-specific insurance, they cannot rebuild without assistance. In 2013, maximum federal loans in the United States totaled $31,900. For most low-income households, choices must be made about rebuilding or relocation. Without assistance from volunteer disaster organizations, many cannot return home. Most will enter into a local case management process and await help from faith-based and civic organizations. In addition, the low cost of mobile homes makes it more likely that people living in poverty will rent or buy this type of housing. As a result, when tornados or hurricanes occur, those that are poor are more likely to be harmed when they take cover within their homes.[39]

Renters encounter similar challenges. After the 1994 Northridge earthquake in California, renters faced extensive displacement due to the time required to rebuild multi-family dwellings and the state of the regional economy.[40] After Hurricane Katrina, public housing in New Orleans was condemned; the process of rebuilding takes years. Rural-urban divides also produce challenging circumstances. Farm families affected by drought, floods, wildfire, or severe storms may lose their livelihoods or be forced to adapt by taking on new economic roles.

Social networks are especially important to low-income families, particularly in neighborhoods where families have lived for some time. Their neighborhood and familial relationships help sustain them. When disasters force relocation, those social resources diminish and life circumstances become even more difficult. This appears to be particularly true for minority communities, especially those with long-held ties to the land, such as Native American households in the United States.

Race and Ethnicity

Although studies find similarities both within and across racial and ethnic groups, important differences exist.[41] Studies of rapid-onset events illustrating these differences have implications for warning those at risk. For example, in a study of a massive tornado that damaged a neighborhood near Birmingham, Alabama, 80% of white residents heard the warning from television compared with only 67% of African-Americans.[42] While the influence of social media may change results, historical data show that Hispanics are more likely to get warning information from the radio or from social networks. They are also the largest minority group living in the United States. New Mexico and Texas will likely become Hispanic majority states by the end of the decade.[43]

Ethnic groups may experience linguistic barriers, such as when warning messages are not distributed in relevant languages.[44] Translation must also be done correctly. As a tornado approached the small town of Saragosa, Texas, in 1987, efforts failed to translate warnings into Spanish correctly. Rather than learning of an approaching risk, the few listening to the radio heard "news" about a tornado.[45] Those watching cable television originating far from their location received no warning. Twenty-nine people died and dozens sustained injuries. After any major disaster, companies may hire low-income workers who are recent immigrants and may not receive appropriate training and protective equipment.

Ethnicity has also been associated with income discrimination and segregation patterns that impede abilities to secure adequate housing in areas safer from local hazards.[46] Lower-income housing tends to fare poorly in areas of high risk. For example, affordable housing is more likely to be located in floodplains and closer to hazardous materials sites. Manufactured housing can fail in the lowest level of tornadoes. In earthquake prone regions, such housing is more likely to lack seismic retrofitting.[22,46] This exposure increases the likelihood of injuries, property loss, and psychological trauma. Minority populations are also less likely to have adequate homeowners' or rental insurance, as well as being less likely to access aid from federal programs, despite experiencing greater effects from disaster.[47]

Gender

The bulk of published vulnerability research concentrates on gender issues. Much of this research has resulted from a concerted effort by investigators who are linked through the Gender and Disaster Network (www.gdnonline.org). Researchers have documented differential results in survival rates as well as in the methods women and men use to respond to and recover from disasters. The 2004 Indian Ocean Tsunami, for example, resulted in approximately 300,000 deaths and displaced at least 1.6 million people across thirteen nations. More than 80% of the fatalities were women and children.[48] This differential impact was due to that, in many nations, women waited on the shore with their children for fishermen to arrive with the daily catch, which they would then clean and sell at market.

As a leading nongovernmental organization reported after the tsunami, "disasters, however 'natural', are profoundly discriminatory. Wherever they hit, pre-existing structures and social conditions determine which members of the community will be less affected, while others pay a higher price. Among the differences that determine how people are affected by such disasters is that of gender."[48] The same is true across the Caribbean, where sex differences result in health risks that increase in disasters. These include sexual abuse and violence as well as "malnutrition, anemia, maternal morbidity and mortality, complications in pregnancy, sexually transmitted diseases, and mental and psychological conditions that cause loss of healthy life and wellbeing among women."[49]

In some contexts, men differentially experience disaster impact. In 1998, Hurricane Mitch generated higher fatalities among Honduran men than women. Gender socialization patterns produced the differential mortality rate, as men felt compelled to remain behind and try to protect livestock and property from storm damage. Hurricane Katrina statistics also demonstrate risks, especially in elderly African-American men, who experienced a disproportionate death rate.[3] Post disaster, gender roles can affect continued exposure to hazards, such as after the Chernobyl incident wherein the majority of soldiers and civilians who helped clean up were men.[50] Gender bias more likely to unequally affect women is evident in other settings. In a shelter environment, for example, women's needs may include maternity support, privacy for hygienic and religious reasons, nutritional supplements, childcare, trauma counseling, and an environment free from violence. Gender differentiation also occurs when warnings are issued, as women appear more likely to disseminate the warning among others, to respond positively when instructions are given, and to gather the family for evacuation.[51-53] Small businesses and home-based enterprises, which are more likely to be owned by women, tend to sustain higher losses.[54-55] Women also tend to be the family member most likely to access recovery assistance and to link older family members to aid.[56]

Response and recovery organizations have been criticized for their failure to include women.[56] In Central America, increasing women's capacities and roles in disaster preparation and aid is strongly recommended. "Women's societal role is multifaceted... [T]his is extremely important in the health field where women are often employed and, at the same time, are generally responsible for family health and well-being."[57] In the Caribbean, sex-based social capital brings local knowledge, social networks, and critical links to others at risk. Vulnerability can be mitigated by leveraging women's resources through increased representation, mobilization, education and training, recognition of their needs, and direct involvement in emergency management activities.[49]

Disability

While disaster-related fatalities in the United States have decreased overall, people with disabilities are disproportionately affected.[58] Historically, individuals with disabilities have been neglected in disaster planning. People with disabilities are less likely to have emergency plans in place, and communities are less likely to have plans that meet the needs of those with disabilities.[59] One study reported that only 23% of emergency managers have received training on the needs of individuals with disabilities during evacuation.[60] According to a January 2004 Harris Poll commissioned by the National Organization on Disability (NOD),[61] 66% of people with disabilities did not know who to contact about emergency plans in their communities; 61% of persons with disabilities had not made plans for quickly and safely evacuating their homes; and among those people with disabilities employed full- or part-time, 32% said that no plans had been made to safely evacuate from their workplaces. After Hurricane Katrina, NOD commissioned a task force to examine issues associated with shelter needs for people with disabilities. Known as the SNAKE Report (Special Needs Assessment of Katrina Evacuees), NOD identified several concerns including those related to intake, inappropriate transfers to "special needs" rather than to general population shelters, loss of durable and related medical equipment, inaccessible shelters, and lack of accommodation for sign language and service animals.[7]

Challenges for persons with disabilities exist across all disaster stages including evacuation, sheltering and reentry into the affected community. In a survey conducted in hurricane-prone states 3 years after Hurricane Katrina, 14% of residents in high-risk hurricane areas lived in households in which a person with a chronic illness or disability would require assistance in order to evacuate. Of this group, 43% did not have accessible help, and 17% were not prepared at all for a major hurricane in the next 6 months compared to 9% of households without persons with chronic illnesses or disabilities. They were also less likely to have a 3-week supply of the necessary prescription drugs (39% versus 30%) or to have a first-aid kit (30% versus 20%).[61]

A study of Hurricane Katrina survivors sheltered just after the disaster found that 38% of the individuals interviewed reported that they did not evacuate because they were physically unable to leave or that they were caring for someone physically unable

to evacuate.[62] According to the Committee on Disaster Research in the Social Sciences: Future Challenges and Opportunities and National Research Council, "Major failures occurred in the provision of evacuation assistance by both governmental and nongovernmental organizations to citizens with limited capacity to evacuate on their own prior to Hurricane Katrina."[63] In addition to the evacuation of persons with disabilities, evacuation plans need to make allowances for transporting and reuniting special equipment, mobility devices, and assistance animals with users.

People with disabilities report difficulties during and after disasters when shelters, shelter restrooms and showers, and other temporary housing are not accessible to them.[64] People with disabilities may be physically unable to enter or clean up their properties, while the assistive services that they require may be lost along with other community infrastructure. In addition, many voluntary organizations may be unfamiliar with effective ways to assist individuals with disabilities or unaware of organizations that provide disability-related assistance.

Workplaces are of similar concern. After the terrorist attacks in 2001, NOD launched an Emergency Preparedness Initiative. Initially, it conducted surveys asking people with disabilities whether evacuation plans were in place at work. In 2001, 50% of the respondents said "yes" followed by a decline to 34% in 2005.[65] Subsequently, NOD crafted a booklet of recommendations for emergency managers and posted downloadable disability-specific preparedness brochures on its website (see Resources list).

From a sociopolitical perspective, many of these problems emanate from a societal failure to structure emergency and disaster procedures with accessibility in mind. U.S. Presidential Executive Order 13347 established that emergency preparedness measures must consider people with disabilities and "increase the rate of participation of people with disabilities in emergency planning... preparedness, response and recovery drills and exercises."[66] Since then, a number of new policies have emerged to address gaps in planning and preparedness (for example, the U.S. Department of Justice shelter protocol and the U.S. National Response Framework).[67] The emphasis is on building capacity among those with disabilities and including people with disabilities, disability organizations, and knowledgeable advocates in the planning process. Better practices encourage independence and provide for equal access, trained staff, appropriate food and equipment support, proper communications, and assistance in keeping people together with their families and service animals.[68]

Partnerships are the key. Disaster resilience can be increased and new insights generated by strengthening individuals through personal preparedness planning and by including disability organizations in the planning process. Risk reduction requires active participation and involvement by those individuals believed to be vulnerable.

Language and Literacy

Language influences the ability to obtain information of all kinds, from warnings on rapid-onset events to the problems of lingering heat waves. Within most nations, this kind of information is usually disseminated primarily in the most commonly spoken language. Efforts to translate information must be made to reach the full population, from people with low levels of literacy to people fluent only in sign language. In addition, weather information language may not be user-friendly to the public as it is intended primarily for other users such as emergency managers. Few weather stations include live interpretation. Scrolls and weather maps may be difficult to understand and meteorologists sometimes obscure closed-captioning. For people who became deaf in later life, following the scroll or understanding sign language may be next to impossible.

Low literacy levels can inhibit proper understanding and response to public health messages. Written materials present obvious problems. The manner in which communication occurs can also impact response. The National Hurricane Center in the United States strives to provide understandable information to the public as well as to emergency managers.[69] Because hurricanes can be unpredictable, forecasts must be issued in terms of probabilities and risks. Understanding probabilities and how they apply to one's personal risks can be challenging. When making a decision to evacuate, understanding those risks is crucial.

During recovery, applying for federal aid requires the ability to understand and complete multiple forms. Social workers and case managers report that low-literacy applicants denied benefits tend not to challenge the decision without encouragement and assistance. Benefit loss among low-literacy applicants appears to be higher as a result, with increases in stress and related illnesses. Similarly, individuals with disabilities often need support in negotiating the post-disaster recovery system and benefit from support from case managers with expertise in supporting people with disabilities.[70]

Sign language varies across geographical areas and nations and must be adapted to incorporate these linguistic differences. As noted in a breakthrough study, warnings often fail to reach people who are deaf or hard of hearing.[71] Although U.S. Federal Communications Commission policy dictates that closed-captioning must occur during emergency news broadcasts, stations frequently fail to provide closed-captioning during rapid-onset events. Meteorologists often turn their backs or their sides to the camera during on-air coverage, which precludes lipreading, and graphics often scroll across closed-captioning. Few schools of meteorology offer instruction regarding vulnerable populations or prepare students to work with the deaf.[71] Thus the problem is not individual culpability, but one reflecting a larger societal problem. Although technologies address some warning distribution issues, the cost of those devices can be prohibitive.

Increasing diversity within the United States has prompted the integration of pre-event messages and interpreters into emergency operations plans. In the San Francisco, California area alone, at least 112 languages are spoken.[72] The most frequently spoken languages include English, Spanish, Chinese (various dialects), Portuguese, and Punjabi. Issues with language and literacy can be addressed. As an example, FEMA issued informational brochures in dozens of languages after September 11, 2001. FEMA then increased its capacities after Superstorm Sandy in 2012. FEMA's Limited English Proficiency (LEP) department conducted outreach in twenty-five different languages and distributed over 900,000 flyers, fact sheets, and other materials. The FEMA telephone registration line was staffed by personnel who could identify languages and then route the caller to the proper staff member. Within 3 months, more than 11,300 people had called and received assistance in 35 different languages. Interpreters also went to nearly sixty community meetings and provided 25 language interpreters at Disaster Recovery Centers in the affected area.

Congregate Facilities

Functional and access needs also exist for those who live in congregate facilities. Such facilities include assisted living, nursing homes, adult day care centers, schools for students who are blind or deaf, and facilities for veterans or adults with cognitive disabilities. However, very little empirical work has been performed on any of these populations in a disaster context.

More is known about nursing homes than other facilities. Transferring such populations to other facilities carries risk; however, failure to evacuate can have fatal consequences, as seen in Japan after the Fukushima radiation disaster and in the United States after Hurricanes Katrina and Rita. The U.S. Government Accountability Office found additional problems. There is no national system to evacuate patients in nursing homes and "states and localities face challenges in identifying these populations, determining their needs, and providing for and coordinating their transportation." Those challenges include identifying transportation resources (vehicles and drivers) and escort staff. It is likely that in a major disaster, the "local demand for transportation would exceed supply" of vehicles.[73]

Hurricane Rita, which occurred shortly after Katrina, prompted massive evacuations and resulted in gridlock on Texas highways. In the worst tragedy of the evacuation, a nursing home bus caught fire and twenty-four patients died. Unlike hurricanes that have some warning, rapid-onset events may not allow for movement to safe rooms, or facilities may lack such shelters. In 2011, a massive, violent tornado tore the roof off a local nursing home in Joplin, Missouri. Sixteen residents and a caregiver died as medical staff tried to protect, cover, and hold on to their patients.

Nursing homes that are most likely to evacuate, particularly in the case of slow-onset events, belong to systems that are capable of providing patient care at alternate facilities. Independent facilities are less likely to evacuate, to have adequate transportation assets to do so, and to have the staff necessary to travel with patients. The evacuation itself can be associated with increased morbidity, including what appears to be a higher potential for death, a reaction called "transfer trauma." Other challenges include the patient's ability for adapting to changes in heat or cold or obtaining proper nutrition, especially in relation to medication protocols. In addition older adults may experience physical challenges that limit their abilities to evacuate or shelter during events like earthquakes or tornados. Statistics indicate that approximately 32% of American adults aged 70 or older report difficulty walking.[74] In addition, facilities face challenges for ensuring that support systems remain in place during evacuation, including transfer of medical records.[75,76] Actions by emergency managers working closely with home healthcare agencies, doctors, and other community organizations to disseminate messages about the impending disaster, transportation options, and shelters were effective during the evacuation for Hurricane Katrina.[73] Studies also recommend that families and patients remain together to provide social support and lessen transfer trauma.[76]

Medical facilities that offer outpatient care can also sustain damage during an event, reducing the availability of crucial services to vulnerable populations. Disruption in treatment can occur for patients receiving dialysis, cancer therapy, and HIV/AIDS–related interventions, as well as for those with significant respiratory conditions who require assistance. In addition, the loss of facilities that provide critical resources such as oxygen and tube feeding highlights the need for rapid restoration of such services. An important factor for those living in congregate care is that caregiver and medical supports are available to provide continuity of care during a disaster event.[77] Similarly, employers who provide supported work environments must consider needs of their employees with disabilities should a disaster occur. In both congregate housing and work environments, designing a disability-accessible area for sheltering-in-place is important.[78]

Immigrants and International Visitors

People who have recently arrived in a new location are among the last to receive disaster information. International students, for example, face different hazards from those in their native country and need to acquire new survival skills. Similarly, recent immigrants require education about local risks and training on appropriate protective actions. Because immigrants may include extended family members, materials should be distributed in multiple languages and with consideration of literacy levels in those languages. An elderly immigrant may never learn the locally or nationally spoken language. Outreach to people who are new to, or unfamiliar with, an area is crucial. These individuals include tourists, convention-goers, exchange students, or medical mission team members. The type of event can make a difference as well. For example, American Muslims experienced violent retributions after the events of September 11, 2001, putting them at considerable risk in some locations.[79]

After the 2013 tornadoes in Oklahoma, recent immigrants who had lost their documents in the storms feared requesting government aid because of a perceived risk of deportation. To address this concern, faith-based organizations provided services where people felt comfortable accessing aid. In 1999, Darwin officials in Australia hosted over 1,800 evacuees from East Timor. Local officials worked with members of the existing East Timorese/Portuguese community out of concern for potential negative consequences resulting from language, religious, and sex differences. Together, they established the Police Ethnic Advisory Group to operate a reception center. For more than 2 years, local fire, police, and Timorese leaders worked as partners to receive evacuees. They used local Timorese representatives to meet new arrivals and use their native language. Their "fellow country" people helped to establish and explain appropriate food preparation, sleeping, religious, and health procedures.[11] As with other groups, involving the "at-risk" population in addressing issues provides crucial resources.

An estimated 11.3 million undocumented immigrants live in the United States, many of whom are Hispanic.[80] After the Southern California wildfires of 2007, reports of mistreatment and discrimination against undocumented individuals included instances of police officers who circulated through shelters, woke up families, asked for identification, and escorted those with no papers out of the shelters.[81] Understandably, these actions dissuaded families without documentation to seek shelter and support during this disaster. Navarrette[80] later reported that at least "half a dozen charred bodies have been uncovered in the ashes-bodies that authorities believe are those of illegal immigrants who did not get out of harm's way fast enough."[82]

People in Rural Areas

Although the population of the United States has become increasingly urban, over 20% of households are located in rural areas.

Rural communities can be more vulnerable than their urban counterparts as they confront unique challenges that affect how they are able to prevent, serve, and respond to the public's needs during disasters.[83] For example, the Bastrop County Complex wildfire occurred in a wildland urban interface area where homesteads and ranches were established in a piney forest. When drought struck Texas in 2011, pine needle drop, lack of moisture, and high winds led to a multiple wildfires that converged and consumed nearly 1,700 homes. Rural residents had to quickly evacuate and many lost livestock and ranching infrastructure in addition to their homes.

Rural communities frequently lack disaster resources and sufficient formal governmental structures that facilitate effective mitigation, preparedness, response, and recovery.[84,85] Additionally, rural areas must plan for a trio of considerations that include common disasters, unique local threats, and urban populations fleeing densely populated areas to the perceived safety of rural America.[85]

Intersected Vulnerabilities

It is difficult to separate demographics and specify that only gender, income, or age create a vulnerable condition. In reality, demographic conditions and the broader social, economic, cultural, and even political conditions in which people live create "entangling effects" that foster and exacerbate vulnerability.[86]

Although specific circumstances and/or conditions may generate vulnerabilities and support needs, overlapping conditions occurring together create vulnerabilities. For example, greater susceptibility to health issues such as osteoporosis means that women may be generally more likely to sustain injuries. Women's vulnerability is further exacerbated by age, which can be aggravated by disability. An elderly woman with a mobility, sensory, or cognitive disability bears disproportionate risk in a disaster and merits a more comprehensive range of intervention strategies.

As another example, elderly men are more likely to live in socially isolated conditions, away from relationships and networks that may provide buffers against the consequences of disasters. In addition, their disability risk increases with age. In the United States, one in five people have a disability, a situation that increases with age.[76] Gender may complicate the intersection of age and disability. For example, older men may receive delayed evacuation information and have difficulty accessing supports that facilitate timely evacuation.

To summarize, one "condition" or population demographic is insufficient to understand vulnerability. Rather, a complex set of conditions, circumstances, and contexts interact to produce vulnerability. Using a simple checklist of possibly affected population groups is a starting point. Understanding the intersected nature of vulnerability informs the concerted efforts needed to address vulnerability reduction.

A Resilience Perspective

In contrast to the concept of vulnerability, scholars and practitioners have endorsed the idea of "resilience." Defined generally as the ability of individuals and communities to recover from adverse circumstances, resilience has been used to describe not only psychosocial hardiness but also the time it takes for a community to reestablish essential services and commerce postdisaster. Medical personnel can facilitate resilience on the individual level by providing psychological treatment resources to disaster survivors. With respect to community resilience, medical personnel can support disaster preparedness of hospitals and clinics. Post-disaster, they are instrumental in providing care and restoring needed medical services. Key actions should focus on mitigation and preparedness, at both the individual and community levels.[87]

Resilient communities take deliberate, meaningful, collective action in response to disasters. An emphasis is placed on connection and caring among community members and organizations.[88] These communities are able to minimize the effects of, and recover quickly from, disasters. A community is only as prepared and protected as its most vulnerable members. The health and safety of traditionally vulnerable populations can be considered an indicator of overall community resilience.

The Life Cycle of Emergency Management

Emergency managers and disaster researchers describe a "life cycle" of emergency management. Most nations organize their disaster activities around the categories described in this cycle. In New Zealand, for example, they are known as the Four R's: readiness, response, recovery, and reduction. In the United States, the National Governor's Association first organized the phases into preparedness, response, recovery, and mitigation activities. Regardless of the terms, the phases have influenced both practice and research. The remainder of this chapter addresses relevant issues and connects each disaster phase to vulnerability. Practical strategies that promote resilience are discussed. To emphasize the importance of these phases, this section begins by addressing legal mandates for emergency managers.

Legal Issues

Individuals with disabilities in the United States are entitled to equal access to emergency services, including evacuation procedures and sheltering. The Stafford Act, which gives FEMA the responsibility for coordinating government-wide disaster efforts, specifies that the needs of individuals with disabilities be included in the components of the National Preparedness System.[89] In addition, Title II of the Americans with Disabilities Act requires modifications to policies, practices, and procedures to avoid discrimination against people with disabilities. This requirement also applies to programs, services, and activities provided through third parties, such as the American Red Cross, private nonprofit organizations, or religious entities. Specifically, entities must make reasonable modifications and accommodations, cannot use eligibility criteria to exclude people with disabilities, and must provide effective communication to individuals with disabilities.[90] Attention on national policies concerning the needs of individuals with disabilities and/or functional and access needs resulted in changes to the Stafford Act, which was amended as the Post-Katrina Emergency Management Reform Act of 2006. Executive Order 13347, Individuals with Disabilities in Emergency Preparedness, "established a policy that the Federal government appropriately support the safety and security of individuals with disabilities impacted by either natural or man-made disasters."[66] Also included in the Executive Order was the establishment of an Interagency Coordinating Council (ICC) to coordinate the federal response to emergency preparedness as it pertains to individuals with disabilities. In 2010, FEMA adopted the functional-needs approach to defining disability-related needs during disaster in its Comprehensive Preparedness Guide 101 and as part of the 2008 National Response Framework (NRF).[91] The NRF is part of the National Preparedness System, mandated in Presidential Policy Directive (PPD) 8: National Preparedness. PPD 8 is aimed at strengthening the security and resilience of the United States through systematic preparation for threats that pose risks to national security. The NRF of 2013 emphasizes a whole community approach to disaster planning and authorizes federal financial assistance for disability-related access and functional needs equipment if funding is available.

Rather than specifying types of disabilities, the functional needs approach uses a five-part taxonomy of requirements in the areas of communication, medical health, functional independence, supervision, and transportation (C-MIST).[2] For example, individuals with auditory limitations may need modifications in how they receive emergency communications, while individuals with memory or decision-making difficulties may require supervision while in a shelter. The C-MIST definition of the functional needs approach to disability is:

> Populations whose members may have additional needs before, during, and after an incident in functional areas, including but not limited to: maintaining independence, communication, transportation, supervision, and medical care. Individuals in need of additional response assistance may include those who have disabilities; who live in institutionalized settings; who are elderly; who are children; who are from diverse cultures; who have limited English proficiency or are non-English speaking; or who are transportation disadvantaged.[91]

Thus, in the United States, all individuals with disabilities, including those who have a life-long disability, as well as those who have acquired a disability, are entitled to equal access and inclusion across all phases of disaster management. The National Preparedness Report of 2013, as one of its key findings, describes that the United States has made important progress in the integration of individuals with disabilities and in access and functional needs over the last several years.[92]

In 2005, the U.S. Congress enacted the "No Pets Left Behind" or Pet Evacuation and Transportation Act (PETS) as an amendment to the Stafford Act. Because of massive loss of life among animals after Hurricane Katrina, Congress said that pets and service animals must be included in evacuations. This protocol may encourage human evacuation, particularly among older populations. Strategies to accommodate pets in shelters include co-establishment of animal and human sites so that owners can care for their pets or separate sites for animals where shelter workers provide care. After the 2013 tornadoes in Oklahoma, the state Department of Agriculture led efforts to rescue, triage, and shelter pets and livestock. Working with local shelters, rescue groups, and the State of Oklahoma Medical Reserve Corps/Animal Response Teams, their efforts saved hundreds of pets, enabled emotional reunions, and ultimately led to adoptive homes for animals that could not be reunited with their owners.

Preparedness

Preparedness is defined as "actions undertaken before disaster impact that enable social units to respond actively when disaster does strike."[86] Actions should be taken at the individual, household, organizational, and community levels as well as within local, state, and federal governments. Activities might include building partnerships, developing and disseminating educational materials, training for specific tasks such as sheltering or triage, evacuation planning, the creation of functional and access needs registries, writing emergency operations plans, and holding exercises. This section examines key areas.

KNOW THE COMMUNITY

Before addressing specific population needs, emergency managers must become familiar with community demographic groups and potential partnership organizations. The U.S. census is a good source of local population data. The census occurs every 10 years with more frequent assessments made through random sampling conducted by the American Community Survey. Both can be accessed at www.census.gov. General information gleaned by geographical location includes overviews of race, ethnicity, languages, gender and age distributions, disabilities, and income levels. A limitation of the census is that it misses key population descriptors, such as recent immigration, literacy levels, and homelessness. Thus the census is only the first step in assessing localized and special needs. For developing nations, census data may be incomplete or never collected. Capturing a sense of the community requires familiarity with the population. Interacting with local organizations provides valuable data.

Thus, the second step in knowing the community is identifying the range of local community-based organizations. From these groups, it is possible to learn more about those present in the community. Agricultural areas in southern Florida and parts of California, for example, have health and advocacy organizations dedicated to both migratory and resident farm workers. Urban locations usually host missions and other places dedicated to the homeless. Faith-based organizations extend services to new immigrants and may offer personnel who speak relevant languages. The local emergency management agency is another key organization. An increasing trend among emergency managers is to establish a "Functional and Access Needs Advisory Panel" or to generate an approach based on the notion of the "Whole Community." Developed by FEMA in the United States, "Whole Community" means that everyone is invited to participate in planning and preparedness, including community, civic, and faith-based organizations. Becoming part of this partnership provides links to organizations with expertise. Relevant groups include disability and rehabilitation agencies, health organizations, and senior networks, as well as other higher-risk populations.

Medical personnel represent a marginally tapped disaster management resource in many communities. Typically, medical staff remain in stationary hospital locations waiting to receive patients. Conversely, outreach by medical personnel into existing or emerging partnerships that address special needs can make a considerable difference. Expertise on disabilities, movement of fragile patients or frail elderly, and insights into child and partner abuse can help emergency managers and other organizations to reduce risks. According to the U.S. Government Accountability Office, physicians and other medical staff played an important role in identifying patients who needed transportation during Hurricane Katrina. A stronger link among individuals, the medical community, and emergency managers can mitigate bad outcomes. Medical personnel who provide services to nursing homes, assisted living facilities, settings for people with cognitive disabilities, and other similar locations can encourage those facilities to train personnel frequently on emergency procedures.

By getting acquainted and working with a broad array of partners, special needs can be identified pre-event.

TRAINING AND EDUCATION

Ongoing education about vulnerable populations is necessary, particularly as policies and procedures are rapidly evolving within the United States alone. The following are useful resources:

- Universities and colleges have developed programs across the United States and in some other nations that include opportunities for stand-alone courses, certificates, or degrees. Many offer distance learning courses available on the Internet. Links to programs can be found at the FEMA Higher Education Project website: http://www.training.fema.gov/EMIweb/edu/collegelist.
- Many states and communities have developed robust Medical Reserve Corps with volunteers from the medical sector.[93] They respond on an as-needed basis when disasters occur and assist with a range of issues including pandemics, shelters, and annual immunizations. For more information, visit www.citizencorps.gov.
- FEMA offers an interactive course at their Independent Study (IS) website. IS197 concerns functional and access needs. See http://training.fema.gov/EMIWeb/IS/is197SP.asp.
- States offer instructor-led functional and access needs training courses. Course materials may be obtained from FEMA at https://training.fema.gov/EMIWeb/pub/register.asp.
- Professional emergency management conferences, such as the National Hurricane Conference or the International Association of Emergency Managers, offer topical workshops and continuing education credits for special needs courses. Organizations such as the International Association of Emergency Managers, the National Emergency Management Association, or the Natural Hazards Center at the University of Colorado-Boulder provide listserves. The latter is available at www.colorado.edu/hazards.
- FEMA hired disability coordinators at their ten regional offices. Contacting them may lead to the initiation or furtherance of important partnerships. FEMA's Office of Disability Integration offers additional information at http://www.fema.gov/office-disability-integration-coordination/office-disability-integration-coordination/office-1.
- Scholarly journals are increasingly publishing research on populations at risk. Key sources include the *Natural Hazards Review, the International Journal of Mass Emergencies and Disasters, Environmental Hazards, Natural Hazards, Disaster Prevention and Management, Disasters, and the Journal of Emergency Management.*

Further information and training resources are available from local, state, federal, and international emergency management agencies. Such entities routinely hold tabletop exercises and community drills. Training should include all levels of personnel working in a medical setting.

Finally and perhaps most importantly, healthcare personnel should engage in cross-training with disaster organizations. The American Red Cross trains shelter managers and provides other disaster courses. For professionals in psychology and psychiatry, the Red Cross requires credentialing before participation in actual disaster response.

U.S. FEMA "Getting Real" Conference Public Education Initiatives

- Educating those at risk about approaches to reduce their own vulnerabilities is essential for preparedness. Medical personnel play an important role in this by providing information to their patients.
- Place informational brochures in waiting rooms. Free, disability-specific brochures can be downloaded from NOD at www.nod.org (select "Emergency Preparedness Initiative"). Provide materials in multiple formats for various languages and literacy levels as well as for people with varying degrees of visual limitations. Offices should also consider purchasing communication boards that include specific languages, pictures, and situations (i.e., denoting bleeding or pain).
- Include individual and household risk assessments during medical histories and annual examinations. Disaster checklists can be obtained at www.ready.gov, www.fema.gov, and similar sites. Focus history taking on the level of individual and household preparedness for an event such as an evacuation. PTSD is more likely among those with previous trauma such as war injuries, interpersonal violence, prior disaster, or severe injuries. Assessment for a history of trauma helps pre-event identification of populations who may benefit from advice and counseling resources.[9,10]
- Advise patients that they should establish an emergency bag or "go kit." Materials that should be included are identified at www.ready.gov and www.redcross.org. Within this kit, it is particularly important that patients include medications, lists of medical routines, a medical history, communication information and preferences, nutritional needs, insurance papers, and contact information for healthcare and pharmacy providers, family, guardians, and caregivers.
- Alert patients to opportunities for obtaining emergency bag items or other information, especially low-income patients and, in the United States, seniors on Medicare Part D (particularly those that are experiencing gap coverage). This might include assisting patients with pharmaceutical programs that provide free or reduced medications.
- Assist families with transitions into assisted living facilities. Immediately orient new residents to emergency procedures and establish a clear means of communication with families about what will happen, how, and under what circumstances.
- Support practices and legislation that mandate safe rooms in schools, day cares, and other locations where large numbers of children may need rapid sheltering.
- Explain to patients the resources that will be available in evacuation shelters. Because individuals with disabilities may be reluctant to evacuate due to the belief that shelters will not be ready, it can be valuable to provide that information to encourage evacuation.[50]
- Send new parents home from the hospital with checklists for emergency procedures in a disaster. Provide emergency bags (formula, diapers, and other key items).
- Target people with disabilities and seniors for special attention. Provide information through both direct contact and accessible-format materials. Medical personnel tend to have high levels of credibility when disseminating information, so these efforts can have considerable impact.
- Link with home healthcare agencies and encourage them to provide disaster information to patients, particularly those in transition from hospital to home. A family leaving the hospital with someone using an oxygen tank for the first time may need special training not only on the medical equipment but also on how to help the family member take appropriate protective actions in a disaster. For example, how a family member can move an individual with mobility limitations without injury.
- Support domestic violence shelters with outreach to individuals experiencing intimate partner violence. Because it appears that domestic violence may increase after disasters, those known to be at risk require additional attention. Medical personnel can provide information and escape options and support the efforts of domestic violence prevention staff.[51]

Other organizations can benefit from cross-training as well. For example, after the 1989 Loma Prieta earthquake in San Francisco, a Latino healthcare organization called Salud Para La Gente cross-trained with the American Red Cross. The benefits were significant. Salud Para la Gente developed an emergency response healthcare plan and the Red Cross expanded its network of providers for the Spanish-speaking community. This partnership likely led to other benefits across the community by demonstrating the value of cross-cultural and interorganizational linkages. The medical community can work with experienced disaster providers to offer training. Shelter managers can benefit from specialized instruction offered by the medical community to help identify evacuees who appear stable, but could deteriorate due to unseen medical conditions, nutritional requirements, and other circumstances. Medical associations can partner with veterinary organizations to deliver joint assistance to people using service animals.

Since 2010, FEMA has organized several "Getting Real" conferences, which have brought together emergency managers, first responders, state emergency planners, and members of disability organizations to discuss factors that place individuals with disabilities or functional and access needs at risk. As part of these conferences, FEMA has provided cross-training for disability content experts on the structure of emergency management, while concurrently providing disability awareness training for emergency management personnel. State and regional partnerships established at these conferences have led to increased dialog between emergency management and disability groups, as well as the inclusion of people with disabilities and their advocates in disaster planning. Medical personnel associated with

Registries[94]

The whole community approach to emergency management requires an informed and shared understanding of a community's risks, needs, and capabilities. Communities often consider using Emergency Assistance Registries as a strategy for gaining such an understanding of their populations with communications, medical, independence, support, or transportation access or functional dependencies. An emergency assistance registry is a specified list or set of lists of identifiable individuals used by a community to plan for and provide emergency services to its enrollees.[1] The U.S. Department of Justice recommends using such registries as a step toward meeting Americans with Disability Act requirements for providing "same access" to emergency services.[2] The State of Florida has made county use of registries a statutory requirement.[3] A 2009 NOD report indicated that 63% of emergency management agencies and 54% of disability organizations maintain emergency assistance registries.[4]

Emergency assistance registries can vary by purpose and by how registry operators collect and store enrollee information. Some registries focus on meeting a single response-related need such as providing evacuation transportation to carless individuals. Others are very comprehensive, collecting information that leads to the community providing a complex mix of preparedness and response support to enrollees. Still others focus on only collecting information to help with community emergency planning efforts. Most registries collect their information by return-mail questionnaires (e.g., postcards, forms), online registration, or from organizations that provide services to people with disabilities and access or functional needs. There are issues with each collection method. Using return-mail questionnaires can be expensive because of postage. The target population's access to computers – which tends to be 75–90% less than the general population for people with disabilities[5] – affects the rate of online registration. The ability to obtain information from service providers is often constrained by privacy laws such as the Healthcare Insurance Portability and Accountability Act (HIPAA). Registries take the form of indexed card decks, tables, spreadsheets, electronic databases, and complex geographic information systems.

Existing studies reveal that registries have benefits as well as limitations. One major benefit of registries is the building of relationships among the groups that work together to maintain them and provide services. They include a wide array of partners from across the community. Limitations and concerns include issues of high operational and staffing costs, difficulties with responder access, and enrollee privacy. One rural Alabama county estimated the cost to operate a registry at between $194 and $199 per enrollee, with predicted operating costs of $123,000 per annum.[6]

Used with permission from Paul Hewett, Argonne National Laboratory.

References

1. Hewett P. *Organizational networks and emergence during disaster preparedness: The case of an emergency assistance registry.* Doctoral dissertation. Stillwater, Oklahoma State University, 2013.
2. U.S. Department of Justice. Emergency management under Title II of the ADA. ADA Best Practices Tool Kit for State and Local Governments. http://www.ada.gov/pcatoolkit/chap7emergencymgmt.pdf (Accessed August 21, 2013).
3. Registry of Persons with Special Needs, Title XVII Florida Statutes § 252.355. http//:www.leg.state.fl.us/STATUTES/index.cfm?App_mode=Disaply_Statute&Search_String=&URL=Ch0252/Sec355.HTM (Accessed August 22, 2013).
4. National Organization on Disabilities. Integrative emergency planning: Voices of emergency management agencies and disability organizations. 2009. http://www.nod.org (Accessed August 21, 2013).
5. Kaye HS. *Computer and Internet use among people with disabilities.* Disability Statistics Report (Report No. 13). Washington, DC, U.S. Department of Education, National Institute on Disability and Rehabilitation Research, 2000.
6. Metz WC, Hewett PL, Mitrani JE, Miller D, Hill DD. *Design and Implementation of Data Maintenance Methods for the Alabama CSEPP Special Needs Population Registry.* Argonne National Laboratory Report to the Alabama CSEPP Operational Assessment Team, 2001.

departments of public health and emergency medical services have been key participants in these conferences and contributed to the resulting initiatives.

REGISTRIES

Functional and access registries are a useful preparedness strategy.

Registries are lists of people who might require assistance in an emergency, such as a person who is blind or someone with limited transportation options. Such listings have been touted as a possible approach to identify those at risk and provide them adequate resources. Registries vary and might be extremely comprehensive, for example, including everyone who lacks transportation. In comparison, others might focus on just those who require paratransit vehicles for people using wheelchairs. Typical groups who work together to maintain registries include emergency managers, home health and related social service agencies, aging organizations, disability organizations, disaster organizations such as the American Red Cross, fire departments, emergency transportation and medical units, paratransit resources, the health department, veterans affairs personnel, disability and rehabilitation services, and interpreters. Issues of confidentiality and access typically arise because of the myriad organizations and agencies that participate. Registries, although certainly a practical strategy, also represent a considerable challenge. For example, a well-funded effort in Alabama for a chemical weapons facility faced annual challenges in updating registrant contact information.[95]

EVACUATION

There are numerous reasons why evacuation is problematic. Many people were stranded or died after Hurricane Katrina due to lack of transportation. A study of Hurricanes Floyd and Dennis discovered that people with disabilities might have assumed that shelters were not prepared for them and therefore would not evacuate.[96] There is no standardized system in place to evacuate massive numbers of people from non-medical congregate facilities. Specific locations face particular challenges. As an example, a domestic violence shelter in New Orleans could not purchase bus tickets when officials closed the bus station during the Hurricane Katrina evacuation. The shelter director eventually found keys to a van and drove the residents to safety in Baton Rouge.[97] The final bus of evacuees to leave Plaquemines Parish below New Orleans was populated with Vietnamese-American fishermen attempting to protect their economic livelihoods and family possessions until the last possible minute.

The large-scale evacuation efforts in New Orleans uncovered several issues. To facilitate rapid movement, those assisting people with disabilities left wheelchairs, assistive devices, and other necessary items behind. The Louisiana Department of Rehabilitation spent 6 months trying to retrieve these items and return them to their owners. Some wheelchairs, costing up to $30,000, were irreplaceable. Paramedics in Texas, Oklahoma, and other locations reported serious problems when evacuated patients arrived at shelters without their support equipment. In some cases, patients were transported on buses for 12 hours or more without stopping. This resulted in both deterioration of existing medical conditions and accumulation of hazardous waste. After the 2010 Haiti earthquake, the number of crush injuries and amputations resulted in tens of thousands of people with new disabilities. A critical lack of assistive equipment left them even more vulnerable and without support to help with transition to independent living.

Because medical professionals represent trusted, credible individuals, it is valuable for them to become involved in evacuation and transportation planning and in issuing warning messages. Medical personnel can also engage in the following activities:

■ Participate in evacuation planning and provide insights on how to transport people with medical conditions in a safe and healthy manner. Ensure that medical records, medications, and support staff stay with those at risk. This includes those who may appear healthy but could deteriorate under conditions of stress, heat, severe cold, and movement to unfamiliar environments.

■ Assist with training evacuation personnel in methods for transporting individuals with different conditions, from someone relying on a ventilator to a patient with a bariatric disorder.

■ Contact patients who might not receive warning, evacuation, and transportation messages, including the deaf, hearing impaired, blind, aged, and those with low levels of literacy or who are non-English speaking. Conduct outreach through health clinics and other facilities that serve low-income individuals. Advocate for these groups and encourage local officials to do the same.

■ Advise patients and local authorities to develop plans for pet evacuation. Seniors seem more likely to evacuate if pets accompany them. Such planning also benefits service animals used by people with functional needs.

■ Encourage local officials to identify multiple sources of accessible transportation. The best efforts to use nongovernmental resources require advance negotiation for liability protections and reimbursements.[98]

■ Ensure that receiving personnel are well trained and organized to manage a variety of conditions when patients or vulnerable groups arrive. These range from medical problems and interpersonal violence to children separated from their parents.

■ Join local officials in planning and advertising locations for general population and "functional and access needs" shelters. Ensure that those in need of such facilities realize that arrangements have been made for their mobility and nutritional and accessibility needs, as well as for their service animals.

■ Request that local officials keep evacuees together with their durable medical equipment, assistive devices, and service animals. Help patients and officials develop personal evacuation plans, protective actions, and communication strategies that keep families, guardians, and caregivers together. Suggest a buddy system, with multiple backups, for those in need of personal transportation assistance.

Response

The emergency response phase focuses on saving lives and reducing damage from an impending or ongoing event. Efforts are made "to reduce casualties, damage and disruption and to respond to the immediate needs of disaster victims."[86] Response activities are likely to include: implementing an emergency response plan and requesting support personnel; initiating search and rescue activity; first aid and emergency medical intervention; opening special needs and medical shelters; and measures such as sandbagging, implementing a plan to operate generators, or opening a distribution center for medications.

Warnings

In the United States, nearly 25% of the population may need some form of assistance or accommodation to receive emergency alerts.[99] At the federal level, Executive Order 13407 stipulates that the U.S. Emergency Alert System should include all Americans, including those with disabilities and those who do not speak English.[96,100] Although evidence suggests that older adults are just as likely to attempt to comply with disaster warnings,[99] they have functional needs that must be considered when developing emergency preparedness plans.[102] Likewise, the needs of adults with disabilities may limit the availability of protective actions such as evacuation if shelters are not equipped with medical equipment or at least have the space to accommodate such equipment.[16] Thus, there is a critical need for the development and testing of warnings that consider the needs of vulnerable populations. These universal approaches to design have collateral benefits in that they typically result in more user-friendly products and environments for people of all abilities.[103] While social media has limitations for certain populations, it is nevertheless a useful resource.

Medical professionals can be part of the alerting process. Doing so is easier when slow-onset events occur and can be anticipated (e.g., hurricanes, heat waves, pandemics, and droughts). In these situations, email alerts, phone calls, personal contact, and agency outreach can help motivate and assist people. For

Using Social Media to Connect to Vulnerable Populations

Social media platforms are being used more frequently during disasters. Social platforms, which include Facebook, Twitter, and YouTube, have been used during search and rescue and for reconnecting loved ones.[1] Additionally, these platforms combined have been used to coordinate resources, volunteers, and donations.[2] Globally, the public used social media platforms after the 2011 Tōhoku Earthquake and Tsunami, the 2010 Haiti earthquake, and the cyclone in Myanmar.[2,3,4] Emergency managers and government agencies use social media platforms during response and recovery efforts.[1,5,6] After Hurricane Sandy in 2012, U.S. government agencies and emergency management organizations used social media more than ever before.[7] One study identified 74% of states (and 45% of cities) currently use social media to disseminate emergency information.[8]

Social media platforms are typically accessed through the use of wireless-, information-, and communication-based technologies such as portable computers, mobile phones, and tablets. The increase in use of these tools and of social media among people with disabilities and older adults suggests that using this technology to disseminate emergency information may prove viable. People with disabilities and older adults often use wireless- and information-based technologies.[5] Madden identified a rise in the number of individuals over 65 that use social media platforms.[9] Other researchers have noted that wireless-based technologies are rapidly becoming a necessity among the deaf and hard of hearing communities.[5] In a study of user needs, the Wireless Rehabilitation Engineering Research Center found that social media use is increasing among people with disabilities. Social media is being used to receive and verify public alerts among individuals with disabilities.[10] After tornadoes struck Alabama in 2011, one emergency agency representative noted that, with the use of social media, they have been able to connect to "often invisible populations [people with disabilities]."[1]

Emergency management agencies and individuals of all ages are using what was originally considered "just a fad" for youth. Given that older populations and people with disabilities are often forgotten during emergency planning, steps can be taken to include these populations when using social media for disasters.[11,12] Emergency managers should seek to include accessible formats in multimedia social media posts.[8,13] Posts that include video content should also have captioning with large fonts, interpretation, or a link to a written transcript. Emergency service agencies should include outreach programs for people with disabilities and older adults.[8,13] Additionally, agencies should investigate the integration of social media training for emergency management offices.[13] Proper training can increase the usefulness of this communication tool and provide a viable link to harder-to-reach populations.

Used with permission from DeeDee Bennett, Georgia Institute of Technology.

References

1. Bennett D. Social Media for Emergency Management. 66th Interdepartmental Hurricane Conference, Charleston, South Carolina, March 2012.
2. Gao H, Barbier G, Goolsby R. Harnessing the Crowd-sourcing Power of Social Media for Disaster Relief. *IEEE Intelligent Systems* 2011. http://wordpress.vrac.iastate.edu/REU2011/wp-content/uploads/2011/05/Harnessing-the-Crowdsourcins-Power-of-Social-Media-for-Disaster-Relief.pdf (Accessed August 22, 2013).
3. Mills A, Chen R, Kee J, Rao HR. Web 2.0 Emergency Applications: How Useful Can Twitter Be for Emergency Response? *J Info Priv & Sec* 2009; 5(3).
4. Yates D, Pacquette S. Emergency knowledge management and social media technologies: A Case Study of the 2010 Haitian Earthquake. *Int J of Info Mgmt* 2011; 31(1): 6–13.
5. Mitchell H, Bennett D, LaForce S. Planning for Accessible Emergency Communications: Mobile Technology and Social Media. 2nd International AEGIS Conference. Brussels, Belgium, 2011.
6. Mileti D. Social Media and Public Warnings. Denver UASI Conference on Shared Strategies for Homeland Security. Boulder, Colorado, 2010.
7. Cohen SE. Sandy Marked Shift for Social Media use in Disasters. *Emergency Management Online* 2013. http://www.emergencymgmt.com/disaster/Sandy-Social-Media-Use-in-Disasters.html. (Accessed August 22, 2013).
8. Laforce S. Social Media, Emergency Communications and People with Disabilities. Wireless RERC Conference, Minneapolis, Minnesota, 2011.
9. Madden M. Older Adults and Social Media. *Pew Research Center* 2010. http://pewresearch.org/pubs/1711/older-adults-social-networking-facebook-twitter (Accessed August 22, 2013).
10. Wireless RERC. SUN: About Wireless Users with Disabilities. 2010. http://www.wirelessrerc.org/publications/sunspot-latest-findings-from-our-survey-of-user (Accessed August 22, 2013).
11. Gooden S, Jones D, Martin KJ, Boyd M. Social Equity in Local Emergency Management Planning. *St & Local Govt Rev* 2009; 41(1): 1–12.
12. Bennett D. State Emergency Plans: Assessing the Inclusiveness of Vulnerable Populations, *Int J Emergency Management* 2010; 7(1): 100–110.
13. Bennett D. Evidence-Based Best Practices for Disability Issues. 37th Annual Natural Hazards Research and Application Workshop, Broomfield, Colorado, July 2012.

more no-notice and rapid-onset events, agencies and medical professionals can play a crucial role in educating people about potential threats, for example, from flash floods or tornadoes. Encouraging people at risk to prepare and plan in advance of disasters is important.

SHELTERS

At least two types of shelters may be established after a disaster: general population shelters and medical shelters. The first is a general population or mass care shelter open to everyone. Traditionally, the American Red Cross operates these facilities in the

United States, although in most disasters, other entities such as faith-based organizations may also manage shelters. In developing nations, nongovernmental organizations may establish relief centers. General population shelters are supposed to accommodate people with disabilities and their service animals, but that is not always the case. During Hurricane Katrina, for example, some general population shelters rejected people with disabilities who could have been sheltered independently at the facility. The massive evacuation also complicated the situation for people who lost or were forcibly separated from their assistive devices, such as hearing aids, and durable medical equipment, for example, walkers. Children, people with acute medical needs, seniors, and people with disabilities were also separated from friends, family, guardians, and caregivers, and were routed to a medical shelter. Similar problems occurred with Superstorm Sandy in the United States, when evacuating seniors could not take their pets. Some elderly patients remained in public shelters because they could not find housing that accommodated their needs. In addition, evacuated individuals lost valuable social networks that supported their ability to preserve independent daily living.

Accommodating most people in a general population shelter is desirable. Keeping evacuees with their own families, personal equipment (e.g., medical, communications), key social support systems, medical records, and medications increases the probability that they will comply with evacuation orders. Medical shelters should be reserved for those who need acute medical care to manage injuries and illnesses. The U.S. Department of Justice offers a shelter-specific Americans with Disabilities toolkit for state and local governments.[104] Key recommendations for shelters include:

- Plan ahead; "a person's health will be jeopardized without access to life-sustaining medication that must be refrigerated."[104]
- Individuals with disabilities, including "those with disability related needs for some medical care, medication, equipment, and supportive services"[104] should use general population shelters with family, friends, and others.
- Deploy trained staff to medical shelters and keep families together in such locations.
- Modify kitchens to allow people with medical conditions, such as diabetes, to have immediate access to food and medications.
- Provide a variety of means to communicate. Consider print versions as well as audio versions of announcements. Make announcements in multiple languages, as appropriate.
- Safeguard residents from further injury by assessing the environment. Consider the needs of individuals with mobility or sensory disabilities such as low vision or blindness.
- Offer a "low-stress" location – particularly valuable to children and to adults with cognitive disabilities.
- Invite people with disabilities to specify their needs and participate in problem solving as they can provide relevant, useful insights.
- Stockpile durable medical equipment and medications.
- Assign cots in the general shelter so that individuals with functional needs can more easily access needed supports. For example, people with mobility impairments should be located nearer to accessible restrooms, those with special dietary needs near the food service areas, and people who need to leave the shelter for frequent dialysis near the exits.

- Ensure electrical access and chargers for those with electric wheelchairs and other durable medical supports requiring electricity.

General population shelters should establish intake procedures to identify specific needs and ascertain whether an evacuee requires further support. Generally, shelters distinguish between those who require minor assistance and can remain in a general population center (e.g., those with asthma or who requiring tube feedings) and those who require advanced care such as continuous intravenous infusions. Other issues to assess include mobility, language and communication preferences, literacy levels, presence and needs of service animals, and availability of family members and translators. If most of these needs are met, the individual can remain in the general population shelter; however, the facility should remain cognizant of the ongoing needs of the evacuee. Confidential questions should be asked in a private setting to encourage disclosure and facilitate appropriate support or intervention.[105] For example, a patient with HIV may fear discovery; however, if that patient were separated from medications required to control the disease, this would be problematic. A similar situation exists with an evacuee at risk for intimate partner violence. Intake staff should be trained to establish a trusting environment to ease collection of crucial healthcare information. The intake process also allows for consideration of potential transfer to a functional and access needs or medical shelter.

Functional and access needs or medical shelters represent a "higher level of care" outpatient facility where those with extensive medical requirements can receive care. Such locations are typically reserved for those with stable medical conditions rather than acute injuries and illnesses. Admission should be based solely on medical eligibility. Most individuals with functional and access needs can be accommodated in general shelters. Medical needs shelters require extensive pre-event planning for staffing, supplies, facility selection, transportation, logistical support, and training on intake and discharge procedures. Medical supervision is mandatory in a medical shelter and should be coupled with adequate staffing and resources including reliable sources of power, water, heat, air conditioning, proper nutrition, and supplies. Placing patients in an existing facility is a simpler option.

In both general population and functional and access needs shelters, discharge planning is required. Those in charge must consider whether the evacuee is able to travel home. Issues to consider include: 1) debris removal from the roads and inside the home; 2) restoration of utilities to necessary levels; 3) proper support to sustain basic needs availability in the home; 4) the evacuee's needs to return home, including transportation, medical care, family support, and power; 5) the evacuee's loss of critical resources that need replacement, including a wheelchair; and 6) needs of the evacuee's service animal. By identifying the problems that must be addressed, a list of possible support organizations can be created including disability and aging organizations, veterans facilities, home health agencies, veterinarians, rehabilitation centers, medical supply companies, and others familiar with the transition from shelter to home.[106]

Recovery

Recovery is a process that involves "putting a disaster-stricken community back together."[107] Activities that might occur during this period include: 1) discharging individuals from shelters; 2) ensuring that persons with disabilities can navigate their damaged living environment when they return home; 3) restoration of utilities and healthcare access; 4) debris removal with adequate safeguards for health risks; 5) major reconstruction of the built environment including roads, ports, bridges, transit, and paratransit systems; and 6) providing both temporary and permanent homes that are accessible. This section examines key areas in which medical personnel can have a significant impact.

RECOVERY PLANNING

Although pre-disaster recovery planning is ideal, it is not commonly done. Consequently, post-disaster recovery planning is needed to develop guidelines and goals for community rebuilding. Often, a recovery planning task force is convened. The broader public may be periodically informed of progress or invited to actively participate. Medical professionals provide unique skills and perspectives to the planning process. They have a social capital that emanates from their status.[108,109] The capital can include insights, ideas, suggestions, procedures, and perspectives that can inform the recovery plan. Because medical professionals also benefit from the respect of the broader community, they are viewed authoritatively and their opinions have a great deal of credibility. Their participation is important, in part, because they can advocate for those lacking a presence on the recovery planning team. Seniors may be unable to travel to a recovery meeting. People with disabilities may be occupied reestablishing basic household, work, and healthcare routines and not have time to attend. New immigrants may not be aware of the meeting or be unfamiliar with how such a process is conducted.

Medical personnel can thus be advocates for those lacking a voice though actions including:

- Emphasize a need for paratransit resources and accessible roads, curbs, bridges and neighborhoods during the rebuilding process.
- Encourage recovery planners to reach out to and include non-English speaking residents.
- Request that recovery meetings are accessible for a wide variety of participants that represent the full spectrum of the community.
- Suggest that recovery meetings be held in accessible locations including senior centers, homeless missions, farm worker labor camps, independent living centers, and public housing units.
- Discuss the value of integrating a holistic recovery design that connects people to the locations they need to visit such as the pharmacy, grocery store, and healthcare facility or fitness center. Ensure that environmental quality is included in the recovery plan so that future generations are less affected by debris management, pollution, or loss of habitat.[110]
- Advocate that a percentage of all new construction be affordable for the affected community.
- Help maintain a wide range of economic opportunities so that people can earn a living in multiple settings including home-based, small businesses, and large-scale industries. Specify that rebuilt businesses must safeguard those at risk with appropriate mitigation strategies.

DEBRIS

Disasters can generate massive amounts of debris that must be handled according to appropriate environmental controls. Due to concerns about air quality and ozone pollution that could exacerbate chronic respiratory conditions, after Hurricane Hugo in 1989, North Carolina officials sought alternatives to burning large amounts of green waste.[109] Their solution was to convert the downed trees into mulch and firewood. The attacks on September 11, 2001, resulted in multiple types of environmental challenges. Monitoring of both short- and long-term health conditions due to inhalation of contaminated air at the World Trade Center is ongoing.[6,112,114] Increased rates of asthma and a condition known as "World Trade Center cough" have emerged as key health concerns, especially among specific groups such as firefighters, truck drivers, and other debris workers. The U.S. Congress passed the James Zadroga 9/11 Health and Compensation Act in 2011 to provide funding for medical care. The act was named in memory of a first responder who died from debris exposure.

Workers cleaning adjacent locations after 9/11 are an additional population at increased risk for negative health effects. A mobile medical screening project reached out to non-English speaking Hispanic workers without health insurance. These workers had not received personal protective equipment (PPE) or training for hazardous waste contact. Medical staff found persistent symptoms that lingered after discontinuing the work including irritated airways, fatigue, headaches, difficulty sleeping, and dizzy spells.[115] Monitoring day laborers over time became impossible due to their mobility and lack of knowledge about the long-term effects of such exposures. One study of expectant mothers found a possible incidence of lower birth weights and shorter duration of pregnancies.[6] The following are useful strategies to support vulnerable populations in disasters that generate debris:

- Question patients about their exposure to any element of debris including dust that settles inside a home, mold that grows from flood waters, and exposure to hazardous household chemicals or more serious toxic waste. Monitor patients appropriately.
- Ask patients to identify their occupations and note any potential exposure to debris. Screen for temporary work assignments and volunteer activities.
- Identify specific work crews that handle debris and establish a procedure to follow their health and record symptoms for an appropriate duration of time. Pay particular attention to those who lack training and may be hired as day laborers.
- Demand protective equipment and training for all debris workers and contact state and federal authorities to provide oversight at work sites. Ensure workers are educated about the need for PPE.
- Work with medical epidemiologists to gather and analyze debris effects. Include a census of people living, working, or traveling in or through the affected area. Identify populations that may bear disproportionate risk due to exposure, and provide appropriate medical interventions.
- Support healthcare and other organizations that manage people who lack routine access to medical care who may have been exposed to hazardous substances. This includes undocumented workers and the homeless.
- The World Trade Center Health Registry is monitoring 8,148 individuals exposed to the debris and other effects after the terrorist attacks for 20 years. Medical providers should remain informed about the longitudinal consequences of debris exposure.[114,116]
- Provide healthcare information in relevant local languages and at varying literacy levels.[115,117]

PSYCHOLOGICAL

While most people have limited psychological consequences from being involved in a disaster, assessment and monitoring to identify groups at risk is important. In a massive meta-analysis of 60,000 disaster victims, the most common psychological symptoms were depression and anxiety.[18,19] PTSD, a form of anxiety, was relatively low. Nonetheless, it was also clear that certain conditions increased vulnerability to psychological symptoms. Prior trauma has been linked to the development of PTSD. Some studies link gender, race, and ethnicity to higher rates, although it is also believed that severity of exposure exacerbates PTSD. People living in inferior housing, which is more prevalent among some populations such as female-headed households, experience higher levels of exposure to damage and injuries and are therefore more vulnerable. Pre-disaster trauma can also increase the potential for post-disaster trauma (e.g., prior exposure to interpersonal violence). Massive collective loss is also associated with higher rates of trauma, such as when an entire community must relocate or suffers significant harm.[118]

More common psychological responses include trouble sleeping and increased use of alcohol, drugs, and smoking, also associated with pre-disaster use.[117,119] Strong interpersonal relationships, pre-trauma counseling, being embedded in a secure social network, and remaining optimistic about the situation may mitigate negative psychological responses to disasters. Medical personnel can screen patients for risk (alcohol and drug use, nicotine addiction, and intimate partner violence history) and offer information and referrals to local counseling and crisis intervention. In the United States, FEMA funds crisis counseling for disaster survivors.

REESTABLISHING MEDICAL FACILITIES

When the Indian Ocean tsunami struck the community of Nagapattinam in the State of Tamil Nadu in 2004, a local hospital with 56 buildings and 300 patients lay in its path. As local villagers raced into the compound with cries of "water, water," staff and family scrambled to carry patients to higher floors. The waves burst through the neonatal unit, surged into most of the buildings above the height of patient beds, and destroyed valuable medical equipment. This represented a significant loss for an impoverished community. Yet not a single patient or staff member died. Medical staff then moved quickly to try to resuscitate victims outside the facility. The futility of this effort, however, soon became clear. Victims either lived or died; there was little middle ground. Just a few months earlier, the staff had experienced disaster training, albeit not for a tsunami. The training transferred to the new context.

As the waters receded, remaining mud and debris further damaged buildings. Over the following year, medical staff worked with the United Nations Children's Fund (UNICEF) and other nongovernmental organizations to secure funds and rebuild the hospital farther inland. The new hospital required water treatment facilities, a kitchen, beds, x-ray and surgical equipment, and offices. Restoration of services was urgent because the hospital was the only medical facility for hundreds of miles.

Hurricane Katrina caused similar damage to healthcare facilities, including Charity Hospital in New Orleans, a facility for indigent patients that will not reopen. Although some hospital and treatment facilities have opened in the damaged areas, low-income healthcare remains disrupted. Reports of limited service to people with disabilities continued more than 4 years later. To maintain services to vulnerable populations, the following are recommended:

- Develop business continuity plans for a medical facility or office.
- Determine the additional number of disaster survivors who can be added to a patient load (surge capacity) and the costs for those services. Consider a sliding fee or tax to fund those services.
- Develop mutual aid agreements with comparable facilities, including cross-credentialing of staff, so they may work at multiple hospitals.
- Prepare memoranda of understanding with area shelters, congregate facilities, and others to provide continuity of care to these locations.
- Plan medical mission teams with stored supplies and funds prior to the event.
- Develop a staff release plan to send medical personnel to affected areas.
- Join international and national efforts like Disaster Medical Assistance Teams before a disaster strikes; acquire training and plans for deployment.
- Support local emergency management efforts to reduce risks through mitigation, planning, and implementation of risk reduction measures.

CONTINUITY OF CARE

Disasters disrupt multiple community functions, including a wide range of medical services needed by vulnerable populations. Post-Hurricane Katrina reports indicate that not only did hospitals close, but other facilities including clinics, mobile outreach units, dental offices, dialysis centers, and cancer treatment facilities ceased operations. Superstorm Sandy cased evacuation of several medical facilities including ones with women in labor. Both Mount Sinai Medical Center and Memorial Sloan-Kettering Cancer Center in New York had to be evacuated. The Hoboken Medical Center in New Jersey was flooded with significant damage to facilities. In Moore, Oklahoma, the local hospital was directly impacted (Figures 10.3 and 10.4).

Although a situation as extensive as Hurricane Katrina or an EF5 tornado occurs rarely in the United States, it is clear that continuity of care to low-income households suffers. On a global level, there are many populations at risk. To ensure that vulnerable populations maintain continuity of medical care, the following are necessary:

- Ensure that medical records can be easily transferred. This requires a system for protecting and duplicating medical records that can survive the disaster itself.
- Develop a crisis plan to expedite prescription refills, potentially from a distant site.
- Store extra supplies, including prescription medications, in an easy-to-access location for distribution to low-income households, especially seniors on fixed incomes. When people must evacuate, it may be useful to help them reestablish contact with a pharmacy and/or pharmaceutical company assistance program.
- Establish and participate in networks among healthcare organizations, public health agencies, and community-based organizations that connect to vulnerable populations. These include groups who are non-English speaking, homeless, and newly arrived immigrants.
- Contact congregate or similar facilities that may need support due to staff reductions or disruption of supplies. Solicit volunteers (best done through pre-disaster memoranda of

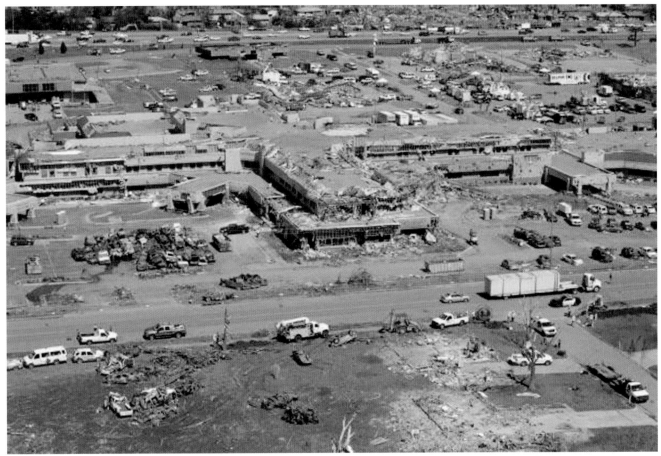

Figure 10.3. Damage to the Moore Medical Center in Oklahoma after the May 2013 Tornado. The center was later demolished. Photo by Jocelyn Augustino, FEMA.

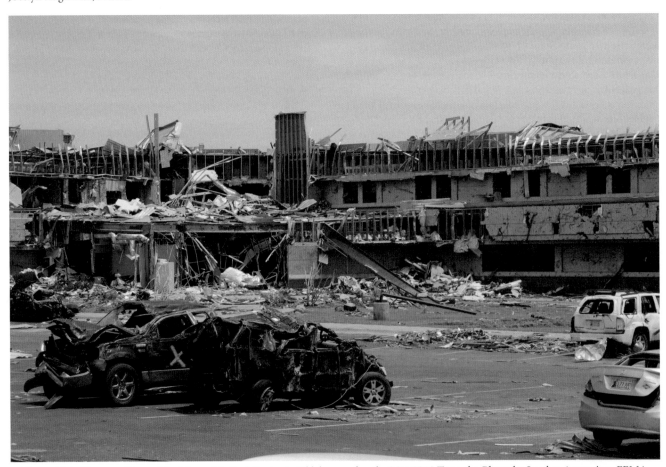

Figure 10.4. Close-up View of the Moore Medical Center in Oklahoma after the May 2013 Tornado. Photo by Jocelyn Augustino, FEMA.

understanding or mutual aid agreements) to serve at veterans' centers, state schools, centers for people with cognitive disabilities, farm worker rest centers, domestic violence centers, adult day care, senior centers, nursing homes, and similar locations. Offer free screening or testing for basic healthcare needs.

■ If healthcare facilities are established during a disaster (including points of distribution for medications for patients exposed to bioterrorism agents or mass vaccination centers), be sure that locations are accessible to people with disabilities, seniors, and others. Offer childcare to encourage single parents to present for medical care.

■ Work with and train shelter staff to identify and assist people experiencing a disruption in healthcare services, including those requiring dialysis, cancer treatment, or HIV management. Plan how to assist these shelter residents prior to the event, particularly those distant from their usual healthcare providers.

■ Be aware that most donations and acts of volunteerism occur during the response period, while the bulk of human needs occur through the extended recovery period.

Mitigation

Mitigation is defined as "sustained action taken to reduce or eliminate the risk to human life and property from hazards."[120] Mitigation can be divided into two main types, structural and nonstructural mitigation. Structural mitigation measures target the built environment and might include shatter-resistant glass in nursing homes, elevating homes above anticipated flood levels, securing bookcases and filing cabinets to the wall to avoid injuries during an earthquake, and safe rooms. Nonstructural mitigation measures include land-use management that disallows development in floodplains or building codes that increase roof resistance to high-velocity winds. Medical offices should create protective action plans for the range of local hazards that could affect patients and staff including ways to help staff affected by the disaster and ways to transport them to patient care facilities.

Medical facilities can be hardened to withstand local hazards and ensure continuity of care. By working with architects and engineers, additional strengthening can be added to secure roofs, retrofit walls for local risks, and prevent projectiles and debris from penetrating windows and doors. To reduce risks to life safety, FEMA recommends that facilities prevent loss of power through purchasing and locating generators in areas safe from hazards and by developing a generator operations plan. Securing medical facilities gives vulnerable populations a greater chance of having access to critical services. Nonstructural mitigation measures would include code compliance, purchasing hazard-specific insurance, and identifying alternate locations for continuing operations should a disaster affect offices and facilities. Avoiding downtime for the facility and reducing the costs of displacement can protect a medical business.

Medical professionals can also support local efforts to safeguard those at higher risk. Trailer parks, which usually house low-income households, rarely offer congregate safe room locations from tornados. Other congregate settings are likewise ill-prepared, a situation that can be improved through supporting new building codes and local land-use planning. In 2008, FEMA funded a grant to the American Red Cross of Baldwin County in the U.S. state of Georgia for construction of the first congregate safe room for people with special needs. The Hazard Mitigation Grant Program provided $3.2 million USD for a 430-person shelter facility. In addition, the grant provided funds to retrofit the Laundry and Life Skills Training Center to increase the capacity of the roof to withstand 320-kph winds. This structural mitigation project protects a previously at-risk population and should be duplicated widely.

Other locations can benefit from mitigation measures that alert people to danger. Sirens, alarms, lighted strobes, vibrating devices, pagers, wireless devices, tactile signs, and evacuation devices can be installed in any workplace including a medical office, home health agency, dialysis center, hospital, or personal home. Physical barriers can be removed to allow for egress by those in wheelchairs and evacuation devices can be purchased and installed pre-event (an extensive list of disability-specific devices can be seen at the Job Accommodation Network[119]).[121] Medical associations should consider partnering with civic organizations to secure funding for placement of such devices in private homes and congregate facilities.

Finally, the time period immediately after a disaster is sometimes referred to by emergency managers as the "window of opportunity." This phrase means that the opportunity exists to introduce measures that reduce further risk during this period. After the 2004 Indian Ocean tsunami, for example, many nations expressed concern about massive epidemics resulting from the many cadavers. Although most researchers suggest that such outbreaks are extremely unlikely, the concern prompted a public health opportunity. Across the affected area within India, both governmental and nongovernmental organizations vaccinated tens of thousands of survivors against cholera, typhoid, hepatitis A, and dysentery.

Emerging Policies and Practices

Several policies and practices have emerged since Hurricane Katrina in the U.S. The U.S. Department of Transportation is developing additional plans for highway evacuation. The Federal Highway Administration is producing guidance for transportation of people with disabilities that provides advice for evacuation of congregate facilities. FEMA, following a lawsuit (Brou v. FEMA),[120,122] is continuing to integrate people with disabilities and disability organizations into their policies and programs and making temporary housing accessible. The National Disaster Housing Strategy and Plan (http://www.fema.gov/national-disaster-housing-strategy-resource-center) acknowledges the valuable partnership that can occur with disability organizations, especially at the state level. The National Council on Disability investigates emergency preparedness issues. Minutes of its quarterly meetings are available on its website.[119,122] In 2013, FEMA's Incident Management Cadre of On-Call Response/Recovery Employees (CORE) Program created disability integration advisors who will serve as reservists by assisting citizens and first responders during disasters or emergency situations. These disability integration advisor reservists will assist in the coordination and integration of persons with disabilities during response and recovery of affected communities.

RECOMMENDATIONS FOR FURTHER RESEARCH

Extensive research remains necessary on vulnerable populations, a circumstance that has not changed significantly since the previous edition of this chapter. More specifically, a number of research questions carry implications for medical professionals. Future research might focus on:

- How various jurisdictions develop, use, and share registries, including the challenges of maintenance and confidentiality.
- Studies of "na-tech" or combined natural and technological events for their impacts on higher-risk populations (such as Fukushima).
- Medical support during the evacuation of residents using general transportation resources including buses, paratransit vehicles, and caravans in a cross-cultural context.
- The development and implementation of checklists and forms usable during life histories to assess risk and document disaster-related health issues.
- Identification of the most effective strategies for keeping families, guardians, and caregivers together during evacuation, sheltering, and return to the home.
- The ways in which disasters create newly vulnerable populations, such as the number of amputations that generated new disabilities from the Haiti earthquake.
- The effects of climate change on vulnerable populations and the communities in which they live.
- Loss of healthcare facilities for low-income households, senior citizens, and people with disabilities, how they regain access, and how communities restore such services.
- The type of medical outreach services most commonly needed for marginalized populations after a disaster and the duration of time those services must be provided (from routine procedures like annual examinations to more detailed care).
- Analysis of communication tools for a full range of vulnerable populations as used by medical professionals.
- The critical role of home health agencies, senior centers, agencies on aging, and others in reaching the homebound with disaster information including pandemics. Comparative research is essential in this area.
- The critical role of the case manager in insuring that vulnerable populations have access to appropriate medical care and health-related supports. Studies of appropriate ways to train and support case managers for long-term commitments and to avoid burnout would be essential.
- The assessment of functional needs and medical shelters, from intake procedures to discharge, and all dimensions of service from routine patient care to medical emergencies, staffing, and logistics, and into recovery of permanent housing.
- The most expedient routes for provision of healthcare access to immigrant populations after disasters, as well as the kinds of healthcare concerns that most commonly arise.
- Improving knowledge about some racial and ethnic groups in disasters, such as Native Americans. Within the Native American population, additional issues may surface such as how elders fare in disasters and whether the impact of proximity to hazardous wastes, newly appearing diseases such as the hantavirus, or long-term exposure to occupational hazards has an effect.
- Comprehensive examinations that span the life cycle of disasters: preparedness, response, recovery, and mitigation.
- Case studies of effective partnerships that span vulnerable populations, engage the broader community, and leverage resources to address unmet healthcare needs after disasters.

- Ways in which medical care providers can participate on long-term recovery committees, which usually address unmet and functional access needs across affected communities.
- Psychological effects of disasters on medical personnel including secondary trauma or compassion fatigue that may result from working with survivors.
- Successful mitigation strategies for a full range of medical facilities including those in developing nations. The loss of medical facilities and medical staff after the 2010 Haiti earthquake serves as an important reminder of their value to a community post-disaster.

Conclusion

Whether involved with public education, emergency response, long-term recovery, or risk reduction, the medical community can support efforts to aid vulnerable populations. From a social vulnerability perspective, risk reduction requires more than healthcare, accessible shelters, or construction assistance. As international disaster humanitarian Fred Cuny wrote, "Vulnerability reduction is ultimately a social problem that requires a lifetime commitment."[122] Civic involvement is necessary to address continuing problems including a lack of affordable and safe housing, intimate partner violence, pollution and environmental degradation, access to jobs, language prejudice, racial discrimination, and exclusionary practices. Such involvement will ultimately reduce risks. By participating in efforts that address public housing issues, promote literacy, reduce intimate partner violence, increase healthcare access, conserve floodplains, retrofit low-income housing, and reach out to new immigrants, society can create more disaster-resilient communities. In the interim, those interested in vulnerable populations can educate patients and providers, secure important facilities, design outreach efforts, partner with other community and advocacy organizations, and be part of the cadre of people dedicated to increasing life safety for all.

Resources

- FEMA offers a variety of training materials, including free online courses (downloadable and interactive) and on-campus courses at its Emergency Management Institute (EMI) location. A list of courses can be obtained from www.fema.gov. From the independent study (IS) course list, select the FEMA IS197 course.
- NOD offers downloadable resources at its Emergency Preparedness Initiative page at https://www.ncd.gov/.
- The National Council on Disability is generating a series of reviews on all phases of emergency management; www.ncd.gov contains updates and copies of minutes from the quarterly meetings.
- The Gender and Disaster Network provides extensive materials including those that apply worldwide at www.gdnonline.org.
- FEMA and the Humane Society offer tips for protecting pets and service animals at www.fema.gov and www.hsus.org.
- FEMA for Kids provides games and downloadable materials at http://www.ready.gov/kids.
- The American Red Cross offers a "Master of Disaster" curriculum that is tied to school content at www.redcross.org.
- Buddy assessments and emergency kit information can be secured in multiple languages at www.preparenow.org.

- A set of papers that include content on vulnerable populations is available at http://understandingkatrina.ssrc.org.
- A large bibliography on social vulnerability can be found along with college course materials at the FEMA Higher Education Website at http://www.training.fema.gov/EMIweb/edu/collegelist
- Project REDD: Research and Education on Disability and Disaster provides an annotated bibliography of research articles on disability and disaster, as well as several products that support individuals with disabilities and their families impacted by disasters at redd.tamu.edu.
- American Health Care Association forms and checklists for home health agencies (Florida) and adult day care facilities, assisted living facilities, ambulatory surgical care centers, hospice centers, and hospitals per Florida statute can be found at http://ahca.myflorida.com/MCHQ/Corebill.
- Educational materials for seniors and people with disabilities can be viewed at www.eadassociates.com. These materials are in the form of "wheels" that can be dialed to reveal hazard-specific preparedness information.
- The 2011 Tōhoku Earthquake and Tsunami is revealed from the perspective of a hospital evacuation in this documentary: http://www.youtube.com/watch?v=cfsevdMsfHg.
- An extensive bibliography on Hurricane Katrina can be accessed at http://lamar.colostate.edu/~loripeek/Katrina Bibliography.pdf.

REFERENCES

1. Thomas, et al. *Social Vulnerability to Disasters*. Boca Raton, FL, CRC Press, 2013.
2. Kailes JI, Enders A. Moving beyond "special needs": A function-based framework for emergency management and planning. *J Disab Pol Studies* 2007; 17(4): 230–237.
3. Fisher S. *Gender based violence in Sri Lanka in the after-math of the 2004 tsunami crisis*. Master's Thesis. United Kingdom, University of Leeds, 2005.
4. Fisher S. Sri Lankan women's organisations responding to post-tsunami violence. In: Enarson E, Chakrabarti P, eds. *Women, gender and disaster: Global issues and initiatives*. New Delhi, Sage Publications Limited India, 2009.
5. Phillips B, Hewett P. Home alone: disasters, mass emergencies and children in self-care. *J Emerg Manage* 2005; 3(2): 31–35.
6. Landrigan P. Health and environmental consequences of the World Trade Center disaster. *Environ Health Perspect* 2004; 112(6): 731–739.
7. National Organization on Disability. *Special Needs Assessment for Katrina Evacuees*. Washington, DC, National Organization on Disability, 2005.
8. American Medical Association. Nearly 1000 People Killed by Hurricane Katrina in Louisiana. http://www.amaassn.org/ama/pub/category/print/20035.html (Accessed January 10, 2009).
9. Sharkey P. Survival and death in New Orleans: an empirical look at the human impact of Katrina. *J Black Studies* 2007; 37(4): 482–501.
10. Laska S. What if Hurricane Ivan had not missed New Orleans? *Natural Hazards Observer* 2004; 1.
11. Tanigawa K, Hosoi Y, Hirohashi N, Iwasaki Y, Kamiya K. Loss of life after evacuation: lessons learned from the Fukushima accident. *Lancet*. March 10, 2012; 379(9819): 889–891.
12. Mitchell L. Guidelines for emergency managers working with culturally and linguistically diverse communities. *Aust J Emerg Manage* 2003; 18(1): 13–18.
13. Enarson E. Social Vulnerability Course. FEMA. http://www.fema.gov (Accessed September 30, 2008).
14. Wisner B. Development of Vulnerability Analysis. FEMA. http://www.fema.gov (Accessed September 30, 2008).
15. Arslan S, Atalay A, Gokce-Kutsal Y. Drug use in older people. *J Am Geriatr Soc* 2002; 50(6): 1163–1164.
16. Flanagan BE, Gregory EW, Hallisey EJ, Heitgerd JL, Lewis B. A social vulnerability index for disaster management. *J Homeland Security Emerg Manage* 2011; 8(1): 1–22.
17. McGuire LC, Ford ES, Okoro CA. Natural disasters and older US adults with disabilities: Implications for evacuation. *Disasters* 2007; 31(1): 49–56.
18. Friedsam H. Older persons as disaster casualties. *J Health Hum Behav* 1970; 1(4): 269–273.
19. Norris F, Friedman M, Watson P. 60000 disaster victims speak: Part II. *Psychiatry* 2002; 65(3): 240–260.
20. Norris F, Friedman M, Watson P, Byrne C, Diaz E, Kaniasty K. 60000 disaster victims speak: Part I. *Psychiatry* 2002; 65(3): 207–239.
21. Bourque LB, Siegel JM, Kano M, Wood, MM. Weathering the storm: The impact of hurricanes on physical and mental health. *Annals Amer Academy* 2006; 604: 129–151.
22. Lindell MK, Perry RW. *Communicating Risk in Multiethnic Communities*. Thousand Oaks, CA, Sage, 2004.
23. Prince-Embury S, Rooney JF. Psychological symptoms of residents in the aftermath of the Three Mile Island accident and restart. *J Soc Psychol* 1988; 128(6): 779–790.
24. Bell BD, Kara G, Batterson C. Service utilization and adjustment patterns of elderly tornado victims in an American disaster. *Mass Emergencies* 1978; 3: 71–81.
25. Poulshock S, Cohen E. The elderly in the aftermath of disaster. *Gerontologist* 1975; 15(4): 357–361.
26. Baylor College of Medicine, American Medical Association. *Recommendations for Best Practices in the Management of Elderly Disaster Victims*. Houston, TX, Baylor College of Medicine, 2006.
27. Peek L, Stough LM. Children with disabilities in the context of disaster: A social vulnerability perspective. *Child Dev* 2010; 81(4): 1260–1270.
28. Peek L, Fothergill A. Displacement, gender, and the challenges of parenting after Hurricane Katrina. *National Women's Studies Association Journal* 2008; 20(3): 69–105.
29. Weber LP, Peek L. *Displaced*. Austin, University of Texas Press, 2012.
30. Peek L, Fothergill A. *Reconstructing Childhood: An Exploratory Study of Children in Hurricane Katrina*. Boulder, CO, Natural Hazards Center, 2006.
31. Fothergill A, Peek L. Surviving catastrophe: a study of children in hurricane Katrina. In: Center NH, ed. *Learning from Catastrophe*. Boulder, CO, Natural Hazards Center, 2006; 97–129.
32. Pfefferbaum B, Call J, Sconzo G. Mental health services for children in the first two years after the 1995 Oklahoma City terrorist bombing. *Psychiatry Serv* 1999; 50(7): 956–958.
33. Fairbrother G, Stuber J, Galea S, Pfefferbaum B, Fleischman A. Unmet need for counseling services by children in New York City after the September 11th attacks on the World Trade Center: implications for pediatricians. *Pediatrics* 2004; 113(5): 1367–1374.
34. Delica ZG. Balancing vulnerability and capacity: women and children in the Philippines. In: Enarson E, Morrow BH, eds. *The*

Gendered Terrain of Disaster. Miami, FL, International Hurricane Center, 2000; 109–113.

35. Stratton SJ. Cholera in Haiti: Redefining emergency public health philosophy. *Prehosp and Disaster Med* 28(3): 195–196.

36. McAdams DE, Stough LM. Exploring the support role of special education teachers after Hurricane Ike: Children with significant disabilities. *J Fam Issues* 2011; 32: 1325–1345.

37. Heinz Center. *Human Links to Coastal Disasters*. Washington, DC, The Heinz Center, 2002.

38. Daley WR, Brown S, Archer P, Kruger E, Jordan F, Batts D, et al. Risk of tornado-related death and injury in Oklahoma, May 3, 1999. *American Journal of Epidemiology* 2005; 161(2): 1144–1150.

39. Comerio M. *The Impact of Housing Losses in the Northridge Earthquake: Recovery and Reconstruction Issues*. Berkeley, Institute of Urban and Regional Development, University of California-Berkeley, 1996.

40. Fothergill A, Maestas EGM, Darlington JD. Race, ethnicity and disasters in the United States: a review of the literature. *Disasters* 1999; 23(2): 156–173.

41. Legates DR, Biddle MD. *Warning Response and Risk Behavior in the Oak Grove-Birmingham, Alabama Tornado of 8 April 1998*. Boulder, CO, Natural Hazards Center, 1999.

42. U.S. Census. 2010. http://www.census.gov/2010census (Accessed August 11, 2015).

43. Santos-Hernandez J., Hearn Morrow B. Language and Literacy. In Thomas D, et al. *Social Vulnerability to Disasters*. Boca Raton, FL, CRC Press, 2013; 265–280.

44. Aguirre BE, Anderson WA, Balandran S, Peters BE, White HM. *Saragosa, Texas, Tornado May 22, 1987: An Evaluation of the Warning System*. Washington, DC, National Academies Press, 1991.

45. Cutter S. The geography of social vulnerability: race, class and catastrophe. Social Sciences Research Council. http://understandingkatrina.ssrc.org/Cutter/printable.html (Accessed January 11, 2009).

46. Bolin R., Stanford, L. Shelter, housing and recovery: A comparison of U.S. disasters. *Disasters* 1991; 15: 24–34.

47. Oxfam. *The Tsunami's Impact on Women*. London, Oxfam International, 2001.

48. Noel G. The role of women in health-related aspects of emergency management: a Caribbean perspective. In: Enarson E, Morrow BH, eds. *The Gendered Terrain of Disaster*. Miami, FL, International Hurricane Center, 2000: 213–219.

49. World Health Organization. Chernobyl's legacy: Health, environmental and socio-economic impacts. 2nd revised version. 2006. http://www.who.int/ionizing_radiation/chernobyl/chernobyl_digest_report_EN.pdf (Accessed June 26, 2013).

50. Enarson E, Morrow BH. Why gender? Why women? An introduction to women and disaster. In: Enarson E, Morrow B, eds. *The Gendered Terrain of Disaster*. Miami, FL, International Hurricane Center, 2000; 1–9.

51. Enarson E, Phillips B. Invitation to a new feminist disaster sociology. In: Phillips B, Morrow B, eds. *Women and Disasters: From Theory to Practice*. Philadelphia, PA, Xlibris, International Research Committee on Disasters, 2008; 41–74.

52. Phillips B, Morrow BH. What's gender got to do with it? In: Phillips B, Morrow B, eds. *Women and Disasters: From Theory to Practice*. Philadelphia, PA, Xlibris, International Research Committee on Disasters, 2008; 27–40.

53. Enarson E. What women do: gendered labor in the Red River Valley flood. *Environ Hazards* 2001; 3: 1–18.

54. Enarson E, Morrow B. A gendered perspective: the voices of women. In: Peacock W, Morrow B, Gladwin H, eds. *Hurricane Andrew*. Miami, FL, International Hurricane Center, 2000; 116–140.

55. Toscani L. Women's roles in natural disaster preparation and aid: a Central American view. In: Enarson E, Morrow BH, eds. *The Gendered Terrain of Disaster*. Miami, FL, International Hurricane Center, 2000; 207–211.

56. National Council on Disability. The Impact of Hurricanes Katrina and Rita on People with Disabilities: A Look Back and Remaining Challenges. 2006. http://www.ncd.gov/policy/emergency_management (Accessed July 8, 2013).

57. Rooney C, White GW. Narrative analysis of a disaster preparedness emergency response survey from persons with mobility impairments. *J Disab Pol Studies* 2007; 17(4): 206–215.

58. White GW, Fox MH, Rooney C, Cahill A. *Assessing the impact of Hurricane Katrina on persons with disabilities*. Lawrence, The University of Kansas, Research and Training Center on Independent Living, 2007.

59. National Organization on Disability. Harris Survey Data. 2006. http://nod.org/about_us/our_history/annual_reports/2006_annual_report (Accessed July 8, 2013).

60. Brodie M, Weltzien E, Altman D, Blendon RJ, Benson JM. Experiences of Hurricane Katrina evacuees in Houston shelters: Implications for future planning. *Am J Public Health* 2006; 96(8): 1402–1408.

61. National Research Council. *Facing Hazards and Disasters: Understanding Human Dimensions*. Washington, DC, The National Academies Press, 2006.

62. Rooney C, White GW. Narrative analysis of disaster preparedness emergency response survey from persons with mobility impairments. *J Disab Policy Studies* 2007; 17(4): 206–215.

63. National Organization on Disability. Harris Survey Data. http://nod.citysoft.org/index.cfm?fuseaction=page.viewPage&PageID=1565&C:\CFusion8\verity\Data\dummy.txt (Accessed January 11, 2009).

64. U.S. National Response Framework. FEMA. http://www.fema.gov/national-response-framework (Accessed August 21, 2013).

65. Twigg J, Kett M, Bottomley H, Tan LT, Nasreddin H. Disability and public shelter in emergencies. *Environ Hazards* 2011; 10: 248–261.

66. The Federal Register. Executive Order 13347 – Individuals With Disabilities in Emergency Preparedness, July 26, 2004. http://www.hhs.gov/ocr/civilrights/resources/specialtopics/emergencypre/eo13347disabilitiesemergencypreparedness.pdf (Accessed August 11, 2015).

67. Phillips B, Morrow B. Social vulnerability, forecasts and warnings. *Natural Hazards Rev* 2007; 8(3): 61–68.

68. Stough LM, Sharp AN, Decker C, Wilker N. Disaster case management and individuals with disabilities. *Rehabil Psychol* 2010; 55(3): 211–220.

69. Wood V, Weisman R. A hole in the weather warning system. *Am Meteorol Soc* 2003; 84(2): 187–194.

70. Hendricks T. Bay Area report: 112 languages spoken in diverse region. *San Francisco Chronicle*. March 14, 2005.

71. Government Accountability Office. *Transportation-Disadvantaged Populations*. Washington, DC, GAO, 2003.

72. McGuire LC, Ford ES, Ajani UA. Cognitive functioning as a predictor of functional disability in later life. *Am J Geriatr Psychiatry* 2006; 14(1): 36–42.

73. Eldar R. The needs of elderly persons in natural disasters. *Disasters* 2007; 16(4): 355–358.

74. Fernandez L, Byard D, Lin C-C, Benson S, Barbera J. Frail elderly as disaster victims. *Prehosp Disaster Med* 2002; 17(2): 76–74.

75. National Council on Disability. Effective emergency management: Making improvements for communities and people with disabilities. 2009. http://www.ncd.gov/policy/emergency_management (Retrieved July 8, 2013).

76. Christensen KM, Collins SD, Holt JM, Phillips CN. The relationship between the design of the built environment and the ability to egress of individuals with disabilities. *Rev Disab Studies* 2006; 2(3): 24–34.

77. Peek L. Becoming Muslim. *Sociol Religion* 2005; 66(3): 215–242.

78. Hoefer M, Riytani N, Campbell C. *Estimates of the unauthorized immigrant population residing in the United States.* Department of Homeland Security Office of Immigration Statistics, January 2006.

79. Stough LM, Villarreal E, Castillo LG. Disaster and social vulnerability: The case of undocumented Mexican migrant workers. In Rivera JD, Miller DS. *Minority resiliency and the legacy of disaster.* New York, Edwin Mellen Press, 2010; 297–315.

80. Navarrette R. Relatively safe refuge. *Hispanic Magazine* December/January 2008; 18.

81. Office of Rural Health Policy. Rural communities and emergency preparedness. 2002. ftp://ftp.hrsa.gov/ruralhealth/ruralpreparedness.pdf (Accessed July, 8, 2013).

82. Quiram BJ, Carpender K, Pennel C. The Texas Training Initiative for Emergency Response (T-TIER): An effective learning to prepare the broader audience of health professionals, *Journal of Public Health Management and Practice* November 2005; S83–S89.

83. Center for Rural Health Practice. Rural health preparedness: What all rural health responders must know about public health emergencies. 2004. http://www.cphp.pitt.edu/upcphp/crhp_textbook.pdf (Accessed July 8, 2013).

84. Tierney KJ, Lindell MK, Perry RW. *Facing the Unexpected: Disaster Preparedness and Response in the U.S.* Washington, DC, Joseph Henry Press, 2001.

85. National Academy of Sciences. *Disaster Resilience: a national imperative.* Washington DC, National Academies, 2012.

86. Pfefferbaum RL, Brand M, Elledge, BL. *Building Community Resilience to Disasters.* Presentation at the National Voluntary Organizations Active in Disaster Conference, Albuquerque, NM, April 2007.

87. Federal Emergency Management Agency. Robert T. Stafford Disaster Relief and Emergency Assistance Act, as amended, and Related Authorities. Public Law 93–288, as amended 42 U.S.C. 5121–5207, and Related Authorities. June 2007.

88. Americans with Disabilities Amendment Act. Public Law 110–325, 122 Stat. 3553. 2008.

89. Federal Emergency Management Agency. Developing and maintaining emergency operations plans. Comprehensive preparedness guide 101. 2010. http://www.fema.gov/pdf/about/divisions/npd/CPG_101_V2.pdf8 (Accessed July 8, 2013).

90. Homeland Security. National Preparedness Report. March 2013. http://www.fema.gov/national-preparedness-report (Accessed on July 9, 2013).

91. Phillips B, Mwarumba N, Wagner D. The Role of the Trained Volunteer. In: Cole L, Connell N, eds. *Local Planning for Terror and Disaster: From Bioterrorism to Earthquakes.* Hoboken, NJ, Wiley and Sons, 2012.

92. Hewett PL, Jr. *Organizational networks and emergence during disaster preparedness: The case of an emergency assistance registry.* Doctoral dissertation. Stillwater, Oklahoma State University, 2013.

93. Metz W, Hewett P, Muzzarelli J, Tanzman E. Identifying Special Needs Households that Need Assistance for Emergency Planning. *Intl J Mass Emerg Disasters* 2002; 20(2): 255–281.

94. Willigen MV. Riding out the storm. *Natural Hazards Rev* 2002; 3(3): 98–106.

95. Jenkins P, Phillips BD. Battered women, catastrophe and the context of safety. *NWSA J* 2008; 20(3): 49–68.

96. U.S. Government Accountability Office. Emergency alerting: Capabilities have improved, but additional guidance and testing and needed. April 2013. http://www.gao.gov/assets/660/654135.pdf (Accessed July 8, 2013).

97. FEMA. Alerting the whole community: Removing barriers to alerting accessibility. Integrated Public Alert and Warning System. 2013/2014. http://www.fema.gov/library/viewRecord.do?id=7762 (Accessed July 8, 2013).

98. U.S. Government Accountability Office. Emergency alerting: Capabilities have improved, but additional guidance and testing and needed. April 2013. http://www.gao.gov/assets/660/654135.pdf (Accessed July 8, 2013).

99. Perry RW, Lindell MK. Aged citizens in the warning phase of disasters: Re-examining the evidence. *Int Journal Aging Hum Dev* 1997; 44(4): 257–267.

100. Lafond R. Emergency planning for the elderly. *Emerg Prep Digest* 1987; 15–21.

101. Vanderheiden GC. Designing for people with functional limitations resulting from disability, aging, or circumstance. In: Salvendy G, ed., *Handbook of human factors and ergonomics.* 2nd ed. New York, NY: Wiley, 1997; 2010–2052.

102. U.S. Department of Justice. 2013. http://www.ada.gov/pcatoolkit/chap7emergencymgmt.htm (Accessed August 21, 2013).

103. Webb G, Tierney K, Dahlhamer J. Businesses and disasters. *Natural Hazards Rev* 2000; 1(3): 83–90.

104. Florida Department of Health. *Resource Guide for Special Needs Shelters.* Tallahassee, FL, Florida Department of Health, 2006.

105. Mileti D. *Disasters by Design.* Washington, DC, Joseph Henry Press, 1999.

106. Nakagawa Y, Shaw R. Social capital: a missing link to disaster recovery. *Intl J Mass Emerg Disasters* 2004; 22(1): 5–34.

107. Uphoff N. *Understanding Social Capital.* Washington, DC, The World Bank, 2000.

108. Natural Hazards Center. *Holistic Disaster Recovery.* Boulder, CO, Natural Hazards Center, 2001.

109. Steuteville R. Hugo sets an example. *BioCycle* 1992; 33: 1030–1033.

110. Centers for Disease Control and Prevention. Self-reported increase in asthma severity after the September 11 attacks on the World Trade Center. *MMWR* 2002; 51: 781–784.

111. Lin S. Respiratory symptoms and other health effects among residents living near the World Trade Center. *Am J Epidemiol* 2005; 162(16): 499–507.

112. Szema A. Clinical deterioration in pediatric asthmatic patients after September 11, 2001. *J Allerg Clin Immunol* 2004; 113: 420–426.

113. Malievskaya E. Assessing the health of immigrant workers near ground zero. *Am J Indust Med* 2002; 42(6): 548–549.

114. http://nyc.gov/html/doh/html/wtc/html/registry/registry.shtml (Accessed January 12, 2009).

115. Santos-Hernandez J, Hearn Morrow B. Language and Literacy. In: Thomas DSK et al., eds. *Social Vulnerability to Disasters.* Boca Raton, FL, CRC Press, 2013; 265–280.

116. Erikson K. *Everything in its Path.* New York, Simon and Schuster, 1976.

117. North CS, Kawaskai A, Spitznagel EL, Hong BA. The course of PTSD, major depression, substance abuse, and somatization after a natural disaster. *J Nerv Ment Dis* 2004; 192(12): 823–829.

118. Godschalk DR. Mitigation. In: Waugh W, Tierney K, eds. *Emergency Management: Practice and Principles for Local Government.* 2nd ed. Washington DC, ICMA Press, 2007; 89–112.

119. Job Accommodation Network. 2013. http://askjan.org (Accessed August 21, 2013).

120. Brou v. FEMA. 2013. http://www.nclej.org/pdf/BrouSettlement .pdf (Accessed August 21, 2013).

121. National Council on Disability. www.ncd.gov (Accessed October 15, 2008).

122. Cuny F. *Disasters and Development.* Dallas, TX, Intertech, 1983.

PART II
OPERATIONAL ISSUES

11

PUBLIC HEALTH AND EMERGENCY MANAGEMENT SYSTEMS

Connie J. Boatright-Royster and Peter W. Brewster

OVERVIEW

Introduction

Emergency management and public health addresses broad systems, components, and practices. An increased focus on concepts such as risk, risk reduction, and resilience has emerged over the past few years. From a global perspective, this has influenced how we view the roles and responsibilities of those who lead and are involved in these fields. The focus has also expanded considerably to include not just traditional "systems," but individuals and communities who, through their actions, are integral elements of the comprehensive emergency management and public health paradigm.

Disasters and the resultant impacts on population health are increasing in frequency and severity in the United States and globally. This chapter examines challenges to emergency management and public health systems in their combined quest to reduce the impacts from health disasters. A health disaster is a precipitous or gradual decline in the overall health status of a community, for which the community is unable to cope without outside assistance.[1]

In the last decade, public health and emergency management systems and practices have become more integrated, likely improving their effectiveness. Included in this chapter are examples of efforts to successfully impact population health outcomes. The chapter concludes with recommendations for improvements in processes to include evidence-based, data-driven monitoring and analysis of disaster trends and their impact on population health. Such assessments are vital in measuring the true effectiveness of emergency management and public health systems.

What Are Emergency Management and Public Health Systems?

In addressing disasters, an emergency management program or system promotes the comprehensive approach of: 1) mitigation (reducing or eliminating impacts from hazards by increasing resiliency); 2) preparedness (building the capacity of organizations to respond to the impacts from hazards); 3) response (acutely reducing or eliminating the impacts from hazards);

and 4) recovery (remediating the impacts from hazards). This is achieved through the full integration of government, the private and non-profit sectors, and the public. As such, "emergency management" is the science of managing complex systems and multidisciplinary personnel to address emergencies and disasters across all hazards, and through the phases of mitigation, preparedness, response, and recovery.[2]

Comprehensive Emergency Management (CEM) is a conceptual framework developed in 1978 by the National Governor's Association that encompasses all hazards and all levels of government (including the private sector). It includes the four phases of mitigation, preparedness, response, and recovery. When the Federal Emergency Management Agency (FEMA) was created in 1980, it used CEM as the basis for its "all-hazards" policy platform. FEMA introduced the Integrated Emergency Management System (IEMS) as a process that could be used to develop CEM programs. The IEMS process included these steps: 1) assessment of the current program status through an audit and the establishment of goals and priorities; 2) an appraisal of hazards including weapons of mass destruction (WMD) and the primary and secondary effects (needs assessment); 3) mitigation activities designed to reduce the effects of those hazards; 4) the development of capabilities (preparedness activities of staff education, planning, training, exercises, and purchase of equipment and supplies); 5) emergency operations (response and recovery); 6) identification of shortfalls in capability (evaluation activities including after-action critiques from exercises or actual events providing the feedback loop to unmet preparedness issues); and 7) a multi-year development plan to guide the overall mitigation, preparedness, response, and recovery activities. The multi-year development plan is reviewed annually and its work increment guided by goals, objectives, and strategies.

With the advent of homeland security after the terrorism experienced in the United States in 2001, changes were made to the structure of traditional emergency management policy (the "four phases" of emergency management). Homeland Security Presidential Directive 8, National Preparedness (2003) introduced the phase of "prevention" and Presidential Policy Directive 8 (2011) updated the HSPD with the purpose to strengthen the security and resilience of the United States through an

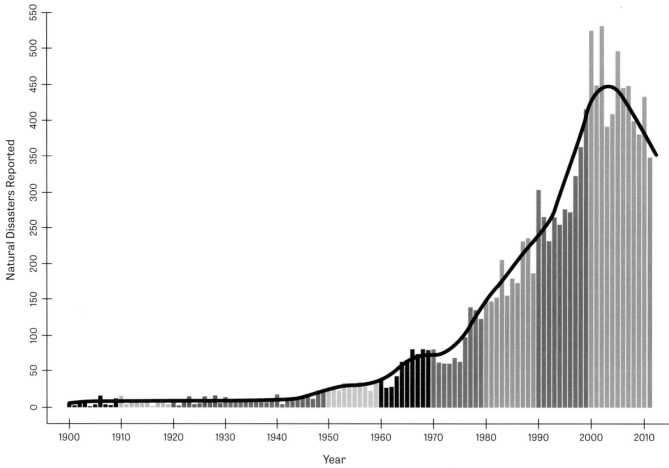

Figure 11.1. Natural disasters reported, 1900–2011.[5]

integrated, nationwide, capability-based approach. A set of "core capabilities" that address the five mission areas that define homeland security and emergency management program activity include: prevention, protection, mitigation, response, and recovery. While the five mission areas may seem to be a departure from the classic "mitigation, preparedness, response, and recovery" orientation, they represent greater unity in the United States between emergency management, law enforcement, public health, business continuity, and social services communities.

"Public health" refers to all organized measures, public or private, to prevent disease, promote health, and prolong life among the whole population. Its activities aim to provide conditions in which people can be healthy and that focus on populations, not on individuals or diseases. Public health is concerned with the total system, not just eradication of a particular disease. Public health's primary functions are:

■ Assessment and monitoring of the health of communities and populations at risk to identify health problems and priorities.
■ Public policies to solve local and national health problems and address priorities.
■ Assurance that all populations have access to appropriate, cost-effective care, including health promotion and disease prevention services.[3]

Disaster health is a term that encompasses the health and medical disciplines and organizations that support the overall management of disasters. These include governmental public health, public and private healthcare delivery including Emergency Medical Services (EMS), and governmental emergency management.[4] Effective emergency management and public health system planning and intervention rely on current and relevant disaster data and information, including reporting on the magnitude, frequency and trends associated with disasters. Disasters are occurring more frequently, as reflected in Figure 11.1, which illustrates reported global natural disasters over the period from 1900 to 2000. Although there is occasional waning, depicted by period with fewer reported disasters, the upward trend over time is evident.

Has There Been an Increase in Risk and Vulnerability of Society to Disasters?

As data and information become available, trends and patterns emerge that are applied as planning assumptions, providing direction for emergency management and public health systems. Table 11.1 depicts trends resulting in increased disaster risk and vulnerability. Although the cited trends address the United States, they are globally applicable as well.

Table 11.1. Trends resulting in increased disaster risk and vulnerability[6]

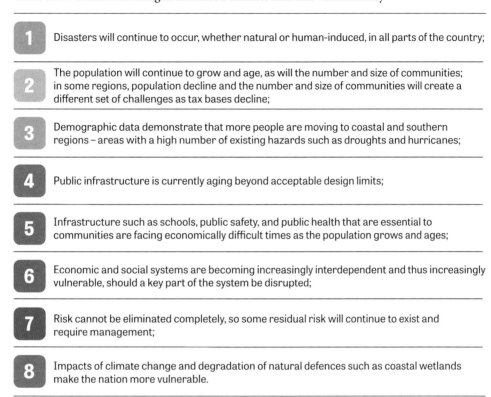

1	Disasters will continue to occur, whether natural or human-induced, in all parts of the country;
2	The population will continue to grow and age, as will the number and size of communities; in some regions, population decline and the number and size of communities will create a different set of challenges as tax bases decline;
3	Demographic data demonstrate that more people are moving to coastal and southern regions – areas with a high number of existing hazards such as droughts and hurricanes;
4	Public infrastructure is currently aging beyond acceptable design limits;
5	Infrastructure such as schools, public safety, and public health that are essential to communities are facing economically difficult times as the population grows and ages;
6	Economic and social systems are becoming increasingly interdependent and thus increasingly vulnerable, should a key part of the system be disrupted;
7	Risk cannot be eliminated completely, so some residual risk will continue to exist and require management;
8	Impacts of climate change and degradation of natural defences such as coastal wetlands make the nation more vulnerable.

The increase in the occurrence of disasters is obviously manifest by an expanding impact on global populations. Contributing factors to this impact include a continuation of population growth and rapid urbanization, the outsourcing of production (and resulting population density) to areas prone to hazards, and the evolving effects of climate change.[7] The public health impact of disasters includes injuries, disease, and death, and a reduced ability to provide shelter, water, sanitation, hygiene, healthcare (including immunizations), public services, and utilities to the impacted population. Reduction in such basic support raises the risk of long-term health consequences, both physical and stress-related.[8] From Figure 11.2, one can presume or deduce types of illnesses and injuries, as well as issues impacting health that are associated with specific categories of depicted events.[9]

Social factors such as educational status, gender-related issues (societal roles, potential for equality compared to males), disparities in income levels, weakening of family and social protection structures, and poor living and working conditions have a profound effect on health and health behavior. These conditions are only exacerbated by disasters. Other disaster-related issues that health systems must address in coming years are care of the aging population, providing health services to the burgeoning urban population (particularly the urban poor), and ensuring readiness to address the effects of climate change.[10]

The risks and vulnerabilities are many, as are factors which, in combination, determine how many people die, become ill, and suffer physical and psychological trauma from disasters and other events. Added to these factors are other issues including:

1) locations of settlements; 2) quality of building construction; 3) advanced hazard warnings; 4) availability of evacuation shelters; 5) level of community expertise to take appropriate action; 6) availability of food, water, and medical and health services; and 7) emergency response systems.[11]

Are There Successful Disaster Health Outcomes as a Result of Public Health and Emergency Management System Interventions?

Utstein[1] defines an outcome as the result of a specific intervention(s) or project(s) relative to their established goals and objectives. The increase in global disasters, combined with the new reality of expanded awareness and connectivity, invites a clarion call to those who examine and seek solutions to the impact of these events. Of particular focus and concern is the public health impact of disasters on global populations. The impact, along with the status, roles, and progress of public health and emergency management systems, determines the extent of successful outcomes in prevention and management of disaster consequences.

Who Is Responsible for Emergency Management and Public Health Systems?

Internationally, the World Health Organization (WHO), an agency of the United Nations (UN), is the lead agency for providing health assistance during humanitarian crises worldwide through the Global Health Cluster (GHC). The mission of the GHC is to build consensus on humanitarian health priorities

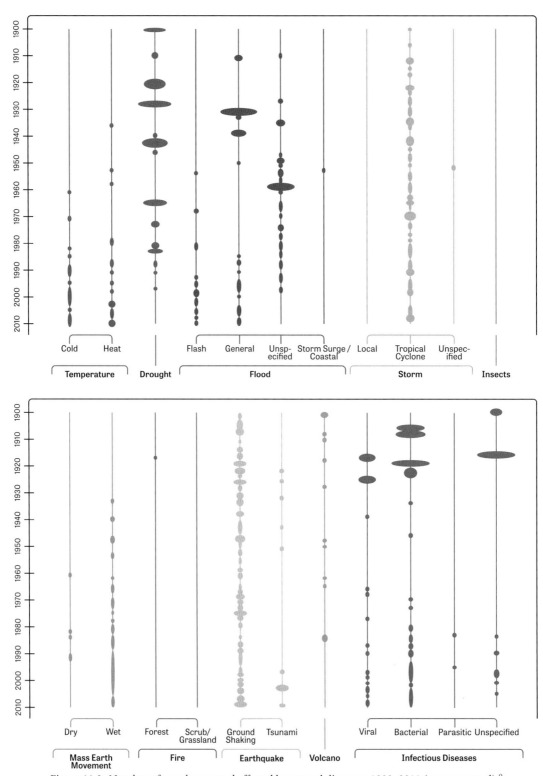

Figure 11.2. Number of people reported affected by natural disasters, 1900–2011 (square rooted).[9]

and related best practices, and strengthen system-wide capacities to ensure an effective and predictable response.[12] Since designating the 1990s as the "International Decade for Disaster Risk Reduction" (IDNDR), the UN has been actively engaged with leading the global community in saving human lives and reducing the impact of disasters. The 1994 Yokohama Strategy and Plan of Action for a Safer World provided a unified direction to IDNDR efforts. It noted that: 1) prevention, mitigation, and preparedness activities are primary to reducing the need for disaster response; 2) prevention and preparedness are integral components of economic development efforts; 3) effective prevention requires the involvement of the whole community; and 4) vulnerability could be reduced through appropriate land use and building design.[13]

In the United States, FEMA has the overall lead for the coordination of federal agencies and the development of emergency management capacity and capability at the state and local levels.[14] The U.S. Centers for Disease Control and Prevention (CDC) is the lead agency for ensuring the nation's public health, and the Office of the Assistant Secretary for Preparedness and Response (ASPR) has the overall lead for ensuring national health security from disasters and other threats.[15] The National Disaster Medical System (NDMS), a program administered by the ASPR, was originally developed in 1984 to provide federal support to states and local jurisdictions. This is achieved through establishment of Disaster Medical Assistance Teams (DMATs), a nationwide network of participating hospitals to receive casualties from the disaster area(s), and an aeromedical transportation system to move casualties to these designated hospitals. The four federal partner departments or agencies that coordinate and support NDMS activities include HHS/ASPR (lead department), Department of Veterans Affairs (VA), Department of Defense, and FEMA. Over the past 30 years, HHS has deployed DMATs and other resources to presidentially declared disasters, the presidential inauguration, the State of the Union address, political conventions, and to large events like the Super Bowl. Another cornerstone of NDMS is the Federal Coordinating Centers (FCCs), located at VA Medical Centers throughout the country. FCCs oversee patient reception teams assembled at the nationwide network of NDMS-enrolled civilian hospitals where disaster victims may be transported to receive definitive care. The program has evolved to also provide states with mortuary and veterinary care teams, and with a patient identification and tracking system.

What Are the Problems, Gaps, or Challenges?

Internationally, universal support within the UN for activities conducted through IDNDR prompted the International Strategy for Disaster Reduction (ISDR) in 2000. A review of the Yokohama Strategy was conducted in 2005, resulting in the Hyogo Framework for Action covering the period 2005–2015. While applauding previous efforts, it identified five areas where gaps or challenges currently exist:

1) Risk identification, assessment, monitoring, and early warning;
2) Reduction of underlying risk factors;
3) Governance: organizational, legal, and policy frameworks;
4) Knowledge management and education; and,
5) Preparedness for effective response and recovery.[16]

Underlying these gaps is a more fundamental problem of insufficient knowledge about the impacts from disasters on population health and the relative effectiveness of interventions designed to increase resiliency, reduce suffering, and restore normalcy. Historically, while both public health and emergency management disciplines have had similar overall goals, conceptual models, and operational methods, in practice these two groups have not always been effective in sharing tools and personnel in preparing for and responding to mass emergencies.[17] Recently, implementation of common frameworks and systems are providing for greater coordination, collaboration, and integration.

STATE OF THE ART

Status and Best Practices

The aforementioned Hyogo Framework for Action identified five areas of gaps and challenges that can serve as a presentation framework for emergency management and public health system status and best practices. Included throughout the following discussion are real world examples, as well as formal and official policies and directives.

Risk Identification, Assessment, Monitoring, and Early Warning

TECHNOLOGY/SOCIAL MEDIA'S IMPACT ON WARNING AND MONITORING

The tremendous access to information about disasters, including their frequency and impact, has been reported widely throughout recent events. Following the 9.0 Tōhoku Earthquake and Tsunami that devastated Japan in March 2011, American Ambassador John Roos led the mission to render America's response support to this unprecedented disaster. He coordinated almost 200 U.S. military ships and aircraft for transport of food and supplies, as well as the U.S. Embassy's response to the Fukushima Dai-ichi nuclear power plant crisis. Noteworthy is his immediate use of Twitter feed to 155,000 Americans residing in Japan, critical during initial hours when event information was scarce.[18]

Response and recovery to the 2010 Haiti earthquake was aided significantly by use of social media and was bolstered through systems like Skype and Ushahidi. These platforms served as a base for volunteers and supported digital volunteers in site-map creation.[19] The World Food Program, U.S. Marine Corps, and U.S. Coast Guard have also used Ushahidi in disaster responses and in the 2011 Japan complex disaster.[20] It is becoming standard practice for the Red Cross and many disaster relief agencies to rely on Twitter and other forms of social media (such as Facebook) to inform the global community of events as they unfold, and to request, acquire, and coordinate disaster resources.

SURVEILLANCE

The use of surveillance is a more scientific approach to predicting the potential health impact of disasters. Surveillance is the systematic collection, analysis, and interpretation of deaths, injuries, and illnesses that enables public health officers to track and identify any adverse health effects in the community. Surveillance allows assessment of the human health impacts of a disaster and evaluation of potential problems in planning and prevention.[21] Both WHO and the World Bank cite health surveillance as an essential function of a public health system.[22] The current WHO perspective is to create an integrated disease surveillance process where all surveillance activities employ a common process that conducts many functions, using similar techniques and types of personnel. Those activities that are well developed in one area may help strengthen other surveillance activities.

Protocols have been developed for the implementation of Integrated Disease Surveillance and Response (IDSR) and all WHO Member States have endorsed the model.[23]

In addition to the WHO IDSR system, assistance and support is available from the international public health sector. The U.S. CDC is an international leader in surveillance. The CDC Disaster Surveillance Workgroup (DSWG) has set standards for data collection, sharing, and reporting during a public health disaster. Through the work of DSWG, morbidity and mortality surveillance tools and training have been developed. They have also created four ready-to-use, standardized morbidity surveillance forms for use in conducting active surveillance during a disaster. These templates can be modified to meet the needs of the specific incident. The CDC Health Studies Branch (HSB) has rigorously engaged in disaster surveillance activities in many disasters including the 2010 Haiti earthquake; the 2009 tsunami/earthquake in American Samoa; and many hurricanes, floods, and other U.S.-based incidents. CDC HSB provides scientific consultation, technical assistance, and disaster epidemiology training to U.S. government, nongovernmental, and academic entities. It is available to (and has assisted) international organizations, public health systems, and governments as well.[24] One of the recent CDC HSB advances is the development of the Community Assessment for Public Health Emergency Response (CASPER) rapid needs assessment toolkit. CASPER can be used by public health practitioners and emergency management officials to determine the health status and basic needs of the affected community in a quick and low-cost manner.[25]

The use of predictive modelling to estimate potential numbers of deaths and injuries has been applied to earthquakes, weather-related calamities, chemical/biological/radiological events, and recently to studying the potential spread of disease such as pandemic influenza.[26–29] This knowledge, aligned with the ability to estimate the broader losses to the public health infrastructure and supply chains, is emerging as an important area of development.

Risk Reduction

TECHNICAL ASSISTANCE

The Pan American Health Organization (PAHO) is the world's oldest international public health agency. It provides technical assistance and cooperation to countries of the Americas, thus mobilizing partnerships to improve health and quality of life. PAHO, a member of the UN system, is the specialized health agency of the Inter-American System and serves as the Regional Office for the Americas of the World Health Organization.[30]

Over the past decade, PAHO has made safe hospitals an issue of central importance. The PAHO/WHO publication *Safe Hospitals – A Collective Responsibility, A Global Measure of Disaster Reduction* proclaims that, "Protecting critical health facilities, particularly hospitals, from the avoidable consequences of disasters, is not only essential to meeting the UN Millennium Development Goals (MDGs), but also a social and political necessity." PAHO affirms that hospitals and other health facilities, particularly in developing countries, offer more than medical care to the sick. They also: 1) support preventive medicine; 2) host public health reference labs; 3) contribute to diagnosis and prevention of HIV/AIDS; 4) are resource centers for public health education; 5) serve as research entities; and 6) signal warnings for communicable disease.

PAHO provides many graphic examples of dire situations resulting from hospitals destroyed by disasters. For example, it captured images of large numbers of injured victims awaiting treatment at makeshift facilities that functioned under primitive conditions. These circumstances resulted from hospital loss after earthquakes in Turkey (1999), Gujarat, India (2001), and Bam, Iran (2003) or cyclones/hurricanes in Grenada, Haiti, and the Philippines in 2004. Such problems continue or are heightened, as the impacted area must attempt to resume treatment of medical emergencies, routine care, and also offer follow-up care to disaster victims.

Beyond the obvious health and medical implications, PAHO frames the issue of destroyed hospitals in multi-faceted terms, declaring the issue as one of sociopolitical and economic significance. Hospitals are core community assets and symbols, especially in developing countries. A destroyed hospital can represent failure of the entire healthcare system and has collective emotional repercussions. Political fallout can occur if residents believe that leaders could have implemented preventative measures but failed to do so. Economic implications are also evident, when one considers the enormous amount of money expended on long-term deployment of mobile hospitals and supporting resources, not to mention the assets damaged or destroyed.[31]

Keeping hospitals operational in normal times consumes almost two-thirds of all public health care spending in Latin America and the Caribbean, and that fact alone is a compelling reason to protect these facilities. This is especially true when one considers the extraordinary amount dedicated to expensive equipment and resources inherent in a hospital. PAHO contends that reducing hospital vulnerability is indeed achievable and provides guidance on how to accomplish this goal. For example, it recommends that new hospital structures comply with the most stringent and modern safety requirements, anti-seismic norms, and other safeguards. The planning for new hospital structures must include a multidisciplinary team, such as disaster risk reduction specialists, engineers, and representatives of the political and economic communities. These individuals all must be involved from the beginning of the planning process. The safety of existing facilities must also be addressed and interventions applied to vulnerable structures. Since the mid-1980s, earthquake affected countries such as Chile, Colombia, Costa Rica, Ecuador, India, Mexico, and Peru have been retrofitting hospitals to correct structural and non-structural deficiencies. PAHO recognizes that it would be cost-prohibitive and disruptive to retrofit all hospitals, but urges that selected facilities correct deficiencies in the most critical areas. These include operating rooms, blood banks, and emergency departments. PAHO cites examples of facilities that have undergone needed correctional processes and have subsequently survived disasters with only cosmetic damage. PAHO concludes that, without reducing the vulnerability of health infrastructure, meeting the MDGs will remain an elusive goal.[31]

READILY AVAILABLE HEALTH INFORMATION

The American Medical Association (AMA), the largest association of physicians and medical students in the United States, has proposed the adoption of a Secure Health Information Card (SHIC) to address health and medical issues associated with disasters. AMA cites several compelling factors leading to this recommendation. It notes that about half of the 2005 Hurricane Katrina evacuees did not carry health and medical information, resulting in delays in receiving healthcare and in lives lost. It also cites that 60% of Médecins Sans Frontières (Doctors Without Borders) consultations following Hurricane Sandy in 2012 were related to prescription refills for diabetic, asthmatic, and hypertension patients. AMA adds that approximately 125 million Americans have at least one chronic illness, making them more vulnerable to adverse health outcomes following a disaster or public health emergency. AMA conducted a detailed multiphase project using focus groups, a prototype card with thirty points of personal/medical information, and evaluation of the SHIC through an exercise. The project involved 707 volunteer participants from six FEMA Regions. The card's value was widely endorsed by those volunteering as patients and responder/caregiver participants. AMA recommends adoption of the SHIC and emphasizes the benefits to improved disaster public health:

- Prompt and accurate identification in emergency/disaster events
- More timely and appropriate care
- Improved surveillance and situational awareness
- Reduced morbidity and mortality in affected populations
- Improved health outcomes in affected populations

It is projected that the use of a SHIC-type device can increase efficiency (saving time and reducing costs) and effectiveness (providing more complete information to providers). AMA adds that a SHIC or similar device is also potentially dual-use and can be applied during more routine healthcare encounters as well as in disasters.[32]

COMMUNITY-BASED RISK REDUCTION PROGRAMS

Beyond programs that are government-initiated, other programs are emerging throughout the United States. The American Red Cross (ARC) is partnering with local citizen groups in community resilience programs. ARC has supported pilot programs in disaster-prone cities such as New Orleans, Miami, and San Francisco and is increasingly engaging in similar initiatives in other areas. ARC, along with the Departments of Emergency Management and Health in Syracuse, New York, and the Food Bank of Central New York, have partnered to coordinate a Resilience Strategy program. Their approach is based on three phases. Phase I identifies disaster preparedness strengths and weaknesses through meetings, town hall discussions, and surveys. Phase II provides emergency equipment for public venues and sheltering items such as cots for neighborhood centers. It also implements neighborhood emergency drills and trainings, and other interventions to fill identified gaps. Phase III establishes performance benchmarks, reconvenes the community for updates and success sharing, and publishes resiliency best practices for other communities.[33]

Governance: Organizational, Legal, and Policy Frameworks

ADVOCACY – SUSTAINABILITY/RESILIENCE AND HEALTH SECURITY

The emerging global trend in disaster management is within the framework of sustainability and resilience. The sustainability or resilience of the population/environment against hazards is its pliability, flexibility, or elasticity to absorb the event.[1] Sustainability is a broad social responsibility of government and of the business community. A primary role and responsibility of emergency management and public health systems leaders and strategists is to strive for sustainability and resilience in the form of health security. Health security from disasters is the goal of governmental efforts including public health, out-of-hospital and alternate care systems, pre-hospital and EMS, hospitals and acute care, and emergency management and public safety sectors.

Following the 2000 UN Millennium Summit, eight MDGs were issued. All 189 UN Member States and more than 23 international organizations agreed to achieve the goals by 2015. Those eight goals are: 1) eradicating extreme poverty and hunger; 2) achieving universal primary education; 3) promoting gender equality and empowering women; 4) reducing child mortality rates; 5) improving maternal health; 6) combating HIV/AIDS, malaria, and other diseases; 7) ensuring environmental sustainability; and 8) creating a global partnership for development.[34] Although not specifically cited as one of the eight MDGs, the area of disaster risk reduction is believed by many to be inherent in and interconnected with the goals. One body that has vigorously acted on that belief is the UN Inter-Parliamentary Union (IPU).

In 2010, IPU and UNISDR published *Disaster Risk Reduction: An Instrument for Achieving the Millennium Development Goals, an Advocacy Kit for Parliamentarians*. The kit assists parliamentarians in playing an active oversight role in building the resilience of their nations and communities to disasters, accelerating progress towards the MDGs. The kit outlines priorities, cites policies and interventions needed to reduce or eliminate disaster risks, and provides examples of work done by many parliaments throughout the world. The document also cites important applicable resolutions adopted by the 122nd Inter-parliamentary Assembly. One such resolution urges "governments to assess all their critical public facilities, such as schools and hospitals . . . making them resilient to earthquakes, floods and storms, and to make disaster-risk reduction a part of poverty reduction and of all planning and programs aimed at achieving the MDGs and the ensuing long-term welfare of the people."[35] The kit emphasizes the risk faced by the health infrastructure and proclaims that the most expensive hospital is the one that fails, adding that destruction and damage to health facilities, their contents, and infrastructure represent very substantial losses of development investment.[35] For instance, the cost from losses to the health sector in the 2005 Kashmir earthquake was equivalent to about 60% of the national health budget for the entire country of Pakistan. In 2009, Typhoon Pepeng damaged 30 hospitals and 100 health centers in the Philippines.[35] Hospitals, primary health centers, and other health facilities are central to sustainable recovery from disaster, and to health-driven development goals. One initiative mentioned in the document, and supported by IPU, is the PAHO focus on Safe Hospitals.[35]

The MDGs, set to expire in 2015, will be replaced by new goals. During the 2013 meeting of the Global Platform for Disaster Risk Reduction, participants advocated for overtly recognizing disaster risk. In addition, they requested that governments take a strong lead in ensuring that disaster risk reduction is incorporated into sustainable development goals. It was suggested that this concept should be part of the post-2015 development agenda, noting that, "it is the poor . . . the most vulnerable who are most affected."[36]

U.S. EMERGENCY MANAGEMENT POLICIES

National governments are increasingly responding to this challenge. Using the United States as an example, three significant

HSPDs were issued in 2003. HSPD 5, Management of Domestic Incidents, established requirements for the National Incident Management System (NIMS), an update to the original National Interagency Incident Management System published in 1983. HSPD 5 also mandated the use of the Incident Command System (ICS) by federal, state, and local government agencies and other organizations involved with domestic incident management.[37] HSPD 7, Critical Infrastructure Protection, required federal and non-federal agencies and organizations to identify and prioritize critical infrastructure along seven sectors, including public health and healthcare.[38] HSPD 8, National Preparedness, called for the development of a national preparedness goal and system, which included a set of metrics and guidance for the development and evaluation of exercises using those metrics.[39] Recently, both critical infrastructure protection and national preparedness have been re-issued by the Obama Administration as PPDs.[40,41] In addition, FEMA has issued new national preparedness metrics, procedures for implementing the metrics, and guidance on the integration of public, non-profit, and private sectors; academia; communities; and individual citizens in preparedness activities.[42–44]

PPD 8 calls on the U.S. Department of Homeland Security to embrace systematic preparation against all types of threats, including catastrophic natural disasters. Because the scope of resilience is sometimes not fully appreciated, some who contemplate national resilience policy think first of the Stafford Act (federal law that regulates U.S. government disaster aid to states and local governments) and its role in disaster response and recovery. Although the Stafford Act does provide guidance for certain responsibilities and actions in responding to a disaster incident, national resilience transcends the immediate impact and disaster response and therefore grows from a broader set of policies. Many of the critical policies and actions required for improved national resilience are also enacted and implemented at the state and local levels.

The National Response Framework (NRF) is a guide to how the United States responds to all types of disasters and emergencies. It is built on scalable, flexible, and adaptable concepts identified in NIMS to align key roles and responsibilities across the nation. This framework describes specific authorities and best practices for managing incidents that range from the serious but purely local to large-scale terrorist attacks or catastrophic natural disasters. NRF describes the principles, roles and responsibilities, and coordinating structures for delivering the core capabilities required to respond to an incident and further describes how response efforts integrate with those of the other mission areas.[45]

A key element of NRF is the fifteen Emergency Support Functions (ESFs). These functions represent the totality of the federal response to disasters (transportation, communication, search and rescue, mass sheltering, etc.) when the NRF is activated. The roles and responsibilities of coordinating and supporting federal departments are outlined for each of the fifteen ESFs. The provision of medical and public healthcare are coordinated by those agencies identified within ESF 8, Public Health and Medical. Some of what ESF 8 provides includes: 1) assessment of public health and medical needs; 2) health surveillance; 3) medical care personnel; 4) equipment, supplies, blood, and blood products; 5) patient evacuation; 6) behavioral healthcare; and 7) mass fatality management.[45]

The National Infrastructure Protection Plan provides the unifying structure for the integration of existing and future critical infrastructure protection efforts and resiliency strategies into a single national program to achieve this goal. The risk management framework is structured to promote continuous improvement to enhance critical infrastructure protection. It focuses on efforts to: 1) set goals and objectives; 2) identify assets, systems, and networks; 3) assess risk based on consequences, vulnerabilities, and threats; 4) establish priorities based on risk assessments and on the cost-effectiveness of mitigating the risk; 5) implement protective programs and resiliency strategies; and 6) measure effectiveness.[46]

The Healthcare and Public Health (HPH) Sector-Specific Plan complements the National Infrastructure Protection Plan by detailing the application of the framework to the unique characteristics and risk landscape of the sector. This plan lays out a collaborative process among government and private enterprise partners to protect the HPH Sector from natural disasters, pandemics, terrorist attacks, and other disasters, referred to collectively as "all hazards." The plan describes current processes and sets a path forward for the sector to cooperatively identify and prioritize its assets, assess risks, implement protective programs, and measure the effectiveness of these protective strategies. The HPH Sector is vast and diverse. The sector employs approximately 13 million personnel and represents an estimated 16.2% ($2.2 trillion USD) of the nation's gross domestic product. It includes not only acute care hospitals and ambulatory healthcare, but also the vast and complex public-private systems that finance that care. It includes population-based care provided by health agencies at the federal, state, local, tribal, and territorial levels, as well as other public health and disease surveillance functions. It incorporates a large system of private sector enterprises that manufacture, distribute, and sell drugs, vaccines, and medical supplies and equipment, as well as a network of small businesses that provide mortuary services. All of these goods and services are provided in and by means of a complex environment of research, regulation, finance, and public policy. The HPH Sector has established four goals in the areas of service continuity:

1. Maintain the ability to provide essential health services during and after disasters or disruptions in the availability of supplies or supporting services (e.g., water, power);
2. Workforce protection (protect the sector's workforce from the harmful consequences of all hazards that may compromise their health and safety and limit their ability to carry out their responsibilities);
3. Physical asset protection (mitigate the risks posed by all hazards to the sector's physical assets); and,
4. Cybersecurity (mitigate risks to the sector's cyber assets that may result in disruption to or denial of health services).[47]

U.S. Public Health and Medical Policies

The U.S. Congress passed the Pandemic and All-Hazards Preparedness Act (PAHPA) in 2006. PAHPA transformed the HHS preparedness and response activities, establishing within the department a new ASPR. PAHPA provided new authorities for a number of programs, including the advanced development and acquisition of medical countermeasures, creation of a focus on at-risk populations, and establishing a quadrennial National Health Security Strategy review.[48]

HSPD 10, Biodefense for the 21st Century (2004), focused on reducing the threat from biological weapons and established the Strategic National Stockpile, the BioWatch program, and the BioShield program.[49] HSPD 21, Public Health and Medical

ACHIEVING NATIONAL HEALTH SECURITY

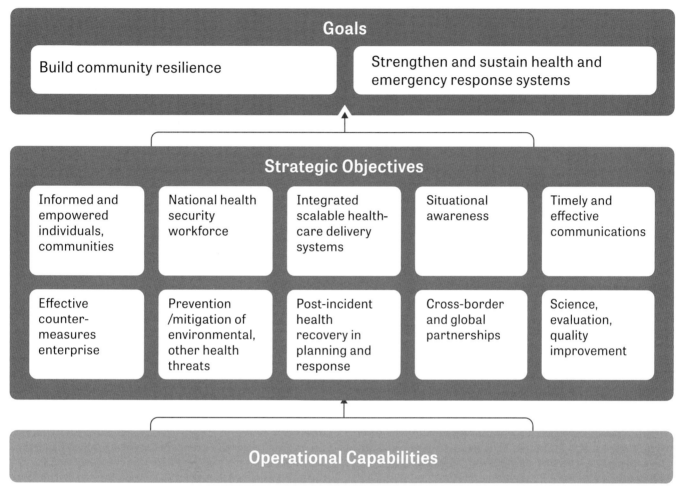

Figure 11.3. The Framework for the U.S. National Health Security Strategy (2009).[50,51]

Preparedness (2007), reaffirmed some key principles in earlier homeland security and health policies, including: 1) all-hazards preparedness; 2) vertical and horizontal coordination across levels of government, jurisdictions, and professional disciplines; 3) a regional approach to health sector preparedness; 4) engagement of the private sector, academia, and other nongovernmental entities; and 5) the important contributions and roles of individuals, families, and communities.[50]

HSPD 21 called for a National Health Security Strategy (NHSS), setting as its goals the building of community resilience and strengthening and sustaining of the health and emergency response systems (see Figure 11.3). The purpose of NHSS is to "refocus the patchwork of disparate public health and medical preparedness, response, and recovery strategies in order to ensure that the nation is prepared for, protected from, and resilient in the face of health threats or incidents with potentially negative health consequences."[52] This refocusing is intended to strengthen the community, integrate response and recovery systems, generate a framework for accountability and continuous quality improvement, and create seamless coordination between all levels of the medical system. It is hoped that NHSS will provide a common vision for the nation in achieving national health security.[50]

Knowledge Management and Education
CITIZEN INVOLVEMENT

Israel has a reputation for a population that is well trained and rehearsed in response to emergencies. The country's history of wars, terrorist attacks, bombings, and threats against its security are influencing factors for vigilance and a robust national preparedness posture. Citizens are highly practiced in drills and real alerts. The population is familiar with responding to air raid sirens by evacuating to the nearest safe room or public shelter. The donning of protective gas masks is familiar to even the youngest citizens.[53]

The Home Front Command, which is the Israeli Defense Force (IDF) regional command responsible for civilian safety and preparedness, routinely conducts drills, including the annual numbered Turning Point exercises. Most of the drills and exercises have focused on the prevalent concern for enemy terrorist attacks. In the fall of 2012, however, the Home Front Command and National Emergency Authority (NEA) launched Turning Point 6, a nationwide event that aggressively addressed another concern, that of earthquakes. NEA, formed in 2007, is the Defense Ministry body responsible for coordinating military and civilian actions during a state of emergency, war or natural disaster. Of note, NEA and the United States have a cooperative agreement.[54]

Many countries and cultures conduct disaster exercises and some label them as national in scope. In the United States, FEMA and DHS have conducted disaster and terrorism exercises several times that span all levels of government, including several iterations of TOPOFF, involving thousands of leaders and responders.[55] Few countries, however, conduct exercises that involve not only all levels of government, health and medical responders, and the private sector, but also fully integrate the nationwide citizenry.

Turning Point 6 was a 5-day nationwide exercise involving the police, fire, Magen David Adom (Israel's national emergency medical services, ambulance, and blood bank system), municipalities, and regular citizens in preparation for a national emergency. Civilians at home, work, and school were notified through the nationwide broadcasting system by television, radio, cellular phones, and other means.[56] The scenario assumed that Yoseftal Hospital in Eilat and Ha'emek Hospital in Afula collapsed due to an earthquake, while Haifa's Rambam Hospital was hit by a tsunami. Paramedics triaged and treated thousands of mock life-threatening injuries. Rescue workers dug through the night to rescue survivors of a collapsed school. Electric wires and mobile phone networks were destroyed, and a prison in Be'er Sheva along with many buildings collapsed. A continuous 24-hour-per-day blood donation drive was initiated and global appeals to the Red Cross and American Blood Centers in the United States tested inter-country agreements.[57]

The scenario utilized government-estimated figures compatible with a devastating earthquake, projecting 7,000 fatalities, tens of thousands of wounded, 170,000 persons displaced and homeless, and devastating damage to infrastructures throughout Israel. The Israeli prime minister and cabinet, serving as examples, evacuated their areas and fully participated throughout, as the media instructed the public. "The main message we seek to convey to the citizens is that via this drill, and other measures, we want to run into homes during a missile attack and to run outside during an earthquake," said the prime minister.[58] The nationwide population of Israel was aware, involved, and engaged in Turning Point 6. This massive full-scale event occurred concurrent with a month-long drill of the IDF and its American military counterparts, affording Israel's leaders and emergency planners an opportunity to assess and revise response systems and actions at all levels, including the citizens at school, work, and home.[58]

WHOLE COMMUNITY

The central theme of FEMA is the involvement of the "whole community" in building resilience and in improving preparedness, response, and recovery efforts.[58] The term "whole community" refers to the larger collective team that includes more than just FEMA. It also includes its partners at the federal, state, local, tribal, and territorial levels; nongovernmental organizations like faith-based groups, non-profit enterprises, and the private sector; and individuals, families, and communities. FEMA's whole community concept aligns with public health's focus on population health and those entities and components, depicted in Figure 11.4, that must be collaboratively engaged to build resilience.[59]

CITIZEN CORPS: GOVERNMENT / CITIZEN PARTNERSHIP

In the past decade, the U.S. government and other entities have adopted a definitive focus on citizen preparedness. As of September 15, 2011, there were 1,083 local, county, and tribal Citizen Corps Councils nationwide, representing more than 178 million people, or approximately 58% of the U.S. population. Cit-

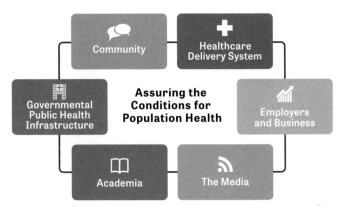

Figure 11.4. The public health system, government, and some of its potential partners.[60]

izen Corps emphasizes personal responsibility for: preparedness; education and training in such areas as first aid and emergency skills; and volunteer support to emergency responders, disaster relief, and community safety. Engaging the whole community to support resilience and all phases of emergency management is a core mission area of the Citizen Corps Councils. Of the 1,083 approved Citizen Corps Councils analyzed, most councils (60%) include representation from the public, private, and volunteer/community sectors, as well as representation by elected leadership (67%). Over half (57%) of councils have representation from youth or youth-based organizations. Recognizing the power of education and training in preparing the public, the councils support programs in multiple locations; 72% of the Citizen Corps groups deliver materials and training in neighborhoods, 71% in schools, 63% in workplaces, and 53% in places of worship. The majority of councils specifically tailor their public education materials for people with disabilities (60%), the frail elderly (57%), pet owners (54%), and youth (54%). The power of citizen involvement in building capacity is evident in the strength of the Citizen Corps volunteer force, where most volunteers have been trained and almost three-fourths have been deployed in support of local responses.[61]

EDUCATION WITHIN THE UNITED STATES
NATIONAL CENTER FOR DISASTER MEDICINE AND PUBLIC HEALTH

The 2009 HSPD 21 called for the creation of a joint program for disaster medicine and public health, housed at the Uniformed Services University of the Health Sciences. This program leads federal efforts to develop and disseminate core curricula, training, and research related to disaster medicine and public health in disasters. The program was to encompass education and research in the related specialties of domestic medical preparedness and response, international health, international disaster and humanitarian medical assistance, and military medicine. Established in 2008, the National Center for Disaster Medicine and Public Health has contributed significantly to the development of disaster health education and training.[62]

COMPETENCIES

Experts have developed several examples of disaster-related competencies for healthcare workers and a hierarchy now exists that aligns the many models. Of note for healthcare personnel are those developed by the George Washington University Institute for Crisis, Risk and Disaster Management in 2007 under contract with the U.S. Veterans Health Administration (VHA). The Healthcare Emergency Management Competencies were developed by multidisciplinary representatives of federal, state, and local agencies as well as hospitals, professional organizations, public health groups, and emergency management entities. The competencies are uniquely categorized by position; for example, healthcare leaders, clinical leadership, clinicians, emergency managers, and non-clinical staff are now in use by VHA and other hospital professionals and personnel throughout the United States.[63] Healthcare emergency management competencies have also been developed and are being applied to other groups, such as public health professionals, physicians, nurses and EMS personnel.[64,65] These and other competencies are addressed in Chapter 2.

FEMA CENTER FOR DOMESTIC PREPAREDNESS

A plethora of emergency management and disaster health-related education and training opportunities exists throughout the United States through on-site and online opportunities. An example of a federal venue that offers a vast selection of on-site, exercise-based education and training is the FEMA Center for Domestic Preparedness (CDP) an Anniston, Alabama. In addition to offering more traditional emergency management training, the CDP offers unique courses in chemical, biological, and radiological agents. The CDP's Noble Training Facility is the only venue of its type in the United States that offers rigorous realistic training and exercises in a mock hospital setting, where a model hospital facility is fully activated for functional-level exercises.[66] More information about various education and training models and programs is contained in Chapter 2.

Education within Afghanistan

Afghanistan exemplifies a developing country with extraordinary challenges in addressing disaster health issues. Disaster health is of great concern when one considers the pervasive threats. The country of almost 30 million residents has a history and cycle of disasters that threatens the health integrity of its people. The mountainous areas experience harsh winters accompanied by heavy snow, resulting in extreme flooding during the spring thaw. In addition, the northeastern Hindu Kush mountain range is a geologically active area, prone to earthquakes almost annually. Landslides and avalanches follow. A 1998 quake killed about 6,000 people in Badakhshan and hundreds more have been killed or injured in subsequent quakes.[67,68] The disaster health status in Afghanistan is complicated by the stark reality of three decades of war. Such conflict-associated injuries and deaths frequently result from terrorist and suicide attacks and landmine detonations.

The Afghanistan health and medical community have made sincere attempts to aggressively manage disaster health issues, but are constrained by the framework in which they operate. These groups must function in a nation where 42% of the population lives below the international poverty line and approximately 70% of the population is illiterate, coupled with infrastructure and communication systems in dire need of improvement and enhancement.[69,70] Such conditions make it difficult to manage what would be ordinarily considered routine health and medical issues. Morbidity, mortality, and disability rates remain high. A multitude of international partners and supporters, such as WHO, IFRC, academic institutions, the United States, and other partners continue to be involved in seeking solutions to these problems.

One successful initiative in the medical education realm is that of the Afghan Armed Forces Academy of Medical Sciences (AFAMS). Each class admits forty students from throughout the Afghan provinces. Those admitted must meet challenging scholastic and physical requirements by the National Military Academy of Afghanistan, AFAMS, and Kabul Medical University. In addition to the standard seven years of medical education and training to become doctors, medical students receive education in leadership, advanced trauma surgery, operational medicine, and medical ethics. Approximately one-fourth of each class is female. Program leaders believe they are developing a new generation of doctors, highly skilled for practicing in war and disaster as well as in peacetime. Other successful initiatives introduced by U.S. medical advisors (and supported by Canadian medical experts) to the Afghan National Army are disaster medicine courses, now included in university-level curriculum for medical, nursing, and allied health students.[71,72]

Preparedness for Effective Response and Recovery

In recent years, both HHS and FEMA have formalized specific focus on at-risk populations (formally known as special needs populations) in disasters and have issued national guidance on identifying and addressing issues for inclusion in disaster planning initiatives. At-risk populations are those having needs in the following functional areas: communication, medical care, maintaining independence, supervision, and transportation. In addition to those individuals specifically recognized by FEMA as at-risk, PAHPA cites at-risk populations as: 1) children; 2) senior citizens; 3) pregnant women; 4) individuals who may need additional response assistance including those who have disabilities; 5) residents living in institutionalized settings; 6) those who are from diverse cultures, have limited English proficiency, or are non-English speaking; 7) citizens who lack access to transportation; 8) persons with chronic medical disorders; and 9) individuals with pharmacological dependency.[73]

While the public health and medical care sector tend to apply the at-risk term to the populations just described, FEMA identifies groups in these same general categories as those with functional needs. In 2010, FEMA published *Guidance on Planning for Integration of Functional Needs Support Services in General Population Shelters*, an important planning document for those managing shelters and populations displaced by disasters.[74] The guidance is compatible with FEMA's whole community perspective, where both the composition of the community and the needs of individual members must be accounted for when planning and implementing disaster strategies regardless of age, economics, or accessibility requirements.[58]

One U.S. system that routinely manages the health and social services needs of patients included in at-risk populations is that of Community Health Centers (CHCs). CHCs serve the primary healthcare needs of more than 22 million patients in over 9,000 locations in the United States. Their focus is to provide care to underserved populations. A large component of their patient population is in the at-risk category of maternal-child health.[75] They also include focus on services to the non-English/limited English populations, offering appropriate translation services. Homeless individuals and those with limited transportation access are also among their patient population. Over the past decade, with guidance from HHS and state health departments, CHCs have become increasingly involved in developing viable emergency management plans, training, and exercises, and are involved in local interagency emergency planning initiatives.

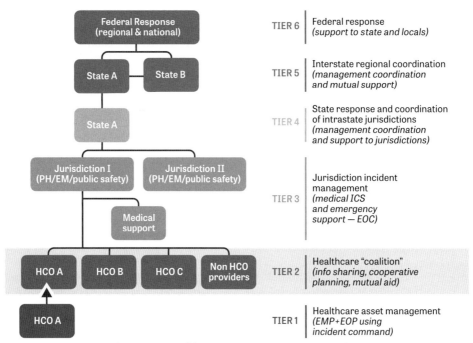

Figure 11.5. Healthcare Emergency Management Tiers.

Healthcare Coalitions

The U.S. government's perspective on the future direction of hospital preparedness is addressed by ASPR in the HHS/ASPR publication *From Hospitals to Healthcare Coalitions: Transforming Health Preparedness and Response in Our Community*. It highlights the need for an increased emphasis on a broader, community-wide, healthcare preparedness approach, including building and strengthening healthcare coalitions. The report also cites that coalitions should enhance the efficiency and effectiveness of preparedness and response in a community or region, and interface with jurisdictional health and public health authorities. It also states that coalitions should be consistent with FEMA's whole community approach, through service to at-risk populations.[76] Figure 11.5 depicts the healthcare coalition, a Tier 2 entity, and its relationship in the overall healthcare emergency management paradigm.[77]

Healthcare Coalitions are an emerging concept in the United States and vary in both organizational management models and mission scope. A successful model that has emerged is that of a public-private partnership. Historically, the government has had the responsibility for public health and welfare during the response to a disaster or other event, although the majority of assets reside within the private sector. A public-private partnership establishes a framework for decision makers to provide services and resources across the disaster continuum and also allow for effective regional planning, data sharing, service coordination, and collaborative policy development.[78] An example of a successful public-private healthcare partnership is the Managed Emergency Surge for Healthcare Coalition (MESH) in Indianapolis, Indiana. Established in 2007 through an HHS/ASPR grant award, MESH is a model of public-private collaboration. Partners and boards of directors are comprised of area hospitals, local and state health departments and emergency management agencies, EMS, academia, and other entities. It provides education and training, healthcare intelligence, preparedness planning, and policy analysis. It functions through many working groups –

such as maternal-child health and community health organizations – that address real-world issues. MESH also serves as the official Medical Multi-Agency Coordination Center (Med-MACC) for the city, county, and surrounding areas. It analyzes and disseminates intelligence; assists with coordination, distribution, and tracking of patients and resources; and provides other services.[79] MESH, along with two other coalitions, the Northern Virginia Hospital Alliance and the Northwest Healthcare Response Network (Seattle, Washington), have established the National Healthcare Coalition Resource Center. This entity provides technical assistance to the many nationwide emerging and established healthcare coalitions and offers workshops and training opportunities for coalitions, local groups, and state agencies.[80]

Partnerships

While international relief organizations were still assembling their deployment strategies, packing supplies, and arranging travel to support Haiti in the aftermath of the devastating 2010 earthquake, the Dominican Republic had already begun providing assistance. Those who are unaware of the history of the two countries may expect nothing less than a supportive response from Haiti's neighbor. The two countries share an island (Hispaniola) east of Cuba and west of Puerto Rico. The Dominican Republic comprises 64% of the island while Haiti makes up the remaining 36%. Figure 11.6 depicts Hispaniola Island, its location, and each country's land portion.

They also share mountain ranges, coast lines, and a similar history of disaster threats (hurricanes, seasons of heavy rainfall and floods, and earthquakes). They even share fault lines. However, the differences between the two countries and cultures are notable. Spanish is the predominant language of the Dominican Republic while French or Creole is spoken in Haiti. While Haiti is one of the most impoverished countries in the Caribbean, by comparison, the Dominican Republic's standard of living is higher (in large part because of tourism). There

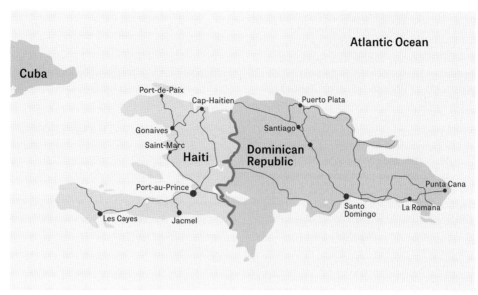

Figure 11.6. Map, Hispaniola.[81]

is a several-generation history of tense relations between the two countries, as well as occupations, massacres, border issues, human and drug trafficking, and other divisive issues. Nonetheless, when the 7.0 earthquake struck southern Haiti in January 2010, the government of the Dominican Republic, along with its healthcare personnel and regular citizens, responded fully and without hesitation.[82] The needs were overwhelming, as Haiti and much of its healthcare infrastructure were severely impacted. Figure 11.7, a photo taken by U.S. responders, portrays a pediatric treatment center, still quasi-operational when the responders arrived a few days after the earthquake. This photo represents the all-too-familiar devastation caused by the temblor.[82]

Dominicans were the first responders, providing critical medical personnel and supplies, logistical support, food and water, transportation, and shelter. Dominican helicopters and vehicles transported injured Haitians across the border for treatment. Santo Domingo served for months as a logistics coordination and entry site for cargo planes. Dominican support in many forms continued for months beyond the initial event.[82] The effects on the Dominican Republic of its collective actions in supporting Haiti have been, in many ways, transformative. While not perfect, the relationship between the two countries and cultures has seemed to become more collaborative and more mutually trusting. The presidents and government representatives of the two countries met and, over time, continued dialogue about

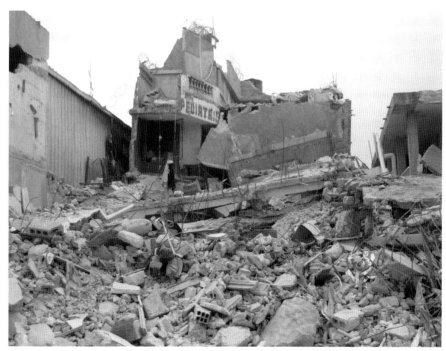

Figure 11.7. A Pediatric Clinic, Devastated by the 2010 Haiti Earthquake.[83]

how they could address mutual concerns. The post-earthquake cholera outbreak found the two countries working together, sharing information more than may have been the case in the past.[82]

There have been other instances where the two countries have collaborated together and conjointly with the international community. The Frontera Verde Project, launched in 2011, is a joint Haiti-Dominican Republic trans-boundary project, funded by the Government of Norway and implemented by the Dominican government, UN Environmental Program (EP), and other partners.[84] In 2013, the two countries' presidents launched "Re-greening Haiti-DR," based on the Dominican experience in forest recovery. Most of Haiti's vegetation has been decimated by human-induced deforestation, putting it at high-risk for severe flooding.[85]

In addition to the seemingly improved relationship and partnership between the Dominican Republic and Haiti, an enhanced appreciation of, and interest in, disaster risk reduction by Dominicans has occurred. The Dominican Republic has endured its share of hurricanes, floods, and earthquakes over the years, and it has been admirable in unselfishly providing to Haiti responsive emergency operations, public warnings, and volunteer response actions. Recognizing the proximity of the devastation just across its border, however, has awaked and expanded focus on the seriousness of vulnerabilities, risk reduction, training, and other strategies. The Dominican government has also become more attuned to the importance of governance in emergency management. The government has issued several regulations, standards, and executive orders designed to address preparedness, prevention, and mitigation. It has also become more engaged in the Caribbean region and the international disaster and risk reduction planning sectors.[82] Many positive changes and new directions resulted from one country assisting a neighbor.

Disaster Stress

It is important that those responsible for emergency management and public health systems acknowledge and apply principles of disaster stress management in planning and implementation programs. The VHA National Post Traumatic Stress Disorder (PTSD) Center, originally developed to address stress-related issues incurred as a result of war, has emerged as a leader in disaster stress management. Through its website, training, and publically available tools, it is a significant resource to those responsible for disaster stress management programs. The center offers the following insight: disasters cause loss of property, possessions, and community and create other stressors that place victims at risk for both physical and emotional health problems.[86] Many factors make it likely that an individual will suffer severe or long-lasting stress reactions following a disaster:

- Severity of exposure: Studies of severe disasters, such as devastating earthquakes and hurricanes, show that at least half of survivors suffer from distress or mental health problems that need clinical care.
- Gender and family: Females usually suffer more negative effects than males. Recovery is more stressful when children are in the home. Marital stress increases after disasters.
- Age: Adults in the 40–60 age range are most likely to be distressed post-disaster. Higher stress in parents relates to worse recovery in children.
- Low or negative social support: Support or lack thereof can be a resilience factor or risk factor. Negative or absent social support is linked to long-term distress in survivors.

- Developing countries: Disasters in developing countries have more severe mental health impact than do disasters in developed countries.
- Survivor characteristics: Recovery is worse if an individual has poor self-esteem, is bereaving the death of a loved one, is displaced or separated from family, is injured, and/or suffers great property loss.

Factors that increase resilience include:

- Social support: Positive support improves well-being, allows sharing of experiences, assists with tips on coping, and increases coping confidence.
- Hope: Better outcomes increase in those who possess optimism and confidence, have a belief in God and believe that others are acting on one's behalf, and generally have good coping skills.

It is important to know that most of those impacted by disaster do recover and sometimes even report positive changes, as they rethink and appreciate what is truly important.[86]

There are many tools available to those affected by disaster and other trauma, and to those working with effected populations. The VHA National PTSD Center posts self-help and coping aides, available online or downloadable, on its public page. It also has a mobile app, "PTSD Coach," available to the public.[87]

RECOMMENDATIONS FOR FURTHER RESEARCH

The development of systems and approaches for the measurement of healthcare delivery during disasters is impeded by difficulties in conducting controlled studies that will identify effective assessment strategies. Obtaining a more objective approach is limited by a lack of expertise, a lack of effective coordination between responding agencies, and a mismatch between established minimum standards, health status indicators, and decision processes.[88] Both in the United States and internationally, however, important steps are being taken.

A key step is establishing common terminology and a universal framework for research and evaluation. The 2003 Health Disaster Management Guidelines for Evaluation and Research in the Utstein Style emphasized the importance of common terms and definitions for the developing field of disaster health.[1] This publication standardized methods for research by public health practitioners to produce sound information about the health impacts of disasters and the effectiveness of interventions. However, little research has been published using this template and it is not yet clear if this approach is valid. More investigations using this tool are needed to determine if it is effective or if it requires further modification.

Another step is the articulation of desired health outcomes and minimum health standards during disasters. WHO is the lead agency for providing health assistance during humanitarian crises worldwide and does so through the GHC. This group is comprised of thirty-eight international health organizations and four observers. The mission of the GHC is to build consensus on humanitarian health priorities and related best practices, and strengthen system-wide capacities to ensure an effective and predictable response. In its 2012–2013 Strategic Framework, the GHC set an objective to demonstrate progress toward agreed-upon health outcomes/impact and service availability to affected populations, and to use data for more effective health cluster advocacy. The GHC has established performance standards for health surveillance, coordination of health organizations, and maintenance of health outcomes in the affected population.[12] Minimum standards in health action were established for the health system and essential health services. These include control of communicable diseases, child health, sexual and reproductive health, injury, mental health, and non-communicable diseases. These standards for international humanitarian disaster health services, tools for the assessment of health needs, and the monitoring of interventions serve as models for the development of an evidence base.[89] More data is needed to demonstrate whether these standards and tools are worthy of support or if different metrics are needed.

Also evolving is the identification of universal data indicators, which serve to enhance collection and analysis capability. Internationally, WHO has developed three systems to support data collection and performance monitoring: initial health assessment, health resource availability mapping, and the health information record.[12] In the United States, web access to some existing health conditions contributes to responders' ability to provide optimal care.[90] NDMS uses a system of records to document patient treatment and tracking and for disaster medical assistance team quality improvement processes.[91] A template for the reporting of the acute medical response in disasters identified fifteen data elements with indicators for both research and quality improvement.[92] Efforts are underway to promote the use of the template for the establishment of an international database.[93]

In the United States, sustained efforts to enhance national preparedness focus on a "secure and resilient nation, with the capabilities required across the whole community to prevent, protect against, mitigate, respond to, and recover from the threats and hazards that pose the greatest risk."[42,94] NHSS seeks to build community resilience by strengthening and sustaining health and emergency response systems through monitoring data on a unified public health and healthcare preparedness capability framework.[51,95,96] The U.S. Veterans Health Administration is establishing a quality management system to support its comprehensive emergency management program that will monitor value through the use of five outcomes: 1) continuity and access to care; 2) medical outcome and functional status; 3) patient satisfaction; 4) readiness and competence; and 5) cost.[97] Evaluation of these policy initiatives through prospective data collection and outcomes monitoring will be important to determine if they actually improve national preparedness, resilience, and the quality of healthcare. In addition, adopting and implementing quality management system processes such as these within the emergency management/business continuity and public health fields will contribute to greater organizational resilience, continuity of service delivery, and societal security.[15–18]

REFERENCES

1. Sundnes KO, Birnbaum ML, Health Disaster Management Guidelines for Evaluation and Research in the Utstein Style. *Prehosp and Disaster Med* 2003; 17(Suppl. 3). http://www.laerdalfoundation.org/dok/Health_Disaste_%20Management.pdf. (Accessed August 14, 2015).

2. ICDRM/GWU Emergency Management Glossary of Terms. The Institute for Crisis, Disaster, and Risk Management (ICDRM) at the George Washington University (GWU), Washington, DC, June 30, 2009. http://www.gwu.edu/~icdrm. (Accessed August 14, 2015).

3. WHO, Trade, Foreign Policy, Diplomacy and Health. Glossary of globalization, trade and health terms. http://www.who.int/trade/glossary/story076/en (Accessed June 7, 2013).

4. *Emergency Preparedness Education and Training for Health Professionals: A Blueprint for Future Action.* Whitepaper for the Assistant Secretary for Preparedness and Response, 2008.

5. EMDAT-CRED. Natural Disasters Reported 1900–2000 graph-increase disasters. http://www.emdat.be/disaster-trends (Accessed June 5, 2013).

6. Committees on Increasing National Resilience to Hazards and Disasters, and Science, Engineering, and Public Policy. *Disaster Resilience: A National Imperative.* The National Academies, 2013. http://www.nap.edu/catalog.php?record_id=13457 (Accessed August 14, 2015).

7. UN Global Assessment Report on Disaster Risk Reduction. 2013. http://www.preventionweb.net/english/hyogo/gar/2013/en/home/GAR_2013/GAR_2013_2.html (Accessed August 14, 2015).

8. Noji E. Public Health Issues in Disasters. *Critical Care Medicine* 2005; 33(Suppl. I): 29–33.

9. EMDAT – CRED. Number of People Reported Affected by Disasters, 1900–2011. http://imgur.com/a/KdyTV#0 (Accessed June 5, 2013).

10. Strengthening National Public Health Systems to Emerging Health Challenges. Report of the Regional Conference of Parliamentarians. WHO, Bangkok, Thailand 2012.

11. Global Platform for Disaster Reduction for Health, 2013. http://www.who.int/hac/techguidance/preparedness/global platform2013/en/index.html (Accessed August 14, 2015).

12. Strategic Framework 2012–2013. Interagency Standing Committee, Global Health Cluster, World Health Organization. Geneva, Switzerland, 2013.

13. Yokohama Strategy and Plan of Action for a Safer World. Guidelines for Natural Disaster Prevention, Preparedness and Mitigation. 1994. http://unpan1.un.org/intradoc/groups/public/documents/APCITY/UNPAN009632.pdf (Accessed June 5, 2013).

14. FEMA mission statement. http://www.fema.gov/medialibrary/media_records/10089 (Accessed June 5, 2013).

15. HHS operating divisions. http://www.hhs.gov/about/foa/opdivs (Accessed August 23, 2014).

16. Hyogo Framework for Action 2005–2015: Building the Resilience of Nations and Communities to Disasters. International Strategy for Disaster Reduction, United Nations, 2005. http://www.unisdr.org/we/coordinate/hfa (Accessed August 17, 2015).

17. Bissell RA. Public Health and Medicine in Emergency Management. In: McEntire DA, ed. *Disciplines, Disasters and Emergency Management.* Springfield, IL, Charles C. Thomas Publisher, 2007.

18. Toman-Miller MA. U.S. Ambassador to Japan Speaks. *Stanford Daily.* November 22, 2011. http://www.stanforddaily.com/2011/11/22/u-s-ambassador-to-japan-speaks-on-%E2%80%9Cworlds-first-megadisaster%E2%80%9D (Accessed February 3, 2013).

19. Meier P. How Crisis Mapping Saved Lives in Haiti. *National Geographic Emerging Explorers in Explorers Journal* July 2, 2012. http://newswatch.nationalgeographic.com/2012/07/02/crisis-mapping-haiti (Accessed August 19, 2015).

20. Heinzelman J, Waters C. *Crowdsourcing Crisis Information in Disaster-Affected Haiti.* United States Institute of Peace, Washington, DC, October 20, 2010. http://www.usip.org/publications/crowdsourcing-crisis-information-in-disaster-affected-haiti (Accessed August 19, 2015).

21. Surveillance Resource Center. CDC. http://www.cdc.gov/surveillancepractice (Accessed June 5, 2013).

22. Nsubuga P, et al. Public Health Surveillance: A Tool for Targeting and Monitoring Interventions. In: *Disease Control Priorities in Developing Countries.* 2nd ed. http://www.ncbi.nlm.nih.gov/books/NBK11770 (Accessed June 5, 2013).

23. Integrated Disease Surveillance and Response (IDSR). http://www.who.int/csr/labepidemiology/projects/diseasesurv/en (Accessed June 5, 2013).

24. Disaster Surveillance. CDC. http://www.cdc.gov/nceh/hsb/disaster/surveillance.htm (Accessed June 5, 2013).

25. Surveillance-Casper Tool. CDC. http://www.cdc.gov/nceh/hsb/disaster/casper.htm (Accessed June 5, 2013).

26. Tabata N, et al. Casualty Estimation Model Based on the Mechanism of Human Injury in Damaged Buildings. Paper No. 729, 13th World Conference on Earthquake Engineering, Vancouver, BC, Canada, August 1–6, 2004. http://www.iitk.ac.in/nicee/wcee/article/13_729.pdf (Accessed June 5, 2013).

27. Sea, Lake, and Overland Surges from Hurricanes (SLOSH). National Weather Service, National Hurricane Center. May 4, 2010. http://www.nhc.noaa.gov/surge/slosh.php (Accessed June 5, 2013).

28. Health Effects and Medical Response. Applied Research Associates. http://www.ara.com/Capabilities/docs/HEMR072310.pdf (Accessed June 5, 2013).

29. A Review of Pandemic Preparedness Plans and Modelling Studies on Pandemic Influenza. The Scientific Committee on Advanced Data Analysis and Disease Modelling, Centre for Health Protection, March 2006. http://www.chp.gov.hk/files/pdf/a_review_of_pandemic_preparedness_plans_and_modelling_studies_on_pandemic_influenza_r.pdf (Accessed June 5, 2013).

30. About PAHO. WHO. http://www.paho.org/hq/index.php?option=com_content&view=article&id=91&Itemid=220&lang=en (Accessed June 5, 2013).

31. Safe Hospitals: A Collective Responsibility A Global Measure of Disaster Reduction. PAHO. WHO. http://www1.paho.org/English/DD/PED/SafeHospitals.htm (Accessed June 5, 2013).

32. Health Security Card. AMA Physician Resources. http://www.ama-assn.org//ama/pub/physician-resources/public-health/center-public-health-preparedness-disaster-response/health-security-card.page (Accessed June 12, 2013).

33. CNY Chapter Helps Launch Community Resilience Strategy. Red Cross. March 2013. http://www.redcross.org/news/article/CNY-Chapter-Helps-Launch-Community-Resilience-Strategy (Accessed June 12, 2013).

34. UN Millennium Development Goals 2015 and Beyond. WHO. http://www.un.org/millenniumgoals (Accessed June 12, 2013).

35. Disaster Risk Reduction: An Instrument for Achieving Millennium Development Goals. IPU-UNISDR. 2010. www.ipu.org/PDF/publications/drr-e.pdf (Accessed June 12, 2013).

36. Post-2015 Framework for Disaster Risk Reduction. *Prevention Web.* May 2013. http://www.preventionweb.net/english/hyogo/mdg/?pid:507&pil:1 (Accessed June 12, 2013).

37. Homeland Security Presidential Directive 5, Management of Domestic Incidents. February 28, 2003. http://www.fas.org/irp/offdocs/nspd/hspd-5.html (Accessed August 19, 2015).

38. Homeland Security Presidential Directive 7, Critical Infrastructure Identification, Prioritization and Protection. December 17, 2003. http://www.dhs.gov/homeland-security-presidential-directive-7#1 (Accessed August 19, 2015).

39. Homeland Security Presidential Directive 8, National Preparedness. December 17, 2003. http://www.fas.org/irp/offdocs/nspd/hspd-8.html (Accessed August 19, 2015).

40. Presidential Policy Directive 8, National Preparedness. March 2011. http://www.dhs.gov/presidential-policy-directive-8-national-preparedness (Accessed July 8, 2013).

41. Presidential Policy Directive 21, Critical Infrastructure Protection. February 12, 2013. http://www.whitehouse.gov/the-press-office/2013/02/12/presidential-policy-directive-critical-infrastructure-security-and-resil (Accessed August 19, 2015).

42. Core Capabilities. FEMA, Department of Homeland Security. 2012. https://www.fema.gov/core-capabilities (Accessed July 8, 2013).

43. National Preparedness System, Executive Office of the President. March 2011. http://www.dhs.gov/presidential-policy-directive-8-national-preparedness (Accessed July 8, 2013).

44. A Whole Community Approach to Emergency Management: Principles, Themes, and Pathways for Action. FEMA. http://www.fema.gov/media-library/assets/documents/23781?id=4941 (Accessed August 19, 2015).

45. National Response Framework. FEMA. May 2013 (revised). http://www.fema.gov/national-response-framework (Accessed August 19, 2015).

46. National Infrastructure Protection Plan (NIPP). FEMA. 2009. https://www.dhs.gov/national-infrastructure-protection-plan (Accessed August 19, 2015).

47. National Health Sector-Specific Plan, An Annex to the NIPP. DHS/HHS. 2010. https://www.dhs.gov/xlibrary/assets/nipp-ssp-water-2010.pdf (Accessed August 23, 2014).

48. Public Health Service Act. Legal Authority. HHS. 2006. http://www.phe.gov/preparedness/legal/pahpa/pages/default.aspx (Accessed August 19, 2015).

49. Homeland Security Presidential Directive 10, Biodefense for the 21st Century. April 28, 2004. http://www.fas.org/irp/offdocs/nspd/hspd-10.html (Accessed August 19, 2015).

50. Homeland Security Presidential Directive 21, Public Health and Medical Services. October 18, 2007. http://www.fas.org/irp/offdocs/nspd/hspd-21.htm (Accessed August 19, 2015).

51. National Health Security Strategy. Assistant Secretary for Preparedness and Response, Department of Health and Human Services. 2009. http://www.phe.gov/Preparedness/planning/authority/nhss/Pages/default.aspx (Accessed July 7, 2013).

52. National Health Security Strategy, U.S. Department of Health and Human Services, Assistant Secretary for Preparedness and Response, Washington, DC, 2015, http://www.phe.gov/Preparedness/planning/authority/nhss/Pages/default.aspx (Accessed August 27, 2015).

53. Soclof A. Gas Masks for Kids in Israel. *Jewish Telegraphic Agency.* January 30, 2013. http://www.jta.org/2013/01/30/news-opinion/the-telegraph/gas-masks-for-kids-in-israel (Accessed July 4, 2013).

54. Fendel I. Israel and U.S. Train Together on Emergency Response. *Arutz Sheva, Israel National News.* May 17, 2010. http://www.israelnationalnews.com/News/News.aspx/137572 (Accessed July 4, 2013).

55. TOPOFF 4 Full Scale Exercise. FEMA-DHS. October 17–19, 2007. http://www.dhs.gov/topoff-4-full-scale-exercise (Accessed July 4, 2013).

56. Matliach M. Earthquake Drill: What to Do in Case of Earthquake. October 20, 2012. http://nofryers.com/israel-earthquake-drill-what-to-do-in-case-of-earthquake (Accessed July 4, 2013).

57. Miskin M. Earthquake Doomsday Scenario: Hospitals Collapse, 4,000 Hurt. *Israel National News.* October 23, 2012. http://www.israelnationalnews.com/News/News.aspx/161229 (Accessed July 4, 2013).

58. Salomon G. Israel drills for regional war, earthquake, tsunami. *English News CN.* October 22, 2013.

59. Whole Community. FEMA. June 16, 2012. http://www.fema.gov/whole-community (Accessed July 15, 2013).

60. Teutsch SM. *Toward Quality Measures for Population Health and the Leading Health Indicators Report.* IOM. July 9, 2013. http://www.iom.edu/Reports/2013/Toward-Quality-Measures-for-Population-Health-and-the-Leading-Health-Indicators.aspx (Accessed August 19, 2015).

61. Citizens Corps. FEMA. http://www.ready.gov/citizen-corps (Accessed July 11, 2013).

62. Compendium of Disaster Health Courses. National Center for Disaster Medicine and Public Health. http://ncdmph.usuhs.edu/Documents/NCDMPH_Compendium_V1.pdf (Accessed June 20, 2013).

63. Barbera JA, MacIntyre AG, Shaw G, et al. *Healthcare Emergency Management Competencies: Competency Framework Final Report.* Institute for Crisis, Risk and Disaster Management, The George Washington University developed under contract with the U.S. Veterans Health Administration, 2007. http://www.va.gov/VHAEMERGENCYMANAGEMENT/Documents/Education_Training/Healthcare_System_Emergency_Management_Competency_Framework_2007.pdf (Accessed August 19, 2015).

64. Core Competencies for Public Health Professionals. The Council on Linkages Between Academia and Public Health Practice. 2010. http://www.phf.org/resourcestools/Documents/Core_Competencies_for_Public_Health_Professionals_2010May.pdf (Accessed September 23, 2014).

65. Schultz CH, Koenig KL, Whiteside M, et al. Development of National, Standardized, All-Hazard Disaster Core Competencies for Acute Care Physicians, Nurses and EMS Professionals. *Annals of Emergency Medicine* 2012; 59: 196–208.

66. Center for Domestic Preparedness. FEMA. https://cdp.dhs.gov (Accessed June 11, 2013).

67. Earthquakes Pose a Serious Hazard in Afghanistan. US Geological Survey Fact Sheet FS 2007–3027. http://pubs.usgs.gov/fs/2007/3027/pdf/FS07-3027_508.pdf (Accessed June 15, 2013).

68. Earthquake Hazards USGS Projects in Afghanistan. US Geological Survey. August 2011. http://afghanistan.cr.usgs.gov/earthquake-hazards (Accessed June 15, 2013).

69. Afghanistan: Food still unaffordable for millions. *IRIN.* March 12, 2009. http://www.irinnews.org/report/83417/afghanistan-food-still-unaffordable-for-millions (Accessed June 15, 2013).

70. Rising literacy in Afghanistan ensures transition. June 3, 2011. http://www.army.mil/article/59541/Rising_literacy_in_Afghanistan_ensures_transition/ (Accessed June 19, 2015).

71. Davis G. The Power of One. In: Firestone CH. *Afghans and Americans United (Telling the Stories of Transforming Lives Halfway Around the World).* Irwindale, CA, 1st Global Graphics Inc., 2011; 82–85.

72. Giddens J. COL, USA (ret), interview re: AFAMS, G. Davis, COL, USA (ret) COL re: Senior Medical Advisor to the Advisor to the Surgeon General of the Afghan Army. August 14, 2013.

73. HHS ASPR. At-risk individuals. http://www.phe.gov/Preparedness/planning/abc/Pages/atrisk.aspx (Accessed June 17, 2013).

74. Guidance on Planning for Integration of Functional Needs Support Services in General Population Shelters. FEMA. 2010. http://www.fema.gov/pdf/about/odic/fnss_guidance.pdf (Accessed August 19, 2015).

75. National Association of Community Health Centers. http://www.nachc.org (Accessed June 21, 2013).

76. From Hospitals to Healthcare Coalitions: Transforming Health Preparedness and Response in Our Community. End-of-Year 2007–2009 Reporting Period of Hospital Preparedness Program, HHS/ASPR. www.phe.gov/Preparedness/planning/hpp/Documents/hpp-healthcare-coalitions.pdf (Accessed on September 23, 2014).

77. Medical Surge Capacity and Capability, A Management System for Integrating Medical and Health Resources During a Large-Scale Incident. 2nd ed. Department of Health and Human Services, 2007. http://www.phe.gov/Preparedness/planning/mscc/Pages/default.aspx (Accessed July 10, 2013).

78. Priest C, Courtney B. Medical Surge Management: Public-Private Healthcare Coalitions. *Domestic Preparedness Journal* May 2011. www.domesticpreparedness.com/DomPrep_Journal (Accessed June 17, 2013).

79. MESH Coalition. http://www.meshcoalition.org (Accessed June 17, 2013).

80. National Healthcare Coalitions Resource Center. http://healthcarecoalitions.org/about-nhcrc (Accessed June 17, 2013).

81. Fry, A. Map Hispaniola. Big Car, Inc. Indianapolis, IN. 2014

82. Mendelson-Forman J, White S. The Dominican Response to the Haiti Earthquake, A Neighbor's Journey. *A Report of the CSIS Americas Program.* Center for Strategic and International Studies, Washington, DC, November 2011.

83. Haiti 2010 Earthquake. Photo, devastated pediatric clinic. Photo taken by, courtesy of BCFS Health and Human Services, Grimm D.

84. Transnational Programme, Frontera Verde Project, UN Environment Programme. Disasters and Conflict. April 2011. http://www.unep.org/disastersandconflicts/CountryOperations/Haiti/TransnationalProgramme/tabid/105715/Default.aspx (Accessed August 23, 2014).

85. Schaaf B. Haiti and the DR Launch Joint Reforestation Project. *Haiti Innovation.* June 6, 2013. http://haitiinnovation.org/en/2013/06/06/haiti-and-dr-launch-joint-reforestation-project (Accessed June 22, 2013).

86. Disaster Risk and Resilience Factors. VA National PTSD Center. http://www.ptsd.va.gov/public/types/disasters/effects_of_disasters_risk_and_resilience_factors.aspe (Accessed August 17, 2015).

87. PTSD Coach. VA National PTSD Center. http://www.ptsd.va.gov/public/pages/PTSDcoach.asp (Accessed July 22, 2013).

88. Bradt DA, Aitken P. Disaster Medicine Reporting: The Need for New Guidelines and the CONFIDE Statement. *Emergency Medicine Australia.* http://onlinelibrary.wiley.com/doi/10.1111/j.1742-6723.2010.01342.x/abstract (Accessed August 19, 2015).

89. The Sphere Handbook, Minimum Standards in Health Action, Humanitarian Charter and Minimum Standards in Humanitarian Response. The Sphere Project, 2011, www.sphereproject.org (Accessed August 27, 2015).

90. Health Indicator Sortable Statistics. Centers for Disease Control and Prevention. http://wwwn.cdc.gov/sortablestats/Report_Docs/PDFDocs/Sortable_Stats_Data_Sources.pdf (Accessed August 27, 2015).

91. System of Records, National Disaster Medical System. Assistant Secretary for Preparedness and Response, Department of Health and Human Services, 2009. No longer on the Internet, hardcopy available from the author.

92. Research Group on Emergency and Disaster Medicine. Utstein Template Project, 2012. http://currents.plos.org/disasters/article/utstein-style-template-for-uniform-data-reporting-of-acute-medical-response-in-disasters (Accessed August 19, 2015).

93. Debacker M. Data Reporting Disasters. Emergency Management and Disaster Medicine Academy, 2012. http://www.cochrane.org/sites/default/files/uploads/Evidence_aid/DEBACKER%20-%20Data%20reporting%20in%20disasters.pdf (Accessed August 19, 2015).

94. National Preparedness Goal. FEMA, Department of Homeland Security, 2012. https://www.fema.gov/national-preparedness-goal (Accessed August 19, 2015).

95. Public Health Preparedness Capabilities: National Standards for State and Local Planning. Centers for Disease Control and Prevention, March 2011. http://www.cdc.gov/phpr/capabilities (Accessed August 19, 2015).

96. Healthcare Preparedness Capabilities: National Guidance for Healthcare System Preparedness. January 2012. (http://www.phe.gov/preparedness/planning/hpp/pages/default.aspx (Accessed September 23, 2014).

97. Performance Improvement Management System. VHA, Office of Emergency Management, 2010. http://www.va.gov/vhaemergencymanagement (Accessed August 19, 2015).

12

LEGISLATIVE AUTHORITIES AND REGULATORY ISSUES

Ernest B. Abbott and Jeffrey H. Luk

OVERVIEW

Catastrophic disasters disrupt the health and medical system in a variety of different ways. The event itself – a hurricane or earthquake – may cause physical damage to medical infrastructure (e.g., hospitals, clinics, doctors' offices, laboratories, pharmacies, and medical suppliers). The event can also disrupt electrical power or communications capabilities such as Internet and computer services. A disaster can also create new requirements for medical care by injuring large numbers of people when buildings or other structures collapse. Similarly, a pandemic outbreak of infectious disease, or widespread exposure to chemical, radiological, or biological contamination, can overwhelm medical infrastructure and medical providers with the number of patients requiring treatment. Finally, as demonstrated by the 2004 Indian Ocean Tsunami, Hurricane Katrina in the United States (2005), and more recently, in 2012, Hurricane Sandy on the east coast of the United States, a disaster can force the evacuation of hundreds of thousands of people who then become separated from their regular medical care network (e.g., doctors, nurses, prescription medications, and medical records). These evacuees arrive in relocation areas with medical systems unprepared to treat the baseline health and medical needs of so many additional patients, in addition to any traumatic and psychological conditions caused by the disaster.

Catastrophic disasters also challenge the legal basis of the health and medical system. Practitioners may be familiar with legal and regulatory requirements applicable to the provision of medical care in normal times, but in a disaster environment, compliance with some legal requirements becomes problematic. Are regulatory requirements relaxed or changed under emergency conditions, or are practitioners left simply to do the best they can and trust that regulators will choose not to enforce standards? The following scenarios illustrate this dilemma:

- In the United States, federal rules require clinicians to perform a medical screening examination and stabilization of any patient who arrives on hospital grounds requesting medical care. How does this regulation apply when there is a physical plant disruption such as a hospital flood or fire, or a chemical, biological, or radiological contamination on site?

- Virtually all sovereign governments ensure the competence of medical professionals by issuing certificates or licenses to those authorized to practice medicine within their respective borders – yet, in a disaster, medical volunteers and medical providers from other jurisdictions will cross state or national boundaries to treat disaster victims. Under what circumstances do their medical or other health professional licenses allow them to treat casualties? Should they be concerned about violating geographic restrictions contained in their professional malpractice insurance policies?

- Sovereign nations, and provincial and states within sovereign nations, bestow on designated officials broad emergency powers over healthcare and public health systems – upon some sort of designation or declaration of a state of emergency or disaster. Yet, exactly what those powers are, who can exercise them, how timely they can be executed, and how those powers affect institutions and professionals providing medical care can vary dramatically.

This chapter will review disaster legal issues primarily from the perspective of persons or institutions – including individual doctors or nurses, medical practices, laboratories, clinics, and hospitals – who collectively provide medical care to patients in the midst of a catastrophic disaster or other public health emergency. This chapter summarizes the key areas where the legal environment of medical care may change as a result of disasters and other catastrophic events. Some of these changes occur in the specific requirements imposed on practitioners by national, state/provincial and, in some cases, local governments and agencies. Providers must be alert to how those changed requirements will be communicated to them.

Providers must also be familiar with how a disaster may create exposure to economic penalties and liabilities where the care provided in emergencies does not meet normal standards of medical practice. This exposure may be experienced, after the fact, through judicial award of money judgments based on malpractice of medical providers. Providers must also be cognizant of requirements existing with third-party payers and private credentialing organizations and vendors.

Despite what some may view as a minefield of legal risks – risks of criminal or civil penalties, revocation of critical licenses or credentials, and malpractice or breach of contract judgments – disaster medicine creates an extraordinary and rewarding opportunity to provide medical care to people when they need it most.

CURRENT STATE OF THE ART

Medical Malpractice and Disaster Medicine

Just as they do during non-disaster times, medical care providers must manage the liability risk (for improper or inadequate treatment) during catastrophic events. In litigious countries like the United States, the tort liability system may have as much or more effect on how medicine is practiced than do regulatory standards imposed by the government. Under this tort system, liability attaches to any persons or institutions who participated in care provided to an individual patient who has suffered a significant injury or illness – *if* the injury or illness can be proven, in court after the fact, to be wholly or partially their "fault." Damages awarded can range in the millions of dollars for individual patients, including both "compensatory damages" (such as current and future medical expenses, lost wages, projected future losses in wages, or a monetary reward for pain and suffering), and, in egregious situations, "punitive damages." The impact of malpractice liability on individual practitioners is reduced in nations where medical care is provided by government. In England and Wales, for example, practitioners employed by the National Health Service (NHS) are indemnified from liability; practitioners outside the NHS must arrange for liability protection through a medical defense society or union, and the NHS itself may be vicariously liable for negligent acts of its practitioners.[1]

The liability system is intended to make "tortfeasors" (the label given to the persons whose improper actions or failure to act caused a patient's injuries and illness) pay money damages to make that patient (or the patient's estate) "whole," to the extent possible. The liability system is also intended to create a strong incentive to persons and institutions to act with appropriate care – that is, prudent and reasonable care in accordance with accepted medical practice in the circumstances in which that care is provided.

Medical care providers are generally familiar with the liability system as it applies to the day-to-day practice of medicine. The same principles also apply to the practice of medicine under disaster conditions. In fact, one of the main issues discussed by public health officials and emergency planners is how to assure that medical providers can assist in the response to a catastrophic event without incurring debilitating liability judgments.[2] Liability systems vary considerably in different nations and even in different states or provinces within nations – but it is useful to provide at least an overview of key characteristics of liability systems. An individual or institution can be found "liable" for an injury to a person if the individual or institution owes a duty to provide treatment, fails to fulfill that duty, and thereby causes harm to that person.[3] In many jurisdictions, however, the government – using doctrines like "sovereign immunity" – has limited or even completely immunized not only itself from liability for actions taken during emergencies, but has also immunized other persons or institutions providing medical care in the midst of emergencies.[4]

The "duty" described previously, whose breach leads to liability, can arise from several sources. These include: 1) an agreement (in which a medical provider promises to perform certain services in a particular manner); 2) statutes (in which the legislature has declared that a person has a duty, or responsibility, to act in a particular way); or 3) "common law" resulting from judgments of courts in individual cases determining or denying liability in particular situations and establishing legal precedents.

For medical malpractice liability, the most significant "duty" owed by a medical provider is a duty to diagnose and treat patients without negligence, in accordance with a standard of care. Normally this is the care which is reasonable for a qualified professional providing treatment in similar circumstances.[5] In "normal," non-disaster times, providers generally manage the risk that they might be found negligent by establishing and following standard procedures and protocols. Following these procedures minimizes the likelihood that their actions could, in hindsight, be characterized as "negligent." Providers also protect themselves by purchasing medical malpractice insurance.[6]

During a disaster, however, medical providers' ability to use non-disaster standard procedures and protocols is severely compromised because:

- Facilities are not fully functional due to infrastructure or operational damage.
- Facilities are crowded.
- Care may be provided under austere conditions and in nontraditional settings like alternate care facilities or even the field.
- Supplies and drugs are in short supply.
- Staff is short-handed and fatigued.
- Staff has been imported from other jurisdictions that use different procedures and protocols.
- Medical records are missing or temporarily unavailable.
- Volunteer medical providers are working in unfamiliar facilities and jurisdictions.

The circumstances under which the conduct occurs determine whether it can be classified as "negligent" medical care. A doctor operating in a tent field hospital established by government officials or in an airport concourse may not have the equipment necessary for certain tests that in "normal times" would be standard medical procedure. It would not be "negligence" for a doctor to treat a patient requiring care during this emergency without using unavailable equipment, even if the patient experienced life-threatening complications that would have been avoided had that equipment been used. Rather, the care provided would be reasonable given the environment and situation.

There are, nonetheless, significant liability risks that providers face in providing care during an emergency. For example, a patient's attorney may agree that a doctor did the best he or she could in the middle of a catastrophic event – but argue that the event became catastrophic because of negligence. For example, a medical facility could be found negligent in the development of its emergency plan which led to the loss of electrical power during a surgical procedure and that *this* negligence – not the heroic efforts taken after disaster had struck – is what led to injury. Proper pre-event preparation might have ensured that necessary test equipment was available or training was provided on substitute tests that did not require the equipment.

Moreover, whether the particular care provided was "negligent" even under emergency conditions will likely be a question that a court would decide after the fact. Some medical providers are, accordingly, concerned that actions taken in a catastrophic environment could lead to large malpractice judgments based not on true negligence, but rather on their inability to provide the care that would be considered appropriate under normal conditions. Even though practitioners are held to the standard that care must be reasonable given the circumstances in which it was provided, this may be insufficient protection. Given the delay inherent in litigation, the memory of emergency conditions will fade long before practitioners will be judged for possible negligence.

Malpractice insurance may not provide protection to providers in the disaster environment. To limit an insurer's malpractice exposure, malpractice insurance is typically written to cover a particular type of practice in a particular geographic location. Yet, in a disaster, medical providers may be needed in other jurisdictions, perhaps even in another state or country. They may be asked to practice in temporary or substandard facilities and may perform procedures that are not normally within their scope of practice. Standard malpractice insurance may exclude from coverage medical care provided under any of these circumstances.

To address some of these concerns in the United States, most states and the federal government have enacted legislation that provides some immunity to medical professionals providing care during disasters. State "Good Samaritan" legislation and the Federal Volunteer Protection Act of 1997[7] provide significant immunity protection. For example, in California's Good Samaritan Law, there is "no liability where the licensee in good faith renders emergency care at the scene of an emergency."[8] In many states, liability protection is also extended to medical professionals who volunteer to help state or local public health or emergency management officials. California also has this type of provision: "health providers . . . who render services during any state of . . . emergency, at the express or implied request of any responsible state or local official or agency, shall have no liability for any injury sustained by reason of such services, regardless of how or under what circumstances or by what cause such injuries were sustained."[9] This immunity does not apply when the injury was intentional or resulted from actions (or failures to act) that were clearly likely to cause harm – that is, where the injury results from a "willful" act or omission. Similarly, the Federal Volunteer Protection Act provides that "no volunteer of a nonprofit organization or governmental entity shall be liable for harm caused by an act or omission of the volunteer if . . . the harm was not caused by willful or criminal misconduct, gross negligence, reckless misconduct, or a conscious, flagrant indifference to the rights or safety of the individual harmed by the volunteer."[10] Note that protection under this law extends only to the actual volunteer – and not to any organization that dispatches or supports the work of volunteers (e.g., nongovernmental organizations such as the American Red Cross).

Furthermore, providers should be aware that the liability protection offered by Good Samaritan legislation and the Federal Volunteer Protection Act typically does not extend to those who receive compensation for their efforts. Is a physician who is part of a group medical practice, and who receives a fixed share of the profits from that practice, even though much of the profits were earned while the practitioner was "volunteering" in a disaster, covered? Could the immunity provided by a Good Samaritan Act be challenged if a medical care provider receives an allowance for meals and living expenses while serving in a disaster field hospital? Is a pharmacist in the employ of a corporation a "volunteer" if the corporation allows the pharmacist, during his paid vacation, to travel to a disaster and serve as a pharmacist at a shelter for evacuees? The answers to these questions are unclear and make the extent of liability risk uncertain.

Immunity is also provided under the laws of some U.S. states to contractors providing emergency response services "in coordination with" or "under contract to" emergency response authorities.[11] Other statutes may provide immunity to responders in particular circumstances – such as in the administration of smallpox vaccine.[12]

There are often limitations on the scope of immunity. For example, no immunity extends to: 1) caregivers receiving compensation; 2) persons who are unlicensed; and 3) for-profit businesses (such as incorporated providers of medical care). Furthermore, the immunity from liability given to government contractors may also be limited. Although contractors are generally not liable when operating under a government contract that precisely describes the required duties, contractors can be liable if they are permitted to use judgment in performing the contracted work.[13] This exception can be significant, because the provision of medical services frequently requires the application of judgment.

Although liability for volunteers practicing disaster medicine is very limited, there is uncertainty about the definition of "volunteer" and the scope of liability protection provided by existing immunity statutes. There is also controversy about whether the public is served by extending immunity from liability to practitioners whose actions are found to have caused unnecessary injury or even death to patients. For example, to address liability (and other issues), a model law called the Uniform Emergency Volunteer Health Professionals Act, was developed in the United States in 2007. While the intent was to encourage states to provide for legislative immunity, 6 years later, the primary provisions of this model act had been enacted in only twelve of the fifty-two U.S. states and territories, and some states rejected the liability provisions.[14] The accelerated pace of legislative changes and the variety of approaches adopted in many U.S. states illustrate the challenges in finding solutions to the many liability issues.

Despite a lack of clarity under existing law, medical providers can take actions that will eliminate or significantly reduce their exposure to liability when providing volunteer medical services in an emergency. Within the United States, virtually all of these solutions require that a medical provider be registered with an official governmental response organization and become a part of the government response. Government officials increasingly view the coordination of volunteer and private sector response efforts (i.e., public–private partnerships) to be a critical part of disaster preparedness and response efforts. In many U.S. states, statutes immunize actions taken at the direction of state emergency management officials.[15] In some state and federal government programs, volunteer individual practitioners are "hired" as temporary employees for minimal or no salary and the government extends its immunity protection to them and becomes the defendant to pay judgments arising from any remaining liability.[16] For example, if an individual is deployed to assist at a disaster site as part of a national Disaster Medical Assistance Team, the provider becomes "federalized" and is allowed to practice in any U.S. state or territory and has federal liability protections.

The liability protections available under current law and under a number of legislative proposals are primarily directed to individuals, and particularly to individual volunteers, rather than to the nonprofit organizations and private businesses that may participate in response efforts. Some of the organizations that will assist in medical care provision during disaster events are not traditionally part of the medical system. For example, during a pandemic influenza event, public health officials may request a major employer in a community to assist in the distribution of pharmaceuticals and administration of vaccines to its employees and their families. Current law may provide only limited protection to these businesses. They may refuse to participate in planning and actual response unless they can obtain liability protection or indemnity.

Registration with an official government response organization provides other important benefits, particularly where medical providers will be working in facilities, communities, and states different from those in which their home practice is located. These benefits – discussed in greater detail later – include recognizing the provider's medical license in the new state, generating identification documents and credentials that allow the provider entry into the disaster area, and logistical support.

Healthcare facilities are also exposed to liability should they fail to provide quality care and meet the needs of their patients after a disaster. One type of negligence is corporate negligence, which hospitals face when managing liability claims. Hospitals have four duties: "[1] a duty to use reasonable care in the maintenance of safe and adequate facilities and equipment; [2] a duty to select and retain only competent physicians; [3] a duty to oversee all persons who practice medicine within its walls; and [4] a duty to formulate, adopt, and enforce adequate rules and policies to ensure quality care for the patients."[17] Accordingly, healthcare organizations that hold these duties may be found liable if they fail to safeguard the welfare and safety of patients, employees, and occupants.

Healthcare facilities are further at risk via vicarious liability in that "the negligent acts of a health care provider may be directly imputed to the hospital in which the care is given."[18] Vicarious liability is based on the legal doctrines of *respondeat superior* and *ostensible agency*. It extends liability to employers based on an assumption that the employer has control over the actions of its employees.[19] Therefore, hospitals may be held liable for the conduct of nurses, residents, interns, and other health professionals. Typically, only negligent acts committed within the "scope of employment" are subject to liability. In addition, most courts will not hold a hospital liable for the negligence of an employee if the contract specifically negates an employment or agency relationship. Accordingly, physicians are considered independent contractors in many instances, and this status shields hospitals from any liable acts that they may commit. However, "courts have found that a hospital's imposition of rules and regulations upon staff physicians is enough to undercut the doctors' independent contractor status and expose the hospital to liability."[20]

Even where there is no actual agency, liability can be based on ostensible agency. This occurs when: 1) the patient looks to the entity rather than the specific physician for care and the patient reasonably believes that the healthcare provider is an agent or employee of the hospital; and 2) the hospital affirmatively "holds out" the doctor as its employee or agent, or knowingly permits the provider to project himself or herself as such. This theory applies to care in the emergency department since patients are unaware of and unconcerned with the technical complexities that define the employment relationship

and generally seek medical treatment without regard to who the physician will be. Accordingly, "public has every right to assume and expect that the *hospital* is the medical provider it purports to be."[21] Consequently, since few patients presenting for care will specifically request an individual physician and patients during a disaster are likely to seek treatment in emergency departments rather than from individual physicians, the *ostensible agency* theory is likely to be relevant in litigation cases arising from crises.

As noted previously, legal protections for volunteer health professionals rarely extend to hospitals and other organizational entities providing healthcare and health services. Some hospitals may possess civil liability protections in their role as government entities or emergency care providers through specific grants of immunity during public health emergencies. These protections would grant these hospitals sovereign immunity because of their status as public institutions or as hospitals affiliated with state government. Sovereign immunity essentially removes the legal routes through which these facilities may be sued. City- or county-run hospitals may be considered state entities by some courts, effectively granting them the same protection from liability as healthcare facilities affiliated with the state. However, other courts consider hospital administration as a corporate undertaking, and therefore not within the sphere of state action and not protected by sovereign immunity. In addition, some states have greatly reduced or even eliminated this type of protection. Furthermore, sovereign immunity is curbed in many states through tort claims acts, which effectively waive sovereign immunity for government actors and agents acting within their official capacities.[22]

As demonstrated by some U.S. states, hospitals do not entirely lack safeguards. In Oregon, designated emergency healthcare facilities enjoy immunity as state agents for any claim arising out of the provision of uncompensated medical care in response to a declared emergency. In Minnesota, the governor can "grant immunity to organizations and individuals providing health care services during a declared emergency when good faith acts or omissions cause harm during emergency care, advice, or assistance." The Department of Health in Hawaii is statutorily empowered to enter into agreements with healthcare providers, including healthcare entities, to control infectious epidemics that require more resources than the department itself can provide. When a hospital acts pursuant to such an agreement, they "are not liable for any personal injuries or property damage resulting from the performance of their duties, absent willful misconduct." The state legislation in Louisiana immunizes hospitals and healthcare entities from liability resulting from injury or damage to people or property during a state-declared emergency, except in cases of gross negligence or willful misconduct. However, the lack of adequate planning for disasters could be considered gross negligence.[23]

Legal Framework for Disaster Medicine and Public Health Emergencies: Public Health Powers

In the United States, the foundation of both the "normal" and "disaster" legal system is the Constitution that created the federal system of government. In this system, it is state governments, and not the federal government, that have primary authority and responsibility to protect public welfare. In the Constitution, states granted enumerated powers to the federal government, including authority over interstate and foreign commerce, national defense, and the right to tax and spend for the public welfare. Yet the states retain their basic police power – the power to place restrictions on people and property and business to protect the public.

The U.S. system of federalism devised by its founders is reflected throughout the medical system. Acting under its police power authority, states have created licensing and certification requirements for hospitals, physicians, nurses, pharmacists, and other medical professionals. State statutes specify rules for reporting of communicable diseases and other public health concerns (such as unsafe conditions in restaurants), and empower public health officials to take action (impose quarantine, or close restaurants) to protect the public. State law is also generally responsible for determining the standards of care applicable to the medical system and these standards are enforced through state court judgments in the medical malpractice system.

The federal government nonetheless also exerts extraordinary power over the medical care system. Communicable diseases can spread across state and international boundaries – allowing the federal government to exercise its power over international and interstate commerce and impose federal rules to prevent transmission of disease. For example, federal legislation authorizes federal quarantine within a state on findings that a state's quarantine efforts are ineffective.[24] Similarly, because pharmaceuticals and medical supplies are sold in interstate commerce, the federal government has authority to regulate drug manufacture and use. Federal taxes fund the Medicare and Medicaid programs that pay for 23% and 17%[25] of the medical care provided in the United States, respectively. As a result, federal requirements placed on medical care providers who treat Medicare or Medicaid patients are enforced by federal civil and even criminal penalties. These requirements include protection of patient records and service obligations in addition to billing and reimbursement procedures.

In the United States, officials at all levels of government have broadly worded authority to take action in the face of "imminent threats," to "save lives, defend property, and protect the public health and safety." This authority can extend to actions that would normally be viewed as blatant violations of constitutionally protected rights to "life, property and the pursuit of happiness." These actions include seizure or destruction of property (including hospitals, medical supplies, or even animals); voluntary or mandatory evacuation of people from (or detention of people in) a facility or geographic area; or even mandatory treatment of persons.[26,27] For some of these actions, the government may be required to provide compensation. For others, the government may provide discretionary disaster assistance, and for still others, individuals and businesses are not provided any additional resources.

Mandatory evacuation may be difficult to enforce in some societies. There are a wide range of enforcement schemes for mandatory evacuation orders. For example, mandatory detention of tuberculosis patients who refuse to complete a drug regimen may include physical restraints. A "mandatory" evacuation in advance of a hurricane or a fire can be enforced by forcibly transporting evacuees to safe areas or by simply notifying residents of the danger and, if they refuse to leave, requesting them to provide authorities with contact information for their next of kin.

As demonstrated during the 2009 H1N1 influenza pandemic, the U.S. federal government has a procedure to waive federal requirements applicable to healthcare facilities during public health emergencies. At the time, President Obama declared H1N1 influenza a national emergency given that "the rapid increase in illness across the Nation may overburden healthcare resources and that the temporary waiver of certain standard Federal requirements may be warranted in order to enable U.S. healthcare facilities to implement emergency operations plans."[28] This declaration, combined with the Department of Health and Human Services (HHS) secretary's declaration of H1N1 as a public health emergency, allowed healthcare facilities to petition HHS under Section 1135 of the Social Security Act[29] for waivers of regulatory requirements implicated by the emergency.

Provider Obligation to Protect Patient Rights

Privacy

The patient-doctor relationship is a sacred trust and medical files contain a great deal of highly personal information. These files contain data not just about the state of a patient's health, but about the patient's habits, family, finances, sexual practices, and sexual orientation. Proper sharing of patient information (with multiple medical specialists and with third-party payers) is critical to achieve appropriate medical care and for successful healthcare system operations. In the United States, however, disclosure without patient consent in accordance with specific provisions is prohibited, frequently by multiple statutory and regulatory provisions. Most medical providers use well-developed procedures to assure that any exchange of patient information complies with law.

During disasters, sufficient resources to comply with these procedures may be lacking. Circumstances may force additional disclosures, and trigger exceptions to "normal" disclosure requirements. For example, in the aftermath of a catastrophic disaster, locating missing persons, while respecting patient privacy, can be difficult. Finding relatives of family members to authorize treatment and determining what medical information to provide family members and the general public are additional challenges. Disaster conditions also require hospitals and medical personnel to operate in stressful, rapidly changing, and uncertain situations. Despite this environment, the need to share information and keep the public informed must be weighed against the privacy rights of patients and their families. Federal and state laws governing the release of patient information are generally unchanged in the setting of a disaster; however, there are provisions for information sharing in emergent settings. Typically, a provider should obtain patients' verbal permission for a disclosure of health information, and patients should be "informed in advance of the use of the disclosure," when possible.[30]

Federal Health Insurance Portability and Accountability Act Requirements and Protected Health Information in the United States

One of the more detailed regulatory systems governing protection of personal healthcare information is that in the United States. A detailed discussion of this system and its provisions for public health emergencies illustrates the issues that any healthcare system must address. The U.S. regulations on confidentiality were developed in the year 2000 pursuant to the Health Insurance Portability and Accountability Act (HIPAA). This act was primarily intended to address difficulties experienced when employees with employer-provided health insurance changed jobs – but this required regulators to address how to protect patient privacy when transferring health records to the new employer. This requirement for protecting privacy while addressing the portability of insurance led to a comprehensive federal regulation governing how participants in the medical care system – care providers, laboratories, and third-party payers, such as insurance companies – maintain, protect, and disclose what is defined as protected health information (PHI). To assure appropriate attention to the privacy interest of patients, HIPAA requires that medical care providers and payers have a documented privacy policy and appoint a privacy official and contact person responsible for training the workforce in PHI privacy policy.[31]

HIPAA allows healthcare providers to share a patient's PHI as necessary to provide treatment, payment, or healthcare operations; this sharing of information applies during disaster events just as it does in "normal" times.[32] Treatment includes coordinating patient care with others, such as emergency relief workers or personnel at potential referral receiving sites. Furthermore, where required or necessary to prevent or control disease, injury, or disability, disclosure to a public health authority is expressly authorized by HIPAA.[33]

State legislation largely echoes the provisions of federal HIPAA regulations. Some states further delineate permissible activities for sharing PHI. For example, California legislation expressly permits the communication of PHI between emergency medical personnel by radio transmission or other means.[34]

Location/Health Status

HIPAA generally permits providers to share very limited information concerning a patient's location and general condition (including death) as necessary to identify, locate, and notify family members or guardians.[35] Therefore, if necessary, a hospital may inform the police, press, or the public at large to the extent necessary to help locate, identify, or otherwise notify family members as to the location and general condition of the patient. Federal regulations also permit the sharing of basic information, including the patient's identity, residence, age, sex, and condition, to disaster relief organizations without patient consent if necessary to facilitate disaster response.[36] Even when disclosures are permitted by HIPAA, however, providers must be aware of any state statutes that might restrict release of patient information. California law expressly permits disclosure of basic patient information to state or federally recognized disaster relief organizations,[37] and Arkansas has adopted basic HIPAA disclosure provisions,[38] but other states have not done so and may have more stringent restrictions on disclosure. There is some confusion about whether HIPAA rules *permitting* disclosures preempt state laws.[39] What is clear is that, under normal circumstances, when a patient incapable of communication arrives at a hospital, the facility must attempt to make contact with a family member or surrogate within 24 hours – a requirement that is suspended during periods of disaster.[40]

Hurricane Katrina in August 2005 in the United States forced the rapid evacuation of more than 1 million residents. In the process of evacuation, many families were separated. Isolated individuals included parents and other caregivers, children, and grandparents. This disaster exposed the challenges associated with effective federal government evacuee tracking and family member reunification. As a result, in the post-Katrina Emergency Management Reform Act of 2006,[41] Congress enacted legislation requiring the Federal Emergency Management Agency

(FEMA) administrator to establish a: 1) National Emergency Child Locator Center (in cooperation with the U.S. Attorney General) within the National Center for Missing and Exploited Children; and 2) National Emergency Family Registry and Locator System. The former provides information about displaced children and serves as a resource for adults who have information about displaced children; the latter focuses on allowing displaced adults to register, furnish personal information to a database, and make this personal information accessible to "those individuals named by displaced individuals."[41] Implementation of this section requires a memorandum of understanding with the Department of Justice, and HHS, the American Red Cross, and "other relevant private organizations."[41] This system should help medical providers in their efforts to locate a patient's next of kin.

Public Health Officials

In the United States, HIPAA allows disclosure of PHI to a "public health authority that is authorized by law to collect or receive such information for the purpose of preventing or controlling disease, injury, or disability, including, but not limited to, the reporting of disease, injury, vital events such as birth or death, and the conduct of public health surveillance, public health investigations, and public health interventions." This authorization also permits disclosures to "a person or entity other than a public health authority" if it can demonstrate that it is acting "to comply with requirements of a public health authority." PHI can also be disclosed to a person who may have been exposed to a communicable disease or is at risk of spreading a disease (for example, sexually transmitted disease), "and is authorized by (state) law to be notified as part of public health intervention or investigation." These specific provisions governing disclosure to public health officials that facilitate public health interventions are even more important during a public health emergency than during "normal" times. The provision in the HIPAA rule authorizing disclosure of PHI to law enforcement officials "to help identify or locate a suspect, fugitive, missing person," and "to provide information related to victim of crime" is even more critical during public health emergencies, particularly those that are triggered by criminal or terrorist activity.[42]

Immediate Danger

HIPAA further permits the disclosure of PHI without consent or prior notification when "necessary to prevent or lessen a serious and imminent threat to the health or safety of a person or the public; and is to a person or persons reasonably able to prevent or lessen the threat, including the target of the threat."[43] This exception is particularly important when communicable disease is involved; it allows disclosure of a patient's communicable disease status without the patient's consent to other persons (such as a patient's spouse or partner) to protect them from exposure.

Reporting and Recordkeeping Requirements

Even where disclosures of PHI are fully authorized, and even if those disclosures are in the midst of a public health emergency, HIPAA requires that the entity making the disclosure track when the disclosure was made, and to whom. Authorities must make this information available to the patient on request.[44] As a result, when developing their emergency plans, medical providers in the United States must pay special attention to ensuring that they will have systems to document the disclosures that they make, whether required or permitted, of a patient's PHI.

Media

A public health emergency or disaster will generate significant media attention. Despite media inquiries, hospitals must maintain confidentiality of PHI. A hospital reporter must have a patient's consent before releasing any personal information. A facility may, however, disclose general information about a disaster response, such as the number of victims treated at the facility and the general types of injuries sustained, so long as this information is not specifically identifiable to an individual. As mentioned previously, a hospital may disclose specific PHI to the media if this disclosure constitutes an effort to locate family members.

Data Storage and Security

The requirements of HIPAA include a stipulation that "covered entities" institute a data recovery plan ensuring continuity of operations in the aftermath of a disaster.[45] A covered entity is a health plan, a healthcare clearinghouse, or a healthcare provider who transmits any health information in electronic form in connection with a HIPAA transaction.[46] Covered entities include doctors, hospitals, laboratories, and pharmacists, and also the insurance companies and other third-party payers that have access to a patient's PHI. This required system must include a data backup plan for the retrieval and restoration of electronic PHI as well as an operations plan that enables the maintenance of privacy and security safeguards over PHI. These plans for data recovery have become increasingly important since the Health Information Technology for Economic and Clinical Health (HITECH) Act was signed into law in February 2009. The act promotes the adoption and meaningful use of health information technology by reducing the cost for covered entities to implement electronic medical records and establishing penalties for covered entities that do not follow security and privacy rules. The act also commits an investment of $20 billion (USD) in health information technology infrastructure.

State regulations may also require data protection and access in a disaster situation. For example, in California, hospital licensing regulations require hospitals to safeguard their medical records against loss or corruption.[47] California also details specific requirements for organizations maintaining only electronic records. These include off-site backup and retrieval systems.[48]

Although it is preferable to anticipate post-disaster challenges and proactively pass enabling legislation, in some situations the legal requirements have been modified post-event. For example, in the aftermath of Hurricane Katrina, the U.S. Secretary of HHS issued a waiver of penalties for violating certain HIPAA privacy provisions that proved impractical in the disaster setting including:

> Sanctions and penalties arising from noncompliance with the following provisions of the HIPAA privacy regulations: (a) the requirements to obtain a patient's agreement to speak with family members or friends or to honor a patient's request to opt out of the facility directory (as set forth in 45 CFR §164.510); (b) the requirement to distribute a notice of privacy practices (as set forth in 45 CFR §164.520); or (c) the patient's right to request privacy restrictions or confidential communications (as set forth in 45 CFR §164.522).[49,50]

HHS provides a fact sheet confirming that HIPAA is not suspended and explaining what provisions may be waived during a national or public health emergency.[51]

Individual Liberty

Decisions on treatment of patients involving such issues as selection of diagnostic tests, therapeutic agents, surgical procedures, drugs, and diets are generally made by physicians and other care providers only with consent after appropriate disclosure of the risks, costs, benefits, and alternatives. This system reflects the privacy and liberty interests that patients have in their own bodies, and it is enforced not only by numerous regulatory requirements, but also by judicial precedents. The provider may be liable after a patient suffers an adverse effect of treatment, if it was a known adverse effect of that treatment, and it was not fully disclosed to the patient. The rules may change during a disaster. To protect the public health, the government is granted significant power to require testing or treatment of individuals, isolation of patients with a communicable disease, and quarantine of those with suspected or known exposure to communicable disease irrespective of the patients' wishes. Exercise of these authorities requires balancing the threat to the public with the risks to the individual. In addition, enforcement of public health orders in pandemic and other public health emergencies – when authorities are overwhelmed with the sheer number of individuals affected – can be very challenging.

Legal Basis of Mandatory Public Health Measures

Governments have a wide variety of legal tools that address communicable disease. Some, such as quarantine, have a history extending back centuries if not millennia. These public health powers may significantly limit individual patient rights, but as illustrated later, U.S. courts have generally provided wide latitude to public health authorities in adopting them.

A seminal case on restricting individual rights to protect the public health is *Jacobson v. Massachusetts*, 197 U.S. 11 (1905). In 1902, the City of Cambridge, Massachusetts, passed an ordinance finding that "smallpox [was] prevalent in the city and continues to increase." The city ordered vaccination of all its inhabitants, except children with a doctor's note saying that they were unfit subjects for vaccination. Henning Jacobson, a charismatic minister who had emigrated from Sweden, refused to be vaccinated. Reverend Jacobson viewed vaccination as unsafe and ungodly. Side effects of the cowpox vaccine used in vaccination were common. He refused to pay the $5 fine specified for violators, and he appealed his fine all the way to the U.S. Supreme Court.[52]

The court responded with a decision supporting the right of communities to use their police powers to protect the public welfare. In the words of Justice Harlan:

> Real liberty for all could not exist if each individual can use his own, whether in respect of his person or property, regardless of the injury that may be done to others.... *Upon the principle of self defense, of paramount necessity, a community has the right to protect itself against an epidemic of disease which threatens the safety of its members.*[53,54]

Justice Harlan also qualified the scope of the power to restrict liberty for public health: "Police power of state must be held to embrace, at least, such *reasonable* regulations established directly by legislative enactment as will protect the public health and safety... *subject, of course, that... no rule... or regulation... shall contravene the Constitution of the United States, or with any right which that instrument gives or secures.*[55,56] In other words, within the United States, public authorities have the right to protect their communities from an epidemic of disease, but the actions taken to do so must be "reasonable," with some rational basis grounded in knowledge about treatment for the disease and its incubation period, virulence, and communicability. The requirement that public health measures – even those taken to protect the community from disease – cannot "contravene the Constitution" or any "right which that instrument gives or secures" is also extremely significant. The fifth and fourteenth amendments to the U.S. Constitution preclude a federal or state government from taking a person's liberty or property without "due process." Mandatory treatment, inoculation, quarantine, and isolation measures clearly restrict the liberty of individuals. Therefore, state and federal government use of these powers must be in accordance with due process, which includes both "procedural due process" (following appropriate *procedures*) and "substantive due process" (requiring that officials have a *substantive* reason and a rational basis for restraining individual liberty).

The case of *Best v. Bellevue Hospital New York* is illustrative of these "due process" principles.[57] Mr. Best was diagnosed with tuberculosis but refused to complete his medication regimen and could have developed a drug-resistant strain. The health department issued an order detaining him and requiring completion of his treatment. Mr. Best filed suit against the health department and the hospital where he was confined. Mr. Best was granted a hearing and the courts assessed whether he was a danger to himself and the community. After a prolonged legal process that included four public hearings, significant attorneys' fees, and at least seven administrative, state court, and federal court orders, the court found that the health department and other defendants had indeed provided the due process required by the Constitution. On procedural due process, the federal appeals court described the factors considered in determining constitutionality of detention procedures:

> First, the private interest that will be affected by the official action; second, the risk of an erroneous deprivation of such interest through the procedures used, and the probable value, if any, of additional or substitute procedural safeguards; and finally, the Government's interest, including the function involved and the fiscal and administrative burdens that the additional or substitute procedural requirement would entail.[58,59]

In general, quarantine and isolation procedures that provide notice and an opportunity for hearing (which can be held after an individual is detained) will satisfy procedural due process requirements. The hearing requirement does not preclude health officers from taking action immediately when there is a risk that the public will be exposed to a communicable disease if a person is not immediately placed in isolation or quarantine.

Courts must also determine whether a public health order violates a person's substantive due process rights; that is, it must review whether the government had a rational, reasonable basis for the order. This analysis involves a balancing of the collective right of self-defense enunciated in *Jacobson* against individual rights to liberty and property. In these cases, courts have traditionally given great deference to the judgment of public health officers. One historical example is provided in an opinion by Judge Hydrick of South Carolina's Supreme Court in 1909: "In dealing with such matters, a wide range of discretion must be allowed the local authorities, and they should not be interfered with, unless it is clearly made to appear that they have abused that discretion to the probable injury to health or life."[60,61]

There are relatively few recent cases defining the Constitutional requirements for mass quarantine; at the time of this writing, the United States has not had occasion to impose a mass quarantine for more than 50 years. In the U.S. legal system, two basic principles that have support in case law can assist public health officials in understanding legal approaches to control of communicable disease. First, the greater the restraint on individual liberty, the greater the responsibility of government to provide for those restrained. For example, when the state confines individuals in prison, or involuntarily commits individuals in a mental health facility, these individuals are no longer able to access their own food or medicines; courts have declared confinement without food or medicine, or in crowded and dilapidated prison conditions to be unconstitutional.[62] When individuals and families are deprived of the ability to meet their basic needs for food, shelter, and medical care by quarantine or other movement restrictions, the state becomes obligated to provide those basic needs.

Second, despite the great deference given public health officials, they cannot justify their orders simply by stating that the actions will prevent the transmission of disease. They must also show that they could not have controlled the spread of disease with different public health measures that would have had less impact on individual liberty. The U.S. Constitution provides that states cannot deprive persons of their "life, liberty, or property without due process." As in the *Best v. Bellevue* case, this language has been interpreted to mean that the public health objective should be achieved with the least restrictive measures possible in all cases, including those for patients with communicable diseases, suspected infections, and known or suspected exposures.[63]

By enforcing "restrictions of movement," the goal of public health officials is to increase the "social distance" between potentially infected persons and uninfected persons. Effectiveness of different movement restrictions in increasing social distance and reducing transmission of disease is highly dependent on disease characteristics. These include incubation period, method of communicability, virulence, treatment options, and whether asymptomatic patients are contagious.

Some U.S. states have adopted statutes that include "the least restrictive means necessary test,"[64] and others have not yet defined the minimum requirements for quarantine. In many cases, strict quarantine procedures are not necessary to reduce disease transmission. Other restrictions of movement that increase social distance, such as school closings, restrictions on public meetings, work quarantine, and wearing of masks or respirators may be just as effective.[65] Because there are a number of less intrusive measures that may be equally or more effective than mandatory detention in a quarantine facility, a public health official may need to provide an affidavit with the quarantine order that explains why these less physically intrusive options were not selected.

Although there are a myriad of measures that reduce disease transmission, some are less intrusive on individual rights than others. For example, restricting public meetings or requiring use of face masks respects individual liberties much more than placing people in involuntary detention in a quarantine center. The decision about which measures to employ has important legal consequences.

Legal preparation for a large-scale quarantine from a pandemic event extends beyond simply developing a notebook of standardized hearing notices and affidavits to be signed by public health officials. Officials and their attorneys must also enhance the procedural readiness of the judicial system, encouraging the courts to think through the following issues:

▪ The systems to be used for handling a large number of hearing requests.
▪ The measures that will be employed to protect the safety of hearing officers and participants from exposure to disease.
▪ Documentation/affidavits that will be required in a mass quarantine environment.
▪ How the court and other officials will communicate to the public.

Consent

Generally, rules for consent do not change in a disaster or public health emergency. The medical care system is accustomed to situations in which it is impossible to obtain consent from patients. For children, or those who are unconscious, mentally disabled, or otherwise unable to make an informed choice, consent is generally obtained from parents, a spouse, or a guardian. In an emergency, whether it involves an individual patient or a whole population during a catastrophic event, patient consent for management of an imminent medical crisis is implied. In this context, an "emergency" is a situation in which delay in immediate care would lead to serious disability or death, or immediate treatment is required to relieve severe pain. Frequently, U.S. state statutes provide specific definitions and requirements.

For example, in California, B&P § 2397 protects a medical care provider from liability when treatment is provided without consent if the patient was unconscious, there was insufficient time to inform the patient, or the patient was without the legal capacity to provide consent and there was no time to obtain consent from the patient's legal representative. The term "capacity" is defined by the statute as "a person's ability to understand the nature and consequences of a decision and to make and communicate a decision." Minor patients lack capacity as a matter of law except when the minor has been given "emancipation" status (e.g., by court order, by military service, by marriage, or because the minor has been determined self-sufficient). In some jurisdictions, there are additional exceptions to the rule that minor patients lack decision-making capacity. For example, in California, a patient twelve years of age or older has the legal capacity to make informed consent decisions with respect to communicable reportable diseases, outpatient mental health, substance abuse, and pregnancy-related treatments.

The specific rules of consent can vary substantially in different states. For example, rules regarding pregnancy-related treatment are frequently controversial and there is no national consensus on the age at which a minor no longer requires parental consent. As a result, if volunteers from one U.S. state provide disaster medical services in another state, they should be aware of the specific consent laws that apply in that state.

Authorization to Provide Medical Care

Licensing and Credentialing

LICENSING

Sovereign nations and, in federal systems, state/provincial governments generally regulate the practice of medicine. Thus, providers must be licensed in the state in which they are providing medical care. State licensing requirements generally extend not only to clinical care providers (e.g., physicians, nurses, pharmacists, veterinarians), but also to institutions (e.g., clinics, hospitals, and nursing homes). To obtain a state license, providers or institutions must demonstrate that they meet particular educational, training, and experience requirements. Medical practice is restricted to those skills and procedures commensurate to the training received and authorized under a professional license, a so-called scope of practice.[66] Requirements are established by state laws and agencies; they vary by state, and licenses authorize professional activities only in the state in which the license is granted. When a disaster covers a broad geographic area, nations, and states may find that their existing resources of medical (and other) professionals are insufficient and that they must rapidly obtain assistance of professionals from other localities. Medical professionals from other areas must be qualified to provide disaster relief services.

On declaration of a disaster or state of emergency in the United States, the governor of a state generally has the power to adjust the state's licensing requirements to allow practice by professionals from out of state. In some states the governor has the power to completely suspend the state's licensing scheme,[67] although in practice this power is not invoked except through procedures that assure professional qualifications. More commonly, a governor will exercise an emergency power that temporarily recognizes professional licenses issued in another state. For example, after declaring an emergency in California, the California Emergency Services Act bestows on the governor broad emergency powers that include the ability to grant "any person holding a license issued by any state for professional skill permission to render aid involving such skill to meet the emergency as fully as if the license had been issued in California."[68] In the United States, the Emergency Management Assistance Compact automatically provides for "cross licensing" to professionals who are deployed to a state as "state personnel" under this agreement. During Hurricane Katrina, existing laws allowing cross-licensing of professionals did not work as quickly or as broadly as needed, and several efforts to broaden these rules were initiated. The Commission on Uniform State Laws developed the Uniform Volunteer Emergency Health Practitioners Act in 2006 and 2007. This act, which is only effective in a state after it is introduced to and enacted by the state, provides automatic cross-licensing of health professionals volunteering through a recognized credentialing system during emergencies.

HOSPITAL CREDENTIALING

In addition to the licensing requirement, practitioners need "privileges" to be permitted to work in a specific healthcare facility. The Joint Commission (formerly known as the Joint Commission on the Accreditation of Healthcare Organizations) is an independent, not-for-profit, U.S.-based organization nationally recognized for setting certain hospital performance standards and granting accreditation and certification to those hospitals meeting these standards. Joint Commission International, established in 1997, "extends The Joint Commission's mission worldwide by assisting international health care organizations, public health agencies, health ministries and others to improve the quality and safety of patient care in more than 80 countries."[69] The Joint Commission's Hospital Accreditation Manual includes standards for administrators to grant disaster privileges (i.e., authorization for practitioners to work in their hospitals). When the healthcare facility emergency management plan has been activated and the hospital capacity is exceeded by the immediate surge in patients, "the CEO or medical staff president or their designee(s) has the option to grant disaster privileges."[70] The official authorized to grant disaster privileges has broad discretion. To receive these privileges, however, the provider must present: 1) a current picture hospital identification card; or 2) a current license to practice issued by any state, federal, or regulatory agency; or 3) identification indicating that the individual is a member of a federal Disaster Medical Assistance Team; or 4) there must be a current hospital or medical staff member with personal knowledge regarding the practitioner's identity.[71] This standard requires that individuals authorized to grant hospital privileges be specifically identified and that there is a mechanism for managing personnel operating under temporary disaster privileges. The requirement further specifies that there must be a means for allowing staff to readily identify these personnel and that verification of credentials and privileges begins as soon as the immediate patient surge has resolved. This process is identical to the process established under Joint Commission standard M.S.4.100 for granting privileges to meet an important patient care need.[72] As an alternate to the Joint Commission process, the executive branch of state government may also have authority to grant hospital privileges in the setting of a declared emergency.

Financial and Reimbursement Issues

Regional disaster plans may include memoranda of understanding between healthcare facilities for staff sharing during emergencies. In some models, the facility requesting assistance provides reimbursement directly to temporary employees; in other systems, the regular employer continues to pay salaries and receives reimbursement from the hospital that benefited from the shared services. For example, the District of Columbia Hospital Association and the District of Columbia Emergency Healthcare Association, both in Washington, D.C., maintain agreements among their members to assist hospitals in emergency management. These agreements address the logistics of personnel and equipment sharing and the transfer of patients. They also assign credentialing responsibilities and legal liability to hospitals receiving assistance from others.[56,73,74]

Federal rules for reimbursement in the United States under Medicare, Medicaid, and state children's health insurance programs were relaxed in the aftermath of Hurricane Katrina. This was primarily because compliance with prior provider enrollment in these programs, recordkeeping, and licensure in the same state in which services were provided was both impractical and counter to public policy. Six days after the storm made landfall, HHS issued a waiver of various requirements for participation in federally funded healthcare programs including:

1. Certain conditions of participation, certification requirements, program participation or similar requirements, or pre-event approval requirements for individual healthcare providers or types of healthcare providers, including as applicable, a hospital or other provider of services, a physician or other healthcare practitioner or professional, a healthcare facility, or a supplier of healthcare items or services.

2. The requirement that physicians and other healthcare professionals hold licenses in the state in which they provide services, if they have a license from another state (and are not affirmatively barred from practice in that state or any state in the emergency area).[75]

Although this post-hoc administrative response was less efficient than having pre-event procedures in place, the government recognized the importance of encouraging flexibility in staffing to provide adequate healthcare delivery in the midst of a mass-casualty incident. To accommodate an increasing patient surge, this waiver also extended to hospital bed classification requirements allowing "non-medical beds" to be used for patients requiring medical services. The government reimbursed these services according to relaxed billing requirements. During the time of disaster relief, paper billing and substitute data were accepted for those records that were destroyed or unrecoverable.

Healthcare Facilities

The Joint Commission standards require hospitals, acute care facilities, and acute care psychiatric facilities to maintain and regularly update disaster plans and to train and test staff preparedness.[76] Medicare in the United States also promulgates federal hospital emergency management plan accreditation requirements. Although Medicare "conditions of participation" for critical care facilities do not contain specific requirements for disaster management plans, the Interpretative Guidelines issued by Medicare to its state survey teams require the adoption of "emergency preparedness plans and capabilities."[77] These guidelines for hospitals include "critical access hospitals" – a safety network of hospitals identified by Medicare to ensure access to healthcare services in rural areas. They require that the hospital formulate and implement a disaster plan to "ensure that the safety and well-being of patients are assured" during a disaster.[77] Such plans must include coordination among all levels of government emergency preparedness authorities with specific identification and response to likely risks in their general areas, such as earthquakes, floods, and so forth.[78] The Interpretative Guidelines are detailed in their list of issues to be addressed in the disaster plan and include consideration for security of walk-in patients; security of supplies (including pharmaceuticals, water, and equipment); communications systems; provisions in the event of gas, power, and water disruptions; and mechanisms for the transfer of patients.

The U.S. Occupational Safety and Health Administration asserts authority to regulate "any reasonably anticipated disaster that could create a hazard for employees" at the workplace.[79] Such hazards include workplace injuries, fires, blood-borne pathogen exposure, and radiation and other hazardous materials exposures.

The U.S. 2006 Pandemic and All-Hazards Preparedness Act (PAHPA) mandates that state and local governments and other eligible entities, such as hospitals, "develop and implement emergency management plans that are consistent with evidence-based benchmarks and standards developed by the Department of Health and Human Services."[80] It authorizes HHS to "withhold emergency preparedness funds from hospitals that do not meet certain benchmark requirements."[81]

HHS also administers the Hospital Preparedness Program (HPP). A major goal of this program is to "strengthen health care partnerships at the community and substate levels."[82] A requirement of the program is that funding for HPP must be directed through state health departments so community response entities work together to develop community emergency management capabilities. Consequently, hospitals are required to participate in regional cooperation to receive funding for the program. In addition, the program encourages hospital involvement in community coalitions and community emergency response networks. HPP is based on capabilities and requires recipients of funding to develop and demonstrate specific benchmarks by the end of the funding cycle. The goal is to create objective and reproducible ways of measuring hospitals' emergency management abilities.

U.S. states also impose hospital disaster plan requirements. For example, California hospital licensing regulations require a "disaster and mass casualty program," which must be approved by the medical staff and administration, practiced by conducting at least two drills per year, and available for review by representatives of the California Department of Health Services.[83] California regulations require the plan to contain a hazard vulnerability analysis, community linkages with an all-hazard command structure, specific procedures during a disaster, a mechanism for plan activation, a process for reporting emergencies to external authorities, a command structure, and a means to notify and activate personnel.[84] Even though hospitals may fulfill these disaster regulations, they could be out of compliance with a multitude of requirements placed on them during non-disaster operational periods. For example, patient–nurse ratio requirements in the State of California (designed to provide individual patients with optimum nursing care) are unlikely to be practical in the setting of mass casualties and may actually be harmful to the affected population. Staffing ratios should not determine hospital capacity, as is often the case in non-disaster settings when nursing shortages frequently dictate the maximum number of patients that may be cared for at a facility. During a disaster, however, it would be difficult to obtain timely waivers of legislated nurse–patient ratios. Hospitals should be encouraged to prepare agreements with its nursing staffs and unions prior to and in anticipation of a patient surge during a disaster. Discussions between hospital administration and nursing should also explore means to increase staffing during emergencies.

Medical Screening Exams in Disasters

The requirement for medical screening varies by country. These differences have implications for the management of disaster victims. Article 25 of the Universal Declaration of Human Rights states that "everyone has the right to a standard of living adequate for the health and well-being of himself and of his family, including food, clothing, housing and medical care and necessary social services, and the right to security in the event of unemployment, sickness, disability, widowhood, old age or other lack of livelihood in circumstances beyond his control."[85] However, it does not specifically mention any universal requirement for the medical screening of individuals who present to a healthcare facility requesting assistance.

In the United States, individuals who present to an emergency department are required to receive a medical screening exam by law. The U.S. Emergency Medical Treatment and Active Labor Act (EMTALA) was passed in 1986 in response to reports that hospitals were refusing to treat individuals with emergency conditions if they did not have insurance.[86] EMTALA requires Medicare-participating hospitals to provide any individual presenting to hospital grounds for care a medical screening, stabilizing services, and appropriate transfer to a higher level of care if indicated. In addition, EMTALA sets forth civil monetary penalties on hospitals and physicians for:

1. Failing to properly screen an individual seeking medical care.
2. Negligently failing to provide stabilizing treatment to an individual with an emergency medical condition.
3. Negligently transferring or releasing from care an individual with an emergency medical condition (including active labor).[87]

Waivers to EMTALA mandates, even in the setting of a mass-casualty event, have not been well developed. Project Bioshield legislation (enacted in the United States in 2004) provides some relief from EMTALA when the federal government declares an emergency.[88] This legislation allows HHS and the Centers for Medicare and Medicaid Services to temporarily waive EMTALA standards relating to:

1. Transfer of unstable emergency patients if required by the circumstances of a declared emergency by a hospital in the emergency area during the period of the emergency; and
2. Directing or relocating patients for medical screening to alternate locations in accordance with the state emergency preparedness plan.

The U.S. federal government issued an EMTALA waiver during Hurricane Katrina that suspended the requirement for hospitals in the designated disaster area to screen and stabilize patients if the disaster situation prevented it, provided that these patients were redirected to another facility for the medical screening examination and stabilization.[89] As the Agency for Healthcare Research and Quality notes, EMTALA requirements are not entirely clear, particularly with respect to transfer or "surge" facilities. The Agency for Healthcare Research and Quality recommends that elements of EMTALA "be reduced/waived for a temporary/limited service surge facility."[90] For example, the benefits of transfer to a surge facility would be to create capacity for other patients needing tertiary hospital services, not necessarily for the benefit of the transferred patient; the patients would not necessarily be asked to consent to transfer to the surge facility.[90]

In the United States, EMTALA regulations could be suspended if a Section 1135 waiver were issued. According to regulation 42 CFR 489.24(a)(2), when an 1135 waiver has been granted, "sanctions . . . for an inappropriate transfer or for the direction or relocation of an individual to receive medical screening at an alternate location do not apply to a hospital with a dedicated emergency department" if certain conditions are met.

Emergency Management and Public Health Systems

Through the end of the twentieth century, there was relatively little effort to connect the public health and medical care systems with the emergency management system. Public health officials worked independently, operating under public health laws and authorities to protect public health and transmission of communicable diseases. Similarly, emergency management officials worked in isolation and were not prepared to assist in response to a major public health emergency such as an epidemic that had the potential to overwhelm the healthcare system. There was rarely coordination of disaster program development between public health, medical, and emergency management officials.

In the United States, there was a major philosophical shift after the terrorist attacks of September 11, 2001. The federal government mobilized massive resources to focus attention on preparing the nation for catastrophic events. Within a year of the attacks, Congress had enacted legislation creating a new federal department, the Department of Homeland Security (DHS), with the mission of protecting the nation from terrorist attacks and other threats. By Executive Order, President Bush directed the new DHS to establish a National Response Plan (later renamed the National Response Framework) that would coordinate emergency response efforts of the entire federal government, in collaboration with states.[91] The president also required DHS to establish a National Incident Management System (NIMS) and directed that *every* federal agency (not just DHS) require state and local governments to be "NIMS compliant" as a condition for receipt of federal preparedness grants.[92] Congress passed legislation adding new emergency healthcare authorities, with particular emphasis on preparation for a bioterrorism event.[93] Federal funding for state and local governments, first responders, and, to some extent, hospitals expanded dramatically to address the healthcare impact of potential terrorist attacks. Applicants for these billions of dollars in preparedness funding[94] had to demonstrate that they were "NIMS compliant." Although the emergency management system had traditionally focused only on *government* actions, legislation passed after September 11, 2001, required that all first responders, including the private owners of critical infrastructure, like hospitals and other medical facilities, be included in any emergency management plans and responses.[95] Other countries also re-examined and updated policies and procedures sometimes using the U.S. system as a model. Nevertheless, there remains no international consistency in approach, and the ministries with the lead for different types of events vary by country.

U.S. Federal Disaster Assistance Programs

If a catastrophic event creates emergency or disaster conditions that exceed the response capacity of state and local governments, the governor of a state may request the president of the United States to declare a "major disaster" or emergency under the Robert T. Stafford Disaster Relief and Emergency Assistance Act (Stafford Act).[96] This declaration, once issued, triggers eligibility for a number of different federal assistance programs, including both grant assistance and direct federal assistance. Several of these programs may be important for medical providers.

First, under the Stafford Act's Public Assistance Program, the federal government will provide a grant to "eligible applicants" of "not less than 75%" of the "eligible cost" of 1) performing certain emergency work to save lives, property, and the public health and safety; and 2) "repairing, restoring, replacing, or reconstructing" any damaged state or local government facilities, and eligible facilities of nonprofit organizations.[96] The Stafford Act's public assistance program, administered by FEMA within the DHS, can be critical to the financial survival of eligible entities affected by a declared disaster event. These include government and nonprofit healthcare providers, such as hospitals, clinics, ambulance services, and nursing homes.

Entities must meet certain requirements to be eligible for FEMA grant assistance. For example, the provision of emergency medical care is considered part of the normal business of a medical facility and the associated costs are not generally eligible for FEMA reimbursement, except in the most catastrophic of events.[97] The cost of creating additional facilities for emergency treatment may, however, be eligible for federal reimbursement during a catastrophic disaster.[98] Disaster assistance grants provided by FEMA are considered federal grants, subject to all of the boilerplate requirements of federal regulations,[99] including a requirement that all contracts for work be competitively bid.[100] Federal support will only be provided to supplement (not replace) assistance available from insurance, including employer-provided and individual policies, and Medicare/Medicaid.

U.S. Government Emergency Powers over Healthcare Facilities

State emergency statutes are drafted extremely broadly and provide enormous power to governors and other designated state officials for emergency response. As previously discussed, the scope of these powers allows substantial restrictions on individual liberties by evoking quarantine, isolation, and mandatory treatment or inoculations. The governors' powers over private property are similarly expansive. For example, in Georgia (and in many other states) the governor may "Commandeer or utilize any private property if he finds this necessary to cope with the emergency or disaster."[101]

Although the power to commandeer property is clear, any exercise of this power is subject to two critical requirements identified in the Fifth Amendment to the U.S. Constitution: "a person shall not *be deprived of life, liberty, or property, without due process of law . . . nor shall private property be taken for public use, without just compensation.*" Thus, an owner can object to seizure of the property and is entitled to due process to determine whether the seizure is justified. Similarly, the owner will be entitled to government compensation, measured by the value (as determined in court) of the property taken. In emergency circumstances, the due process and compensation hearings will occur after the government has taken possession of the property.

Although it may be authorized in law, commandeering of property in emergencies is highly disfavored. Effective catastrophic response by governments requires development of response plans, training of those who will implement them, and exercising those plans to ensure that they work. Governments recognize that the voluntary involvement of the private sector is fundamental to effective disaster response. In fact, the U.S. Congress has added a number of amendments to federal emergency management laws since Hurricane Katrina, directing FEMA and other agencies to include the private sector in emergency response plans and exercises. These statutory directives are repeated in Presidential Directives on National Preparedness.[102] Moreover, the emphasis in emergency planning is to identify emergency response needs in advance of the disaster and, if private sector response resources are required, to invite bids and proposals for contracts under which resources will be provided in an emergency. The cooperation from the private sector that is necessary for effective emergency planning and response is incompatible with any plan that relies on commandeering of property except in the most unusual of events – where a need could not have been anticipated, and circumstances precluded negotiation of contractual arrangements.

Emergency Waiver of U.S. State Laws

In addition to commandeering property, governors in many U.S. states have authority to temporarily suspend state laws and regulations that may interfere with the response or that become impossible to implement due to emergency conditions. California law states that "the Governor may suspend any regulatory statute . . . or the orders, rules, or regulations of any state agency . . . where he declares that compliance would . . . in any way prevent, hinder, or delay the mitigation of the effects of the emergency."[103] This provision can be applied to procedural and paperwork requirements of agencies, to medical staffing or other state regulatory requirements governing medical care, to substantive licensing provisions, or virtually any regulatory statute. For example, during the 2004 hurricane season (after Florida was struck by Hurricanes Charlie, Francis, Ivan, and Jean), Florida's state coordinating officer (with authority delegated from the governor) issued sixty-one Supplemental Orders that overrode statutory and regulatory requirements encompassing such varied subjects as property valuations for ad valorem taxes (taxes based on the value of real estate or personal property), the cancellation of homeowners' insurance policies, staffing requirements for home care services, and the reconstruction of facilities for cattle auctions.[104] Medical providers should be aware of this provision so that they can request waiver or suspension of requirements if necessary during a catastrophic event.

RECOMMENDATIONS FOR FURTHER RESEARCH

Comparative Research on Public Health Emergency Laws

The legal and regulatory issues that arise in catastrophic events are highly dependent on the particular legal system of the jurisdiction in which the catastrophe occurs. There are necessarily significant differences in the legal requirements faced by medical practitioners in a country with a national healthcare system (such as the United Kingdom), than in a country (such as the United States) where medical care is provided by private practitioners and healthcare facilities, albeit with heavy government involvement as insurer and regulator.

Despite these differences, each healthcare system needs to address the underlying legal issues discussed in this chapter during catastrophic events:

■ How do the powers of government over healthcare practitioners and healthcare facilities change in catastrophic events?

■ How does a nation or state modify its licensing and credentialing systems to allow practitioners, arriving from beyond its borders in the midst of an emergency, to help the nation's overwhelmed medical system in providing care to disaster victims?

■ How does a nation protect the privacy of individual patients and their medical records when care is provided in catastrophic events?

■ What limitations are there on the state's authority to order mandatory actions against consent of individuals and families (e.g., quarantine, isolation, evacuation, cordon sanitaire, mandatory treatment, mandatory inoculations, closure of gathering places)?

■ How does the state modify its liability to assure that medical practitioners volunteer to assist in catastrophic events – without jeopardizing incentives to act with care under the circumstances?

This chapter focuses primarily on the ways in which the United States and its constituent states have addressed these issues. In the years since the September 11 terrorist attacks and Hurricane Katrina, the United States has dedicated extraordinary resources and attention to improving disaster readiness. Much of the guidance cited in this chapter was prepared by or partially funded by the U.S. DHS and HHS, including CDC.

Other nations will necessarily follow a different path in addressing these critical questions. Some of the practices of the United States may be unique to its peculiar, mixed public and private, fee for service, insurance-centric medical system – mixed together with a highly litigious legal system. But all nations either explicitly or implicitly, directly or by default, have laws, rules or practices that determine how the authorities of government over the medical care system change in emergencies, how catastrophic events will impact individual rights with respect to movement and treatment, and how medical practitioners and providers work together with health authorities to provide treatment to those in need.

Accordingly, an important area for future research is a comparative study of how different nations address the key issues faced in public health emergencies. This will help inform which legal regulatory issues in emergencies are a function of a particular legal or medical system – and which are simply a function of the challenge faced by *any* medical and legal system when its resources and facilities are damaged and overloaded in catastrophic events.

Public Health Emergency Legal Drills and Exercises

Whatever the form of the national medical system, it is critical that those participating in it understand the rules prior to the event that overwhelms the medical system. An emergency plan cannot guide response consistent with law, and protect medical responders from legal violations, if the rules that apply in emergencies are not known. Legal issues encountered in catastrophic events are extremely dependent on who is the client and how that client may be affected by the event – either as a person or entity suffering loss, as a government seeking to protect the welfare of residents and businesses, or as a medical worker providing services on a contract or volunteer basis to assist those in need.

The kinds of legal issues encountered include "zero sum gain" situations where different individuals or entities seek to redistribute the cost or pain of the catastrophe by imposing liability so that negligent providers must pay the injured patient for the loss caused by their acts. This can include nonmonetary or regulatory issues, where those subject to regulatory requirements are simply trying to ensure that they do not run afoul of the law when their world has been disrupted by a catastrophic event.

To reduce ambiguity in the aftermath of a disaster, it is useful to clarify the rules prior to an event. It is harder to act confidently if liability is a concern. The knowledge that authorities will grant a waiver of a rule when a disaster has rendered compliance much more difficult would improve a responder's ability to care for patients. A directive by the Uniform Law Commission to develop and then encourage legislative adoption of a Uniform Emergency Healthcare Practitioners Act is one example of a project that addresses these issues. Changing legislation may not be the most important challenge. The U.S. CDC's Public Health Law Program convened a group of experts to develop a National Action Agenda for Public Health Legal Preparedness.[105] Although summit participants identified some areas in which new laws would be useful, they did not believe that developing new law was the first priority. Instead, they maintained that those who make, use, and are affected by the laws should become more familiar with the scope, substance, and application of existing laws.

Attention should not be limited to the written rules and laws that provide authority for officials to act. In the United States, after the ineffective management of Hurricane Katrina, studies found that the government may have had adequate legal *authority* to manage public health emergencies. However, public health and medical personnel may have had an inadequate *understanding* of existing laws and how they could be applied in the unusual environment of a public health emergency. Furthermore, even in cases when providers do comprehend the statute, existing laws have not necessarily been enacted with consideration for scenarios in which patient care needs massively exceed available medical and health resources, creating a scarce resource environment. Further work is needed to define an effective approach to these circumstances.[106,107]

Healthcare personnel will attempt to provide the best possible care during a disaster. Through the ethical principles of beneficence and non-malfeasance, medical providers aim to care for patients to the best of their abilities despite the lack of usual resources that exists during catastrophes. Accordingly, even if providers do comprehend existing laws, it is most likely not in the forefront of their minds when caring for the patients in front of them. In order to increase awareness of possible legal issues during disasters, exercises such as tabletop or full-scale drills need to be completed before the event.

These simulations serve to test emergency plans, train emergency responders, and familiarize all organizations that will be involved in emergency response with the other organizations, governments, and businesses with whom they will work during a catastrophic event. In most of these exercises, relatively little attention is paid to the kind of legal issues that are important to the government response – let alone that by private and non-profit organizations. Future research in the area of legal issues in disasters will be significantly advanced through the careful development of a legal issues tabletop exercise.[108] Here, a potential public health emergency scenario is presented, and participants drawn from organizations that must respond determine what regulations and laws might interfere with providing medical care effectively. The result of the tabletop exercise would be the identification of legal obstacles that are as yet unresolved and require further research.

Acknowledgments

The authors express their sincere thanks to Douglas P. Brosnan, MD, JD for his valuable contributions as the co-author for this chapter in the first edition.

REFERENCES

1. Medical Malpractice Liability. United Kingdom (England and Wales). Law Library of Congress, prepared by Prepared by Clare Feikert, Senior Foreign Law Specialist, May 2009, at http://www.loc.gov/law/help/medical-malpractice-liability/uk.php. http://www.loc.gov/law/help/medical-malpractice-liability/uk.php (Accessed June 7, 2013).

2. "Legal Issues" Report identified in a study for HHS's Emergency System for the Advance Registration of Volunteer Health Professionals, September 2006 Draft. http://www.publichealthlaw.net/Research/PDF/ESAR%20VHP%20Report.pdf (Accessed November 13, 2013).

3. Hoffman S. Responders' Responsibility: Liability and Immunity in Public Health Emergencies. *Georgetown Law Journal* 2008; 96: 1913–1969.

4. This doctrine of sovereign immunity, which originates from English common law during the feudal period, premised on the maxim that the "King could do no wrong" persists as a basic principle of sovereignty. See 74 Fordham L. Rev. 2927, April 2006. The Federal Tort Claims Act, 28 USC § 1346(b), provides limited exception to the doctrine of sovereign immunity only under certain circumstances.

5. Koenig KL, Cone DC, Burstein JL, Camargo CA. Surging to the Right Standard of Care. *Acad Emerg Med* February 2006; 13(2): 195–198.

6. Malpractice insurers in turn manage their risk by requiring that insured practitioners and institutions establish systems and procedures that will reduce the likelihood of malpractice judgments.

7. 42 U.S.C. § 14503.

8. Cal. B&P § 2395.

9. Cal. GC § 8659.

10. 42 U.S.C. § 14503.

11. Fla. Stat. § 252.51.

12. 42 U.S.C. § 239(2).

13. In the World Trade Center Disaster Site Litigation, 521 F.3d 169 (2d Cir. 2008), at pages 196–198 (Finds no immunity of government contractor for health damages suffered by employees who did not wear effective masks to protect lungs from toxic substances at disaster site, because government did not require contractor to abandon normal safety procedures.).

14. The Commission on Uniform State Laws has approved the Uniform Volunteer Emergency Health Practitioners Act. This "Uniform Act" – which becomes "law" in a state only when adopted by state legislatures – includes alternate provisions on liability with varying protection. The model act's text and the current status of efforts to adopt are Volunteer Health Practitioners, at http://www.uniformlaws.org/Act.aspx?title=Emergency (Accessed June 7, 2013).

15. See Hoffman S. Responders' Responsibility: Liability And Immunity In Public Health Emergencies, Case Research Paper Series in Legal Studies, Working Paper 07–29, September2007, pages 29–32 and statutes cited therein, at http://papers.ssrn.com/sol3/papers.cfm?abstract_id=1017277 (Accessed June 7, 2013). In Florida, a person is not liable for civil damages arising out of care or treatment in emergency situations, including declared emergencies. Fla. Stat. § 252.51.

16. Under 42 U.S.C. §§ 300hh–15, the federal government extends immunity to "Intermittent Disaster-Response Personnel" appointed by the secretary, to assist the corps in carrying out duties during a public health emergency. Applicable protections of Section 2812 shall apply to such individuals. PAHPA PL109–417, December 19, 2006, 120 Stat. 2831.

17. Hoffman S. Responders' Responsibility: Liability and Immunity in Public Health Emergencies. *Georgetown Law Journal* 2008; 96: 1913–1969.

18. Hodge JG, Calves SH, Gable LA, Meltzer E, Kraner S. Risk Management in the Wake of Hurricanes and Other Disasters: Hospital Civil Liability Arising from the Use of Volunteer Health Professionals During Emergencies. *Michigan State University College of Law Journal of Medicine and Law* 2006; 10: 57–86.

19. *Id.*
20. Hoffman S. Responders' Responsibility: Liability and Immunity in Public Health Emergencies. *Georgetown Law Journal* 2008; 96: 1913–1969.
21. Pozgar G. *Legal essentials of health care administration.* Jones and Bartlett Publishers, 2009, Su dbury, MA, p. 59.
22. *Id.*
23. *Id.*
24. 42 USC § 264 is the principal federal quarantine statute. HHS has proposed revised quarantine regulations, but these have not been finalized at the time of this writing. 70 Fed. Reg. 71892 November 30, 2005.
25. Health Care Spending and the Medicare Program: A Data Book, June2012, Medicare Payment Advisory Commission, Page 5.
26. Matthews G. Preparedness for Public Health Emergencies. In: Homeland Security and Emergency Management: A Legal Guide for State and Local Governments, ABA Press, 2010. Misrahi J, Matthews G, Hoffman R. Legal Authorities for Interventions in Public Health Emergencies. In: Law in Public Health Practice, 2nd ed. Oxford Press, 2006; Gostin L. Restrictions of the Person: Autonomy, Liberty, and Bodily Integrity. In: Public Health Law, University of California Press, 2000.
27. *Id.*
28. President Barack Obama. Declaration of a National Emergency with Respect to the 2009 H1n1 Influenza Pandemic. The White House. October 24, 2009. Accessed June 14, 2013 at http://www.whitehouse.gov/the-press-office/declaration-a-national-emergency-with-respect-2009-h1n1-influenza-pandemic-0.
29. 42 USC §1320b-5.
30. 45 CFR § 164.510.
31. 45 CFR § 164 et seq.
32. *Id.*
33. 45 CFR § 164.512(b).
34. CA Civil Code § 56.10.
35. 45 CFR § 164.510(b)(3).
36. 45 CFR § 164.510(b)(4).
37. CA Civil Code § 56.10(c)(15).
38. Arkansas C.A § 20–27–1706: "Pursuant to the Health Insurance Portability and Accountability Act of 1996, disclosure of protected health information is allowed for public health, safety, and law enforcement purposes."
39. Cohen B. Reconciling the HIPAA Privacy Rule with State Laws Regulating Ex Parte Interviews of Plaintiffs' Treating Physicians: A Guide to Performing HIPAA Preemption Analysis. Houston Law Review, Vol. 43, No. 1091, 2006, 1091–1142.
40. California Probate Code § 4717.
41. 6 U.S.C. § 774.
42. 45 CFR § 164.512(f)(2). Disclosure to law enforcement officials is also authorized where it is pursuant to a court subpoena or order. 45 CFR § 164.512(f)(l)(ii).
43. 45 CFR § 164.512.
44. 45 CFR §164.515, Accounting for disclosures of protected health information.
45. 45 CFR § 164.512.
46. 45 CFR § 160.103.
47. 22 Cal. Code Regs. § 70751 et seq.
48. Health and Safety Code § 123149.
49. Congressional Research Service Report for Congress, Hurricane Katrina: HIPAA Privacy and Electronic Health Records of Evacuees, October 28, 2005, at http://assets.opencrs.com/rpts/RS22310_20051028.pdf (Accessed July 1, 2013).
50. *Id.*
51. U.S. Department of Health & Human Services. Is the HIPAA Privacy Rule suspended during a national or public health emergency? http://www.hhs.gov/ocr/privacy/hipaa/faq/disclosures_in_emergency_situations/1068.html (Accessed August 16, 2015).
52. Parmet, Wendy. Individual Rights versus the Public's Health – 100 Years After Jacobson v. Massachusetts. *N Engl J Med* 2005; 352: 7.
53. *Jacobson v. Massachusetts*, 197 U.S. 11, 25 S. Ct. 358 (1905), emphasis added.
54. *Id.*
55. *Id.*, emphasis added.
56. *Id.*
57. *Best v. Bellevue Hospital New York.* 115 Fed. Appx. 459. C.A.2 (N.Y.), 2004. After this 2-year saga, the federal court declared that in order to detain a patient under the health code, New York had to comply with both procedural due process ("the right to a particularized assessment of an individual's danger to self or others") and substantive due process ("the right to less restrictive alternatives").
58. *Id.*
59. *Id.*
60. *Kirk v. Wyman*, 83 S.C. 372 at 394 (1909)(dissenting).
61. *Id.*
62. *Wellman v. Faulkner*, 715 F.2d 269. In this case, the judge held that inadequate medical care and overcrowding in prison was unconstitutional.
63. *Best v. Bellevue Hospital New York*, 115 Fed. Appx. 459. C.A.2 (N.Y.), 2004.
64. The Georgia provision was adopted after review of the Model State Emergency Health Powers Act.
65. In *Moore v. Morgan*, 922 F.2d 1553 (11th Cir. 1991), a county failed to satisfy constitutional responsibility in maintaining the county jail by delay in rectifying overcrowded conditions and was held liable for damages, as provided under 42 U.S.C. § 1983 and U.S. Const. amend. VIII.
66. The Joint Commission MS 4.110.
67. In disasters other than minor ones, the declaration also constitutes authority for medical practitioners licensed in other jurisdictions to practice in Florida, subject to such conditions as the declaration may prescribe. FLA. Stat. 252.36(3)(c)(1) (2004).
68. California Emergency Services Act § 8850 et seq.
69. Joint Commission International. http://www.jointcommissioninternational.org/about_us/fact_sheets.aspx, at http://www.jointcommissioninternational.org (Accessed August 17, 2015).
70. The Joint Commission Standard MS4.110 (amended January 2004).
71. *Id.*
72. *Id.*
73. DC Hospital Association, Mutual Aid Memorandum of Understanding, Sept 27, 2001. https://www.healthlawyers.org/Members/PracticeGroups/THAMC/EmergencyPreparednessToolkit/Documents/V_EMAC/C_DCHAMutualAidMemo Understanding.pdf (Accessed August 17, 2015). Hodge JG, Gable LA, Cálves SH. The Legal Framework for Meeting Surge Capacity through the Use of Volunteer Health Professionals during Public Health Emergencies and Other Disasters. *J Contemp Health Law Policy* Fall 2005; 22(1): 5–71.
74. *Id.*
75. Congressional Research Service Report for Congress, Hurricane Katrina: HIPAA Privacy and Electronic Health Records of Evacuees, October 28, 2005, at http://www.policyarchive.org/handle/10207/bitstreams/4258.pdf (Accessed July 1, 2013).
76. The National Fire Protection Association (NFPA) § 1600 provides disaster and emergency management and business continuity programs and the criteria to assess current programs or to develop, implement, and maintain aspects for prevention, mitigation, preparation, response, and recovery from emergencies.

Voluntary private sector compliance with NFPA § 1600 recommendations was strongly encouraged by the U.S. Congress in passing the 9/11 bill, P.L. 110–53, 6 U.S.C 321k. However, The Joint Commission standards supersede any NFPA recommendations.

77. SOM, Appendix A, Interpretive Guidelines for Hospitals (guidance for § 482.41) and Appendix W, Interpretive Guidelines for Critical Access Hospitals (§ 485.623).

78. Id.

79. 29 U.S.C § 651.

80. Sauer LM, McCarthy ML, Knebel A, Brewster P. Major influences on hospital emergency management and disaster preparedness. *Disaster Med Public Health Prep* 2009; 3(2 Suppl.): S68–S73.

81. Hodge JG, Jr., Garcia AM, Anderson ED, Kaufman T. Emergency legal preparedness for hospitals and health care personnel. *Disaster Med Public Health Prep* 2009; 3(2 Suppl.): S37–S44.

82. Sauer LM, McCarthy ML, Knebel A, Brewster P. Major influences on hospital emergency management and disaster preparedness. *Disaster Med Public Health Prep* 2009; 3(2 Suppl.): S68–S73.

83. Title 22, Cal. Code Regs. §§ 7(a), 71539(a), and 72551.

84. Id.

85. The Universal Declaration of Human Rights, Article 25. http://www.un.org/en/documents/udhr/index.shtml#a25 (Accessed August 17, 2015).

86. Centers for Medicare & Medicaid Services, HHS. Medicare Program: Clarifying Policies Related to the Responsibilities of Medicare-Participating hospitals in Treating Individuals with Emergency Medical Conditions. *Federal Register* September 9, 2003; 68(174), at https://www.federalregister.gov/articles/2003/09/09/03-22594/medicare-program-clarifying-policies-related-to-the-responsibilities-of-medicare-participating

87. 42 CFR § 489.24.

88. 42 U.S.C. § 1320b-5.

89. Congressional Research Service Report for Congress, Hurricane Katrina: HIPAA Privacy and Electronic Health Records of Evacuees, October 28, 2005, at http://www.policyarchive.org/handle/10207/bitstreams/4258.pdf. (Accessed July 1, 2013).

90. Hassol A, Zane R. Reopening Shuttered Hospitals to Expand Surge Capacity. Prepared by Abt Associates Inc., under IDSRN Task Order No. 8. AHRQ Publication No. 06-0029. Rockville, MD: Agency for Healthcare Research and Quality. February 2006.

91. HSPD 5, at http://training.fema.gov/EMIWeb/IS/ICSResource/assets/HSPD-5.pdf. (Accessed July 1, 2013).

92. HSPD 8. This Bush Administration directive has been superseded by President Obama's Presidential Policy Directive 8, National Preparedness (PPD 8), at http://www.dhs.gov/presidential-policy-directive-8-national-preparedness (Accessed August 17, 2015).

93. Public Health Security and Bioterrorism Preparedness and Response Act of 2002, Pub. L. No. 107–88, 116 Stat. 594; see also Pandemic Flu and All-Hazards Preparedness Act, Pub. L. No. 109–417.

94. The consolidated appropriations act for fiscal year 2012 appropriated $1.7 billion for FEMA preparedness grants, $1.28 billion less than requested. See Pub. L. No. 112–74, 125 Stat. 786, 960 (2011).

95. 42 USCA § 5122.

96. P.L. 93–288, as amended, 42 USC §§ 5121–5206 and related authorities.

97. FEMA Recovery Policy 9524, at http://www.fema.gov/9500-series-policy-publications.pdf/government/grant/pa/9525_4.pdf. (Accessed July 1, 2013).

98. Id.

99. 44 CFR Part 13, "Uniform Administrative Requirements for Grants and Cooperative Agreements to State and Local Governments."

100. 44 CFR § 13.36.

101. Ga. Code Ann., § 38–3–51. The California statute is even broader: it provides that the governor may "commandeer or utilize any private property or personnel deemed by him necessary in carrying out his responsibilities and the state shall pay the reasonable value thereof." California Emergency Services Act, GC § 8572. The power granted to commandeer personnel is unusual in emergency management statutes, and the limitations on exercise of this authority are unclear.

102. Obama Administration: PPD 8, National Preparedness, at http://www.dhs.gov/presidential-policy-directive-8-national-preparedness and Bush Administration: HSPD 5; HSPD 8. http://www.dhs.gov/presidential-policy-directive-8-national-preparedness (Accessed July 1, 2013).

103. California Emergency Services Act, GC § 8571.

104. Bragg A. Experiencing the 2004 Florida Hurricanes: A Lawyers Perspective. In: Abbott E, Hetzel O, A Legal Guide to Homeland Security and Emergency Management for State and Local Governments, ABA Press, 2005.

105. Legal Preparedness for Public Health Emergencies: A Model for Minimum Competencies for Mid-Tier Public Health Professionals, Last Updated September 17, 2012, Editor: Montrece McNeill Ransom, JD, MPH, Associate Editor: Acasia B. Olson, MPH, CDC http://www.cdc.gov/phlp/docs/legal-preparedness-competencies.PDF (Accessed August 17, 2015).

106. Chang EF, Backer H, Bey TA, and Koenig KL. Maximizing Medical and Health Outcomes after a Catastrophic Disaster: Defining a New "Crisis Standard of Care." *Western Journal of Emergency Medicine* 2008; 9(3): Article 18, at http://repositories.cdlib.org/uciem/westjem/vol9/iss3/art18. (Accessed November 25, 2008).

107. "American Lawyers" Public Information Series; Community panflu preparedness: A checklist of key legal issues for healthcare providers. 2008 American Health Lawyers Association, p. 20, fn 45, at http://www2a.cdc.gov/PHLP/docs/Pan-Flu08.pdf and http://www.healthlawyers.org/panfluchecklist (Accessed August 17, 2015).

108. A "tabletop" is so named because it does not try to recreate an emergency event by simulating the event and actually deploying response resources (ambulances, helicopters, doctors, nurses, and so forth); rather, a scenario is presented to participants representing their organizations. These participants – perhaps while sitting around a table – think through and describe how they would respond to an event and interact with other organizations. One such tabletop was conducted by the University of the District of Columbia's National Legal Preparedness Program in 2009; the report of this effort is "The Law and Catastrophic Disasters, Legal Issues in the Aftermath" by Ernest B. Abbott and Otto J. Hetzel. One segment of this Exercise focused on Public Health and Medical Care.

13

Syndromic Surveillance

Gary A. Roselle

OVERVIEW

Syndromic surveillance has been defined by the U.S. Centers for Disease Control and Prevention (CDC) as "a process that regularly and systematically uses health and health-related data in near 'real-time' to make information available on the health of a community."[1] Based on its original definition, the purpose of syndromic surveillance would be to prevent morbidity and mortality by early identification of case clusters in which mitigation would affect the outcome of the disease's natural course. This original definition was designed for early event detection and became prominent in the public domain after the September 11, 2001 terrorist attacks in the United States and the subsequent anthrax illnesses and deaths. Since 2001, syndromic surveillance systems have been implemented during mass gatherings, such as the 2012 London Olympic and Paralympic Games. Elliot identifies syndromic surveillance as the collection, analysis, interpretation, and dissemination of health-related data, typically on a real-time (or near real-time) basis, to determine the early impact (or absence of impact) of potential human or veterinary public health threats that require effective public health action.[2]

With a heightened sense of urgency related to the so-called war on terror, many systems were put into place within the United States for the protection of the public health. These included such diverse programs as vaccine initiatives (BioShield), static detectors located throughout large cities to identify specific organisms of interest in the air (BioWatch), and the beginning and sustainment of a national syndromic surveillance system for early detection of outbreaks (BioSense). These three initiatives were designed for the following reasons, respectively: 1) prevention of disease if a terrorist attack occurred; 2) early identification of airborne pathogens during the asymptomatic phase of such disease; and 3) early identification of illness prior to definitive diagnosis that would be confirmed either by culture or laboratory tests. These government initiatives were complemented by independent, non-federal syndromic surveillance systems that were designed primarily for early identification of naturally occurring illnesses but were adaptable for use in bioterrorism surveillance. Other countries, such as the United Kingdom, have also heightened the evaluation of syndromic surveillance systems for

response to early detection of bioterrorism events.[3] In addition, there are other syndromic surveillance initiatives in Europe and Asia (Taiwan)[4–6,7].

These systems are largely based on surveillance of existing data, such as help line calls and emergency department visits. For such population-based reporting, several factors must be defined if the surveillance system is to be useful. The system must provide initial detection such as finding an event as early as possible. It must quantify the event by defining the number of people who are potentially ill and identifying the location for the source of infection with enough granularity to allow for specific intervention. In addition, it would be useful if the surveillance system incorporated other supportive data such as provider and laboratory testing, and permitted early, computer-based investigation of possible case clusters by using such items as patient demographics. At least in theory, this should allow for initial outbreak management, such as confirming existing cases and tracking new ones. It would also facilitate timely countermeasure administration such as individual or community isolation, antimicrobial prophylaxis, and vaccination. In addition, if maximal utilization of data is the goal, then bioterrorism surveillance systems should also identify naturally occurring outbreaks and case clusters, because this will be the most frequent use of the data on an ongoing basis.[8–16]

For such data usage, there are multiple components of a surveillance system that should be defined prior to its implementation (see Table 13.1). Such questions as "What is the population under surveillance?", "What is the time period for data collection?", and "What data will be collected and who provides it?" are essential components that should be decided in the planning phase. For personal data security purposes, the issue of information transfer and storage is absolutely critical. Some assortment of personal identifiers is mandatory even if only regional mail code, age, and sex are used. The issue of data analysis is also critical, particularly: 1) who will analyze the data; 2) what methodology will be used and how often; and finally, 3) how will the reports be disseminated, to whom, and by what method. Although all of these factors may appear to be self-evident, there are no accepted and universally available standards for syndromic surveillance that would make the answer to these questions simple. Added to

Table 13.1. Components of surveillance systems to be determined before development

Theme	Examples of Questions to Consider for Surveillance
Who	Who is the population under surveillance?
	Who uses the data and for what purposes?
What	What data are being collected?
Where	Where is the geographic location for consideration?
When	When is the time period of data collection?
Why	Why is the data collection important?
	Why is personally identifiable data needed?
How	How is the data being collected?
	How is the data being stored?
	How will the data be analyzed and distributed?
	How will the conclusions be conveyed?

these complexities would be the need for data validation, which may or may not be possible based on the need for reporting timeliness. The quantification of uncertainty may be required for optimal use of data by decision-makers.

With an increased emphasis on surveillance for non-intentional events to augment the usefulness of expensive bioterrorism surveillance systems, the term "situational awareness" has moved from the military to the public health community. Thus, for a system to be fully operational, it should go beyond the possibility of early signal event detection and define the location, extent, and progression of multiple disease clusters and outbreaks that can occur at different times. For this mission, it may be important to evaluate a greater variety of data sources beyond traditional symptom syndromes. It may require more well-defined geographic locations for individuals (for example, including all five numbers in a zip code vs. just the first three numbers in the United States, or specific geo-tagging, particularly in rural or low-density population areas). More rapid reporting that would approach real-time may be necessary, meaning instantaneous transmission of any data point as soon as it is available with instantaneous analytic processing and report generation and distribution.

Last, the traditional use of symptoms for syndromic surveillance may not be adequate to accomplish all of these missions, including early event detection and situational awareness. A variety of other data sources have been suggested and investigated. Examples include over-the-counter medication sales, prescription drug purchases, number of phone calls to pediatricians' offices, absenteeism from schools or work, and ambulance emergency runs. This so-called augmented syndromic surveillance could allow for greater specificity of signals that define true clusters or outbreaks versus statistical anomalies that would otherwise require large increments of time by public health authorities for investigation.[17]

CURRENT STATE OF THE ART

The concept of syndromic surveillance is relatively straightforward, although the proof of concept and/or value is yet to be shown. In its simplest terms, data that can be immediately obtained prior to definitive diagnostic testing (e.g., microbiology culture or laboratory serology) are transferred to a central repository. Examples of these types of data include healthcare diagnostic or procedural coding, such as International Classification of Diseases (ICD-10) or Current Procedural Terminology (CPT-5) codes, or emergency department chief complaints. After receipt at the repository, the data are parsed into groupings related to established syndromes, such as respiratory, neurological, or gastrointestinal. The philosophy of syndrome grouping such as this rests on the assumption that, although errors may be made in specific diagnostic or procedural codes or chief complaints, the general group of the codes should be correct and allow early analysis of data. In addition, even if ICD-10 or CPT-5 coding is not possible, natural language interpretation of chief complaints can be used with specific trigger words to allow assignment of a syndromic grouping. As an example, identification of the possible spread of avian influenza is an important public health issue. In support of this effort, syndromic surveillance is considered an important component for early detection of avian flu infecting humans. Patients potentially infected with the virus will be categorized as having an "influenza-like illness" or "respiratory" syndrome using the syndromic surveillance model. It should be noted, however, that with the greater availability of molecular testing and other rapid diagnostic modalities, the use of surrogate markers such as ICD-10 coding and natural language readers may decrease or, for certain diseases, become unnecessary.

Additional data can be added such as blood pressure or temperature to improve the predictive value of any signal derived from statistical analysis of the syndrome groupings. For instance, if evaluating traditional respiratory syndromes, the blood pressure of most patients arriving at a healthcare facility would be reasonably normal, even during cold and flu season. On the other hand, if an airborne anthrax attack were to occur, there may be a significant increase in patients with a respiratory syndrome, high fever, and very low blood pressure. A more robust response by the public health community may be required when confronting such a severe syndrome as defined by augmented syndromic surveillance. However, it remains unclear whether such a robust approach would provide added value since the severity of illness and multiple patients presenting with similar signs and symptoms would likely alert the clinicians and public health authorities that an event had occurred.

There are multiple syndromic surveillance systems in use around the globe and across the United States. Often more than one is visible to regional public health entities for use as a stand-alone system or in conjunction with other local alerting systems, such as ambulance runs, to determine priorities for public health investigation and intervention. Syndromic surveillance contrasts with the "knowledgeable intermediary," the single clinician who, recognizing that a patient or group of patients arriving for care displays an unusual set of signs or symptoms, alerts public health authorities. Such knowledgeable intermediaries were evident in the anthrax attack in the United States and the sarin gas attack in Tokyo. Syndromic surveillance is also different from standard notification of reportable diseases to public health. In the latter, such disease reporting is often made after a diagnosis is confirmed, such as with hepatitis B, meningococcal meningitis, or tuberculosis. Although such reporting is important, it generally lacks the timeliness necessary for mitigation in the case of an intentional biological event. Syndromic surveillance, therefore, is a methodology designed to gain the advantage of earlier

Table 13.2. Examples of Surveillance Systems

System	Owners/Stakeholders	Description
BioSense	CDC	Used at the local, state, and national level by health officials; cloud computing environment that has analytical capabilities.
Epi-X	CDC	Used by CDC officials, state and local health departments, poison control centers, and public health to access and share preliminary health information.
National Electronic Disease Surveillance System (NEDSS)	CDC	Used by hospitals and healthcare systems to submit surveillance data to public health departments, which is then submitted to the CDC. Currently forty-six states, New York City, and Washington, DC, use NEDSS-based systems.
Electronic Surveillance System for the Early Notification of Community-based Epidemics (ESSENCE)	Department of Defense (DOD) and Johns Hopkins University	A web-based application to monitor and provide alerts on rapid and usual increases in the occurrence of infectious diseases and biological outbreaks. DOD outpatient data is monitored worldwide.
Real Time Outbreak and Disease Surveillance (RODS)	University of Pittsburgh	Real-time public health surveillance system that is used by multiple cities, states, and countries. The National Retail Data Monitor (NRDM) monitors 30,000 retail stores for over-the-counter medication sales throughout the United States
The European Surveillance System (TESSy)	European CDC	Used by all Member States of the European Union and European Economic Area countries for the reporting of communicable diseases.
Global Outbreak and Alert Response Network (GOARN)	WHO	Global network for technical support for outbreak surveillance. IHR 2005 expanded the role of GOARN for increased surveillance and response.

detection (by days) of a biological attack or other infectious illness. This may facilitate: 1) earlier interventions to stop the spread of disease; 2) rapid initiation of appropriate treatment for affected individuals; and 3) perhaps, by increasing such timeliness, an enhanced probability of apprehending the perpetrators of an intentional biological event.

The current state of the art in syndromic surveillance is a rapidly moving target. There are a multitude of surveillance systems available. One review of the literature identified 36 surveillance systems and U.S. health departments alone have implemented syndromic surveillance systems at more than 100 sites since 2003.[14,18] This, coupled with the shift from early event detection to situational awareness, the development of large city systems individualized for specific geographic areas, and the creation of new technologies, necessitates using exemplary systems of syndromic surveillance in this discussion. In fact, for public health entities that are better resourced, multiple systems are often used simultaneously to differentiate true case clusters or outbreaks compared with anomalies identified by the syndromic surveillance system. Improving this signal-to-noise ratio allows for optimum use of public health resources for investigation and mitigation as needed. This point receives particular emphasis in the paper by Buehler where multiple interviews indicate that syndromic surveillance was best utilized as a component of multiple data inputs at the local level.[19] The author also notes the trend for syndromic surveillance away from early detection to situational awareness. In contrast, however, the American Reimbursement and Recovery Act of 2009 provides financial incentives to individual physicians to fully use an electronic medical record.[20,21] Participating in activities such as syndromic surveillance reporting to electronic data systems may give the opportunity to enhance the value of syndromic surveillance as a component of an overall early identification or situational awareness plan. Table 13.2 gives a brief listing of several U.S. surveillance systems, past and present, using a variety of methodologies to achieve the previously stated goals.

Surveillance Systems – A World View

Perhaps the most significant change in surveillance systems of all types, including syndromic surveillance, is the appreciation that a broader perspective on biosurveillance is needed. Of particular importance is the World Health Organization (WHO) issuance of the revised International Health Regulations in 2005 (IHR 2005). This was to take effect in 2007 with compliance by member countries by 2012. It calls for international cooperation for surveillance, detection, reporting, and response to biological threats. While this may seem self-evident to those in public health and epidemiology, it may not have been so clear to others with a less defined mission. With the rise in international travel, long-distance transportation of goods and services, and particularly the movement of food commodities, the need for internationalization of biosurveillance must certainly be highlighted.

The United States provides an excellent example of a distributed system for syndromic surveillance. Chen provides comments on thirteen different systems that use a variety of inputs for biosurveillance purposes.[22] For the most part, these do not interconnect, but instead utilize varying input models and a multitude of statistical methodologies to provide outcome data. While not surprising, the usefulness of the data for decision-makers will be limited by the narrow scope of the data provided.

Regarding the systems deployed in the United States, two are perhaps the most well-known, the BioSense system from the CDC and the Electronic Surveillance System for the Early Notification of Community-Based Epidemics (ESSENCE) from the U.S. Department of Defense (DOD). For BioSense, the primary initial daily inputs for the system originally came from the electronic medical records of the DOD and the U.S. Department of Veterans Affairs (VA). This has been widely expanded to other facilities in the private sector as well as laboratory results. While BioSense has gone through several years of testing and updates, BioSense 2.0 is the current iteration for general use. It is available to public health authorities and has the advantages of incorporating a large data set, containing analytic tools, and possessing the imprimatur of the CDC. The system in general does not require data input by practitioners and relies heavily on the electronic medical record. For the current iteration, local and state health departments are able to store, analyze, and control data in a government-certified cloud environment, which provides analytical tools to the health departments.[23]

The second system, ESSENCE, was developed to monitor the health status of military healthcare beneficiaries around the world. It relies heavily on diagnostic billing codes (ICD-10), now expanded to increase data inputs from a variety of additional sources and statistical algorithms to define outliers. It is relatively user-friendly, but is generally not a system for country-wide use and does not support national decision making.

Other systems found in the United States such as the Real-Time Outbreak Detection System (RODS), Early Aberration Reporting System (EARS), and others provide information with varying emphasis on such topics as spatial and temporal data monitoring systems, visualization methodologies, and data modeling. Any of the systems may be extremely useful for health authorities, but likely will be used as adjuncts to locally adapted approaches and in combination with other procedures used to collect information. This will be particularly important since valid signals from each of the models may be difficult to separate from the inevitable "noise" commonly found in such widely disparate data sets.

Emphasizing the need for a more global approach and for greater information organization from varying sources, the ProMed, HealthMap, and Argus projects monitor open source information using a variety of data monitoring infrastructures. Argus uses primarily web-based technology to capture information for biologic events and outbreak severity. Using this methodology, worldwide information can be accrued and made available across the globe. HealthMap also uses disparate data sources with a variety of inputs, including those with varying reliability such as official alerts from WHO, accounts from ProMed mail alerts (also containing animal health data), and open news sources. While validity of these systems may vary, they do provide a more global perspective that can support not only immediate interventions, but also the consideration of future needs as diseases travel from continent to continent.[23–25]

As the United States has progressed with syndromic surveillance, so have Europe and other parts of the world. Over the last several years, Europe and member states of the European Union have examined many syndromic surveillance systems methodologies across the continent, and perhaps the need for a new definition for syndromic surveillance.[4] The goal appears to be defining a more formal network of syndromic surveillance activities. One of the European Syndromic Surveillance Systems (Triple-S) project deliverables was an inventory of the current existing syndromic surveillance systems. This was followed by questionnaires, country visits, and framework discussions. Some of the same issues seen in the United States are also of concern in Europe, such as communication, minimum data sets that are available at multiple sites, evaluation criteria, and methods for data collection and analysis. In addition, veterinary syndromic surveillance systems were also reviewed. While as many as forty-five systems may be in use, very few are fully operational; many are still in the developmental stage. Looking at animal-human biosurveillance synergies is being considered.[4] While many individual European states and governmental entities have their own syndromic surveillance systems, some are not convinced about

the value of syndromic surveillance as a strategy. Overall, the issue of interoperability remains critical. Open source software provides infrastructure that may be applicable to the needs of areas with limited resources. These assets help breech part of the gap between the developed and developing worlds.[26,27] Such software can provide aggregation systems, statistical analysis components, and mapping capabilities. In addition, they can provide some interoperability that is necessary when dealing with multiple surveillance systems. This is critical since diseases do not respect international boundaries and move freely among countries around the globe.

In comparison to the developed, city-based environment, surveillance in the developing world, particularly in rural areas, presents different challenges. Of particular note, these regions lack capability for rapid, specific diagnostic testing for infectious diseases, either traditional or emerging. Compounding this problem is a high prevalence of infectious diseases, case clusters, and outbreaks that occur in these settings due to a variety of socioeconomic and geopolitical issues. In the past this might have generated a localized focus of cases. However, with massive amounts of travel, movement of goods, and perhaps even changes in weather patterns, localized case clusters can easily expand to involve larger cities, different countries, and span continents, as occurred with severe acute respiratory syndrome (SARS). Currently, China is testing a web-based integrated surveillance system for early detection of infectious diseases. This will include standard syndromic surveillance coupled with at least school absenteeism and over-the-counter drug sales, and will be compared with the traditional case reporting systems. Multiple algorithms and statistical methodologies will be tested. While results are not yet available, this sort of innovation is critical for control of the onset and movement of infectious diseases.[28]

Data Integration

The addition of nonhuman data might also add further value to any syndromic surveillance system. For instance, data on national or international water systems, unusual illnesses or deaths in animals, or unusual occurrences affecting plants or food crops might also increase the positive predictive value of any clusters of human cases found by syndromic surveillance.[29]

However, the complexity of integrating systems that are dramatically diverse, such as those involving plants, animals, BioWatch sensors, and human data, is daunting. In addition to the different types of data elements, there is also the question of differences in information technology architecture among the variety of datasets or between countries. Although there is variable architecture in human datasets, this situation is accentuated when automated data systems are implemented for plants, animals, or other more technical datasets such as BioWatch sensors.[30–32] The information technology architecture of the originating datasets will be important if such large amounts of diverse data are to be electronically delivered, sorted, initially analyzed, and outliers defined. Developing a specific platform architecture that has been clearly defined for all of these diverse datasets remains a challenge.

In August 2007, the U.S. government established the National Biosurveillance Integration Center (NBIC). Subsequently, this center developed and provides oversight for the National Biosurveillance Integration System (NBIS).[33] This system is designed to track and integrate data received electronically from individual U.S. Government agency liaisons. Such agencies include the CDC, the U.S. Environmental Protection Agency, the Department of Agriculture, and many other national and international sources. It will use these data to generate reports on the level of risk to the public health and nurture further collaboration among the government entities. In addition to the difficult task of electronic data interpretation, NBIS will also require human analysts to integrate the algorithmic quantifiable data and the more opaque threat data obtained from a variety of intelligence systems. Such sources include U.S. Embassies and other electronic surveillance traffic. Although this is groundbreaking technology, it will take significant time to fully implement and an even longer period to determine whether it is effective.

Data Analysis

There are a variety of mathematical data analysis formulae in place in the extant syndromic surveillance systems.[34–48] These methods include everything from cumulative sum scores, smart scores, and anomaly detection algorithms to trends, proportions, expected to observed frequency, standard deviations, and other more descriptive statistics. At this time, system designers have not demonstrated that any of the statistical methodologies are definitively and clearly superior to any of the others, or that they define specifically which outliers are critical for investigation.

With limited resources provided to the public health community, the critical element in a syndromic surveillance system is the ability to define which outliers are sufficiently important to generate an on-the-ground investigation and determine whether a biological event has occurred. This so-called signal-to-noise ratio is one manner of defining the validity of the syndromic surveillance system. If alerts are generated very frequently with little or no outcome from laborious investigation, the system will go unused and thus have little value. If, on the other hand, the surveillance system is correct every time it defines an abnormal signal, then it is likely that such extreme specificity will not allow for sufficient sensitivity. It may allow other critical signals to go undetected at some unknown rate. Although mathematicians, statisticians, and modelers are critical to the process of syndromic surveillance analysis, the most essential element will be in the hands of the public health and epidemiologic community where the signal-to-noise ratio will truly be defined.

Technology and Social Media

In general, "social media" can be described as the use of web- and/or mobile-based technologies to support interactive dialogue among the public, public health authorities, and other subject matter experts. With reference to syndromic surveillance, such social media can be used for rapid accumulation of data that is much different from the tradition of ICD-10 codes, natural language readers, forms submissions, and other modestly useful methodologies. There are two types of technology and/or social media that should be highlighted. The first is trend analysis based on web browsing and examination of other general electronic modalities. This approach looks for key elements and words and, more recently, evaluates the flow of electronic traffic. The second is the interactive use of mobile devices for data transmission. The subjects of these transmissions include specific illnesses, blogs related to illness topics, and tweets regarding public health or disease topics. These communications could involve any other interactive system that establishes a link between the general public and a data gathering site that would digest and trend the information.

Probably the most noteworthy example of social media trend analysis would be the effort to follow the spread of influenza in the United States.[49] A method was developed to look at large numbers of Google search engine queries to track influenza-like illness in the population. Using that technology, investigators could actually estimate the current level of weekly influenza activity in each region of the United States. They were able to compare these data with those reported to the CDC's traditional influenza reporting system. The positive correlation was remarkable. Similar data were found with other diseases such as *Salmonella*.[50] Positive findings were also published by Corley et al. using blog posts that discussed influenza.[51] Again these results correlated well with CDC's influenza-like illness data. These positive outcomes may not be sustainable, however, since they can be influenced by disease specific publicity, fear related to new organisms or strains or type of influenza, and availability or shortage of vaccine.[52]

Although similar to web-based systems in some areas, the use of mobile technology presents different challenges and different opportunities for syndromic surveillance. Such mobile systems may not require an Internet connection at all, but only mobile or satellite phone connectivity, particularly with short messaging service. Reporting systems using mobile technology have the advantages of portability, simplicity, and value in the developing world where mobile or satellite phone connectivity may be replacing wired telephone and other interactive devices. There are multiple existing systems that vary in complexity from simple text messaging to transmission of geocoded photographs.[53,54] The term "crowdsourcing" was coined for groups of participants who are willing to answer queries that are timely and require a rapid response. While some of these may provide just a snapshot of a specific activity, such as influenza-like illnesses, they could be extended to daily or weekly reporting by sentinel groups of individuals.

Combinations of technologies may also be of interest. Yang et al. searched websites related to social media using a fairly complex system of keyword algorithms, filtering methods, and analytic tools to look for infectious diseases in China.[55] Kool et al. used a combination of reporting methodologies for syndromic surveillance in the Pacific Islands.[56] These included data extraction from log books, short questionnaires by triage nurses, computer data entry screens, and mobile phones. While these represent initial explorations, they do point to a direction for further evaluation of validity and usefulness. In fact, it is far more likely that a combination of systems will be required rather than a single, "one size fits all" approach for worldwide use.

Twitter, Facebook, and other similar social media platforms present special functionalities and pitfalls for syndromic surveillance. These social media enterprises encourage disclosure and expression of thoughts, opinions, and random details related to people's lives.[57] While often these thoughts are idiosyncratic and personal, they do provide a window into the experiences of individuals and a mechanism for interaction with persons or groups. In fact, since many users of these modalities are in younger age groups, the opportunity exists to engage a different, youthful population that is often loath to visit the hospital or an individual medical practitioner. This provides a more accurate assessment (larger numerator and denominator), resulting in better correlation with disease states, earlier identification of certain illnesses, and perhaps a more precise measurement of an intervention's effectiveness. Pitfalls, however, are ubiquitous. Specifically, data validity and accuracy must be defined. As evidenced with Google Flu in 2012–2013, systems that work one day may not work the next.[52] This can be related to multiple external forces such as publicity. One such example would be an illness in a celebrity generating multiple news reports, tweets, and blog traffic.

Forecasting/Predictive Analysis

In addition to early warning and situational awareness, forecasting future trends (predictive analysis) in both disease type and severity is a critical element for decision-makers. Such predictions can improve preparation and deployment of resources that may be critical for mitigation of disease. These mitigation interventions may include slowing spread of disease, or perhaps preventing a cluster of cases from becoming a larger geographic outbreak.

While many diseases have been studied, dengue fever probably provides some of the best current data. Potts et al. published a paper predicting disease severity in pediatric patients in Thailand using early clinical laboratory indicators.[58] The diagnostic algorithm had a 97% sensitivity to identify patients who went on to develop a shock syndrome while correctly excluding 48% of non-severe cases using relatively straightforward diagnostic testing at time of admission. This may be important since early identification of those patients who will develop severe illness allows optimum resource utilization for patient-specific intervention that may prevent morbidity and/or mortality.

Gharbi et al. looked at predicting daily dengue incidence in Guadalupe, French West Indies.[59] Historical disease data and weather variables including relative humidity, minimum temperature, average temperature, and rainfall were reviewed to define a predictive model that would allow early warning of increased dengue incidence. Relative humidity, and more importantly temperature, significantly affected the model for dengue incidence forecasting. This may well be related to the life cycle of the mosquito. Rainfall, however, did not contribute substantially to the model. It was felt by the authors that adequate early warning could lead to mitigation of the increases in disease. The authors note that factors such as breeding sites for mosquitoes that may be impacted by human activity play a critical role in dengue. Early warning could lead to increased efforts at mosquito control by raising community awareness and other methods.

The Department of Veterans Affairs has also looked at predictive analysis for dengue in Puerto Rico, where a VA hospital and outpatient clinics serve the population. Periodicity of dengue incidence and lag times between outpatient and inpatient disease were determined using a rather complex mathematical model based on historic disease data. Future mathematical modeling will add weather parameters to enhance predictive analysis for management decision making.[60]

China is the country most seriously affected by hemorrhagic fever with renal syndrome (HFRS); 90% of HFRS cases reported globally occur in China. Historical data and mathematical modeling were used by Liu et al. to forecast HFRS incidence.[61] They showed that accurate forecasting of the HFRS incidence is possible using historical data. They further postulate that the need for monitoring incidence and predictive analysis is critical to enhance reduction of the substantial morbidity and mortality caused by the disease.

Privacy/Ethics

The privacy issues surrounding patient data transmission, information storage, and population surveillance are not new. There is a long history of illness reporting by public health with the need for community protection outweighing any potential privacy issues related to the patient. This becomes a much more complex and ill-defined issue when syndromic surveillance is involved. It may be necessary to individually identify patients to follow up potential case clusters categorized by syndrome, while the individual patient may not have the illness in question at all. It is well recognized, however, that the methodology inherent in syndromic surveillance has difficulty with the signal-to-noise ratio. It is, therefore, inevitable that individual patient information will be used to follow up signals that may not be related to true case clusters. As such, the benefit to the public good may or may not outweigh personal privacy. This is particularly significant since it is not clear at what level data are valid in any individual syndromic surveillance system. As algorithms are adjusted over time, data availability changes, and resource availability at the local level may alter the threshold required to initiate syndrome cluster alert review.

As far back as 2007, experts were reviewing the issues of privacy, confidentiality, and other legal and ethical concerns related to syndromic surveillance.[62] Certain items were noted that amplify the dilemmas regarding privacy and confidentiality. The first is the trend toward digitalization of medical records. This process was in the initial stages of implementation in 2007, but is now moving forward rapidly and most facilities will soon have electronic medical records. This makes the transmission of data much easier and requests for information much larger. The second trend is a growing public health emphasis on an expanding array of diseases including noninfectious conditions. The push toward syndromic surveillance will allow for more access to digitized information for the theoretic public good, and could include noninfectious diseases. One example is the number of fractures identified in a geographic region following a tornado. The third trend is the increasing role of the U.S. federal government in public health. In the past, most surveillance was done at the local and state jurisdictional levels. Now the trend is toward the collection of "big" data at the national level. The classic example of this is CDC's BioSense program that involves the transfer of large volumes of data from participating facilities to the federal government.

These three trends may lead to increased opportunities for loss of privacy and a critical intrusion into private healthcare issues. Francis et al. suggest that the specific healthcare data set could threaten confidentiality and the individual person's control over the information obtained.[63] All of this is usually done without the knowledge or consent of the patient. The authors also point out that on the international level, IHR 2005 went into effect in the last decade. It is not clear whether the surveillance noted in IHR 2005 includes the capacity for syndromic surveillance, particularly since the validity of syndromic surveillance data may be in question. This is especially important if the IHR 2005 are to be implemented in a transparent and non-discriminatory manner despite the use of non-diagnostic data.

RECOMMENDATIONS FOR FURTHER RESEARCH

Syndromic surveillance remains a relatively new concept, and a myriad of opportunities exist for research and development (see Table 13.3). It is clearly necessary to automate data transfer and initial data screening if syndromic surveillance is to be timely, available without transcription errors, and useful without primary review by an individual. This will require investigation into proper and safe methodologies for data transfer (although some of this has been accomplished). Defining the most useful algorithms for initial screening is needed since simple algorithms may be inadequate, and may not support the timeliness required by the decision-makers for effective use of the information. Investigation is also needed into methodologies for combining and aligning disparate data types from a variety of sources. Inherent in this need will be research identifying the minimum data set required for specific indications to avoid the conglomeration of "big" data that may or may not have value. It must be noted that types and sources of data should be considered when creating a minimum data set that may include pharmacy data, syndromic surveillance data, physician/nurse phone traffic, and other sources yet to be determined.

Investigation into mathematical methods and models will be critically important for validity testing of syndromic surveillance data. Once the data are validated, further investigations will be needed to optimize the signal-to-noise ratio. Otherwise, public health resources will be strained unrealistically in responding to multiple signals that yield no useful information. It is understood that public health authorities cannot expect all signals to represent accurate identification of real disease. However, the ratio of signal-to-noise must be acceptable.

It will be necessary to investigate the use of data that is potentially individually identifiable to address the concerns regarding privacy, confidentiality, and ethics. The first question is whether the collection of identifiable data is actually necessary, and the second is who has access to the data. For example, uniquely identifiable data may be necessary for a local jurisdiction to investigate potential case clusters of public health importance. From a national perspective, however, aggregate data reported on a regional level, such as a city or county, might be adequate, with further inquiries made to the local public health authority as needed. Such graduated access will require research into both the methodology for such access as well as which jurisdictions need what type of information to protect the public health.

Lastly, at the regional, national, and international levels, political officials must make decisions based on the data given to them. These decision-makers, however, may or may not have expertise in public health concepts, medical illnesses, and the complexities of disease transmission. Because of this situation, research is necessary to mathematically quantify the uncertainty associated with the validity of collected data and the modeling used in analyzing these data. Clear communication of such information to a variety of stakeholders is required, since many will have little medical background. When data are provided in the form of a traditional medical diagnosis, the information is more straightforward and somewhat familiar to most audiences. On the other hand, when the data are based on syndromic surveillance or predictive analysis, uncertainty is inevitable. This uncertainty should be quantifiable and explainable to the decision-makers as well as the general public.

In conclusion, syndromic surveillance is a methodology that has yet to be firmly integrated into public health or specific patient care systems throughout the United States and the world. While syndromic surveillance is often used as a component of public health surveillance, its specific value may vary depending on how it is used by the public health authorities in various regions and countries. Since this technique is a tool, not an outcome, it is incumbent on the medical and political communities to continue syndromic surveillance research and development to fully define its value, optimal use, and validity.

Table 13.3. Further Research Needs

Category	Additional Research Needs and/or Future Considerations
Data	■ Automation of data – collating data from various systems for analysis ■ Methods for data transfer – ensuring ethical and privacy issues ■ Signal-to-noise ratio – identifying data of value for analysis
End Users	■ Consideration of workflow and the impact on day-to-day operations ■ User education – training on using syndromic surveillance systems
Ethics & Privacy	■ Individually identifiable data needed versus aggregate-level data ■ Determination of who needs access to individual-level data, circumstances, etc.
Decision-Makers	■ Consideration of level of expertise of individuals making decisions, without having background and/or depth of knowledge in medicine and/or public health ■ Drawing conclusions from data given a level of uncertainty from analysis and generalizing the results ■ Quantitative evaluation of validity and reliability of data and data analyses to communicate to the decision-makers

Acknowledgments

The author wishes to thank Ms. Meredith Ambrose for her assistance with research and editing and Ms. Darlene Cooper for her administrative support of this work.

REFERENCES

1. Centers for Disease Control and Prevention. Public Health Information Network. PHIN Messaging Guide for Syndromic Surveillance: Emergency Department, Urgent Care, Inpatient and Ambulatory Care Settings. ADT Messages A01, A03, A04 and A08. Optional ORU^R01 Message Notation for Laboratory Data. HL7 Version 2.5.1 (Version 2.3.1 Compatible) Release 2.0. April 21, 2015. http://www.cdc.gov/nssp/documents/guides/syndrsurvmessagguide2_messagingguide_phn.pdf
2. Elliott AJ, Hughes HE, Hughes TC, et al. Establishing an emergency department syndromic surveillance system to support the London 2012 Olympic and Paralympic Games. *Emerg Med J* 2012; 29(12): 954–960.
3. Smith GE, Cooper DL, Loveridge P. A national syndromic surveillance system for England and Wales using calls to a telephone helpline. *Eurosurveillance* 2006; 11(12): 220–224.

4. Triple S Project. Assessment of syndromic surveillance in Europe. *Lancet* 2011; 378(9806): 1833–1834.

5. Josseran L, Nicolau J, Caillère N, et al. Syndromic surveillance based on emergency department activity and crude mortality: two examples. *Euro Surveil* 2006; 11(12): 225–229.

6. Rockx B, van Asten L, van den Wijngaard C, et al. Syndromic surveillance in the Netherlands for the early detection of West Nile virus epidemics. *Vector Borne Zoonotic Dis* 2006; 6(2): 161–169.

7. Wu TSJ, Shih FYF, Yen MY, et al. Establishing a nationwide emergency department-based syndromic surveillance system for better public health responses in Taiwan. *BMC Public Health* 2008; 8: 18.

8. Bravata D, McDonald K, Smith W, et al. Systematic review; surveillance systems for early detection of bioterrorism-related diseases. *Ann Intern Med* 2004; 140(11): 910–922.

9. Green M, Kaufman Z. Surveillance for early detection and monitoring of infectious disease outbreaks associated with bioterrorism. *Isr Med Assoc J* 2002; 4(7): 503–506.

10. Irvin C, Nouhan P, Rice K. Syndromic analysis of computerized emergency department patients' chief complaints: an opportunity for bioterrorism and influenza surveillance. *Ann Emerg Med* 2003; 41(4): 447–452.

11. Begier E, Sockwell D, Branch L, et al. The National Capitol Region's Emergency Department Syndromic Surveillance System: do chief complain and discharge diagnosis yield different results? *Emerg Infect Dis* 2003; 9(3): 393–396.

12. Platt R, Bocchino C, Caldwell B, et al. Syndromic surveillance using minimum transfer of identifiable data: the example of the National Bioterrorism Syndromic Surveillance Demonstration Program. *J Urban Health* 2003; 80(2 Suppl. 1): i25–i31.

13. Lober W, Trigg L, Karras B, et al. Syndromic surveillance using automated collection of computerized discharge diagnoses. *J Urban Health* 2003; 80(2 Suppl. 1): i97–i106.

14. Buehler J, Berkelman R, Hartley D, Peters C. Syndromic surveillance and bioterrorism-related epidemics. *Emerg Infect Dis* 2003; 9(10): 1197–1204.

15. Centers for Disease Control and Prevention. What is syndromic surveillance? *MMWR* 2004; 53(Suppl.): 7–11.

16. Centers for Disease Control and Prevention. New York City syndromic surveillance systems. *MMWR* 2004; 53(Suppl.): 25–27.

17. Centers for Disease Control and Prevention. Progress in understanding and using over-the-counter pharmaceuticals for syndromic surveillance. *MMWR* 2004; 53(Suppl.): 117–122.

18. Hope K, Durrheim DN, d'Espaignet ET, Dalton C. Syndromic surveillance: is it a useful tool for local outbreak detection? *J Epidemiol Community Health* 2006; 60: 374–375.

19. Buehler JW, Whitney EA, Smith D, et al. Situational uses of syndromic surveillance. *Biosecur and Bioterror: Biodefense Strategy, Practice, and Science* 2009; 7(2): 165–177.

20. International Society for Disease Surveillance. Syndromic Surveillance for meaningful use: background and resources. *ISDS Brief.* April 2012. www.syndromic.org (Accessed November 16, 2012).

21. Lenert L, Sundwall DN. Opportunity Forged by Crisis: Public Health Surveillance and Meaningful Use Regulations: A Crisis of Opportunity. *Am J Public Health* 2012; 102(3): e1–e7.

22. Chen H, Zeng D. Yan P. Public Health Syndromic Surveillance Systems. In: *Infectious Disease Informatics: Syndromic Surveillance for Public Health and BioDefense*, Springer Science + Business Media, LLC, New York, 2010. http://www.springer.com/us/book/9781441912770 (Accessed August 20, 2015).

23. Centers for Disease Control and Prevention. BioSense 2.0. http://www.cdc.gov/biosense/biosense20.html (Accessed July 16, 2014).

24. Chan EH, Brewer TF, Madoff LC, et al. Global capacity for emerging infectious disease detection. *Proceedings of the National Academy of Sciences of the United States of America* 2010; 107(50): 21701–21706.

25. Donahue DA, Jr. BioWatch and the Brown Cap. *Journal of Homeland Security and Emergency Management* 2011; 8(1): Article 5.

26. Campbell TC, Hodanics CJ, Babin SM, et al. Developing open source, self-contained disease surveillance software applications for use in resource-limited settings. *BMC Med Inform and Decis Making* 2012; 12: 99.

27. Lewis SL, Feighner BH, Loschen WA, et al. SAGES: A suite of freely-available software tools for electronic disease surveillance in resource-limited settings. *PLoS One* 2011; 6(5): e19750. DOI: 10.1371/journal.pone.0019750.

28. Yan W, Nie S, Xu B, et al. Establishing a web-based integrated surveillance system for early detection of infectious disease epidemic in rural China: a field experimental study. *BMC Med Inform and Decis Making* 2012; 12: 4.

29. Vourc'h G, Bridges V, Gibbens J, et al. Detecting emerging diseases in farm animals through clinical observations. *Emerg Infect Dis* 2006; 12(2): 204–210.

30. Centers for Disease Control and Prevention. Information system architectures for syndromic surveillance. *MMWR* 2004; 53(Suppl.): 203–208.

31. Forslund D, Joyce E, Burr T, et al. Setting standards for improved syndromic surveillance. *IEEE Eng Med Biol Mag* 2004; 23(1): 65–70.

32. Mandl K, Overhage JM, Wagner M, et al. Implementing syndromic surveillance: a practical guide informed by the early experience. *J Am Med Inform Assoc* 2004; 11(2): 141–150.

33. Department of Homeland Security. National Biosurveillance Integration Center. http://www.dhs.gov/national-biosurveillance-integration-center (Accessed July 16, 2014).

34. Reis B, Mandl K. Time series modeling for syndromic surveillance. *BMC Med Inform Decis Making* 2003; 3: 2.

35. Kleinman K, Lazarus R, Platt R. A generalized linear mixed models approach for detecting incident clusters of disease in small areas, with an application to biological terrorism. *Am J Epidemiol* 2004; 159(3): 217–224.

36. Reis B, Mandl K. Syndromic Surveillance: The effects of syndrome grouping on model accuracy and outbreak detection. *Ann Emerg Med* 2004; 44(3): 235–241.

37. Feinberg S, Shmueli G. Statistical issues and challenges associated with rapid detection of bio-terrorist attacks. *Statist Med* 2005; 24: 513–529.

38. Hutwagner L, Thompson W, Seeman G, Treadwell T. A simulation model for assessing aberration detection methods used in public health surveillance for systems with limited baselines. *Statist Med* 2005; 24: 543–550.

39. Centers for Disease Control and Prevention. Bivariate method for spatio-temporal syndromic surveillance *MMWR* 2004; 53(Suppl.): 61–66.

40. Centers for Disease Control and Prevention. Role of data aggregation in biosurveillance detection strategies with applications from ESSENCE. *MMWR* 2004; 53(Suppl.): 67–73.

41. Centers for Disease Control and Prevention. Scan statistics for temporal surveillance for biologic terrorism. *MMWR* 2004; 53(Suppl.): 74–78.

42. Centers for Disease Control and Prevention. Approaches to syndromic surveillance when data consist of small regional counts. *MMWR* 2004; 53(Suppl.): 79–85.

43. Mandl KD, Reis B, Cassa C: Measuring Outbreak-Detection Performance by Using Controlled Feature Set Simulations. Centers for Disease Control and Prevention, *MMWR* 2004; 53(Suppl): 130–136. http://www.cdc.gov/mmwr/preview/mmwrhtml/su5301a26.htm (Accessed August 20, 2015).

44. Centers for Disease Control and Prevention. Benchmark data and power calculations for evaluating disease outbreak detection methods. *MMWR* 2004; 53(Suppl.): 144–151.

45. Kleinman K, Abrams A, Kulldorff M, Platt R. A model-adjusted space-time scan statistic with an application to syndromic surveillance. *Epidemiol Infect* 2005; 133(3): 409–419.

46. Centers for Disease Control and Prevention. Use of multiple data streams to conduct Bayesian biologic surveillance. *MMWR* 2005; 54(Suppl.): 63–69.

47. Centers for Disease Control and Prevention. Deciphering data anomalies in BioSense. *MMWR* 2005; 54(Suppl.): 133–139.

48. Najmi A-H, Magruder S. An adaptive prediction and detection algorithm for multistream syndromic surveillance. *BMC Med Inform Decis Making* 2005; 5: 33.

49. Ginsberg J, Mohebbi MH, Patel RS, et al. Detecting influenza epidemics using search engine query data. *Nature* 2009; 457(7232): 1012–1014.

50. Brownstein JS, Freifeld CC, Madoff LC. Digital Disease Detection – Harnessing the web for public health surveillance. *N Engl J Med* 2009; 360(21): 2153–2157.

51. Corley CD, Cook DJ, Mikler AR, Singh KP. Using web and social media for influenza surveillance. *Adv Exp Med Biol* 2010; 680: 559–564.

52. Butler D. When Google got flu wrong. *Nature* 2013; 494(7436): 155–156.

53. Freifeld CC, Chunara R, Mekaru SR, et al. Participatory epidemiology : use of mobile phones for community based health reporting. *PLoS Medicine* 2010; 7(12): e1000376.

54. Fuller S. Tracking the global express: new tools addressing disease threats across the world. *Epidemiology* 2010; 21(6): 769–771.

55. Yang M, Li Y-J, Kiang M. Uncovering social media data for public health surveillance. PACIS 201 Proceedings, Paper 218. 2011. http://aisel.aisnet.org/pacis2011/218 (Accessed November 16, 2012).

56. Kool JL, Paterson B, Pavlin BI, et al. Pacific-wide simplified syndromic surveillance for early warning of outbreaks. *Global Public Health: An International Journal for Research, Policy and Practice* 2012; 7(7): 670–681.

57. Paul MJ, Dredze M. You are what you tweet: analyzing Twitter for public health. Proceedings of the 5th International AAAI Conference on Weblogs and Social Media. Association for the Advancement of Artificial Intelligence. 2011. http://www.aaai.org/ocs/index.php/ICWSM/ICWSM11/paper/view/2880/3264 (Accessed August 20, 2015).

58. Potts JA, Gibbons RV, Rothman AL, et al. Prediction of Dengue disease severity among pediatric Thai patients using early clinical laboratory indicators. *Negl Trop Dis* 2010; 4(8): e769.

59. Gharbi M, Quenel P, Gustave J, et al. Time series analysis of dengue incidence in Guadeloupe, French West Indies: forecasting models using climate variables as predictors. *BMC Infect Dis* 2011; 11: 166.

60. Gamage S, Mohtashemi M, Simbartl L, Kralovic S, Wallace K, Roselle G. Analysis of dengue in Department of Veterans Affairs (VA) patients in Puerto Rico. *Emerging Health Threats Journal* 2011; 4: 11184.

61. Liu Q, Liu X, Jiang B, Yang W. Forecasting incidence of hemorrhagic fever with renal syndrome in China using ARIMA model. *BMC Infect Dis* 2011; 11: 218.

62. Stoto MA, Dempsey JX, Baer A, et al. Expert meeting on privacy, confidentiality and other legal ethical issues in syndromic surveillance. Report from an International Society for Disease Surveillance Consultation, Washington, DC, October 4–5, 2007. *Advances in Disease Surveillance* 2009; 7(2). http://faculty.washington.edu/lober/www.isdsjournal.org/htdocs/articles/6217.pdf (Accessed August 21, 2015).

63. Francis LP, Battin MP, Jacobson J, Smith C. Syndromic surveillance and patients as victims and vectors. *Bioethical Inquiry* 2009; 6: 187–195. http://papers.ssrn.com/sol3/papers.cfm?abstract_id=1517420 (Accessed August 21, 2015).

14

TRIAGE

Christopher A. Kahn, E. Brooke Lerner, and David C. Cone

OVERVIEW

Introduction

One of the hallmarks of a disaster is that the immediate needs of the affected population exceed currently available resources. Intuitively, this leads to the question of how limited resources can be used to optimize patient outcomes. Triage is the allocation of limited resources during a disaster. Although the concept of triage is applicable to all resources, the most commonly discussed and most studied application is to patient care. In this context, triage is the rapid evaluation of patients to determine the most appropriate level of care and treatment, given the limited resources at hand. For the remainder of this chapter, triage shall refer specifically to identifying the appropriate level of care for patients during a mass-casualty incident.

Although researchers have investigated this type of triage more extensively than the triage of equipment or other resources, even patient triage is not well studied. As with many topics encompassed by disaster medical sciences, it is extremely difficult to conduct randomized, controlled trials during an actual event; the use of other comparative study designs is also challenging. As a consequence, there is no high-quality evidence indicating which triage systems provide optimal resource utilization or maximal outcomes, or even whether any of the existing triage systems are of any value in managing the scene, optimizing resource allocation among patients, or ensuring maximal outcomes. The majority of studies on disaster triage focus on how well triage systems can be applied, how well they work in drills, or how they can be modified for specific scenarios. These studies are usually conducted with simulated scenarios, and are often performed on paper rather than using real or simulated victims.[1-3] Studies and reports describing the performance of triage systems during actual disasters are scarce and until recently anecdotal; comparative and outcomes studies are mostly lacking, although a few retrospective analyses have been conducted on individual patients comparing outcomes using different triage systems.[4-6] In fact, some of the basic assumptions underlying the use of triage in mass-casualty situations have not been tested. For example, there is no solid evidence to support the claim that triage systems provide improved outcomes related to morbidity or mortality when compared with randomly assigned or "first come, first served" methods. Further, it is not clear that various triage levels closely correlate with severity of illness or injury. These assumptions are, however, commonly accepted a priori, and provide a base from which a closer evaluation of triage systems can begin. Accordingly, this chapter will describe the existing triage systems, along with recommendations for their evaluation and implementation.

History of Mass Casualty Triage

It is generally accepted that triage was invented during the Napoleonic Wars by Dominique Jean Larrey, surgeon-in-chief of Napoleon's army from 1797 to 1815. Although the concept of "inventing" resource allocation is dubious, Larrey can be credited with codifying a system for sorting battle casualties into categories based on urgency of evaluation. It is from the French verb *trier*, meaning "to sort," that the word triage is derived.

Following this initial development of a casualty sorting system, triage continued to evolve as a consequence of wartime experience for over a century. The first civilian triage systems were developed in the latter half of the twentieth century. Now, approximately 200 years after Larrey's initial work in the field, several dozen systems exist worldwide, employing over 120 different types of triage labels and tools.

CURRENT STATE OF THE ART

Vignette

On April 15, 2013, two bombs exploded near the finish line of the Boston Marathon. Three people were killed as a result, and well over 200 suffered injuries. A medical tent at the finish line, only a few hundred yards from the explosions, was quickly transformed to serve as a casualty collection point and initial triage station. An emergency medical services fellow from the University of Massachusetts Medical School was working in the tent, and described the role of triage in the evaluation and management of the victims:

208

Within moments of the bombing, patients came in a steady stream of casualties. Because of the nature of the devices, there were a tremendous amount of extremity injuries. Almost no one was 'walking wounded.' There was need for immediate triage and management of what became an acute shortage of resources. An *a priori* thought process was required and the ability to distinguish those who needed immediate transport and those who could wait for more resources to arrive on scene. A system familiar to providers on scene was SMART triage. From a legacy of training elsewhere, people were able to utilize this consistent means of dialogue from provider to provider regardless of agency or training. Triage as a system and means of communication amongst prehospital professionals saved lives that day.

– Adam Darnobid, MD

The preceding example illustrates several difficulties with the implementation and evaluation of mass-casualty triage systems. First, actual disasters and mass-casualty events are often quite different from simulations and training exercises. Protocols developed without field testing may be difficult to apply or seem less relevant in a field situation. Second, the possibility of secondary events (such as additional explosions) or contamination may complicate a triage situation. Third, the need to rapidly evaluate a large number of persons to promptly find those most in need of immediate care almost certainly leads to a baseline level of inaccuracy in triage; there is no evidence to define an "acceptable miss rate," which is likely both situation- and agency-dependent. Further, even the outcomes that would define accurate triage have not been universally accepted, although some have been identified.[7] With these caveats in mind, we examine the individual triage systems in more detail.

Triage Systems

Despite the large number of triage systems extant throughout the world, most have several features in common. A majority of these systems use a "walking filter" to quickly identify less-severely injured patients and remove them from the immediate disaster zone. Patients not expected to survive are usually tagged "expectant," "morgue," or "black." Remaining patients are then categorized into the remaining triage levels. The use of color codes – generally black (deceased), grey (expectant), red (most severe), yellow (intermediate severity), and green (least severe) – to identify differing severity levels is common. The primary differences between systems rest in how patients are triaged to each level. Additionally, some systems use supplemental levels, colors, or classifications to further stratify victims. To date, no system has been shown conclusively to be better than any other in terms of patient outcomes, scene management, or resource allocation. Little information is publicly available about some triage systems known to be in use worldwide, particularly in Europe. What follows is a description of the triage systems that had sufficient available information to describe and discuss. These systems include START (Simple Triage and Rapid Treatment), Homebush Triage Standard, CareFlight Triage, Triage Sieve, the Sacco Triage Method, the CESIRA (Italian abbreviations for Unconscious, Hemorrhaging, Shock, Insufficient respirations, Broken bones, Other injuries) Protocol, SALT (Sort, Assess, Lifesaving measures, Treat/Transport), and Military/NATO (North Atlantic

Treaty Organization) Triage. We also include a brief discussion of the Model Uniform Core Criteria, which was introduced in the United States in 2011 and is a list of core principles that should be followed to promote interoperability and standardization of the mass-casualty triage process. We provide a separate discussion of the secondary triage systems SAVE (Secondary Assessment of Victim Endpoint) and Triage Sort, as well the pediatric specific systems, JumpSTART and Pediatric Triage Tape (PTT).

START

Simple Triage and Rapid Treatment (START) is the most commonly used triage system for handling multi-casualty emergencies in the United States, and has been adopted by components of the federal government.[8] START is also used in Canada, Saudi Arabia, and parts of Australia and Israel. The START system was developed by the Newport Beach Fire and Marine Department and Hoag Hospital in Orange County, California, in the early 1980s, and is based on the NATO triage classification system.

START uses physiologic parameters, and is designed to make a patient assessment within 60 seconds or less and identify the patients with immediate medical needs. Each patient is assessed and assigned to one of four color categories depending on his or her injuries (see Figure 14.1).

A visible triage tag or ribbon is placed on each victim, identifying the patient's category for rescuers who will collect, treat, and/or transport them. START is based on ability to obey commands, respiratory rate, and capillary refill.

Following a mass-casualty incident, START triage begins with directing ambulatory victims (often referred to as the "walking wounded") to move to a safe area. These patients are tagged as

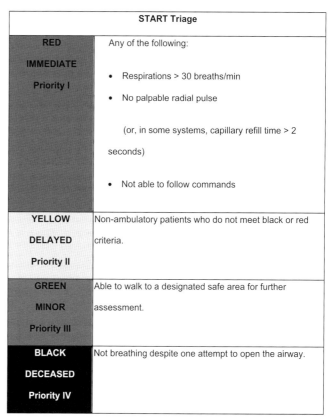

START Triage	
RED **IMMEDIATE** **Priority I**	Any of the following: • Respirations > 30 breaths/min • No palpable radial pulse (or, in some systems, capillary refill time > 2 seconds) • Not able to follow commands
YELLOW **DELAYED** **Priority II**	Non-ambulatory patients who do not meet black or red criteria.
GREEN **MINOR** **Priority III**	Able to walk to a designated safe area for further assessment.
BLACK **DECEASED** **Priority IV**	Not breathing despite one attempt to open the airway.

Figure 14.1. START Triage.

"minor" using a green label and, typically, are more thoroughly assessed following assessment of the remaining, more seriously injured victims. Triage continues in a systematic manner for the remaining patients. Triage categorization is based on three observations: respiration, perfusion, and mental status. An easy mnemonic, RPM, has been created as a memory aid. Patients with no spontaneous respirations receive airway repositioning; if they remain apneic, they are tagged "deceased" using a black label and receive no further interventions. Patients with respirations greater than 30 breaths per minute, lack of a palpable radial pulse (or capillary refill longer than 2 seconds), or unable to follow simple commands are tagged "immediate" using a red label. The remaining patients are tagged "delayed" using a yellow label.

Some areas use variations of the START triage system. For example, the Israeli triage system uses two additional categories and colors: blue for children, and grey for combined injuries such as chemical contamination and physical trauma.[9] Additionally, most agencies use a "no radial pulse" criterion rather than "capillary refill time longer than 2 seconds" to compensate for difficulties in determining capillary refill time in cold or dark condition. Few agencies continue to use capillary refill for determination of circulatory status.

START only allows for two interventions to be made during the triage process: direct pressure for bleeding control (preferably applied by another victim to keep the rescuer free for further triage), and basic airway opening maneuvers. It is also recommended that repeat assessments are made as often as possible since patient conditions may change. Use of START triage has been described for two terrorist incidents: the attack on the World Trade Center in New York in 2001, and the bombing of the Alfred P. Murrah Federal Building in Oklahoma City in 1995.[10–12] Use of START for two additional U.S. disasters, Hurricane Andrew in 1992 and the Northridge earthquake in 1994, has also been described.[13] However, there are no data in these descriptive papers regarding whether the system was used correctly or improved outcomes for patients in any of these events; a description of the 2001 World Trade Center attacks describes limitations of START due to concerns regarding personnel and structural safety, but does not describe triage accuracy for the few rescued patients.[10]

Some of these concerns were subsequently addressed for the first time in a research article by Kahn et al., investigating the use of START at a 2002 train collision. The analysis compared assigned triage levels with patients' actual acuity based on a priori criteria.[7] After evaluation of 148 patient records, the authors determined that all critically ill patients were successfully identified and triaged as immediate; 94.7% of the patients triaged as minor did, in fact, meet the minor triage criteria. However, while undertriage (the assignment of a higher acuity patient to an inappropriately lower acuity triage category) was minimal, there was a significant amount of overtriage (assignment of a lower acuity patient to an inappropriately higher acuity triage category).

Homebush Triage Standard

The Homebush Triage Standard methodology was developed in Australia in 1999 as an attempt to unify varying triage protocols across the country.[14] It is based on the START and SAVE triage systems. It includes a fifth triage category called "dying" which is given a white label. This category is meant to separate the dead (labeled black) from the dying, so that comfort care

HOMEBUSH TRIAGE STANDARD		
RED Immediate	ALPHA	Any of the following: • Respirations > 30 breaths/min • No palpable radial pulse • Not able to follow commands
YELLOW Urgent	BRAVO	Non-ambulatory patients who do not meet black, white, or red criteria.
GREEN Non-urgent	CHARLIE	Able to walk to a designated safe area for further assessment.
WHITE Dying	DELTA	Dying patients; may have a pulse, but no spontaneous respirations.
BLACK Dead	ECHO	Not breathing despite one attempt to open the airway.

Figure 14.2. Homebush Triage Standard.

can be provided to those patients who are dying. The red category is assigned to patients who have no palpable radial pulse, are unable to follow commands, or have respirations > 30 breaths per minute. Non-urgent and urgent patients are determined identically to START's minor and delayed patients, respectively. This system also uses geographic location rather than triage tags to indicate the patients' condition. In other words, patients are physically moved to the "level white" area, rather than placing a tag on their body to indicate their triage assignment. In addition to a color, each category also has a designated standard phonetic alphabet code (e.g., alpha, bravo, charlie, delta, and echo) to facilitate radio communication (see Figure 14.2).

Finally, in addition to primary triage, this system includes a secondary patient assessment to evaluate the extent of injuries and consider them in light of the available resources. This secondary system is used to prioritize order of transport to the hospital.

Use of the Homebush Triage System was documented in the Bali bombing on October 12, 2002, but again, only descriptive information is provided, with no data regarding triage accuracy or effect on any particular outcome.[15] Although it is not clear which triage system, if any, was used at the scene, the Homebush taxonomy was modified and used on board the first aircraft repatriating patients to Australia.

CareFlight Triage

The CareFlight system is a triage tool used in parts of Australia. Presence of breathing, level of consciousness, and presence of radial pulse determine the triage priority. This system is similar to START, with the notable exceptions that respiratory rate is not evaluated in CareFlight, and that assessment of mental status (ability to follow commands) is done prior to assessment

CareFlight Triage	
RED **Immediate**	Any of the following: • Not able to follow commands • No palpable radial pulse
YELLOW **Urgent**	Non-ambulatory patients who do not meet black or red criteria.
GREEN **Delayed**	Able to walk to a designated safe area for further assessment.
BLACK **Unsalvageable**	Not breathing despite one attempt to open the airway.

Figure 14.3. CareFlight Triage.

TRIAGE SIEVE	
Priority I **Immediate**	Any of the following: • Respirations < 10 or > 29 breaths/min • Capillary refill time > 2 seconds OR pulse > 120 beats/min
Priority II **Urgent**	Non-ambulatory patients who do not meet dead or immediate criteria.
Priority III **Delayed**	Able to walk to a designated safe area for further assessment.
Priority IV **Dead**	Not breathing despite one attempt to open the airway.

Figure 14.4. Triage Sieve.

of circulation. CareFlight also uses a four-color system to identify patients who should be triaged as unsalvageable, immediate, urgent, and delayed (see Figure 14.3).

A retrospective 2001 study by Garner et al. compared START, modified START, and Triage Sieve with CareFlight and determined CareFlight to be more specific for critical injury (as defined by modified Baxt criteria) and faster to administer.[5] However, this difference was minimal, with the difference between the upper limit of the 95% confidence interval for specificity of the modified START system (using radial pulse) and the lower limit of that for CareFlight being only 1%. Although Triage Sieve was significantly less sensitive (with roughly equivalent specificity) for critical injury in this study, some have noted that failure to include Triage Sort (the secondary triage system that is meant to follow Triage Sieve) as part of this algorithm may limit the applicability of these results to actual disasters.

Triage Sieve

Triage Sieve has been widely adopted in the United Kingdom, parts of Europe, and parts of Australia, and is accepted by NATO. Triage Sieve is similar to START in that a preliminary walking filter is followed by the use of respiratory rate and capillary refill or heart rate to classify patients into triage categories. Patients able to walk are classified as "delayed" priority III; patients who do not breathe following an attempt to open the airway are classified "dead" priority IV; and patients with a respiratory rate of <10 or >29, capillary refill time of >2 seconds, or heart rate

of >120 beats/minute are classified "immediate" priority I. All other patients are considered "urgent" priority II. Triage Sieve does not measure level of consciousness (see Figure 14.4).

Use of Triage Sieve was documented in the London bombings of July 7, 2005.[16] In general, Triage Sieve is used as a primary "triage-to-treatment" algorithm, and is followed by a secondary "triage-to-transportation" algorithm, Triage Sort.

Sacco Triage Method

The Sacco Triage Method was developed in the United States by conducting a logistic regression analysis using data from a statewide trauma registry. The Delphi technique was then used to estimate the chances of victim deterioration by obtaining consensus among a group of six experts based on changes in physiologic parameters of the patient.[17] This triage system is intended to account for both the patient's physiologic parameters and the available resources.

The Sacco Triage Method first requires on-scene personnel to enter available resource information into a computer database. A physiological score is then computed mathematically for each patient. This score considers the patient's respiratory rate, pulse rate, and best motor response, assigns each variable a coded value, and then sums these values to calculate the Sacco Score (see Table 14.1).[18]

Prehospital personnel can calculate this score manually or using the computer. After data entry, the developers report that this score can be determined and a triage category assigned within 45 seconds. The victims are tagged and organized into groups

Table 14.1. Sacco Triage Score

Sacco Score

	Coded Values	0	1	2	3	4
R	Breaths per minute	0	1–9	36+	25–35	10–24
P	Beats per minute	0	1–40	41–60	121+	61–120
M	Response to stimulus (motor response)	None	Extension or flexion	Withdraws	Localizes	Obeys commands

CESIRA Protocol		
Red	**C**oscienza	Unconscious
	Emorragie	Hemorrhaging
	Shock	Shock
	Insufficienza respiratia	Insufficient Respiration
Yellow	**R**otture ossee	Broken bones
	Altro	Other injuries
Green		Walking

Figure 14.5. CESIRA Triage Protocol.

Table 14.2. Military/NATO Triage

P1	T1	IMMEDIATE: Life threatening injuries must be treated within first hour. Good chance of survival.
P2	T2	DELAYED: Delay in treatment, can wait a few hours. Stabilization
P3	T3	MINIMAL: Walking, treatment may be delayed for several hours.
P1 – Hold	T4	EXPECTANT: Significant resources needed to treat patient. Signs of impending death.
Dead	Dead	Dead

according to the score. Triage tags have a large clock face with numbers representing the score. The triage officer contacts a central dispatcher and provides information on number of victims, the Sacco Scores, ambulance processing rate at the scene, and number of landing sites for helicopters. These data are entered into the proprietary software, which then produces the optimal triage strategy. This strategy defines the order in which victims are transported and treated and to which hospitals they are sent. The system can also alert the hospitals to the number, severity, and scheduled arrival of patients. The Sacco Triage Method is proprietary, and accordingly, the specific details of how triage and transport decisions are determined are not publicly available for review, research, or independent confirmation. Reliable information on current deployment and field success is not available. The developers report that the Sacco Score accurately predicts a patient's survivability from trauma, although this has not been prospectively validated.[19]

CESIRA Protocol

The CESIRA Protocol, developed in Italy in 1990, has three basic categories: red, which includes patients who are unconscious, hemorrhaging, in shock, or having respiratory insufficiency; yellow for patients with broken bones and other injuries; and green for victims able to walk. CESIRA is the Italian acronym for the words describing these injuries (see Figure 14.5).

CESIRA does not contain a "dead" category; non-physicians are not legally authorized to declare death in Italy, and the system is designed for prehospital use when physicians are not present.

Military/NATO Triage

The main objective of military triage is to treat and return injured soldiers to the front lines as soon as possible. For those who cannot return to duty, medical focus is on wound debridement, limb salvage, and preservation of life. Military triage is based on the North American Treaty Organization (NATO) triage classification, a subjective categorization based on expected survival and resource utilization. All NATO member countries follow a standardized triage system for their military operations providing consistency for multinational operations. Military triage begins with the immediate sorting of patients according to type and severity of injury and likelihood of survival, and the establishment of priority for treatment and evacuation to assure

optimal medical care to the largest number of casualties. Most military triage systems use the "T" (treatment) system: T1, T2, T3, T4, and dead. Others such as the British Military use the "P" (priority) system: P1, P2, P3, and P1-hold.[20] Holding areas are set up for the victims according to their injuries following initial evaluation. Patients are treated and stabilized until they can be transported to a medical facility. The classification scheme is subjective, based on the experience of the triage provider rather than specified physiologic criteria (see Table 14.2).

SALT Triage

A U.S. government funded project to examine existing triage systems has resulted in the development of the SALT Triage system. After determining that no existing system had enough scientific support to recommend its use, a workgroup used the limited existing data and expert opinion to develop the SALT Triage system, attempting to incorporate the best features of the existing systems. SALT is intended to serve as a national all-hazards mass-casualty initial triage standard for all patients (e.g., adults, children, special populations).[21]

SALT begins with a global sorting of patients to prioritize them for individual assessment. Patients who are able to walk are instructed to walk to a designated area, and are assigned last priority for individual assessment. Those who remain are asked to wave or are observed for purposeful movement. Those who do not move (i.e., are still) and those with obvious life threats are assessed first, since they are the most likely to need lifesaving interventions (LSIs).

The individual assessment begins with limited LSIs that are only performed if the intervention is within the responder's scope of practice, and only if the equipment is immediately available. The recommended LSIs include controlling major hemorrhage, opening the airway, providing chest decompression, and using auto injector antidotes. If the patient is a child and not breathing, the provider can consider giving two rescue breaths.

After any needed LSIs are provided, patients are prioritized for treatment and/or transport by assigning them to one of five categories. Patients who are not breathing even after LSIs are attempted are triaged as dead. Patients who have mild injuries that are self-limited if not treated, and can tolerate delays in care without increasing their risk of mortality, are triaged as minimal. Patients who do not obey commands, do not have a peripheral pulse, are in respiratory distress, or have uncontrolled major hemorrhage are triaged as immediate. Within this group of immediate patients, however, providers should also consider if a patient has injuries that are likely to be incompatible with life

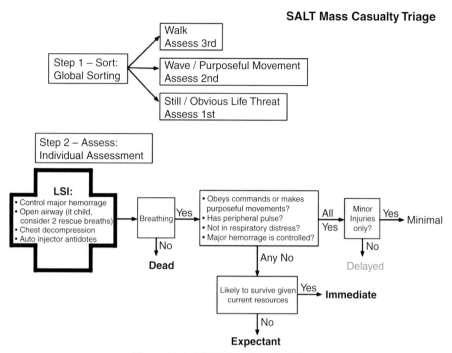

SALT Mass Casualty Triage

Figure 14.6. SALT Mass Casualty Triage.

given the currently available resources. If so, then the provider triages that patient as expectant rather than immediate. The remaining patients are triaged as delayed (see Figure 14.6).

To assist with identification of patients, SALT recommends that the deceased be symbolized by the color black, expectant by gray, immediate by red, delayed by yellow, and minimal by green.

Standardizing the Structure for Disaster Triage

As is evident from the previous discussion, a lack of standardization exists across multiple mass-casualty triage platforms. Development of guidelines to promote interoperability and standardization in disaster triage would be a significant advancement. This has recently been achieved in the United States with the creation of the Model Uniform Core Criteria (MUCC). These Core Criteria review the science on mass-casualty triage and promulgate a set of principles that should be adhered to by whatever mass-casualty triage system is being used in a community. They were developed by expanding the work group that created SALT Triage using funding from the CDC.[22] The concept of the Core Criteria is to allow local agencies to develop or modify their response plans in accordance with a national guideline that sets standards and creates interoperable terminology and definitions, while maintaining the local control required to ensure an appropriately flexible response.

There are four general categories of criteria in the MUCC: general considerations, global sorting, lifesaving interventions, and assignment of triage categories. While it is clear that there is a lack of scientific evidence to support most of the current components of mass-casualty triage – for example, only two of the twenty-four criteria listed in the MUCC are supported by direct science – the Core Criteria do provide a framework in which existing triage systems can be modified to ensure that even when working in different jurisdictions, emergency responders will have the basic knowledge needed to successfully perform triage.

The U.S. government recently approved an implementation plan for ensuring that the Model Uniform Core Criteria are adopted nationwide.

One limitation of the Core Criteria is that the group creating them first developed SALT Triage. Therefore, potential bias exists in favor of SALT by the Core Criteria. To address this potential flaw, it might be useful to expand this concept to the global community using a group of international experts. Creating international guidelines standardizing disaster triage across countries could improve the effectiveness of response teams from multiple countries deployed to the same event.

Secondary Triage Systems

In situations where time to definitive care is extensively prolonged, or when resources are insufficient to meet demand, secondary triage systems may be used to further categorize victims for prioritization of transport or treatment. In severely resource-constrained environments, these systems are designed to consider the likelihood of a positive outcome in addition to the urgency of treatment and the amount of medical supplies and equipment required. Consequently, the resulting priority decisions for transport and other resource utilization may not be in complete concordance with the primary triage. Importantly, there has been even less research done to examine these systems compared to primary triage.

SAVE Triage

SAVE Triage is used with the START triage algorithm. This system uses objective and subjective individualized criteria to estimate victim survival probability and resource utilization, thus directing limited treatment options in the field and prioritizing transport of patients who are most likely to benefit from advanced care. SAVE is designed to limit use of medical resources by identifying victims with poor prognoses and those whose outcomes are unlikely to be affected by immediate care. Also, consideration is given to healthcare workers and other special categories of victims who, with minimal treatment (e.g., splinting of a sprained ankle), could assist in the disaster response and increase the available personnel resources for patient treatment. Medical care is prioritized toward victims whose likelihood of survival (given treatment) is over 50% and who would benefit from immediate intervention. These likelihoods are calculated based on prognostic tools including a limb salvage score, the Glasgow Coma Scale, and data on survivability after burns. The full details of this system are too extensive to present here, but can be found in the original 1996 manuscript.[23]

Triage Sort

Often paired with Triage Sieve, Triage Sort is a secondary triage system that uses the Revised Trauma Score (based on Glasgow Coma Scale, blood pressure, and respiratory rate) to categorize patients into immediate, urgent, and delayed categories. This system is generally first applied to patients initially "sieved" into the immediate category to further stratify them when transportation is limited. Attention is then given to urgent, and then delayed patients.

Pediatric Triage Systems

The physiological and anatomical differences between children and adults are significant. Children are more prone to head injuries, airway obstruction, and hypothermia. They have proportionally less blood volume than adults, and very young children may be unable to walk, communicate verbally, or cooperate with instructions. Care providers may have difficulty obtaining blood pressure readings on children, and the act of triaging children may cause emotional challenges to rescuers beyond the already stressful scenario of disaster triage. With these differences in mind, several triage systems have been developed specifically for use with pediatric patients. However, like the general triage systems, some of which are intended for use in children and adults (e.g., SALT, Sacco), there are presently no validated pediatric triage tools.

JumpSTART

JumpSTART is designed to be an objective, physiologically appropriate tool for triaging children. It is intended for use in pediatric mass-casualty victims who are generally younger than 8–10 years of age. Victims who appear to be adolescents or older should be triaged using the prevailing adult triage method. JumpSTART was developed by Romig in 1995 and modified in 2001, and is a modification of the START triage system.[24] Four key changes were made to the START system based on children being more likely to suffer respiratory arrests than adults, having different respiratory rates, and young children being unable to follow commands or walk.

In the JumpSTART system, when a child is identified as not breathing, the rescuer is instructed to reposition the airway. If this does not result in spontaneous respirations, and the child has a palpable pulse, the rescuer then gives five mouth-to-barrier rescue breaths (called "jumpstart" breaths). A child who is still not breathing after the rescue breaths is labeled dead, while a child whose breathing is present at this point is labeled immediate.

JumpSTART Triage	
RED **IMMEDIATE**	Any of the following: • Spontaneous respirations after upper airway positioning or the 5-breath ventilatory trial • Respirations < 15 or > 45 breaths/min • No palpable pulse • Inappropriate response to pain (posturing) or unresponsive to stimuli
YELLOW **DELAYED**	• Respirations > 15 or < 45 breaths/min • Palpable pulse • Alert, verbalizes, or appropriate pain response
GREEN **MINOR**	Able to walk to a designated safe area for further assessment, or not able to walk at baseline but with no external evidence of significant injury after having been evaluated by the remainder of the algorithm.
BLACK **DECEASED**	Not breathing despite one attempt to open the upper airway and, in patients with a palpable pulse, provision of 5 rescue breaths to open the lower airway.

Figure 14.7. JumpSTART Triage.

When deciding whether a child should be triaged into the immediate or delayed category, responders must recognize the different values for age-adjusted normal and abnormal respiratory rates and the limited ability to follow commands in the pediatric population. For children, a respiratory rate less than 15 or greater than 45 indicates that the immediate category should be assigned. If the respiratory rate is between 15 and 45, additional assessment is needed to determine the appropriate triage designation. While normal respiratory rates in children vary by age, this simplified rule accounts for those variations while limiting the information that must be memorized. For assessing mental status, young children may lack the capability of responding to commands, or may be too upset to comply with instructions. Therefore, JumpSTART uses the AVPU (Alert/Verbal/Painful/Unresponsive) tool rather than response to commands for the mental status component of the algorithm. A child who is unresponsive or demonstrates an inappropriate pain response is placed in the immediate category. Absent other indications for triage to the immediate group, individuals who are alert, able to verbalize, or demonstrate an appropriate pain response will be designated as "delayed (see Figure 14.7)."

The JumpSTART scheme also recommends that children who are carried to the minimal area should be the first to be evaluated during secondary triage (or earlier if possible), as they may have serious injuries. Children who are developmentally or otherwise unable to walk at baseline should proceed through the entire JumpSTART algorithm; if they reach the delayed decision point and do not have any external evidence of significant injury, they may be considered minimal for the purposes of further evaluation.

Pediatric Triage Tape

The PTT is derived from Triage Sieve. It is used throughout the UK and parts of Europe, India, Australia, and South Africa. The PTT is designed to work with any existing triage labeling system. If the child is walking or an infant is alert and moving all limbs, use of the tape is not necessary, and the patient is labeled "delayed" (green). If a child is not walking or moving appropriately, the tape is used to measure the length of the child, similar to the Broselow Tape or other length-based algorithms. The PTT is divided into five length blocks; each block contains the algorithm for Triage Sieve, modified for age-appropriate respiratory and heart rate parameters.[25,26]

Comparison of Pediatric Triage Systems

CareFlight triage can be used in both children and adults. In a study by Wallis et al., CareFlight, PTT, START, and Jump-START were compared in 3,461 injured children presenting to the Trauma Unit of the Red Cross Children's Hospital in Cape Town, South Africa.[4] The same modified Baxt criteria employed in the Garner comparative study was used to define critical injury. Overall, CareFlight showed the best performance in sensitivity and specificity. However, the 95% confidence intervals for sensitivity overlapped with PTT, CareFlight, and START. The 95% confidence intervals for specificity overlapped only with PTT and CareFlight, with JumpSTART very slightly lower. Sensitivity was very poor (approximately 1%) for JumpSTART, compared with approximately 39–46% for the other algorithms. Unfortunately, this is the only published report that could be identified comparing pediatric triage systems. Therefore, it is currently not possible to recommend any of the pediatric triage systems as superior to any of the others.

Use of Common Scales for Triage

One might ask whether any of the individual assessment items contained in some of the previously discussed triage systems might provide comparable sensitivity and specificity in identifying the more seriously injured patients. It seems reasonable to assume that if assessment of a single "score" or feature were as accurate as assessment of a multi-feature triage system, the former would be simpler and more rapid, and thus preferable. The most studied of these is the motor component of the Glasgow Coma Scale (GCS). A 1998 study first demonstrated that the major discriminatory power of the GCS lies in the motor component. In this retrospective study correlating mortality with the first GCS score obtained in the field in approximately 1,200 patients, the motor score alone performed slightly better than the summed three-part GCS.[27] Several large studies have subsequently supported this finding.[28–31] A retrospective study of almost 30,000 patients from a state trauma registry suggests that separating patients into those who can follow simple commands (Glasgow motor score = 6) from those who cannot (Glasgow motor score from 1 to 5) provides the best discriminatory capability, perhaps providing a simple and elegant alternate to a multi-step triage algorithm.[29] Research has demonstrated that a GCS motor component score of 5 or less is correlated with worse outcomes in trauma patients.[30]

Respiratory rate is another commonly used trauma triage criteria. There is limited evidence to support its use in the trauma setting, although it may have greater utility for triaging patients with medical ailments. The frequently used cutoff of 30 breaths per minute as the respiratory criterion is arbitrary and not supported in current literature; it appears that lowering this cutoff to the mid-20s may improve overall triage performance.[32]

Finally, assessment of a victim's ability to walk as part of a global sorting mechanism does have some support in current literature.[7] This criterion is widely used as part of several triage schemes.

Outcome Measures for Triage Research

Although a large number of mass-casualty triage systems exist worldwide, many with similar features, there are no currently accepted reference standards that define key outcome measures. There are essentially two categories of outcomes that could be used in assessing how triage affects patient outcome: patient-based scoring systems, such as Injury Severity Score (ISS) (e.g., does triage system "x" appropriately assign all patients with an ISS greater than "y" to the "red" category?), and resource-based systems (e.g., did all patients who required surgery or a blood transfusion in the first two hours after arrival at the hospital get correctly assigned to the "red" category?). In 1990, Baxt et al. defined a set of criteria based on resource utilization within 2 days of arrival at the hospital to define a patient's level of serious injury, in an attempt to correlate resource utilization to the ISS.[33] He found that the ISS underestimated the resource requirements of trauma patients. These Baxt criteria were modified by Garner et al. in 2001 to more accurately reflect which patients in the prehospital setting were truly in need of immediate care. This landmark study retrospectively examined individual trauma patients to evaluate how each of four systems (Care-Flight, START, modified START, and Triage Sieve) performed. A major limitation of this investigation is that the subjects were not disaster victims. While some triage algorithms performed well on this population, these patients do not represent the typical individuals seen in disasters nor did they present in the overwhelming numbers encountered in catastrophes. Therefore, the value of this model remains unclear. In fact, only one study has been published that examines the real-time performance of any mass-casualty triage system with reference to these a priori criteria. A 2009 article by Kahn et al. discussed the performance of START Triage at a train collision involving approximately 150 victims; the authors found that the "walking filter" appeared to function well in defining less-severely injured patients.[7] This manuscript may represent the first truly outcomes-based study of mass-casualty triage performed during an actual disaster.

Some researchers suggest that scored scales, such as the ISS and Revised Trauma Score (RTS), could be used as reference criteria for validation of triage instruments. It remains unclear which of these scores, if any, accurately predict outcomes or need for resource utilization in the mass-casualty setting. Further, there is no agreement within specific scores as to which cutoffs should be used to define "correct" use of a triage instrument (e.g., in the previous paragraph, what would "y" be in the example using ISS?). In addition, comparing the accuracy of various triage algorithms using a number scale to define correct triage may provide a statistically significant difference but not necessarily translate into a clinically significant one. A good example of this concern is represented by the Second National

Acute Spinal Cord Injury Study (NASCIS) trial reported in the United States in 1990. Spinal cord injury patients receiving high-dose methylprednisolone demonstrated a statistically significant improvement in a neurologic outcome score, but a clear improvement in clinically relevant outcomes was difficult to identify.[34] Although the reproducibility and applicability to a wide range of trauma patients makes tools such as ISS and RTS attractive, their validity in assessing outcomes in the mass-casualty setting is unknown.

Lastly, some investigators have proposed using predicted mortality as an outcome parameter to measure triage accuracy. Given most triage systems were designed to determine acuity and not mortality, the effectiveness of this outcome measure remains unknown. It is also problematic how medics would use this information to prioritize patient assessment and care. It may not be appropriate in a constrained resource environment to treat patients with high predicted mortality, as they are likely to die regardless of intervention and will consume significant amounts of limited resources in the process.

Criteria other than clinical patient outcome may be important in judging and comparing trauma systems. Such potentially significant issues include: 1) how efficiently scarce field resources are used; 2) how quickly patients are transported to hospitals; and 3) the costs of training, program implementation, and competency maintenance for personnel in a given system. Essentially no work has been done to examine or define these non-clinical outcomes.

At this time, no specific recommendation based on strong evidence can be made to support any one triage system over another, although the MUCC (when implemented) will likely bring some standardization to the process. While not studied, it seems likely that use of a single standard system across an entire region is likely to improve interoperability during mass-casualty responses. In the absence of additional evidence to recommend a particular methodology, choice of this system will likely be based on existing resources, the need for retraining, and flexibility in the face of the local hazard vulnerability analysis.

Other Triage Considerations

Differentiation of Disaster Triage from Other Triage Modalities

It is important to distinguish disaster triage from other types of triage, including daily emergency department triage, single-patient trauma triage, and multi-casualty incident triage when resources are not exceeded. Single-patient trauma triage (the process of determining whether a given single trauma patient, such as a motor vehicle crash victim, needs transport to a trauma center or not, often using the Field Triage Decision Scheme developed jointly by the American College of Surgeons and the CDC) attempts to match the patient's clinical needs with the correct resources (trauma center vs. a hospital that is not a trauma center).[35] Unlike the mass-casualty setting, however, this type of triage does not weigh the relative needs of several patients to determine who will get a limited resource, but instead helps determine whether a single patient might benefit from the resources of the trauma center.

When personnel in the prehospital setting or emergency department are confronted by multiple patients, these providers are forced to prioritize care for individuals based on their acuity. In multiple casualty situations, as well as in daily emergency department triage, the goal is to determine which patients can

Table 14.3. Patient Care Focus Based on Number of Victims

Incident Type	Triage Goal	Difference
Single-patient incident	Optimize individual patient outcome by providing all resources required to meet the patient's needs	No consideration of other patients
Multiple casualties	Prioritize patients for appropriate treatment/transport so they receive needed resources in sufficient time to reduce morbidity and mortality	Resources are devoted to patients according to priority, but patients receive all the care they need
Disaster	Prioritize patients for appropriate treatment/transport so they receive needed resources in sufficient time to reduce morbidity and mortality, but also ensure that scarce resources are utilized to provide the best outcome at a population level	
	Resources are devoted to patients according to priority, but patients who are unlikely to survive given the available resources are given a low priority for treatment/transport	

wait for treatment without increasing their risk for morbidity and mortality.

In disaster situations when demand for care exceeds supply, the need to prioritize patients must also include a rationing of resources, shifting the focus from ensuring that each individual receives the best possible care to ensuring the population as a whole experiences the best possible outcome. In other words, the focus is on providing care for the greatest number of people (see Table 14.3).

In some cases, this will include identifying patients who are not expected to survive, and making the decision that no resources beyond comfort measures be used for these individuals.

Context-Specific Triage

While the majority of disasters to date have resulted in traumatic injuries from explosions, collisions, collapses, and other releases of kinetic energy, other scenarios that involve chemical, biological, radioactive, or nuclear agents (CBRN), or even a combination of agents, are also possible; responders must be prepared to respond to any type of event. Most of the triage systems described here focus on triage of trauma victims where kinetic or thermal energy is the only cause of their injury. It is possible that applying these triage systems to other types of events may not be feasible and may not improve patient outcomes. Developing an all-hazards triage algorithm may be difficult since it must be scientifically valid for all types of threats while remaining simple to use, accurate, reproducible, and rapid. A 2005 manuscript proposed a basic triage algorithm, based on START Triage, with simple modifications made for each category of CBRN event.

These modifications address the need for further triage to maximize patient outcomes while protecting response personnel.[36] A small pilot test of this system has been described; no further study or validation has been published.[37] SALT Triage is also intended to be an all-hazards triage method. In addition, timing of decontamination versus transport may be of critical importance in balancing patient care needs with personnel protection, and is an important component of mass-casualty triage protocols for CBRN events.

Additional considerations require implementation of triage in nontraditional situations. Typically, mass-casualty triage is initiated in situations with a more defined relationship between victims and responders, where decisions are made after individual person-to-person contact. However, in a biologic or weather-related disaster, there may be a large number of casualties spread over a wide region. In these cases, triage methods where an entire population may be impacted require consideration. Rather than a single, large peak of acutely injured individuals, response personnel may be faced with a prolonged presentation of victims in addition to the baseline number of patients already evaluated. Accordingly, a system that groups patients by exposure status may be necessary instead of a system that triages strictly by acuity. Such a strategy has been proposed by Burkle and advocates triaging patients into five groups: 1) susceptible but not exposed; 2) exposed but not yet infectious; 3) infectious; 4) removed by death or recovery; and 5) protected by vaccination or prophylactic medication.[38] Triage tools for population-based events require development in concert with infectious disease, public health, and other experts in epidemiology and mass patient care. These tools may eventually take the form of telephone screening or broadcast messages for self-evaluation in affected areas. It is possible that referral to hospitals for triage evaluation may not be prudent, due to risk for spreading a contagion or issues with transportation such as during a flood. Given the broad uncertainty in population-based triage, and the substantial differences between triage tools useful for a defined incident scene, further discussion of these tools is deferred, but it is important to note that some incidents may use a combination of mass-casualty triage and population-based triage. For example, a hurricane that results in a building collapse will need mass-casualty triage at the scene of the collapse, but if the area is subsequently flooded and travel is inhibited, population-based triage will be needed to assist in getting people to treatment.

RECOMMENDATIONS FOR FURTHER RESEARCH

Current triage systems suffer from significant limitations:

- lack of scientific validation;
- lack of standardization and interoperability;
- absence of flexibility in addressing non-traumatic disaster scenarios.

It is vital that methodologically sound outcomes-based research be conducted to address these limitations. In particular, specific questions that should be addressed within the field of disaster triage include:

- What is the appropriate outcome measure for studying triage systems?
- Using this measure, which system (if any) is superior?

- What is the best way to rapidly sort large numbers of non-traumatic victims for prioritization of treatment and transport? This population includes not only victims of chemical, biological, or radiological attack, but also the large number of medical patients seen daily at healthcare facilities.
- Is it possible, or even desirable, to have a "one size fits all" algorithm that would cover all of these possibilities, or are the differences between event types too pronounced?
- Can simulation strategies be identified that accurately reproduce field conditions such that triage protocols can be realistically evaluated without the need to test them in an actual disaster?

In the meantime, it is recommended that each community select the triage system that is most appropriate for its circumstances, keeping in mind that interoperability within a region will be enhanced by using a standardized triage system. Further, whichever triage system is selected, it should be used and practiced regularly, and whatever tools are needed for its use should be readily accessible and familiar to the providers who will use it.

REFERENCES

1. Sanddal TL, Loyacono T, Sanddal ND. Effect of JumpSTART training on immediate and short-term pediatric triage performance. *Pediatr Emerg Care* November 2004; 20(11): 749–753.
2. Risavi BL, Salen PN, Heller MB, et al. A two-hour intervention using START improves prehospital triage of mass casualty incidents. *Prehosp Emerg Care* April–June 2001; 5(2): 197–199.
3. Schenker JD, Goldstein S, Braun J, et al. Triage accuracy at a multiple casualty incident disaster drill: the Emergency Medical Service, Fire Department of New York City experience. *J Burn Care Res* September-October 2006; 27(5): 570–575.
4. Wallis LA, Carley S. Comparison of paediatric major incident primary triage tools. *Emerg Med J* June 2006; 23(6): 475–478.
5. Garner A, Lee A, Harrison K, et al. Comparative analysis of multiple-casualty incident triage algorithms. *Ann Emerg Med* November 2001; 38(5): 541–548.
6. Cross KP, Cicero MX. Head-to-Head Comparison of Disaster Triage Methods in Pediatric, Adult, and Geriatric Patients. *Ann Emerg Med* June 2013; 61(6): 668–676.
7. Kahn CA, Schultz CH, Miller KT, et al. Does START triage work? An outcomes assessment after a disaster. *Ann Emerg Med* September 2009; 54(3): 424–430.
8. *Domestic Preparedness Training Program: Instructor Guide.* Edgewood Arsenal, Maryland. U.S. Army Chemical and Biological Defense Command, Department of Defense, 1998.
9. Mor M, Waisman Y. Triage principles in multiple casualty situations involving children – the Israeli experience. August 2002. http://www.pemdatabase.org/files/triage.pdf (Accessed October 20, 2013).
10. Asaeda G. The day that the START triage system came to a STOP: observations from the World Trade Center disaster. *Acad Emerg Med* March 2002; 9(3): 255–256.
11. Cook L. The World Trade Center attack. The paramedic response: an insider's view. *Critical care (London, England)* December 2001; 5(6): 301–303.
12. Teague DC. Mass casualties in the Oklahoma City bombing. *Clinical Orthopaedics and Related Research* May 2004; 422: 77–81.
13. Schultz CH, Koenig KL, Noji EK. A medical disaster response to reduce immediate mortality after an earthquake. *N Engl J Med* February 15, 1996; 334(7): 438–444.

14. Nocera A, Garner A. An Australian mass casualty incident triage system for the future based upon triage mistakes of the past: the Homebush Triage Standard. *Aust N Z J Surg* August 1999; 69(8): 603–608.

15. Tran MD, Garner AA, Morrison I, et al. The Bali bombing: civilian aeromedical evacuation. *Med J Aust* October 6, 2003; 179(7): 353–356.

16. Hines S, Payne A, Edmondson J, et al. Bombs under London. The EMS response plan that worked. *Jems* August 2005; 30(8): 58–60, 62, 64–57.

17. Sacco WJ, Navin DM, Fiedler KE, et al. Precise formulation and evidence-based application of resource-constrained triage. *Acad Emerg Med* August 2005; 12(8): 759–770.

18. Lindsey J. New triage method considers available resources. *Jems* July2005; 30(7): 92–94.

19. Sacco WJ, Navin DM, Waddell II, RK, et al. A new resource-constrained triage method applied to victims of penetrating injury. *J Trauma* August 2007; 63(2): 316–325.

20. Hodgetts TJ. Triage: a position statement. *European Union Core Group on Disaster Medicine*(2002). http://ec.europa.eu/echo/files/civil_protection/civil/prote/pdfdocs/disaster_med_final_2002/d6.pdf (Accessed August 16, 2015).

21. SALT mass casualty triage: concept endorsed by the American College of Emergency Physicians, American College of Surgeons Committee on Trauma, American Trauma Society, National Association of EMS Physicians, National Disaster Life Support Education Consortium, and State and Territorial Injury Prevention Directors Association. *Disaster Med Public Health Prep* December 2008; 2(4): 245–246.

22. Lerner EB, Cone DC, Weinstein ES, et al. Mass casualty triage: an evaluation of the science and refinement of a national guideline. *Disaster Med Public Health Prep* June 2011; 5(2): 129–137.

23. Benson M, Koenig KL, Schultz CH. Disaster triage: START, then SAVE–a new method of dynamic triage for victims of a catastrophic earthquake. *Prehosp Disaster Med* April–June 1996; 11(2): 117–124.

24. Romig LE. Pediatric triage. A system to JumpSTART your triage of young patients at MCIs. *Jems* July 2002; 27(7): 52–58, 60–53.

25. Wallis LA, Carley S. Validation of the Paediatric Triage Tape. *Emerg Med J* January 2006; 23(1): 47–50.

26. Hodgetts TJ, Hall J, Maconochie I, et al. Paediatric triage tape. *Prehospital Immediate Care* 1998; 2: 155–159.

27. Jagger J, Jane JA, Rimel R. The Glasgow coma scale: to sum or not to sum? *Lancet* July 9, 1983; 2(8341): 97.

28. Al-Salamah MA, McDowell I, Stiell IG, et al. Initial emergency department trauma scores from the OPALS study: the case for the motor score in blunt trauma. *Acad Emerg Med* August 2004; 11(8): 834–842.

29. Meredith W, Rutledge R, Hansen AR, et al. Field triage of trauma patients based upon the ability to follow commands: a study in 29573 injured patients. *J Trauma* January 1995; 38(1): 129–135.

30. Ross SE, Leipold C, Terregino C, et al. Efficacy of the motor component of the Glasgow Coma Scale in trauma triage. *J Trauma* July 1998; 45(1): 42–44.

31. Healey C, Osler TM, Rogers FB, et al. Improving the Glasgow Coma Scale score: motor score alone is a better predictor. *J Trauma* April 2003; 54(4): 671–678, discussion 678–680.

32. Husum H, Gilbert M, Wisborg T, et al. Respiratory rate as a prehospital triage tool in rural trauma. *J Trauma* September 2003; 55(3): 466–470.

33. Baxt WG, Upenieks V. The lack of full correlation between the Injury Severity Score and the resource needs of injured patients. *Annals of Emerg Med* December 1990; 19(12): 1396–1400.

34. Bracken MB, Shepard MJ, Collins WF, et al. A randomized, controlled trial of methylprednisolone or naloxone in the treatment of acute spinal-cord injury. *Results of the Second National Acute Spinal Cord Injury Study. N Engl J Med* May 17, 1990; 322(20): 1405–1411.

35. Sasser SM, Hunt RC, Faul M, et al. Guidelines for field triage of injured patients: recommendations of the National Expert Panel on Field Triage, 2011. *MMWR Recomm Rep* January 13, 2012; 61(RR-1): 1–20.

36. Cone DC, Koenig KL. Mass casualty triage in the chemical, biological, radiological, or nuclear environment. *Eur J Emerg Med* December 2005; 12(6): 287–302.

37. Cone DC, MacMillan DS, Parwani V, et al. Pilot test of a proposed chemical/biological/radiation/ nuclear-capable mass casualty triage system. *Prehosp Emerg Care* April–June 2008; 12(2): 236–240.

38. Burkle FM, Jr. Population-based triage management in response to surge-capacity requirements during a large-scale bioevent disaster. *Acad Emerg Med* November 2006; 13(11): 1118–1129.

15

PERSONAL PROTECTIVE EQUIPMENT

Howard W. Levitin

OVERVIEW

Personal protective equipment (PPE) refers to protective garments (clothing, boots, or gloves), goggles, helmets, respirators, or other equipment designed to shield the wearer's body from exposure to toxic agents. Its primary purpose is to reduce a user's exposure to hazards when other measures are not feasible or effective enough to decrease these risks to acceptable levels. PPE is limited by the fact that it does not eliminate the hazard, may result in injury to the wearer if the equipment fails, or may itself cause harm if not worn or used correctly.[1]

Emergency responders and healthcare personnel risk occupational exposure to various chemical, biological, or radiological agents when responding to emergencies. These dangers persist during victim transport, or when receiving and treating those individuals who may have been injured, contaminated, or made ill from the incident. In a chemical release, the adverse signs and symptoms of exposure or contamination (skin irritation, cough, shortness of breath, or eye irritation) are often more apparent than those from exposure to biological or radiological agents, which may be delayed or go unrecognized.

Occupational exposure risk can be reduced through a combination of interventions. These are generally referred to as engineering controls, safe work practices, administrative practices, and the use of PPE. Engineering controls, such as building ventilation systems and deluge showers, are the first priority and most effective means of reducing occupational exposure risks. Safe work practices are the second order of protection and include general workplace rules and other operation-specific requirements that are typically regulatory-based, such as respiratory protection and blood-borne pathogens standards. The third tier of protection is administrative controls. Administrative controls are changes in workplace processes or procedures that are designed to reduce or eliminate worker exposure to hazards. Examples include: 1) product labeling; 2) using the least toxic chemicals in the smallest quantity possible; 3) training staff to manage chemicals safely and how to respond appropriately if a spill occurs; and 4) having well-established protocols supported by staff training. This last component should address provider response to contaminated patients, identification of specific iso-lation areas, and procedures for performing decontamination including the use of PPE.

PPE is considered the least desirable within this hierarchy of controls because of dependence on the individual to select and consistently use the equipment correctly. In a 2009 study of hazardous substances released during 3,458 events in the United States, only 97 of 475 employee victims (20.4%) and 33 of 74 responder victims (44.6%) wore PPE. Of those who wore PPE, most ensembles did not include respiratory protection.[2]

The selection of PPE can be challenging and should be based on several factors: 1) the environment in which the hazardous agent is deployed; 2) the concentration and toxic properties of the agent; 3) the type of threat encountered (infectious particle, solid, liquid, vapor, or radiation); and 4) the anticipated duration of an individual's exposure to the hazardous substance. Additionally, one's level of training, physical fitness, health, and habitus also influence who can safely wear certain types of PPE and impacts the type of equipment selected. For example, not all respirator designs can be worn by all users (i.e., anything that prevents the face mask from fitting tightly against the face, such as a beard or long sideburns, may cause leakage). Industrial hygienists, safety professionals, and manufacturers should be consulted when selecting PPE.

Additional challenges are associated with the use of PPE. In many circumstances, the presence of a hazardous substance may not initially be recognized. Even if it is detected, its identity may remain unknown. PPE may not be accessible or circumstances may lead responders not to use PPE even if it is available. An initial investigation of the incident or information based on a previously performed hazard assessments can be used to determine the need and level of PPE required. However, such approaches include a margin of error that may not be universally tolerated. Therefore, the appropriate and consistent use of PPE requires sound planning that should be the first line of defense in all types of emergencies. By tailoring emergency plans to reflect the reasonably predictable worse-case scenario under which public safety and hospital personnel might work, emergency managers can develop plans that guide PPE selection, training, and use.[3]

The objective of this chapter is to provide an overview of PPE that guides the reader in the practical selection and use of this equipment. The goal is to maximize protection of those whose work environment may expose them to hazardous materials. The discussion will focus on protection against primarily chemical, biological, and radiological hazards that may be encountered in the pre-hospital and hospital setting. Only civilian PPE will be addressed.

CURRENT STATE OF THE ART

Background

The purpose of PPE is to shield or isolate an individual from the various hazards that may be present in the workplace or response environment. The hazardous agent's predominant physical, chemical, or toxic properties dictate the type and degree of protection required. For example, protection needed against a liquid corrosive compound is different from one that releases a highly toxic vapor. The type of job activity and probability of exposure must also be considered when specifying the use of PPE. As with the selection of a proper respirator, the hazards encountered must be thoroughly assessed before deciding on the protective clothing to recommend.[4] Once the specific hazard has been identified, appropriate equipment can be selected. Several factors must be considered, most important being the safety of the individual. The level of protection assigned must at least match the hazard confronted. Other factors to be considered are cost, availability, compatibility with other equipment in the ensemble, suitability, and performance.[1,4]

Protective equipment ensembles range from safety glasses, hardhats, and steel-toed safety shoes to fully encapsulating, gas-tight, chemical resistant suits with a supplied source of breathing air. The variety of clothing includes disposable coveralls and gowns, fire retardant clothing, and chemical splash suits. Different materials and combinations of materials are used to provide a protective barrier against the hazard.[1] No single type of PPE can protect against all hazards and its incorrect use can cause harm to the wearer. In general, the greater the protection afforded by the PPE, the higher the associated risks experienced by the wearer. Therefore, the level of PPE selected needs to provide appropriate balance between risk and protection.[3]

Firefighters and soldiers in battle have been using protective clothing of various types and configurations for centuries. The first fire helmet was invented in the 1730s and was constructed of leather with a high crown and wide brim. By the mid-1800s, the same helmet design was reinforced with a front shield and brim rolling to a long back tail for added protection. The firefighters' uniform at that time was made primarily of wool and included leather boots. After World War I, this PPE began to incorporate long rubber trench coats, tall rubber boots, and the traditional fire helmet design used today. After World War II, PPE standards were developed to shield the firefighter from excessive heat and water exposure and included gear to protect their feet and hands.[5]

Historical records on the use of respiratory protective devices to reduce or eliminate hazardous exposures to airborne contaminants date back to the Romans (circa AD 23–79). They considered the use of loose-fitting animal bladders by mine workers as protection against inhalation of red oxide of lead. During the eighteenth and nineteenth centuries, in the United States and Europe, firefighters were required to have a full beard that was soaked with water and then clamped within their teeth before entering a smoke-filled area in order to block out large airborne particulates.[6] During this time period, the predecessor of the modern atmosphere-supplied respirator was being developed based on two basic principles: 1) purifying the air by removing contaminants before they reach the breathing zone of the worker; or 2) providing clean air from an uncontaminated source.[5]

In 1814, a particulate-removing filter encased in a rigid container was developed – the predecessor of modern filters for air-purifying respirators. By 1854 it was recognized that activated charcoal could be used as a filtering medium for vapors. During World War I, with the use of chemical warfare, improvements in the design of respirators were necessary and included a moveable diaphragm that allowed soldiers to communicate with others. In 1930, the development of a resin-impregnated dust filter made efficient, inexpensive filters available that had good dust-loading characteristics and low breathing resistance.[5,7]

Today, PPE manufacturing and testing must comply with specific national standards, ensuring that they meet stringent performance requirements. The selection, training, and usage of PPE are typically regulated country by country through various agencies. Examples include: 1) The United States – the National Institute for Occupational Safety and Health (NIOSH), the Occupational Safety and Health Administration (OSHA), the Environmental Protection Agency (EPA), and the National Fire Protection Association (NFPA); 2) Europe – the European Council (EC) Directive; 3) Canada – the Canadian Centre for Occupational Health and Safety; 4) Argentina – the Instituto Argentino de Normalizacion y Certificacion (IRAM); and 5) Australia – the Occupational Health, Safety, and Welfare Act of Australia. To meet these standards, protective suits and equipment are exposed to harsh conditions, simulating the actual threats wearers may face when using the PPE, such as extreme temperatures, chemical exposures, and abrasion.

Routes of Exposure

Individuals may become ill or injured through direct contact with chemical agents in their vapor, gas, liquid, or solid state. Mucous membranes of the eyes, nose, and mouth are particularly effective as a portal of entry for chemicals because moisture promotes the absorption of these substances. Ingestion, injection, and skin absorption are less common routes of exposure for chemical agents.

For infectious pathogens such as tuberculosis and plague, exposure is more likely to occur from inhaling aerosolized particles produced by coughing, sneezing, or mechanical means (bronchoscopy, intubation, and suctioning). Exposure to anthrax also occurs via aerosolized material but is not transmitted human to human. The more common contagious diseases such as influenza and viruses that cause the common cold spread primarily by droplets of moisture expelled from the upper respiratory tract through sneezing or coughing. They travel short distances from the infectious individual to susceptible mucosal surfaces of a recipient.[8] Mucous membranes or breaks in the skin are also vulnerable to viruses and bacteria and require standard barrier protection to offset the risk of disease.[9,10]

Individuals exposed to ionizing radiation (for example from an X-ray) do not emit radiation and therefore pose no risk to others. Those who become contaminated with a radioactive material (on their clothing, skin, or hair) can expose others to the harmful effects of these agents. Radiation contamination can also occur internally through inhalation, ingestion, and injection.[11]

Types of PPE

PPE components are categorized in several ways. These include: 1) type of garment (suit, boots, gloves); 2) area of the body protected (head, eyes, skin, hands, or feet); 3) type of hazard encountered (chemical, biological, or radiological); 4) performance required (particulate protection, liquid-splash protection, or vapor protection); or 5) service life (single use, limited use, or reusable). A common classification scheme used in the United States by EPA/OSHA employs the letters A through D to categorize PPE ensembles in order of decreasing levels of protection (Table 15.1).[1,11,12] For discussion purposes, this section will focus primarily on chemical protective clothing (CPC) and respirator ensembles used in hazardous materials operations. PPE requirements unique to radiological and biological hazards will also be addressed.

CPC is designed to shield the wearer from skin contamination and airway exposure. The garment prevents skin contact with the toxic agent and the respirator protects parts of the face and airway from inhaled hazardous vapor or harmful particles. There is a wide selection of PPE available with varying protection levels, styles, sizes, types of construction, comfort levels, and ease of use. The incident commander or purchasing entity should choose an ensemble that will protect the wearer in the most reasonably foreseen emergency.

Chemical Protective Clothing

The purpose of CPC is to shield or isolate an individual from the chemical, physical, and biological hazards that may be encountered in a hazardous materials incident. During chemical operations it is not always apparent when exposure occurs. Many chemicals pose invisible hazards and offer no warning signs. As a result, appropriate procedures must be followed and protective clothing must be worn whenever the wearer faces the potential of being exposed to a hazardous agent. This includes the response phase of a hazardous materials incident, victim triage, decontamination, site cleanup, and waste disposal.[1,12]

CPC is part of a PPE ensemble that may include other equipment items such as inner and outer gloves, boots, and eye protection. These items must be easily integrated with the CPC to provide both an appropriate level of protection and allow the wearer to carry out various activities demanded in the response. In addition, the ensemble may require the deployment of a cooling system when working in hot, humid weather, or a communications device. Each of these ensemble components must support the mission of the wearer and not interfere with mobility, dexterity, vision, or donning requirements.[1]

For hazardous substances, the protective clothing ensemble typically includes a chemical resistant, multi-layered coverall type suit, two layers of gloves, and boots or flexible overboots to go over shoes. No single material protects against all chemicals, combinations of chemicals, or against prolonged exposure, so a multi-layered garment composed of different materials should be considered. The choice of composite materials should provide protection against a variety of known chemicals stored, used, or transported in the community as well as offering the broadest chemical resistance against the widest range of unknown chemicals. The material(s) selected must also resist degradation, permeation, and penetration by the respective chemicals.[1]

- **Degradation** involves physical changes in a material that occur through direct contact with chemical substances, use of the garment, or ambient conditions (e.g. sunlight). Such contact may cause the suit's material to crack, become brittle, discolor, or deteriorate.
- **Permeation** is a process in which a chemical diffuses or dissolves through a garment's material on a molecular basis. The rate of diffusion varies depending on the chemical concentration; material composition and thickness; and the humidity, temperature, and pressure of the surrounding environment. Most material testing is done with 100% pure chemical over an extended exposure period. The time it takes the chemical to permeate through the garment material is the breakthrough time. An acceptable material is one where the breakthrough time exceeds the expected period of garment use. It is required that the suit's manufacturer provide information on a suit's permeation or breakthrough time.
- **Penetration** is the movement of chemicals through an opening in the suit, specifically at seams or zippers, and from faulty manufacturing.

The selected protective ensemble should be comfortable to wear while allowing the user to perform vital tasks. It must: 1) be economical; 2) decontaminate easily (disposal should also be simple); 3) comply with regulatory standards; and 4) possess key physical properties such as functionality in extreme environmental conditions and strength (resist physical hazards, tears, and weather extremes). A series of questions should be asked or considered when assessing the material properties of a particular type of CPC:[1,11]

- Is the material sufficiently durable to withstand the physical demands of the tasks at hand?
- Will the material resist tears, punctures, cuts, and abrasions?
- Will the material withstand repeated use after contamination and decontamination?
- Is the material flexible or pliable enough to allow end users to perform needed tasks?
- Will the material maintain its protective integrity and flexibility under hot and cold extremes?
- Are garment seams in the clothing constructed so they provide the same physical integrity as the garment material?

In addition to evaluating these material characteristics, the CPC selected needs to match the type of protection desired. If liquid-splash protection is required, then the wearer's entire body may require coverage using a suit, boots, gloves, and face protection (goggles and a mask, face shield, or full-face respirator or hood). Applying tape at suit/boot/glove/zipper/respirator interfaces provides additional splash protection but does not make the suit vapor protective.[1] The nature of the hazards and the expected exposure will determine if the clothing should provide partial or full body protection. Splash protective suits guard against liquids and particulates, while vapor protective suits provide vapor, liquid-splash, and particulate protection. A totally encapsulated suit provides particulate and liquid-splash protection but may not universally offer gas-tight integrity. Demonstration of this capability requires the performance of a pressure or inflation test and a leak detection test of the respective suit (to assess the adequacy of the seams or closures).[1,11]

Most chemical protective suits require additional items to complete the ensemble. A vapor-protective, totally encapsulated

Table 15.1. Decontamination suit ensembles Levels A–D

	Description	Advantages	Disadvantages	Example
Level A	Fully encapsulated suit with self-contained breathing apparatus (SCBA)	The highest level of protection, offers protection against contact and inhaled hazards	The expense, training, and program maintenance restricts the use of this level to specialized hazardous response teams. The lack of mobility and the heat/physical stresses in the ensemble limit the air supply and personnel who can utilize this capability.	
Level B	Suit with sealed seams, supplied air respirator, or SCBA	A high level of protection. Utilized in an unknown environment. This ensemble offers more dexterity and mobility then Level A.	The Level B ensemble is dependent on an airline or limited air supply. Expense, training, and program maintenance are a limiting factor. Heat/physical stresses remain an issue. Fit testing is required for this ensemble.	
Level C	Splash suit and air-purifying respirator	Mobility is significantly increased; heat/physical stresses are reduced. Operational time in the ensemble is increased with a high level of protection against a limited number of chemical agents. Fit testing is not required if hood is utilized. Moderate expense and training.	The Level C ensemble is not adequate for high concentration levels, high splash contamination, and low oxygen atmospheric levels.	
Level D	Work clothes with standard precautions (gloves and splash protection.	Highest mobility, low heat/physical stresses, operational time unlimited. Expenses and training minimal.	No protection against chemical and other hazardous materials.	

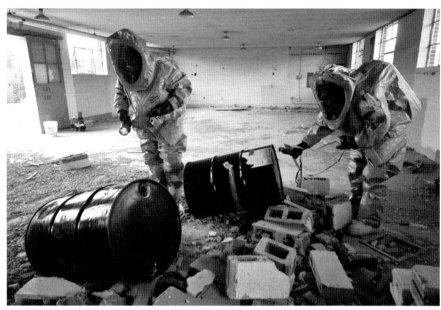

Figure 15.1. Self-contained breathing apparatus (SCBA) shown in association with level A suits.

suit will often have attached boots and gloves but still require the wearer to don a pair of inner gloves and boots. Liquid splash-protective suits are generally sold with or without an attached hood, shoe covers, or gloves. Missing items require separate purchases and must match or exceed the performance and protection level of the primary garment.

The gloves and boots selected should protect against a wide range of substances that might be encountered. Gloves and boots manufactured from either nitrile or butyl rubber ought to provide adequate protection in most circumstances. Other material options include neoprene, polyvinyl chloride, and natural rubber. Various glove thicknesses and lengths are available; with increased thickness comes greater degradation time but loss of manual dexterity. Double gloving of different materials offers enhanced hand protection and may reduce the need for thicker gloves. Frequent glove changes or glove decontamination are important when working with patients who were not fully decontaminated (e.g., those who self-refer to the emergency department or who arrive by transport with life- and limb-threatening injuries).[11] Some adjustments in glove and boot fit can be made with the use of chemical or duct tape.

Information on the protective clothing's chemical resistance, permeation rates, breakthrough times, and other testing data can be obtained from the manufacturer. If needed information is absent, the manufacturer should be asked to supply the missing data. Only suits certified by organizations such as NFPA or the European Committee for Standardization (CEN) should be considered for purchase. Organizations should obtain, inspect, and train using samples of CPC in which they are interested prior to purchase. Discussing various options for the ensembles with individuals experienced in their use should ensure that the appropriate PPE has been selected.

Respiratory Protection

A respirator is a protective device that covers the nose and mouth or the entire face and head to guard the wearer against hazardous atmospheres. Respirators are available as either air-purifying or atmosphere-supplying and may be tight fitting or loose fitting. A tight-fitting respirator includes half masks that cover the mouth and nose and full facepieces that cover the face from the hairline to below the chin. They create an air-tight seal around the area of contact. Loose fitting respirators utilize hoods or helmets that cover the head completely. An air-purifying model removes contaminants from the ambient air using filters or canisters while an atmosphere-supplying respirator provides clean, breathable air from an uncontaminated source such as a high-pressure cylinder. As a general rule, atmosphere-supplying respirators are used for more hazardous exposures. Specific examples of respirator types include the following:[1,12,13,14]

▪ **Self-contained breathing apparatus (SCBA)** consists of a full facepiece connected by a hose to a portable air tank of breathing-quality compressed air worn by the user and provides the highest level of respiratory protection (Figure 15.1).

▪ **Supplied-air respirators (SAR)** consist of a tight-fitting mask or a hood connected to a distant air source via an air hose. Because supplied-air respirators are less bulky than SCBAs (no tank is worn) and are typically connected to a larger air source, they can be used for longer periods of time (Figure 15.2).

▪ **Powered air-purifying respirators (PAPR)** deliver filtered air under positive pressure to a tight-fitting mask or loose-fitting helmet/hood. Because PAPRs function under positive pressure, they provide a higher degree of respiratory protection as compared to a negative pressure mask. Hooded PAPRs are popular at hospitals because they minimize the administrative burdens associated with other types of respirators such as maintaining an appropriate air source and requiring annual fit testing (Figure 15.3). They can also be worn by people with facial hair and eyeglasses and are usually more comfortable for people who are not accustomed to regularly wearing respirators. For hazardous material (non-CBRN) operations, PAPR air filtering canisters used should include high efficiency (HE) particulate filters plus organic vapor (OV) and acid gas cartridges that together will protect

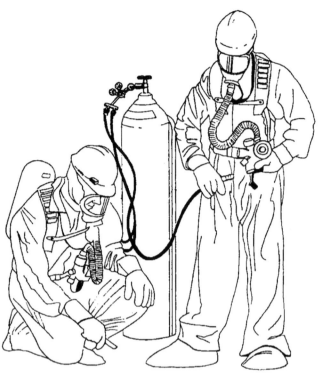

Figure 15.2. Atmosphere-supplying respirators: SCBA and SAR shown with Level B suits.

against many of the more common airborne hazards that might be encountered (toxic dusts, biologicals, radioactive particulates, pesticides, and solvents).[15]

■ **Air-purifying respirators (APR)** consist of a tight-fitting mask worn over the mouth and nose with filters that work to reduce exposure of particulates or hazardous vapors present in ambient air before inhalation. APRs operate under negative pressure and are dependent on the inhalation effort of the wearer to draw air through a filter. All APRs are limited by the adequacy of their face seal and the efficiency of the filters (Figure 15.3).

Levels of PPE

PPE ensembles are generally divided into various types, classes, or levels based on the certifying country, agency, and degree of protection afforded. The European system for chemical protective clothing designates CPC as Types 1–6 with corresponding standards describing the requirements on the products. Type 1 clothing provides the highest level of protection against solids, liquids, and gases (gas-tight); Type 2 provides similar protection but are not gas-tight; Type 3 provides liquid-tight protection; Type 4 are spray-tight protective clothing; Type 5 protects against particulates; and Type 6 is reserved for CPC that provides protection from liquids.[16]

NFPA, an international nonprofit organization with membership representing nearly 100 nations, issues standards for hazardous materials response teams, fire services, and first responders. NFPA certifications are only issued for complete ensembles (garments, boots, gloves, and respirators). Individual protective elements are not considered unless used as part of a complete and certified ensemble. An NFPA Class 1 ensemble provides the highest level of protection against toxic vapors, liquids, and particulates during hazardous materials incidents. The use of Class 1 suits is indicated in any environment where the concentration of a substance will exceed its immediately dangerous to life and health (IDLH) limits. The term IDLH refers to the maximum concentration level of a substance from which an individual could escape within 30 minutes of exposure without incapacitation or irreversible toxic effects. For example, the IDLH limit for hydrogen sulfide is 300 parts per million. The protection offered by an NFPA Class 1 ensemble includes specific chemical and biological agents in vapor, liquid-splash, and particulate environments during CBRN terrorism incidents. The ensemble consists of a suit with attached gloves that totally encapsulates the wearer and breathing apparatus.[17]

Class 2 NFPA ensembles include a suit or garment with attached or separate hood, attached or separate gloves, attached footwear or booties, outer protective boots, and SCBA. This ensemble is selected when the agent or threat has generally been identified and the actual release has subsided. It may also be used in terrorist incidents involving vapor or liquid chemical or

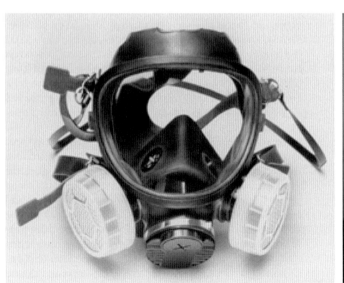
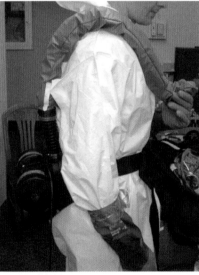
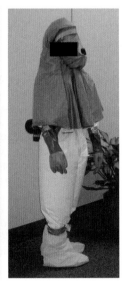

Figure 15.3. APR and PAPR with hood.

particulate hazards where concentrations are at or above IDLH levels.[17]

NFPA Class 3 is intended for use long after the hazardous substance release has occurred or in the peripheral zone of the release scene. This includes terrorism incidents involving low levels of vapor or liquid chemical hazards where concentrations are below IDLH levels and includes non-encapsulating CPC with either an APR or PAPR. A Class 4 NFPA ensemble is the least protective and designated for use in situations involving potential exposure to biological aerosols or particles and low-level radiological particles.[17] Typical Class 4 ensembles have not been tested for protection against chemical vapor or liquid permeability, gas-tightness, or liquid integrity. An APR or PAPR are permitted but not required.[11]

In the United States, CPC ensembles are also classified as levels A through D. These levels are EPA/OSHA recommendations for skin and respiratory protection and do not describe the clothing in detail. The various levels are described in the OSHA Hazardous Waste Operations and Emergency Response Standard (HAZWOPER), 29 CFR 1910.120 Appendix B.[12] Each level consists of a combination of respiratory protection and clothing that guards against varying degrees of inhalation, eye, or skin exposure. Within each level of PPE, individual adjustments of ensemble components can be made (e.g., gloves and types of air purifying respirator protection selected) to align better aligned with the hazard assessment.[12]

Level A gear should be worn when the highest level of respiratory, skin, eye, and mucous membrane protection are required and corresponds to NFPA Class 1. The Level A suit is mandatory in an IDLH environment. A typical Level A ensemble is worn by hazardous material entry teams and includes a positive pressure (pressure-demand) SCBA or positive pressure SAR with an escape SCBA. The chemical protective suit is fully encapsulating and the wearer typically dons an inner and outer pair of chemical resistant gloves along with steel-toed, chemical resistant boots. Such a vapor-tight ensemble inhibits physiological cooling mechanisms, reduces mobility, and the limited air supply restricts the personnel who can utilize this capability. Responders working in a typical Level A ensemble, depending on ambient temperature and humidity, air capacity of the SCBA, and conditioning of the individual, are only able to remain in this gear for up to 20–30 minutes.

Level B should be selected when the highest level of respiratory protection is needed but a lesser level of skin and splash protection is required. This level is comparable to NFPA Class 2 and is the minimum protection recommended for initial site entry teams when the hazard has not been identified or defined by monitoring, sampling, and research. A typical Level B ensemble utilizes the same respiratory protection used with Level A along with non-encapsulating chemical resistant clothing, inner and outer chemical resistant gloves, and boots. This protective ensemble may offer more dexterity and mobility than Level A but remains dependent on an airline or limited air supply. Heat and physical stresses remain an issue and fit testing of the respirator is required.

A Level C ensemble provides the same level of splash protection as Level B, with a lower level of respiratory protection. It is comparable to NFPA Class 2 and is selected when the type and concentration of airborne substances are known and criteria for using an APR are met. Periodic air monitoring should be performed to ensure ongoing adequacy of the respirator and filter selected. The Level C ensemble includes a full-face or half-mask,

Table 15.2. Hospital Decontamination Zone

Conditions necessary for hospitals to rely on the PPE selection presented in Table 15.4

1. Thorough and complete hazard vulnerability analysis (HVA) and emergency management plan (EMP), which consider community input, have been conducted/developed, and have been updated within the past year.

2. The EMP includes plans to assist the numbers of victims that the community anticipates might seek treatment at this hospital, keeping in mind that the vast majority of victims may self-refer to the nearest hospital.

3. Preparations specified in the EMP have been implemented (e.g., employee training, equipment selection, maintenance, and a respiratory protection program).

4. The EMP includes methods for handling the numbers of ambulatory and non-ambulatory victims anticipated by the community.

5. The hazardous substance was not released in close proximity to the hospital, and the lapse time between the victims' exposure and victims' arrival at the hospital exceeds approximately 10 minutes, thereby permitting substantial levels of gases and vapors from volatile substances time to dissipate.

6. Victims' contaminated clothing and possessions are promptly removed and contained (e.g., in an approved hazardous waste container that is isolated outdoors), and decontamination is initiated promptly upon arrival at the hospital. Hospital EMP includes shelter, tepid water, soap, privacy, and coverings to promote victim compliance with decontamination procedures.

7. EMP procedures are in place to ensure that contaminated medical waste and wastewater do not become a secondary source of employee exposure.

And

8. The decontamination system and pre-decontamination victim waiting areas are designed and used in a manner that promotes constant fresh air circulation through the system to limit hazardous substance accumulation. Air exchange from a clean source has been considered in the design of fully enclosed systems (i.e., through consultation with professional engineer or certified industrial hygienist) and air is not re-circulated.

Source: http://www.osha.gov/dts/osta/bestpractices/html/hospital_firstreceivers.html

APR or hooded PAPR with the same clothing, boots, and gloves as described for Level B. This protective ensemble provides for greater mobility and the associated heat and physical stresses are reduced. Operational time in the ensemble is increased with a high level of protection afforded against a limited number of chemical agents. Fit testing is not required if a positive-pressure respirator and hood combination are used. Level C does not provide adequate protection against exposure to toxic substances at high concentration levels (exceeding IDLH) or in low oxygen atmospheric environments.

In the United States, Level C protection is deemed appropriate for hospital personnel (first receivers) receiving and treating victims from mass-casualty incidents involving the release of unknown hazardous substances as long as certain criteria are met: 1) the hospital is not the release site or adjacent to it; 2) at least 10 minutes have elapsed between the time of victim exposure and arrival to the healthcare facility; and 3) the hazardous substance is not known (Tables 15.2–15.4). To use this level of

Table 15.3. Hospital Post-Decontamination Zone

Conditions necessary for hospitals to rely on the PPE selection presented in Table 15.4

1. EMP is developed and followed in a way that minimizes the emergency department (ED) personnel's reasonably anticipated contact with contaminated victims (e.g., with drills that test communication between the hospital and emergency responders at the incident site to reduce the likelihood of unanticipated victims).

2. Decontamination system (in the hospital decontamination zone) and hospital security can be activated promptly to minimize the chance that victims will enter the ED and contact unprotected staff prior to decontamination.

3. EMP procedures specify that unannounced victims (once identified as possibly contaminated) disrobe in the appropriate decontamination area (not the ED) and follow hospital decontamination procedures before admission (or re-admission) to the ED.

4. Victims in this area were previously decontaminated by a shower with soap and water, including a minimum of 5 minutes under running water. Shower instructions are clearly presented and enforced. Shower facility encourages victim compliance (e.g., shelter, tepid water, reasonable degree of privacy).

5. EMP procedures clearly specify actions ED clerks or staff will take if they suspect a patient is contaminated. For example: 1) do not physically contact the patient; 2) immediately notify supervisor and safety officer of possible hospital contamination; and 3) allow qualified personnel to isolate and decontaminate the victim.

And

6. The EMP requires that if the ED becomes contaminated, that space is no longer eligible to be considered a hospital post-decontamination zone. Instead, it should be considered contaminated and all employees working in this area should use PPE as described for the hospital decontamination zone (Table 15.4).

Source: http://www.osha.gov/dts/osta/bestpractices/html/hospital_firstreceivers.html

protection, hospitals must first complete a hazard assessment that carefully considers an employee's role in such an incident, the hazards that might be encountered, and the level of training required. In addition, the hospital must address the steps they will take to minimize the extent of the employee's contact with hazardous substances. This OSHA PPE best practice is not universally applied to all hazardous materials releases. If the hazard assessment indicates the potential need for a higher level of protection (i.e., CBRN threat), then that PPE must be provided.[3]

Level D consists of standard work clothes without a respirator and is used when no respiratory protection is required and only minimal skin protection is necessary. This ensemble is comparable to NFPA Class 4. In the hospital setting, Level D PPE consists of a surgical gown or coverall, splash protective mask, and surgical gloves (universal precautions). In an emergency decontamination operation (EDO), this level of protection is appropriate for support personnel who may either set up and oversee the operation, aid entry personnel in donning and doffing their PPE, or assist in the cleanup operation. Level D provides minimal to no protection against chemicals and a variety of other hazardous materials, but in comparison offers the highest mobility, low heat and physical stress, and operational time is unlimited.

The European and U.S. standards for PPE described herein are typically the ones most frequently referred to internationally. There are some national standards and specifications that apply to limited locations, although these have had little impact outside their region. Such local standards and specifications can be found in countries such as Russia, Japan, Germany, and Poland. There is an international standard, ISO 16602, which specifies a system of clothing with protection levels that are practically the same as in Europe.[18,19]

PPE in Radiation Emergencies[11]

For first responders, the level of PPE recommended for radiation emergencies depends on: 1) the environment that they are entering; 2) their expected roles in the response; 3) the anticipated impact of on-scene hazards (radioactive and environmental) on their response activities; and 4) the overall risk of radiation contamination (internal, external). Many PPE ensembles can guard against external contamination (alpha particles and most beta particles), internal contamination (via inhalation, ingestion, or absorption through open wounds), and other physical hazards (e.g., debris, fire/heat, or chemicals). However, most PPE cannot protect against exposure from high-energy, highly penetrating forms of ionizing radiation associated with most radiation emergencies.

In an environment with lower toxicity, less restrictive PPE ensembles can be chosen. For example, in a radiation-only event with a high risk of radioactive contamination but no risk from other non-radiation hazards (e.g., after detonation of a radiological dispersal device), Level C PPE usually provides sufficient respiratory and skin protection. If a radiation incident is combined with a chemical or biological hazard, however, a higher level of protection should be considered (Level A or B).

PPE for first receivers in a radiation emergency should protect against the anticipated hazards. In general, Level C PPE should provide a sufficient level of respiratory and skin protection when delivering care to externally contaminated victims, including triage and decontamination. In these circumstances, a full-facepiece APR or hooded PAPR with a P100 or HEPA filter should suffice. A surgical mask or fitted N-95 will not provide sufficient protection when caring for contaminated victims. If the likelihood of external contamination is low or if victims are suspected to be internally contaminated, then Level D PPE (standard precautions attire) should be adequate. The use of lead aprons may not be beneficial in scenarios involving high-energy, highly penetrating ionizing radiation and can actually increase tissue damage if beta radiation is present.

Regardless of the PPE selected, the ensemble should include a personal radiation dosimeter whenever there is a concern about exposure to penetrating ionizing radiation. The dosimeter measures environmental levels of penetrating, ionizing radiation and is used to determine if an area is safe to enter. It also measures the amount of one's radiation exposure over time (radiation absorbed dose – RAD). Environmental testing and hazard assessment by a radiation safety professional can help identify hazards and risk levels and direct choices of permissible PPE.

PPE in Biological Emergencies

Like chemical and radiological hazards, emergency responders and healthcare personnel may be exposed to biological agents through multiple routes including inhalation, ingestion, direct

Table 15.4. Minimum PPE for hospital-based first receivers of victims for mass-casualty incidents involving the release of unknown hazardous substances

SCOPE AND LIMITATIONS *This Table applies when:*	
■ The hospital is not the release site. ■ Prerequisite conditions of hospital eligibility are already met (Tables 15.2 and 15.3).	■ The identity of the hazardous substance is unknown.

Note: This table is part of, and intended to be used with, the document entitled *OSHA Best Practices for Hospital-based First Receivers of Victims from Mass Casualty Incidents Involving the Release of Hazardous Substances.*

ZONE	MINIMUM PPE
Hospital Decontamination Zone ■ All employees in this zone (Includes, but not limited to, any of the following employees: decontamination team members, clinicians, set-up crew, cleanup crew, security staff, and patient tracking clerks.)	■ PAPR that provides a protection factor of 1000. The respirator must be NIOSH-approved. ■ Combination 99.97% high-efficiency particulate air (HEPA)/OV/acid gas respirator cartridges (also NIOSH-approved). ■ Double layer protective gloves. ■ Chemical resistant suit. ■ Head covering and eye/face protection (if not part of the respirator). ■ Chemical protective boots. ■ Suit openings sealed with tape.
Hospital Post-Decontamination Zone ■ All employees in this zone	■ Normal work clothes and PPE, as necessary, for infection control purposes (e.g., gloves, gown, appropriate respirator).

Source: http://www.osha.gov/dts/osta/bestpractices/html/hospital_firstreceivers.html

contact with the mucous membranes of the eyes or nasal tissues, and penetration of the skin through lesions or abrasions.[20] The selection of PPE against biohazards (naturally occurring or intentionally released) must be made through planning that includes an assessment of hazard and exposure potential, respiratory and dermal protection needs, entry conditions (i.e., are other hazards present), exit routes (i.e., can escape occur quickly and unobstructed), and decontamination strategies.

From a healthcare provider's perspective, the type of protection selected should also take into consideration the intensity of patient care they must deliver (routine verses critical), fit characteristics of the wearer, and the agent's anticipated transmission pattern. The specific pathogen should also be considered, along with the method of aerosol generation anticipated (cough vs. sneeze vs. aerosol-generating procedure), the age and health of the provider, and the stage of the patient's illness.[8] During high-risk procedures, such as suctioning, bronchoscopy, and intubation, where an aerosol may be generated, a higher level of protection should be considered.[20]

Examples of diseases that may be caused by inhalation of airborne organisms include tuberculosis (TB), hantavirus, anthrax, plague, influenza, SARS, pertussis, and pneumonia. Biohazards may become airborne as the agent itself (e.g., anthrax spores) becomes airborne or rides on some other material that becomes airborne such as dusts, mists, or droplet nuclei. Inhalation of these infectious agents may be reduced by wearing a respirator, while the use of surgical masks may reduce the spread of exhaled aerosols if worn by infected people. The use of safety glasses and face shields may also protect the wearer from disease by shielding their mucous membranes (eyes, nose, and mouth).[21,22]

For airborne infectious biological particles (i.e., bioterrorism), their concentration in air will depend on the method used to release the agent, the initial amount of agent in the dispersal device, the particle size (very small particles often remain suspended in the air for prolonged periods while large particles tend to fall out of the air more quickly), and the elapsed time since the release.[8,21] The PPE selected should be based on the anticipated exposure risk associated with different bioaerosols and the likelihood of a concurrent or secondary (intentional) release of other types of hazards such as chemicals or radiologicals. For example, emergency response entry teams should consider the use of a Level A (NFPA Class 1) protective ensemble in a suspected bioterrorism scenario when the offending agent and dissemination method are unknown, the dissemination is via an aerosol-generating device, or conditions exist that present a vapor or splash hazard.[20]

Responders may use Level B (NFPA Class 2) in a bioterrorism scenario if the suspected agent is no longer being generated or a splash hazard is present. Level C (NFPA Class 3) may be appropriate if the suspected biological aerosol is no longer being generated, its hazard level has been defined, or the dissemination was by a letter or package than can be easily bagged.[20]

When a risk assessment has been conducted by qualified safety and health experts, responders may use alternate PPE, including non-CBRN Level C protective ensembles with a full facepiece particulate respirator (N100 or P100 filters) or PAPR with HEPA filters, in conjunction with disposable hooded coveralls, gloves, and foot coverings as appropriate.[20] In certain specialized situations, half-mask filtering facepiece respirators (Figure 15.4) in conjunction with reduced levels of dermal protection may be considered, after appropriate fit testing, but it should be recognized that this level of PPE may not provide sufficient exposure reduction for many situations. Several parameters must be assessed when making a decision to downgrade

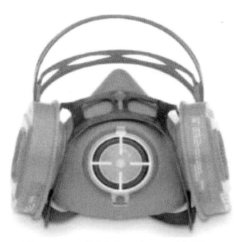

Figure 15.4. NIOSH respirator with HEPA filters.

the ensemble. These include knowledge of the source and extent of contamination, the level of uncertainty in the risk assessment, specific activities to be conducted, investigator experience, contingency/backup plans, length of time in the contaminated area, and availability of and provision for immunization and post-exposure prophylaxis. A decision of this nature should be carefully evaluated and made by industrial hygiene, safety, and medical personnel in conjunction with the incident commander and other appropriate public health authorities.[20]

In the healthcare setting, under normal circumstances, the PPE worn for the care of an infectious patient should follow standard infection control guidelines developed to manage the transmission of specific diseases, including airborne, droplet, and contact precautions.[20] This includes good hand hygiene along with the wearing of gloves, a gown, facemask, and goggles or face shield to protect against the potential splash or spray of blood, respiratory secretions, or other body fluids. If available, a fit-tested N95 or higher level of respiratory protection (Figure 15.5) should be used for potential exposure to infectious agents transmitted via the airborne route (e.g., TB, anthrax, and plague).[23,24,25] An engineered release of a weaponized biological agent or emergence of a highly infectious one may require a higher level of respiratory protection than what is used routinely in standard precautions. Such considerations were made during the SARS outbreak in China and Canada where common use of N95 and PAPRs occurred.[26,27,28]

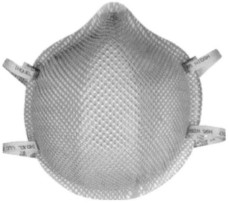

Figure 15.5. NIOSH-approved N95 respirator.

A hospital's ultimate decision on the type of respiratory protection to provide comes down to risk. As long as inhalation of infectious particles is a possible mode of disease transmission, healthcare personnel are at risk if not properly protected. During an investigation of the 2003 SARS outbreak in Canada, the final report concluded that the most important concept emerging from the study was that the precautionary principle – the principle that safety comes first and that reasonable efforts to reduce risk need not await scientific proof – should be heeded.[8,28]

Special PPE Considerations

How can the level of PPE be reduced in the hospital setting?

For hospitals, training and equipping large numbers of personnel with specialized PPE in preparation for hazardous materials and CBRN incidents may be an unrealistic and unworkable approach to staff protection. Hospitals should instead consider implementing procedural controls that minimize the level of PPE required and then train a core group of staff to wear more specialized gear. In most emergency decontamination operations, only a small number of personnel will need to wear an advanced level of protection at any given time.

The level of PPE, especially respiratory protection, can be minimized by allowing contaminated individuals to decontaminate themselves whenever possible. Having them remove and contain their own clothing markedly reduces the presence of contamination and lowers the risk of secondary exposure. This also allows protected first receivers to concentrate their efforts on decontaminating those non-ambulatory patients who are unable to care for themselves.

What are the hazards associated with using PPE?

The use of PPE may itself create hazards to the wearer. The equipment can produce: 1) physical and heat stress; 2) impair visibility, mobility, and communication; and 3) cause psychological stress (i.e., claustrophobia). These problems are more commonly associated with higher levels of personal protection in which the user is totally encapsulated within the PPE. The proper selection of equipment and appropriate training (along with periodic retraining) may significantly reduce these problems. Because of the potential hazards associated with wearing advanced levels of PPE, employers must keep accurate training and medical records for all of their workers.

What are medical surveillance requirements for wearing PPE?

First responders and first receivers who wear CPC and a respirator should first have an occupational medical evaluation by a licensed healthcare provider. A screening medical evaluation questionnaire (available in most countries through their occupational health agency) should be completed and reviewed before any fit testing or use of a respirator takes place.

An examination of the employee's medical history should screen for preexisting medical conditions (hypertension, heart or lung disease, or diabetes) or occupational exposures that might preclude or limit one's ability to wear certain types or levels of PPE. The employee evaluation should also assess any limitations an individual may have to wearing PPE such as facial hair, the need to wear corrective lenses, hearing problems, panic disorder, and lung disease. The examining healthcare professional should confidentially review the evaluation results with the employee and provide written notice of their fitness for wearing a respirator and any physical limitations. This evaluation should be repeated when: 1) an employee reports signs and symptoms that are related to the ability to use a respirator; 2) the individual conducting a fit test indicates that an employee needs to be reevaluated; or 3) when a change in workplace conditions occurs (i.e., temperature, amount of physical work required, or the additional use of protective clothing) that may result in a substantial change in the physiological burden placed on an employee.[1,4,12]

Any time respirators are used to shield workers from hazards, a respiratory protection program should be implemented. This program includes procedures for: 1) selecting the appropriate respirator; 2) performing a medical evaluation of employees required to use respirators; 3) fit testing (if applicable); 4) proper use and maintenance of respirators; 5) employee training; and (6) regularly evaluating the effectiveness of the program.

What are the logistical constraints of wearing PPE in biohazard event?

Due to the need to don and doff PPE after each patient encounter, the amount of protective gear (gloves, gown, and N95 mask and eye protection or PAPR-type respirator) required per clinical provider in a standard 8-hour shift could quickly become overwhelming. In a hypothetical scenario in which a hospital nurse provided care twice an hour to four patients with smallpox, a minimum of sixty-four changes of PPE during a shift would be necessary. If each period of dressing and subsequent removal of the PPE takes only 2 minutes, the nurse in this scenario will spend over 4 hours of an 8-hour shift doing nothing more than changing and disposing of equipment. These conservative estimates will only increase in a large-scale bioterrorist attack that requires nurses to care for more patients and work longer shifts. When the PPE needs of physicians, ancillary personnel, and non-clinical staff are included in the equation, the inventory requirements and associated costs could quickly overwhelm the capacity of most if not all hospitals.[29]

How should PPE be maintained, inspected, and stored?

The individual using the PPE should be responsible for ensuring that their ensemble will perform as expected. During an actual incident is not the time to discover that one's needed PPE is not available, the PAPR's batteries are not fully charged, or that there are defects in the material. Protective clothing should be stored in a well-ventilated area based on manufacturer's recommendations to prevent damage from exposure to dust, moisture, sunlight, chemicals, temperature extremes, and impact. Protective clothing should either be packaged and stored as various sized ensembles or packaged and labeled by clothing (boots, gloves, suits, etc.) and material types (e.g., nitrile, butyl, or rubber gloves). Clothing should be folded or hung in accordance with manufacturer instructions. It should also be kept separate from street clothes and potentially contaminated clothing and gear.[1,30]

PPE should be inspected and operationally tested upon receipt, prior to actual usage, and after use or training. In addition, PPE requires periodic inspection during storage based on the manufacturer's guidelines and when a question arises concerning the functionality or appropriateness of the selected equipment. This inspection process should be formalized and procedurally focused.

Before newly purchased equipment is placed in inventory, a designated individual should determine that the clothing material is appropriate for the specific task at hand. The gear should be visually inspected to identify imperfect seams, non-uniform coating, tears, cracking, and malfunctioning closures. Garments and gloves should be examined for pinhole leaks. This is achieved by holding the garment up to light and by pressuring the gloves. Cracks can be exposed by flexing the material. If the product has been used previously, inspect inside and outside surfaces for signs of chemical damage, discoloration, swelling, and stiffness.

During use, one should periodically inspect the ensemble for evidence of chemical damage such as discoloration, swelling, stiffening, and softening of the CPC's material (keep in mind, however, that chemical permeation can occur without any visible effects). In addition, evidence of closure failure, tears, punctures, and seam discontinuities should also be sought.

If PPE is used in a decontamination event, responders/receivers should go through self-decontamination to ensure that excess amounts of contaminants do not remain on the exterior of the suit, boots, gloves, or respirator. This step reduces the potential of secondary contamination to those individuals assisting the wearer when doffing the gear. In all circumstances, specific doffing procedures should be developed and closely followed to minimize risk of contact with the exterior of the equipment. Once removed, the contaminated PPE should immediately be placed in an appropriate receptacle for proper storage and/or disposal.

If equipment is designed to be reused, it must be thoroughly decontaminated, sanitized, and inspected for wear before it can be placed back in service. Non-reusable PPE must be disposed of in accordance with local and national mandates in conjunction with the agent of exposure. Equipment maintenance should only be performed by those individuals who have specialized training and equipment. No repair should be made without checking with the person at your department or facility that is responsible for CPC maintenance.[1,30]

RECOMMENDATIONS FOR FURTHER RESEARCH

PPE is one of the vital components in a system of controls and administrative processes designed to protect staff from job-related hazards. In many circumstances, the hazard may be unknown or unrecognized until adverse health effects result. Instead of waiting for the hazard to be identified, its route of transmission defined, and exposure risks calculated, proper PPE should be worn routinely and used correctly. This requires users to have a working knowledge of why this gear is necessary, ready access to the equipment (in various sizes, designs, and configurations), appropriate training, and institutional support that values worker safety. Staff safety can only be enhanced if workers actually use the required protective equipment. Despite these expert recommendations and the existence of high-risk conditions in the work environment, the routine use of PPE does not occur. The reasons for this should be explored. Additional research is needed to help guide manufacturers in designing protective equipment that is less challenging to wear and encourages use. As a consequence of donning PPE, verbal communications and interactions with patients and victims becomes more difficult. Tactile sensitivity and dexterity are reduced or lost when thicker gloves or double gloving is required. Respirators increase the work of breathing and some designs limit visibility while protective suits and boots impair mobility. In addition, the one size fits all design of current gear is a misnomer and does not address the spectrum of end users. In general, protective suits are designed and sized for men, not women. Yet women make up much of the workforce in EMS and hospitals and are often the providers donning this gear in a hospital-based emergency decontamination operation. In addition, current protective ensembles are designed for a healthy, young, physically fit, compliant workforce rather than for the varying body sizes, physical capabilities, and fitness levels of those actually using the gear. Future investigators need to examine and better define interventions that improve PPE adherence rates. In the hospital environment, for example, workers typically wear protective gloves (adherence rates greater than 90%) but less commonly wear masks and eye protection or routinely perform appropriate hand hygiene. Reasons cited for noncompliance with PPE usage include lack of time to comply, job hindrance, physical discomfort, and perception that PPE is an unnecessary barrier to patient care. In addition, surveyed workers complain that wearing PPE makes communicating and recognizing others difficult and creates a sense of isolation when wearing the gear. PPE compliance was also found to be inversely proportional to the experience and training level of the user. Although counterintuitive, researchers have suggested that this trend is due to an increased sense of invulnerability as a possible explanation. Effective methods to reverse these trends will require additional exploration.[31]

Researchers also need to examine enhancements in good PPE fit, comfort, and functionality. Ensembles with multiple components that are designed to be used individually may tempt workers to remove or improperly use one component or the other. Manufacturers need to look at designing PPE ensembles that work well together, in terms of fit and comfort, and can be customized for certain industries, indications, and user profiles. In particular, PPE designed specifically for hospital personnel are needed. It should be developed, manufactured, and certified (i.e., Level H ensemble) so that it is styled and sized appropriately for both men and women. It should also be engineered with enhanced tactile capability to support the need for invasive procedures (i.e., the starting of intravenous lines and advanced airway management), include wireless electronic devices to facilitate responder communication, and afford the highest level of respiratory protection without encumbering the various tasks required of the wearer. Finally, future research in facilitating PPE usage and compliance should assess methods to improve training and institutional support that creates a culture of safety. How frequently should training be provided? What format or method of training is most efficient and cost-effective? Can online education, email, or use of text, Twitter, and other social media be used to increase awareness, understanding, and PPE compliance? Would a top-down (administrative driven) or bottom up (employee driven) approach to PPE usage be more effective in enhancing compliance? What policies, procedures, management support, and resources are necessary to enhance an organization's commitment to safety? What developments in prevention and safety, environmental and engineering controls, and administrative practices reduce the need for PPE? What are the individual, environmental, and institutional factors that impact PPE use and how can they be enhanced? What are the primary cost drivers associated with PPE usage and how can they be curtailed without impacting safety and compliance?[31]

In the end, the use of PPE is about enhancing staff safety. The equipment selected must balance cost, functionality, practicality, and usability. In addition, the appropriate incentives should be in place to ensure that the equipment is actually used when indicated and the wearer is able to accomplish all medical tasks in the most efficient and cost effective manner.

Acknowledgments

Special appreciation to Stanley "Skeet" Dickinson, Dr. Paul D. Kim, Frank J. Denny, and Sarah J. Salk-Pope.

REFERENCES

1. Occupational Safety & Health Administration. OSHA Technical Manual, Section VIII, Chapter 1, Chemical Protective Clothing. Available at: http://www.osha.gov/dts/osta/otm/otm_viii/otm_viii_1.html (Accessed April 8, 2013).

2. Agency for Toxic Substances and Disease Registry. *Hazardous Substances Emergency Event Surveillance (HSEES), Annual Report* 2009. Available at: www.atsdr.cdc.gov/HS/HSEES/annual2009.html (Accessed April 8, 2013).

3. Occupational Safety and Health Administration. *OSHA Best Practices for Hospital-Based First Receivers of Victims from Mass Casualty Incidents Involving the Release of Hazardous Substances.* U.S. Department of Labor, OSHA 3249–08N, 2005. Available at: http://www.osha.gov/dts/osta/bestpractices/firstreceivers_hospital.pdf (Accessed April 8, 2013).

4. Occupational Safety and Health Standards. Personal Protective Equipment, 1910.132, General Requirements. Available at: http://www.osha.gov/pls/oshaweb/owadisp.show_document?p_table=STANDARDS&p_id=9777 (Accessed April 8, 2013).

5. The History of PPE. The Fire Call. Spring 2010. Available at: http://www.iafpd.org/PDFs/The%20History%20of%20PPE.pdf (Accessed April 8, 2013).

6. Herris WP. How Regulation and Innovation Have Shaped Respiratory Protection. *EHS Today.* January 1, 2009. Available at: http://ehstoday.com/print/ppe/respirators/regulation_innovation_shaped (Accessed April 8, 2013).

7. Smart J. History of Chemical and Biological Warfare: An American Perspective. In: *Textbook of Military Medicine, Warfare, Weaponry, and the Casualty.* Washington, DC, Office of the Surgeon General, Department of the Army, 1997; 9–86.

8. Harriman KH, Brosseeau LM. Controversy: Respiratory Protection for Healthcare Workers, *Medscape.* April 28, 2011. Available at: http://www.medscape.com/viewarticle/741245_1 (Accessed August 16, 2015).

9. Centers for Disease Control and Prevention. Precautions to Prevent the Spread of MRSA in Healthcare Settings. Available at: http://www.cdc.gov/mrsa/healthcare/clinicians/precautions.html (Accessed August 16, 2015).

10. Bell DM, Kozarsky PE, Stephens DS. Clinical Issues in the Prophylaxis, Diagnosis, and Treatment of Anthrax. *Emerg Infect Dis* February 2002; 8(2): 222–225. Available at: http://europepmc.org/articles/PMC2732453 (Accessed April 8, 2013).

11. U.S. Department of Health & Human Services. Radiation Emergency Medical Management; Guidance on Diagnosis & Treatment for Health Care Providers; Personal Protective Equipment (PPE) in a Radiation Emergency. Available at: http://www.remm.nlm.gov/radiation_ppe.htm (Accessed April 8, 2013).

12. Hazardous Waste Operations and Emergency Response. Vol 29 CFR Part 1910.120: U.S. Department of Labor, OSHA. Available at: http://www.osha.gov/pls/oshaweb/owadisp.show_document?p_table=standards&p_id=9765 (Accessed April 8, 2013).

13. Respiratory Protection. OSHA 3079, US Department of Labor. 2002 (Revised). Available at: http://www.osha.gov/Publications/osha3079.pdf (Accessed April 8, 2013).

14. Yeung RSD, Chan JTS, Lee LLY, Chan YL. The use of personal protective equipment in Hazmat incidents. *Hong Kong Journal of Emergency Medicine* July 2002; 9(3): 171–176. Available at: http://www.fmshk.org/database/articles/v09n03012.pdf (Accessed April 8, 2013).

15. Centers for Disease Control and Prevention. The Emergency Response Safety and Health Database. Available at: http://www.cdc.gov/niosh/ershdb/default.html (Accessed April 8, 2013).

16. Occupational Safety & Health. Global Classification Systems for Chemical Protective Apparel. Available at: http://ohsonline.com/Articles/2011/08/01/Global-Classification-Systems-for-Chemical-Protective-Apparel.aspx (Accessed April 8, 2013).

17. National Fire Protection Agency. Standards 1991, 1992, and 1994. Available at: http://www.nfpa.org/aboutthecodes/list_of_codes_and_standards.asp (Accessed April 8, 2013).

18. Chemical Protective Clothing. Available at: http://protective.ansell.com/en/knowledge/standards/chemical-protective-suits (Accessed April 8, 2013).

19. Certified Safety: Understanding EN and NFPA standards for chemical protective suits. *CBRNe World.* August 14, 2012. Available at: http://www.cbrneworld.com/news/certified'safety'understanding'en'and'nfpa'standards'for'chemical'protectiv#axzz2PuEHw31l (Accessed April 8, 2013).

20. Centers for Disease Control and Prevention. Recommendations for the Selection and Use of Respirators and Protective Clothing for Protection Against Biological Agents. Available at: http://www.cdc.gov/niosh/docs/2009-132 (Accessed August 16, 2015).

21. Centers for Disease Control and Prevention. Prevention Strategies for Seasonal Influenza in Healthcare Settings. Available at: http://www.cdc.gov/flu/professionals/infectioncontrol/healthcaresettings.htm (Accessed April 8, 2013).

22. Loeb M, Dafoe N, Mahony J, et al. Surgical Mask vs N95 Respirator for Preventing Influenza Among Health Care Worker; A Randomized Trial. *JAMA* 2009; 302(17): 1865–1871. Available at: http://jama.jamanetwork.com/article.aspx?articleid=184819 (Accessed April 8, 2013).

23. Derrick JL, Gomersall CD. Protecting Healthcare Staff From Severe Acute Respiratory Syndrome: Filtration Capacity of Multiple Surgical Masks. *J Hosp Infect* 2005; 59: 365–368.

24. Derrick JL, Chan YF, Gomersall CD, Lui SF. Predictive Value of the User Seal Check in Determining Half-Face Respirator Fit. *J Hosp Infect* 2005; 59: 152–155.

25. Cluster of Severe Acute Respiratory Syndrome Cases Among Protected Health-Care Workers – Toronto, Canada. *MMWR Morb Wkly Rep* April 2003; 52: 433–436.

26. Loeb M, McGeer A, Henry B, et al. SARS Among Critical Care Nurses, Toronto. *Emerg Infect Dis* 2004; 10: 251–255.

27. Teleman MD, Boudville IC, Heng BH, et al. Factors Associated with Transmission of Severe Acute Respiratory Syndrome among Health Care Workers in Singapore. *Epidemiol Infect* 2004; 132: 797–803.

28. Ontario Health Care Health and Safety Committee Under Section 21 of the Occupational Health and Safety Act. Guidance Note for Workplace Parties #5. Application of Hazard Control Principles, including the Precautionary Principle to Infectious Agents. October 2011. Available at: http://www.healthandsafetyontario.ca/HSO/media/PSHSA/pdfS/HCS21_HazardControlPrinciples_Eng.pdf (Accessed April 8, 2013).

29. Grow RW, Rubinson L. The Challenge of Hospital Infection Control During a Response to Bioterrorist Attacks. *Biosecur and Bioterror: Biodefense Strategy, Practice, and Science* 2003; 1(3): 215–220.

30. Chemical Protective Clothing (Inspection, Storage, and Maintenance). OSHA Technical Manual, Section VIII: Chapter 1. Occupational Health and Safety Administration, United States Department of Labor. Available at: https://www.osha.gov/dts/osta/otm/otm_viii/otm_viii_1.html (Accessed August 16, 2015).

31. Goldfrank LR, Liverman CT. Using PPE: Individual and Institutional Issues. In: *Preparing for an Influenza Pandemic: Personal Protective Equipment by Healthcare Workers.* Institute of Medicine, Washington, DC; The National Academies Press, 2008; 113–146.

16

DECONTAMINATION

Howard W. Levitin and Christopher A. Kahn

OVERVIEW

Hazardous materials, in various quantities and configurations, are ubiquitous throughout the world. They are key ingredients of thriving economies in the form of agriculture, manufacturing, food production, and sanitation. They are readily found in commercial and retail establishments, medical facilities, and laboratories, as well as in various configurations in the home. Communities and residences located near industries that use or store hazardous materials are at a higher risk of experiencing a hazardous material incident.

Hazardous materials move throughout the world by truck, rail, ship, and pipeline. In the United States alone, 1.7 million railway shipments of hazardous materials occur yearly, of which 100,000 are toxic chemicals prone to becoming airborne in an accident.[1] World chemicals shipments in 2008 were €2,257 billion; €883 billion in Asia, €537 billion in Europe, €529 billion in the North American Free Trade Agreement (NAFTA) countries, and €157 billion in Latin America.[2] Modern societies must use hazardous materials to produce goods and services vital for healthy living and a robust economy. An often-overlooked byproduct of this economic growth is the creation of hazardous waste. The United Nations and other agencies estimate worldwide annual waste production at more than 1 billion tons, and some estimates go as high as 1.3 billion.[3]

The potential for an environmental release of a hazardous material is significant. In the United States there are approximately 850,000 facilities that manufacture, store, or use hazardous or extremely hazardous substances. Many of these sites are located in urban areas with populations at risk exceeding 1 million.[4] In the first 6 months of 2009, 4,074 acute releases of hazardous materials were reported to the U.S. Agency for Toxic Substances and Disease Registry (ATSDR) in 13 states participating in the study. During this reporting period, 439 events (12.7% of all reported events) resulted in a total of 1,050 victims, 44 of whom (4.2%) died.[5] Similarly, the Health Protection Agency recorded 1,015 chemical incidents in England and Wales in 2007, up 5% from the previous year. As a result of these incidents, approximately 27,970 people were exposed to hazardous agents with 6,220 reporting symptoms. More than 1,000 people were exposed in each of six separate events. There were nine fatalities as a result of chemical incidents.[6] The twenty-seven-nation European Union reports twenty to thirty-five major chemical accidents yearly.[7]

The actual incidence of chemical events in a particular locale, where the public is placed at risk of ill health, is unknown because reporting of such incidents is not internationally mandated, but globally such events are not rare. Most are a direct result of human error during the handling, manufacturing, and transportation of the hazards. The deliberate release of chemicals by terrorists (e.g., sarin attacks in Matsumoto in 1994 and on the Tokyo subway system in 1995), the intentional military attacks by Serbia on large chemical plants in the Balkans (1992), and the nuclear fallout in Japan after the 2011 Tōhoku Earthquake and Tsunami, reinforces the scope of potential hazardous materials incidents and their associated decontamination complexity.

Decontamination is any process, method, or action that leads to the reduction, removal, or inactivation of a hazardous substance on or in the patient to mitigate or prevent adverse health effects. The procedure's primary objective is timely removal of the offending agent by the best means available; chemical destruction (detoxification) of the hazard is a desirable secondary objective. Physical removal is imperative because none of the chemical means of destroying these agents do so instantaneously. Rapid toxin removal also serves to protect emergency first responders, hospital first receivers, facilities, vehicles, equipment, and others from secondary contamination.[8–11]

CURRENT STATE OF THE ART

Introduction

The process of decontamination should be viewed as a nonlinear spectrum of activities that progress from scene evacuation and clothing removal to full body showering designed to quickly limit a patient's exposure and the toxicity that follows from contamination. Although an essential procedure, the actual act of performing decontamination should not delay other lifesaving interventions.[11]

The need for and type of decontamination performed varies depending on the nature of the release, availability of resources, number of victims, capability of responding and receiving personnel, environmental conditions, exhibited signs and symptoms, initial toxicology information, and perceived patient needs and desires. When executed, it should be performed upwind, uphill, and at enough distance away from the release location to prevent recontamination.

The decision on which method or methods of decontamination to perform becomes more challenging when the initial identification of the responsible agent is unknown, victims present with varying signs and symptoms of exposure, or the sheer number of individuals seeking care overwhelms the local capability. As a result, a one-size-fits-all approach to decontamination is insufficient; rather it should include a flexible cadre of tools and approaches that can be scaled accordingly. Under certain circumstances, self-evacuation, wiping visible contaminants from skin and clothing, and personal showering at home may be all that is needed (self-care). Other types of incidents may require varying combinations of self-care, victim clothing removal at the scene and mass washing (gross decontamination), and/or thorough soap and water showering at the hospital (technical decontamination).[4,8,10–12]

In general, removing and bagging a victim's clothing eliminates much of the contaminant (depending on the extent of clothing worn at the time of exposure) and minimizes the risk of spreading the toxic agent to others. This initial step in the decontamination process should always be performed, when possible, regardless of the agent or setting. When additional decontamination is required, the patient should be thoroughly rinsed with water.[4,8,10–12]

The decision to perform decontamination is often subjective, commonly undertaken without knowledge about the agent, and based on a historical premise that early intervention reduces short-term morbidity and mortality, helps prevent delayed health consequences, and protects others against unnecessary harm. This standard approach is not without risk since the procedure itself can cause injury (e.g., applying water to reactive metals produces a volatile exothermic reaction, showering in freezing temperatures causes hypothermia and mechanical injuries, and performing decontamination can exacerbate underlying psychological disorders due to the stress associated with the procedure). Objectivity to this risk-based response decision can be enhanced by taking into account the presence or absence of exposure signs and symptoms, visual evidence of contamination, location of the patient relative to the site of release, site-specific data, and any available toxicology information. This offers decontamination personnel flexibility in adopting response capabilities and decontamination methods to dynamic situations. Such risk-based decision making requires decontamination team leadership to have the knowledge, experience, and access to information necessary to make appropriate response determinations.[4,8,10–13]

In this chapter, discussion will be limited to the decontamination after exposure to a hazardous substance. Issues related to regulatory standards, personal protective equipment (PPE), toxicology, and training are addressed elsewhere (see Chapter 15).

Background

Individuals may become contaminated through direct contact with hazardous substances in their various physical states (vapor, gas, mist, liquid, or solid) or from others who are already contaminated. The contamination risk is low when gases are involved because they tend to dissipate rapidly once the individual has been removed from the source. Liquids and solids (particles, dust) are more likely to cause contamination and spread to others because they tend to persist on the patient until medical attention is received.[13–15] The overall likelihood of secondary contamination is directly related to the volatility of the substance. Agents that are less volatile are more persistent and therefore more prone to remain on the contaminated victim. Chemical agents can persist on patients' hair, skin, and clothing. If there is significant delay between exposure and symptom onset (latency), victims may be unaware of their contamination and therefore more apt to spread the hazard to others, especially if they are self-presenting to the hospital.[16]

In most cases of airborne releases, simply evacuating persons from the source and removing their outer clothing when possible is sufficient to prevent further exposure or injury.[13–15] Clothing can act like an occlusive dressing; failure to remove it quickly after chemical exposure may prevent the evaporation of volatile skin contaminants.[9] In chemical mass-casualty incidents, where aerosolized substances are more commonly the causative agent, procedures geared toward detaining ambulatory victims near the scene in order to direct them through a mass showering field decontamination system (e.g., tents or ladder sprayers) can needlessly delay evacuation and treatment. This often-practiced approach may inadvertently increase the potential for harm to the victims as well as those caring for these individuals by congregating them and vital response resources in the contamination zone ("hot zone").[13,17]

Those contaminated with liquids or solids require copious skin lavage and wound irrigation with water within minutes of skin contact to minimize the degree of injury. Rinsing the patient with a high-volume, low-pressure water source dilutes, neutralizes, and helps rid the skin of reactive surface contaminants. In the case of corrosive agents, decreasing the duration of skin contact helps restore tissue to its normal pH, thereby reducing the incidence of full-thickness burns.[13,18,20–24] Using soap to help emulsify fat soluble agents and a soft brush, sponge, or cloth to mechanically remove any remaining solid materials may also be beneficial.[4,8–10,19]

The intensity of chemical injury is based on a number of factors including: route of exposure, concentration and reactivity of the agent, pH, duration of skin contact, and the integrity of the skin.[13,22,24–26] When the duration of skin contact is prolonged, the potential for tissue damage, agent absorption, and systemic toxicity is increased. Pesticides, hydrogen fluoride, and phenolic substances rapidly penetrate the skin and enter the general circulation (e.g., Malathion penetrates the skin almost immediately on contact).[25] Corrosives and solvents damage the outer skin layers within minutes, yet beneficial effects of decontamination by dilution have been seen even when irrigation was delayed up to 1 hour.[13,19] It appears that treatment within 1 hour of injury is critical in reducing the severity of burns, a timeline that may also be applicable to hazardous substance contamination in general.[13,18,19] Decontamination beyond this "golden hour" appears to be most beneficial in reducing the risk of secondary contamination of emergency personnel, and may offer some psychological benefit to exposed patients.

Water reacts exothermically when combined with metallic substances such as sodium, potassium, lithium, cesium, and rubidium. Other substances such as white phosphorus, sulfur, strontium, titanium, uranium, zinc, and zirconium will ignite on contact with air. If any of these uncommon sources of contamination are present or suspected, they have the potential to react with the ambient air and the moisture on the victim's skin until they can be physically removed with forceps and secured in a container filled with mineral oil. After these exposures, despite the potential for reactivity, quickly removing the victim's clothing and flushing them with large volumes of water should minimize the injury.[27]

The process of decontamination for radiological agents is similar to the one used for other hazardous substances but should incorporate radiological survey instruments. Patients should have their clothing removed and double bagged with date and time of collection recorded on a radiation warning label, followed with a soap and water showering. Unstable victims, or those with life-threatening injuries, should have gross decontamination (i.e., clothing removal) performed quickly so lifesaving interventions can be offered. The presence of radioactive materials should not delay these activities.

Specialized detectors can confirm and measure the presence of radiation as well as serve as a guide to the effectiveness of the decontamination process. Not uncommonly, at least two decontamination cycles are performed in order to demonstrate a decrease in the external contamination to a level of no more than two times the background radiation level. Attempts to remove all contamination from skin may not be feasible or desirable since some radioactivity may remain trapped in the outermost layer of skin. Covering areas of residual contamination with a waterproof dressing may help limit the spread of contamination. Persistent elevated levels of radiation may be due to internal contamination.[29]

The proper decontamination procedure for biological agents has not been established. Historically, these agents were considered non-volatile and thought not to exhibit absorption capability in the presence of intact skin. They were also believed to pose a minimal risk of re-aerosolization. This premise changed after the intentional release of anthrax using envelopes mailed through the U.S. Postal Service in 2001, in which twenty-two individuals became ill and five died from exposure to the spores.[30] In general, a biological agent exposure does not require decontamination, although it is worthwhile to instruct patients to remove and wash their clothing at home and take a shower. If dermal or mucous membrane contamination is suspected, the area should be thoroughly irrigated with water.

The science of decontamination is limited and rarely evidence-based, with procedural recommendations extrapolated from military guidelines and field experience. Military and fire services from several countries (Australia, Canada, Israel, Japan, the United Kingdom, and the United States) have contributed considerably to the procedural approach to the contaminated patient. However, research designed to advance knowledge on the proper care of the contaminated patient does not lend itself to placebo-controlled, double-blind studies. As a result, the advantages of using water in the decontamination process are derived indirectly from burn studies. This research demonstrated the benefits of hydrotherapy on cutaneous skin pH and clinical outcomes when experimental skin models were contaminated with harsh chemicals.[18,20–22] The urgency of decontamination after exposure is derived from measuring chemical absorption rates in animal skin models.[22,23,25] Finally, the essential role of clothing removal in the decontamination process is based in part on studies using clothed mannequins where evaporation rates and exposure levels of volatile agents are easily measured.[28]

Initial Approach to Contaminated Patients

The primary objectives in a hazardous material incident include limiting victim exposure by quick removal from the contamination zone, containment of the hazard to prevent ongoing contact with the agent, and patient treatment (via decontamination) to minimize harm, all without jeopardizing the safety of first responders/receivers. With contamination reduction, the level of PPE required by staff can be downgraded to a point that will better facilitate patient care (preferably standard precautions).

The essential (although not necessarily sequential) approach to decontamination consists of several key steps:

- Recognition of a hazardous material exposure
- Identification of the contaminant (or its basic properties if identification is not immediately possible)
- Prevention of further contamination
- Stabilization of acute medical conditions
- Removal of contaminant from victims
- Preservation of evidence (when required)
- Removal and disposal of contaminant and runoff

Recognition of a Hazardous Material Exposure

Recognizing the necessity for decontamination is the first critical step to successfully managing a hazardous materials event. Several clues may help first responders/receivers determine that victims of an event are contaminated. These include patient history and associated complaints (e.g., eye irritation, cough, or shortness of breath), their location relative to the release, the presence of hazardous material odors or vapor clouds, identification of a constellation of signs and symptoms (i.e., toxidrome) that suggest a specific class of poisoning, observation of suspicious materials, previous warnings of a contamination event, or labels identifying contaminating agents as present in the incident area. On recognition or high suspicion of a contamination event, first responders/receivers should activate a coordinated, planned response, which rapidly removes victims from the contaminated area and the hazardous material from the victims. These steps should occur while providing for stabilizing medical care and protecting personnel.

It is also incumbent to recognize that victims may present with suspicious signs and symptoms yet no known exposure exists. In the initial aftermath of an exposure, it may be difficult to determine whether patients have actually been contaminated or are merely manifesting illness signs and symptoms that have no organic etiology. In other cases, individuals may request decontamination even if the presence of a toxic substance is unlikely.[29] An appropriate and timely response in a non-judgmental and professional manner may help prevent the escalation of these symptoms and their rapid spread to others (mass psychogenic illness). As a result, resources must be available for and allocated to patients who have not been truly exposed as well as for those who have.

Identification of the Contaminant

Although general decontamination measures can proceed without contaminant identification, determination of the specific agent can focus decontamination methods and make the process more efficient. In some cases, it can also increase safety for victims and staff. For example, certain metals are explosive when mixed with water; as water is the most common choice of decontamination agent, failure to identify these metals as the contaminant could prove dangerous.

The most reliable method for identifying a contaminant is to have advance knowledge of the hazardous agents present in the environment where the exposure occurred. This is feasible in the context of manufacturing, distribution, agriculture, laboratory, or research settings where chemical inventories are commonly known, as well as incidents involving properly labeled shipments of hazardous materials or those occurring at regulated industrial sites. However, in the setting of a criminal act or a release at an unregulated site, it is unlikely that first responders/receivers will have advance knowledge of the contaminant.

Detectors for various chemical and biological agents exist, but currently suffer from imperfect reliability. Recognition of a specific toxidrome is potentially the most reliable method for rapidly identifying the class to which a particular chemical contaminant belongs. Biological contaminants, by virtue of causing disease, may be more recognizable retrospectively by the presentation of victims with similar illness symptomatology; however, their usually delayed presentation may make overall recognition of a biological release event more difficult. Radiological contaminants can be easily identified by the use of radiological detectors such as Geiger-Müller counters.

If witnesses to the contamination event are able to identify the physical state of the toxic agent (i.e., solid, liquid, or vapor/gas), its container, or its associated warning placard, the decontamination and hazard identification process can be further streamlined. Resources such as poison control centers, Internet and telephone-accessed chemical databases, and government agencies can also be contacted to help guide decision making as it relates to decontamination, PPE selection, and waste disposal requirements.

Prevention of Further Contamination

A basic tenet of emergency response is ensuring scene safety; failure to ensure the well-being of personnel and other nearby persons risks the creation of additional victims. The decontamination corridor should be strategically arranged to separate contaminated persons and items from clean areas, utilities, and unprotected staff. Patient flow through the corridor should be clearly marked and supervised. Appropriate levels of PPE should be used at all times (discussed further in Chapter 15). Guidelines from several countries state that when faced with an unknown contaminant, the highest available level of PPE should be used.[32–34] Identification of the contaminant will likely allow the use of a lower level of PPE. There is no current consensus on which PPE level should be used when medical procedures are urgently indicated on contaminated patients. Studies have been performed indicating that higher-level protection may significantly impair the ability of medical personnel to perform lifesaving procedures such as airway stabilization or obtaining intravenous access for medication administration. The creation of a hospital-specific category of PPE to help maximize procedural ability while minimizing risks to hospital staff has been suggested.[8]

Stabilization of Acute Medical Conditions

The decision to provide emergent medical care (e.g., intravenous access, airway management) to a contaminated patient prior to decontamination must be balanced against the need to protect staff and their ability to provide interventional care while dressed in advanced levels of PPE. Intuitively, the sicker the patient, the greater the perceived need for emergent care. However, if the victim's critical injuries or state of distress is a direct result of hazard exposure, the provider must don appropriate PPE prior to providing care or they themselves may become victims. This key principle is counterintuitive to the normal desire to provide immediate aid to the victim.

When appropriately trained and protected resources are available, emergent patient care can be provided simultaneously with decontamination. However, the advanced level of protection required in most decontamination scenarios dramatically affects the caregiver's ability to render such care. In most circumstances, basic life support skills such as maintaining a patent airway, stabilizing a fracture, and controlling significant bleeding can be accomplished concurrently with providing decontamination. Advanced life support techniques, however, must often be delayed until immediately after decontamination when caregivers can wear a reduced level of protective attire (e.g., standard precautions) that allows them greater mobility, dexterity, sight, and hearing.

If a treatment cannot be provided without contaminating and therefore endangering responders and other persons, that treatment should be withheld until safety can be reasonably assured. Treatment that can be reasonably deferred should be delayed until the patient has been decontaminated.[11]

Removal of Contaminant from Victims

Several resources exist to describe the various approaches to decontamination as well as individual decontamination methods for specific agents.[35–38] The focus here will be on gross and technical decontamination principles.

Koenig coined the term "strip and shower" to describe the most common decontamination method, the use of soap and water after removal of all clothing and other items from a contaminated victim.[8] While considered largely effective, and relying on inexpensive materials, several logistical concerns are raised when employing this method. Patient throughput (the number of patients that can be decontaminated per hour) may be limited by the availability of private areas with access to running water. In cold weather, stripping and being washed may cause mechanical and thermal injuries to patients, personnel, and equipment, and could result in hypothermia if decontamination is prolonged, particularly if warm water is unavailable.

Having a reliable water source at the scene to perform decontamination may necessitate the use of high-pressure systems (such as fire apparatus) that require pressure-reducing manifolds to manage water flow and prevent potential injuries to equipment and victims. Decontamination at a fixed facility requires the acquisition of decontamination equipment, heaters, water containment systems, and shelters that need ongoing maintenance and capital investment. Maximizing victim privacy through the decontamination process, addressing communication difficulties involving staff wearing PPE, proper handling of at-risk populations, and logistical matters are also issues to address. Despite these concerns, this technique of clothing removal followed by showering remains the most common decontamination method in use today.

Dry powder decontamination is an alternate approach used in some countries to absorb liquid substances. After removal of clothing, a dry powder such as Fullers Earth (a highly absorbent, claylike earthy material) is applied to the victim. The adsorbent nature of the powder helps remove contaminant remaining on the skin. This method is more cumbersome to apply and requires the availability of the powder. However, it is an option to consider when the contaminant is a thickened agent, when access to water is limited, or when the agent is known to be reactive with water.

Foam is a more recent innovation for decontamination and is available commercially. Advantages include less production of waste products, a potential for enhanced skin coverage, and increased activity against a broad range of agents. Disadvantages include expense and the need to store large quantities of this decontamination agent.

Whatever decontamination method is used, orifices, mucous membranes, and injured areas require special attention. Uptake of radioactive material may be faster through body orifices and mucous membranes than through intact skin.[29] In general, these areas should be decontaminated first before washing intact skin but after cleaning open wounds to minimize the continued absorption and effects of the contaminant. Water-based methods are the most rapid and appropriate means of decontaminating these areas.

Cotton-tipped applicators can be used to clean the nose and ears, and used to assess orifice contamination in the presence of radioactive material. Gentle irrigation of the ear canal with a syringe (ensuring first that the tympanic membrane is intact) and encouraging tooth brushing with frequent mouth rinsing is recommended. Gargling with water or 3% hydrogen peroxide may also be beneficial for pharyngeal contamination.[29] Decontaminated wounds should be covered with waterproof dressings or drapes to limit the spread of the toxic substance and to prevent recontamination during the full body decontamination process.

Preservation of Evidence

Contamination incidents may occasionally result in investigation by either occupational health and safety agencies or law enforcement. In either case, contaminated items may be crucial pieces of evidence to assist the investigation. Although preservation of evidence is clearly a lower priority than safeguarding life and health, evidence should be retained by identifying, isolating, and maintaining the chain of custody for evidentiary items whenever possible. Since evidence preservation is resource intensive and may not be necessary for a given event, determining the desirability for evidence collection should be made early in conjunction with the appropriate agencies. Procedures may include the removal of personal items from contaminated victims and sealing them in a nonreactive container (a plastic bag will often suffice). Containers should be labeled and maintained in a secure area or, if possible, with the patient.

Removal and Disposal of Contaminant and Runoff

After completing decontamination and adequately addressing the medical needs of victims, designated individuals should begin a more thorough assessment of the incident scene and surrounding environs. Although responsible groups will almost certainly conduct environmental restoration at a future time, first responders can mitigate this later work by their initial actions. For example, directing the flow of contaminated water runoff into storage drums or collection pools minimizes entry into watersheds and storm drains, limiting contamination of the environment. As with evidence collection, environmental concerns are a lower priority than the preservation of life and safety during the initial phase of the emergency response, but should be addressed once conditions stabilize.

To assist with environmental protection, medical and health workers should dispose of contaminants and contaminated items in a fashion consistent with safe practice. In most countries, specialized contractors and governmental agencies are generally better equipped and more familiar with regulatory issues regarding disposal of hazardous waste than individuals, small agencies, or medical facilities. Any waste disposal should be performed with careful attention to regulatory guidance.

One particular issue regarding disposal of contaminants is management of wastewater produced during water decontamination. In general, it is preferred that water be contained for later treatment or disposal; however, in the United States, the Environmental Protection Agency has issued guidance that in emergency situations with no other alternatives, discharge of wastewater into sewers is acceptable in order to preserve life. Specifically, avoidance of contaminated water runoff "should not impede necessary and appropriate actions to protect human life and health."[39]

Decontamination in Healthcare Facilities

Although many community decontamination plans describe methods for providing decontamination at the site of exposure, it has been demonstrated that after a mass-casualty contamination event, many victims will spontaneously present at medical facilities distant from the event for treatment.[9] Initial evaluation and treatment of contaminated victims has resulted in injuries to facility medical staff.[40–42] It is imperative that medical facilities have a decontamination program, both for the case in which they receive contaminated victims from a distant location and also for situations where they are the site of exposure.[43]

Decontamination in the hospital or other healthcare facility setting follows the same principles delineated previously. A crucial step is to reduce the risk to other patients and to facility staff by minimizing exposure. Decontamination should occur in a designated area with staged equipment to allow for mitigation of the contaminant without the need to move the patient through other areas of the hospital. The designated decontamination area should have restricted access.

Special Considerations

HOW CLEAN IS CLEAN?

An objective endpoint for determining when decontamination is complete is not reliably available. The goals of decontamination are to terminate a substance's harmful effects on the patient (eliminate continued absorption), reduce the risk of secondary exposure/contamination to other people, and eliminate the need for an advanced level of PPE (beyond standard precautions) for caregivers working in the treatment area. Yet it is difficult to determine when decontamination efforts are sufficient to achieve these goals and can therefore be stopped. This concept has been expressed by the phrase "How clean is clean?"

There is a lack of scientific data to provide consistent guidance in this area. Eliminating evidence of visual contamination or reducing reported signs and symptoms is the only current means to establish evidence of contamination reduction. This approach is generally accepted despite the knowledge that some agents have a clear latency between local symptomatology and systemic illness (e.g., blistering agents and VX nerve agent). In other cases, antidote treatment may be required before symptoms can be reduced via decontamination.[11]

In most instances, a thorough washing with soap and water accomplishes the clean objective. However, some insoluble chemicals are resistant to soap and water decontamination and other primary decontamination agents must be identified. For example, tars and heavy oils require the use of petroleum-based solvents (e.g., petroleum jelly, mineral spirits, vegetable oil) to degrade the agents; followed quickly by standard soap and water cleansing.

Clinical determination of the effectiveness of decontamination is unreliable since signs and symptoms may be inconsistent with the actual chemical exposure and may persist despite adequate technique. Likewise, victims cannot be continuously decontaminated until symptoms resolve. The longer they remain in the system, the more wastewater is generated and the more resources are consumed. Furthermore, responders cannot wear advanced levels of PPE indefinitely since it impacts body temperature, hydration status, and stress levels, and may lead to injuries such as falls. An unnecessary prolongation of the decontamination process may divert personnel resources from other critical services.

Current literature supports the need to irrigate contaminated tissue quickly to positively influence the outcome for the patient.[18,20–26] Recommended showering intervals vary between 30 seconds and 5 minutes depending on the water temperature, pressure, and volume. Some chemicals, such as ammonia and chlorine, are highly water-soluble and will virtually disappear within the first few minutes of decontamination. Other agents will continue to penetrate the skin despite irrigation but at a lower rate. Nonetheless, human senses may still detect the presence of various agents even though the actual skin concentration is well below a harmful threshold as confirmed by studies of swab samples from specific areas of victims' bodies pre- and post-decontamination.[44]

The process of decontamination also influences its effectiveness. Washing in a head-to-toe manner reduces the likelihood of drawing contaminants from the lower extremities back into vital areas such as the face, eyes, and airway. Also, irrigating open wounds first and then covering them with water occlusive dressings reduces the amount of contaminated wash flowing into the wound. Similarly, a thorough washing of the victim's hair and other body recesses reduces the retention of contaminants.[11]

All devices applied to the patient at the initial site of exposure (e.g., cervical collars, splinting devices, backboard, and intravenous lines) should be considered contaminated and ought to be either replaced or cleaned during the decontamination process. It is clearly disadvantageous to focus efforts solely on decontaminating the patient's skin while contaminants may still remain on these devices.

Decontamination effectiveness is presumably enhanced when: 1) a corridor is properly established and maintained by trained personnel, maximizing patient safety and equipment usage; 2) expectations and procedural guidance are well communicated; 3) language barriers are minimized; and 4) the actual decontamination procedure is observed to ensure thoroughness. Individuals who are able to walk into a shower and clean themselves probably receive a more thorough decontamination than non-ambulatory individuals. The addition of soap may increase the efficacy of showering in some circumstances. Although detectors are available for chemical and biological agent identification, they play a very limited role in determining the effectiveness of decontamination. Radiological detectors, on the other hand, are more prevalent and have a defined role in decontamination.

Other agents such as bleach and specialized soaps have not been shown to significantly impact the overall effectiveness of decontamination. Current evidence clearly indicates that water alone or in combination with soap is the most effective and readily available decontamination solution. Non-abrasive liquid soap should be used and should not contain perfumes, lanolin, or other additives.

In addition to soap, water temperature dramatically impacts the effectiveness of decontamination. Cold water reduces victim compliance and may make some agents more viscous and difficult to remove. Showering in cold water may also trap volatile contaminants in constricted skin pores, increasing the likelihood that these agents will continue to be released from the skin (i.e., off-gassing) once the victim is removed to a warmer environment such as the emergency department. On the other hand, victims suffering from skin lesions or burns may not tolerate hot water. Water at an elevated temperature may also cause pores to open, thereby increasing the skin's surface area and absorption rate of the agent. Tepid water is the ideal temperature for optimum results.[4,8–13]

WHO SHOULD PERFORM DECONTAMINATION?

With a proper system in place, the vast majority of contaminated victims are ambulatory and can be guided to remove their own clothing, package and manage their personal valuables, and thoroughly wash themselves. Creating an environment where decontamination can be self-administered is essential. Some individuals, however, are debilitated to the point where responders must assist or intervene in the decontamination process.

Although some patients require total assistance, others may have only minimal injuries or preexisting conditions that inhibit their ability to ambulate through the decontamination process. Placing these individuals on backboards and accompanying them through decontamination is labor intensive, potentially dangerous to the caregivers and victims, and may be a less effective means of fully removing the contaminants as compared to aggressive self-decontamination.

Patients who can walk with assistance and sit unattended can be categorized as semi-ambulatory. These individuals may be placed in chairs inside the decontamination unit and in most circumstances can thoroughly wash all accessible areas themselves with minimal intervention or assistance. Decontamination team members in appropriate PPE should wash those areas of the body that are not readily accessible to the patients themselves. Once complete, victims can then be assisted out of the decontamination area to an awaiting wheelchair or other mobility device. This simple procedure reduces the physical demands placed on responders and may be inherently safer for the patient.

IN WHAT ORDER SHOULD PATIENTS BE DECONTAMINATED?

Decontamination of multiple casualties is an enormous task. The process requires a large dedication of personnel, equipment, materiel, and time. Even with appropriate planning and training, the process itself demands a significant contribution of resources.

In a multiple casualty scenario, the order in which patients are sequenced through the decontamination process impacts the success of the operation. This decision needs to go beyond the normal patient triage and assessment protocols to include chemical information, patient mobility levels, and the availability of resources.[11] In addition, the timing of victim presentation in relation to when the decontamination area is established and team members don protective gear also plays a role in deciding who is decontaminated first. The sequencing approach should be aligned with the philosophy of doing the greatest good for the greatest number of people. That philosophy should be supported in advance with a decontamination corridor that can be configured for ambulatory, semi-ambulatory, and non-ambulatory casualties.

Ambulatory patients are able to self-administer decontamination, starting with outer clothing removal. Therefore consideration should be given to proceeding with these individuals first while the decontamination team is preparing for the potentially more serious, labor intensive, non-ambulatory patients. In most instances, multiple ambulatory patients can be verbally directed through the decontamination process once the corridor is configured. Decontamination can occur even while responders are still in the process of donning their PPE. This approach expedites the decontamination process in multiple casualty events and reduces the amount of time the response team must spend wearing advanced levels of PPE. If all ambulatory patients are made to wait until decontamination is completed on all semi-/non-ambulatory casualties, the response team becomes adversely fatigued and non-operational, and bottlenecks will occur. Once the response team is readied, the decontamination of high-priority casualties (those with the highest level of contamination and/or acuity), regardless of their mobility level, should be addressed.

HOW SHOULD PEDIATRIC PATIENTS BE DECONTAMINATED?

Children present unique challenges that must be addressed in order to make the decontamination process successful. There are sparse data on the frequency of children involved in hazardous material incidents. Data on 2009 incidents in the United States where ages were recorded showed that 2.9% of injuries occurred in individuals less than 5 years of age, 7.4% of injuries were aged 5–14, and 5.6% were 5–19 years old.[5]

The principles of decontamination (disrobe, shower if needed, treatment) remain the same regardless of the victim's age. However, to effectively decontaminate children, the response team must be very cognizant of the nuances of the process. For example, children develop significant anxiety and may become inconsolable when separated from their caregiver, making them less cooperative during the decontamination process. Older children may resist or be difficult to handle out of fear, peer pressure, and modesty issues, even in front of their parents or caregivers.[45]

Children's skin is thinner as compared to adults, thereby offering less protection against and greater absorption of toxic chemicals. Children also have faster respiratory rates and their breathing zones are situated closer to the ground, which increases their potential for injury from vapor-prone agents. Finally, children are less able to maintain their core body temperature, which allows hypothermia to occur much faster when it is cold outside and water temperature is below 37°C. This risk is highest when they are unclothed and wet.[45]

Pediatric victims of a multiple casualty chemical incident may arrive separated from their parents and unable to articulate their identity, symptoms, medical history, or needs. In addition, it is very difficult for staff to communicate with children, let alone handle them, while wearing PPE.

Experts recommend that response initiatives be closely tied to the age of the child. Children less than 2 years of age should be managed with their caregiver whenever possible to help disrobe, jointly shower, and move the patient through the decontamination process. Placing infants and young toddlers in a laundry basket reduces the risk of dropping them. Responders should ensure that water temperature in the shower doesn't drop below 37°C and that children are dried off and warmed quickly after decontamination.

Children 2 to 8 years of age should also be disrobed and showered with their caregiver whenever possible. Non-ambulatory patients should be escorted through the process with their caregiver. The issue of hypothermia needs to be addressed as described previously. Privacy will be a bigger issue for children between 8 and 18 years of age, so steps should be taken to protect modesty as much as possible.[45]

Other issues to consider include astute observation of respiratory status, proper removal and containment of contaminated clothing, and patient tracking. The most effectively prepared decontamination teams will conduct realistic drills using infant-sized dolls, toddlers, and pre-teen volunteers to fully address the special needs of children.

WHAT ARE IMPORTANT CONSIDERATIONS IN DECONTAMINATION OF AT-RISK POPULATIONS?

A successful decontamination operation relies on the free flow of information between personnel and between staff and patients.[11] In a hectic, demanding environment, any breakdown in communication makes the decontamination process more arduous and hazardous. Despite best intentions, there are a number of barriers to effective communication that must be considered and addressed in order to enhance the outcome of an emergency decontamination operation and increase victim compliance. Examples of these barriers include communication, disability, and culture.

An at-risk population includes individuals who may have additional needs before, during, and after an incident in functional areas, including but not limited to: maintaining independence, communication, transportation, supervision, and medical care. Individuals in need of additional response assistance may include those who have disabilities, residents of institutionalized settings, the elderly, children, persons from diverse cultures, those with limited local language proficiency, or persons who lack transportation.

There are over 6,000 living languages spoken in the world.[46] In addition to spoken language barriers, 35 million Americans are affected by hearing loss and 16% of adult Europeans have hearing impairment great enough to adversely impact their daily lives.[47] Planning and training initiatives focusing on communication barriers should also consider the various visual inputs inherent in the decontamination process and how they may impact its effectiveness for those with impaired sight.[48,49] Lastly, decontamination readiness activities must also address local cultural sensitivities as related to clothing removal, modesty, male/female interactions, and other expected norms. A number of steps can be taken to better improve communication and address cultural sensitivities during decontamination. For example, clearly demarcating each stage of the decontamination process with signage that uses pictograms to illustrate the expected activity (e.g., clothing removal and use of privacy garment, showering, drying off, and donning a gown), theatrical demonstration of the activity expected at each station, strategic placement of interpreters, and the distribution of pre-event printed, multilingual information sheets can improve communication. Recognizing the inherent need for modesty through adequate use of privacy screens, separate showers for men, women, and children, and gender segregation of staff is also important to consider. Understanding that personal space varies among cultures and that eye contact is not always appropriate should be stressed in training. Staff should be attuned to a patient's apparent comfort level when making direct eye and physical contact.[11]

For many patients, allowing a friend, relative, or support person to accompany them through the decontamination process may enhance their calmness and cooperation. Wheelchair patients can perform their own transfers as appropriate. In many cases, wheelchair, walker, and cane dependent patients may need guidance through the decontamination process using a chair or other mobility device. Proper positioning of occupational and physical therapists may prove very valuable. Service animals should be decontaminated with the patient. Finally, patients should not be rushed through decontamination. Forcing an uncomfortably rapid pace may promote feelings of anxiety and confusion. This is especially true with pediatric and elderly patients.[48,49] Enhancing communication with patients during decontamination or any other encounter will enhance the healthcare experience for all involved. Success requires planning, training, practice, patience, and consistency.

RECOMMENDATIONS FOR FURTHER RESEARCH

There is still much that needs to be learned about patient decontamination, but clinical experience and scientific studies are coming together to enhance the efficacy of the procedure. Future research should focus on the following: How does one measure the adequacy of decontamination? Should this determination be based on victim symptomatology, length of showering time, measurements made from new promising technology, or other parameters? Is traditional soap and water showering appropriate decontamination for victims of a chemical mass-casualty incident? How frequently should healthcare facility staff be trained to maintain their knowledge, skills, and abilities as it relates to the use of PPE and patient decontamination? Is annual training sufficient (as dictated by U.S. federal standards) or does knowledge quickly wane after the initial instruction period? Who should be trained? How does one maintain a decontamination capability with reduced funding? Does currently available PPE and decontamination equipment adequately address the needs of both sexes, various age groups, and the unique demands of the hospital? What medical interventions (e.g., airway management, intravenous catheter placement) should staff wearing PPE be expected to perform?

Conclusion

An effective decontamination capability must be multidisciplinary and integrated. It requires planning, training and retraining, equipment acquisition and maintenance, frequent exercises, and teamwork. The fact that an exposure has occurred must be recognized early. First responders, first receivers, and facilities must be adequately protected, and decontamination must be performed quickly, safely, and efficiently. The involvement of multiple categories of personnel (e.g., EMS, fire, hazmat, medical staff, administrators, trainers, security personnel, regulatory officials) demands a unified approach and collaborative, detailed planning. An incident command system, such as that promulgated by the U.S. National Incident Management System (NIMS), is an excellent framework within which the structure of a decontamination response can be formed. Ongoing training and exercises will help ensure that response team members are familiar with their roles and are capable of achieving the goal of rapid contaminant removal and victim stabilization while protecting themselves and the public from injury.

REFERENCES

1. Wald ML. Tighter Rule on Hazardous Rail Cargo Is Ready. *New York Times.* December 15, 2006. www.nytimes.com/2006/12/15/us/15rail.html?_r=0&pagewanted=print (Accessed March 14, 2013).

2. The Future of the European Chemical Industry, KPMG International, 2010. www.kpmg.com/Global/en/IssuesAndInsights/ArticlesPublications/Documents/future-european-chemical-industry.pdf (Accessed March 12, 2013).

3. Malone R. World's Worst Waste. *Forbes.* May 24, 2006. www.forbes.com/2006/05/23/waste-worlds-worst-cx_rm_0524waste.html (Accessed March 14, 2013).

4. Levitin H, Siegelson H: Hazardous materials emergencies. *Disaster Medicine.* Philadelphia, PA, Lippincott, Williams, and Wilkins, 2002; 258–273.

5. Department of Health and Human Services, Agency for Toxic Substances and Disease Registry, Hazardous Substances Emergency Event Surveillance Annual Report. 2009. www.atsdr.cdc.gov/HS/HSEES/annual2009.html (Accessed March 14, 2013).

6. Health Protection Agency: Health Protection Agency Records an Increase in Chemical Incidents. May 20, 2008. www.hpa.org.uk/NewsCentre/NationalPressReleases/2008PressReleases/080520ChemIncidents (Accessed March 12, 2013).

7. Baumgarten S. European Chemical Accidents Fall Further on EU Seveso Directive. *ICIS News.* August 17, 2010; 20: 09. http://www.icis.com/resources/news/2010/08/17/9385916/european-chemical-accidents-fall-further-on-eu-seveso-directive/ (Accessed August 21, 2015).

8. Koenig KL. Strip and shower: the duck and cover for the 21st century. *Ann Emerg Med* September 2003; 42(3): 391–394.

9. *OSHA Best Practices for Hospital-Based First Receivers of Victims from Mass Casualty Incidents Involving the Release of Hazardous Substances. Occupational Safety and Health Administration.* U.S. Department of Labor, OSHA 3249–08N, 2005. https://www.osha.gov/dts/osta/bestpractices/firstreceivers_hospital.pdf (Accessed August 21, 2015).

10. Cox RD. Decontamination and management of hazardous materials exposure victims in the emergency department. *Ann Emerg Med* 1994; 23: 761–770.

11. Patient Decontamination in a Mass Chemical Exposure Incident: National Planning Guidance for Communities. Department of Health & Human Services. Draft / For Public Comment, v. 17, February 21, 2014.

12. Guidelines for Mass Casualty Decontamination During a Terrorist Chemical Agent Incident. U.S. Army Soldier and Biological Chemical Command (SBCCOM), Aberdeen Proving Grounds, Maryland, January 2000. http://www.au.af.mil/au/awc/awcgate/army/sbccom_decon.pdf (Accessed August 21, 2015).

13. Levitin H, Siegelson H, Dickinson S, et al. Decontamination of Mass Casualties – Re-evaluating Existing Dogma. *Prehosp and Disaster Med* July–September 2003; 18(3): 199–207.

14. Hurst G. *Decontamination. Textbook of Military Medicine, Warfare, Weaponry, and the Casualty. Medical Aspects of Chemical and Biological Warfare.* Office of the U.S. Surgeon General, Department of the Army, 1997; 351–359.

15. Lake W. Chemical Weapons Improved Response Program. *Guidelines for Mass Casualty Decontamination During a Terrorist Chemical Agent Incident.* Domestic Preparedness Program, U.S. Soldier Biological and Chemical Command, 2000.

16. Clarke S, Chilcott, R, Wilson J, et al. Decontamination of Multiple Casualties Who Are Chemically Contaminated: A Challenge for Acute Hospitals. *Prehosp and Disaster Med* March–April 2008; 23(2): 175–181.

17. Institute of Medicine. National Research Council. *Chemical and Biological Terrorism. Research and Development in Improved Civilian Medical Response*, Washington, DC, National Academy Press, 1999: 97–109.

18. Gruber R, Laub D. The effect of hydrotherapy on the clinical course and pH of experimental cutaneous chemical burns. *Plast Reconstr Surg* 1995; 55(2): 200–204.

19. Amlot R, Larner J, Matar H, et al. Comparative Analysis of Showering Protocols for Mass-Casualty Decontamination. *Prehosp and Disaster Med* September–October 2010; 25(5): 435–439.

20. Leonard L, Scheulen J, Munster A. Chemical burns: Effect of prompt first aid. *J Trauma* 1982; 22(5): 420–423.

21. Moran K, O'Reilly T, Munster A. Chemical burns. A ten-year experience. *Ann Surg* 1987; 53(11): 652–653.

22. Fredrikson T. Percutaneous absorption of parathion and paraxon. *Arch Environ Health* 1961; 3: 67–70.

23. Brown V, Box V, Simpson BJ. Decontamination procedures for skin exposed to phenolic substances. *Arch Environ Health* 1975; 30: 3–6.

24. Correri P, Morris M, Pruitt B. The treatment of chemical burns: Specialized diagnostic, therapeutic, and prognostic considerations. *J Trauma* 1970; 30: 634–642.

25. Wexter R, Malbach H. In-vivo percutaneous absorption and decontamination of pesticides in humans. *J Toxicol Environ of Health* 1985; 16: 25–37.

26. Weber L, Zesch, Rozman K. Decontamination of human skin exposed to 2,3,7,8-tetrachlorodibenzene-p-diuain (CDD) in vitro. *Arch of Env Health* 1992; 47(4): 302–308.

27. Nocera A, Levitin H, Hilton M. Dangerous Bodies: A case of fatal aluminum phosphide poisoning. *Med J of Australia* 2000; 173(3): 133–135.

28. Schultz, M., Cisek, J, Wabeke R. Simulated exposure of hospital emergency personnel to solvent vapors and respirable dust during decontamination of chemically exposed patients. *Annals Emerg Med* September 1995; 26(3): 324–329.

29. U.S. Department of Health and Human Services, Radiation Emergency Medical Management, Guidance on Diagnosis & Treatment for Health Care Providers, Decontamination Procedures. www.remm.nlm.gov/ext_contamination.htm (Accessed on March 14, 2013).

30. Centers for Disease Control and Prevention, Emerging Infectious Disease. Investigation of Bioterrorism-Related Anthrax, United States, 2001: Epidemiologic Findings. http://wwwnc.cdc.gov/eid/article/8/10/02-0353_article.htm (Accessed March 12, 2013).

31. Bartholomew RE. Mystery illness at Melbourne Airport: toxic poisoning or mass hysteria? *Med J Aust* December 5–19, 2005;183(11–12): 564–566.

32. Hazardous Waste Operations and Emergency Response. Occupational Safety & Health Administration Vol 29 CFR Part 1910.120, U.S. Department of Labor. http://www.nps.gov/policy/DOrders/HAZWOPR.pdf (Accessed August 21, 2015).

33. Designing an Effective PPE Program. Canadian Centre for Occupational Health and Safety. January 2011. www.ccohs.ca/oshanswers/Prevention/ppe/designin.html (Accessed March 14, 2013).

34. Ordinance on Industrial Safety and Health, Ministry of Labour Ordinance No. 32 & 212, Chapter II. Japan International Center for Occupational Safety and Health, Government of Japan. https://www.jniosh.go.jp/icpro/jicosh-old/english/law/IndustrialSafetyHealth_Ordinance/index.html (Accessed August 21, 2015).

35. Centers for Disease Control and Prevention. Emergency Preparedness and Response. http://www.bt.cdc.gov (Accessed March 12, 2013).

36. U.S. Army Medical Research Institute of Infectious Diseases (USAMRIID). http://www.usamriid.army.mil (Accessed March 12, 2013).

37. US Department of Homeland Security. http://www.dhs.gov/index.shtm (Accessed March 12, 2013).

38. Agency for Toxic Substances and Disease Registry. http://www.atsdr.cdc.gov/Mhmi/mmg166.html (Accessed March 12, 2013).

39. Chemical Safety Alert: First Responders' Environmental Liability Due To Mass Decontamination Runoff. United States Environmental Protection Agency, Office of Solid Waste and Emergency Response, EPA 550-F-00–009. July 2000. http://www2.epa.gov/sites/production/files/2013-11/documents/onepage.pdf (Accessed August 21, 2015).

40. Auf der Heide E. Disaster planning, Part II. Disaster problems, issues, and challenges identified in the research literature. *Emerg Med Clin North Am* 1996; 14(2): 453–480.

41. Okumura T, Suzuki K, Fukuda A, et al. The Tokyo subway sarin attack: disaster management, Part 2: Hospital response. *Acad Emerg Med* 1998; 5(6): 618–624.

42. Okumura T, Takasu N, Ishimatsu S, et al. Report on 640 victims of the Tokyo subway sarin attack. *Ann Emerg Med* 1996; 28(2): 129–135.

43. Koenig KL, Boatright CJ, Hancock JA, et al. Healthcare facility-based decontamination of victims exposed to chemical, biological, and radiological material. *Am J Emerg Med* 2008; 26(1): 71–80.

44. Lavoie FW, Coomes T, Cisek JE, et. al. Emergency department external decontamination for hazardous chemical exposure. *Vet Hum Toxicol* 1992; 34: 61–64.

45. Freyberg C, Arquilla B, Fertel B, et.al. Disaster Preparedness: Hospital Decontamination and the Pediatric Patient – Guidelines for Hospitals and Emergency Planners. *Prehosp and Disaster Med* March–April 2008; 23(2): 166–173.

46. Languages throughout the World. University of Pennsylvania Department of Linguistics. http://www.ling.upenn.edu/courses/ling001/world_languages.html (Accessed January 9, 2013).

47. Hearing Loss Numbers in Different Countries. Hear-it AISBL. http://www.hear-it.org/Hearing-loss-in-different-countries (Accessed March 12, 2013).

48. Bulson J, Bulson TC, Vande Guchte KS: Hospital-based special needs patient decontamination: Lessons from the shower. *Am J Disaster Med* 2010 November–December; 5(6): 353–360.

49. Taylor K, Balfanz-Vertiz K, Humrickhouse R, et.al. Decontamination with At-Risk Populations: Lessons Learned. *The Internet Journal of Rescue and Disaster Medicine* 2008; 9(1). http://ispub.com/IJRDM/9/1/12519 (Accessed August 21, 2015).

17

QUARANTINE

James G. Hodge, Jr. and Lawrence O. Gostin

OVERVIEW

Quarantine is one of the oldest known public health powers. Its primary objective is to prevent the introduction, transmission, and spread of communicable diseases. Together with other social distancing measures designed to exclude persons with infectious conditions from work, school, or other public settings[1] (notably isolation and civil commitment), quarantine has been used for centuries. The result is to sequester potentially infectious individuals and groups until they no longer present risks to others, and thus may safely circulate in society. The legal authority to quarantine exists within many nations globally, and pursuant to state and local laws in the United States. When practiced efficiently, appropriately, and consistent with best public health practices, quarantine can be highly efficacious in limiting the spread of communicable diseases, especially those spread easily through airborne transmission.

In practice however, protocols on time and distance necessary to contain diseases via quarantine are often missing; and effectiveness of differing levels of separation is not well documented. Clear and convincing evidence to support the use of quarantine is sometimes difficult to establish (especially in emergencies) raising concerns over potential violations of civil liberties.[2] The history of quarantine internationally is marked with well-documented human rights abuses and infringements of legally protected individual rights. Criteria for the use of quarantine have often been subjective or based on discriminatory practices. Groups of individuals and entire communities have been cast away from society for years and denied access to essential services.

Quarantine enforcement in the modern era poses challenges due in part to the rapid transmission of infectious diseases throughout a global population that is constantly on the move. Even when quarantine is necessitated, there are few effective options for how to provide or pay for its secondary effects, including lost wages, impact on business contracts and services, and logistical support related to providing sustenance, medical services, and communications for those individuals confined. Beyond these adverse impacts on individuals, whole societies can be impacted by reductions in trade and tourism.

As noted by the World Health Organization (WHO), crude methods of quarantine lacking public health justification are ineffective and abusive. Successful implementation of quarantine requires adherence to best practices and refined guidelines. Current international guidelines focus containment strategies on real-time epidemiology and evidence-based data, rather than resorting to quarantine and border control.[3] Clarifying objectives, defining terms, and establishing realistic policies through quarantine, however, are thought to reduce the impact of contagious disease outbreaks.

This chapter reviews the complexities of quarantine related to three interlinked perspectives: 1) scope and effectiveness; 2) legal authority; and 3) ethical and logistical challenges of implementation.

CURRENT STATE OF THE ART

Defining Quarantine

The essential premise of quarantine (i.e., separating those with exposure to communicable disease from the healthy) dates back to Biblical and Koranic references that include isolation of lepers. The term quarantine may have originated from practices dating back to the 1400s AD when ships were detained for 40 days outside of Italian ports to protect against foreign diseases. The word is derived from the Italian *quaranta* meaning "forty."[4]

In modern times, quarantine is sometimes used interchangeably with similar public health powers of isolation and civil commitment however, there are major differences. The U.S. Centers for Disease Control and Prevention (CDC) distinguishes quarantine from isolation and provides additional data on legislative authorities, enforcement, and historical uses of quarantine within the United States. According to CDC, quarantine is defined as "the restriction of activities or limitation of freedom of movement of those presumed exposed to a communicable disease in such a manner as to prevent effective contact with those not so exposed."[5] Quarantine applies to the separation of exposed (potentially infected) persons from unexposed persons. Conversely, "isolation" refers to the "separation of a[n infected] person or group of persons from other persons to prevent the spread of infection." Simply stated,

Table 17.1. Efficacy of Differing Civil Confinement Strategies

Type	Pros	Cons	Efficacy	Control
Isolation	■ Known infectious patient ■ Closely monitored	■ Lack of capacity for large-scale events	Widely accepted as effective	Compulsory or voluntary
Home Quarantine also called: ■ self-quarantine ■ sheltering in place	■ Less onerous ■ Logistically simpler ■ Socially and politically acceptable	■ Difficult to monitor and enforce ■ May place family members at risk ■ Requires significant logistical support, e.g., for medical care, heating, food, and water	Thought to be effective	Voluntary but could be compulsory
Work Quarantine (generally for healthcare workers: permitted to work, but restricted to home when not working)	■ Keeps essential employees at their jobs ■ Closely monitored	■ Risk of transmission of infection to vulnerable persons congregated together	Unknown	Voluntary but could be compulsory
Travelers' Quarantine	■ Addresses the risk of transmission from areas with suspected disease ■ Population is confined to the transport vehicle	■ Confines unexposed without confirmation of suspected disease ■ Cohorting may expose susceptible individuals to disease ■ Entails potential economic harms to the traveler	Unknown	Compulsory
Institutional Quarantine (applies to institutions or geographic areas)	■ Cohorting is easier than assessing individuals ■ May increase surge capacity	■ Rapid spread of disease in confined and crowded areas	Unknown	Compulsory
Cordon Sanitaire also called: ■ Perimeter quarantine ■ Geographic quarantine	■ Restricts travel into or out of an area	■ May restrict unnecessarily	Unknown	Compulsory

quarantine involves "exposed" populations, whereas *isolation* restricts movement of "ill" persons. Civil commitment is different from both practices. It refers to the "detention of an individual, usually in a hospital or other health care setting, for the purposes of providing care and treatment." Table 17.1 illustrates the efficacy of different forms of these civil confinement strategies.

Modern public health laws authorize the practice of quarantine and isolation in routine and emergency settings. In the United States, the Model State Emergency Health Powers Act (MSEHPA),[6] which applies to state-based declared emergencies, and the Turning Point Model State Public Health Act, which applies to routine settings in public health practice, properly reflect the distinctions between quarantine and isolation (Figure 17.1).[7]

Per MSEHPA, *quarantine* is defined as "the restriction of the activities of *healthy* persons who have been exposed to a case of communicable disease during its period of communicability to prevent disease transmission during the incubation period if infection should occur."[6] Thus, *quarantine* refers to the physical separation and confinement of an individual or groups of individuals who are or may have been exposed to a contagious or possibly contagious disease but who do not show signs or symptoms of infection. Given that persons can be contagious prior to exhibiting symptoms, the purpose of such separation is to prevent or limit the transmission of the disease to non-quarantined individuals. Thus, for diseases that are not contagious prior to symptom onset, quarantine would not be a scientifically supported public health strategy. Despite this, sociopolitical factors have resulted in forced quarantine in some settings, such as

The Model State Emergency Health Preparedness Act. Developed after the U.S. anthrax incidences of 2001, and in an effort to address the emergence of future biologic threats, this guidance was offered to assist states in updating antiquated public health law. It addresses:

Purposes and definitions
Planning for a public health emergency
Measures to detect and track public health emergencies
Declaring a state of public health emergency
Special powers during a state of public health emergency: control of property
Special powers during a state of public health emergency: control of persons
Public information regarding a public health emergency

The Turning Point Model State Public Health Act. Adopts a systematic approach to the implementation of public health responsibilities and authorities, presents a broad mission for state and local public health agencies, and balances the protection of the public's health with respect for the rights of individual and groups. It addresses:

Purposes and definitions
Mission and functions
Public health infrastructure
Collaboration and relationships with public and private sector partners
Public health authorities/powers (including quarantine and isolation)
Public health emergencies
Public health information privacy
Administrative procedures, civil and criminal enforcement, and immunities

Figure 17.1. The Model State Emergency Health Powers Act and Turning Point Model State Public Health Act.

Table 17.2. The International Health Regulations (2005)

Developed by WHO, the IHR is a legally-binding international agreement providing a framework for the coordination of the management of events that may constitute a public health emergency of international concern (PHEIC). It was designed to improve the capacity of countries to detect, assess, notify and respond to public health threats. Member states are urged to build, strengthen, and maintain the required capacities identified in the IHR, collaborate to ensure their effective implementation, and develop the necessary public health capacities and legal and administrative provisions within the regulation. IHR provisions address:

Definitions, purpose and scope, principles, and responsible authorities
Information and public health response
Recommendations
Points of entry
Public health measures (including quarantine)
Health documents
Charges
General provisions
IHR roster of experts, the emergency committee, and the review
  committee

during the 2014 Ebola epidemic.[8] Quarantine restrictions can be voluntary or involuntary, the choice of which raises different legal, social, financial, and logistical challenges.[9]

Isolation is defined in MSEHPA as "the separation, for the period of communicability, of *known* infected persons in such places and under such conditions as to prevent or limit the transmission of the infectious agent."[6] In this context, *isolation* refers to the physical separation and confinement of an individual or groups of individuals who are infected or reasonably believed to be infected with a contagious or possibly contagious disease. Its purpose is to prevent or limit the transmission of the disease to non-isolated individuals.

On the global scale, the International Health Regulations (IHR), revised in 2005 by the World Health Assembly (Table 17.2), and implemented on June 15, 2007, serve as the model for global health security. The IHR – containing sixty-six articles organized into ten parts, with nine annexes – is among the world's most widely adopted treaties, with 194 state parties.[10] The IHR reflect enhanced practices in global health, international security, epidemic alert and response, travel restrictions, and use of quarantine. WHO's strategic plan has evolved to a proactive risk management process focusing on source containment, active surveillance, prompt detection, isolation of new cases, and rapid tracing of contacts. In addition, the plan calls for building capacity to cope with an inevitable pandemic.[11] The IHR focuses on early identification and interventions based on appropriate decision making and evidence-based data,[12] to "prevent, protect against, control and provide a public health response to the international spread of disease in ways that are commensurate with and restricted to public health risks, and which avoid unnecessary interference with international traffic and trade."[13]

Quarantine in Theory and Practice

In theory, separating highly contagious individuals from susceptible persons is a sound method for limiting the spread of infection. Research suggests that quarantine can be effective given a compliant community and appropriately managed resources.[14] However, in practice it is difficult to maintain complete sep-

aration of individuals or groups during the time of infectivity. While comprehensive containment strategies to limit the impacts of emerging infectious diseases should include elements of physical separation, quarantine alone will not prevent the spread of disease. Effective emergency planning within the larger context of disease outbreak requires multiple approaches. Global travel, enforcement, employment and financial considerations, and population medical needs of a physical or psychological nature can all complicate a quarantine plan. Appropriate logistical support for affected individuals and healthcare workers caring for them are critical to ensure effective quarantine.[15]

Historically, crude quarantine measures have been largely ineffective. At the turn of the twentieth century, for example, San Francisco's Board of Health quarantined a predominantly Chinese neighborhood in response to nine reported cases of plague. Although all known infected persons were limited to a seven-block radius, the quarantine reached twelve blocks; implicating thousands of otherwise healthy Chinese-Americans. In a resulting case, *Jew Ho v. Williamson*, the court opined not only that such action was insufficient to quell disease, but also a direct violation of equal protection principles via the Fourteenth Amendment of the U.S. Constitution.[16]

Modern examples demonstrate how quarantine can thwart the spread of disease. Flying home from Africa in April 2012, Lisa Sievers reported to her mother about a rash similar to one she noticed on her newly adopted son from Uganda. Concerned, Ms. Sievers's mother contacted a local hospital.[17] Unable to confirm the severity of the rash, the hospital immediately contacted CDC, activating a series of measures to prevent the spread of what was thought to be monkeypox, a rare viral disease with a rash similar in appearance to the rash of smallpox. CDC ordered the plane to land in Chicago, and in collaboration with local public health authorities, temporarily quarantined passengers to determine whether the rash posed a real threat to the public's health. Ultimately, it was determined that the rash presented no such danger. However, the expeditious resolution of the hazard demonstrates the modern capacity for government to rapidly prevent the spread of disease through quarantine.[18]

Improved public health responses worldwide, including better sanitation, mass immunization, and skilled epidemiological investigations, have greatly reduced the prevalence of infectious diseases, and therefore their ability to spread. While controversial, countries have employed travel restrictions as a first line of defense against the spread of disease. During the 2003 SARS global outbreak, for example, WHO administered unprecedented travel restriction advisories, halting nearly all non-essential travel in Hong Kong, Guangdong province, Beijing, Shanxi province, Tianjin, Inner Mongolia, Taiwan, and Toronto, Ontario, Canada.[19] Similar efforts in select jurisdictions were also deployed by specific countries, including China, in response to the 2009/2010 H1N1 pandemic.[20]

With increased ability for persons to travel globally, the threat of cross-border spread of disease is high. Figure 17.2 depicts the worldwide spread of H1N1 influenza in an 8-month period from April to November 2009. Notwithstanding some nationally issued travel restrictions (noted previously) and related travel advisories from WHO, the virus reached every continent and caused hundreds of thousands of cases and many deaths. This illustration highlights the potential need for social distancing measures like quarantine to restrict travel of individuals who are exposed and isolation of those who present symptoms of infectious disease to help thwart a global outbreak.

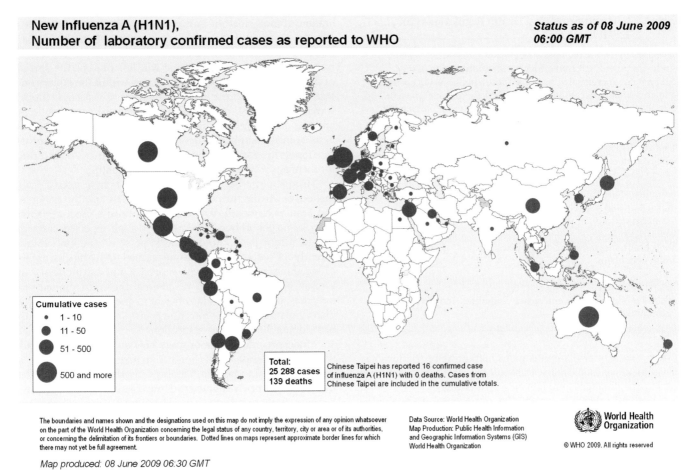

Figure 17.2. Global Spread of H1N1, 2009.

As noted in a study by Pourbohloul and colleagues, contact network modeling suggests that simultaneous case–patient isolation and quarantine of close contacts can substantially improve disease containment.[21] With the addition of ring vaccination – a strategy where individuals who may come into direct contact with an infected person or group are identified and vaccinated–[22] quarantine can prevent the spread of disease. Data are conclusive as to the potential to improve public health outcomes by eliminating contacts between infected and susceptible persons. However, study authors note the need for strong surveillance, reliable rapid diagnostic tests, and social acceptance of quarantine measures; all of which may be unavailable or contested in specific countries or settings depending on available resources and commitment to compliance with IHR standards.

In limited instances where vaccines or other countermeasures are not available or capable of thwarting the spread of infectious diseases, quarantine may be needed. Actual separation of infectious persons from noninfectious individuals through social distancing measures, including isolation and quarantine, may be the only major course of public health intervention. Strategies to prevent the spread of disease inevitably include quarantine, but should also focus on augmenting surge capacity to optimize population outcomes. An outbreak is a dynamic type of public health emergency and strategies must be flexible to account for the influx of either more patients or of more resources (e.g., vaccines and other countermeasures).

Healthcare facilities have isolation procedures and methods for separating infectious patients from the general hospital (or other healthcare entity) population. In the United States, The Joint Commission, which accredits healthcare facilities, requires hospitals and other entities to specify facility responsibilities when governmental authorities establish quarantine.[23] CDC's Pandemic Influenza Plan identifies isolation of infectious patients in private rooms or cohort units as a measure of controlling disease transmission in healthcare facilities.[24] Coordinating healthcare workers assigned to an outbreak unit is needed, as is consistent training in implementing quarantine measures.[25] In addition, caution must be exercised to prevent cohorting that exposes persons without the disease of concern to infected patients who may be contagious.

In 2003, quarantine practices were integral to controlling the spread of SARS. Still, such practices reportedly caused transmission of SARS to healthy individuals in Canada when those without the disease were exposed and confined with infected cohorts.[26] Multiple studies have reviewed containment strategies but not quantified the full impact and effectiveness of quarantine alone. Voluntary compliance with quarantine orders during SARS was greater than 90% among most populations; generalized studies indicate that 100% compliance may not be necessary.[27]

In 2014, while not evidence-based,[52] quarantine measures were implemented with varying effectiveness to combat the spread of Ebola virus disease (EVD) in West Africa. Due to the lack of effective EVD treatments and vaccines, public health responses centered on quarantine, isolation, contact tracing, and disinfection.[28] Unlike past Ebola outbreaks, researchers suggested that the use of sanitary burial practices alone was insufficient to control transmission rates, requiring the concurrent use of quarantine and other social distancing measures.[29] Because EVD symptoms may appear up to 21 days after first exposure,[30] quarantine measures had a finite end point. Yet, due to the high morbidity and mortality rates of EVD, some experts suggested they had to be stringently enforced to prove effective. Mandatory enforcement can lead to significant negative consequences on quarantined individuals.[8]

In September 2014, a Liberian, Thomas Eric Duncan, entered the United States. Despite being asymptomatic for EVD during his air travel, Duncan presented to a Dallas-area hospital with symptoms shortly after arriving in Texas.[31] Duncan eventually succumbed to EVD in early October, leaving behind multiple exposed contacts subject to mandatory quarantine including family members, healthcare workers, and emergency medical providers. While none of the contacts contracted Ebola, their lives were significantly impacted by the quarantine through social stigma and public fear, the inability to return to work or school,[32] and difficulty in finding suitable housing.[33]

Legal Issues Underlying the Use and Implementation of Quarantine

Public health powers to quarantine individuals and groups exist at all levels of governance in most countries and many provinces or states. The complexity of governance creates numerous overlaps as well as gaps in containment of disease spread. Cross-jurisdictional issues require clear guidance and defined lines of authority to enable authorities to execute appropriate powers.

The aforementioned IHR's purpose is achieved at both the national and international level through: 1) routine public health protection – ongoing surveillance and response to disease threats within countries and at their borders; and 2) coordinated and proportionate global detection and control of transnational disease threats. The regulations strive to balance public health with trade and human rights, ensuring that all three are respected.

The IHR require administering states to develop capacities for surveillance and response, including an adequate public health law infrastructure. States have sovereignty to exercise public health powers, such as quarantine, but WHO's director-general can issue recommendations, such as the appropriateness of containment measures, or declaration of a PHEIC. Member states are required to use a decision instrument to determine whether they have a duty to report cases or outbreaks to WHO (Figure 17.3).[34]

On the national level, laws authorizing quarantine can be antiquated and fail to reflect current evidence-based disease management.[35] This observation, in part, led to the development of the aforementioned MSEHPA and Turning Point Act to provide modern legislative/regulatory language for the use of quarantine. These models not only define quarantine, but also provide effective language on its proper use, consistent with a balance of individual constitutional rights and other civil liberties.[36] More than forty U.S. states and the District of Columbia have adopted some portion of MSEHPA, including twenty-eight states that have updated their quarantine laws.[37]

Canada updated its national Quarantine Act[38] following its experience with SARS. Much like other countries, its legal guidance was dated since its initial enactment in 1872. Influenced by MSEHPA and corresponding draft guidance in the IHR, Canada amended its quarantine legislation on June 22, 2007. Conse-

quently, representatives of the Ministry of Health have broad powers to limit the spread of infectious disease, including the capacity to order treatment[39] and detain non-compliant individuals.[40]

In the United States, protecting the public's health via quarantine is largely the responsibility of state and local governments. However, the federal government is authorized to engage in quarantine powers.[41] Federal legislation authorizes the U.S. surgeon general to direct all national quarantine stations, designate their boundaries, and appoint officers to manage them. The secretary of the Department of Health and Human Services (HHS) is authorized "to make and enforce regulations that in [his or her] judgment are necessary to prevent the introduction, transmission, or spread of communicable diseases."[42] Federal authorities govern the introduction of diseases, both foreign and interstate, pursuant to quarantine rules.[43] The federal government can also assist states with execution of their quarantine laws. Although courts have upheld states' primary responsibility for quarantine,[44] the federal government can preempt state power if necessary to control disease spread across state or international borders.[45]

The U.S. CDC's Division of Global Migration and Quarantine operates quarantine stations as part of the comprehensive quarantine system network. Stations are located at twenty ports of entry and land-border crossings focused on the arrival of international travelers. CDC health officers determine appropriate measures to address an ill, or potentially ill, person attempting to enter the country. CDC officials may isolate an individual showing symptoms of contagious disease. If diagnosed with a disease subject to quarantine, CDC authorities permit its officers to detain, admit to a hospital, or confine individuals until the threat of spread is contained or averted.[46] Although legally clear as to CDC's power, an Institute of Medicine (IOM) study found that "most practices of the quarantine stations and their surrogates lack a scientific basis" and were based primarily on "experience and tradition." IOM recommended development of "scientifically sound tools to measure the effectiveness and quality of all operational aspects of the quarantine system."[47]

While CDC proposed significant revisions to communicable disease control regulations in late 2005,[48] including quarantine powers, at the time of this writing, these proposed rules have not been finalized.[49] Specific diseases subject to quarantine must be authorized by Executive Order of the President (Table 17.3),[50] thus requiring amendments to the order each time a new disease emerges (e.g., SARS in 2003).[51] This is inefficient and potentially catastrophic if the legal process cannot move rapidly enough to formally add a condition to the federal list. A more effective approach would include using language such as "any contagious infectious disease that could be a threat to the public health and safety" (like that used in the IHR and MSEHPA) instead of a specific listing of known conditions.[52]

Although broad ranging, neither federal, state, nor local quarantine laws in the United States may unduly infringe on constitutional rights, including due process, right to travel, freedom of religion, or equal protection interests. For example, use of quarantine authority without justification may impinge an individual's right to travel. A government must have some compelling argument that clearly demonstrates that an individual's travel to or from an infected area puts the greater population in danger before it may quarantine the person.

In 2007, a well-publicized case involving an attorney, Andrew Speaker, based in CDC's home jurisdiction (Atlanta, Georgia),

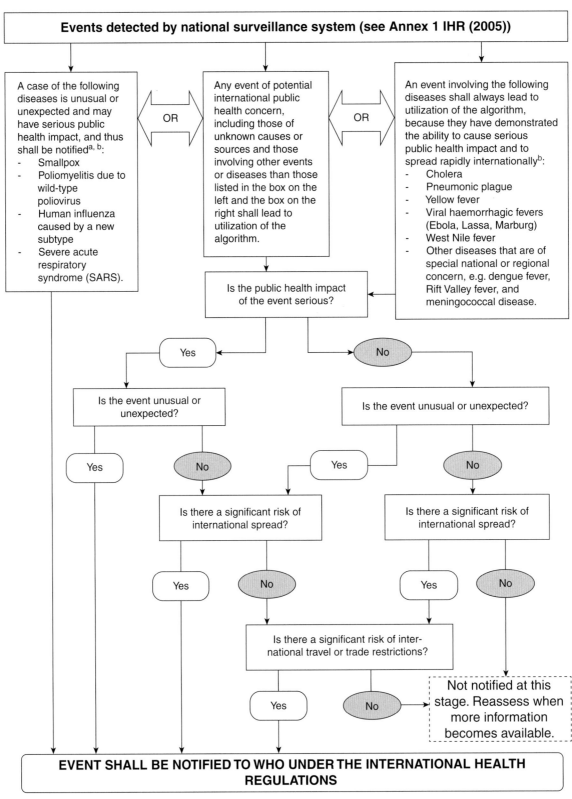

Figure 17.3. Decision Instrument for the Assessment and Notification of Events that May Constitute a Public Health Emergency of International Concern, IHR 2005. *The World Health Report 2007: A Safer Future, Global Public Health Security in the 21st Century.* Geneva: WHO.

Table 17.3. Diseases Subject to U.S. Federal Quarantine as of 2013*

- Cholera
- Diphtheria
- Infectious tuberculosis
- Plague
- Smallpox
- Yellow fever
- SARS
- Viral hemorrhagic fevers
    - Lassa
    - Marburg
    - Ebola
    - Crimean-Congo
    - South American
    - Others not yet isolated or named
- Influenza (caused by novel or reemergent influenza viruses that are causing, or have the potential to cause, a pandemic)

* Defined in Executive Order 13295

tested the efficacy and constitutionality of U.S. quarantine policy. After receiving an initial diagnosis of tuberculosis (TB), Speaker was asked by local health authorities to limit his travel. However, Speaker managed to depart from Atlanta's airport for an extensive European trip to attend his wedding and honeymoon. During the course of the trip, CDC determined that Speaker may have had an extremely drug-resistant form of tuberculosis (XDR-TB). CDC authorities asked Speaker to immediately identify himself to Italian health authorities. Speaker refused. Following an international media storm and questions of whether the privacy of his protected, identifiable health information had been compromised, Speaker eventually returned to the United States days later by flying into Canada and driving across the border into New York State.

When CDC learned of his presence back in the United States, it issued its first federal quarantine order since a suspected smallpox carrier was quarantined in 1963.[53] Speaker surrendered to public health authorities and received treatment in an isolated room at a Denver, Colorado, hospital known for its care of TB cases. Multiple persons close to Speaker during his extensive travel were placed under quarantine for limited duration to ascertain whether they too had contracted TB. Eventually it was determined that Speaker never had XDR-TB, but rather a more common type of the disease that presents less risk to others because it can be more easily treated.

Similar compliance issues impeded quarantine efforts to combat the spread of Ebola during the 2014 outbreak in West Africa. In October 2014, U.S. nurse Kaci Hickox resisted a quarantine order on her return from treating Ebola patients in Sierra Leone.[54] While Hickox exhibited no symptoms of Ebola when arriving at Newark Liberty International Airport, Governors Andrew Cuomo in New York and Chris Christie in New Jersey had implemented automatic quarantine procedures for any healthcare worker returning from West Africa that had contact with Ebola patients, exceeding CDC recommended guidance. After New Jersey rescinded its mandatory quarantine procedure, Hickox returned to her home in Maine where she faced a court-ordered quarantine sought by the state commissioner of health. Hickox contested the order, arguing that automatic quarantines of asymptomatic individuals would discourage health-

care workers from providing aid in Ebola affected countries. State officials in Maine defended the quarantine as a public health necessity. Ultimately, the Maine District Court dismissed the request for mandatory quarantine, allowing Hickox to move about freely, submit to self-monitoring, and report any upcoming travel. She never contracted Ebola and all restrictions were lifted at the end of her twenty-one-day monitoring period. Her case, however, illustrates the effects that inconsistencies at the federal and state levels may have on the efficacy of quarantine measures.

The events surrounding Andrew Speaker and Kaci Hickox not only illustrate the difficulties of issuing and implementing modern quarantine orders, they also demonstrate the complex balance of public and private interests (including strong media influences that dictated, in part, some of the public health interventions undertaken) concerning public health powers like quarantine.

Ethical Issues

Against a backdrop of legal challenges and at times specious empirical support for the use of quarantine in the modern era, core ethical issues arise. Adhering to ethically supported practices in the implementation of quarantine requires government to routinely balance the need for potentially intrusive quarantine measures against the individual's legal rights[55] and ethical interests. Consistent with principles of public health ethics, public health authorities must establish that a significant risk of transmission exists before detaining individuals against their will via quarantine or isolation.[56] Quarantine or isolation is only warranted if based on known, identified public health risks and if there are no other, less restrictive measures that can be taken to adequately abate these risks. When quarantine is ethically justified under these standards, authorities must also provide to the fullest extent possible adequate sustenance, medical treatment, appropriate sanitary conditions, and logistical and psychosocial support for persons under quarantine.[57]

During public health emergencies potentially affecting the health of thousands of people, adherence to these sorts of ethical requirements may arguably be outweighed by the need to implement quarantine measures en masse. In reality, however, failure to subscribe to these and other basic ethical norms, even during emergencies, may ultimately counter the goal of protecting the public's health. To the extent that government must rely on public participation in reasonable and efficacious quarantine measures, public support is required. Unethical practices at the core of quarantine implementation may undermine such support, leading to mistrust of government and societal rejection of specific public health efforts. In this way, attending to ethically sound practices is often synergistic with achieving enhanced public health outcomes.

RECOMMENDATIONS FOR FURTHER RESEARCH

Despite limited empirical data, emergency managers and public health authorities will continue to use quarantine together with other countermeasures to curtail the spread of infectious diseases. Recommendations for further research must focus on realistically achievable results. The following points identify critical areas of study that would contribute to enhanced, effective strategies.

- Improved modeling is needed concerning operational challenges for managing large numbers of displaced individuals. Basic elements of delivery of sustenance, medical services, and support are often missing. Additional needs for communications, financial support, and family integrity must be addressed.
- Timelines must be developed to reflect the duration of optimal separation via quarantine to reduce contagion. Criteria are needed to determine whether the potentially infected population can be identified soon enough to achieve physical separation and limit transmission.
- New metrics may more accurately measure the role of quarantine as an effective strategy within an increasingly mobile, global society.
- Clearly delineated and modern legal authorities must be developed that enable clinicians to act and political figures to decide on the appropriate timing and use of quarantine powers.
- A realistic assessment should be developed regarding the impact of other social distancing measures (e.g., school closure, curfews, evacuations) in conjunction with quarantine.
- Enhanced understanding is needed of the increasing role of media and social networking toward the issuance, implementation, and monitoring of quarantine measures through public and private collaborations in emergencies.
- Quarantine enforcement options should be identified and applied in culturally respectful ways.

Quarantine is an important tool to protect the public's health, especially in the face of a significant threat stemming from highly infectious and potentially deadly diseases. The efficacy, legality, ethicality, and logistical challenges of quarantine implementation are each critical factors, the resolution of which may help to decrease morbidity and mortality during global disasters involving infectious diseases.

REFERENCES

1. Centers for Disease Control and Prevention. Menu of Suggested Provisions For State Tuberculosis Prevention and Control Laws. *July* 6, 2011. http://www.cdc.gov/tb/programs/laws/menu/social.htm (Accessed August 17, 2015).
2. Gostin LO. *Public Health Law: Power, Duty, Restraint*. 2nd ed. Berkeley, University of California Press, 2008.
3. WHO. *The World Health Report 2007: A Safer Future, Global Public Health Security in the 21st Century*. Geneva, 2007.
4. World Health Organization. *The World Health Report 2007: A Safer Future, Global Public Health Security in the 21st Century*. Geneva: WHO.
5. CDC. Smallpox Response Plan. March 2003. http://www.bt.cdc.gov/agent/smallpox/response-plan/files/guide-c-part-2.pdf (Accessed January 14, 2009).
6. Network for Public Health Law. The Model State Emergency Health Powers Act, Summary Matrix. June 2012. http://www.networkforphl.org/_asset/80p3y7/Western-Region–MSEHPA-States-Table-8-10-12.pdf (Accessed December 18, 2009).
7. The Centers for Law and the Public's Health: A Collaborative at Johns Hopkins and Georgetown Universities. The Turning Point Model State Public Health Act. January 27, 2010. http://www.publichealthlaw.net/ModelLaws/MSPHA.php (Accessed December 18, 2012).
8. Koenig KL. Health Care Worker Quarantine for Ebola: To Eradicate the Virus or Alleviate Fear? *Annals Emerg Med*, March 2015; 65(3): 330–331.
9. CDC. Public Health Guidance of Community-Level Preparedness and Response to Severe Acute Respiratory Syndrome (SARS) Version 2, Supplement D: Community Containment Measures, Including Non-Hospital Isolation and Quarantine. January 8, 2004. http://www.cdc.gov/ncidod/sars/guidance/D/pdf/d.pdf (Accessed January 14, 2009).
10. WHO. International Health Regulations (2005), Annex 2. http://www.who.int/csr/ihr/WHA58-en.pdf (Accessed January 14, 2009).
11. WHO. The World Health Report 2007: A Safer Future, Global Public Health Security in the 21st Century. Geneva, WHO, 2007.
12. Fidler DP, Gostin LO. The New International Health Regulations: An historic development for international law and public health. *J Law Med Ethics* 2006; 33(4): 85–94.
13. WHO. Frequently asked questions about the International Health Regulations. 2005. http://www.who.int/csr/ihr/howtheywork/faq/en/index.html#whatis (Accessed January 14, 2009).
14. WHO. *The World Health Report 2007: A Safer Future, Global Public Health Security in the 21st Century*. Geneva, WHO, 2007.
15. Barbera J, Macintyre A, Gostin L, et al. Large-scale quarantine following biological terrorism in the United States: scientific examination, logistic and legal limits, and possible consequences. *JAMA* 2001; 286: 2711–2717.
16. *Jew Ho v. Williamson*, 103 F. 10 (C.C.N.D. Cal. 1900).
17. All-Clear Given for Plane Quarantined at Midway. April 26, 2002. http://www.nbcchicago.com/traffic/transit/ohare-international-airport-delta-flight-quarantine-149141115.html (Accessed August 20, 2015).
18. CDC. Have you Heard? CDC Response to Sick Passenger on Delta Plane in Chicago. April 26, 2012. http://www.cdc.gov/media/haveyouheard/2012.html (Accessed August 20, 2015).
19. Gostin LO, Bayer R, Fairchild AM. Ethical and legal challenges posed by severe acute respiratory syndrome: implications for the control of severe infectious disease threats. *JAMA* 2003; 290: 3229–3237.
20. Hodge, JG. Global legal triage in response to the 2009 H1N1 outbreak. *Minnesota Journal of Law, Science, and Tech* 2010; 11(2): 599–628.
21. Pourbohloul B, Meyers LA, Skowronski DM, Krajden M, Patrick DM, Brunham R. Modeling control strategies of respiratory pathogens. *Emerg Infect Dis* 2005; 11: 1249–1256.
22. Kretzschmar M, van den Hof S, Wallinga J, van Wijngaarden J. Ring vaccination and smallpox control. *Emerg Infect Dis*; May 2004; 10(5): 832–841. http://wwwnc.cdc.gov/eid/article/10/5/03-0419_article.htm (Accessed December 18, 2012).
23. Standing Together: An Emergency Planning Guide for America's Communities. Joint Commission. 2005. http://www.jointcommission.org/assets/1/18/planning_guide.pdf (Accessed August 20, 2015).
24. U.S. Department of Health and Human Services. Pandemic Influenza Plan Supplement 4 Infection Control. http://www.hhs.gov/pandemicflu/plan/sup4.html (Accessed January 14, 2009).
25. Nathawad R, Roblin P, Pruitt D, Arquilla B. Addressing the gaps for preparation in quarantine. *Prehosp and Disaster Med* 2013; 28(2): 132–138.
26. WHO. Weekly Epidemiological Record. May 30, 2003. http://www.who.int/docstore/wer/pdf/2003/wer7822.pdf (Accessed January 14, 2009).
27. CDC. Public Health Guidance of Community-Level Preparedness and Response to Severe Acute Respiratory Syndrome

(SARS) Version 2, Supplement D: Community Containment Measures, Including Non-Hospital Isolation and Quarantine. January 8, 2004. http://www.cdc.gov/sars/guidance/d-quarantine/lessons.pdf (Accessed August 20, 2015.)

28. Pandey A, et al. Strategies for Containing Ebola in West Africa. *Science* 2014; 346(6212): 991–995.

29. *Id.* at 995.

30. CDC. Ebola Virus Disease, Signs and Symptoms. http://www.cdc.gov/vhf/Ebola/symptoms/index.html (Accessed November 2, 2014).

31. Details of Duncan's Treatment Reveal a Wobbly First Response to Ebola. *New York Times.* October 25, 2014. http://www.nytimes.com/interactive/2014/10/25/us/ebola-dallas-timeline.html (Accessed August 19, 2015).

32. Sack K, Healy J, Robles F. Life in Quarantine for Ebola Exposure: 21 Days of Fear and Loathing. *New York Times.* October 18, 2014. http://www.nytimes.com/2014/10/19/us/life-in-quarantine-for-ebola-exposure-21-days-of-fear-and-loathing.html (Accessed August 19, 2015).

33. Schmall E. Ebola Victim's Fiancée Struggles to Rebuild Life. *Associated Press.* October 31, 2014. http://bigstory.ap.org/article/cdccd2330e06495686f626621398a9a2/ebola-victims-fiancée-struggles-rebuild-life (Accessed August 19, 2015).

34. Gostin LO. *Global Health Law: International Law, Global Institutions, and World Health.* Cambridge, MA, Harvard University Press, March 2014. http://www.hup.harvard.edu/catalog.php–isbn=9780674728844 (Accessed August 19, 2015).

35. Gostin LO, Burris S, and Lazzarini Z. The Law and the Public's Health: A Study of Infectious Disease Law in the United States. *Columbia Law Review* 1999. https://litigation-essentials.lexisnexis.com/webcd/app?action=DocumentDisplay&crawlid=1&doctype=cite&docid=99+Colum.+L.+Rev.+59&srctype=smi&srcid=3B15&key=95d4cbe647d743f96b2078d262aca3f0; January, 1999, 99 Colum. L. *Rev.* 59. Reich DS. Modernizing Local Responses to Public Health Emergencies: Bioterrorism. Epidemics, and the Model State Emergency Health Powers Act. *Journal of Contemporary Health Law and Policy* 2003; 19: 379–414.

36. Hodge JG, Gostin LO, Gebbie K, Erickson DL. Transforming public health law: The turning point model state public health act. *J Law, Med & Ethics* 2006; 33(4): 77–84.

37. Network for Public Health Law. The Model State Emergency Health Powers Act, Summary Matrix. June 2012. http://www.networkforphl.org/ asset/80p3y7/Western-Region–MSEHPA-States-Table-8–10–12.pdf (Accessed December 18, 2009).

38. Quarantine Act, S.C. 2005, c. 20. http://laws-lois.justice.gc.ca/PDF/Q-1.1.pdf (Accessed February 4, 2013).

39. Quarantine Act, S.C. 2005, c. 20, s. 26.

40. Quarantine Act, S.C. 2005, c. 20, s. 28.

41. U.S. Code, Title 64. http://www.publichealthlaw.net/Resources/ResourcesPDFs/4quarantine.pdf (Accessed January 14, 2009).

42. 42 U.S.C. § 264 (2012).

43. An Act Granting Additional Quarantine Powers and Imposing Additional Duties upon the Marine Hospital Service. See *Compagnie Francaise de Navigation a Vapeur v. State Board of Health, Louisiana,* 186 U.S. 380, 395–96 (1902).

44. *Hennington v. Georgia,* 163 U.S. 299 (1896) (holding that state police power regulation affecting commerce is valid until super-seded by Congress); see also Cowles, WH. State quarantine laws and the federal constitution. *Am L Rev* 1891; 25: 45–73.

45. *Gibbons v. Ogden,* 22 U.S. 1, 205–206 (1824) ("congress may control the state [quarantine] laws…for the regulation of commerce."); *Compagnie Francaise De Navigation a Vapeur v. Louisiana State Board of Health,* 186 U.S. 380 (1902); *United States v. Shinnick,* 219 F. Supp. 789 (1963).

46. CDC. U.S. Quarantine Stations Fact Sheet. December 2007. http://www.cdc.gov/ncidod/dq/resources/Quarantine_Stations_Fact_Sheet.pdf (Accessed January 14, 2009).

47. IOM. Quarantine Stations at Ports of Entry Protecting the Public's Health, Executive Summary. September 2005. http://www.iom.edu/CMS/3783/22845/29602.aspx (Accessed January 14, 2009).

48. Public Health Service Act §§361–368 (42 U.S.C. 264–271) (authorizing HHS secretary to make and enforce regulations to prevent the introduction or transmission of communicable diseases from foreign countries and from one state into another); U.S. Department of Health and Human Services, Control of Communicable Diseases (Proposed Rule), 42 CFR Parts 70 and 71 (November 30, 2005).

49. Gostin, LO. Federal Executive Power and Communicable Disease Control: CDC Quarantine Regulations, *Hastings Center Report* 2006; 36(2): 10–11.

50. Executive Order 13295 as amended, Revised List of Quarantinable Communicable Diseases. Code of Federal Regulations, Title 3 (2003); Executive Order No. 13375 of April 1, 2005: Amendment to Executive Order No. 13295 Relating to Certain Influenza Viruses and Quarantinable Communicable Diseases. Code of Federal Regulations, Title 3 (2005).

51. Executive Order No.13295, 68 Fed. Reg. 68 (April 4, 2003). http://www.gpo.gov/fdsys/pkg/FR-2003–04–09/pdf/03–8832.pdf (Accessed August 19, 2015).

52. Barbisch D, Shih F, Koenig KL. Is There a Case for Quarantine? Perspectives from SARS to Ebola. *Disaster Medicine and Public Health Preparedness* 2015; 9(5): 547–553.

53. Fidler DP, Gostin LO, Markel H. Through the Quarantine Looking Glass: Drug-Resistant Tuberculosis and Public Health Governance, Law, and Ethics. *J Law, Med & Ethics* 2007; 35: 526–533.

54. Bidgood J, Philipps D. Judge in Maine Eases Restrictions on Nurse. *New York Times.* October 31, 2014. http://www.nytimes.com/2014/11/01/us/ebola-maine-nurse-kaci-hickox.html (Accessed August 19, 2015).

55. *Vitek v. Jones,* 445 U.S. 480, 491 (1980) (holding that an inmate was entitled to due process before transfer to mental institution); see *Addington v. Texas,* 441 U.S. 418, 425 (1979) (holding that civil commitment is a "significant deprivation of liberty").

56. Burris S. Fear itself: AIDS, herpes and public health decisions. *Yale Law and Policy Review* 1985; 3: 479–518. See *Kansas v. Crane,* 534 U.S. 407 (2002) (to commit repeat sex offenders, the state must demonstrate "proof of serious difficulty in controlling behavior" which can distinguish a committable offender from a typical recidivist).

57. WHO. *The World Health Report 2007: A Safer Future, Global Public Health Security in the 21st Century.* Geneva, WHO, 2007.

18

MASS DISPENSING OF MEDICAL COUNTERMEASURES

Susan E. Gorman

The findings and conclusions in this chapter are those of the author and do not necessarily represent the views of the Centers for Disease Control and Prevention.

OVERVIEW

Following a terrorist incident or other large-scale public health emergency, the need to distribute antibiotic prophylaxis or vaccinations rapidly to a large population may be necessary. To successfully accomplish this task, a significant amount of planning and preparation must occur in advance. The ability to respond in the initial phase of an infectious disease outbreak at the local, regional, state, national, or international levels is a key component of public health preparedness. This was demonstrated in the United States in 2001, when more than 30,000 people were advised to take antibiotics during the anthrax incident.[1] Although the need for planning for mass dispensing is essential, many areas have not engaged in the process. A survey in one U.S. state showed that fewer than half of 138 community health centers polled in 2004 had begun to address bioterrorism issues in their planning efforts; only 19% surveyed were included in their county's mass prophylaxis plan.[2] In the same survey, only 46% had sufficient space to create a mass immunization or vaccination area, and 23% had plans to communicate bioterrorism incidents with the public and media.[2] Results such as these emphasize the need for continued and enhanced planning. With the reduction in public health infrastructure funding that has occurred since this poll was taken, emergency preparedness efforts may decline further as available resources are used to maintain necessary daily functions. The inability of a community to dispense needed pharmaceuticals efficiently and effectively to its population may result in significant morbidity and mortality. Therefore, the development of clinics for mass dispensing and mass vaccination should be incorporated into community disaster plans.

Historical Perspectives

Information gathered from past experiences can be applied to future preparations for mass vaccinations and mass pro-

phylaxis. Past mass vaccination campaigns that successfully halted outbreaks have demonstrated areas for improvement. In 1947, New York City conducted a mass vaccination campaign that successfully halted an outbreak of smallpox. Although incomplete vaccine tracking and record keeping make it difficult to establish the exact number of individuals vaccinated in April 1947, it is estimated that more than 2.5 million persons received a smallpox vaccine. This vaccination campaign also dealt with vaccine shortages and little public health information, such as vaccine side effects, was provided to the general populace.[3]

In an effort to halt a smallpox outbreak that began with an infected person returning from a pilgrimage to Mecca, the Federal Epidemiologic Commission organized a larger mass vaccination campaign in Yugoslavia in 1972. Over a period of 3 weeks, they vaccinated 18 million persons out of a population of 20.8 million. The epidemic included 175 cases and 35 deaths and was declared under control in 6 weeks. This mass vaccination campaign noted unsuccessful vaccination uptakes and included the use of strict isolation and quarantine as well as declaration of martial law to restrict population movement into affected areas.[4]

A historical review of the 1976 swine flu vaccination program may also prove informative for current mass vaccination planning efforts. In February 1976, serologic studies of personnel at Fort Dix, New Jersey, suggested that over 200 persons had been infected with a strain of virus similar to the one that caused the 1918 influenza pandemic. By March of that year, public health authorities decided to launch a mass vaccination program to prevent the effects of a possible pandemic. Information gathered from this campaign applies directly to current mass dispensing and mass vaccination planning. This includes addressing the following issues: 1) consideration of special populations when formulating vaccines or antimicrobials; 2) liability issues related to medical countermeasures; 3) interagency cooperation at various levels of government; 4) establishment of surveillance systems for adverse events; and 5) provision of appropriate and timely public health messaging.[5]

CURRENT STATE OF THE ART

Examples of International Efforts

Given the ease of international travel and the potential for rapid spread of disease, a public health emergency in one country has the propensity to become an international issue. Many countries are preparing to undertake mass vaccination or mass dispensing campaigns. For example, Israel has stockpiled enough smallpox vaccine for its population and visitors. Supervision of mass vaccination occurs under the direction of Public Health Services within the Ministry of Health. This group anticipates operating vaccination clinics 24 hours a day. District health officers would determine the clinic locations.[6] Clinic sites might include schools, large existing ambulatory care centers, or other appropriate community buildings.

The United Kingdom anticipates using Smallpox Management and Response Teams, whose members have been vaccinated prior to the event, to assist with the initial management of a smallpox incident. If an outbreak occurred, initial cases and contacts would be vaccinated; however, it is planned that sufficient vaccine will be available to vaccinate the entire country's population should it be deemed necessary. In the event of multiple attacks, mass vaccination would be considered if new cases were identified without an epidemiological link to previously identified cases, or if triggered by overwhelming public demand in the face of an increasing threat. Regional epidemiologists are responsible for identifying, training, and vaccinating individuals who would then serve on regional response teams. In addition, these epidemiologists are also responsible for identifying vaccination centers and training vaccinators. Vaccination centers could be activated and operational within 24 hours.[7] Vaccinia Immune Globulin would be delivered along with vaccine to local authorities within 48 hours of the decision to begin a mass vaccination campaign.[8]

The Public Health Agency of Canada maintains a 24-hour response capability through their National Emergency Stockpile System. This program provides health and social service supplies during an emergency when provinces and territories are overwhelmed. This stockpile system covers emergencies ranging from pandemic influenza to terrorism incidents and natural disasters, and includes assets such as antibiotics, antivirals, and other supplies and equipment.[9]

The World Health Organization (WHO) recognizes the need for developing countries to have access to certain medical countermeasures that may be part of a mass dispensing or mass vaccination campaign. In order to preempt a possible influenza pandemic, the pharmaceutical company Roche donated 3 million treatment courses of antiviral medication in 2005 for use in containment strategies addressing human cases of avian influenza. Logistical considerations for the WHO stockpile include the ability to deliver a portion of this stockpile within 24 hours to countries where assistance will most likely be needed.[10]

WHO distributed more than 2.4 million doses of antivirals to 72 countries during the H1N1 influenza pandemic in 2009. Since then, Roche has donated an additional 5.65 million doses of antiviral medication to replenish depleted stocks. Through the Global Outbreak Alert and Response Network, WHO can also provide rapid technical assistance in managing an outbreak, including clinical guidelines for the use of antiviral prophylaxis or disease treatment. As part of the containment strategy, WHO estimates that the amount of antivirals needed includes enough treatment courses for 25% of the population and enough prophylaxis courses for the remaining 75% of the population.[11] WHO is developing procedures for the distribution of antivirals within the outbreak area.

WHO is also in the process of developing a smallpox vaccine stockpile and will build this strategic stockpile in Geneva. Countries are invited to donate and maintain additional stocks pledged to WHO that would be dispatched to where they are most needed in the event of an emergency. Progress on this reserve is being made steadily, with 2.5 million doses in Geneva, and more than 32 million additional doses donated or pledged by various countries, including 20 million doses from the United States, 5 million from France, 4 million from the United Kingdom, 2 million from Germany, 1 million from Japan, and 10,000 from New Zealand.

Examples of Federal Assistance from the U.S. Model: Strategic National Stockpile and Cities Readiness Initiative Programs

In a large-scale public health emergency requiring mass antibiotic prophylaxis or vaccination, federal assistance may involve procuring necessary medications from several sources. In the United States, the Strategic National Stockpile (SNS) is a federally managed repository of antibiotics, vaccines, antitoxins, antivirals, medical supplies, and equipment that is available to supply affected areas once local, state, or regional resources are depleted or when systems are overwhelmed. The U.S. Centers for Disease Control and Prevention (CDC), part of the Department of Health and Human Services (HHS), manages the SNS program. This repository of medical countermeasures and supplies is maintained in 12-Hour Push Packages and in Supplier Managed Inventory (SMI). The 12-Hour Push Packages are dispatched when the threat is unknown or when rapid delivery is essential. Each 12-Hour Push Package weighs approximately 45 metric tons and is made up of more than 100 different line items. One 12-Hour Push Package is designed for transport without repackaging either on eight semi-tractor trailers or on one wide-body cargo jet. The 12-Hour Push Packages are packed in specialized cargo containers prior to an incident and are strategically located across the United States with the goal to reach any state or territory within 12 hours of a federal decision to deploy assets.

SMI consists of large amounts of palletized material, and is generally delivered after the 12-Hour Push Packages are deployed. SMI can also be used as an initial response when the type of threat is known, as it can be configured for a specific identified incident. The delivery timeframe for SMI may vary, but for most incidents, it is estimated to be 24–36 hours after the federal decision to deploy assets is made. SNS personnel determine the optimal method of transportation for both the 12-Hour Push Package and SMI based on weather, safety, security, and other incident-specific factors at the time of the event.

Included in the SNS are antibiotics in 10-day unit of use bottles. These are dispensed directly to members of the public, thereby saving the time needed to remove the antibiotics from bulk bottles and place them into individual containers. Vaccines for smallpox and anthrax are also included in the SNS, but would be shipped only when clinically indicated, in the event of a smallpox case or widespread public exposure to aerosolized anthrax. Federal planning and response efforts continue to evolve as more scientific data are collected and modeled, and inventory contents and quantities in the SNS change based on an annual review of these new data (Figure 18.1).

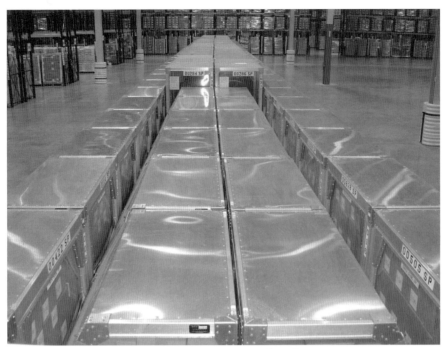

Figure 18.1. SNS 12-Hour Push Package.

Within the United States, the governor of an affected state (or a designee) may contact CDC directly to request SNS assets. A Presidential Disaster Declaration is not required to request SNS support, and activation of the National Response Framework is not necessary; however, procedures for requesting assets may change once there is federal-level involvement. Materiel requested from the SNS will be shipped either by air or ground transport to the nearest safe receipt, store, and stage (RSS) location designated by the state health department. RSS sites are designated warehouses where the 12-Hour Push Package or other assets will be delivered, off-loaded, and organized for further distribution. From the RSS location, the distribution of assets to individual hospitals, clinics, or points of dispensing (PODs) is the responsibility of the state or city. It is therefore recommended that contingency plans be made with shipping companies or other partners to provide local transportation. CDC has program consultants who collaborate on a regular basis with state planners to address how to receive, store, stage, distribute, and dispense assets from the SNS.

Other resources for antibiotics and vaccines should also be explored at the local and state level, as activation of federal assets will only occur after regional resources are depleted. Potential sources can include the normal supply chain, wholesale distributors, manufacturers, local or state stockpiles, or other vendors. Memoranda of agreement (MOAs) with neighboring communities and states should be established prior to a public health emergency. Local planners should consider factors such as immediate availability, timeliness, and security when developing these agreements. Additionally, neighboring regions or countries may enter into mutual aid agreements to share products and provide assistance. Disaster planners should be aware of what inventories are available to them domestically and internationally before a disaster occurs. Some medical countermeasures may be in short supply, necessitating difficult allocation decisions as to who will receive them. Three broad ethical issues related to handling public health emergencies include rationing, restrictions, and responsibilities.[12] Policymakers may benefit from including ethicists in their discussions regarding allocation of scarce resources.[13,14] A triage or tiered process should be developed to determine the order of need for such supplies.[15]

Once antibiotics, vaccines, or other assets are received by the affected area, they must be dispensed to the patient population in a timely manner. Assets from the SNS are delivered to the local receiving authority, which are then responsible for distributing the medical material to hospitals or PODs. Depending on the type of incident, the timeframe for providing effective prophylaxis or vaccination may vary. The Cities Readiness Initiative (CRI) is a federal program established by the U.S. HHS and Department of Homeland Security (DHS) to assist cities with delivering or dispensing medications during large-scale public health emergencies. CRI is in alignment with Presidential Policy Directive 8 (PPD 8) and the National Preparedness Goal, and is directly related to one of the top four national priorities – to strengthen medical surge and mass prophylaxis capabilities. The goal of CRI is to enhance preparedness at federal, state, and local levels of government by using a consistent national approach and response to a catastrophic incident requiring mass antibiotic prophylaxis with assets from the SNS. Federal funding is provided to participating cities that were chosen based on population and location. In 2004, the original program included twenty-one cities; in 2006, the program expanded to encompass seventy-two cities and their metropolitan statistical areas. Approximately 56% of the U.S. population resides in a CRI jurisdiction (personal communication, Stephanie Dulin, Centers for Disease Control and Prevention, March 20, 2007).

The planning scenario for each CRI jurisdiction is to initiate prophylaxis for the entire city population within 48 hours of an anthrax release. To accomplish this, three different mechanisms could be used individually or in combination: 1) methods developed and created by the city or state; 2) delivery of medicines and supplies by the U.S. Postal Service (USPS); or 3) setting up and running PODs. HHS, along with DHS, has negotiated with USPS to provide home delivery of initial doses of antibiotics at any time. This would serve as a stopgap measure while states or cities activate their PODs, and would permit the use of an existing and reliable delivery mechanism while allowing people to shelter-in-place after an incident. Not all U.S. states have chosen to use the USPS delivery option in their planning.

Planning for Points of Dispensing

Dispensing medication or administering vaccines to a large population in a public health emergency will most likely occur at PODs. These have also been called dispensing/vaccination clinics by some authors.[16] PODs and points of distribution may or may not mean the same thing. A point of distribution can be a holding area from which assets are further distributed before being dispensed. The goals for a mass dispensing program are two-fold: 1) reducing the overall risk of the population becoming ill; and 2) providing public health information to the general public and healthcare providers.[17]

Mass vaccination is usually performed to rapidly increase population immunity in the setting of an outbreak.[18] During a smallpox or other contagious infectious disease outbreak, surveillance and containment may be implemented. If multiple cities experience simultaneous cases of a contagious disease or multiple near-simultaneous releases of a biologic agent, it is possible that voluntary mass vaccination may be implemented.[19] In the United States, dispensing or distributing medications or vaccinating patients is mainly a local-level public health responsibility. Since dispensing laws, policies, procedures, and expectations may differ between states, it is important for state disaster planners to provide assistance and guidance for local planners to ensure a consistent approach throughout their jurisdiction.

Planning for PODs should take into account such logistical issues as design, operation, staffing, and activation and deactivation.[20] The number of persons needing prophylaxis or vaccination and the time necessary to implement effective prophylaxis or vaccination strategies will help determine how many PODs are required for any particular incident. Using a full 48-hour window of time for providing prophylaxis to the entire population will allow planning for worst-case scenarios. Plans can then be adjusted to fit the size and scope of the emergency. This flexibility is important since it is impossible to have a set of throughput measurements for every possible scenario.[21]

POD throughput may be defined as the number of persons receiving prophylaxis per unit of time. The number of PODs required can then be determined using the formula:

$$TP \div (HPP - S) \div PPH = PODs$$

where TP is the total population needing prophylaxis, HPP is the number of hours to provide prophylaxis to the population (i.e., 48 hours), S is the amount of time needed to establish the POD once the decision is made to do so, and PPH is the number of persons per hour who are provided prophylaxis (i.e., throughput). This equation has limitations in that it makes several assumptions that may not be correct, including: a 24-hour-a-day operation; an equal distribution of population among the PODs; equivalent types of PODs within a jurisdiction; POD performance at 100% capacity; adequate staffing; and a constant flow of people into and out of the POD.[16,20]

To ensure adequate facilities are available, it is prudent to identify such resources in advance of any emergency and establish written agreements (i.e., MOAs). Such agreements should address immediate use of the facility during an incident, periodic access for building inspections, 24-hour contact information, security, compensation or liability/indemnification agreements (if applicable), and authority to use the facility for exercises or drills. The MOA should also clearly identify the entity having responsibility and authority for managing response operations.

Points of Dispensing Site Selection

Facility site selection is critical to a successful response effort. Publicly owned facilities such as schools, universities, community recreation centers, firehouses, polling places, and armories are usually well known to the community, easy to find, have adequate parking, and are accessible by public transportation or private vehicle. The problem with use of these locations includes possible disruption of their regular functions and potentially enduring stigmatization of the site due to a gathering of "exposed" people. Alternate locations may include aircraft hangers and shuttered public areas such as hospitals no longer in use. Although military installations may have available space, heightened security during a terrorist incident or other public health emergency may result in restricted access to these sites.

Hospitals, commercial pharmacies, or other healthcare institutions may be overwhelmed with additional patient loads created by the incident and may not be the best choice to locate PODs. Although a recent survey indicated the willingness of private industry to partner with public health entities for administration of medications or vaccines, concerns regarding liability remain.[22] In the United States, liability protection is provided to covered persons who administer a covered countermeasure as defined through the Public Readiness and Emergency Preparedness Act.[23] This takes effect after the U.S. Secretary of HHS declares a public health emergency that requires administration of such countermeasures as identified by the secretary.[23] Section 224(p) of the Public Health Service Act also specifically addresses the liability concerns associated with administration of smallpox countermeasures.[24] Fewer liability protections exist for institutions responding to emergencies compared with available protection for individuals.[25]

Commercial facilities such as grocery stores, wholesale clubs, or retail stores may be useful vaccine administration settings because many of these organizations host annual influenza vaccination clinics. Use of such nontraditional settings for influenza vaccination campaigns is becoming a more common practice.[26] Nontraditional settings have positive cost/utility ratios, and their convenience and desirable locations increase their value as potential vaccination sites. Ninety-five percent of the U.S. population resides within 5 miles of a retail pharmacy.[27]

Retail stores and other non-clinical community establishments in the United States administer upwards of 30 million influenza vaccinations annually, along with third-party logistics providers and health service providers.[22] Because of increased use of such facilities, guidelines have been established to define quality standards for immunizations in nontraditional settings.[28] Although there have been some concerns regarding safety, one study assessed over half a million persons vaccinated in nontraditional settings and found that adverse events were extremely rare, totaling only 112 occurrences, most of which resolved within minutes.[26]

Physical characteristics of the POD location should include the ability to accommodate hundreds or even thousands of people at one time, while keeping them protected from adverse weather conditions. Communities have used a varying range of POD sizes, ranging from 1,670 to 5,500 square meters. Desirable features include heating and air conditioning, adequate

Table 18.1. POD Equipment and Supplies

Name badges	Batteries	Large trash bags
Badge strap clips	Calculators	Waste cans
Badge neck straps	Clipboards	Regular trash bags
Vests	Dry-erase boards	White copy paper
Whistles	Dry-erase markers	Scotch tape
Bullhorns	Adult scales	Paper towels
Red barrier tape	Bike flags	Kleenex
Traffic cones	Red ink pens	Duct tape
Portable copy machines	Black ink pens	Accordion folders
Emergency alert radios	Walkie-talkies	Colored paper
Extension cords	Blankets	Biohazard bags
Power strips	Hand sanitizer	Sharp containers
Flashlights	Surgical masks or N95 respirators	Disposable cups
Sign easels	Label makers	Labels
Thermometers	Candy (simulated medicine)	Staplers
Paper clips	Permanent markers	Highlighters
Post-it notes	Lanterns	Gloves
Trash cans with wheels	Toilet paper	Pencils

bathrooms, water and electricity, handicap access with a minimum of stairs, a public address system, an unloading area for receipt of supplies, parking, a helicopter landing site, and a break room/canteen. Good security, including the ability to control access, is a requirement. These physical characteristics will provide the security team sufficient space to coordinate traffic, manage parking, maintain crowd control, and protect staff and assets.[29]

Equipment for Points of Dispensing

Adequate equipment and supplies will be useful at the POD. Table 18.1 describes equipment and supplies that should be considered. This is not a comprehensive list and each city or state may identify additional items that are useful. Some areas have developed a "go-kit" of items that can be easily transported to POD locations, have multiple uses during different types of disasters, are easily stored at room temperature, and are packaged pre-event according to different POD functions.[30]

Points of Dispensing Operations

All PODs within an affected area should be uniform in their medication delivery system, patient flow process, staff roles, operating procedures, projected throughput, hours of operation, information products, and policies. Uniformity of PODs will make it easier to share personnel between PODs if needed, and will avoid the public perception of better service at one location versus another.[17,31] Distributing the population evenly among the PODs will be a challenge. To optimize the chances for success,

a robust public information campaign is necessary. This can include distribution of the population by first letter of last name, postal code, census tract, school district, or neighborhood. POD sites should nevertheless be prepared for greater than anticipated numbers of people because the population may be unable or unwilling to follow instructions despite an aggressive public information campaign.

Each POD must designate an on-site director (incident commander) capable of managing large numbers of people under difficult circumstances and who is familiar with the specific needs of the community. Although POD management is a local responsibility, POD locations, sizes, operations, and leaders are often chosen after collaboration between local, state, and regional health agencies. The Incident Command System (ICS) and National Incident Management System (NIMS) are both well recognized command and control systems in the United States that may be used in POD management.[16,31,32] Using these command and control systems facilitates establishing clear leadership roles and chains of command, as well as the delegation of duties. Such processes are necessary to support effective reporting systems and recordkeeping.

PODs may be organized in one of two primary ways using a segmented or non-segmented structure. This organizational plan will have a direct impact on transportation and traffic management surrounding the POD. In a segmented POD, greeting/information, triage, or registration is performed in a central location with medication and/or vaccine dispensing conducted at another location. Segmented PODs allow the public to gather at staging sites accessible by public transportation and that also provide adequate parking. Examples include stadiums and sporting arenas, convention centers, and shopping malls. At the initial site, the exposed population is screened, triaged, and given information before being transported to the actual dispensing location. Symptomatic patients can be transported or directed to treatment facilities. Advantages to a segmented POD include a reduction in traffic congestion and parking at the actual POD location; improved security; a potential decrease in the number of people presenting to the POD who do not need prophylaxis; a regulated flow of people; and the ability to triage symptomatic patients away from the POD. Disadvantages include the need for large parking facilities at the staging site, the necessity of utilizing transportation assets to shuttle people to the POD, a potential lack of understanding by the public of where to go, more difficult just-in-time (JIT) training for staff in two locations, a greater security burden, and an increase in staffing requirements. Figures 18.2 and 18.3 depict segmented POD operations.

In contrast, non-segmented PODs conduct all operations in a single location. Advantages to this type of operation include reduced requirements for staffing and security. Disadvantages include the need for increased parking, the risk of having symptomatic patients in proximity to those who were exposed but are not yet symptomatic, and the potential for secondary disease transmission (for example, pneumonic plague) as a result of crowded conditions. Figure 18.4 depicts a non-segmented POD operation.

Points of Dispensing Functional Areas

There are four basic functional areas to a POD: intake, screening, dispensing, and exit. Intake includes the processes, procedures, stations, and personnel involved in introducing people into the POD. Paperwork such as medical history can be completed at

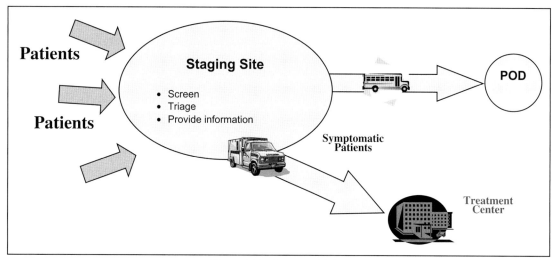

Figure 18.2. Segmented POD.

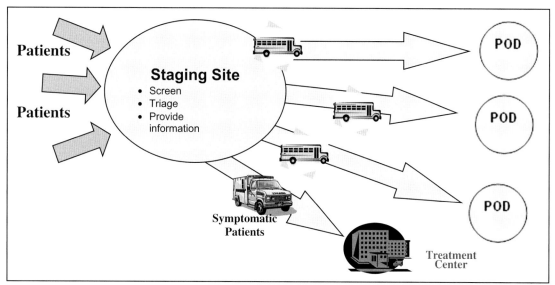

Figure 18.3. Segmented POD with one staging area feeding multiple PODs.

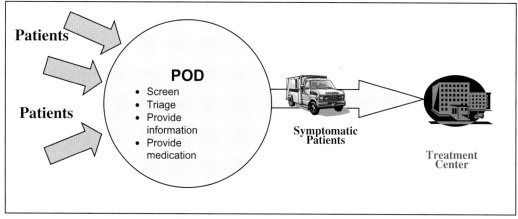

Figure 18.4. Non-Segmented POD.

this stage, with patients being appropriately directed to receive the correct medication. Patient information collected at this time can be used for monitoring medication compliance and adverse events, as well as tracking dispensed medication in case of a drug recall. The amount of information collected is a decision made by state and local planners but should be concise and useful. In certain circumstances, there may be federal requirements as well. Such data can be collected and transmitted on paper forms, computer databases, telephones, or faxes.[33] Throughput of the POD will decrease as the amount of paperwork or data increases; therefore, forms should be short, simple, and specific. Many U.S. states have developed templates for information collection, both for individuals and for heads of household.[34–37]

Public health information and education must be conveyed at the POD. This may be accomplished during intake with written materials; however, other methods such as television, newspaper, Internet, video, or recordings may be used, and would lessen the burden of replicating printed materials at the time of an incident. If written patient information is used, a small inventory of previously printed sheets or electronic master templates can be distributed initially, followed by additional information sheets that may be generated through contingency contracts with local printing or photocopy businesses. Other functions that may be necessary at this step include traffic management, security, greeting, registration, and triage.

Screening encompasses sorting and classifying individuals to optimize resources and maximize patient survival. This step may involve a variety of functions including greeting, sorting, roaming (helping with any task), first aid delivery, medical transport, providing social services, and mental health counseling.

Dispensing involves the processes and procedures for preparing and distributing medications to the public. Various methods of dispensing may be used. Certain populations may be unable to access PODs and will, therefore, require different dispensing methods. These groups include prison inmates, nursing home or other institutionalized long-term care patients, workers at large industries operating 24-hour-a-day schedules, hospitalized or homebound patients, homeless persons, and undocumented immigrants. Dispensing methods for these populations may include deliveries to large corporations or universities that have occupational health clinics or medical staff on site. These sites may serve as "closed PODs" that take care of employees and their families to further relieve the burden on regular PODs. Other alternatives may include: mobile dispensing clinics, "drive-through" clinics, or the USPS delivery system previously described.[17] Drive-through clinics have been tested in some states and offer advantages such as alleviation of crowding and a decrease in risk for disease transmission. Noted pitfalls of this dispensing method included confusing traffic flow and congestion, long processing times, and limited access to parking or restrooms.[38] Distributing or "pushing" medical countermeasures out to these special populations could be faster and may cover a larger area, but does not allow for the medical evaluation of patients for adjustment of medication dosing or addressing drug contraindications. Also, the push method is not feasible for mass vaccinations.[16] Transporting or "pulling" people into PODs for prophylaxis or vaccination more efficiently uses healthcare workers and resources and facilitates medical evaluation and centralized data collection. Logistical delays and establishing multiple PODs are the disadvantages of pulling people into POD locations. A combination of both pushing and pulling methods may be most useful.

Permitting a single individual to accept medications for an entire household is a decision that should be made in advance by the local jurisdiction. This practice has the potential advantage of decreasing the number of people at the POD and increasing throughput. If dispensed medications are for children, individuals collecting the drugs must provide an accurate body weight, to ensure accurate pediatric dosing. Providing other medical information on family members, such as allergies, current medications, or existing disease states may also be necessary. The type of information or evidence required to justify the number of regimens for a family should be decided before an incident and should be made known to the public so they can provide appropriate documentation for family members. POD staff should be prepared to answer questions about the risk of disease, transmission between humans, the risk to pets, and whether prophylaxis would be provided for pets. It is unlikely that prophylaxis would be provided to pets with the exception of service animals. The U.S. Department of Agriculture maintains a National Veterinary Stockpile that may have applicability to certain animal diseases in the event of an impending economic disaster involving cattle or livestock.[39]

Exiting includes moving the public out of the POD and providing any necessary follow-up information. Useful avenues for providing additional information to patients regarding compliance, adverse effects, or other questions include: 1) hotlines established through the local or state health department; 2) poison control centers or nurse advice lines; 3) implementing a community phone bank; 4) creating a website; and 5) providing information to primary care physicians.

Security and patient education permeate all four phases of a POD operation and should be addressed throughout. Every step of the POD process may be used to provide patient education. At the intake step, fact sheets, handouts, or videotapes may be used to provide information. Such information should be prepared in multiple languages as appropriate to the community. During screening or dispensing, drug and individual patient-specific information may be shared through a variety of means. At the exit, follow-up information can be provided. Security should be present at each step of the POD as well as outside of the POD. Security should address crowd and traffic control inside and outside of the POD, and protection of staff and assets. All staff should wear badges identifying them as such. Plans for security should be addressed in preparation for an incident, because local law enforcement will likely be performing other duties as a consequence of the incident and not be available. This is especially important as unprotected PODs are at increased risk for theft of supplies in situations where resources are limited. In addition, PODs could become sites of secondary terrorist attacks. All POD workers should be made aware of security concerns and know how to report suspicious individuals or activities. POD locations with controllable entry and exit points will assist security with traffic flow. An evacuation route for patients and personnel should be part of the disaster plan of the POD itself.

In streamlining POD operations, a simple assembly line concept may help improve efficiency and increase throughput. If standing in lines is culturally feasible, using multiple parallel lines rather than a single line is likely to increase throughput. In a mass-casualty situation requiring mass dispensing, a thorough individual-based medical practice approach will not be practical. The focus shifts from individual patient medical care to population healthcare. Ensuring continual movement of patients through the system to eliminate bottlenecks will allow for a more effective mass dispensing POD model.

If necessary, a high throughput rate (increasing the numbers of persons per hour moving through the POD) may be achievable by shortening or foregoing orientation, simplifying medical forms, and eliminating secondary medical screening and a final quality assurance check. Patients requiring specialized attention for any reason may be moved to remote stations outside of the POD. This could include individuals with specific medical, safety, mobility, psychiatric, or communication needs. Typical groups consist of: children; the medically fragile; those with physical disabilities; migratory and homeless persons; those with language, culture or literacy barriers; and disruptive persons.[40] These groups may require additional attention in order to understand public information messages. Options include translating messages and fact sheets, using on-site translators, and implementation of color coding and pictograms.

Identifying bottlenecks and adding additional resources to relieve these congested locations may also be helpful.[41] Bottlenecks at PODs may occur when: 1) too many people are allowed into the POD at a time; 2) too many people arrive at one particular station; 3) too few staff are operating a station; or 4) staff have too many activities to perform for each person presenting. These obstructions can be alleviated by having "express lanes" for those with no complications, by properly estimating the number of staff and individuals at each POD, and by having a flexible command and control system in place that allows for modification of staff and type of PODs.[16,17] Prophylaxis of POD workers should be addressed before the POD is open to the general public.

Staffing and Training for Points of Dispensing

It is the responsibility of each public health jurisdiction to conduct both first response and ongoing community-wide mass antibiotic dispensing and vaccination campaigns that can be federally supported.[16] Local mass prophylaxis activities will probably be underway before any federal assets arrive. In addition, federal and state assistance will likely not include sufficient personnel to supplement POD staff, particularly if the incident encompasses a wide geographical region such as multiple states or counties. Even after federal assets arrive, POD operations will probably remain under local control, and POD operations may continue well after the departure of state or federal assistance.[16]

Adequate staffing is paramount in running a successful POD, and will require people with the correct skill sets who can be trained to fulfill specific tasks. Trained staff should be able to quickly establish the POD and ensure its operation at maximal efficiency with the highest possible throughput. Staffing the PODs has been accomplished in many different ways depending on historical successes for a particular city or state.[21,33,42–44] A general guiding principle is to require various types of staff, such as professionals (physicians, nurses, pharmacists, public health workers, and social workers), volunteers (trained and untrained), and management support staff familiar with the facility or general POD operations. Volunteers or non-clinical staff should be used for any appropriate jobs to unburden professional staff and maximize efficiency of POD operations. Volunteers may be recruited before an event occurs. However, expect that others will present unannounced at the time of the incident. The enormous task of training volunteers should be conducted, to the extent possible, before an incident occurs. This task is easier if roles and responsibilities are kept consistent throughout the state or region.[17] Maintaining a statewide registry of trained volunteers may also be helpful. Trained volunteers with special skill sets such as translation and sign language abilities, and those from the Red Cross, can provide invaluable assistance.[31] Untrained volunteers may be found in community civic or fraternal organizations, or as spontaneous volunteers.

When planning for staffing, considerations should also include having enough people to support two or three shifts per day. Some exercises conducted by states and cities have shown a rapid onset of staff burn-out, so planning for additional shifts or rotating staff between several different duty stations may be useful.[42]

During an emergency, professionals will be in high demand to perform other jobs or tasks. However, potential sources for accessing professional services include: 1) commercial pharmacies; 2) state licensing agencies; 3) professional associations; 4) nursing, pharmacy, or medical schools; 5) the DHS Emergency Coordinator for the region; 6) the HHS regional health administrator; and 7) programs such as the U.S. Medical Reserve Corps.[45] Federal staff support for dispensing efforts may be obtained through the U.S. Public Health Service, National Pharmacy Response Teams, National Nursing Response Teams, and Disaster Medical Assistance Teams. These federal personnel assets may be available depending on the situation, such as when a Federal Disaster Declaration is in effect. Table 18.2 lists possible roles for healthcare professionals and volunteers.

Training of POD staff will help shape the success of the POD operation. Training should include orientation to their particular tasks or roles, the physical layout and flow of the POD, other team members, and forms and other paperwork. It may be helpful for planners to maintain a database of those who have received training. Ideally, training would be conducted before an incident occurs; however, due to staff turnover, skill degradation, and updates or changes in procedures, this would require periodic refresher training and eventually may be too costly or time consuming. Another option is to provide JIT training, where staff would not be trained until they were needed. New people could be trained in the POD at their own workstations with a straightforward job action sheet. This method has been used successfully in a number of exercises.[37,42,46]

A third option is to train enough staff ahead of time (along with refresher training) to comprise the first shift of a POD and provide JIT training for subsequent shifts. JIT training should include the person's role, the forms or paperwork that will be used, the physical layout and flow of the POD, shift hours, information about related POD functions and how the trainee integrates into the process, to whom to report any problems, and emergency evacuation procedures.[47] POD managers can address issues such as staff shortages, medication shortages, or other problems that arise.

Drills and exercises will be the most beneficial way to determine whether a given POD will be successful. A number of dispensing campaign and POD-specific tasks, objectives, and performance metrics can be evaluated. These include: 1) unlocking and opening the facilities; 2) locating lights, circuit breakers, and alarms; 3) preparing the facility by assembling chairs, tables, rope lanes, and portable toilets; 4) providing food and water; and 5) implementing POD staffing. After drills or exercises have taken place, after-action reports or briefings can help identify areas for improvement.

Table 18.2. Suggested Roles for Healthcare Professionals and Volunteers

Assignment	Staffing	Tasks
Intake		
Greeting/Entry	Volunteer with standardized script	Greet, direct, answer nonmedical questions
		Assist disabled persons
		Orient the public
Forms Distribution	Volunteer	Distribute medical history forms
		Explain form completion with a script
		Check completion of forms
Briefing	Trained volunteer	Translate dispensing-site procedures and policies to persons who do not understand English, are hearing impaired or illiterate.
	Volunteer with task specific training	Hand out medical record forms and provide instruction on completing them
	Volunteer with script	Educate and orient people standing in line
	Health professional or video	Provide information about drugs, including pediatric medicines
	Volunteer with script	Advise about importance of adhering to regimen instructions
		Warn about danger of overmedicating
		Confirm date to return for additional medication if needed
Screening		
Triage	Professional	Perform initial health screen
		Redirect symptomatic people to treatment facility
	Volunteer	Assist seriously ill persons to transport vehicles
Mental Health Screening and Counseling	Health professional and social worker	Watch for signs of anxiety, fear, impatience
		Provide counseling
Medical Evaluation	Professional	Perform health examination and assessment
Healthcare Center Transport	Volunteer	Drive ambulance or other vehicle
Drug Triage	Professional	Screen for contraindications for drugs or medical conditions
		Answer questions or prescribe alternate drug
Dispensing		
Express Drug Dispensing	Pharmacist supervisor	Oversee dispensing process
	Volunteer	Weigh children under 5
	Volunteer	Dispense regimens depending on state regulations
	Pharmacist or pharmacy technician	Dispense regimens
Assisted Drug Dispensing	Pediatrician or pediatric nurse practitioner	Examine infants and small children
		Dispense proper medication
Exit		
Collection and Review of Medical Data	Volunteer with professional supervision	Check for completeness of forms
		Distribute patient information sheets
		Explain importance of compliance with regimen
		Stress danger of overmedicating
		Note date to return for additional medications if needed

Adapted from *Receiving, Distributing, and Dispensing SNS Assets: A Guide for Preparedness.*[20]

Table 18.3. Software and Programming for POD Modeling

BERM, the Weill Cornell Bioterrorism and Epidemic Response Model	http://archive.ahrq.gov/research/biomodel.htm
Clinic Planning Model Generator	http://www.isr.umd.edu/Labs/CIM/projects/clinic
Maxi-Vac software program	http://emergency.cdc.gov/agent/smallpox/vaccination/maxi-vac
SNS TourSolver	https://snstoursolver.c2routeapp.com/about.html
MEDS/POD	See note 44
RealOpt ©	See note 48

More research is needed to develop effective POD management models that will ensure high throughput to meet the 48-hour goal for dispensing. However, several computer-generated management models have been created to help with POD planning efforts for both antibiotic distribution and vaccinations.[16,20,48–52] CDC has also published guidance for establishing large-scale smallpox vaccination clinics.[53] In addition, a number of webcasts are available to assist planners with POD operations.[17,40,41,54]

Using these tools will allow officials to formulate realistic plans. POD staffing levels for entry screening, triage, medical evaluation, and drug dispensing stations may be determined using various bioterrorism response scenarios.[49] The number of staff needed to provide prophylaxis for the entire population within 48 hours can also be determined.[17] Other approaches allow for simulation and decision support for planning large-scale emergency dispensing clinics by offering clinic design and staffing models, including scenarios for smallpox or influenza vaccination and antibiotic dispensing.[49–52] Most of the software or programming is free to planners and access links can be found in Table 18.3.

Many states and cities have conducted exercises and drills to test their preparedness plans and their dispensing or vaccination capabilities.[21,32,37,42–44,46,55–60] Vaccination clinics were also tested beginning in 2002, when President George W. Bush instituted a smallpox vaccination program for military and civilian medical first responders.[61] President Bush's two-pronged program called for HHS to immunize a cohort of healthcare workers and first responders, and for the Department of Defense to vaccinate the military population.[62] Military administration of anthrax vaccine has also followed the vaccination clinic model.[63] Annual influenza vaccination clinics are another good source of testing mass vaccination protocols.[31,64] Additionally, testing mass vaccination programs with influenza vaccine provides the opportunity to enhance pandemic preparedness while achieving annual prevention goals.[31] These exercises have produced similar information; some of the most important recommendations are highlighted in Table 18.4.

To be effective, POD operations should address the needs of different patient groups. These include otherwise healthy people with no complications who require prophylaxis, people with existing medical conditions who require prophylaxis, or those already suffering from illness as a result of the exposure.[17] The goal for those with symptoms is rapid transport to a healthcare facility. Those exposed with no complications should receive appropriate prophylaxis medications quickly, and those with complicated medical histories need proper evaluation to

Table 18.4. Important Guidelines for Effective POD Management

Limit medical histories	Defined responsibilities
Clear signage	Clarity of mission
Collaboration with law enforcement	Defined line of authority
Hotline/phone bank	Partnerships
Good communication	Liability
Redistribution of resources	Just-in-time training
Transportation arrangements	Chain of custody
Streamlined triage	Regulate entrance/exit to limit flow
Multiple languages/translators	Limit distractions
Patient education	How to obtain refills
Directions for leftover medication	Procedures for special cases

determine any contraindications or dosage adjustments before receiving prophylaxis. Some patients may be directed to an alternate care site, particularly if they are less ill than others. In some previously practiced scenarios, healthcare facilities could not provide care for all patients with symptoms.

Secondary goals for PODs may include crisis or mental health counseling, recordkeeping, or patient tracking. PODs should have direct communications channels with hospitals and other facilities where symptomatic individuals or those who experience adverse reactions can be evaluated. Successful operation of PODs may decrease the number of people who initially present to a healthcare facility; successful vaccination or mass antibiotic dispensing may reduce the number of individuals who become ill and require subsequent treatment.

PODs should be ready for use in an emergency once sites are selected, staffing determined, training provided, and exercises conducted. In the activation of a dispensing campaign, implementation of PODs could occur in four phases as listed in Table 18.5.[17,20] Providing prophylaxis or vaccination to critical infrastructure personnel and their families may improve work attendance by these responders because they and their families have been protected. Critical infrastructure personnel may include healthcare workers, first responders, law enforcement personnel,

Table 18.5. Four Phases of POD Activation

Phase 1	Notify and recall all staff necessary to initiate dispensing campaign
Phase 2	Provide prophylaxis or vaccination to critical infrastructure personnel and their families
Phase 3	Set up POD network – obtain staff, set up the PODs, print forms, unpack inventory
Phase 4	Public notification and opening of PODs

government leaders, and others who are necessary to support the essential infrastructure of the affected area. Local supplies may be available to accomplish this while SNS or other assets are being delivered.

Public Information Delivery Related to Points of Dispensing

Providing timely, accurate public information is one of the most critical elements of a successful dispensing campaign. One key factor is to address the information needs of the public, first responders, healthcare workers, and other stakeholders in an effective manner. The process should identify the risks they face and actions they can take to protect themselves and others.[40] Messages should be designed to instill trust as well as provide the motivation and reassurance to do what is recommended.[65,66]

Once PODs are ready to open, the public should be informed. If feasible, planners should wait until all PODs within a region are ready for opening before notifying the public, so as not to overwhelm any one site. If information regarding PODs is released too far in advance, people may form long lines well before the PODs are open or functional. The media may be used as a first level of triage in addition to public address systems outside of the POD, with announcements telling those who have recently become ill to go to the nearest hospital or other designated healthcare site.[41]

A variety of media outlets may be used to disburse messages to the community, including newspapers, radio, television, Internet, social media, telephone hotlines such as poison control centers or nurse advice lines, and press conferences. The Public Broadcast System or other emergency broadcast systems may also be used. Local media outlets should be alerted regarding the potential for opening PODs to ensure consistent messages across all levels of government. The media can be helpful during an incident and they should have a designated area at the POD location. A media kit prepared before an event occurs will be a useful tool. It should discuss: 1) background information on threat agents; 2) characteristic signs and symptoms resulting from exposure to an agent; 3) information about the medical products that may be used as prophylaxis or treatment; and 4) information about the communication plan used during a disaster along with contact information. Monitoring of media reports will be essential to ensure that critical information is relayed accurately and to determine if changes, corrections, or updates are necessary.[17]

Points of Dispensing Deactivation

Once an emergency enters the recovery phase, implementing a plan for deactivation of PODs is important. PODs may be deactivated individually or in groups, but this should be accomplished in a staggered fashion. This allows the community to retain some capability while people continue to receive medications, in case renewed activity is warranted. Sites most needed for community resilience, such as businesses or schools, should be deactivated first. Information and data from the PODs, including throughput figures, staffing hours, expenses, and comments from staff for improvements as well as what went well, should be gathered. Some people may have difficulty adjusting after an emergency or mass-casualty incident, so counseling should be provided for staff as well as the public.

Special Considerations

Drug Formulations for Patients at Extremes of Age

Small children or elderly persons may have difficulty swallowing tablets or capsules as part of a post-exposure prophylaxis campaign. The U.S. National Advisory Committee on Children and Terrorism recommends that suspension formulations be available for children aged 9 and younger and the SNS contains a limited quantity of such suspensions.[67] The quantity of recommended suspensions required to fulfill a 60-day prophylactic antibiotic course (i.e., for anthrax) greatly exceeds the manufacturing capacity and storage capabilities of most countries. Additionally, suspension formulations have a relatively short shelf life, may be costly to produce, and may have a small (or non-existent) annual usage. For these reasons, alternate methods for creating suitable formulations for children have been explored.

One potential avenue is to compound the needed suspension from pills, as could be accomplished in a pharmacy setting. This method is very time consuming, and when performed on a large scale, pharmacies may be subject to regulatory implications imposed by the U.S. Food and Drug Administration (FDA) such as those applying to a manufacturer. Another option is to crush tablets in the home setting and add the crushed medications to a food or liquid which would then be administered to the child. Informal testing of the initial guidelines provided by the FDA revealed that they were too confusing for some parents to follow. In addition, some of the oral dosage forms have an extremely bitter taste that is difficult to conceal. Current guidelines are being updated to make them easier to understand and execute. Those related to the crushing of doxycycline tablets are a good example. The doxycycline guidelines are available on the FDA website (http://www.fda.gov); others are under consideration and will be made available on completion.

Dispensing Laws – The U.S. System

The label of a drug must have certain information according to U.S. federal law [Food Drug and Cosmetic Act (FDCA) Section 502 (21 U.S.C. § 352)] and the Code of Federal Regulations [(CFR) (21 C.F.R. Part 201)]. These laws state that the label of a drug should include (but is not limited to): established name of drug; name and address of manufacturer, packer, or distributor; quantity of contents (weight, measure, or numerical count); lot number; expiration date; and adequate directions for use. Additionally, under federal law [FDCA Section 503(b)(2) and 21 U.S.C. § 353(b)(2)], the label of a dispensed prescription drug must include: name and address of the dispenser; serial number; date of prescription or of its filling; name of prescriber; name of patient if stated on prescription; directions for use; and cautionary statements, if contained in the prescription. State laws may also impose further requirements on the label of a dispensed drug.

These labeling regulations were originally developed to support day-to-day needs of medication dispensing. Planners may want to explore options for attaining regulatory relief (from state and federal regulations) on the labeling requirements for pharmaceutical medications dispensed during an emergency incident.

There are also dispensing requirements for prescription drugs. Under U.S. federal law [FDCA Section 503(b)(1) and 21 U.S.C. § 353(b)(1)], prescription drugs must be dispensed only with a written prescription, an oral prescription (which is reduced promptly to writing), or by refilling a prescription. State laws also impose requirements on the dispensing of prescription drugs.

The size and scope of an emergency may dictate that personnel other than pharmacists or physicians dispense medication to the public. Disaster planners may need to investigate existing legislative authorities such as the Emergency Powers Act and possibly regulatory relief that would allow individuals other than pharmacists to dispense prescription drugs during an emergency. It is also recommended that disaster planners become familiar with state laws surrounding these issues. Currently, all fifty states allow pharmacists to administer vaccines, and thirty states allow pharmacy students to vaccinate individuals under the supervision of a pharmacist. Although it would require authorization for an expanded scope of practice in some states, trained paramedics may be an untapped source for vaccine administration and may provide the benefit of having access to underserved populations.[68]

Investigational New Drugs

If a pharmaceutical or biological product has not yet been approved by the FDA, or when a product is approved by the FDA but not for a particular indication, its use may require an Investigational New Drug (IND) protocol. Drugs that are administered under the IND process can only be given to individuals according to the Institutional Review Board (Ethics Committee) approved protocol, which is maintained by the principal investigator and approved by the FDA. The principal investigator may have co-investigators who are also able to administer the protocol. Pharmaceuticals or biological agents used under IND protocols require informed consent from each person receiving the drug. A few examples of such products integrated into the SNS include smallpox vaccine diluted in a 1:5 ratio, colony-stimulating factors for the treatment of radiation-induced neutropenia, and anthrax immune globulin to treat symptomatic anthrax patients. Obtaining informed consent can be a tedious process especially during a disaster involving mass casualties.

To better serve the population in a time of disaster, the U.S. Project BioShield Act was passed in 2004 to help provide new tools to assist in protecting Americans against terrorist threats involving chemical, biological, radiological, or nuclear materials.[69] Oversight of Project BioShield lies with the secretaries of HHS and DHS. One key aspect of the legislation gives the FDA the ability to rapidly offer promising treatments in emergency situations.[70] The Project BioShield Act permits the FDA Commissioner, on official declaration of an emergency, to authorize the use of medical countermeasures for the diagnosis, treatment, or prevention of serious or life-threatening conditions for which there are no adequate, approved, or available alternatives. This process is known as an Emergency Use Authorization (EUA). The EUA is an authorization by the FDA to allow use of medical products during a real or potential emergency. This may include either unapproved products (those that are not yet approved under sections of the Federal Food, Drug, and Cosmetic Act or the Public Health Service Act), or unapproved uses of approved products (drugs, biological agents, or devices).

One example of an unapproved use for an approved product may be administration of an antibiotic for post-exposure prophylaxis to viruses or bacteria not included on the approved labeling for the drug. It may also encompass dispensing of prescription drugs by an unlicensed healthcare provider. The following criteria must be met before the FDA Commissioner may issue an EUA:

▪ A serious or life-threatening condition could result from the agent specified in the emergency declaration
▪ It is reasonable to believe the product may be effective in diagnosing, treating, or preventing the serious or life-threatening disease or condition based on the total scientific evidence available
▪ The known and potential benefits outweigh the known and potential risks of the product when used to diagnose, prevent, or treat the serious or life-threatening disease or condition;
▪ There are no adequate, approved, or available alternatives to the product.

Informed consent is not required for products used under an EUA; however, recipients must be still be informed and provided with general information regarding the risks and benefits. Use of an EUA, granted by the FDA at the time of the emergency, may be a more expeditious way of dispensing investigational countermeasures than the IND approach. Not all investigational or IND products will qualify or be approved for use under an EUA. Additional information on EUA and a current list of active EUAs may be found on the FDA website at http://www.fda.gov/EmergencyPreparedness/Counterterrorism/ucm182568.htm.

In 2013, Section 564 of the Federal Food, Drug, and Cosmetic Act was further amended by the Pandemic and All-Hazards Preparedness Reauthorization Act (PAHPRA). This act facilitates preparedness and rapid deployment of medical countermeasures and clarifies FDA's existing authority. Enhancements include allowing FDA to issue an EUA before an emergency, or based on the HHS Secretary's determination that a potential emergency exists due to a chemical, biological, radiation, or nuclear incident An example would be the EUA currently in place permitting use of oral formulations of doxycycline products for the post-exposure prophylaxis of inhalational anthrax.[71] This was issued after a determination by the Secretary of Homeland Security that a significant potential exists for a domestic emergency involving a heightened risk of attack with *Bacillus anthracis*. Subsequently, the HHS Secretary declared that present circumstances justify emergency use authorization for all oral formulations of doxycycline, accompanied by emergency use information. PAHPRA permits federal, state, and local governments to position medical countermeasures in anticipation of an EUA, facilitating faster movement and dispensing of assets. It also provides a mechanism to use certain medical countermeasures without an EUA and without the need for individual prescriptions, if permitted by state law or under an order by the HHS Secretary.

Adverse Events

Medication-related adverse events may be seen in varying numbers as part of a mass dispensing or mass vaccination campaign. Using medical products under an IND or an EUA may require public health officials to capture medication-related adverse events data. This can be accomplished using existing mechanisms available for passive reporting of adverse events such as the Vaccine Adverse Event Reporting System hosted by CDC, or MedWatch, which is sponsored by FDA. Further research, however, is needed to determine the capabilities of these systems to manage large magnitude events. Additionally, the details of who is responsible for adverse event reporting during a mass-casualty situation require further definition. The timing and peak number of clinically significant medication-related adverse events will likely be related to the duration of the mass prophylaxis campaign, with short campaigns having the greatest potential to overwhelm the capacity of emergency departments, clinics, or PODs.[72] States may also have their own reporting mechanisms in place such as toll-free numbers that patients may call to report medication-related adverse events.

Cold Chain Management

Cold chain management is defined as maintaining the quality of temperature-sensitive pharmaceuticals throughout transportation, product handling, and storage. Dispensing sites must maintain the temperature of the drugs or vaccines they provide to the public, in accordance with the package insert of the products. In some cases, vaccines may be frozen at temperatures of $-20^{\circ}C$ or may be refrigerated at $2-8^{\circ}C$. Some vaccines have strict thawing guidelines. Deliveries of assets to the POD locations should not be left outside, both for security and for proper storage reasons. Each POD location should have the appropriate equipment such as forklifts or pallet jacks to move deliveries, as well as sufficient equipment to provide cold chain storage as needed.

Ancillary Supplies

For successful mass vaccination and dispensing, ancillary supplies must be available for administration of POD assets. Alcohol swabs, bandages, syringes, and needles should be procured in advance to ensure that vaccines can be administered in a timely fashion. These supplies may not automatically be provided with the vaccines when ordered from vendors or requested from stockpiles. Planners need to consider other additional supplies that may be critical to dispensing, including water for reconstitution of pediatric medications and devices to accurately measure pediatric dosage.

RECOMMENDATIONS FOR FURTHER RESEARCH

Although advances in the areas of mass dispensing and mass vaccination continue to accumulate, progress has been slow.[73] Opportunities for future research include: 1) the development of standardized policies governing the use of businesses (partnerships and agreements) during a public health response; 2) clarifying potential liability issues and solutions that vary from state to state and are sub-optimally explained in the U.S. Public Readiness and Emergency Preparedness Act of December 2005; 3) providing guidance and funding to encourage public and private organizations to partner with public health entities; 4) improving communication with local communities regarding partnerships and plans between public health and private industry; and 5) encouraging state authorities to establish legal authorization and regulatory guidelines (for example, allowing pharmacists to vaccinate and providing guidance on who can dispense).[73]

Additional guidance at the federal level is needed to assist state and local emergency planners with understanding the details of PAHPRA, and to identify data collection requirements for products distributed under an EUA. Standardization of data collection forms for gathering patient information before dispensing or vaccination should be considered.

More research is required to obtain licensed indications for pediatric or other special populations in product labeling. Creation of alternate dosage forms for pediatrics would help relieve the shortage and storage costs associated with antibiotic suspensions and may also increase compliance. Development of alternate vaccination forms such as a transdermal patch would simplify administration and decrease storage needs.[74]

Additional work is needed on mass dispensing models for vaccinations and medication distribution to help communities streamline their operations and provide prophylaxis to their populations in a timely manner. More innovation is required to meet the challenge of providing prophylaxis or vaccination to large populations in a short time while maintaining adherence to appropriate regulations. Mass dispensing and vaccination should be tailored to the available local, regional, national, and global resources.

Finally, given the rapidity with which a public health emergency could become a national or international incident, it is imperative that preparedness, training, and exercise participation continue at every level. There is a need for continued funding to maintain an acceptable level of readiness. Building a more robust basic public health infrastructure would not only benefit the national and international communities on a daily basis, but would also provide the foundation for conducting a response to a large-scale public health emergency.

REFERENCES

1. Inglesby T, O'Toole T, Henderson D, et al. Consensus statement–anthrax as a biological weapon, 2002 update recommendations for management. *JAMA* 2002; 287(17): 2236–2252.

2. Clawson A, Menachemi N, Beitsch L, Brooks RG. Are community health centers prepared for bioterrorism? *Biosecur Bioterror* 2006; 4(1): 55–63.

3. Sepkowitz KA. The 1947 smallpox vaccination campaign in New York City, revisited. *Emerg Infect Dis* 2004; 10(5): 960–961.

4. Fenner F, Henderson DA, Arita I, Jezek Z, Ladnyi ID. *Smallpox and Its Eradication*. Geneva, World Health Organization, 1988.

5. Sencer DJ, Millar JD. Reflections on the 1976 swine flu vaccination program. *Emerg Infect Dis* 2006; 12(1): 29–33.

6. Slater PE, Anis E, Leventhal A. Preparation for an outbreak of smallpox in Israel. *Israel Med Assoc J* 2002; 4: 507–512.

7. Harling R, Morgan D, Edmunds WJ, Campbell H. Interim Smallpox Guidance for the United Kingdom. *BMJ* 2002; 325(7377): 1371–1372.

8. United Kingdom Department of Health. Smallpox vaccination: an operational planning framework. 2005. http://www.scotland.gov.uk/Publications/2005/09/20160232/02340 (Accessed September 17, 2014).

9. Public Health Agency of Canada. National Emergency Stockpile System. http://www.phac-aspc.gc.ca/ep-mu/ness-eng.php (Accessed September 17, 2014).

10. World Health Organization. Pandemic Influenza Preparedness Framework for the Sharing of Influenza Viruses and

Access to Vaccines and Other Benefits. 2011. http://whqlibdoc .who.int/publications/2011/9789241503082_eng.pdf (Accessed September 17, 2014).

11. World Health Organization. WHO Pandemic Influenza Draft Protocol for Rapid Response and Containment. 2006. ftp://ftp.cdc.gov/pub/phlpprep/Legal%20Preparedness %20for%20Pandemic%20Flu/4.0%20-%20International/4.1.2 %20WHO%20Pandemic%20Flu%20Protocol.pdf (Accessed September 17, 2014).

12. Wynia MK. Ethics and public health emergencies: rationing vaccines. *Am J Bioeth* 2006; 6(6): 4–7.

13. Moodley K, Hardie K, Selgelid MJ, Waldman RJ, Strebel P, Rees H, Durrheim DN. Ethical considerations for vaccination programmes in acute humanitarian emergencies. *Bull World Health Organ* April 1, 2013; 91(4): 290–297.

14. Timbie JW, Ringel JS, Fox DS, et al. Systematic review of strategies to manage and allocate scarce resources during mass casualty events. *Ann Emerg Med* 2013; 61(6): 677–689.

15. Hick JL, O'Laughlin DT. Concept of operations for triage of mechanical ventilation in an epidemic. *Acad Emerg Med* 2006; 13(2): 223–229.

16. Hupert N, Cuomo J, Callahan MA, Mushlin AI. *Community-based Mass Prophylaxis: A Planning Guide for Public Health Preparedness.* Rockville, MD, Agency for Healthcare Research and Quality, 2004.

17. Centers for Disease Control and Prevention. Mass Antibiotic Dispensing: A Primer. Webcast. Atlanta, GA. June 24, 2004. http://www2a.cdc.gov/tceonline/registration/detailpage .asp?res_id=996 (Accessed September 17, 2014).

18. Heymann DL, Aylward RB. Mass vaccination: when and why. In: Plotkin SA, ed. *Mass Vaccination: Global Aspects–Progress and Obstacles. Current Topics in Microbiology and Immunology.* Berlin Heidelberg, Springer, 2006; 1–16.

19. Lane JM. Mass vaccination and surveillance/containment in the eradication of smallpox. In: Plotkin SA, ed. *Mass Vaccination: Global Aspects–Progress and Obstacles. Current Topics in Microbiology and Immunology.* Berlin Heidelberg, Springer, 2006; 17–29.

20. Centers for Disease Control and Prevention. *Receiving, Distributing, and Dispensing Strategic National Stockpile Assets: A Guide for Preparedness.* Version 10. Atlanta, GA, CDC Division of Strategic National Stockpile, 2005.

21. Giovachino M, Calhoun T, Cary N, et al. Optimizing a District of Columbia Strategic National Stockpile dispensing center. *J Public Health Manage* 2005; 11: 282–290.

22. Lien O, Maldin B, Franco C, Gronvall GK. Getting medicine to millions: new strategies for mass distribution. *Biosecur Bioterror* 2006; 4: 176–182.

23. Cohen H. Pandemic Flu and Medical Biodefense Countermeasure Liability Legislation: Division C of P.L. 109-148 (2005), 42 U.S.C. §§ 247d-6d, 247d-6e. Washington, DC. http://www .hrsa.gov/gethealthcare/conditions/countermeasurescomp/ covered_countermeasures_and_prep_act.pdf (Accessed August 25, 2015).

24. Department of Health and Human Services Office of the Secretary. Amendment to extend the January 24, 2003 declaration regarding administration of smallpox countermeasures as amended on January 24, 2004, January 24, 2005, and January 24, 2006. *Fed Reg* 2007; 72(18): 4013–4014.

25. Hodge JG. Assessing the legal environment concerning mass casualty event planning and response. In: *Providing Mass Medical Care With Scarce Resources: A Community Planning Guide.* Rockville, MD, Agency for Healthcare Research and Quality, 2006; 24–37.

26. D'Heilly SJ, Blade MA, Nichol KL. Safety of influenza vaccinations administered in non-traditional settings. *Vaccine* 2006; 24: 4024–4027.

27. Hearings before the House Committee on Energy and Commerce Subcommittee on Health, Subcommittee on Oversight and Investigations. Testimony of Carlos A. Ruiz, Pharmacy Director, Navarro Discount Pharmacies. March 10, 2003. http://www.gpo.gov/fdsys/pkg/CHRG-108hhrg86053/html/ CHRG-108hhrg86053.htm (Accessed September 17, 2014).

28. Centers for Disease Control and Prevention. Adult immunization programs in non-traditional settings: quality standards and guidance for program evaluation: a report of the National Vaccine Advisory Committee. *MMWR* 2000; 49(RR-01): 1–13.

29. Baccam P, Willauer D, Krometis J, Ma Y, Sen A, Boechler M. Mass prophylaxis dispensing concerns: traffic and public access to PODs. *Biosecur Bioterror* 2011; 9(2): 139–151.

30. May L, Cote T, Hardeman B, et al. A model "go-kit" for use at Strategic National Stockpile points of dispensing. *J Public Health Manage* 2007; 13: 23–30.

31. Schwartz B, Wortley P. Mass vaccination for annual and pandemic influenza. In: Plotkin SA, ed. *Mass Vaccination: Global Aspects–Progress and Obstacles. Current Topics in Microbiology and Immunology.* Berlin Heidelberg, Springer, 2006; 131–152.

32. Phillips FB, Williamson JP. Local health department applies incident management system for successful mass influenza clinics. *J Public Health Manage* 2005; 11(4): 269–273.

33. Karras BT, Huq S, Bliss D, Lober WB. National pharmaceutical stockpile drill analysis using XML data collection on wireless java phones. *Proc AMIA Symposium* 2002; 365–391.

34. Mass dispensing authorization to pick up medicine form. http://www.madisonct.org/emergency/docs/forms/MASS %20DISPENSING%20AUTHORIZATION%20TO%20PICK %20UP%20MEDICINE.pdf (Accessed on September 17, 2014).

35. Philadelphia Department of Public Health. Head of household form. Point of Dispensing (POD) Operations Manual 2006. http://www.naccho.org/toolbox/_toolbox/POD %20operations%20manual_1.pdf (Accessed on September 17, 2014).

36. Missouri Strategic National Stockpile public health dispensing assessment form. http://health.mo.gov/emergencies/sns/pdf/ DrugDispensingProtoco.pdf (Accessed September 17, 2014).

37. Stergachis A, Wetmore CM, Pennylegion M, et al. Evaluation of a mass dispensing exercise in a Cities Readiness Initiative setting. *Am J Health-Syst Ph* 2007; 64(3): 285–93.

38. Zerwekh T, McKnight J, Hupert N, Wattson D, Hendrickson L, Lane D. Mass medication modeling in response to public health emergencies: outcomes of a drive-thru exercise. *J Public Health Manage* 2007; 13: 7–15.

39. U.S. Department of Agriculture. National Center for Animal Health Emergency Management. http://www.aphis.usda .gov/wps/portal/aphis/ourfocus/animalhealth/sa_emergency_ management (Accessed September 17, 2014).

40. Centers for Disease Control and Prevention. Mass Antibiotic Dispensing: Using Public Information to Enhance POD Flow. Webcast. Atlanta, GA. December 1, 2005. http://www2a.cdc.gov/ TCEOnline/registration/detailpage.asp?res_id=1981 (Accessed September 17, 2014).

41. Centers for Disease Control and Prevention. Mass Antibiotic Dispensing: Streamlining POD Design and Operations. Webcast. Atlanta, GA. April 14, 2005. http://www2a.cdc.gov/ TCEOnline/registration/detailpage.asp?res_id=1863 (Accessed September 17, 2014).

42. Beaton RD, Stevermer A, Wicklund J, Owens D, Boase J, Oberle MW. Evaluation of the Washington state National

Pharmaceutical Stockpile dispensing exercise, part II: dispensary site worker findings. *J Public Health Manage* 2004; 10(1): 77–85.

43. Blank S, Moskin LC, Zucker JR. An ounce of prevention is a ton of work: mass antibiotic prophylaxis for anthrax, New York City, 2001. *Emerg Infect Dis* 2003; 9: 615–622.

44. Andress K. A postevent smallpox mass vaccination clinic exercise. *Disaster Manage Response* 2003; 1(2): 54–48.

45. Office of the Surgeon General. Medical Reserve Corps. http://www.surgeongeneral.gov/mrc (Accessed September 17, 2014).

46. Banner G. The Rhode Island medical emergency distribution system (MEDS). *Disaster Manage Response* 2004; 2: 53–57.

47. Durante A, Melchreit R, Sullivan K, Degutis L. Connecticut competency-based point of dispensing worker training needs assessment. *Disaster Med Public Health Prep* 2010; 4(4): 306–311.

48. Young D. Pharmacist's software design aids mass dispensing clinics. *Am J Health-Syst Ph* 2006; 63: 400–402.

49. Hupert N, Mushlin AI, Callahan MA. Modeling the public health response to bioterrorism: using discrete event simulation to design antibiotic distribution centers. *Med Decis Making* 2002; 22(Suppl.): S17–S25.

50. Washington ML, Mason J, Meltzer MI. Maxi-vac: planning smallpox vaccination clinics. *J Public Health Manage* 2005; 11(6): 542–549.

51. Aaby K, Abbey RL, Herrmann JW, Treadwell M, Jordan CS, Wood K. Embracing computer modeling to address pandemic influenza in the 21st century. *J Public Health Manage* 2006; 12(4): 365–372.

52. Lee EK, Maheshwary S, Mason J, Glisson W. Decision support system for mass dispensing of medications for infectious disease outbreaks and bioterrorist attacks. *Ann Oper Res* 2006; 148(1): 25–53.

53. Centers for Disease Control and Prevention. Smallpox Vaccination Clinic Guide Template. http://www.bt.cdc.gov/agent/smallpox/response-plan/files/annex-3.pdf (Accessed September 17, 2014).

54. Centers for Disease Control and Prevention. Mass Antibiotic Dispensing-Managing Volunteer Staffing. Webcast. Atlanta, GA. December 2, 2004. http://www.naccho.org/toolbox/tool.cfm?id=81&program_id=18 (Accessed September 17, 2014).

55. Young D. Iowa pharmacists dispense from Strategic National Stockpile during drill. *Am J Health-Syst Ph* 2003; 60: 1304–1306.

56. Partridge R, Alexander J, Lawrence T, Suner S. Medical counterbioterrorism: the response to provide anthrax prophylaxis to New York City US Postal Service employees. *Ann Emerg Med* 2003; 41: 441–446.

57. Pine AE. Vaccination ventures: explanation and outcomes of a mass smallpox vaccination clinic exercise held June 17, 2003. San Francisco Department of Public Health Communicable Disease Prevention Unit, 2005.

58. Beaton RD, Oberle MW, Wicklund J, Stevermer A, Boase J, Owens D. Evaluation of the Washington state National Pharmaceutical Stockpile dispensing exercise. Part I: patient volunteer findings. *J Public Health Manage* 2003; 9: 368–376.

59. Taylor L, Tan CG, Liu S, Miro S, Genese CA, Bresnitz EA. New Jersey's smallpox vaccination clinic experiences, 2003. *J Public Health Manage* 2005; 11(3): 216–221.

60. Osterholm MT. How to vaccinate 30,000 people in three days: realities of outbreak management. *Public Health Rep* 2002; 116(Suppl. 2): 74–78.

61. Gibson WA. Mass smallpox immunization program in a deployed military setting. *Am J Emerg Med* 2004; 22: 267–269.

62. Poland GA, Grabenstein JD, Neff JM. The U.S. smallpox vaccination program: a review of a large modern era smallpox vaccination implementation program. *Vaccine* 2005; 23: 2078–2081.

63. Folio LR, Lahti RL, Cockrum DS, Bills S, Younker MR. Initial experience with mass immunization as a bioterrorism counter-measure. *J Am Osteopath Assoc* 2004; 104(6): 240–243.

64. Fontanesi J, Hill L, Olson R, Bennett NM, Kopald D. Mass vaccination clinics versus appointments. *J Med Practice Manage* March/April 2006; 288–294.

65. Rinchiuso-Hasselmann A, Starr DT, McKay RL, Medina E, Raphael M. Public compliance with mass prophylaxis guidance. *Biosecur Bioterror* 2010; 8(3):255–63.

66. Steelfisher G, Blendon R, Ross LJ, Collins BC, Ben-Porath EN, Bekheit MM, Mailhot JR. Public response to an anthrax attack: reactions to mass prophylaxis in a scenario involving inhalation anthrax from an unidentified source. *Biosecur Bioterror* 2011; 9(3): 239–250.

67. National Advisory Committee on Children and Terrorism. Recommendations to the Secretary. 2003. https://www.hsdl.org/?view&did=437514 (Accessed September 17, 2014).

68. Walz BJ, Bissell RA, Maguire B, Judge JA. Vaccine administration by paramedics: a model for bioterrorism and disaster response preparation. *Prehosp Disast Med* 2003; 18(4): 321–326.

69. The White House. President details Project BioShield. http://georgewbush-whitehouse.archives.gov/news/releases/2003/02/20030203.html (Accessed September 17, 2014).

70. The White House. Fact sheet: progress in the war on terror. http://www.whitehouse.gov/news/releases/2004/07/print/20040721–9.html (Accessed September 17, 2014).

71. Courtney B, Sherman S, Penn M. Federal legal preparedness tools for facilitating medical countermeasure use during public health emergencies. *J Law Med Ethics* 2013; 41 (Suppl. 1): 22–27.

72. Hupert N, Wattson D, Cuomo J, Benson S. Anticipating demand for emergency health services due to medication-related adverse events after rapid mass prophylaxis campaigns. *Acad Emerg Med* 2007; 14: 268–274.

73. Trust for America's Health. *Ready or Not? Protecting the Public's Health from Diseases, Disasters, and Bioterrorism.* Washington, DC, Trust for America's Health, 2006.

74. Glenn GM, Kenney RT. Mass vaccination: solutions in the skin. In: Plotkin SA, ed. *Mass Vaccination: Global Aspects–Progress and Obstacles. Current Topics in Microbiology and Immunology.* Berlin Heidelberg, Springer, 2006; 247–268.

19

MANAGEMENT OF MASS GATHERINGS

Michael S. Molloy

Some people think football is a matter of life and death. I don't like that attitude. I can assure them it is much more serious than that.

Bill Shankly
Liverpool Football Club Manager,
in Sunday Times (UK) *1981*

OVERVIEW

Introduction

Mass gathering medical care is a very important subspecialty of disaster medicine and quite a challenging one. Such care is generally provided in unfamiliar environments and often without access to familiar hospital structures and resources.

Medical management of mass gatherings encompasses a wide range of activities due to the varying types of events and baseline medical and health infrastructures where the events are held. Terrorist attacks are becoming an ever increasing concern for organizers of mass gatherings. Stratton highlights the importance of recognizing potential sources for violence at mass gatherings, particularly in light of the events that took place at the 2013 Boston Marathon.[1] The Boston Marathon bombings in April 2013 highlighted how preparedness can mitigate effects of terrorist attacks.[2,3] This event also highlighted how an organized EMS system, well versed in triage and supported by a large number of local trauma centers, can distribute the patient load effectively and efficiently to maximize outcomes.[4] Caterson describes how teamwork on scene and in the emergency department and operating theatres contributed to beneficial outcomes for patients.[5]

Emergency physicians are ideally trained to provide direct patient care services at mass gathering sites. They can also provide leadership in planning the organization of routine emergency medical care and potential disaster response to such events. The American College of Emergency Physicians (ACEP) published a position paper in 1976 on the role of emergency physicians in mass casualty/disaster management, emphasizing that their training prepares them for these unique roles.[6] In 1998, the Council of the European Society for Emergency Medicine

suggested that "specific training in preparedness for disasters is required for all emergency physicians." The Council recommended that members of the specialty should participate in disaster planning at local, regional, national, and international levels.[7] Mass gatherings are a form of organized disaster. A large group of patrons are in a defined area where an adverse event would affect a significant number of attendees and require activation of the region's emergency management plan. Since mass gatherings occur sporadically, they are not routinely included in local authority or regional disaster plans. Lund proposes that mass gathering medicine provides a practical means of enhancing disaster preparedness for the Canadian medical workforce at municipal, provincial, and national levels.[8] Event-specific planning and appropriate training at the local and regional levels are important. Hsu, in a review of the effectiveness of mass-casualty incident training, highlighted that although preparedness at the hospital level has increased, the effectiveness of training still requires evaluation.[9]

In many countries, routine prehospital care is the domain of emergency medical technicians and paramedics. In others, a mixed model exists with physician involvement and occasionally physician direction. While nomenclature is inconsistent across countries, this chapter will use the term "medical director" to denote the physician in charge of medical management at a mass gathering.

Mass gathering medicine involves a spectrum ranging from additional prehospital resources being directed to a specific area for a short time (a sports events taking place on a single afternoon) to very sophisticated models where resources remain in place over a number of months. The world's largest and longest duration mass gathering is the Kumbh Mela, which takes place in India over 55 days every 12 years. Tens of millions of pilgrims visit this 58-square-kilometer holy site to bathe. A temporary city is created to house the more than 1 million "permanent residents" for the event in a floodplain that is dry at this time of year.[10] Millions of Muslim pilgrims have gathered annually for centuries at Mecca, Saudi Arabia, to participate in sacred rituals known as the Hajj. There are around 1.6 billion Muslims worldwide who have an obligation to attend the Hajj at least once in their lifetimes. This forms the largest annually recurring mass gathering event in the world. It involves conversion of empty fixed hospital facilities into full service sites that are equipped solely for the gathering. These are staffed by 15,000 medical, nursing, and paramedical staff who provide care for hundreds of thousands of persons for periods lasting from 1 day to 4 weeks or more.[11] The recurring nature of this event has led Saudi Arabia to develop sophisticated safety, security, travel, and illness/injury prevention strategies.

A mass gathering event site may be a temporary facility or a modified fixed facility where the standard emergency plan is insufficient. The standard event plan focuses on event logistics and not on managing a major incident. For this reason, scheduled mass gatherings should have emergency plans of their own, separate from the event plan. Mass gathering medical care is likely to become increasingly important in the current world climate as governments and other statutory authorities place more emphasis on emergency planning.

Community public health plays an important role in mass gathering medicine, providing guidance on such topics as sanitation, disease surveillance, water supply, and food safety.[12] In 2004, Levett described the growing awareness of public health issues that had developed in the timeframe between the Atlanta and Sydney Olympic games.[13] He noted that "prevention and preparation more than ever are necessary for organized society, and effective planning demonstrates that future uncertainty can be reduced."[13] He further stated that public health should be an integral part of the planning process for the Athens games and that a dual strategy of supporting a successful event and also improving the quality of life of the Greek population would be desirable.

Medical textbooks that describe illnesses and novel treatments generally transcend borders and will provide useful information for clinicians treating patients irrespective of their locations. Conversely, while basic principles apply globally, mass gathering medicine varies according to applicable laws and variable health systems. In a career focus article in the *British Medical Journal*, Hearns outlines the qualities, training, and benefits associated with event medicine or mass gathering medical care.[14] Many physicians provide mass gathering medical care on a voluntary basis for sports clubs or societies where they are also the team physician, thereby mixing roles. Some sports specify that there be a physician present prior to the game starting, while others specify that there must be a separate "crowd" doctor in addition to the team physician when the crowd is over a certain size. Whether the physician is paid or acting as a volunteer does not change the "duty to care" or "standard of care" for the patients. Physicians must be appropriately trained prior to serving as medical directors for mass gatherings. The Gibson report in the United Kingdom (UK) published in 1990 made recommendations about medical care at football matches. Gibson emphasized that the specific requirements should include communication skills and command and control procedure training for major incident management. In the *British Journal of Sports Medicine* in 1999, Kerr noted that 9 years after publication of the Gibson report, 44% of doctors providing medical services at sports events remained unaware of the major incident plan for their stadiums.[15] Nearly three-quarters (72%) of the doctors Kerr questioned had received no training in major incident management and 61% indicated they had not attended Advanced Cardiac Life Support (ACLS), Advanced Trauma Life Support (ATLS), Pediatric Advanced Life Support (PALS), or other British Association for Immediate Care (BASICS) resuscitation courses. These results are for a country that has placed considerable emphasis on major incident training and mass gathering medical care as a result of football match incidents, and therefore may underestimate training deficits in other countries.

Some events that should be considered "mass gatherings" for the purposes of medical management have not traditionally been considered as such. For example, certain religious events are some of the biggest regular mass gatherings (the papal gatherings for the Catholic church and the Hajj for Muslims).[16,17] It is not unusual for half a million people or more to participate in papal gatherings.[18,19] The Hajj has over 2.5 million annual pilgrims, more than 80% of whom travel from 183 countries to Saudi Arabia to fulfill their obligations at the holy site at Mecca.[11] Kumbh Mela is an Indian religious festival where up to 70 million participants congregate over 55 days to bathe in holy waters and live in temporary facilities constructed in dry floodplains (Figure 19.1).

Medical planners may underestimate the numbers who will require medical attention at such events.[20] Avery describes the planning for a papal visit to Coventry in 1982, and suggests that for any gathering of up to 350,000 people, significant planning will be required.[18] In 1979, Pope John Paul II held a papal audience in Phoenix Park, Dublin, Ireland, that was attended by more than 1 million people (about one-third of the population). This was one of the highest percentages of a nation's population in attendance in a confined area for a single event. While data are incomplete, there was only a single fatality recorded at the event that night, a security guard on patrol.

Millions travel to Mecca for the Hajj annually. Every able-bodied Muslim who can afford to do so is obliged to make the pilgrimage to Mecca at least once. More than 2 million persons participate annually and there are excellent data on the various medical aspects of the pilgrims and the additional impact on hospital admissions during Hajj.[21–23] Over the years, there have been significant numbers of deaths associated with crushing injuries as the crowd surges across the bridge. Planners have redesigned the bridge as a mitigation strategy.[24]

Definitions

There is no international standard definition of a mass gathering. The concept of mass gathering medical management has only been described for four decades, possibly because physicians have not had full-time roles in the area. In the United States, ordinances dating from 1974 in North Carolina recognized that "The mass gatherings of people for an extended period of time at one place within Union County, without proper care being taken for the protection of said persons and the public, can create conditions which are detrimental to the health, safety and welfare of the citizens of this County and the peace and dignity of this County."[25]

To provide for the protection of public health, property, public welfare, and safety, the Union County Board of Commissioners in North Carolina adopted ordinances that: 1) define mass gatherings and require that permits are obtained; 2) specify creation of detailed maps showing the location of emergency ingress and egress routes and emergency medical facilities; and 3) mandate services must be organized in advance. The ordinance states: "Mass Gathering means the congregation or assembly in which admission is charged or other contributions are solicited, accepted or received, all in reasonable contemplation of profit, of more than 200 people in an open space, or open air for a continuous period of at least six hours."[25]

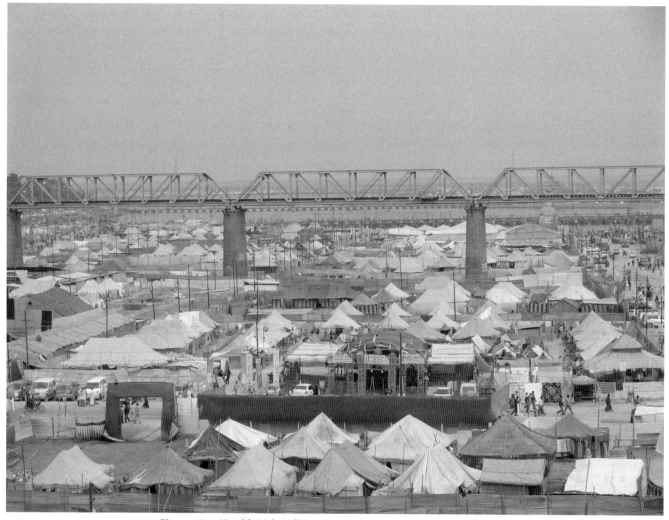

Figure 19.1. Kumbh Mela Religious Festival accommodations on floodplain.

Alleghany County, also in North Carolina, enacted similar ordinances in 1975 that increased the number of people required to define a mass gathering to 300.[26] The Arkansas State Board of Health defined 1,000 persons in one place for more than 12 hours as a mass gathering.[27] Most authors, when discussing mass gatherings in a modern setting, refer to congregations of more than 1,000 people, although others define a mass gathering as being greater than 25,000 persons.[28,29] The precise number must be placed in the context of where the event takes place and what exactly the available medical resources are pre-event. In determining the intensity of care, the level of practitioner staffing, and the type of equipment required at an event site, one needs to consider the following: duration of the event, spectator type, participant numbers and demographics, geography, terrain, and transfer time to access definitive medical care. In 1999, Jaslow published a review of U.S. state legislation and found that only six states had specific EMS legislation governing mass gathering medical care: Connecticut, Iowa, New York, Oregon, Pennsylvania, and Wisconsin.[30]

For this chapter a mass gathering will be defined as an event that requires special planning to assure capacity and capability for the provision of appropriate medical care to attendees without adversely affecting medical care in the host community. This is similar to the World Health Organization definition of "any occasion, either organized or spontaneous, that attracts sufficient numbers of people to strain the planning and response resources of the community, city or nation hosting the event."[31]

The nature of the event, including its size and duration, the numbers and demographics of participants, and its geographic location are important considerations. In contradistinction to the sample ordinances, this definition deliberately avoids using numbers to classify a mass gathering. Consistent with the philosophy of this book, the key consideration is the functional impact of the event rather than the absolute number of people involved.

To determine effects on baseline medical services, events must be considered within the context of the involved community. Medical resources must be planned to mitigate any potential negative effects on routine medical care during the mass gathering.

Classification of Mass Gatherings

A classification system for mass gatherings can aid in the planning process internationally and also achieve a commonality of language for describing future events. Although using numbers of participants alone has limitations, some authors have suggested this approach to determine the resources required for planning (Table 19.1). The majority of physicians involved in

Table 19.1. Mass Gathering Classification Scheme as proposed by Molloy

Mass Gathering Classification

Class	Subclass	Numbers Involved	Resources Required	Example	Planning Process
Mass gathering	Small	200–1,500	Local	Local fair	1–2 months
	Medium	1,500–10,000	Local	Local sports game	1–2 months
	Large	10,000–100,000	Local + Country	Concert/sports game	6–12 months
Major Mass Gathering		100,000–250,000	Regional +/− National	Large music festivals	>12 months
Super Mass Gathering		250,000–500,000	National	Motor sports events	>12 months
Extreme Mass Gathering		500,000–1,000,000	National +/− International	Religious festivals	12–24 months
Mega Mass Gathering		1,000,000+	National + International	Papal visits, Haji	12–24 months

providing mass gathering medical care will participate in events that have less than 100,000 attendances. There are considerable differences between providing care at a local community event where the attendance will be less than 1,500 compared to providing medical support in football stadiums or rock concerts where the attendance will be up to 100,000. However, the commonality between small, medium, and large mass gathering events is the recurrence of such events on sites within the community and institutional memory aiding in preparations for the following week's, month's, or year's events.

Larger events identified as "major mass gatherings" have been defined as those with an attendance between 100,000 and 250,000. These are associated with the added difficulties of mass transit, creation of suitable treatment and potential accommodation facilities, and public health issues for those in attendance. These events typically can last a number of days.

"Super mass gatherings" are those with attendance between 250,000 and 500,000. Commonly these will be sporting events with mass attendance such as NASCAR, Formula 1, the Olympic Games, or football world cups. These will require significant coordination of medical teams where events are longer than 1 day in duration.

"Extreme mass gatherings" and "mega mass gatherings" require significant planning and commonly will be religious events, state funerals, significant political party conventions, inaugurations, or political demonstrations. The majority of these will be planned events for which there will be considerable warning. Recurrent religious festivals such as Hajj and Kumbh Mela will have significant event history and year-round preparations for the next iteration of the event. The true spontaneous events of such size will be political demonstrations such as have occurred in recent years in Egypt. State and political funerals leave little time for preparation but will have significant state and regional involvement in their planning.

Some mass gatherings reduce emergency department visits, probably due to spectators remaining in their homes watching the event on television.[32,33] Events that are recurring (local annual fairs, the Hajj, Kumbh Mela) yield historical data useful for planning future iterations. Planners can estimate resource needs for major sports events like American football, athletics, NASCAR, baseball, golf, rugby, or soccer that recur regularly in the same location.[34–38] Using the same team for each event recurrence reduces training requirements and can enhance team dynamics in the disaster setting. McCarthy et al. outline how community disaster resilience can be enhanced through effective planning for mass sporting events.[39]

This cycle of event, analysis, training, planning, and new event should be the goal for those involved in organizing mass gathering medical care. One drawback of frequent events is that they can lead to complacency. A varied training program emphasizing elements of trauma; cardiac, pediatric, and major incident care; and specific hazards will help mass gathering staff remain vigilant to potential threats.

History of Mass Gathering Medicine

Mass gathering medicine is a relatively new concept. The first mention in the modern UK literature was a short piece entitled "The Price of Pop" in *Lancet* in 1971.[40] The author describes the effect of a pop festival on a small island community with a population of about 120,000. Attendance at the festival was estimated to be 250,000 people at maximum. This temporary tripling of the population created traffic, noise, food supply, and sanitation problems. The author suggests: "Open-air pop festivals lasting two or three days may be a passing phase, but other fashions may encourage similar gatherings and conditions."[40] Mass gatherings have grown in frequency and size since this initial description. Kumbh Mela has been described in medical journals such as the *British Medical Journal* as far back as 1895, when 2 million pilgrims attended the event and specific mitigation strategies were developed to prevent the spread of cholera. However, no other descriptions of medical preparations were identified.

Provision of organized mass gathering medical care in the United States dates back to at least the 1960s. After the death of two spectators at a university football stadium in the state of Nebraska, organizers instituted a system whereby staff and equipment were strategically placed within the stadium to facilitate a rapid emergency response.[41] As a result of historic disasters in the UK and Ireland, procedures for treating urgent casualties have been in place for almost a century in many sports venues (Table 19.2). Initially the focus was on protecting participants rather than spectators. In the 1960s, disaster planners created the forerunner to BASICS with the goal of providing medical assistance to ambulance services at scenes of accidents, emergencies, or major incidents such as mass-casualty events. In 1977, healthcare leaders founded BASICS, a system that provides regional teams for disaster response throughout the UK.[42] Many of its members provide mass gathering medical care at stadiums.

Table 19.2. Deaths in United Kingdom Football Stadiums

Year	Stadium	Cause	Deaths	Injuries
1888	Valley Parade, Bradford	Railings collapse	1	3
1902	Ibrox Park, Glasgow	Terrace collapse	26	550
1939	Rochdale Athletic Ground	Roof collapse	1	17
1946	Bolton	Crushing	33	400
1957	Shawfield, Glasgow	Barrier collapse	1	50
1961	Ibrox Park, Glasgow	Crush on staircase	2	50
1968	Dunfermline	Barriers collapse	1	49
1971	Ibrox Park, Glasgow	Crushing	66	145
1985	St. Andrews, Birmingham	Wall collapse	1	20
1985	Valley Parade, Bradford	Fire	56	hundreds
1989	Hillsborough, Sheffield	Crushing	96	400+
1993	Cardiff Arms Park	Distress rocket	1	0

The Hillsborough Disaster in Sheffield, England, in 1989 is a well-known example of an incident at a mass gathering. At the Football Association Cup semi-final, the opening of a large gate was required to allow those arriving late to enter.[43] This resulted in a rapid buildup of supporters on a terrace that was already crowded. There was no escape at the front due to a crowd control ring fence. Large numbers of the crowd suffered asphyxia.[44,45] Ninety-six people lost their lives, 81 on-site and 15 more subsequently in the hospital.[46] The two local emergency departments received 159 casualties, 155 of these in the first 90 minutes after the incident. All the severely injured were received within 45 minutes and 81 patients were subsequently admitted to the hospital. DeAngeles described a similar incident in the United States that resulted in eighty persons being injured by crushing or trampling during a crowd surge at a college football game.[47] On this occasion, eighty-six people were transported to the hospital, ten were admitted for traumatic asphyxia, two had musculoskeletal injuries requiring admission, one patient had a liver injury, and six others were admitted for observation. Several stadium factors were identified that resulted in crush-related injury. Appropriate changes in crowd control policies were implemented.

Another famous historic event is the Bradford City fire disaster in 1985, resulting from a flash fire that consumed one side of the Valley Parade football stadium in Bradford, England.[48] The fire engulfed old wooden stands in less than 4 minutes and 53 people died, with more than 250 additional people injured.[49] Some of the crowd were so badly burned that they could only be identified from dental records.[50] Sharpe wrote about the treatment and triage of multiple burn victims arriving almost simultaneously at the local hospital and the sequence of internal coincidences that ultimately minimized the consequences.[51]

He subsequently coined the mnemonic COMMUNICATION to help educate other plastic surgeons who may be faced with a similar mass gathering disaster:[52]

C = Chaos
O = Order
M = Most experienced plastic surgeon
M = Make available adequate resources
U = Update casualty figures at regular intervals
N = No points for economizing
I = Inpatient needs
C = Capitalize on goodwill
A = Accommodation
T = Team leader
I = Invite outside help
O = Outpatients
N = Nursing officer

Although this mnemonic was directed at plastic surgeons working in a burn unit, the principles could be adapted to other settings such as the Boston Marathon bombing. Communication failures have been noted as being a major factor limiting effectiveness of response to major disasters. Highlighting the phrase should focus attention on this problem during the response phase.

Internationally, football-related mass gathering disasters (or soccer, as it is known in the United States) have resulted in more morbidity and mortality than most other sports (Table 19.3). Data are derived from multiple sources, and in many cases, it is difficult to determine exact numbers of casualties and deaths. One reason for this is that less seriously injured persons were evaluated by their general practitioners rather than assessed at the site of the event. In some instances, officials blocked media coverage of the disasters and, as was the case with the 1982 football match in Moscow, when dozens of sport spectators were crushed to death, the true magnitude of the disaster did not became evident until many years later, even to those on-site. Morbidity and mortality numbers have been substantial, prompting major changes in the way events are planned and organized. Some of these disasters have occurred in older stadiums where walls, ceilings, or roofs have collapsed. Football authorities have instituted a team licensing system to help prevent this from recurring.

In the 1970s and 1980s, football hooliganism was widespread throughout Europe. During the last 15 years, law enforcement communities have successfully cooperated to minimize such activities. Nevertheless, civil unrest before, during, and after games still contributes to significant numbers of deaths.

Types and Sites of Mass Gathering Events

> I went to a fight the other night, and a hockey game broke out.
>
> Rodney Dangerfield

Mass gathering events may take many formats. Researchers have described event-specific aspects of medical care for the following:

- Local fairs[53]
- Music events[40,54–58]
- School and university gatherings[59]
- Stadium sports events[15,60–63]
- Summer Olympics[64–66]

Table 19.3. Deaths and Injuries during International Football Disasters

Year	Stadium	Cause	Deaths	Injuries
1961	Ibague, Colombia	Stand collapse	11	15
1961	Santiago, Chile	Crushing	5	300 approx.
1964	Lima, Peru	Riot	318	1,000+
1967	Kayseri, Turkey	Riot	48	602
1968	Buenos Aires, Argentina	Crushing	73	150 approx.
1974	Cairo, Egypt	Crushing	49	50
1976	Port au Prince, Haiti	Firecracker/crush/Shooting	6	0
1979	Hamburg, Germany		1	15
1979	Lagos, Nigeria	Riot	24	27
1980	Calcutta, India	Riot	16	100
1981	Athens, Greece	Crushing	21	54
1982	San Luis, Brazil	Shot in riot	3	25
1982	Cali, Colombia	Stampede	24	250 approx.
1982	Algiers, Algeria	Roof collapse	10	600 approx.
1982	Moscow, Russia	Crushing	340+	0
1985	Heysel, Brussels	Riot/wall collapse	38	437
1985	Mexico City, Mexico	Crushing	10	100+
1987	Tripoli, Libya	Riot/wall collapse	20	0
1988	Katmandu, Nepal	Stampede in hailstorm	93	700 approx.
1989	Lagos, Nigeria	Crushing	5?	0
1990	Mogadishu, Somalia	Shot in riot	7	18
1991	Orkney, Johannesburg, South Africa	Crushing/fighting	42	50
1991	Nairobi, Kenya	Stampede	1	24
1992	Bastia, France	Stand collapse	17	1,300 approx.
1996	Lusaka, Zambia	Crushing	9	52
1996	Guatemala City, Guatemala	Crushing	78	180
1997	Lagos, Nigeria	Locked exits – crushing	5	0
1997	Cludad del Este, Paraguay	Roof collapse	30+	200 approx.
1998	Kinshasa, Dem Republic of Congo	Troops fire on crowd	4	0
1999	Alexandria, Egypt	Crushing	8	14
2000	Harare, Zimbabwe	Crowd fleeing tear gas	13	0
2000	Rio de Janeiro, Brazil	Crushing	104	0
2001	Johannesburg, South Africa	Crushing	43	89
2001	Seville, Spain	Fence collapse	28	0
2001	Lubumbashi, Congo (Zaire)	Crowd fleeing tear gas	10	51
2001	Sari, Iran	Roof collapse	2	284
2001	Ivory Coast	Riot	1	39
2001	Accra, Ghana	Crowd fleeing tear gas	126	93
2001	Labe, Guinea	Crushing	2	0

- Winter Olympics[67]
- Major football championships (World Cup, Union of European Football Associations Championship)[38,68,69]
- Marathons[2,70–72]
- Rugby World Cup[73,74]
- Cricket World Cup[75]
- Motorsports[36,76,77]
- Water sports
- Political demonstrations[53,78,79]
- Religious events[18]
- World expositions[80]

Modern arenas or stadiums are equipped with medical facilities built to be compliant with community health and safety standards. In many countries, local governments build municipal stadiums that are licensed to various sporting bodies for use in their particular events. These stadiums are frequently used to host rock concerts and some religious gatherings. Since they are designed as multipurpose stadiums, the basic medical kits and facilities are standardized. For contact sporting events (boxing, mixed martial arts fighting), large rock concerts, or long duration mass gatherings, additional temporary facilities must generally be constructed to meet the increased medical and health needs.

Figure 19.2 shows an example of a well-bounded stadium with wide access and egress routes to prevent crushing at entrance or exits. From this aerial shot, one can see the access roads, free space in the venue, the local town, and the "backstage" area (distant from the stage) in the foreground. This venue accommodates an attendance of approximately 25,000. There are standard first aid areas in all such facilities in Ireland and in many other locations in Europe.

The Union of European Football Associations (UEFA), the European football regulatory authority, has requirements specifying what facilities must exist to license clubs for competition nationally and throughout Europe, such as in the champions league. These regulations are available at www.UEFA.com or from the national football governing body of the specific country.[81] More commonly, a large event takes place in a venue without planned medical facilities, so these must be created de novo.

Figure 19.3 shows an aerial view of Slane Castle, the site of the U2 homecoming concert in 2001. The final qualifying game for the 2002 soccer World Cup was also broadcast live from this venue. Slane Castle is one of Europe's most scenic natural amphitheaters. De novo facilities were created to manage all aspects of the event, from sanitation to medical care. One of the access roads and one of the gates are visible in the foreground. At this late time of day, the lines are short; however it would not be unusual to have a 1.5-kilometer queue of people outside the stadium waiting for gates to open. The castle itself is in the mid-ground and has been host to many of Ireland's most memorable rock concerts since 1981. Evident in the photograph is the natural slope from the entrance on the road to the river over 150 meters gradient below. This particular slope can result in significant numbers of traumatic injuries on challenging underfoot conditions in inclement weather. Murphy described the effects on regional hospitals after an event when eighty-eight patients presented to the two local emergency departments with thirteen fractures, six requiring manipulation under anesthesia or formal open reduction and internal fixation.[82] The river in the background is another hazard. It is deceptively fast and has claimed

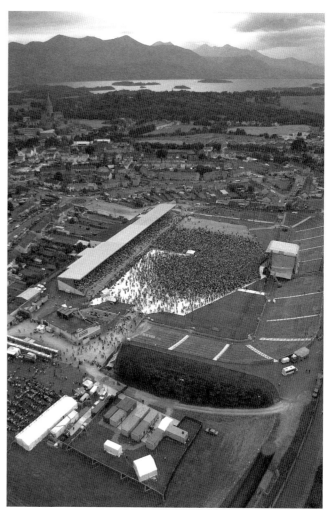

Figure 19.2. Killarney GAA Stadium: Summerfest 2006. *Credit:* macmonagle.com.

lives over the years as concert-goers attempted to swim its course and gain entry for free. In this photograph, more than 84,000 people are located in a very confined space with identifiable access and egress routes. Thus, crowd density would be another potential hazard. This example illustrates the types of challenges that are encountered globally due to geography, topography, and insufficient local medical infrastructure.

CURRENT STATE OF THE ART

Mass Gathering Event Planning

"Tuas maith, leath na hoibre"
An old Irish phrase meaning "a good start is half the work"

International guidelines for mass gathering event planning are lacking. Countries with well-developed emergency medical systems, such as the United States and the UK, have national guidelines that could be applied in other jurisdictions. In most countries, the demand for medical resources at mass gatherings is sporadic and fulfilled on an ad hoc basis. Requests to physicians and other medical workers are increasing in frequency.[61] An ad hoc request made the evening before an event

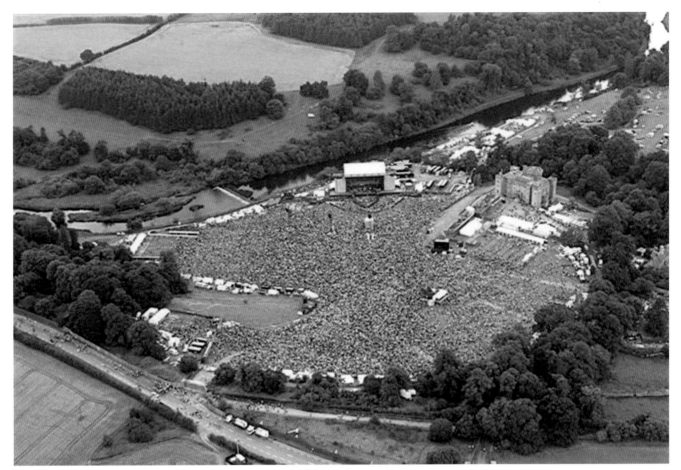

Figure 19.3. Slane Castle 2001: U2 concert.

indicating "the need for a doctor for insurance purposes" leaves the physician unprepared. This may be the first time the physician has been asked to provide medical services. No information may be offered on the layout of the venue, the size of the crowd or number of event employees, what medical facilities will be present, or the level of training and equipment carried by the EMS service (which may be a voluntary provider) on that day. Other important elements to know in advance include historical information such as: How many patrons have needed medical attention? Have there been any fatalities? What were the crowd demographics? How many patients were transferred to hospitals?[83–85]

For large venues, mass gathering event planning may begin up to 2 years prior and should occur no later than 1 year before the expected start date. In some jurisdictions, the event may require licensing by the local authorities or formal planning permissions when the event involves significant change of use for the venue. Examples include a race course transformed to host a large pop festival for 100,000 patrons with on-site camping for 70,000 for 3 days. Considerations include how many medical practitioners would normally work in a town that size and how many would be on call at any specific time. The UK Event Safety Guide has staffing guidelines.[86] The tables estimate a minimum number of staff who should be on-site at all times; when considering staffing levels over a 24-hour period, this is paramount. A medical director should be identified at the planning stage and remain involved in the process to ensure that med-

ical matters are addressed and to mitigate any predicted medical risks.

Event planning for a specific mass gathering begins within the organizing body. Once the basic plan is complete, relevant statutory and voluntary agencies are folded into the planning process. Agencies who should be involved early in the planning process include, but are not limited to, those named in Table 19.4. Nations, states, and smaller jurisdictions such as counties may have different requirements for planning and varying processes for appeals when an application for an event license is refused. As a result, timelines for planning must be tailored to local circumstances. In 1996, the ACEP EMS Committee produced guidelines for the provision of emergency medical care for crowds.[87] These can be applied in most countries. The National Association of EMS Physicians (NAEMSP) also promulgated guidelines.[88] One key NAEMSP planning document is Jaslow's medical directors checklist.[89]

Event Planning Timeline

Local Planning Authority

Plans are only good intentions unless they immediately degenerate into hard work.

Peter Drucker (1909–2005)

Calabro and colleagues produced a precise event planning schedule for ACEP in *Provision of Emergency Medical Care for Crowds*.[87]

Table 19.4. Agencies to Involve in Event Planning

Event promoter

Local planning authorities

Local public service transport companies

Police

Fire services

Ambulance services (public and private)

Voluntary services (e.g., fire and ambulance)

Civil defense

Local health services

Emergency planning/management agency

Local hospitals

Site owners

Event medical officer/command physician and deputy

Public relations/media

A modified sample event timeline is shown in Table 19.5. A new template is used for each event and planners provide periodic reports to the director. To allow flexibility in accounting for unanticipated delays earlier on the timeline, some index times have few or no specific tasks assigned to them, such as at 14 days, 4 days, and 3 days in this model.

The event planning schedule illustrates the intensity of resources needed and the complexity of organizing a successful mass gathering event from the medical perspective. For regular events such as weekly or bi-weekly football games, planning may become routine. The event planning timetable for such regular mass gathering events can be further modified by designating index games such as first pre-season, first in-season, and a mid-season game as full detailed planning events and using a shortened 2-week timescale for the others. For regular events, a year-long timescale is impractical prior to the first event in the series. Rather, a permanent stadium back room management team for the professional club can be formed to assist in the planning stages, compress timescales, and serve as part of the overall event medical team. When the event is annual, each task takes more time and the medical director will have a more time consuming role. Effects on the routine work schedules in the weeks leading up to each mass gathering event for both the director and the team members should be considered.

The following sections provide additional detail for each step in event planning as outlined in Table 19.5 (modified from *Provision of Emergency Medical Care for Crowds*[87]).

DEFINE EVENT
■ Agencies involved
■ Type of event
■ Duration
■ Alcoholic beverages: permitting or banning sales, age policy for sales, and volume per sale
■ Screening for drugs at entrances
■ Attendance levels
■ Demographics of attendees (will minors be admitted and are elderly or disabled expected?)

■ Expected methods of transportation for attendees
■ Event history, if applicable, with specific details of:
  ■ medical usage rates
  ■ patient presentations per thousand attendees
  ■ number of hospital transports
  ■ names and locations of hospitals
  ■ outcomes of those transferred
  ■ numbers of medical, paramedical, and nursing staff
  ■ reports from voluntary aid societies
  ■ after action reports
■ Provide site map/local area map for event planning team

WALK EVENT SITE
■ Identify topography
■ Estimate site diameters/circumference
■ Plan location of access/egress routes for patrons (Use Google Maps for aerial plans)
■ Identify likely location of main and secondary stages for multistage events
■ Based on information previously listed, plan location for first aid posts, roaming medical teams, and on-site hospitals
■ Plan location of access/egress routes for ambulances
■ Identify potential hazards and mitigate them
■ Identify likely location of campsites if applicable
■ Repeat site visit during adverse weather conditions

As can be seen in Figure 19.4, understanding the topography and distances can be vital when planning sites for treatment facilities, on-site transport, and staffing numbers. The site in the figure is from an event with 80,000 attendees, 50,000 of which are in multiple campsites situated around the venue. There are two large open stage areas with capacity of more than 30,000 each and also four marquis facilities with capacities from 2,000–8,000.

EVENT PLANNING MEETINGS / GET SITE PLANS

Regular meetings will take place prior to the event. Some entities like the local emergency planning unit, government health service, and fire and police services will assign a full-time person to this role. For medical personnel, event planning activities will likely represent extra duties. Medical professionals seeking compensation for these additional activities may find it useful to review the planning timeline and calculate a projected time commitment in advance of accepting the position.

Early review of the event site plan allows an analysis of the potential roles for existing medical facilities and ambulance services. Event planners must advocate for using assets that are the most likely to provide necessary medical resources to support the event and not simply use alternate resources that may be more convenient for existing entities.

DESIGNATE AND AGREE ON RESPONSIBILITIES
■ Traffic management
■ Site management
■ Health and safety
■ Voluntary aid
■ Communications
■ Transport to site
■ Transport within site
■ Campsite (if present)

Table 19.5. Event Planning Schedule. Modified from Provision of Emergency Medical Care for Crowds: American College of Emergency Physicians[87]

Task	1yr	6mo	3mo	1mo	14d	7d	4d	3d	2d	1d	Event	Post-event	1d	3d	5d	1wk-1mo
Define Event	X	X		X		X			X	X	X				X	
Visit site + Walk	X			X		X			X	X	X					
Event planning meetings	X	X	X	X	X	X			X	X	X					
Get site plans	X	X		X		X			X		X					
Designate + agree responsibilities	X	X		X		X			X		X					
Designate medical/admin controllers	X			X		X				X	X					
Develop event medical plan	X	X		X	X	X			X	X	X	X			X	
Develop site emergency plan	X	X		X	X	X			X	X	X	X			X	
Liaise local ED/EMS/trauma units	X			X					X	X	X	X		X		
Ride-alongs to local ED/venue				X		X			X		X					
Obtain indemnity/malpractice/insurance	X	X		X												X
Confirm financial arrangements	X	X		X					X		X				X	
Confirm attendance figures	X			X					X		X					
Confirm camping arrangements & review	X			X		X			X		X	X				
Confirm VIP arrangements & review				X		X			X	X	X	X			X	
Recruit staff + check experience	X	X	X	X		X			X							X
Generate outline rosters & review				X		X			X	X	X				X	
Procure + check communications	X			X		X			X	X	X					
Develop medical protocols/SOPs	X		X	X		X			X	X	X	X			X	
Medical staff meeting + agency heads	X		X	X		X				X	X	X			X	
Agree event documentation standard		X	X	X		X				X	X	X			X	
Credential Staff				X		X			X		X	X			X	
Top up Training		X	X	X					X						X	
Procure + check clothing	X		X	X		X			X						X	
Procure + check equipment	X	X	X	X		X			X	X	X	X			X	
Check medical facilities siting				X		X			X	X	X	X			X	
Assign staff roles	X		X	X		X			X	X	X	X			X	
Procure site credentials & review				X	X	X			X	X	X	X			X	
Set Up + build facilities						X			X	X	X					
Pre-event briefing						X				X	X				X	
Debrief/Hotwash												X			X	
Break up event												X	X			
Post-event audit													X		X	
Plan next event																X

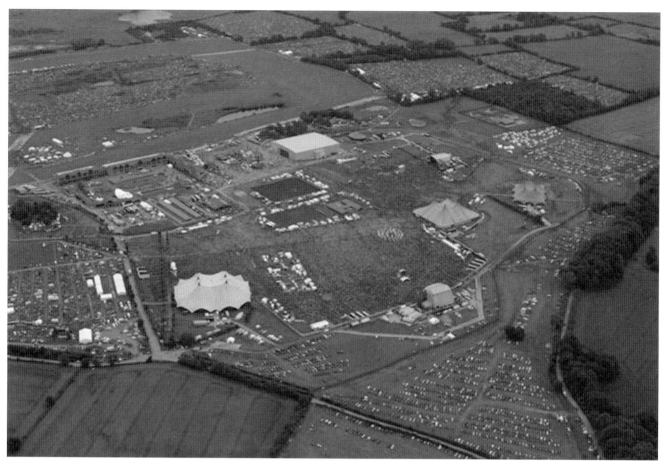

Figure 19.4. Aerial view of Oxegen Music Festival 2007 showing main arena and large tents for other concurrent stage performances with multiple campsites in mid-ground and background for up to 70,000 People.

Occupational health and safety is an important responsibility for the duration of the event. For large gatherings, there may be 5,000 staff on-site and even larger numbers with mega events. In some jurisdictions, medical personnel are required to inform the statutory authorities of industry-related accidents. Thus, a process should be in place to clearly identify medical records specific to staff presentations for work-related injuries. It is important to liaise with the command structures of voluntary aid organizations prior to the event to determine their roles, duties, responsibilities, and reporting relationships.

Specific policies and procedures requiring clarification include: 1) under what authority do accompanying physicians work; 2) who is responsible for the medical actions of non-physicians; and 3) if a major medical incident occurs during the event, how will volunteer workers receive direction from the event medical director.

DESIGNATE MEDICAL AND ADMINISTRATIVE CONTROLLERS

The event medical director and deputy should be identified and trained at least 1 year prior to the start of the event for major mass gatherings. A person without hospital-based responsibilities during a major disaster should be selected to avoid competing priorities at event and hospital sites.

On-site management follows similar principles to the incident command system. For large events, the administration section is a key component. Appropriate types and numbers of

records must be provided and distributed to the various venue posts. An administrator ensures that required paperwork or electronic data input are completed at all levels and that essential data are seamlessly communicated between various medical facilities. Patient tracking is important and a system should be in place that enables workers to provide information to friends and relatives regarding inquiries on victims' locations. Privacy of medical records must be maintained at all times.

DEVELOP EVENT MEDICAL PLAN

Few people have real-life experience with mass gathering event planning. For personnel new to the process, communicating with others who have managed similar events and observation of the planning process are useful approaches. Specific planning needs vary by jurisdiction; however, there are several basic areas that should be addressed.

- Event and audience demographics
- Event medical history
- Proximity to definitive care
- Contact information for medical staff/event managers/safety officers
- Contact information for local hospitals/ambulance services
- Event medical command structure
- Proposed location of field hospital(s) and level of care offered
- Proposed location of satellite units and level of care offered

Table 19.6. METHANE Message Pneumonic to Identify Critical Initial Information to Communicate Regarding an Event

Major incident notification

Exact Location

Type of incident

Hazards involved (if any)

Access to site

Number of casualties

Emergency services required

- Proposed location of ambulances and level of care offered
- Proposed location of staff and parking facilities
- Duties and responsibilities of medical staff
- Duties and responsibilities of medical director/site medical officer
- Communications chain/structure/contact information/procedures
- Documentation and flow of documentation
- Procedure for hospital referrals
- Stand down details (return to baseline operational level)

DEVELOP SITE EMERGENCY PLAN

The site emergency plan differs from the routine medical plan in that it describes the procedures to follow in the event of a disaster. A standard phrase should be determined that will communicate to all staff that an incident has occurred. Event staff should be capable of performing the following tasks in case a disaster is declared:

- Identify staging points
- Establish triage protocols
- Delineate roles and responsibilities for
  - Medical incident officer
  - Triage officer
  - Casualty clearing station officer
  - Nursing incident officer
  - Ambulance incident officer
- Identify designated hospitals and liaisons
- Establish casualty clearing stations
- Find and liaise with other commanders/incident officers (unified command)
- Gather data for METHANE message (Table 19.6)
- Log events carefully
- Identify resource requirements

LIAISE WITH LOCAL EMERGENCY DEPARTMENTS/EMERGENCY MEDICAL SERVICES/TRAUMA UNITS

Many EMS systems have designated specialty receiving hospitals for patients meeting certain criteria. Examples include trauma, burn, cardiac, and stroke centers. Protocols in other systems mandate that patients be transported to the closest ED or to the hospital of patient choice. Advanced coordination with ambulance services and local emergency departments will help ensure integration with non-event-related emergency resource needs and appropriate distribution of patients if a disaster occurs.

RIDE-ALONGS TO LOCAL EMERGENCY DEPARTMENTS/VENUES

The event medical director should be familiar with local EMS transport times to effectively make an assessment of needed transport resources. Site visits to meet local ED leaders are also important to identify key personnel and understand respective responsibilities and resources prior to an event. Local hospitals may provide information critical to event planning.

CONFIRM INDEMNITY/MALPRACTICE/INSURANCE

Liability is a key concern for physicians and other providers working at a mass gathering. Although some countries have no-fault compensation systems, most general insurers are reluctant to provide medical liability coverage for mass gathering events. In some countries, physicians have malpractice insurance; in others, they possess medical indemnity (discussed in more detail later). For maximal legal protection, medical workers should inform their primary employers and insurers ahead of the event about their expected activities and qualifications to work in such environments.

CONFIRM FINANCIAL ARRANGEMENTS/ATTENDANCE/CAMPING/VIP ARRANGEMENTS

Providing financial compensation for event workers will make recruitment easier. Budget calculations and work agreements must be prepared ahead of time.

Projected attendance estimates, including those camping on-site, are necessary to determine medical workforce requirements, particularly for the night shifts. Staffing projections should account for changes in attendees specific for day of the week and time of day (such as campsite overnight).

If significant numbers of VIPs (dignitaries, etc.) are expected, the medical director needs to know in advance. Some categories of VIPs have special security requirements, such as presidents or their families, high-profile politicians, royal families, or other non-performing musical celebrities. Plans must be in place to manage illnesses and injuries if they occur among this group. This is particularly relevant for presidents, as access to services in specific hospitals may be blocked for other patients if a president is being treated.

RECRUIT STAFF AND CHECK EXPERIENCE/TRAIN AND CREDENTIAL STAFF

Staff recruitment, training, and credentialing is extremely time consuming. It is important to ensure that event personnel do not have higher priority competing obligations such as a duty to report to the hospital after a major incident. Community-wide planning is essential to confirm that hospital resources and other components of the healthcare system are not depleted so provision of staff to the event site is possible. If identified staff are not sufficiently trained and certified, the event medical director may need to arrange specific training for the team well in advance of the event. Depending on the jurisdiction, hospital-based physicians may be required to obtain specific medical licensure for prehospital events or may require licensure in another jurisdiction when events occur in multiple countries. The director should consult with local medical licensing authorities to ensure that requirements are met in a timely manner.

DEVELOP MEDICAL PROTOCOLS AND STANDARD OPERATING PROCEDURES

The director, deputy director, and medical team should develop, publish, and distribute medical protocols for medical staff in advance of the event. Standard operating procedures (SOPs) should also be promulgated for first aid and voluntary aid, delineating levels of care and when additional medical help should be requested.

PROCURE CLOTHING

Safety clothing is essential for mass gathering events. Team members should be provided with personal gear including safety boots, gloves, and high-visibility clothing. The event organizers should provide event-specific items such as high-visibility vests, caps, and light rain jackets. Logistical considerations, such as ensuring garments fit correctly for all team members, must be made in advance to guarantee timely delivery of specific seasonally appropriate clothing.

PROCURE EQUIPMENT

The medical director should consult with staff on-site for the event and organizers of prior similar events to determine what type and quantity of equipment will be needed. Once requirements are determined, the medical director should make a request to the event organizer to provide funds for purchase or lease of such equipment for the duration of the event.

GENERATE ROSTERS/ASSIGN ROLES/PROCURE PASSES AND CREDENTIALS

After calculating the expected number of attendees and the expected population variations over time, staff scheduling by area should begin. The UK Event Safety Guide is a valuable resource for estimating staff requirements.[86] Numbers of physicians needed on-site will depend on the training level of volunteers and EMS personnel. Event insurers may also impose requirements distinct from individual physicians' medical liability providers.

Photographic identification is required at most mass gathering events. It should be collected 7 days in advance of the event to ensure distribution to individual team members (unless the team is travelling together to the venue). Identification should allow access to all areas. If team members are travelling separately, they will need parking passes and route-access passes for any roads that are closed to the public.

ESTABLISH EVENT/BEGIN CONSTRUCTION/CHECK ADEQUACY OF MEDICAL FACILITIES

The first phase of preparing for events classified as large mass gatherings begins 7 days prior with staging equipment in containers for transportation to the venue. The day prior to the event, equipment should be moved to the site and secured overnight. Controlled substances must be kept in double locked containers, preferably off-site until medical staff are present to receive them. A system should be in place to account for restricted drugs and ensure continuous supervision with a responsible worker at shift change. Most events start early in the morning. The medical team should arrive on-site 2 hours before the event and remain at the venue until at least 1 hour after the event closes. The team should take a walk-through tour of the site to familiarize themselves with the locations of their duty stations and their access route to the next higher level of care.

PRE-EVENT BRIEFING

On the day of the event, the medical director should organize a briefing for the on-site team that includes information regarding:

■ Use of radios and channel numbers for communications
■ Channels of communications to other services
■ Individual cell phone numbers
■ Roles and responsibilities
■ Chains of command
■ Top medical priorities
■ Identifying transferring physicians if required to accompany patients
■ Interaction with other service providers
■ Importance of documentation
■ Site orientation
■ On-site transport possibilities
■ Location of main medical facility and satellites
■ Staff rest periods with meals

The briefing should also give instructions on procedures in the event of a disaster/major incident that includes:

■ Code words to identify a major incident has occurred
■ Assembly point for re-tasking
■ Triage protocols
■ Communication channels
■ Roles of individual physicians and assigned posts

DEBRIEFING

Mass gathering medical care regulations vary by country and individual locality. In Ireland and the UK, legislation requires medical teams to remain on-site at their posts for a minimum of 1 hour after the event has concluded. For music events, the conclusion of festivities is defined as when the band leaves the stage; for sports events, this definition is met when the teams leave the field. The intent of this requirement is to ensure that an appropriate level of medical care is available for patrons who may suffer a medical event in the process of exiting the mass gathering. In large events, 1 hour may be insufficient for complete egress of patrons, particularly if they must drive from a remote parking facility under crowded conditions. In other confined stadiums, 1 hour may be ample time as patrons walk away from the stadium and board public transport. During this period, it is important for personnel to do a perimeter sweep to ensure that ill or injured patrons are not missed when the event closes.

As the event is closing, there is generally ample time for a roving medical director and deputy to perform a quick debriefing of the medical teams at their posts. Key areas of assessment should include:

■ What went particularly well?
■ Were there any areas of concern?
■ Were the facilities appropriate?
■ Was the provided equipment appropriate?
■ What are the areas for improvement?
■ Were there any patient safety issues?
■ Were there any staff safety issues?

By visiting staff posts, the medical director can determine whether there are any structural issues that need correction before the next day's events or for future events. Photographic reminders are useful to document recommendations. Following the debriefing, the director or designee should prepare a written summary of the event that includes patient demographics for the day.

For prolonged events with on-site camping, some staff will be on night shifts. An overlap period with the day shift is helpful to assist night staff with understanding event operations. The director or deputy should be available for debriefing when overnight staff are going off duty. This allows overnight staff to highlight any issues that need attention during the day and to report on the patients treated overnight. Patterns of injury or illness that may be related to recreational drug use, sanitation facilities, or foodborne pathogens should be sought and the public health services alerted in a timely fashion. WHO recently released a very comprehensive "key considerations" document in relation to communicable diseases and response for mass gatherings. It details risk assessment and management, surveillance and alert systems, outbreak alert and response systems, and cross-discipline considerations such as training, logistics, and communication systems.[90]

DISMANTLE EVENT

Event dismantling procedures should mirror the assembly phase. Containers should be repacked, inventoried, locked, and prepared for transport. A detailed inventory of stock used will assist with planning for similar events in future and will also highlight what additions may be needed for the following day at multiple-day events. Any supplies or equipment left on-site at the conclusion of the event (or end of the day for prolonged events) must be appropriately secured. Procedures should be in place to maintain accountability for controlled medications.

The medical director should collate and secure all medical records. Some jurisdictions require a copy of the medical records be submitted to the regional health service authority. Local ordinances or the permit issued for the mass gathering will clarify requirements. For events with camping at locations remote from the main medical facility, establishment of additional medical posts may be needed overnight. Depending on the flow of patrons, these posts may not be in operation during the day when few attendees are expected to remain at campsites.

Medical Reconnaissance

It is a bad plan that admits of no modification.

Publilius Syrus (∼100 BC)

A site visit by the medical director and deputy can reveal a number of details that may not be evident from reviewing planning applications, architect drawings, or aerial photographs. Venue location, access routes, and topography should all be assessed. Google Maps is a useful tool for generating aerial diagrams of venue sites for the majority of countries worldwide. Maps can show access routes overlain with rail networks. Driving to the event site during peak traffic conditions is useful to estimate transport times to the venue. Per licensing requirements, the start time for the event may be delayed until the medical team arrives. Extra time should be allowed because police and other authorities may alter access routes and change normal traffic flow on event days. For example, roads which may have been bi-directional may only be one-way. The medical director and deputy should remain informed about planned traffic routes to ensure that their team has priority access to routes if such exists. Special parking passes may be required for vehicles and should be secured in advance.

Pre-event visits will also allow the director and deputy to plan ambulance transports from the venue. For large venues, there may be a significant period of on-site travel from the various first aid posts to an ambulance, then another period of travel on-site before the ambulance gets to the access road. At a venue with remote parking or a town nearby, there may be large numbers of attendees walking along the roads to the venue, which may further increase ambulance transport times. These factors affect overall transport times to hospitals. The UK Event Safety Guide has a useful model for predicting resource requirements, including a scoring system for proximity to definitive care.[86]

Planning should account for the fact that transport times may increase dramatically from baseline during mass gathering events. In addition, some mass gatherings take place in remote venues where the nearest ED may be small and have few resources. Even for a moderately sized facility with an annual ED volume of about 36,000 (less than 100 patients per day), a requirement to transport 100 patients over a 24-hour period would likely exceed surge capacity in that institution. Ryan and Nix in their papers from Ireland in 1994 and 2006, respectively, describe the effect on attendance at local and regional emergency departments for a 3-day festival and a large single-day rock concert.[57,91] In Nix's case, there were 1,355 visits for medical attention on-site over a 2-day festival (3 nights camping at the venue). This represented 1.7% of those in attendance at the event. Milsten in 2003 discussed variables influencing medical usage rates (MURs) and described the term MUR as being the number of presentations for medical care per ten thousand attendees (PPTT).[92] For the Nix event, this would result in an MUR of 171, a significant number when compared to Milsten's own average figures of 4.85 for baseball games, 6.75 for football games, and 30 for rock concerts. Ryan's MUR of 10 is still significant but was for a much shorter event than Nix's and resulted in only eighteen patients being transported. Nix reported seventy-two transports during a 3-day event. This represented a 45% increase in workload for the local ED. What is not clear from either report is the number of secondary transfers that occurred from the local ED to regional trauma centers or other specialty facilities due to the need for intensive care services.

The number of physicians deployed at the event may be significantly greater than the number staffing the local ED. What may seem like a small number of referrals from the venue, taking the crowd size into account, may actually overwhelm the local ED, forcing them to go on diversion. This would significantly increase transport and turnaround times with the consequent loss of on-site physicians for longer periods when they accompany patients during transport to more distant hospitals. The local ED may also be unable to accept intubated or other types of critical patients. To guide transport decisions, the site medical director needs to know the current capacity and capability of the local healthcare resources throughout the duration of the event. Historical information as described by Arbon is useful for repeat events.[29] This complex model predicts the requirements for patient transports. Requirements for a physician to accompany transported patients must be clearly understood in advance so that staffing levels can be adjusted accordingly. Air evacuation procedures should also be delineated if applicable.

The medical director should communicate with the venue owner or facility manager regarding the site itself, its current usage, drainage patterns, whether tractors have rolled down the grass fields, internal access routes, and use of chemicals on the land. Rolled fields will help prevent ankle injuries. Facilities which have been sprayed with chemicals may result in allergic-type ophthalmological presentations, especially in summer. Hay fever exacerbations may increase in number when large open fields have been cut in advance of the event. Some facility managers may cover the playing surface in a stadium with a temporary surface in order to protect it from damage. This procedure can create inversion effects with microclimates of increased temperature over specific areas and result in increased demands on medical services. In a review article, Milsten described this phenomenon at a rock concert in Denver, Colorado, where a black tarp caused a local rise in temperature of 17°C.[93]

Additional considerations include the drainage capacity of the land and the locations of internal walkways. If there are areas where water is likely to pool, these should be highlighted on event maps and at campsites; access routes and medical facilities should not be located there. Thousands of patrons could potentially be stranded when attempted to leave the event if parking is situated in an area prone to flooding. If this parking location is unavoidable, contingency plans should be in place for this possibility.

Both director and deputy should walk the site to assess timing of foot travel between the clinical areas, around the circumference of the site, and between the campsite (if present) and the main arenas. In a football stadium, this may be a simple task. In a large open site racecourse, however, where multiple venues and a campsite accommodating over 50,000 people may exist, medical personnel may need on-site transport equipment. Such transportation should be season- and weather-appropriate. As an example, golf carts are unlikely to be useful in muddy or marshy conditions.

VIP care, including access and evacuation plans, should be discussed during the planning stages. In the recent past, Ireland had the highest proportion of helicopters per capita in the world and these were used frequently for VIPs to attend mass gatherings. The event medical plan should address potential hazards from helicopters if they are used. If the VIP area is distant from the on-site medical facility, it may be necessary to establish a separate VIP medical area. Often event promoters will specify this as part of the arrangements from the outset. If this is implemented, support for these facilities should be in addition to the planned numbers required to staff the event.

Local authorities and law enforcement are good sources of information regarding the potential for violence or issues related to drug misuse. They may require the presence of a physician during the search of attendees' possessions at entry to the venue. This is necessary to verify that tablets and drugs are for legitimate medical use, particularly if they are not in their original dispensed containers. Posters that display the common drugs of abuse can be a useful reference aid at this location.

A reconnaissance visit to the local hospitals and potential referral sites in advance may help to ease the transfer process during the event. The local ED may be small and the addition of 80,000 event attendees may result in significant increases in patient visits.[57,82] In some areas, another local hospital may be the best option for referrals. In others, standards may exist for bypassing local facilities and transporting certain types of

Table 19.7. Issues Requiring Negotiation in the Contracting for a Mass Casualty Event

Liability coverage

Compensation

Site access

Required resources

Command and control issues

Safety

Communications

Transport

Housing on-site (if applicable)

Media issues

VIP medical care

Documentation

Post-event debriefing/reporting requirements

patients to specialty receiving hospitals like trauma centers. On-site physicians must be familiar with these policies.

Negotiations

The medical director should ensure that negotiations take place at an early stage. Issues for discussion are listed in Table 19.7. The medical director should negotiate compensation for all staff providing medical services. This should include appropriate compensation for the director and deputy for the planning, preparatory work, and medical direction during the event. Recruiting additional appropriately trained medical staff for the event will be easier if the compensation package is understood. In systems where mass gathering medical care is provided by the local health authority, hospital staff may be offered additional compensation to provide medical services to the event. This arrangement can be advantageous for the event organizer as many of the employment and liability issues will be covered by the hospital.

Site access should also be negotiated in advance. At large event sites, patron access levels vary from highly restrictive to all-access pass. Even the highest level of patron pass may not include access to certain secure areas of the site. Medical personnel should be granted access to all areas to ensure an effective patient care response, even if this includes the ability to traverse a restricted area. On-site security employees must permit healthcare workers access when they are responding to medical emergencies. Other important access issues are car parking and route access. If special venue route access passes exist, medical teams need them to ensure that they can transport medical equipment to the site.

A system of identifying medical, nursing, and paramedical personnel is required and should be coordinated with other event workers. Identifying clothing such as polo shirts, T-shirts, sweatshirts, and rain jackets with pockets to store medical items should be provided. Team members should provide their own PPE such as safety boots, trousers, gloves, and high visibility jackets with appropriate identification for overnight work. Shift duration should be no longer than 12 hours for very high-intensity work or 16 hours for low-intensity work. For events lasting multiple days, on-site lodging may be the most practical and time-efficient arrangement for the team. This would reduce the risk of motor vehicle collisions driving home from the event late at night. For overnight work, accommodations may also be required for on-call staff to allow short rest periods and sleep if possible. Even small amounts of anchor sleep can improve performance.

VIP medical care procedures need to be negotiated in advance. At some large events, there is a specific VIP area that may be backstage or otherwise separated from the rest of the attendees. Placing a dedicated physician in this area may prevent problems related to patrons or the media trying to access the medical tent where a VIP is being treated. If the promoters request a separate physician dedicated to VIPs, this individual should be added to the numbers already required to staff the event, as per the local template used to estimate staffing levels or the UK Event Safety Guide.[86]

Airway problems represent some of the most sensitive issues related to mass gathering medical care. Although anyone with emergency airway experience (such as an emergency physician) can act as an airway manager, event promoters often specify that an anesthesiologist be among the medical team in attendance. Staffing levels as suggested in the Event Safety Guide refer to the number of generic physicians required to staff an event in the UK.[86] If physicians with specific training and experience are required, they should be in addition to the generic number of physicians calculated. The medical director and deputy for large events should focus on administrative aspects of event management. Therefore, they will not be available to provide direct medical care.

On-site transport issues should be addressed during the advance negotiations. For indoor venues and sports stadiums with structural perimeters, it is unlikely that on-site transport will be required. However, for large unbounded events at locations such as city parks, racecourses, marathons, or music festivals with large campsites on-site, transport is essential. For very large events, promoters may need to identify a significant number of golf carts or all-terrain vehicles in advance. The medical director should ensure that adequate types and numbers of transportation vehicles are dedicated to medical staff. Vehicle type should be appropriate to the terrain and weather conditions. Some event sites are only accessible by foot. As an example, patrons hiked through mud baths every day at the Glastonbury Festival of Contemporary Performing Arts in England to reach the concert venue from the campsite. For flat venues with long transport distances, it may be necessary to secure carts that can accommodate spine immobilization boards for transporting patients with suspected spinal injuries.

Level of Care

The level of care provided on-site will depend on a number of factors including:

- Local legislation, ordnances, and licensing rules
- Event size
- Presence of on-site camping
- Estimated effects on local EMS infrastructure
- Whether the site is remote from local hospitals
- Whether the local area is urban or rural
- The capacity of the local ED to treat trauma patients and admit intubated patients

Local designations of provider level may include emergency first responder, first aid personnel, and emergency medical technician. Patients should be assessed by the most appropriate person based on their medical needs. In the setting of mass gatherings, significant numbers of internal transports of patients from satellite facilities to stations where there are nurses and physicians or to the site hospital facility may be required. The level of care plan should address early defibrillation goals and how these will be achieved on a dispersed site. In generic terms, the level of care provided should mimic what is available in the community and should not drain community resources needed for non-event-related emergency care.

The level of care plan should address the ABCDEs of mass gathering management as follows:

A

- Airway – assessment of compromise and management
- Allergic reactions/anaphylaxis
- Altered mental status
- Arrhythmias

B

- Breathing assessment and management
- Bites
- Burns
- Bones
- Back pain

C

- Circulatory problems – assessment and management, including chest pain, strokes

D

- Disability assessment – headaches
- Drug ingestions, exposures, overdoses
- Diabetic emergencies
- Drowning

E

- Electrocution
- Environmental emergencies
- Eye and ENT presentations

S

- Soft tissue injuries
- Psychiatric emergencies
- Syncope
- Seizures
- Spinal assessments in trauma

Airway management is one of the issues causing the greatest concern for event promoters. The medical team on-site at mass gatherings should be skilled in emergency airway management. All members of the medical team should know the location of the nearest equipment (if it is not carried on their person). At least some types of rescue airway devices such as the bougie, supra-glottic airway devices (the laryngeal mask airway [LMA], iGel, and intubating LMA), and Airtraq single-use intubation assistant should be available.[94–96]

Medical Oversight

The event plan, not the medical plan, defines requirements for medical oversight. In many jurisdictions, this is the document submitted for licensing or permits. It should contain specific roles and responsibilities for both the medical director and deputy and indicate which position will have the primary medical command officer role in the event of a major incident. The event plan may also specify the various training requirements, certifications, and indemnity/malpractice or insurance required of the medical director and deputy. The medical team provides both indirect and direct medical control. The medical director's indirect role refers to designing the site medical plan and ensuring that standardized levels of care are present throughout the site. There must also be a mechanism for medical supervision of all activity on-site either directly in the same vicinity or indirectly by protocol or SOP.

Direct medical oversight refers to the director's supervisory role during the event. The director should be easily recognizable by uniform. Jaslow outlines these roles in detail in the U.S. context in *Mass Gathering Medical Care: The Medical Directors Checklist.*[89]

Medical Staff Selection

Medical staff selection should take place as early as possible because significant orientation and training is necessary for personnel without prior experience in mass gathering medicine. On-site providers should not be given the false expectation that they will have the opportunity to enjoy a free sporting or music event. Rather, their primary mission will be to support and provide medical care for the event.

The director should identify the numbers and types of staff needed, using appropriate tools. Depending on crowd numbers, there may be a requirement for first aid or more advanced medical tents spread over a large area. Thus, some practitioners will be expected to work alone at times and must know the indications and procedures for accessing more advanced medical care. If possible, staff recruitment should begin 1 year prior to the event for large mass gatherings, particularly in rural locations where resources may be needed from outside the local area.

Medical Staff Training

All those delivering medical care at the event should be qualified to provide appropriate levels of life support. A board-certified emergency physician with extensive experience in resuscitation during routine duties probably does not need additional clinical training, but may need training in jurisdictionally relevant incident command systems. For certain levels of providers, additional certifications may be desirable or required. Depending on roles, responsibilities, and provider level, these could include a combination of the courses listed in Table 19.8.

Completion of the stadium management or advanced Major Incident Medical Management and Support (MIMMS) courses is desirable for event medical directors. Advanced degree programs (MSc, MPH, MBA, and PhD) that focus on disaster and emergency management are becoming increasingly available and

Table 19.8. Courses Offering Certification in Various Disciplines that May Be Useful or Required for Medical Providers at Mass Gathering Events

Basic Life Support	BLS
Advanced Cardiac Life Support	ACLS
Advanced Trauma Life Support	ATLS
Prehospital Trauma Life Support	PHTLS
International Trauma Life Support	ITLS
Advanced Disaster Life Support	ADLS
Major Incident Medical Management and Support	MIMMS
Safe Transport and Retrieval	STAR
Advanced Life Support in Obstetrics	ALSO
Neonatal Resuscitation Program	NRP
Hazardous Incident Medical Management	HAZIMMS
Advanced Pediatric Life Support	APLS
Advanced Resuscitation and Emergency Aid	AREA
Standard Procedures for Resuscitation and Trauma in Sport	SPoRT

would be useful for physicians pursuing a career in this field. One unique program conceived in 1998 is the European Master in Disaster Medicine (MSc DM), a second-level master's degree awarded jointly by the Free University of Brussels and The University of Eastern Piedmont in Italy (http://www.dismedmaster.com). This is a 1-year interactive distance-learning program in which students from around the world complete course work, online examinations, a publishable thesis, and a concentrated 2-week residential program that includes a full-scale major disaster exercise.

The Royal College of Surgeons in Edinburgh, Scotland offers a diploma (DipIMC) and Fellowship examination (FIMC) in immediate medical care. The training provides a solid framework for medical practitioners and advanced paramedics in many of the skills needed for mass gathering medical care. Sporting bodies such as the Football Association (FA) in the UK sponsor a course in rapid emergency management called the AREA course. The FA also offers a stadium management course, the Crowd Doctors Course, which addresses all aspects of crowd medical care. The Rugby Football League, based in Leeds, England, provides a course entitled Immediate Medical Management on the Field of Play, designed for doctors who are providing medical care to teams and in stadiums at rugby league events. It is mandatory for physicians providing on-field services to rugby league teams to be currently certified. In Ireland, the Faculty of Sport and Exercise Medicine has designed the SPoRT course for team and ground physicians.

If the event is likely to recur, the director should consider developing a training schedule for a pool of dedicated staff. This can provide practical experience as a team member in mass gathering medical care for resident physicians and disaster medicine fellows, and the ability for those with an interest to train as a deputy medical director.

Triage

Triage has existed since the days of the Napoleonic wars as a method to ration medical resources when demand exceeds supply (see Chapter 14). Triage is a complicated process and most triage systems are developed with traumatic injuries in mind, not illnesses.[97]. Turris and Lund have developed the University of British Columbia Mass Gathering Medicine Triage Acuity Scale, but this has yet to be tested and published. Most triage systems have an initial filter for ambulatory wounded patients (termed "minor" or "green"). The remaining patients are then categorized according to reproducible scales. Several dozen triage systems exist and use various tools, labels, and even colored hair bands or clothes pins to sort patients by priority of either medical need or order for transport to definitive care sites. Separate systems exist for pediatric triage and should be considered if applicable to the event demographics. Besides the START protocol in the United States, few data exist that validate any of the multiple triage systems. Therefore, choosing a system familiar to local providers may be the best option.

Medical staff at all levels should be trained on the chosen triage system. For those with no prior triage experience in this setting, exercises should take place in advance with mock patients to simulate working with the selected triage system. Some experts recommend that the triage method be published in team member guidelines and that there be an early practice session for all team members on the opening day of the event. Another suggestion is that posters explaining the triage system be developed and distributed to medical facilities (including receiving hospitals), casualty clearing stations, and each first aid post.

Required Resources

Management of a mass gathering from the medical perspective requires human resources, medical equipment, pharmaceuticals, and medical facilities with sufficient examining rooms on-site. For very large events, a dedicated logistician would be useful. In 2000, Jaslow, on behalf of NAEMSP, produced a document entitled *Mass Gathering Medical Care: The Medical Directors Checklist*.[89] This is a valuable comprehensive resource for anyone involved in directing medical care at mass gatherings. It contains great detail regarding medical equipment needs, including essential and desirable components for basic and advanced medical interventions.

Estimating Medical Resources

> Don't live in a town where there are no doctors.
> Jewish Proverb

There are no international standards for the numbers of physicians, training requirements, or level of care that should be provided at mass gatherings. Even the presence of physicians is not an international standard, as some systems rely on the usual EMS provider or even volunteer services to deliver assistance at mass gatherings. While not necessarily evidence-based, event licensing regulations or local statutes and ordinances may specify required numbers of medical personnel. If they exist, such ordinances or statutes specify minimum levels of physician or provider coverage, and have usually not been updated to account for increased duties and medical developments locally, nationally, or internationally. Estimating medical resources required for any mass gathering is an inexact science and may involve real-time adjustments to ensure that sufficient resources are present on-site. For the first iteration of an event, it is better to overestimate staffing and equipment requirements than to risk the consequences of understaffing or under resourcing. Once experience is gained from the same or similar events on multiple occasions, patterns will emerge that allow for a more valid estimate of the true requirements for human resources, equipment, and transport assets. Even when good data are available, it is prudent to provide more than just the minimum numbers of staff and to have a system for surge capacity in case of a sudden increase in health and medical demands.

Organized planning for mass gatherings at stadiums is relatively new, beginning over the last two decades. Retrospective analysis of attendance rates on-site for medical treatment, medication and equipment use, transport to hospitals, and audit of medical records provides planning guidance for minimum requirements for an event of similar size in the same jurisdiction. Although generic planning elements are similar, no two mass gatherings have identical requirements even when planned for the same site, crowd number, and activities. Resource requirements are dependent on a variety of factors including:

- Jurisdiction and legal safety standards
- Level of care in local EMS systems
- Distance to definitive medical care
- Time period before outside assistance arrives (how long does the stadium need to be self-sufficient?)

The total medical resources required to manage medical services at a mass gathering include but are not limited to:

- Ambulance personnel and on-site ambulance officer
- Communications officer(s)
- EMS director
- Paramedics
- First aid workers, volunteers, and first responders
- Nurses
- Physicians, including medical director and deputy director(s)
- Ambulance service managers
- Support units
- Ambulances
- On-site transport vehicles
- Event safety officer and event controller (provided by event organizer)

Since health systems vary widely, there is no uniform matrix to calculate staff numbers, grades, or types of services required for providing medical coverage at a mass gathering. In some countries, voluntary first aid organizations such as the Red Cross, the St. Johns Ambulance, or the Order of Malta may provide medical services without an on-site physician. In other regions, local referral hospitals operate temporary facilities on-site in an attempt to prevent unmanageable patient volumes from being transported to their existing fixed facilities.

The UK Health Services Executive, in conjunction with the Home Office and Scottish Office, published *The Guide to Health, Safety and Welfare at Pop Concerts and Other Similar Events* in 1993. This was updated in 1999 to reflect changes in UK health and safety law and to update best practices. The UK Event Safety Guide was developed in consultation with an event industry working group and is the standard for managing health and safety at such events.[86] Although it has no legal

Table 19.9. Estimating Resource Requirements – Event Nature

(A) Nature of event	Classical Performance	2
	Public Exhibition	3
	Pop/rock concert	5
	Dance Event	8
	Agricultural/country Show	2
	Marine event	3
	Motorcycle display	3
	Aviation	3
	Motorsport	4
	State occasions	2
	VIP visits/summit	3
	Music festival	3
	Bonfire/pyrotechnic display	4
	New Years' celebrations	7
	Demonstrations/marches/political events	
	Low-risk of disorder	2
	Medium-risk of disorder	5
	High-risk of disorder	7
	Opposing factions involved	9
(B) Venue	Indoor	1
	Stadium	2
	Outdoor, confined location (e.g., park)	2
	Other outdoor (e.g., festival)	3
	Widespread public location in streets	4
	Temporary outdoor structures	4
	Includes camping	5
(C) Standing/seated	Seated	1
	Mixed	2
	Standing	3
(D) Audience profile	Full mix, in family groups	2
	Full mix, not in family groups	3
	Predominately young adults	3
	Predominately children, teenagers	4
	Predominately elderly	4
	Full mix, rival factions	5
Add (A)+(B)+(C)+(D)	Total score for Table 19.9	=

Table 19.10. Estimating Resource Requirements – Event Intelligence

(E) Past history	Good data low casualty rate previously (<1%)	−1
	Good data medium casualty rate previously (1–2%)	1
	Good data high casualty rate previously (>2%)	2
	First event, no data	3
(F) Expected numbers	<1,000	1
	<3,000	2
	<5,000	8
	<10,000	12
	<20,000	16
	<30,000	20
	<40,000	24
	<60,000	28
	<80,000	34
	<100,000	42
	<200,000	50
	<300,000	58
Add (E)+(F)	Total score for Table 19.10	=

basis in Ireland, it is regularly referenced in planning meetings in conjunction with the Codes of Practice for Safety at Sports Grounds, Safety at Outdoor Pop Concerts, and Safety at Indoor Concerts, which are government-sponsored documents.[98–100] These are examples of country-specific documents that outline basic levels of care and resources that attendees can expect to receive at music and sports events.

The UK Event Safety Guide contains tables that are helpful for estimating a reasonable level of resources that should be provided at events. These guidelines provide a good framework; however, they were developed based on the levels of care available in a particular jurisdiction and may not be applicable in all countries. Data from Tables 19.9, 19.10, and 19.11 can be combined to provide a scoring system which can be applied to Table 19.12 to calculate recommended resource requirements. These four tables were modified or taken directly from the Event Safety Guide.[86]

Equipment

A useful approach in determining the equipment needed for a mass gathering is to coordinate with the local ambulance services. Many ambulance services have disaster/major incident-specific equipment in significant quantities with procedures for rapid restocking when necessary. This equipment can be staged either directly on-site or in close proximity. Planners should be prepared for unanticipated changes in requirements and develop flexible command and control systems that can accommodate unexpected events.

It is difficult to estimate the exact quantity of required pharmaceuticals. Planners should develop a restocking agreement

Table 19.11. Estimating Resource Requirements – Sample Additional Considerations

(G) Expected queuing	<4 hours	1
	>4 hours	2
	>12 hours	3
(H) Time of year (outdoor events)	Summer	2
	Autumn	1
	Winter	2
	Spring	1
(I) Proximity to definitive care (nearest suitable ED)	<30 minutes by road	0
	>30 minutes by road	2
(J) Profile of definitive care	Choice of ED	1
	Large volume ED	2
	Small Volume ED	3
(K) Additional Hazards	Carnival	1
	Helicopters	1
	Motorsport	1
	Parachute display	1
	Street theatre	1
(L) Additional on-site facilities	Suturing	−2
	X-ray	−2
	Minor surgery	−2
	Plastering	−2
	Psychiatric/GP facilities	−2
Add (G)+(H)+(I)+(J)+(K)+(L)	Total score for Table 19.11	=

Table 19.13. List of Potential Field Hospital or Medical Aid Station Supplies and Resources

Access to power	Patient ID bracelets
Beds/cots/trolleys	Patient report forms
Blankets	Pen and paper
Drapes	Phone
Fax	Pillows
Flashlights, large and small for examination	Printer
Floor lamps	Refrigerator
Hazardous waste bins	Safety pins
Head lamps	Sheets
Laptop computer	Sink
Lockbox for pharmaceuticals	Spare batteries (multiple sizes)
Near access to bathroom	Tables and chairs
Non-hazardous waste bins	Towels

with a local pharmacy or the local health service. Some medications require refrigeration. Controlled substances should be appropriately secured. One approach is to designate one of the medical teams as being responsible for sign-out of controlled drugs with signature policies on a named patient basis.

Additional field hospital supplies and resources could include, but are not limited to, the items in Table 19.13. The same applies to the specific medical equipment listed in Table 19.14.

Pharmaceuticals

Drugs can be categorized according to the ABCDEs of mass gatherings as described previously. Even with this comprehensive approach, it is likely that medical needs will occasionally exceed immediate resources. For this reason, planners should develop

Table 19.12. Estimating Resource Requirements – Medical Resource Calculations

Score	Ambulance	First aider	Ambulance personnel	Doctor	Nurse	NHS ambulance manager	Support unit
< 20	0	4	0	0	0	0	0
21–25	1	6	2	0	0	visit	0
26–30	1	8	2	0	0	visit	0
31–35	2	12	8	1	2	1	0
36–40	3	20	10	2	4	1	0
41–50	4	40	12	3	6	2	1
51–60	4	60	12	4	8	2	1
61–65	5	80	14	5	10	3	1
66–70	6	100	16	6	12	4	2
71–75	10	150	24	9	18	6	3
> 75	15+	200+	35+	12+	24+	8+	3

Table 19.14. List of Possible Medical Equipment for Field Hospitals or Medical Aid Stations

12-lead EKG machine, paper stock, skin razors	Needle cricothyroidotomy kit and supplies	Airway equipment
Automated blood pressure monitors	Needle thoracostomy kit/portable chest drain kit	Ambu bags
Bandages/gauze pads/band-aids/zinc oxide tapes	Neonatal resuscitator	Laryngoscope blades & batteries
Betadine	Thermometers	Airways ET, nasal/oropharyngeal
Blankets	Observation monitors	Laryngeal Masks/iGel
Blood glucose strips, monitor, ketone measuring strips	Ophthalmoscope	Pulse oximeters
Broselow pediatric tapes	Otoscope	Oxygen masks & tubing
Burn dressings	Oxygen tanks, regulators, masks, nasal cannulae	End tidal CO_2 monitor
Cotton balls	Portable ventilators	
Defibrillator – AED (numbers dependent on site layout)	Prescription pads	Skin closure devices
Delivery pack for obstetrics	Ring cutter	Steri strip
EZ IO intraosseous access device	Snellen charts/Eye patches	Skin glue
Face masks	Spinal boards	Skin clips
Intravenous fluid infuser	Splints – multiple sizes/slings/dynacast/crutches	Suture kits
Intravenous fluid warmer	Stethoscope (electronic)	Sutures
Intravenous fluids	Suction device, suction catheters	
IV devices and tubing	Trauma scissors	Gloves
Multiple cervical collars – adult and pediatric	Urinalysis strips	sterile/nonsterile
Nasogastric tubes	Vaseline gauze and tubs	latex/non latex

policies for medication restocking, using local pharmacists as an option. The classes of drugs listed in Table 19.15 represent a potential pharmacy cache that should be available on-site.

Transport (On- and Off-Site)

Transportation vehicles can include golf carts for football stadiums and quad-cycles for rougher terrain, particularly when there are large distances over open spaces with a potential for boggy ground with precipitation. In Ireland, St. Johns Ambulance Brigade volunteers use specially designed mountain bikes as personal means of transportation to move around some sites.

Mass gatherings can encompass large areas and difficult environments. For example, in the annual Glastonbury Festival, the distance from one of the campsites to the main arena is large and could include muddy areas. Without proper vehicles, it would be nearly impossible to move patients under such conditions. Standard heavy ambulances will not easily traverse this terrain. Alternate vehicles such as quad-cycles or SUV-type ambulances would be needed, especially in very muddy conditions. In some situations, tractors will be required. If not anticipated in advance, it may be difficult to secure environmentally appropriate vehicles. Staffing levels should be sufficient to ensure timely responses to critical areas in venues spanning large geographic areas or events with multiple stadiums.

The local ambulance service typically organizes transport from the event site to local EDs. There may be delays in ambulances returning to the venue, for example, if there are prolonged patient handovers at the local ED or ambulances are needed for secondary transfer of patients to a higher level of care. Staffing

and transportation resources must account for such situations, particularly if an event physician is accompanying a patient off-site or during an inter-facility transfer.

Medical Indemnity – Medical Malpractice

Physicians providing medical coverage at mass gathering events need protection from liability. Although event promoters generally have public liability, weather, and "no-show" insurances, they are unlikely to provide medical liability coverage. The system of medical malpractice or medical indemnity, as it is termed in Europe, is generally based on an individual practitioner's specialty and routine medical practice, and not occasional work such as that performed at a mass gathering event.

There is a significant difference between the two terms and it is important that physicians know which variant they possess. Malpractice insurance, or liability coverage as it is called in the United States, means the physician has an insurance product that covers the financial cost of a malpractice incident or the cost of defending a negligence claim. To obtain such coverage, individual physicians detail their work plans including specific information on their involvement in medical activities outside their primary specialty (such as mass gathering medical care). This is then factored in to the cost of the liability coverage. If an event has not been prospectively included in the work plan, the physician must make a separate request to the liability insurer for coverage.

Medical indemnity, on the other hand, is not an insurance-based product. Physicians become members of mutual medical societies such as the Medical Defense Union and the Medical Protection Society. The organizations were founded in the

Table 19.15. List of Potential Drug Classes that Should Be Available On-Site

Airway	Disability assessment – stroke, headaches
Bronchodilators	Analgesics
Induction agents	Antibiotics
Nebulized and oral steroids	Drug ingestion/drug exposure/drug overdose/diabetic emergencies/ drowning
Paralytic agents	Activated charcoal
Allergic reactions/anaphylaxis	Antidotes to common poisons
Epinephrine	Antiepileptic medications
Oral and topical steroids	(lorazepam/diazepam/midazolam)
Oral and topical antihistamines	Antihistamines – topical, oral, and parenteral
Analgesics	Dantrolene (for MDMA poisoning with hyperpyrexia)
Aspirin (also for chest pain)	50% dextrose solution
Acetaminophen	Glucagon
Antacids (proton pump inhibitors, H2 blockers)	Induction agents
Anti-inflammatory medications	Insulin
Non-steroidal anti-inflammatory agents	Steroids – oral and parenteral
Opioid analgesics	Electrocution/environmental emergencies/eye and ENT presentations
Other non-narcotic analgesics	Topical anesthetics
Breathing	Topical antibiotics (ophthalmological preparations)
Antibiotics	Topical antibiotics (aural preparations)
Bronchodilators	Irrigating solutions
Bites/burns/bones/back pain	Mydriatic agents
Point of care tests for tetanus immunity	Fluorescein dye (strips or drops)
Vaccines – anti-tetanus/hepatitis passive and active immunization	pH strips
Water gel/silver sulfadiazine cream or similar	Soft tissue injuries/skin problems/psychiatric emergencies/syncope/ seizures/spinal assessments in trauma
Analgesics as shown in previous section	Antiepileptics (lorazepam/diazepam/midazolam)
Local anesthetic	Anxiolytics
Circulatory problems – ACLS medications	Skin closure aids (steri strips/skin glue/staples and sutures)
Adenosine	Topical
Amiodarone	antihistamines/steroids/antibiotics/antifungals
Atropine	Oral and systemic antibiotics
Beta blockers	Sedatives
Calcium chloride	Local anesthetic
Calcium channel antagonists	Other
Digoxin	Antidiarrheal agents
Epinephrine	Emergency contraception
Lidocaine	Sunscreen
Nitroglycerin	Aftersun (Sunburn treatment cream)
Sodium bicarbonate	
Vasopressor agents	

nineteenth century as not-for-profit bodies that assist members with financial, legal, and ethical problems arising from clinical practice. The benefits of membership are discretionary. Although rare, these organizations may elect not to assist with the financial consequences of a claim against a member.

Mass gathering medical care is a new concept and liability insurers and indemnification bodies have little experience with it. Therefore, when getting liability coverage, it is advisable to carefully define physician roles and responsibilities (including during a major incident or disaster).

In Ireland, Medisec is one of the bodies involved. It now has an insurance policy for its members specifically stating that for general practitioners (family physicians), the policy will not indemnify GP's for any liability arising from or caused by advice and/or treatment not coming within the range of services normally provided by a general practitioner. The policy specifically excludes acting as an event doctor (medical director) who is responsible for crowd control, ambulance services, provision of appropriate medical equipment, and other related activities. This significantly limits the number of doctors in Ireland who can operate in such roles.

Few if any physicians work full-time in mass gathering medical care. More typically, this activity reflects a small portion of a physician's overall medical practice. Thus, limited case law is available to insurers for decision making. In addition, a physician who provides medical services at an event needs different types of liability coverage than a physician in the role of event medical director who is involved in planning and organizing medical care. The level of responsibility for a medical director or medical incident officer in case of a disaster is much greater than for a physician providing direct medical care at the event.

In the UK and Ireland, large medical indemnity bodies such as The Medical Union and The Medical Protection Society advise physicians against accepting positions at such events where they are operating in roles not part of their normal practice. Examples include physicians without regular trauma experience who assess patients injured at events, or physicians without toxicology training and experience who manage overdose patients at a mass gathering. In instances when physicians must perform such services outside their normal scope of practice, it might be advisable to maintain certification in the relevant courses like ATLS, ACLS, MIMMS, or pediatric trauma management.

Table 19.16. The 10 Best Practice Points Recommended by the Medical Protection Society for Doctors Providing Services at Sports Events

1. Ensure your skills are up to date and that qualifications are appropriate to those required for a specific event.

2. Acquire sufficient knowledge of the sport being played. You should be aware of the risks involved and the likely nature and severity of possible injuries.

3. Be prepared for all medical emergencies, including those which are not sports-related.

4. Ensure that you have access to the appropriate medical equipment and resources that your risk assessment has identified as being required.

5. Know and follow the guidance published by the sport's governing body.

6. Be familiar with the local emergency services and ensure you are aware of and comfortable with the level of support available.

7. Arrange appropriate professional indemnity.

8. Ensure that the extent of your responsibilities are defined and agreed with the event organizer in advance. Specifically, are you responsible for spectators and event staff as well as the participants?

9. You may wish to speak to the referee/umpire regarding arrangements for stopping play if necessary.

10. If you are dissatisfied with the support facilities and resources available, you should bring this to the attention of the event organizer and consider objecting to the event proceeding until the situation has been rectified.

The ten best practice points recommended by the Medical Protection Society for doctors providing services at sports events are listed in Table 19.16.

Medical Records

Maintaining medical records is important but can be challenging because mass gatherings are infrequent events. Voluntary bodies such as the Red Cross, Red Crescent, the St. John Ambulance Brigade, and the Order of Malta have decades of experience providing medical care at mass gatherings and have produced their own standardized medical records. In general, these are single-sided A4-sized pages, occasionally in triplicate form. These records contain information on basic demographics, nature of incident, and nature of treatment given with a record of whether the patient was discharged, referred for more senior opinion, seen by a physician, or transported to a hospital. Although additional detail is desirable for a mass gathering event medical record, documentation will never be as detailed or comprehensive as a hospital chart given the pragmatic considerations of the situation. At the time of this writing, most events use paper records because electronic medical records and Wi-Fi transmission of data on-site are not yet fiscally viable options for organizers of most small-scale events. Records should be kept for 30 years or longer, consistent with local guidelines and regulations. Ranse and Hutton, in *Prehospital and Disaster Medicine*, proposed a minimum data set for mass gathering health research and evalu-

ation.[101] WHO has created a discussion group on mass gathering medical care to develop the concept further and attempt to define an agreed international data set. At a minimum, four forms of documentation are required:

1. Patient Medical Record (PMR)
2. Injured Staff Medical Record (ISMR)
3. Patient Transfer Record (PTR)
4. Cumulative tally of patients treated, patients transported, and the resources used.

The ISMR is important for a number of reasons. Such documentation helps ensure workplace health and safety. If common patterns of illness and injury emerge, these must be identified early, particularly when such staff may be involved in food preparation or event safety and security

Patient Medical Record (PMR)

The essential data set should include:

- Day of week
- Date
- Venue
- Event name
- Medical post designation
- Transfer on-site: identification of post-receiving transfer
- Transfer off-site: destination, hospital name
- Location of incident (if injury)
- Time of incident (if injury)
- Level of healthcare provider (first aider, EMT, paramedic, nurse, physician)
- Name of healthcare provider
- Name of patient
- Date of patient's birth
- Cell phone number of patient
- Details of transport to venue (arrangements may be required for transfer home after hospital treatment)
- Detail of illness or injury
- Past medical history (if relevant)
- Current medications (if relevant)
- Incident related to alcohol ingestion
- Incident related to illicit drug ingestion, name of drug, quantity taken, description of drug (color/shape/symbols)
- Observations (vital signs, pupil size and response, oxygen saturation, 12-lead EKG, if applicable)
- Physical examination
- Differential diagnosis
- Treatments given, including:
  - Airway management required? yes/no (type)
  - Intravenous line required? yes/no
  - Fluids administered intravenously? yes/no
  - Medication names and doses
  - Splint required? yes/no

A triplicate form is used by some event planners. The treating physician receives a copy at the end of the event to maintain a record of patients treated. A second copy is given to the voluntary agency involved in treatment, if any. The third copy is maintained by the event medical director as an overall record of the patients treated. This allows for record maintenance and audit of medical service requirements to assist in post-event report writing. In the absence of triplicate forms, a photocopier should be part of the equipment brought to the event.

In some jurisdictions, event promoters provide branded notepaper for use as medical records and argue that because they own the paper they also own the record. They claim they need records to protect against potential future litigation. Although medical recordkeeping is important for clinicians providing direct medical care, it would be better to provide anonymous summary statistics for the event promoter. If actual records are later required for litigation, the medical director can produce the original. Local medical licensing authorities can assist with ensuring systems are in place to protect confidential patient health information.

Injured Staff Medical Record (ISMR)

In addition to the previously described elements, the ISMR should include the following:

▪ Nature of the injury
▪ Was PPE being used? yes/no
▪ If not, why not?
▪ Staff title and role
▪ Able to resume work? (yes/no)

A separate file should be kept on injured staff, particularly if there is mandatory reporting of workplace accidents.

Patient Transfer Record (PTR)

In addition to the information on the basic PMR, the PTR should include:

▪ Reason for transfer
▪ Details of accompanying persons/cell phone numbers
▪ Physician's name and contact details

Treatment Facilities

During the planning phase, the medical director, in conjunction with the ambulance service, should determine the number, location, and size of medical facilities including first aid stations provided on-site. If there is more than one medical facility, the director should designate a field hospital or medical center. A facility should also be designated as a casualty clearing station for field triage in the event of a major incident.

Satellite medical facilities should be highly visible and easily identifiable from a distance to roaming medical staff. The satellite medical facilities and first aid posts should be located at the peripheries of the audiences in the main arenas to enable unrestricted access and egress for ambulances. Maps should be available for all medical and first aid staff to ensure that they know response locations after receiving a radio call. Generally, a medical facility will be located at one or both sides of the main stage, as this is where the largest crowd concentration will be. Historically, the greatest numbers of crowd crushing injuries have occurred at the areas of highest patron density.

At large sites, consideration should be given to having mobile response teams with the skill mix to provide initial resuscitation to unconscious patients with unprotected airways. Teams should operate in pairs.

Medical facilities should not permit smoking; in the absence of legislation, however, this may be difficult to impose. If oxygen is used in the main medical facility, patrons must be detained if they are trying to gain entry while smoking. The number of treatment gurneys will depend on the estimated crowd size, but a minimum of six ambulance stretchers or examination tables should be provided. Local ordinances may specify exact sizes, materials used in construction, and required utilities. For example, in Ireland, the minimum size for a main medical facility is 25 square meters for crowds in excess of 15,000 and 15 square meters for smaller crowds. Facilities must contain hot and cold running water, a telephone with outside line capability, heating, lighting, ventilation, electrical sockets, and examining couches. They should be staffed by nurses and doctors experienced in accident and emergency work and first aid providers to assist with observation of patients. Emergency vehicles must have ready access to the sites. Toilets restricted from general public use must be available proximate to the medical facility.

Doorways should be large enough for wheelchair access. Although equipment lists are not specified, it would be standard to provide defibrillators both in the facility and situated around the venue, usually automated or semi-automated external defibrillators (AEDs). Several experts have suggested mathematical formulae to assist in determining the number of AEDs needed at mass gathering sites. Crucco derived a formula based on stadium area, severity of slopes, stairway distances, and horizontal distances to achieve certain targeted response times.[102] At the University of North Carolina, Motyka completed a similar study in the football stadium (capacity 60,000) and the basketball stadium (capacity 21,444).[103] Multi-venue events with pass access restrictions and variable crowd densities along the routes present additional challenges. In these situations, roving teams with portable defibrillators in addition to fixed-site AEDs can decrease time to defibrillation.

Communications

Numerous studies, including one by Valesky et al., have highlighted that communication systems need improvement for mass gatherings.[104] Communication requirements will depend on the event setting and the number of people present. If not already available at the stadium, the event promoter usually provides communication systems. For events situated in remote areas, wireless phone services for voice communications are unreliable because the local cell will likely be overloaded by the volume of calls for the duration of the event. There are systems such as Access Overload Control that permit authorities, in the event of an emergency, to request any particular mobile phone cell be shut down to all voice traffic except for those on pre-registered handsets for emergency services. This can be very expensive, as the requesting authority has to compensate the communications provider for lost revenue, which is calculated from the average traffic in that cell over a reference period. This may be inexpensive in remote areas with low usage volumes on non-event days. Text messaging is another possibility and has been proposed by Lund et al. in Canada as a strategy to address limits of audio-based communications during mass gathering events with high ambient noise.[105] This may guarantee message clarity, but timely message delivery cannot be guaranteed in an overloaded cell network. Even with limited bandwidth or weak signals, there are protected channels for text communications. This system would ensure the existence of an audit trail for communications. Whatever system of communication is used, there should be a back-up in case of failure.[106] Chan has proposed wireless local area networks as a possible solution to telecommunications failures.[107]

The choice of communications technology should be made in conjunction with local authorities (police, fire, medical, and health) and should conform to community codes of practice for such systems. There should be a central control area on-site for the relevant service commanders where they can regularly update each other on developments. This area should have a good view of the event site, including the use of closed-circuit television if necessary. There should be a capability to communicate on two-way multi-channel radio sets to event controllers, security, promoters, medical and ambulance services, first aid workers, welfare personnel, and law enforcement. Two-way communications are preferred from the medical perspective because with one-way communication, other users on the same channel cannot hear a colleague's appeal for help; they will only hear the control room response.

Even with very high-quality equipment, it can be difficult to hear radio communications within the main arena or close to a noisy stage. Limited communication may be possible using brief hand signals or, alternatively, runners may be used to bring messages directly from place to place with requests for supplies or assistance.

Audit

In the aftermath of the event, it is important to perform an audit of the on-site medical care to facilitate quality improvement. Specific areas to address include quality issues, whether appropriate skill mix levels existed on-site, levels of care, patient demographics, presentations related to alcohol and drugs, and the effects on off-site health service resources. Analysis of these factors will assist with planning for future similar events to include providing data on appropriate staffing levels to safely manage a mass gathering.

The following represent important data elements that the medical director should collect to facilitate continuous quality improvement:

■ Number of patients treated and demographics
■ Number of patients treated per medical aid station
■ Number of patients who received care from the appropriate provider
■ Number of patients who were referred to see a more experienced or specialty practitioner
■ Number of transfers off-site to other medical facilities and reasons for transfer
■ Average return-to-site times for team members accompanying patients off-site
■ Number of hospital admissions and reasons for admission
■ Number of drug-related presentations and drugs involved
■ Numbers of alcohol-related presentations
■ Number of assaults
■ Number of patients treated per hour
■ Time first patient seen
■ Time last patient seen
■ Number of staff seen as patients
■ Numbers and types of injuries occurring in staff
■ Top ten medical presentation list
■ Medications used and doses
■ Medical equipment used
■ Time to defibrillation

RECOMMENDATIONS FOR FURTHER RESEARCH

The science of mass gathering medicine is in its infancy. Much of the early academic focus has been on descriptive research, including reports of medical involvement at single events.[108,109] Publication of NAEMSP's *Medical Directors Checklist* provided a valuable resource beyond the previously published descriptive studies. The *Lancet* infectious diseases journal supported by the WHO Health Cluster recently ran a series of articles on mass gatherings health. One of the papers featured a research agenda call to action with a significant focus on public health emergencies.[31] Mackway-Jones and Carley in the UK completed a three-round Delphi study of twenty-two experts identified as investigators in the area to determine the research needs in major incident management.[110] This group reached consensus on seventy-four research priority topics with the strongest themes within the topics related to education and training, planning, and communication. Lund, in *Prehospital and Disaster Medicine*, describes the creation and early implementation of an online event and patient registry.[111]

Several authors have emphasized the importance of drills, exercises, advanced preparation, and education. However, more work is needed on improving patient outcomes via training and preparedness for team members at all levels.[9,112–117] A critical review of the efficacy of current physician training for mass gathering medical care would be valuable.

In recent years, a number of mass gathering literature reviews have been published, most notably by Michael and Milsten. Zeitz published a model predicting the workload at a mass gathering.[118] Michael, in a 25-year review published in *Prehospital and Disaster Medicine*, suggests that a uniform classification scheme is necessary for future prospective studies of mass gatherings.[119] Milsten produced a comprehensive literature review examining the variables that can affect patient presentations at events.[93] He found that weather; environmental factors; event type and duration; and crowd mood, attendance, density, age, and alcohol/drug use were prominent factors.

In 2007, Arbon published a comprehensive review of the evidence for mass gathering medical practice and future directions for research.[120] He identifies the lack of a consensus definition for mass gathering and suggests using a description that includes nontraditional mass gatherings such as mass transit systems, shopping complexes, airports, and cruise ships. He delineates accepted principle goals of mass gathering medical care, specifically:

1. Establishing rapid access to ill or injured patients and providing triage
2. Effective and timely stabilization and transportation of seriously injured or acutely ill patients
3. Providing on-site care for minor injuries and illnesses

Arbon argues that there is a lack of uniform standards for the provision of health services at mass gatherings with a foundation based on relatively low levels of evidence. This over-reliance on "expert level of evidence" leads to marked variations in standard and legislation. Expert level of evidence is an example of "eminence-based" as opposed to "evidence-based" medicine. He recognizes the need for consensus among the word experts in creating commonality of language with respect to data collection. Examples include the use of PPTT, transfer to hospital rate (TTHR), patient presentation rate (PPR), and MUR. Until there is an agreed standardized data set that is collected at mass gathering events, there will be no consistency in data collection and it will be impossible to compare similar events. The minimum data set as proposed by Ranse and Hutton would seem to be an excellent beginning in achieving consensus in data collection instruments.[101] In summary, there is an immediate need for new primary research that focuses on:

- Appropriate timelines for event planning
- Liability issues
- Education and training of medical personnel without prior mass gathering medicine experience
- Comparison of medical patient visit rates for similar events
- Appropriate levels of care delivered at mass gatherings and benefits of on-site versus off-site treatment
- Alternatives to hospital transports for diagnostic access
- Treat and release protocols for non-physician providers
- Standardized data sets
- Standardized definitions for events, interventions, and records
- Best practice documentation strategies
- Utilization of tools for on-site electronic documentation/reporting
- Global positioning system (GPS)/radio frequency identification (RFID) tagging for large unbounded events (as an example, to locate roaming teams with critical patients)
- Mitigation strategies
- Outcomes of care provided at mass gatherings
- Appropriate staffing requirements for medical, nursing, and other paramedical personnel based on national scope of practices
- Reduction of effects on local health services
- VIP care strategies
- Impact of licensing legislation in different jurisdictions on patient visits
- Staff presentations for medical care

As mass gatherings become more frequent, more experts must be trained and more research performed to ensure continued reduction in morbidity and mortality among those attending or managing such events.

> The world is a dangerous place, not because of those who do evil, but because of those who look on and do nothing.
> Albert Einstein

> A goal without a plan is just a wish.
> Antoine de Saint-Exupery

REFERENCES

1. Stratton SJ. Violent sabotage of mass-gathering events. *Prehosp and Disaster Medicine.* August 2013; 28(4): 313.
2. Bluman EM. Boston marathon bombing. *Foot Ankle Int* August 2013; 34(8): 1053–1054.
3. Mitchell EL. Finish line becomes front line at Boston marathon. *Ann Emerg Med* November 2013; 62(5): 543–544.
4. Hupp JR. Important take-aways from the Boston marathon bombing. *J Oral Maxillofac Surg* October 2013; 71(10): 1637–1638.
5. Caterson EJ, Carty MJ, Weaver MJ, Holt EF. Boston bombings: a surgical view of lessons learned from combat casualty care and the applicability to Boston's terrorist attack. *J Craniofac Surg* July 2013; 24(4): 1061–1067.
6. The role of the emergency physician in mass casualty/disaster management. ACEP position paper. *Jacep* November 1, 1976; 5(11): 901–902.
7. Manifesto for emergency medicine in Europe. Council of the European Society for Emergency Medicine. *Eur J Emerg Med* December 1, 1998; 5(4): 389–390.
8. Lund A, Gutman SJ, Turris SA. Mass gathering medicine: a practical means of enhancing disaster preparedness in Canada. *CJEM/JCMU* July 2011; 13(4): 231–236.
9. Hsu E, Jenckes M, Catlett C, Robinson K, Feuerstein C, Cosgrove S, et al. Effectiveness of hospital staff mass-casualty incident training methods: a systematic literature review. *Prehosp Disaster Med* July 1, 2004; 19(3): 191–199.
10. Greenough PG. The Kumbh Mela stampede: disaster preparedness must bridge jurisdictions. *BMJ* 2013; 346: f3254.
11. Memish ZA, Stephens GM, Steffen R, Ahmed QA. Emergence of medicine for mass gatherings: lessons from the Hajj. *Lancet Infect Dis* January 2012; 12(1): 56–65.
12. Abubakar I, Gautret P, Brunette GW, Blumberg L, Johnson D, Poumerol G, et al. Global perspectives for prevention of infectious diseases associated with mass gatherings. *Lancet Infect Dis* January 2012; 12(1): 66–74. http://eutils.ncbi.nlm.nih.gov/entrez/eutils/elink.fcgi?dbfrom=pubmed&id=22192131&retmode=ref&cmd=prlinks (Accessed August 25, 2015).
13. Levett J. A new opportunity for public health development: Athens 2004. *Prehosp Disaster Med* April 1, 2004; 19(2): 130–132.
14. Mcdonald R. Career Focus: Event Medicine. *BMJ Classified* 2001; 323(7324).
15. Kerr GW, Wilkie SC, McGuffie CA. Medical cover at Scottish football matches: have the recommendations of the Gibson Report been met? *Br J Sports Med* August 1999; 33(4): 274–275.
16. Bashir El H, Rashid H, Memish Z, Shafi S. Meningococcal vaccine coverage in Hajj pilgrims. *Lancet* April 21, 2007; 369(9570): 1343.
17. Morrison D. Heatstroke on the Hajj. *Lancet* April 26, 1980; 1(8174): 935.
18. Avery J, Chitnis J, Daly P, Pollock G. Medical planning for a major event: the Pope's visit to Coventry Airport, 30 May 1982. *Br Med J (Clin Res Ed)* July 3, 1982; 285(6334): 51–53.
19. Federman JH, Giordano LM. How to cope with a visit from the Pope. *Prehosp and Disaster Med* April 1997; 12(2): 86–91.
20. Schulte D, Meade DM. The papal chase. The Pope's visit: a 'mass' gathering. *Emerg Med Serv* November 1993; 22(11): 46–49, 65, 75–79.
21. Ahmed Q, Arabi Y, Memish Z. Health risks at the Hajj. *Lancet* March 25, 2006; 367(9515): 1008–1015.
22. Madani T, Ghabrah T, Al-Hedaithy M, Alhazmi M, Alazraqi T, Albarrak A, et al. Causes of hospitalization of pilgrims in the Hajj season of the Islamic year 1423 (2003). *Ann Saudi Med* September 1, 2006; 26(5): 346–351.
23. Al-Ghamdi S, Akbar H, Qari Y, Fathaldin O, Al-Rashed R. Pattern of admission to hospitals during Muslim pilgrimage (Hajj). *Saudi Med J* October 1, 2003; 24(10): 1073–1076.
24. Steffen R, Bouchama A, Johansson A, Dvorak J, Isla N, Smallwood C, et al. Non-communicable health risks during mass gatherings. *Lancet Infect Dis* February 2012; 12(2): 142–149.
25. Ordinance pertaining to mass gatherings. The Union County Board of Commissioners, State of North Carolina. September 1, 1974; (224): 224–227, Docket 12. Accessed August 26, 2015.

http://www.co.union.nc.us/Portals/0/Ordinances/Volume1/ Vol1_Ord01.pdf

26. An Ordinance for the regulation of mass gatherings in Alleghany County. Ordinances of Alleghany County, North Carolina, 1975; 1–29. http://alleghanycounty-nc.gov/ordinances/ 1–29.pdf (Accessed August 26, 2015).

27. Mass gathering regulations. Arkansas State Board of Health, Arkansas, 1973.

28. Arnold J, Levine B, Manmatha R, Lee F, Shenoy P, Tsai M, et al. Information-sharing in out-of-hospital disaster response: the future role of information technology. *Prehosp Disaster Med* July 1, 2004; 19(3): 201–207.

29. Arbon P, Bridgewater FH, Smith C. Mass gathering medicine: a predictive model for patient presentation and transport rates. *Prehosp Disaster Med* July 2001; 16(3): 150–158.

30. Jaslow D, Drake M, Lewis J. Characteristics of state legislation governing medical care at mass gatherings. *Prehosp Emerg Care* October 1999; 3(4): 316–320.

31. Tam JS, Barbeschi M, Shapovalova N, Briand S, Memish ZA, Kieny M-P. Research agenda for mass gatherings: a call to action. *Lancet Infect Dis* March 2012; 12(3): 231–239.

32. Best J, McIntosh A, Savage T. Rugby World Cup 2003 injury surveillance project. *Br J Sports Med* November 1, 2005; 39(11): 812–817.

33. Cheng D, Yakobi-shvili R, Fernandez J. Major sport championship influence on ED sex census. *Am J Emerg Med* May 1, 2005; 23(3): 408–409.

34. Roberts D, Blackwell T, Marx J. Emergency medical care for spectators attending National Football League games. *Prehosp Emerg Care* July 1, 1997; 1(3): 149–155.

35. Moreno Millan E, Bonilla F, Alonso J, Casado F. Medical care at the 7th International Amateur Athletics Federation World Championships in Athletics 'Sevilla '99'. *Eur J Emerg Med* February 1, 2004; 11(1): 39–43.

36. Bock HC, Cordell WH, Hawk AC, Bowdish GE. Demographics of emergency medical care at the Indianapolis 500 mile race (1983–1990). *Ann Emerg Med* October 1992; 21(10): 1204–1207.

37. Ma O, Millward L, Schwab R. EMS medical coverage at PGA tour events. *Prehosp Emerg Care* 2002; 6(1): 11–14.

38. Morimura N, Katsumi A, Koido Y, Sugimoto K, Fuse A, Asai Y, et al. Analysis of patient load data from the 2002 FIFA World Cup Korea/Japan. *Prehosp Disaster Med* July 2004; 19(3): 278–284.

39. McCarthy DM, Chiampas GT, Malik S, Cole K, Lindeman P, Adams JG. Enhancing Community Disaster Resilience through Mass Sporting Events. *Disaster Med Public Health Prep* December 1, 2011; 5(4): 310–315.

40. The price of pop. *Lancet* September 25, 1971; 2(7726): 696–697.

41. Carveth S. Eight-year experience with a stadium- based mobile coronary-care unit. *Heart Lung* September 1, 1974; 3(5): 770–774.

42. Fisher J. The British Association for Immediate Care (BASICS). Its experience in major disasters, with special reference to the role of the medical incident officer. *Injury* 1990; 21(1): 45–48, discussion 55–57.

43. Slater D. Hillsborough television drama. *BMJ* March 22, 1997; 314(7084): 901–902.

44. Wardrope J, Hockey M, Crosby A. The hospital response to the Hillsborough tragedy. *Injury* 1990; 21(1): 53–54, discussion 55–57.

45. Heller T. Personal and medical memories from Hillsborough. *BMJ* December 23, 1989; 299(6715): 1596–1598.

46. Walker E. Not all those who died after Hillsborough did so by 3 15 pm. *BMJ* April 26, 1997; 314(7089): 1283.

47. DeAngeles D, Schurr M, Birnbaum M, Harms B. Traumatic asphyxia following stadium crowd surge: stadium factors affecting outcome. *WMJ* October 1, 1998; 97(9): 42–45.

48. Sivaloganathan S, Green M. The Bradford Fire Disaster. Part 1. The initial investigations: who died, where and how? *Med Sci Law* October 1, 1989; 29(4): 279–283.

49. Sivaloganathan S, Green M. The Bradford Fire Disaster. Part 2. Accident reconstruction: who died, when and why? *Med Sci Law* Oct 1, 1989; 29(4): 284–286.

50. Ayton F, Hill C, Parfitt H. The dental role in the identification of the victims of the Bradford City Football Ground fire. *Br Dent J* October 19, 1985; 159(8): 262–264.

51. Sharpe D, Roberts A, Barclay T, Dickson W, Settle J, Crockett D, et al. Treatment of burns casualties after fire at Bradford City football ground. *Br Med J (Clin Res Ed)* October 5, 1985; 291(6500): 945–948.

52. Sharpe D, Foo I. Management of burns in major disasters. *Injury* 1990; 21(1): 41–44, discussion 55–57.

53. Leonard RB. Medical support for mass gatherings. *Emerg Med Clin North Am* May 1996; 14(2): 383–397.

54. Schlicht J, Mitcheson M, Henry M. Medical aspects of large outdoor festivals. *Lancet* April 29, 1972; 1(7757): 948–952.

55. Brock S, Schlicht J. Medical aspects of large outdoor festivals. *Lancet* May 27, 1972; 1(7761): 1178.

56. Ounanian L, Salinas C, Shear C, Rodney W. Medical care at the 1982 US Festival. *Ann Emerg Med* May 1, 1986; 15(5): 520–527.

57. Nix C, Khan I, Hoban M, Little G, Keye G, O'Connor H. Oxegen 2004: the impact of a major music festival on the workload of a local hospital. *Ir Med J* June 1, 2006; 99(6): 167–169.

58. Grange J, Green S, Downs W. Concert medicine: spectrum of medical problems encountered at 405 major concerts. *Acad Emerg Med* March 1, 1999; 6(3): 202–207.

59. O'Keefe J, Kheir J, Martin M, Leslie L, Neal J, Edlich R. Balcony collapse at the University of Virginia graduation: what hath Jefferson wrought? *J Emerg Med* March 1, 1999; 17(2): 293–297.

60. Martinez J. Medical coverage of cycling events. *Curr Sports Med Rep* May 1, 2006; 5(3): 125–130.

61. Grange JT. Planning for large events. *Curr Sports Med Rep* June 2002; 1(3): 156–161.

62. Mortelmans L, Van Rossom P, Bois Du M, Jutten G. Carbon monoxide load in indoor carting. *Eur J Emerg Med* June 1, 2003; 10(2): 105–107.

63. De Lorenzo R, Gray B, Bennett P, Lamparella V. Effect of crowd size on patient volume at a large, multipurpose, indoor stadium. *J Emerg Med* July 1, 1989; 7(4): 379–384.

64. Baker WM, Simone BM, Niemann JT, Daly A. Special event medical care: the 1984 Los Angeles Summer Olympics experience. *Ann Emerg Med* February 1986; 15(2): 185–190.

65. Thackway S, Delpech V, Jorm L, McAnulty J, Visotina M. Monitoring acute diseases during the Sydney 2000 Olympic and Paralympic Games. *Med J Aust* September 18, 2000; 173(6): 318–321.

66. Wetterhall S, Coulombier D, Herndon J, Zaza S, Cantwell J. Medical care delivery at the 1996 Olympic Games. Centers for Disease Control and Prevention Olympics Surveillance Unit. *JAMA* May 13, 1998; 279(18): 1463–1468.

67. Larkin M. Medical teams geared up for winter Olympics. *Lancet* February 2, 2002; 359(9304): 412.

68. Morimura N, Takahashi K, Katsumi A, Koido Y, Sugimoto K, Fuse A, et al. Mass gathering medicine for the First East Asian Football Championship and the 24th European/South American Cup in Japan. *Eur J Emerg Med* April 2007; 14(2): 115–117.

69. Madzimbamuto F. A hospital response to a soccer stadium stampede in Zimbabwe. *Emerg Med J* November 1, 2003; 20(6): 556–559.

70. Tang N, Kraus C, Brill J, Shahan J, Ness C, Scheulen J. Hospital-based event medical support for the Baltimore marathon, 2002–2005. *Prehosp Emerg Care* July 1, 2008; 12(3): 320–326.

71. Rajabali A, Caton H. A tale of two physicians: reflections on the Boston Marathon bombing. *BMJ* 2013;346:f2993. http://www.bmj.com/content/346/bmj.f2993.full.pdf+html (Accessed August 26, 2015).

72. Guermazi A, Hayashi D, Smith SE, Palmer W, Katz JN. Imaging of blast injuries to the lower extremities sustained in the Boston Marathon bombing. *Arthritis Care Res* 2013; 65(12): 1893–1898.

73. Al-Shaqsi S, McBride D, Gauld R, Al-Kashmiri A, Al-Harthy A. Are we ready? Preparedness of acute care providers for the Rugby World Cup 2011 in New Zealand. *Emerg Med J* 2011; 200293. http://emj.bmj.com/content/early/2011/10/31/emermed-2011-200293.full.pdf+html (Accessed August 26, 2015).

74. Moody WE, Hendry RG, Muscatello D. Were attendances to accident and emergency departments in England and Australia influenced by the Rugby World Cup Final 2003? *Eur J Emerg Med* April 1, 2007; 14(2): 68–71.

75. Boisson EV, Imana M, Roberts P. Cricket World Cup: a stress test for the surveillance system in the Caribbean. *West Indian Med J* January 2012; 61(1): 84–89.

76. Bowdish GE, Cordell WH, Bock HC, Vukov LF. Using regression analysis to predict emergency patient volume at the Indianapolis 500 mile race. *Ann Emerg Med* October 1992; 21(10): 1200–1203.

77. Nardi R, Bettini M, Bozzoli C, Cenni P, Ferroni F, Grimaldi R, et al. Emergency medical services in mass gatherings: the experience of the Formula 1 Grand Prix "San Marino" in Imola. *Eur J Emerg Med* December 1997; 4(4): 217–223.

78. Auerbach P, Gelb A, Turns J. Emergency medical services at the 1984 Democratic National Convention. *Ann Emerg Med* July 1, 1985; 14(7): 709–711.

79. Kade KA, Brinsfield KH, Serino RA, Savoia E, Koh HK. Emergency medical consequence planning and management for national special security events after September 11: Boston 2004. *Disaster Med Public Health Prep* October 2008; 2(3): 166–173.

80. Yi HH, Zheng'an YY, Fan WW, Xiang GG, Chen DD, Yongchao HH, et al. Public Health Preparedness for the World's Largest Mass Gathering: 2010 World Exposition in Shanghai, China. *Prehosp Disaster Med* December 1, 2012; 27(6): 589–594.

81. The Football Association of Ireland – Club Licensing Manual. 2004; 118.

82. Murphy D, Jabbar N, Eldin M, Gillen P. Audit of the impact of a major pop concert on the workload of two regional hospitals. *Ir Med J* 2001; 94(1): 15.

83. Zeitz KM, Schneider DPA, Jarrett D, Zeitz CJ. Mass gathering events: retrospective analysis of patient presentations over seven years. *Prehosp Disaster Med* July 2002; 17(03): 147–150.

84. Chambers J, Guly H. The impact of a music festival on local health services. *Health Trends* 1991; 23(3): 122–123.

85. Grange JT, Baumann GW, Vaezazizi R. On-site physicians reduce ambulance transports at mass gatherings. *Prehosp Emerg Care* July 2003; 7(3): 322–326.

86. Bacon J. The Event Safety Guide: A Guide to Health, Safety and Welfare at Music and Similar Events. Her Majesty's Stationery Office, Norwich, United Kingdom, 1999. http://www.sportandrecreation.org.uk/sites/sportandrecreation.org.uk/files/Event-Safety-Guide.pdf (Accessed August 26, 2015).

87. Calabro J, Krohmer J, Rivera-Rivera E, Balcombe D, Reich J. Provision of Emergency Medical Care for Crowds. American College of Emergency Physicians EMS Committee 1995-96, American College of Emergency Physicians, 1996. http://www.acep.org/workarea/downloadasset.aspx?id=4846 (Accessed August 26, 2015).

88. Jaslow D, Yancy A, Milsten A. Mass gathering medical care. National Association of EMS Physicians Standards and Clinical Practice Committee. *Prehosp Emerg Care* 2000; 4(4): 359–360.

89. Jaslow D, Yancy A, Milsten A. Mass Gathering Medical Care: The Medical Director's Checklist. National Association of EMS Physicians Standards and Clinical Practice Committee, National Association of EMS Physicians, Lenexa, Kansas, 2000.

90. World Health Organization. Communicable disease alert and response for mass gatherings: key considerations. Geneva, WHO, 2008, pp. 32–33. http://www.who.int/csr/Mass_gatherings2.pdf (Accessed August 26, 2015).

91. Ryan J, Noone E, Plunkett P. Review of a mobile accident and emergency unit at a rock concert. *Ir Med J* September 1, 1994; 87(5): 148–149.

92. Milsten AM, Seaman KG, Liu P, Bissell RA, Maguire BJ. Variables influencing medical usage rates, injury patterns, and levels of care for mass gatherings. *Prehosp Disaster Med* October 2003; 18(4): 334–346.

93. Milsten AM, Maguire BJ, Bissell RA, Seaman KG. Mass-gathering medical care: a review of the literature. *Prehosp Disaster Med* July 2002; 17(3): 151–162.

94. Black J. Emergency use of the Airtraq laryngoscope in traumatic asphyxia: case report. *Emerg Med J* July 1, 2007; 24(7): 509–510.

95. Maharaj CH, Costello JF, Higgins BD, Harte BH, Laffey JG. Learning and performance of tracheal intubation by novice personnel: a comparison of the Airtraq and Macintosh laryngoscope. *Anaesthesia* July 1, 2006; 61(7): 671–677.

96. Timmermann A, Russo S, Rosenblatt W, Eich C, Barwing J, Roessler M, et al. Intubating laryngeal mask airway for difficult out-of-hospital airway management: a prospective evaluation. *Br J Anaesth* August 1, 2007; 99(2): 286–291.

97. Turris SA, Lund A. Triage during mass gatherings. *Prehosp Disaster Med* December 2012; 27(6): 531–535.

98. Code of Practice for Safety at Indoor Concerts. Government of Ireland, The Stationery Office, Dublin, Ireland,1998. http://www.ssi.ie/docs/Code%20of%20Practice%20for%20Safety%20at%20Indoor%20Concerts.pdf (Accessed August 26, 2015).

99. Code of Practice for Safety at Outdoor Pop Concerts and other Outdoor Musical Events. Government of Ireland, The Stationery Office, Dublin, Ireland, 1996. http://www.ahg.gov.ie/en/Publications/ArtsPublications/safety%20at%20outdoor%20pop%20concerts%20and%20other%20outdoor%20musical%20events.pdf (Accessed August 26, 2015).

100. Code of Practice for Safety at Sports Grounds. Government of Ireland, The Stationery Office, Dublin, Ireland,1996. http://www.dttas.ie/sites/default/files/publications/sport/english/safety-sports-grounds/safety-sports-grounds.pdf (Accessed August 26, 2015).

101. Ranse JJ, Hutton AA. Minimum data set for mass-gathering health research and evaluation: a discussion paper. *Prehosp Disaster Med* December 1, 2012; 27(6): 543–550.

102. Crocco TJ, Sayre MR, Liu T, Davis SM, Cannon C, Potluri J. Mathematical determination of external defibrillators needed at mass gatherings. *Prehosp Emerg Care* July 2004; 8(3): 292–297.

103. Motyka TM, Winslow JE, Newton K, Brice JH. Method for determining automatic external defibrillator need at mass gatherings. *Resuscitation* June 2005; 65(3): 309–314.

104. Valesky W, Silverberg M, Gillett B, Roblin P, Adelaine J, Wallis LA, et al. Assessment of hospital disaster preparedness for the 2010 FIFA World Cup using an Internet-based, long-distance tabletop drill. *Prehosp Disaster Med* June 2011; 26(3): 192–195.

105. Lund A, Wong D, Lewis K, Turris SA, Vaisler S, Gutman S. Text Messaging as a Strategy to Address the Limits of Audio-Based Communication During Mass-Gathering Events with High Ambient Noise. *Prehosp Disaster Med* 2013; 28(1): 2–7.

106. Adini B, Goldberg A, Laor D, Cohen R, Zadok R, Bar-Dayan Y. Assessing levels of hospital emergency preparedness. *Prehosp Disaster Med* 2006; 21(6): 451–457.

107. Chan TC, Killeen J, Griswold W, Lenert L. Information technology and emergency medical care during disasters. *Acad Emerg Med* November 1, 2004; 11(11): 1229–1236.

108. Duffin C. Glastonbury: mud, sweat and tears. *Emerg Nurse* July 1, 2007; 15(4): 10–15.

109. Britten S, Whiteley M, Fox P, Goodwin M, Horrocks M. Medical treatment at Glastonbury Festival. *BMJ* October 16, 1993; 307(6910): 1009–1010.

110. Mackway-Jones KK, Carley SS. An international expert delphi study to determine research needs in major incident management. *Prehosp Disaster Med* July 31, 2012; 27(4): 351–358.

111. Lund AA, Turris SAS, Amiri NN, Lewis KK, Carson MM. Mass-gathering medicine: creation of an online event and patient registry. *Prehosp Disaster Med* December 1, 2012; 27(6): 601–611.

112. Galante J, Jacoby R, Anderson J. Are surgical residents prepared for mass casualty incidents? *J Surg Res* May 1, 2006; 132(1): 85–91.

113. Goldman B. Spectator events: medical preparation a must. *CMAJ* January 15, 1988; 138(2): 164–165.

114. Madge S, Kersey J, Murray G, Murray J. Are we training junior doctors to respond to major incidents? A survey of doctors in the Wessex region. *Emerg Med J* September 1, 2004; 21(5): 577–579.

115. Mann N, MacKenzie E, Anderson C. Public health preparedness for mass-casualty events: a 2002 state-by-state assessment. *Prehosp Disaster Med* July 1, 2004; 19(3): 245–255.

116. Rubin A. Safety, security, and preparing for disaster at sporting events. *Curr Sports Med Rep* June 1, 2004; 3(3): 141–145.

117. Rutherford W. The place of exercises in disaster management. *Injury* 1990; 21(1): 58–60, discussion 63–64.

118. Zeitz KM, Zeitz CJ, Arbon P. Forecasting medical work at mass-gathering events: predictive model versus retrospective review. *Prehosp Disaster Med* May 2005; 20(3): 164–168.

119. Michael JA, Barbera JA. Mass gathering medical care: a twenty-five year review. *Prehosp Disaster Med* October 1997; 12(4): 305–312.

120. Arbon P. Mass-gathering medicine: a review of the evidence and future directions for research. *Prehosp Disaster Med* March 2007; 22(2): 131–135.

20

TRANSPORTATION DISASTERS

Ulf Björnstig and Rebecca Forsberg

OVERVIEW

The Red Cross defines a disaster as an event causing 10 or more deaths and/or 100 injuries. According to the Red Cross World Disaster Report, transportation-related disasters are a major source of morbidity and mortality, causing 45% of all disaster-related deaths in Africa. During the 1990s, approximately 80,000 people were killed in different disasters in the world each year.[1] This number may be compared with the "low virulent epidemic" of road fatalities that annually kill approximately 1.2 million people (16.1/100,000 inhabitants) and injure 50 million people to such an extent that they require medical attention.[2] In India and China, 100,000 road users are killed each year (2012 data). In the United States, the number is about 32,000 (2011 data).[3]

Since the year 2000, approximately 600–700 people have been killed annually in commercial aircraft crashes. This number has steadily decreased over the years since the 1970s. In sea disasters, the events are more infrequent, but may sometimes involve a few thousand victims each. A few major train incidents are reported annually with sometimes hundreds of fatalities. Bus and coach crashes kill fewer people in each incident, but seem to be increasing in frequency. A common feature is that many of these incidents occur in rural and remote areas, creating special rescue problems.

In most of these categories, both unintentional and intentional injury events have been reported. More and more frequent suicide attacks have introduced a new dimension of intentional violence, rendering many previous preventive strategies ineffective.

A structure that helps organize the approach to these events is the Haddon Matrix. Originally created to examine road traffic trauma, it is now widely used throughout the transportation industry. Dr. Haddon identified several factors that contribute to injury events and disasters. These factors are human, vehicle/equipment, physical environment, and socioeconomic environment. These elements contribute to injury events in three phases: 1) pre-event; 2) event; and 3) post-event (Table 20.1).[4] In referring to rescue work in the post-event phase, this chapter will use the structure from the British Major Incident Medical Management System (MIMMS).[5] This system is widely used

Table 20.1. The Haddon Matrix is used to organize the analysis of an injury event and possible mitigation strategies

Haddon Matrix				
Phases	Factors			
	Human	Vehicle/ Equipment	Physical environment	Socioeconomic environment
Pre-crash				
Crash				
Post-crash				

in Europe, Australia, and several other countries in both civilian and military contexts. MIMMS nomenclature for disaster management includes "preparation" (planning, equipment, and training) and "on-scene command." The command structure is described by the mnemonic CSCATTT (Command, Safety, Communication, Assessment, Triage, Treatment, and Transport). In summary, this chapter will use the Haddon Matrix to describe the disasters affecting each mode of transportation and MIMMS to illustrate how these events are managed.

CURRENT STATE OF THE ART

The following sections will discuss disasters involving aircraft, vessels at sea (ship and ferry), railcars (train/railway), and road motor vehicles (bus/coach).

Air Disasters

Incidence Data

During the "Zeppelin era" from 1913–1937, the number of fatalities due to dirigible crashes was fourteen to fifty-two per event. This period ended in 1937 when the Hindenburg exploded, killing thirty-six of the ninety-seven people on board. In the modern aviation era, from 1970–2012, the number of annual passenger airline crashes with human fatalities has declined from about seventy to ten. This shift toward lower numbers is especially evident after the year 2002. The fatality rate has decreased from 2,500 annually during the 1970s to about 600–700 from 2002–2012. The number of fatalities per million departures has decreased from approximately 290 fatalities per million departures from 1970–1974 to less than 50 during the years 2002–2012.[6–8]

Injury Events: Historical Perspective

The track record on fatality rates varies considerably by airline. The following numbers for major airlines are current through 2012. Qantas Airlines has been free from fatal injury events since 1952. Cathay Pacific has been free from deaths since 1972. All Nippon Airways, British Airways, and Lufthansa are among the carriers with low fatal injury rates per flight. Before 2010, the commercial aircraft with the best crash records that had logged more than 2 million flights were: the Boeing 777, with no fatalities, followed by current versions of the Boeing 737 600–900, the Airbus 318–321, and previous Boeing 737 300–500, with rates of 0.09–0.19 plane loads killed per million flights.[7,9]

Most crashes per time unit occur during takeoffs and landings, but some aircraft have experienced problems during flight, mostly related to technical or weather problems.[6] In this business, most incidents are unintentional, but intentional events are also a real threat to flight safety. During the 1980s, an epidemic of aircraft hijacking initiated new passenger and baggage control systems, which have been developed further during the twenty-first century due to special factors introduced by the suicide terrorist threat.

Injury Events: Current Perspective

The geographical distribution of fatal crashes from different parts of the world for the years 2008–2012 involving commercial aircrafts with ten or more passengers on board is as follows: Asia 29%, Sub-Saharan Africa 18%, South and Central America 18%, Russia and former Soviet Republics (on the European side) 18%, Middle East and North Africa 8%, North America (4%), Europe 4% and Australia (0%).[7–9] A trend toward more local/regional airline crashes in low- and middle-income countries is observed during this period. Looking at the eighteen crashes in 2008–2012 involving fifty or more fatalities, 28% happened in the Middle East and North Africa, 22% in Asia, 17% in Africa, and 17% in Russia/Kazakhstan. The most severe crash in the 2008–2012 period, in terms of the number killed, was the Air France crash of 2009 in the Atlantic Ocean, on a flight between Rio de Janeiro and Paris, which claimed 228 lives.[10]

The most disastrous incident involving civilian aircraft is the September 11, 2001, terrorist attack in the United States, when four airliners were hijacked and crashed into the World Trade Center buildings in New York, the Pentagon in Washington, DC, and a field in Virginia. The human losses were approximately 3,000 dead. This incident was extreme and is well-described elsewhere.[11]

Because prevention is the first choice in disaster mitigation, it may be beneficial to more closely examine factors contributing to air disasters.[1] The following are selected incidents that illustrate typical factors and sequences of events found in airline crashes. Each event was thoroughly investigated and documented in reports published by different countries' accident investigating boards (in the United States, this agency is the National Transportation Safety Board).[12]

Errors: Human-Machine Interface
2009 CRASH IN THE ATLANTIC OCEAN

Six and a half hours after departure from Rio de Janeiro, an Air France Airbus A330, flying on autopilot, began a slight turn to the left. Flying in clouds, the aircraft encountered some turbulence at 11,700 meters over the mid-Atlantic Ocean, between South America and Africa. The captain disconnected the autopilot and began a series of controlled maneuvers. Airspeed indications were strongly fluctuating or invalid, the stall warning sounded, and oscillations with pitch attitude of up to 40° were recorded, as well as roll movements. The flight recorder data indicated a vertical speed (downwards) of 3,350 meters per minute (11,000 feet per minute) just before the aircraft struck the surface of the sea. Two and a half minutes later, all 228 on board were dead.[10]

Floating debris was found within a week, but it took nearly 2 years before the submerged major sections of aircraft wreckage were located on the ocean floor by a search vessel using unmanned submarines. The flight data recorder and the retrieved debris provided information to support the crash investigation team's conclusions.

Obstruction of the pitot tube (external device that measures airspeed) by ice crystals resulted in a loss of airspeed information. It was thought that pilots could rapidly diagnose such an event and manage the problem through precautionary measures on pitch attitude and thrust. However, in the actual situation, pilots received inconsistent speed measurements from three different sources. This possibility was not well understood by the aviation community at this time. As a result, the crew probably never understood what was actually transpiring. They were not trained to respond to this situation in flight at high altitude, in clouds, and during turbulence. The aircraft went into a sustained stall (loss of lift force due to low speed and severe angle of ascent). In addition, the stall warning did not generate the expected pilot behavior. Consequently, the crew's failure to diagnose the stall situation and the lack of adequate inputs that would have made it possible to recover from the stall were the basic causes of the crash. Other contributing factors included the lack of a clear display in the cockpit delineating the airspeed inconsistencies identified by the computers.[10]

AMSTERDAM 2009

A similar mismatch between the behavior of automatic avionic equipment and the pilots' response to it caused a crash during the landing procedure in a Boeing 737. Basically, the left altimeter provided incorrect input data, which triggered a sequence of more or less inappropriate automatic measures. The crew failed to recognize the error and did not react quickly. The aircraft finally stalled and crashed onto farmland before reaching Schiphol Airport. Nine people were killed and 126 survived the crash.[13]

Errors: Human Factors and Communication during Fog Conditions
TENERIFE, SPAIN

With regard to number of fatalities, the worst crash in history happened on the island of Tenerife in 1977. Two Boeing 747 jumbo jets (from Pan Am and KLM) collided on the runway in heavy fog. A total of 624 people were involved, of whom 583 died and 41 survived.[7–8]

The following represents the pre-crash sequence. The Pan Am crew was instructed to taxi behind the KLM jet, but to turn left off the runway and into a taxiway before reaching the end of the runway. As the KLM aircraft turned to depart on runway 12, its captain immediately powered up for takeoff. The first officer corrected him, saying, "No, we don't have our air traffic control clearance yet." The captain responded with, "I know that, you call for it." As the first officer was repeating his request for departure clearance, the captain initiated takeoff despite the fact that the control tower had not granted permission for this action. At the same moment, the Pan Am 747 crew was looking through the thick fog for their assigned runway turn-off, and saw the lights of the KLM aircraft approaching at takeoff speed. Just after the nose lifted, the KLM aircraft struck the Pan Am jet just behind the cockpit, climbed to a height of 30 meters, and then crashed on the runway. Both aircraft caught fire.

MILAN, ITALY

In 2001, a crash in heavy fog occurred at Linate Airport in Milan. An MD-87 was cleared for takeoff on a runway with visibility limited to 225 meters. At approximately the same time, a business jet was cleared to taxi, but this plane entered the active runway by mistake and was impacted by the MD-87 during takeoff. Both aircraft skidded along the runway and caught fire before they finally hit a baggage hangar, which partially collapsed and also caught fire. All 118 on board the two aircraft and 4 people on the ground died. Ironically, ground radar equipment had been in storage at the airport for years but was not installed. A number of administrators and controllers at the facility were later sentenced to several years in prison for neglect.[14]

Errors: Aircraft/Equipment Failure
THE BRITISH COMET

Metal fatigue (localized, progressive structural damage that occurs during cyclic loading) is a recognized problem in modern aviation airframes and a difficult issue to resolve. The well-known crashes of the British Comet jet aircrafts in the 1950s first brought this problem to the attention of civil aviation authorities. These aircraft broke up in flight due to a design flaw causing metal fatigue around the aircraft's windows.

CHICAGO, ILLINOIS

A DC-10 lost its left engine during takeoff in Chicago in 1979 due to metal fatigue. When the engine separated from the aircraft, it flew up and over the wing, falling onto the runway. When it separated, the hydraulic lines to the rudder and slots systems were disrupted, making the aircraft impossible to steer. All 270 on board were killed.

UNITED STATES: JAMMED VALVE

In 1991, the first of three Boeing 737 incidents occurred, caused by the same type of servo valve jam and dysfunction. All twenty-five on board died in the first violent crash, which happened during the approach to an airport. When the pilots turned into their final approach at an altitude of 300 meters, the aircraft went out of control and plunged steeply into the ground within 10 seconds. The investigators were confused and could not establish the cause. Another crash of a Boeing 737 in 1994 showed a similar course of events. The aircraft rolled out of control, despite the pilot trying to compensate by opposite rudder deflection. The dive became steeper and the aircraft

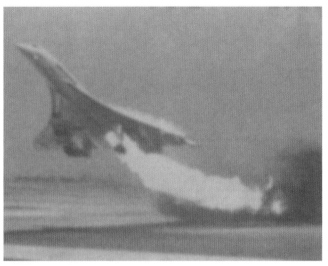

Figure 20.1. Concorde's last flight in 2000. A piece of metal on the runway caused a tire explosion. Debris from the tire punctured the wing fuel tank and the fuel caught fire. Used with permission from Scanpix.

fragmented into small pieces in the violent crash, killing 132 people. This also made the investigation very difficult, and it seemed destined to remain one of few unsolved crashes. In 1996, a third Boeing 737 suffered similar problems. After having gone out of control twice in the same pattern as with the two previous crashes, the pilots finally managed to regain control of the aircraft and land it. This gave the investigators an undamaged aircraft to inspect. They finally came to the conclusion that a servo valve in the steering system had jammed, causing the problem. The jam came after rapid temperature changes, typically during descent from cold temperature at high altitude. These findings explained the unexpected and reversed movements of the rudders that all three aircraft had suffered. After modifying the servo valve, no further incidents of this type have occurred.[7,8,12]

Errors: Physical Environment, Debris on Runway, and Hostile Weather
PARIS, FRANCE

The Concorde crash in 2000 ended the Concorde supersonic era in civil aviation. The aircraft caught fire during takeoff from Charles de Gaulle Airport (Figure 20.1). The pilots lost control and the plane crashed into a hotel, killing all 109 on board and an additional 5 people on the ground. The Concorde had run over a metal strip dropped earlier from another aircraft during departure. This metal strip caused a tire explosion and debris punctured the wing fuel tank.[8]

TORONTO, ONTARIO, CANADA

An Airbus 340 crashed in Toronto in 2005 during inclement weather (Figure 20.2). The aircraft touched down on the 2,700-meter long runway but was unable to stop before reaching the end of the landing strip. It finally came to rest approximately 180 meters from the runway, with its fuselage split into several pieces. Four minutes later, the Airbus was burning furiously; however, all 297 passengers and 12 crewmembers escaped the aircraft without major injury before the fire started. In this crash, the evacuation procedures worked well, and the 4-minute time

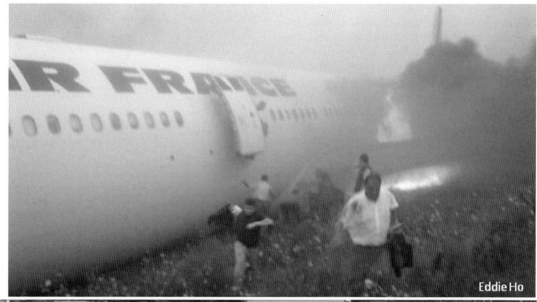

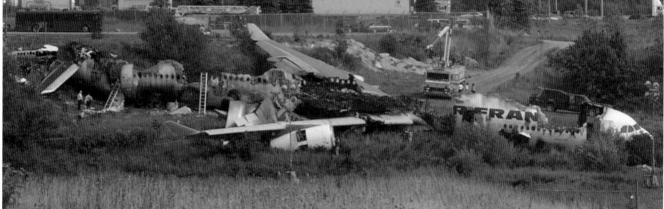

Figure 20.2. The top photo, taken just after the crash, shows the evacuation in progress with the fire beginning. No evacuation slide is seen, however, at the emergency exit. Used with permission from Eddie Ho. The bottom photo was taken a few minutes later. Used with permission from Scanpix.

period before the aircraft caught fire was sufficient for a successful evacuation.[7]

Errors: Socioeconomic Environment and Failure in the Organization
STOCKHOLM, SWEDEN

A 1991 crash of an MD-81 aircraft in Stockholm was caused by lack of proper ground crew procedures and insufficient information in the pilot's flight manual.[15] After departure from Arlanda Airport on a winter day in December, an abnormal noise was heard shortly after the plane became airborne. In clouds, after 25 seconds of flight, clear ice was pulled from the wing into the right engine, which triggered a surge in thrust. The captain throttled back on that engine but the surging did not cease. After 50 seconds, the engine shut down. This same series of events occurred almost simultaneously with the left engine. The captain made an emergency landing in a field and 17,000 liters of jet fuel spilled out. Wet snow on the ground probably prevented a post-crash fire. All on board survived.

The Swedish Board of Accident Investigation concluded that the crash was caused by inadequate company instructions to both the pilots and to ground personnel. It is necessary to climb up and directly inspect the upper wing surface to identify the presence of clear ice. This was not done. Furthermore, the pilots lacked training in identifying and correcting engine surges in an aircraft equipped with an automatic thrust regulation (ATR) system. In this case, the pilots were unaware the aircraft they were flying contained an ATR system and information on ATR was not included in their flight manuals. The ATR automatically increased the engine thrust, ultimately causing engine shutdown, even though the throttles were pulled back to abort the engine surge. As such, the pilots did not anticipate or understand the events as they unfolded.

Crashes Caused by Shootings and Terrorist Attacks
SAKHALIN, RUSSIA

In 1983, a Korean Boeing 747 jumbo jet was shot down by a Soviet fighter plane over the Russian island of Sakhalin and 269 were killed.

IRISH SEA

An Indian Boeing 747 was the target of a terrorist bomb over the Irish Sea in 1985. All 329 people on board were killed, making it the sixth-deadliest incident prior to 2013.

IRAN

In 1988, an Iranian Airbus A300 passenger aircraft was mistakenly shot down by a missile from the American war ship USS Vincennes, which was patrolling the Persian Gulf. All 290 people on board were killed, making it the eighth-deadliest crash prior to 2012.

LOCKERBIE, SCOTLAND

The Lockerbie incident in 1988, in which a Libyan terrorist bomb killed 270 people in a Boeing 747, is also a well-known act of terrorism. A Libyan man was later convicted for this action in 2001. This crash is also among the ten most deadly.

MOSCOW, RUSSIA

In 2004, two domestic Russian aircraft suffered attacks by suspected female suicide bombers during flight. The events occurred within 1 hour of each other, causing forty-six and forty-three fatalities, respectively.

Intentional Crashes: Suicide

Crashing an airliner in an act of suicide is probably a rare event. In a few situations, however, suspicion of such a possibility has been raised, as illustrated by the following case. Half an hour after takeoff from New York, an aircraft with 200 passengers on board steeply descended from approximately 10,000 meters into the Atlantic Ocean in 36 seconds. The data flight recorder showed that the autopilot had been disconnected just before the dive and no technical explanation or malfunction was found.[7]

The Disappearance of Malaysian Airlines Flight MH 370

A Malaysian Airlines Boeing 777 with 239 people on board disappeared suddenly during a night flight from Kuala Lumpur to Beijing on March 8, 2014. "Good night, Malaysian 370" was the last voice message from the aircraft to the Malaysian Air Traffic Control Center 38 minutes after departure. A few minutes later, the automatic radar transponder signal from the aircraft was lost. This happened at a position over the South China Sea. The circumstances surrounding this series of events remain confusing in many ways. Even after investigators collected extensive multinational data from radio, radar, and satellite systems, they were not able to identify an explanation for the events. The most probable crash site (after analysis of all available evidence) is assumed to be in the southern part of the Indian Ocean, 2,000 km west of Perth, Australia. This is a vast area difficult to search effectively. No debris has been found. This is an area with no possible landing sites. In the first 6 months after the disappearance of MH 370, the most extensive search and rescue activity in modern aviation history failed to provide a cause for the incident. The search activities were scheduled to continue for up to an additional year. Many theories exist regarding the cause of MH 370's disappearance. Several have been discussed by the media and include passenger, crew, or cargo factors. However, no clear explanation has been found to date (2016).

What the Human Body Can Survive

The miraculous survival of 22-year-old Yugoslavian flight attendant Vesna Volovic in 1972 is an interesting anecdotal story, indicating what the human body can withstand under advantageous conditions. She was a crewmember aboard a JAT Airways aircraft when it exploded at an altitude of approximately 10,000 meters. She was found in a mountain area, in her chair, unconscious. She suffered severe spine and lower-extremity injuries and

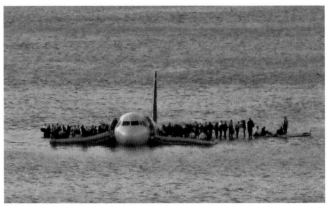

Figure 20.3. A miraculous emergency landing and rescue on the Hudson River in New York City, after double engine failure after takeoff. Used with permission from Scanpix.

was in coma for 1 month, with no memory of the incident when she awoke. After an 8-month hospitalization, she returned as a crew member to JAT Airways, where she worked until her retirement. During World War II, at least three cases were reported of airmen surviving falls without a parachute from altitudes of 5,000–7,000 meters. A common factor is landing on a cushioning surface such as in a tree, on snow, or in a marsh. A similar story is also reported from South America, in which a 10-year-old girl survived a fall from 4,000 meters after a suspected bomb explosion on board her aircraft. She landed in soft marshland, injured but conscious.

PREPARATION

What are the chances of finding survivors after an aircraft crash? In some cases, the crash is so violent that all on board are obviously killed; however, even a violent impact such as the Boeing 747 crash into a Japanese mountain in 1985 can produce survivors. In that case, the aircraft lost its tail fin (a weakness caused by an earlier faulty repair) during flight. It remained airborne for approximately half an hour before it violently crashed into a mountain. Four people survived in the rear section of the cabin, but the other 520 people on board all died, making it the deadliest single aircraft crash on record through 2012. This crash put heavy demands on the rescue teams that had to negotiate hostile terrain.

In approximately half of all airliner crashes, everyone on board is killed. However, in the remaining half, individuals survive, although the numbers vary significantly. In a few of these latter cases, there may be only one or two survivors among hundreds killed.[7] In contrast, a spectacular incident with a pleasant outcome occurred in January 2009 when a US Airways Airbus A320 with 155 people on board crashed into the Hudson River in New York City shortly after takeoff (Figure 20.3). The crash presumably resulted after a flock of geese disabled the engines. The experienced pilot was credited with a safe water landing and this, coupled with the rapid actions of the well-trained crew and local rescuers, resulted in all passengers surviving.[9]

PLANNING

Airport rescue resources must adapt to local circumstances. In 1985, a Boeing 737 caught fire while accelerating down the runway in Manchester, England. Due to the fire, the pilot aborted the takeoff and brought the aircraft to a stop. The fire spread rapidly and filled the cabin with smoke. In an attempt to combat the violent blaze, which ultimately killed fifty-four people, firefighters tried spraying water into the cabin via the emergency doors. This action actually hindered the evacuation of passengers, exacerbating the already deadly situation. The consequences of attempting to extinguish the fire by pumping water through the exit doors was not foreseen, and argues for better planning and training.

There are few areas in modern society where planning for an incident is more rigorously regulated than in aviation. Commercial airports should have rescue resources ready for deployment to a crash site so they arrive within 1.5 minutes of the event and they should have the capacity to extinguish a fire within 30 seconds after arrival. An aircraft must be designed to permit complete evacuation within 1.5 minutes by using half of the emergency exits (experience from the Manchester crash with fire on one side). The International Civil Aviation Organization regulates many of these standards.[16]

EQUIPMENT

Substantial emergency equipment such as emergency slides, flotation devices, life rafts, and emergency oxygen are carried on board. Automatic fire extinguishers for engine fires have been mandatory for decades. Smoke hoods for passengers were recommended after the Manchester crash but have not been introduced.

TRAINING

The aviation workforce receives more training and is better prepared for handling emergencies than the workforces in most other industries. The cost-effectiveness of the substantial rescue resources assigned to commercial airports might be questioned, but obviously there are cases in which lives have been saved because of this investment in response capability.

Scene Response

COMMAND

Crashes that do not occur at airports often generate debris fields covering large areas, such as the downing of a Pan Am 747 over Lockerbie, Scotland. This causes significant command and control problems for the incident officers in the different task forces. Still more problematic was the management of the post-crash events, debris, and human remains after the Malaysian Airways MH 17 downing by a Russian missile in 2014. This occurred in the war zone of eastern Ukraine and resulted in the deaths of 298 people.

SAFETY

Establishing a safe environment at the crash site is sometimes difficult. When the aircraft has crashed in hostile terrain, the safety of rescuers and survivors may be compromised. Spilling fuel and the magnesium–aluminum metal structure may catch fire and burn intensively. Modern composite-rich aircraft may not catch fire as easily as previous planes, but the smoke is expected to be more toxic.

COMMUNICATION

Overload of all types of communication systems has been reported, despite the fact that individuals within the aviation industry are well trained and prepared to manage communication issues. Radio signal interference has compromised rescue operations, even near an international airport as in the Stockholm-Arlanda crash.[15] Hopefully modern communication systems will improve the situation.

Furthermore, implementation of a well-developed communication plan after an aviation incident facilitates transmission of information to all participating agencies. Because international flights often carry passengers from many countries on a single aircraft, those in charge of communicating information must account for time differences, variations in cultures, and multiple languages.[6] All these factors were exposed during the month after the disappearance of flight MH 370, with many Chinese families staying at hotels in China, or even flying to Malaysia, to obtain more information about the aircraft search.

ASSESSMENT

The number of dead and injured may be difficult to assess after crashes in remote areas or at sea. First, it may be difficult to find the crash site, especially in darkness; second, it may be difficult to reach the site if it is located in hostile terrain. Nonetheless, survivors can be expected in half of all crashes, even when they are catastrophic. One example of a difficult situation is the Air France crash in the middle of the Atlantic Ocean, where the first debris was found after 5 days. As such, the assessment must be done very cautiously, and search and rescue efforts should not be withdrawn prematurely.

TRIAGE

The injury spectrum associated with airline crashes is dominated by trauma, burns, and smoke inhalation injuries. Because post-crash fires are quite common, these mechanisms of injury require special attention. More deaths are caused by smoke inhalation than by the flames (such as in the Manchester crash) and this mechanism may complicate the triage process among survivors.

TREATMENT AND TRANSPORT

"Load and go" principles have been used most commonly in takeoff and landing crashes because the transport times are often quite short. Sometimes, this policy can create problems if ambulance dispatch is not well coordinated. In areas without roads, other transport modes must be sought, and in these situations, the military or civil defense forces may provide support.

SEA DISASTERS

Incidence Data

The number of lives lost when the *Titanic* sank was approximately 1,500. The worst single civilian ship disaster ever occurred in January 1945, at the end of World War II. Approximately 9,000–10,000 people died when the German cruise ship *Wilhelm Gustloff* was struck by a Russian torpedo and sank in the Baltic Sea. Many passengers were trapped in the sinking ship. Even those who escaped subsequently perished due to the extremely cold air temperature of $-18°C$; however, approximately 1,200 survived.

The large losses in sea disasters have often been related to warfare. In the civilian context, significant sea disasters occur infrequently. During the years 2000–2012, three incidents occurred with more than 500 victims, and fourteen incidents transpired with 100–500 documented deaths. These are probably conservative figures and may only represent data for better regulated sea transport incidents; some shipwrecks that happened while transporting refugees may be unreported.[8,17]

The world distribution of these incidents has been quite even. In areas such as Indonesia, the Philippines, and Malaysia (with thousands of islands), and in other countries with fast-growing populations and economies, reports of ferry or boating incidents are increasing in number. In these countries, where millions of often poor people rely on ferries for transportation between their archipelagos, overloading of ferries is a frequently reported factor contributing to shipwrecks. The worst incident in Asian waters with respect to the number killed (4,400), and the worst ferry incident in the world, was the collision between the *Dona Paz* and a small oil tanker in Philippine waters in 1987.[18] The *Dona Paz*, constructed with modern safety equipment on board, was built for 1,518 passengers and was probably heavily overcrowded. It caught fire immediately and sank within minutes. Twenty-one survivors had to swim underwater to escape the flames from the burning oil on the water. No lifeboats were launched. The deadliest maritime disaster in African waters occurred in 2000. The Senegalese ferry *Joola*, built for 550 passengers, was also overcrowded and sank, killing 1,200–1,863 people (64 survived).[19] Smuggling migrants on board vessels that are barely seaworthy has also caused hundreds of deaths. In the twenty-first century, pirate attacks are being reported in places such as Somalia.

Injury Events: Historical Perspective

From the beginning of the twentieth century, the most frequent types of incidents involving vessels were: 1) sinking in storms or typhoons; 2) fires and explosions; and 3) collisions with other vessels, icebergs, and submerged structures. Better navigation aids, especially radar and global positioning systems, have reduced collisions and navigational errors on ships equipped with such technology. With modern shipbuilding techniques, ferries and other vessels have become less susceptible to inclement weather.

Injury Events: Current Perspective

After 1970, overturning/sinking and fires have been the most frequent types of incidents, with a component of overloading involved in Asian and African ship disasters. Changes in ship and ferry design are one factor in this development. Ferries that permit cars to drive on and drive off in the same direction have an apparent design weakness in that they contain openings in the front and rear. If water flows into the vehicle deck in rough seas, this can change the center of gravity so the ferry becomes unstable, overturns, and sinks.

The construction of ever-larger cruise ships has increased their vulnerability to fire and other incidents. With many people on board, not only does the potential for careless acts increase, but these vessels may also become potential targets for hostile acts. A fire may erupt spontaneously, but may also be intentionally set, as in the *Scandinavian Star* incident (discussed later).

Errors: Human and Design Shortcomings

Two similar European incidents caused by the increased risk imposed by bow and stern openings in drive-on/drive-off ferries happened during the 1980s and 1990s. The main difference between these two incidents lies in the environmental circumstances, which made the rescue operations quite different. The first happened 1987 in Zeebrugge in Belgium (MS Herald of Free Enterprise), close to a harbor with excellent rescue resources, and in great weather. The second shipwreck – the *Estonia* – occurred in the Baltic Sea, during a storm with 6–8-meter waves, far from shore and with long flight distances for the rescue helicopters.[20]

On an evening in the fall of 1994, the ferry *Estonia* left Tallinn, bound for Stockholm. The weather was bad, with strong winds and waves of 6–8 meters high.[20] Around midnight, a loud noise was reported from the bow opening, and soon thereafter, the ferry rolled heavily 30° when water flushed into the vehicle deck. At 12:20 AM, an emergency call was sent. Ten minutes later, the *Estonia*'s radio went silent and the ferry sank at approximately 12:50 AM. The evacuation was not well organized due to the hull's list, the heavy storm surge, and the speed at which events unfolded. It was later estimated that approximately 200 people escaped the ferry before the ship sank. The incident happened in international waters between Finland, Estonia, and Sweden, so the Maritime Rescue Coordination Centre (MRCC) in Turku, Finland, was in charge of the rescue operations. Helicopters from Finland and Sweden were dispatched to the incident area, as well as ships and ferries. The captain of the Silja Europa ferry was appointed on-scene commander. The Swedish MRCC, however, did not receive the first request for assistance until 40 minutes after *Estonia*'s first emergency call.

Ships and ferries arriving at the site found many people in the water; however, most of the vessels were not able to launch lifeboats because of the stormy conditions. Helicopters lifted some victims from the water and placed them on board the vessels, and some were hoisted on board by other means. Of nearly 1,000 people on board, 137 survived and 838 died. The lowest reported core body temperature in a survivor was 26.5°C. Most of the survivors were men. People did not have time to put on clothing and most of those in the sea were not wearing their life jackets properly.

Errors: Human Factor – Command Failure

The *Costa Concordia* disaster was the partial sinking of an Italian cruise ship in 2012, with the loss of thirty-two lives (Figure 20.4).[21] The ship, carrying 3,206 passengers and 1,023 crewmembers from all over the world, was on the first leg of a cruise around the Mediterranean Sea. It struck a reef during an unofficial near-shore salute to the local islanders. The captain had deviated from the ship's computer-programmed route to perform this maneuver. The collision with the reef (8 meters deep at this point) could easily be heard on-board and caused some panic. A few minutes after the impact, the head of the engine room reported that the hull had a breach of about 70 meters through which water had entered, submerging the generators and engines.

The captain, having lost control of the ship, initially made no attempt to contact the nearby harbor to request assistance. Finally, he had to order evacuation when the ship grounded at 10:44 PM after an hour of listing and partly drifting. Meanwhile, the harbor authorities had been alerted by worried passengers, and vessels were sent to provide rescue assistance. The *Costa Concordia* is one of the largest passenger ships ever abandoned. The Italian Coast Guard testified that the final grounding of the ship was only a fortunate coincidence of winds and tides, which prevented the ship from sinking in deep water.

Some passengers jumped into the water to swim ashore. Others, ready to evacuate the vessel, were delayed by the multinational crew for up to 45 minutes, as they resisted initial attempts to lower the lifeboats. However, during a 6-hour evacuation, most passengers were brought ashore. The search for missing people continued for several months, with all but two ultimately being located. No lifeboat passenger evacuation drill had

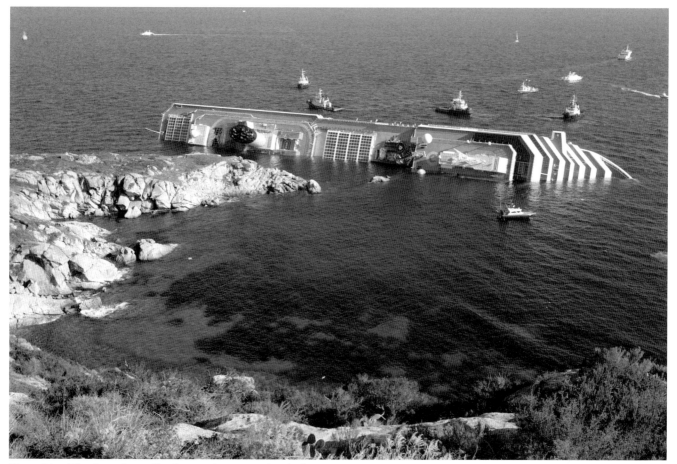

Figure 20.4. The *Costa Concordia* after running aground and taking on water very near the shore. The bottom of the sea was quite steep and the ship had a tendency to slide down into deeper water. The first strategy was to stop this slide by anchoring it to land. Used with permission from Scanpix.

taken place for the approximately 600 passengers who had just embarked.

According to investigators, the captain left the ship around 11:30 PM. In telephone calls from the Coast Guard, the captain was repeatedly ordered to return to the ship from his lifeboat and take charge of the ongoing passenger evacuation. One of these calls occurred as late as 1:46 AM.

The captain was arrested on multiple charges of manslaughter in connection with causing a shipwreck, failing to assist 300 passengers, and failing to be the last individual to leave the wreck. He was also charged with failing to describe to maritime authorities the scope of the disaster and with abandoning incapacitated passengers.

There were immediate fears of an ecological disaster, as the partially submerged wreck was in danger of slipping into much deeper water. This would increase the risk of a fuel oil leak and subsequent area pollution that would have devastated this popular tourist zone.

Following this incident, the Cruise Lines International Association, the European Cruise Council, and the Passenger Shipping Association adopted a new policy requiring all embarking passengers to participate in lifeboat passenger evacuation drills (muster drills) before departure. Previously, all passenger ships, including the Costa Concordia, were subject to two major International Maritime Organization requirements: 1) to per-

form muster drills with passengers within 24 hours after their embarkation; and 2) to launch lifeboats sufficient for the total number of persons aboard within 30 minutes from the time the abandon-ship signal is given. Passenger ships must be equipped with lifeboats for 125% of the ship's passenger and crew maximum capacity, among which at least 37% of that capacity must consist of lifeboats constructed of solid material as opposed to inflatable ones. Launching systems must enable the lowering of the lifeboats under 20° of list and 10° of pitch.

Errors: Shipwreck and Delayed Rescue
AL SALAM BOCCACCIO

This Egyptian drive-on/drive-off ferry, with 1,400 people and 220 vehicles on board, sank during a night in February 2006 in the Red Sea.[22] The ferry caught fire and capsized after only 10 minutes of fire suppression activity. One explanation for why the ship capsized was that the seawater used to fight the fire collected in the hull because the drainage pumps were not working. An emergency call via satellite was received in Scotland, from where it was passed on to the Egyptian authorities. Poor weather conditions hampered the search and rescue operation, and the first rescue vessels did not arrive until 10 hours after the incident. President Mubarak expressed concern that the absence of safety procedures contributed to the loss of 1,000 lives. Rescuers ultimately saved 314 passengers.[22]

Errors: High-Speed Vessel and Bad Weather Navigation

SLEIPNER

The cause of this shipwreck was a combination of navigational error, a high vessel speed, severe wind, and large waves.[23] The high-speed catamaran MS *Sleipner*, on its daily route along the Norwegian coast in November 1999, drifted off course and ran aground on a rock in bad weather and rough seas. The rock damaged the bottoms of both hulls extensively, and due to poor design, the water flooding the hulls could not be controlled. Strong winds soon pushed the vessel off the rock and it sank after half an hour with all on board ending up in the cold water. The crew lost control of the vessel's evacuation. Only one of the vessel's four life rafts was deployed and it landed upside down. Only four passengers managed to get inside the raft, and two managed to remain there until rescued. Many of the vessel's passengers reported difficulty putting on the life jackets. Some of life vests came loose in the water and some nearly strangled the wearer. A total of sixty-nine people were rescued and sixteen died. Hypothermia was a severe problem. These experiences illustrate the following principles.

- Evacuation routes should be adapted to conform with people's behavior in life-threatening situations. Evacuation information must identify alternate routes and be delivered in the local language and in English.
- Life rafts must be designed so they automatically turn right side up in the water. Life jackets must be easy to don, have sufficient buoyancy to keep the victim's head above water, and must also turn an unconscious person into the correct position with the face upward.
- The response time of 1 hour for rescue helicopters during off hours is too long in case of an emergency. Fifteen minutes or less would be ideal. Prioritization principles for managing hypothermic patients must be developed.

Errors: Intentional Incident – Fire on Board

SCANDINAVIAN STAR

One night in 1990, fires were started on board the cruise ship *Scandinavian Star* while traveling between Oslo, Norway, and Fredrikshavn, Denmark.[24] There were 99 crewmembers and 383 passengers on board. The first fire started at 2:00 AM when the ship reached open water. Bedclothes and carpets in a corridor were set on fire. The fire was discovered and extinguished, but a second fire started in another corridor. Within a few minutes, the fire and heavy smoke spread through the corridor and up to the next deck. Only a few of the fireproof doors were activated. A "mayday" message was sent at 2:24 AM. The position was incorrectly given as Norwegian territory, and consequently the Norwegian MRCC was appointed to lead the rescue work (the correct position was in Swedish territory). During the first 30 minutes, several helicopters, vessels, and rescue units were dispatched from Norway, Sweden, and Denmark.

At 2:50 AM, the first two ships arrived. By this time, the *Scandinavian Star* was burning heavily aft. An hour and a half after the fire began, the captain announced that he and the crew were in a lifeboat and that all people had left the ship, which was completely false. The crew was exhausted and lacked knowledge of the ship, its emergency equipment, and the emergency plan. In addition, they had not made any real attempt to control the fire. These factors contributed to the death of 159 people including a number of children. Sweden has an organization of specialized firefighters

(called smoke divers), trained to work in a toxic smoky environment, who are ready for deployment to burning ships, but these resources were not dispatched until later. The post-incident investigation estimated that these firefighters could have arrived 2 hours earlier if dispatched initially. Ultimately, only six people died from burns; the rest died of a combination of hypoxia, carbon monoxide poisoning, and hydrogen cyanide inhalation. It is probable that rescue coordinators could have saved many more lives had they sent the smoke divers immediately. Two-thirds of the fatalities were found in their cabins, one-fourth of them in the bathroom with a towel over their faces. One-third were found dead in the corridors, many of them near locked fire doors they were unable to open.

Preparation

In many incidents at sea, the majority of passengers have been saved, but in a number of the large disasters, most have died. As shown previously, faster and more effective rescue efforts have the potential to improve survival for many victims. In the initial response phase, the on-board crew needs to take responsibility for the rescue effort.

PLANNING

Sea transportation and rescue are tightly regulated areas in many aspects.[25] National authorities standardize the safety of ships, vessel traffic on open waterways, and rescue operations. In addition, the policies of international insurance companies such as Lloyds of London, affect maritime safety. National MRCCs manage emergencies and their planning is often rigorous and well structured. Of course, economic factors influence the availability of rescue resources, such as the number of helicopters and their response times.

EQUIPMENT

It is not unusual that a ship or ferry sinks during bad weather or in rough seas. Therefore, it is critical that safety and rescue equipment function effectively. In the cases referred to previously, the emergency equipment performed poorly. Mistakes were avoidable. Crew members could not launch lifeboats, life rafts turned upside down when deployed, and life jackets failed to automatically keep the heads of unconscious and hypothermic victims in an upright position to prevent drowning.

Rescue helicopters appropriately equipped and rapidly available are essential for saving people at sea. In the Estonia incident, the helicopters dispatched to the scene had inferior quality winches and rescuers lost potential survivors during the process of lifting them from the water. Several arriving helicopters could not participate at all in the rescue efforts for this reason. This disaster suggests that a revision of the guidelines governing the types and quality of resources used in such rescue operations is indicated.

TRAINING

An incident at sea often happens far from land and from emergency and rescue resources. This is why the ship's crew must fill the critical role of first responder during such events. This necessitates extensive training in managing different emergencies. In addition, the training with rescue equipment such as lifeboats and rafts should include experience using these resources under severe weather conditions. Participation by cruise ship passengers in emergency training or drills is equally important.

The use of young, inexperienced persons, such as those fulfilling their military service commitment, is not appropriate for emergency operations such as surface rescue at sea. In the Estonia incident, inexperienced individuals were assigned the demanding position of surface rescuers on Air Force helicopters. It was psychologically stressful for these young people to participate in the response to a deadly disaster, attempting to rescue victims in darkness, with poorly functioning equipment, while enduring extremely high waves.[23]

Scene Response

COMMAND

Effective rescue operations for an incident of this kind involve practically the entire chain of command, from the individual to the government level. All require training specific to their roles to manage the situation properly. Many sea disasters occur in international waters. The MRCC in charge of the rescue effort is normally determined by the rescue zone in which the vessel is located. A rescue mission must be well planned from both the tactical and organizational perspective. Examples include identifying the captain of the first suitable ship arriving at the site as the on-scene commander, and automatic dispatch of the appropriate units. The error of not immediately dispatching smoke divers to the site of the Scandinavian Star fire probably caused additional deaths and suggests commanders experienced lapses in judgment during a stressful situation.[24] Air traffic command and control is also essential when many rescue helicopters are in the air.

SAFETY

Safety precautions for response personnel and crew are a first priority during a rescue mission but may be in conflict with the sometimes extremely difficult conditions under which they must work. To minimize the risks, responders systematically review all safety factors under the category of "preparation," including planning, equipment, and training. In addition, emergency drills at the beginning of a voyage may potentially reduce the risk to passengers. Improving the safety of all involved also mandates the use of emergency equipment that is effective under all conditions, including rough seas.

COMMUNICATION

It may be difficult to communicate the status of passengers to relatives and the press in the initial phase of rescue operations because of the huge numbers of victims. The Al Salam Boccaccio incident is one example in which the delayed release of information regarding survivors created a public outcry; similar reactions have been reported in other incidents. It would be wise for the sea transport industry to have a well-prepared communication plan to reduce these problems.

ASSESSMENT

The initial assessments regarding the number of dead and injured in the previously referenced incidents contained a large degree of uncertainty.[20,22,24] The final assessments, however, were usually quite accurate. Notable exceptions include some Asian and African ferry incidents, where the number on board was not clearly determined. One seriously incorrect assessment was the message from the captain of Scandinavian Star that "all had abandoned the ship." In reality, more than 160 were still on board and this erroneous report may have contributed to the high death toll in the fire.

TRIAGE AND HYPOTHERMIA

Hypothermia may be a complicating factor that is not taken into account in common triage systems. In the aforementioned incidents, hypothermic victims were common. Hypothermia may make it difficult for rescue personnel to know who is truly dead and who is actually alive but profoundly hypothermic. After the Estonia incident, it was observed that the commonly used guidelines regarding survival times in water of different temperatures may be conservative estimates.[26] Young fit men with strong survival instincts seem to survive longer.[20] It is essential to account for these findings when deciding to terminate a search.

TREATMENT

Fire victims and passengers who have ingested or aspirated petroleum products, as in the Dona Paz incident, may need urgent treatment. Hypothermic victims must be handled cautiously (so as not to induce ventricular fibrillation), and should ideally be extricated (or hoisted, if a helicopter is involved) in a horizontal position. This is due to cold-induced diuresis and resultant hypovolemia that can cause hypotension if the patient is placed in the vertical position.

TRANSPORT

Helicopter transport to the nearest appropriate facility is indicated for severely ill patients, such as those suffering from burns, serious traumatic injuries, and profound hypothermia. One limiting factor in the rescue operation is the time helicopters can remain airborne, which is often approximately 3 hours, exclusive of reserve fuel. In practical terms, if it takes a helicopter 1 hour to arrive at the incident site and requires 1 hour or more to reach a medical facility, the time to accomplish the rescue mission at the site may be very limited. In these cases, the tactic may be to hoist people to a ship in the vicinity, and in this way, save as many as possible, as in the Estonia incident. This would, however, not be optimal for severely ill victims.

Rail Disasters

Incidence Data

During the nineteenth century, the number of train crashes that produced a significant number of fatalities was low, as train speed was limited. In the twentieth and twenty-first centuries, the speed and density of rail traffic increased. In many countries, however, railway infrastructure has not kept pace and has become alarmingly worn and overburdened. Despite extensive crash avoidance systems, severe railway events still occur around the world.[27] These crashes which are actually becoming more frequent, cause mass casualties to the extent that they can be classified as disasters (≥ 10 killed and/or ≥ 100 non-fatally injured). Throughout the last 100 years, the number of rail disasters, fatalities, and injured passengers has increased. This is particularly true during the last four decades (1970–2009) when 88% of all train disasters occurred in the world (Figure 20.5).[28] In 2010–2012 there were twenty-five disasters globally, compared with twenty-three during the three preceding years (2007–2009), indicating that the problem persists and may be increasing.[27] The number of fatalities per railway disaster has nevertheless decreased steadily throughout the years.[28]

Moreover, railway transportation facilities have become a preferred target for hostile acts. The system is vulnerable: it is open and accessible to all, generally without individual access controls or passenger identification, and utilized by large

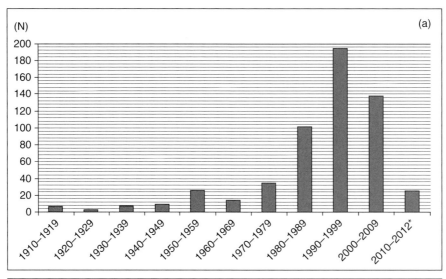

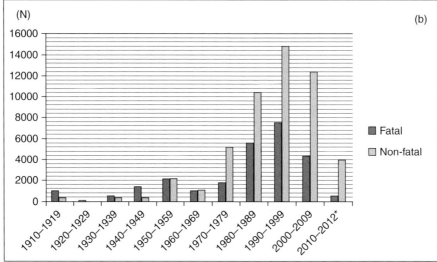

Figure 20.5. (a) Number of global rail disasters with ≥10 fatalities and/or ≥100 non-fatal injuries, 1910–2012; (b) Number of passengers killed and injured in rail disasters, 1910–2012. * Note that this time bracket only consists of 3 years. Data from: EMDAT: The OFDA/CRED International Disaster Database. www.em-dat.net. Université Catholique de Louvain, Brussels, Belgium.

numbers of people. The attempted terrorist attack on a passenger train in Canada in April 2013 is a recent example. The attacks in Tokyo in 1995, Madrid in 2004, London in 2005, Mumbai in 2006, and Russia, including events in 2007, 2009, and 2010, are examples of completed attacks that had enormous consequences. The evolution toward a considerable increase in number of victims injured by attacks on rail-bound traffic is also clear.[29]

Preparation

PRE-EVENT PLANNING

The trends indicate that emergency response organizations should plan for a severe rail incident since these have the potential to produce mass casualties. Further, the complex nature of responding to such events makes pre-event planning essential. This extends to the rail personnel and passengers. A well-prepared train crew is a factor that can affect the outcome. If passengers have not been provided with appropriate safety-critical information, they cannot be expected to know how to handle the situation.

EQUIPMENT

Rescue personnel are exposed to many different hazards when working at a train crash site. This makes the use of adequate PPE mandatory. Staff must also be provided with communication equipment that operates in tunnels and subways. In addition, it is important to investigate whether current rescue tools are effective against the rugged steel construction of today's trains. In a collision in Hamburg, Germany, passengers were trapped inside the railcars and needed extrication. This required the extensive use of cutting torches and rendered the rescue very difficult. In addition, rescue operations could not be properly initiated until the carriages had been securely stabilized, which consumed significant time.[30] Other incidents have demonstrated the difficulty in evacuating passengers due to factors such as a lack of roof hatches (when carriages have overturned) or due to carriage height. Therefore, it is important to test different solutions to facilitate victim rescue and minimize the evacuation time. Using ladders that allow responders to slide a victim down from a window on the stretcher is one effective solution. Another

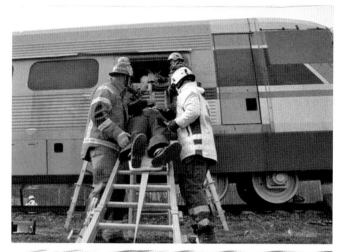

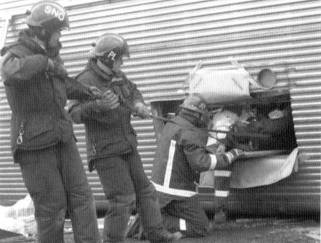

Figure 20.6. The use of ladders allows rescue personnel to slide the victims down from an elevated window (top picture). When a rail carriage has overturned, one effective solution to facilitate evacuation is creating access through the roof (bottom picture).

is to create access in the roof when carriages have overturned (see Figure 20.6).

TRAINING

It is important that rescue personnel receive education and training in tactics and techniques that minimize the delay in delivering medical care to injured passengers. Studies from train crashes have shown the importance of rapid extrication and evacuation of trapped casualties, as passengers have died from injuries that should not have been fatal.[30–32] In the Amagasaki crash in Japan, rescue personnel responding to the event had previously received training in confined-space medical techniques. This experience proved to be most useful. Without this training, the two victims who remained trapped in a railcar for up to 22 hours would probably have died.[33] Prehospital personnel also need training to identify and manage potential threats resulting from train incidents and learn how to manage the situation if the disaster results from a hostile act.

Pre-Incident

Investigators have proven that the "human factor," which denotes the tendency by individuals to misunderstand, miscal-

culate, or act inappropriately, has clearly contributed to several train crashes. The 1999 crash in Ladbroke Grove, UK, is one example where a train derailment was caused by an engineer failing to stop at a red signal.[34] Another example is the head-on collision between a freight train and a Metrolink commuter train in Los Angeles in 2008 when the freight train ran through a red signal. The train's engineer was distracted by sending text messages while on duty. The crash killed 25 passengers and injured 135.[35] A speed limit violation by engineers in the 2005 Amagasaki, Japan, crash caused the train to derail as it travelled along a curved section of track, killing 107 passengers and injuring another 549.[33] Miscalculations or infringements by automobile drivers at intersections where rail lines cross roadways are another common cause of crashes.[36]

Carriage and equipment failure was the reason for the 1998 train crash in Eschede, Germany, when the Intercity Express (ICE) traveling at 200 km/h derailed and collided with a bridge due to a wheel failure (Figure 20.7).[37] A similar example is the 2010 train crash in Skotterud, Norway, which resulted in the injury of forty passengers.[38] Non-user-friendly instruments, tools, and inadequate equipment design (driver safety systems) inside trains are other causes of crashes because these flaws increase the risk for human error.[39]

Physical environment factors can also be reasons for crashes or exacerbate the situation. The environment proved to be of great importance in the July 2013 high-speed crash just outside Santiago de Compostela, Spain. A passenger train derailed due to high speed (approximately 190 km/h) after entering a curve. Alongside the railway track was an aqueduct with a sharp edge that opened some coaches like a tin can, causing 79 deaths and approximately 140 injuries. Improved materials and performance of railway tracks have reduced the number of crashes resulting from such causes as climate, heat distortions of tracks or ice formations, and problems created by snow.[40–42] However, the rail disaster with the highest death count in history occurred in Sri Lanka in 2004, and was caused by the tsunami following the Indian Ocean Earthquake. More than 1,700 people were killed.[43] Crashes related to locations where railroad tracks cross roadways (level crossings) are a high priority issue. The number of European level crossing crashes between 1990 and 2009 has remained the same in relation to the number of passenger kilometers travelled, despite the fact that the existing level-crossings have been improved and the construction of new ones has been minimized. [36,44,45]

Within the socioeconomic environment, multiple factors are put into a larger context. Train crashes are seldom tied to a single causal factor, but could be the result of systematic failure.[34] Lack of a safety culture may be the effect of mismanagement, resulting in deficient train maintenance. This is speculated to have caused the train crashes in Buenos Aires, Argentina. In 2012, concerns related to possible brake failure were repeatedly dismissed. The negligence led to 51 fatalities and more than 700 injuries when a passenger train experienced brake failure and hit the buffers at Once Station (Figure 20.8). In 2013, a passenger train travelling in the morning rush hour was unable to stop and collided with an empty stationary train, killing 3 people and injuring more than 300.

Also, unfavorable company policies regarding work schedules may cause fatigue, stress, and low motivation and may contribute to crashes.[46] In this regard, experts have debated a wider causal perspective questioning the impact of privatization on railway safety. Nevertheless, there is no evidence that the 1994

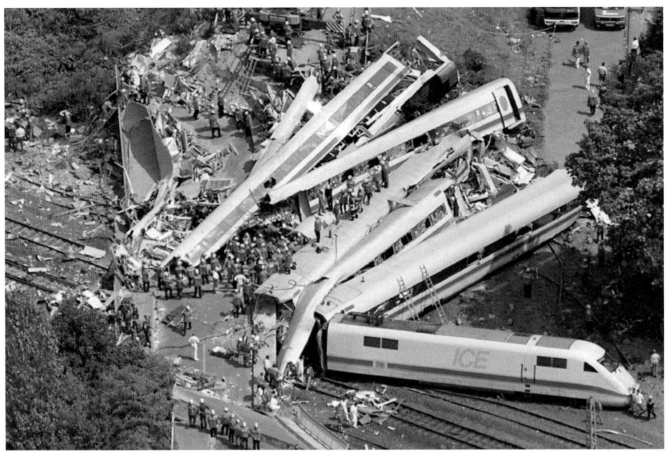

Figure 20.7. The Eschede, Germany, train crash is one of the world's worst high-speed train disasters. The carriages jack-knifed into each other during impact, claiming 101 lives and injuring 103 passengers. Used with permission from Scanpix.

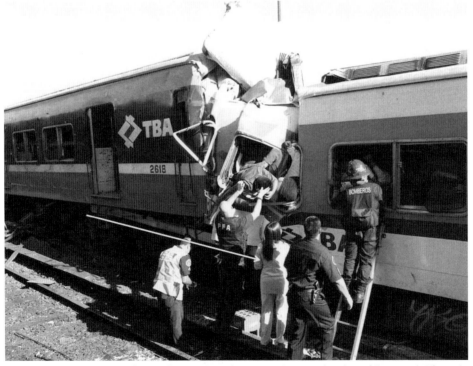

Figure 20.8. One carriage telescoped approximately 6 meters into another (see white arrow). The train crash killed fifty-one passengers in Buenos Aires, Argentina in 2012. The train ran into the buffers at Once Station when the brakes failed. Used with permission from Scanpix.

privatization in the UK or similar action in Japan in 1987 have increased the risk of train crashes.[47,48] In fact, work done by Elvik in 2006 found that deregulation was associated with improved rail safety.

Incident

In the crash phase of an event, the term "human factors" refers to the forceful thrusting of passengers around the interior of the carriage during impact and the subsequent injuries that occur. In a crash, energy will be transferred to the human body by the deceleration of the train. Modern trains run at increasingly high speeds, increasing the kinetic energy that must be absorbed. Passengers sustain injuries when train carriages deform or partially collapse and passengers are thrown as projectiles inside the carriages or are hit by flying objects such as luggage.

Vehicle/equipment factors refer to train carriage crashworthiness and interior design. The improvements in train construction and crashworthiness have been remarkable over the years. In the nineteenth century, carriages were made of wood and simply disintegrated in a collision. A French crash in 1933 demonstrates this reality. In thick fog, a locomotive struck a slow-moving wooden passenger express from behind and managed to run through almost its entire length, killing 230 people.[42] This phenomenon is called "telescoping" (Figure 20.9). Crashes during this time were also very often followed by fire. This resulted from various factors: steam locomotives providing a source of ignition (i.e., hot coals and sparks), the wooden construction and the presence of other combustible materials, the use of flammable paints and varnishes, and the use of gas lighting. Fortunately, train fires are not as common today and collisions and derailments are rarely followed by fire. Fires caused by malicious action are nevertheless a major and growing problem.[49]

Metal train carriages were introduced in the first part of the twentieth century and by the 1950s, had essentially replaced wooden carriages worldwide. The use of modern materials and construction, including steel-framed and aluminum-sided carriages, and the replacement of steam locomotives, has gradually reduced the risks of fire. However, the incidents at Ladbroke Grove, England, in 1999 and on the Kaprun Funicular Railway in Austria in 2000 have shown that, despite the implementation of rigorous safety measures, the risks have by no means been eliminated.[49] Metal carriages often minimize the telescoping problem but inadvertently create another dangerous phenomenon, "overriding" (Figure 20.9). As an example, three morning trains collided in Clapham, England, in 1988. One train overrode the other and crashed down on the passengers below, killing thirty-five people.[41] After this event, experts worked to develop new approaches to carriage design. Deformation zones were created using corrugated metal plates. These structures, which make the carriages hook together in the crash, were fitted to the ends of each rail carriage. These designs decreased the risk of vertical movement that could develop into overriding. One remaining serious collision phenomenon called "jack-knifing" or "lateral buckling" (Figure 20.9) was highlighted by the train crash in Germany in 1998 (Figure 20.7). On impact, the train carriages derailed and collided into each other's sides. The weak side walls collapsed inward.[37] One approach to countering this problem was making the couplings between carriages stronger and more stable to prevent the railcars from buckling either sideways or vertically.

Changes in the design of the train exterior continue to evolve in an effort to provide better passenger protection. This is seen

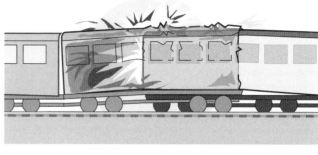

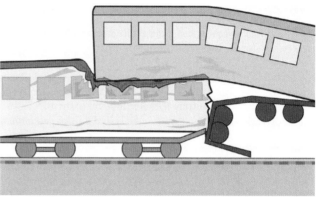

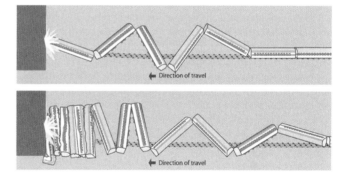

Figure 20.9. Different crash-phenomena: telescoping, overriding, and jack-knifing/lateral buckling. Illustrated by Gunilla Guldbrand.

in numerous articles published in the engineering literature.[50,51] These innovations have improved the crashworthiness of train carriages; however, even with such enhancements, the railcars cannot always withstand the higher energies produced in today's high-speed train crashes. The front carriages often take the brunt of the impact. Thus, sitting in the front carriages proves to be most dangerous; causing the most severe injuries and greatest number of fatalities.[30,32,52] In Washington during 2009, one train collided with another stopped ahead of it. Carriages telescoped over the rear car of the stationary train, killing 9 passengers and injuring approximately 80.[53] Moreover, some countries are still using older carriages, such as Argentina. In the crash in Buenos Aires, one carriage tore completely through another for several meters (telescoping), despite the low speed of 26 km/h. All fifty-one of the passengers killed were in the carriage that experienced telescoping, with additional surviving passengers trapped inside (see Figure 20.8). It can be expected that these crash phenomena will continue to a greater or lesser extent, depending on how fast new carriages are developed.

Relatively little research has been conducted concerning internal carriage design. Rail carriage seats are not equipped with seat belts; thus, passengers are thrown against various structures and into each other during a crash, sustaining significant injuries.[52,54,55]

Studies have also shown that passengers who travel in a rear-facing position have high rates of whiplash injuries.[52,54] In March 1994, a train with a speed of 85 km/h collided with the back of a stationary passenger train, north of Aarhus, Denmark. All of the resulting injuries were related to victims striking structural elements inside the carriages.[56] Passengers can even be thrown through the train windows and land beneath the carriage.[55] Seats or seat structures coming loose in a crash also cause injuries.[55,57] Ilkjær and Lind in a 2001 study also found that passengers received injuries from tables. Folding tables increased the risk of facial injuries significantly and tables located between chairs are a risk factor for thoraco-abdominal injuries. Similar findings were also identified by Forsberg et al. (in press). A collision in Placentia, California, in 2002 is another example. A freight train missed a signal and smashed head-on into a passenger train. Two people died from hitting the table in front of them.[58] Unlike airplanes, train carriages do not have sealable luggage hatches, which allows suitcases to fly around like missiles and cause injuries.[55–57,59–60]

The physical environment, such as bridges or steep embankments, can further aggravate the consequences of a crash. In 2007, a passenger train derailed in Cumbria, UK. All nine carriages left the track, and eight of them subsequently slid down the steep embankment injuring more than eighty passengers.[61] In 2011, a fatal collision on China's high-speed network killed 39 passengers and injured nearly 200. The situation was aggravated when four of the six carriages fell from a bridge.[62]

Formal demands and regulations belong to the socioeconomic environment factor and are important in the crash phase. For instance, if there is no law mandating seat belts in trains or formal requirement for safe storage of luggage, these considerations will not be reflected in the interior construction of railcars.

Post-Incident

When considering human factors in the post-crash phase, many individuals with varying responsibilities are present at a train incident scene. Their actions might improve or weaken both the rescue effort and the well-being of survivors. Besides the physical injuries, and perhaps irrespective of their severity, train crashes affect the whole person (psychological, social, and existential). Acute medical care and subsequent rehabilitation efforts must, therefore, incorporate these aspects. Depending on the circumstances, assistance from family, friends, fellow passengers, media coverage, and visiting the event site may be helpful for dealing with the traumatic event.[63] On the other hand, media coverage can also add to survivors' grief, causing a secondary victimization.[64]

The vehicle/equipment factors involve structural features that can facilitate or hinder a clear and effective evacuation. In an article published in 2005, Weyman et al. demonstrated that serious shortcomings in such functionality existed in the rail crash at Ladbroke Grove, including deficient emergency exits and evacuation equipment. Displaced luggage also increased the difficulties in evacuating passengers. Moreover, the design did not facilitate access through windows in overturned carriages. The doors, which were now located upwards, were impossible

for a single individual to open.[59] Braden stated that the interior design and the lack of roof hatches were the factors that most hampered evacuation. Additionally, evacuation can be impeded by narrow stairways, trapping survivors in upper compartments in double-decker carriages.[65]

Scene Response

COMMAND

Command and control at the scene of a rail incident with injured victims scattered throughout the large site is a challenge. Following the train collision in Eschede, the disaster site encompassed an area over 450 meters long, making it difficult to maintain control over the incident. As a consequence, medical teams had to act independently.[66] The 2004 terrorist attack in Madrid, resulting in 101 deaths and 1,500 injuries, involved four separate incident sites, illustrating the difficulty in obtaining a comprehensive view of the disaster.[67]

SAFETY

Rescue efforts adjacent to railway tracks expose response personnel to great risks. Electrical, kinetic, thermal, and chemical hazards are the most common dangers encountered by workers at a rail incident site. Some parts of trains are extremely hot and it is not uncommon for emergency personnel to receive burns during their rescue work. Power lines in the area may carry up to 25,000 volts of electricity. Maintaining a safe distance of 3 meters from live cable is recommended. It is necessary to wait until the power is disconnected and the cables are grounded.[68] From full speed, a train needs over 2 km to stop. Unless railway supervisors have given clearance, it may be very hazardous to approach the tracks. Bridges, tunnels, and narrow cuttings may further contribute to an unsafe environment on one or both sides of the track. Gaining access to the interior of carriages can be difficult, owing to their height and heavily reinforced construction. Use of ladders and the need to walk on sloped surfaces also contributes to the hazards. Concrete cable ducts are covered by small paving stones. Responders may fall when walking on these stones because they are often unstable. In addition, crossties are often covered in oil and can be slippery. Another danger is the moving blades of switch tracks because they can be operated remotely and could trap a foot without warning. Old trains still contain chemical substances that can be very toxic if ignited in a fire, and the huge array of chemicals that are transported as freight further complicates the issue.

In the Eschede crash, the carriages had a tendency to slide and it was difficult to lift the carriages without causing further damage.[66] Additionally, it is not always possible to use the metal cutters and other rescue equipment due to the high risk of igniting a fire. At the Amagasaki crash, gasoline leaked from vehicles in the garage struck by the train. This precluded the use of these devices and the rescue teams were forced to work with hand-operated tools.[33]

Another major safety issue is emergency evacuation. The stairways within double-decked carriages are small and often destroyed in a crash, trapping passengers on the upper deck. The sliding doors that serve as dividers between the vestibules and seating compartments are also problematic. The doors can jam on impact and prevent passengers from escaping.[59,69] At the Ladbroke Grove rail incident in 1999, passengers were trapped as a result of these flaws and subsequently died in the fire that followed the collision. What the Ladbroke Grove incident highlighted was how difficult it is to evacuate from an overturned

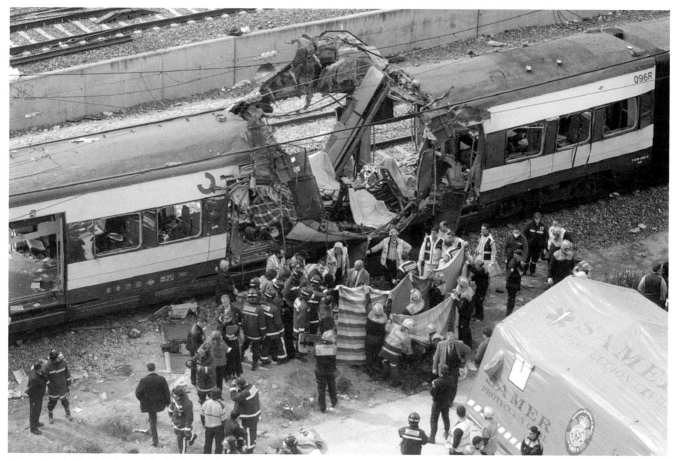

Figure 20.10. The 2004 attack in Madrid is the worst terrorist event in Spain's history. Ten bombs exploded in four different locations, killing 101 passengers and wounding more than 1,500. Ambulance services established a field hospital close to the railway track, placing themselves and the injured passengers in an area at risk for further bomb explosions.

rail carriage. The doors normally used for carriage access are too heavy for many passengers to open, if they can reach them at all in an overturned carriage. Seat cushions, suitcases, and clothes obstruct exit routes and make the evacuation even more difficult. The implementation of airplane-style luggage racks and installation of emergency escape routes would facilitate evacuation.

Lastly, terrorism has also become a hazard. At the 2004 Madrid bombings, the ambulance service established field hospitals close to the railway track, placing themselves and the victims in an area at risk for further bomb explosions (Figure 20.10). One of four backpacks containing unexploded bombs was brought to a police station. The bomb was discovered when someone called the telephone in the backpack. The phone was connected to the detonator via the alarm function; fortunately, the timer was incorrectly set to detonate the bomb 12 hours later than the others.[67]

COMMUNICATION

Communication problems are exacerbated when the incident occurs in a tunnel or a subway. This is a situation in which communication is particularly important. To facilitate communication and the rescue work on an incident site involving several carriages, the different railcars can be marked with numbers or letters using tape or spray paint.

ASSESSMENT

Making an initial assessment of the number and severity of injuries at the disaster site can be very difficult, especially if the incident is in a tunnel or a subway. Moreover, the rail transport industry lacks passenger lists, which makes it difficult to know how many individuals were on board a given train. Since it is quite challenging to estimate the number of fatalities or injured passengers trapped in the debris, experience from the Amagasaki train crash indicates that decisions regarding the withdrawal of rescue activities should be made carefully.[33]

TRIAGE

Performing triage in a cramped train carriage with loose luggage everywhere and victims often lying on top of each other can be extremely difficult, sometimes even impossible. The decision regarding the use of triage must therefore be adapted to each unique situation. In many rail disasters, emergency personnel lack experience using common medical triage protocols and perform triage poorly at the site.[33,66,70] In the 2004 Madrid bombings, 191 people were killed and more than 1,500 were injured. Reasons given for the absence of triage in Madrid were: "it was so obvious who had minor or severe injuries" and "we didn't have enough triage tags."[67] The Amagasaki train derailment, on the other hand, marked the first use of on-site mass casualty triage in a Japanese crisis. The quality of triage was high, and preventable deaths were few. Nevertheless, it was logistically impossible to assign green tags to all of the hundreds of victims with minor injuries.[33]

TREATMENT

In a rail crash, it is common that passengers become trapped by debris. At the crash in Amagasaki, the Japanese physician teams used confined space medical techniques when treating trapped survivors. It took almost 22 hours to extricate the last injured passengers. During that time, the doctors secured intravenous lines in tight spaces and administered fluids to prevent crush syndrome. Other advanced treatments performed at the site included endotracheal intubation, rapid fluid infusion, and needle decompression of tension pneumothoraces.[33] In cold climates and situations in which long evacuation times can arise due to transport over great distances, a reasonable approach might be to reject the goal of immediate evacuation and instead give treatment inside the carriages.

TRANSPORT

After a railway incident, it can be very difficult to even reach the crash site, much less to transport personnel and materials to the location and then evacuate the victims to hospitals. Railway crashes might happen far from roads, as was the case when two trains collided head-on due to a signal malfunction in Japan in 1991. The rural setting of the crash hampered rescue efforts. Forty-two passengers died and 614 were injured.[71] In 2005, a passenger train collided with a truck in Israel. The collision caused a multiple-scene mass-casualty incident in an area characterized by difficult access and a relatively long distance from trauma centers. The crash resulted in 289 injured passengers and 7 fatalities.[72] An attack in Russia using explosives devastated a train travelling from Moscow to St. Petersburg, killing more than twenty-five people. The explosion took place deep in the forest. Around thirty rescue vehicles were immobilized in the mud as they struggled over country roads to reach the wounded. Because the area was so remote, people from nearby towns arrived at the site hours before rescue workers.[73]

Road Motor Vehicle Disasters

Comprehensive data on highway disasters may be more difficult to find than corresponding data on more regulated sectors such as air, sea, and rail. This is not surprising, considering that even an event with a death toll of 50–100 could be considered small within the overall context of the worldwide total of at least 1.2 to 1.3 million deaths annually in motor vehicle crashes. It might also be possible that a major incident could be missed in countries with immature systems for collecting road injury data.

Injury Incidents: Historical Perspective

The number of fatal motor vehicle incidents and the number of casualties associated with them varies considerably. There are many incidents with approximately 25 dead, fewer with approximately 50 dead, and incidents with 100 or more dead do occur but are quite rare. A majority of the events involve buses. Seven road "disasters" with more than 100 killed were reported from 1970 through 2012. In three of these cases (Afghanistan, Spain, and Nigeria), a gasoline tanker collision and subsequent fire were the factors responsible for the deaths of 120–2,000 people. The other cases (106–127 killed) involved a bridge collapse (Nepal), a bus that crashed into a bridge (Kenya), and a bus that drove

into an irrigation canal (Egypt). The worst incident occurred in the Salang tunnel in Afghanistan during the Soviet occupation in 1988. Although details remain obscure, this event is probably the deadliest tunnel fire in history. One hypothesis regarding the incident mechanism is that a fuel tanker crashed into an ammunition truck in a Red Army convoy. The casualty figure is uncertain and varies between 1,000 and 2,000 killed, most of them Afghan civilians. Many died from exposure to toxic gases and smoke. Lethal tunnel fires have also occurred in the Alps. In 1999, some thirty-nine people died when a truck caught fire in the middle of the 12-km Mont Blanc tunnel. The fire reached an estimated temperature of 1300°C, and 53 hours elapsed before it was finally extinguished.[74]

The focus of this section will be on the most probable type of traffic mass-casualty event that rescue forces will encounter, that is, a bus or coach crash. As these crashes often occur in rural or remote areas, their management is challenging for ambulance and rescue organizations.[75] The majority of bus incidents are unintentional; however, intentional attacks, such as the suicide bombings experienced in Israel beginning in the 2000s, and the London bombings in 2005, have highlighted the problem of hostile acts directed against public transportation systems.[6]

To simplify terminology, the word "bus" will be used to represent all types of motor vehicles carrying more than nine people. This term includes the following types of buses: commuter, school, intercity, motor, and tour coaches.

Typical Injury Incidents: Current Perspective

Crashes are the most common incidents affecting buses, but these vehicles may also catch fire, either as a consequence of a collision or spontaneously. These fires can be deadly if passengers are unable to evacuate the bus quickly.

One of the worst bus incidents in the United States with respect to the number killed was the 1988 Carrollton bus disaster, when a tour bus caught fire after a collision and twenty-seven people died.[76] Another crash resulting in many deaths occurred in rural Finland in 2004 when a frontal collision between a heavily loaded tractor trailer and a tour bus claimed twenty-three lives. Many crashes with more than ten fatalities each have been reported from Asia, Africa, South and Central America, and Europe. However, most originate in countries such as Albania, China, India, Iran, Mexico, Nigeria, and Thailand. Most of them have been single vehicle crashes, with a bus plunging into a ravine or down from a bridge. In a 1976 Swedish incident, a tour bus on a shopping tour caught fire due to overheated brakes. The evacuation was a delayed as passengers attempted to collect personal belongings in the bus. The fire and smoke were so intense that fifteen people died within minutes.

Buses Using Compressed Natural Gas (CNG)

Buses powered by CNG may introduce new risks. These buses are becoming popular for use in urban locations due to their perception as environmentally friendly vehicles. Crashes investigated by the Accident Investigation Boards in the Netherlands and Sweden have exposed fire risks caused by low resistance to crash forces in the gas system and limited effectiveness of the automatic fire suppression system. In addition, a secondary fire risk exists when the safety valves of gas tubes on the roof open and the venting gas catches fire and burns for up to 20 minutes with a 10–15 meter flame. New tactics for handling these incidents are needed.

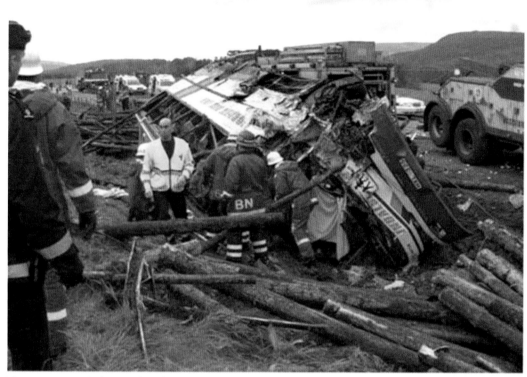

Figure 20.11. A timber truck with trailer suffered a front tire blow out and became so difficult to steer that it crashed into an oncoming school bus in rural northern Sweden in 2001. Timber entered the bus and made the rescue effort extremely difficult. Six of the forty-two involved died. Used with permission from Sundsvalls tidning.

Seat belts are mandatory on buses manufactured after 2005 in the European Union. The impact of this change remains difficult to estimate, in part because the presence of seatbelts does not necessarily imply they will be used. Nonetheless, the combined data from actual crashes and simulations of typical single vehicle rollover events indicate that the potential for reducing moderate to severe injuries is approximately 50% with lap belts only and 80% with three-point restraints.[77]

Single bus crashes in Sweden are characterized by several common elements: 1) they involve intercity and tour buses; 2) events occur during winter, in rural areas under windy conditions; and 3) the buses finally come to rest after a 90° rollover to the right, with the door side down and the doors blocked. Arriving ambulance and rescue personnel often discover numerous injured people lying on top of each other inside the bus, as few passengers use their seat belts. Responders often have difficulty managing the scene. Fatalities typically result from two mechanisms of injury: victims are ejected through the large windows and crushed under the side of the bus as it rolls over; and passengers are crushed between the roof and seat back as the bus overturns and the roof collapses. Extrication of victims is complicated and requires a rapid response and the correct equipment. Research, including wind tunnel tests, has shown that high-profile buses can blow off the road. Ten such cases have been reported from Sweden.[78] Although this is especially true in windy winter conditions, simulation studies have also shown that on a dry road, a bus may deviate 1 meter or more sideways in wind gusts.

As the Swedish Accident Investigation Board has repeatedly concluded, these crashes illustrate the need for improved tac-tics, methods, and rescue equipment. Responders must be better prepared to manage challenging crash scenes. Examples of such difficult scenarios include an incident involving a frontal collision between a timber truck and a school bus (Figure 20.11), or a Finnish crash killing twenty-three people. In this second event, the driver of a tractor trailer lost control of the vehicle and collided with a tour bus on a cold winter night, on a rural road, filling it with paper bales weighting 800 kg.

Fires can result from fuel spills in connection with a crash, but most fires originate in the engine compartment, wheel housing, or from failed electrical and hydraulic components. Tests have shown that up to fifty-two passengers can evacuate a double-decker bus in 1 minute. This rate of egress is usually sufficient to safely evacuate a vehicle on fire in most cases. A disabled person, an individual with a baby carriage, or the accumulation of too many personal belongings in the passenger compartment can, however, delay the process significantly. Vehicle fires in buses or minibuses are one major cause of multi-fatality road incidents.

Bus incidents that illustrate some of the factors in the Haddon Matrix are discussed next.

Errors: Human, Vehicle, and Regulation Factors

The Carrollton bus disaster in the United States incorporates multiple causative factors: a drunk driver, vehicle construction that enhanced the potential for fire, and a flaw in federal safety regulations.[74] The coach involved in this disaster was originally designated as a school bus with chassis construction regulated by older federal standards. Nine days after chassis assembly began, the federal government issued new regulations; however, buses already under construction were exempt and the vehicle was not

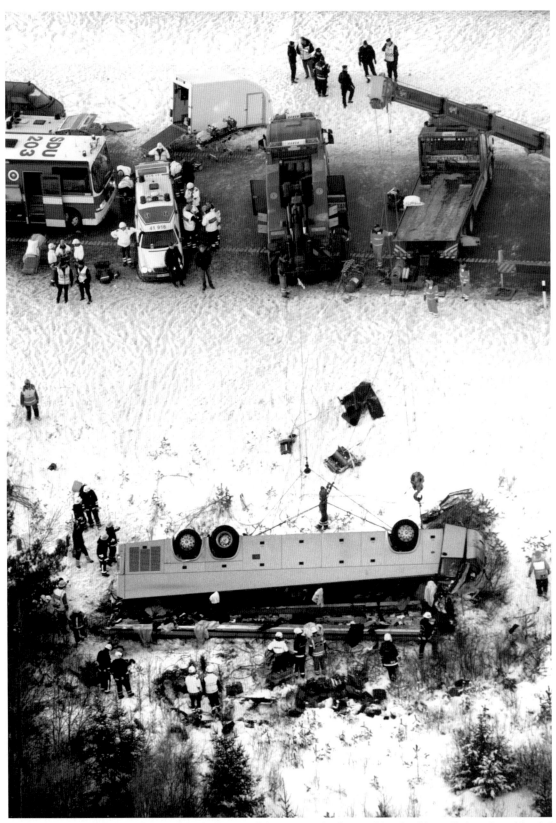

Figure 20.12. This tour bus drove off the highway and down an embankment, hit a boulder, rolled 180°, and landed on the roof that subsequently collapsed. Nine passengers died, but only two had lethal injuries. Six were jammed between the roof and interior structures (usually a seat back), and suffocated due to immobilization of the chest. It took 3.5 hours to extricate the surviving passengers. Used with permission from Scanpix.

upgraded to the better standards. These new standards mandated better fuel tank guard frames, emergency exits, and several other features.

This bus was eventually used by a church youth group. At 11:00 PM, the bus with sixty-six passengers on board was hit almost head-on by a pick-up truck at high speed, driven by an intoxicated driver moving in the wrong direction on the road. The impact fractured the bus's suspension and drove pieces into the unprotected fuel tank. Fuel immediately leaked out and quickly caught fire. The fire spread into the bus and thick noxious smoke filled the passenger compartment. The front door jammed shut in the crash and fire blocked the path forward. All tried to evacuate through the single rear emergency door because victims could not open the windows or break them. A beverage cooler in the aisle contributed to problems with evacuation. The congestion of passengers at the rear emergency door also delayed egress from the vehicle. After approximately 4 minutes, the entire bus was on fire. Twenty-seven people died in the fire and thirty-four were injured, ten of whom suffered severe burns. All suffered emotional trauma and survivor guilt syndrome. This bus had no window emergency exits or roof exits, as newer commercial and school buses have. If the bus had been classified for non-school usage, the applicable standards would have required more emergency exits.

Errors: Human and Rescue Factors

In the winter of 2005, a previously healthy bus driver traveling at approximately 100 km/h suffered a short absence seizure while behind the wheel. As a consequence, the bus veered off the road and down an embankment, struck a large boulder, flipped over, and landed upside down (Figure 20.12). The roof collapsed and all the windows broke. The unrestrained passengers (59%) careened around the inside of the bus and a number of belted and unbelted victims became trapped between the roof and interior structures, mostly the seat backs. Extricating the passengers was extremely difficult and neither the rescue nor ambulance personnel had the training and equipment necessary for an optimal effort. Traditional "heavy rescue" training was of little use in this situation, as even small degrees of carriage movement caused increased or decreased pressure on trapped victims. The ambulance crews working in the overturned bus had significant difficulties extricating people in the confined space. In addition, personnel had to evacuate the bus each time the rescue service tried to lift or move the bus. It took 3.5 hours to remove all survivors from the bus wreck, exposing victims to cold temperatures for a very long time. The last extricated living victim had a core temperature of 32°C when arriving at the hospital, and she later died.

Autopsies performed on the nine dead passengers revealed important findings. Only two of the nine victims had clearly lethal injuries. The remaining seven survived the initial crash. The forensic pathologist determined the subsequent cause of death was suffocation, caused by immobilization of the chest wall in six of the seven with estimated survival times to be from 10 minutes to more than 1 hour. At least four victims could have been salvaged if extrication had proceeded more expeditiously (within 0.5 hours). It was not possible to determine whether the lethal compressing force resulted from deformations associated with the crash itself or from the subsequent rescue efforts.

The Swedish Accident Investigation Board recommended the following actions.

- The National Road Administration should install guardrails preventing vehicles from driving off the road and down steep embankments.
- The National Road Administration should advocate for improvement in the European Union's safety standard for bus roof deformation in cases of a rollover. (Author's comment: The current standard with which manufacturers must comply is that the passenger space should not be compromised when a stationary bus is tipped over sideways from a height of 80 cm. As it must be quite rare for a stationary bus to roll over, the test hardly reflects real highway conditions. This crash demonstrated quite clearly how easily the roof collapses when a longitudinal force is applied.)
- The Swedish Rescue Service Agency should improve its tactics, methods, and equipment for handling this type of bus crash.

Errors: Vehicle and Environmental Factors

In 2001, in windy winter conditions and with a light snowfall, an intercity bus emerged from a woodland area into an open field at a speed of approximately 90 km/h. The driver states, "an invisible hand forced the bus to the right." The vehicle ran over and became entangled with a pre-bridge guardrail.[78] The left front wheel followed the guardrail to the middle of the bridge before the bus tipped over and landed as "a bridge" over the creek. Twelve of thirty-four people on board were unconscious after the crash. This crash was linked to the wind sensitivity of high-profile buses by using an algorithm developed from wind tunnel tests. The wind was blowing at a steady 13 m/s with 21 m/s wind gusts.

Errors: Environmental Road Factor

The 2012 Sierre Tunnel bus crash in Switzerland occurred when a Belgian bus collided with a concrete wall returning from a skiing resort, carrying fifty-two people.[79] Twenty-eight people were killed: both drivers, four teachers, and twenty-two of the forty-six children aged 10 to 12. This was Switzerland's second-worst road crash in history and the country's worst in a motorway tunnel.

The bus veered slightly from the normal roadway and collided with a perpendicular part of a concrete wall at the end of an emergency turnout area (Figure 20.13). The front of the bus was severely damaged, initially preventing survivors from evacuating. Emergency personnel had to break the side and rear windows of the coach to gain access to the trapped passengers. Rescuers had a difficult task removing dead and injured children from the wreckage. Eight air ambulances and a dozen road ambulances were used to transport victims to several hospitals.

Post-crash investigations found that the driver was not intoxicated with alcohol, did not suffer a heart attack or other sudden illness, and was not exceeding the 100 km/h speed limit. Police reported that the bus was a modern and well-maintained vehicle, and that the children had all been wearing seat belts.

The design of the turnout area, which ended abruptly in a concrete wall, caused the terrible outcome. Such a design would probably not pass a decent road safety review in any country with an audit system. This crash was similar to a 1988 event in Norway, when a Swedish bus carrying school children crashed into a concrete barrier at the exit of a long and very steep tunnel after brake failure. Seventeen passengers were killed in that crash.

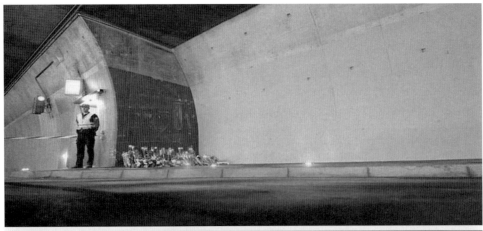

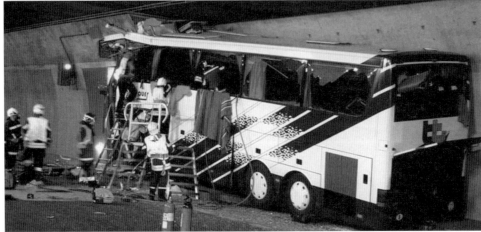

Figure 20.13. The flawed design of the emergency exit in the tunnel, with a concrete wall perpendicular to the driving direction, caused the abrupt stop and severe impact to the front end of the bus. Used with permission from Scanpix.

Preparation

PLANNING

A well-developed plan for a major traffic injury event is needed. Problems may arise, however, when individuals believe a plan is in place but have not examined its contents (the Swedish experience). As these crashes usually occur during winter, equipment to protect victims from hypothermia must be included. Incorporating these assets in the plan avoids delays in deployment of appropriate resources.

EQUIPMENT

Equipment for heavy rescue is needed, but is not always available to smaller rescue organizations in rural areas. Procuring equipment that can quickly lift an overturned bus that has crushed victims underneath is a priority. A 2-year development project in Sweden on the management of crashes with buses overturned 90° or more has come to a number of conclusions.

■ A bus built with stable steel bodywork may be lifted by hydraulic cylinders at the corners of the emergency roof hatches within 3 minutes (Figure 20.14).
■ A bus built from aluminum cannot be lifted by the roof hatches (too weak), but may be lifted with short hydraulic cylinders against the lateral longitudinal beams, as long as the contact points are not too narrow.

■ Two airbags can be used to lift both types of buses, but the lifting time will be more than three times as long as with the hydraulic cylinders.
■ For rescue efforts inside the bus, low-profile equipment is preferred. A spine board can be difficult to maneuver.
■ A completely overturned bus on its roof may be managed by carefully (with support from large airbags) turning it back on its side if possible. Then it will be much easier to manage the evacuation.

TRAINING

During development of the bus rescue program, standardized extrication tests were created using a realistic case scenario involving twenty-two non-ambulatory injured passengers (eight priority-1 cases and fourteen priority-2 cases). In the first test, the extrication time averaged between 40 and 50 minutes. After a formal training program, the same rescue personnel successfully evacuated all victims within 9.5 minutes. New skills learned by the responders included the critical action of rapidly cutting an extra opening in the roof (requiring <2 minutes). This is just one example of the impact that standardized training has on performance and may give an indication of the potential for improvement with effective instruction.

Fig 10 D4

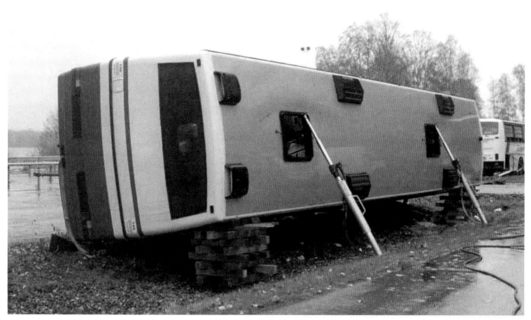

Figure 20.14. If people are trapped under a bus constructed of steel, it can be quickly lifted with extended hydraulic cylinders in the corners of roof hatches or with two airbags.

Scene Response

COMMAND

In motor vehicle incidents, the area of the crash site is usually small. The officers from the ambulance, rescue, and police forces can easily communicate with everyone from a command post established on, or near, the highway. It is an advantage if the personnel from the ambulance and rescue teams act in close cooperation to facilitate extrication of the injured.

SAFETY

Ensuring the safety of rescue personnel from the threat of post-event fires, structural collapse, and oncoming traffic is important. The safety of survivors is a constant concern, especially if they are trapped under or inside the bus. In these situations, a conflict may exist between rescuer safety and providing rapid extrication of victims.

COMMUNICATION

As with command, problems with communication are generally minimal. The most significant concern is the availability of communication from crash sites in remote areas to dispatch centers, hospitals, and higher levels of command.

ASSESSMENT

In developed countries, the potential for death or injury from a motor vehicle incident is usually limited to the estimated maximum number of passengers in the actual vehicles. Accurately estimating the number of injured passengers in highway crashes is generally easier than in other types of transportation-related events.

TRIAGE

In reality, triage prior to extrication has seldom been performed at an incident site. There may be several reasons for this:

it is "forgotten"; it is deemed unnecessary as sufficient ambulance personnel are on-scene; or responders believe the best way to extricate victims is to remove them in the order they are found. Many professionals advocate this latter strategy, arguing that it is the fastest and most effective method. In addition, they believe that for some situations, it might be the only method. To address this controversy, a Swedish study evaluated both strategies (triage vs. extrication in the order found) using a standardized injury model characterized by eight priority-1 cases and fourteen priority-2 cases. (All priority-3 cases are capable of walking out by themselves according to MIMMS triage). Given that a victim's deterioration is related to the number of minutes the person remains trapped in the bus, the total number of person-minutes was used as the outcome variable. Investigators compared extrication time for the triage group (removing priority-1 patients first and priority-2 thereafter) to those extricated in order they were found. The researchers found that evacuation time for priority-1 patients, when using the triage strategy, was 20 person-minutes shorter than when using the alternate method. Extrication time for the priority-2 victims, however, was 150 person-minutes longer in the triage group than for those extricated using the alternate strategy. These results raise additional questions. It is possible that priority-2 cases may deteriorate to a priority-1 status as a result of the additional delay. One compromise would be to evacuate in order of priority, but if a priority-2 victim obstructs the evacuation process, that victim should be removed first.

TREATMENT AND TRANSPORTATION

In a typical single vehicle crash, head and upper-extremity injuries are the most common, followed by chest and abdominal injuries. Neck injuries are rare in single crashes but occur frequently (~50%) in multi-vehicle collisions. In a frontal impact crash, the typical movement of passengers regardless of restraint

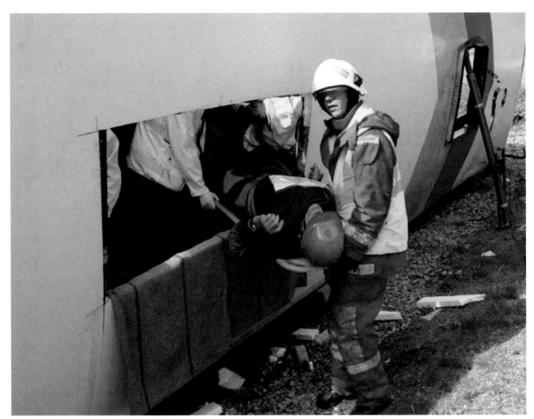

Figure 20.15. Cutting an opening in the roof, which is feasible in 2 minutes with a circular saw, facilitates evacuation. This intervention permits ambulance personnel to effectively work in the passenger compartment and to evacuate victims using the most appropriate exit pathways.

status is forward, head first, into the seat back in front of them resulting in extension of the neck. In a rear impact collision, especially in a bus with low seat backs, nearly all passengers would suffer neck hyperextension and subsequent painful injuries. People may also be wedged under seats, or found in difficult positions in a restricted space. In these situations, a simple cloth lift technique may be fastest and safest. Some of the trapped victims may require treatment on-site; confined-space medicine techniques would be beneficial.

In a typical bus crash, the vehicle is usually found on its side after a 90° roll to the right. An effective rescue approach is to cut openings in the roof, providing extra evacuation routes (Figure 20.15). The optimal responder configuration is four ambulance personnel in the front half of the bus and four in the rear half. This permits each group to evacuate victims by using separate routes, avoiding interference with each other. Evacuation through existing roof hatches is possible, but these openings are so narrow (50 × 80 cm) on many buses, that it is difficult to maneuver a spine board and patient out through these emergency exits.

RECOMMENDATIONS FOR FURTHER RESEARCH

Air Disasters

1. Mistakes, misunderstandings, and management errors continue to cause aircraft crashes, as well as failures in the human–machine interface. Behavioral scientists and others must address these problems and find ways to further minimize their occurrence. A potential solution might be implementation of an anonymous incident reporting system to help identify risk factors, such as the system now implemented for European civil aviation by a European Union directive. The aim of these anonymous reports is to find system shortcomings, not to punish individuals. A system that shares some of these features is also used in the United States. Further research on this promising concept is indicated.

2. The frequent post-crash fires remain a challenge. Increasing utilization of carbon fiber structures within airframes that is now underway in the aircraft industry will make these parts more fire-resistant than the magnesium–aluminum alloy currently in use. When these carbon structures do catch fire, however, they produce very toxic fumes. Further research is needed to develop other non-flammable materials. As toxic smoke kills most people in aircraft fires, new strategies are needed to improve passenger survival. Potential solutions include supporting them with oxygen (an aircraft carries significant amounts of emergency oxygen), or through use of smoke hoods, as the Manchester crash investigators recommended.[16] Finding solutions to these problems remains a challenge for scientists and engineers.

3. The use of rear-facing seats would probably distribute crash impact forces more favorably, but scientific evidence from commercial aviation is scarce. In contrast, this seating configuration is used widely in space aviation to distribute forces.

4. After the British Broadcasting Company aired some concerning programs in 2006 on aircraft crew's alcohol consumption,

the aviation industry examined the issue of substance abuse by their employees more closely. Some companies have introduced random testing programs. The effectiveness of these programs, as well as compulsory testing of all personnel, requires careful evaluation.

Sea Disasters

1. The basic construction flaw with drive-on, drive-off ferries must be resolved, with respect to both reducing the risk of water intake through the bow and stern openings and reducing the movement of large water masses on the vehicle deck should water intrusion occur.
2. Better measures are needed to mitigate the threat of fires, including implementation of fire prevention and suppression strategies and interventions that reduce injury. Automatic sprinkler systems and other measures aimed at reducing and extinguishing fires are necessary and should be required on all vessels.[25] Because most deaths result from exposure to toxic smoke, it is critical to develop methods that will deliver breathable air to passengers and protect them from inhaling toxic fumes.
3. Lifeboats, life rafts, and life jackets (even those placed on modern vessels) have functioned poorly in rough seas, which is the typical condition when vessels are wrecked. Problems have also plagued helicopter winches. These experiences suggest more research and development is needed to ensure this equipment works appropriately.

RAIL DISASTERS

1. Current knowledge about rail incidents is insufficient. To create a significant factual basis for use in further research and improvements, it is necessary to collect data and experiences from rail incidents in a structured international database.
2. Despite extensive crash avoidance systems, train crashes continue to be highly relevant today. Interior structures, such as tables, seats, internal walls, and glass have a large impact on the injury panorama, as do luggage and unbelted passengers. There is still insufficient emphasis on the reduction of passengers' injuries related to these factors. More research is therefore needed to investigate carriage interior design and its injury-inducing effect.
3. Studies from rail crashes show that passengers die as a consequence of non-lethal injuries due to delays in evacuation. Therefore, the need to ease evacuation routes through intelligent design applications is obvious. Further research and development concerning tactics, techniques, and equipment are also needed.
4. Improvement of level crossings should be a high-priority issue, since collision with vehicles at level crossings is a common cause for injury events.
5. There are some shortcomings in company policies and existing safety rules within the train sector. For example, legal mandates are lacking that: require seatbelts for train travel; make formal demands on the design of train interiors (except as regards fire safety); and require more secure stowage of luggage. It remains unclear why such safety flaws persist and what distinguishes the rail sector from the aviation and automotive industries in terms of safety. This should be explored further.

6. Recent history has shown that the railway sector is vulnerable to hostile acts. Therefore, it is critical to identify measures that reduce the rail transport system's vulnerability. This could be done by reducing opportunities to launch an attack, minimizing the consequences of an attack, and facilitating the discovery of additional unexploded devices. Lastly, training programs that assist responders to better manage a rescue operation involving terrorist attacks with explosives and chemical agents is a priority.

Motor Vehicle Disasters

1. The stability problems, especially of high-profile buses with engine and cargo compartments in the rear, should be highlighted. This configuration results in a center of gravity displaced to the vehicle's rear with relatively less weight on the front wheels. These buses are extremely wind sensitive and their speed should be restricted in windy weather. The development of monitoring devices that can warn drivers of potentially dangerous wind gusts would improve bus safety.
2. The effectiveness of two- and three-point seat belts should be established and optimized, as well as the most beneficial type of locking mechanism. If such data were available, this information could facilitate legislation and subsequent production of such devices. In addition to regulatory solutions, studies of human behavior to determine how to achieve compliance with seat belt use in buses would be beneficial.
3. In case of bus bombings, a strategy to divert the shock wave away from passengers requires investigation. It might be presumed that an explosion in the upper compartment of a double-decker vehicle may be less damaging than one in the lower compartment (supported by the experience from the Madrid train bombing referred to previously).
4. Bus fires remain a persistent and serious threat. Fire indicators and automatic extinguishers in the engine compartment have the potential to substantially mitigate this danger, but so far, it has been difficult to enforce installation of these devices. Better bus construction to prevent fuel spills in case of a crash, such as installing crash safe fuel tanks similar to those in helicopters, would be a substantial improvement and justifies further investigation.
5. Rescue techniques and equipment require further improvements that will permit responders to manage incidents more rapidly and effectively when buses have landed upside down. Vehicles constructed with emergency exits and entry openings for emergency personnel would also minimize the time to rescue passengers. The management of incidents involving CNG-powered buses could also be improved by additional investigation. All these issues need further refinement through more research and development.

Common Challenges: All Modes of Transportation

Every method of transportation has its own specific problems; however, it seems all modes are at a growing risk from terrorist attacks. Suicide bombing has invalidated traditional security strategies. The approach to addressing this problem has been fundamentally different within the airline industry compared with other modes of transportation. Extensive and intrusive control of airline passengers is accepted in a way that probably would be questioned in other transport modes. It is also extremely expensive, not only with respect to direct costs, but also the cost of time air travelers lose waiting in the airport security lines. Therefore, this approach would be very difficult, if not impossible, to implement on public ground transport systems such as a subway in a major city used by millions of people every day. The London and Madrid bombings are examples of the disastrous impact terrorist attacks can have on commuter trains. The number of lost lives and injuries generated may be greater than from an attack against an aircraft (excluding the unusual attack on September 11, 2001, in the United States). New solutions to this problem must be identified such as: 1) strategies that reduce the opportunity to place bombs in critical locations; and 2) new methods to mitigate the impact of an explosion in case of detonation.

A second problem shared by all members of the transportation industry is the issue of alcohol and/or drug intoxication involving those who drive or pilot the various vehicles, vessels, and aircraft. It is well known that those in the transportation industry represent a group at risk for addictive behavior. Some companies have instituted random drug and alcohol testing programs, but verification is needed as to whether these interventions will be sufficient to improve safety or whether mandatory testing of all personnel is required.

A final common problem is that transportation disasters occur relatively infrequently, making it difficult to study them. This situation could be substantially improved if the world's experience with such disasters were available for investigation. This suggests a potential solution: incorporating the global experience with these events into a common, well-structured database. The existence of this repository could serve as a basis for significant future research.

Acknowledgment

Professor Ulf Björnstig acknowledges and appreciates the general contributions to this chapter and specific authorship of the section on rail disasters by Rebecca Forsberg, Ph.D., RN, and BA in Peace and Conflict Studies.

REFERENCES

1. World Disasters Report 2003. International Federation of Red Cross and Red Crescent Socieities, Geneva, 2003. https://www.ifrc.org/Global/Publications/disasters/WDR/43800-WDR2003_En.pdf (Accessed August 26, 2015).

2. Injury: A leading cause of the global burden of disease. World Health Organization, Geneva, 1999. http://apps.who.int/iris/bitstream/10665/66160/1/WHO_HSC_PVI_99.11.pdf (Accessed August 26, 2015).

3. Fatal Accident Reporting System. 2007. www.fars.nhtsa.dot.gov (Accessed July 15, 2007).

4. Haddon W. A logical framework for categorizing highway safety phenomena and activity. *J Trauma* 1972; 12: 193–207.

5. Advanced Life Support Group. *Major Incident Medical Management and Support.* 4th ed. Bristol, British Medical Journal Publishing Group, 2000.

6. Levinson J, Granot H. *Transportation Disaster Response.* 1st ed. San Diego, CA, Academic Press, 2002.

7. Accident database. http://www.airdisaster.com/cgi-bin/database.cgi (Accessed July 15, 2007).

8. List of disasters. http://www.en.wikipedia.org/wiki/List_of_disasters (Accessed June 23, 2013).

9. Aviation Safety Network. www.aviation-safety.net/database (Accessed June 26, 2013).

10. Final report on the accident on June 1, 2009 to the Airbus A330–203 Air France Flight 447. Bureau d'Enquêtes et d'Analyses pour la sécurité de l'aviation civile; Government of France, 2012. http://www.bea.aero/en/enquetes/flight.af.447/rapport.final.en.php (Accessed August 28, 2015).

11. Wikipedia. September 11, 2001 attacks. http://en.wikipedia.org/wiki/September_11_2001_attacks (Accessed June 23, 2013).

12. NTSB. Aviation, accident database. http://www.ntsb.gov/aviation/aviation.htm (Accessed July 15, 2007).

13. Aviation Safety Network. Amsterdam. http://aviation-safety.net/database/record.php?id=20090225–0 (Accessed June 23, 2013).

14. SHK. Final report: ACCIDENT INVOLVED AIRCRAFT BOEING MD-87, registration SE-DMA and CESSNA 525-A, registration D-IEVX Milano Linate airport October 8, 2001. http://www.havkom.se/virtupload/reports/FINALREPORTA-1–04Linate.pdf (Accessed June 23, 2013).

15. Laurell L, Lorin H, Lundin T, Dammström B-G. Air traffic accident at Gottröra, Sweden December 27, 1991 (in Swedish with English abstract). *KAMEDO Report 63.* Stockholm, National Board for Health and Welfare, 1994.

16. Fries H. The aeroplane fire in Manchester August 22, 1985 (in Swedish with English abstract). *KAMEDO Report 58.* Stockholm, National Board for Health and Welfare, 1991.

17. Brandsjö K. *Katastrofer och räddningsinsatser (in Swedish).* 1st ed. Stockholm, Informationsförlaget, 1996.

18. Hooke. *Norman: Maritime Casualties, 1963–1996.* London, Lloyd's of London Press, 1997.

19. Map Report. World Sea Disasters. httm://www.mapreport.com/century/subtopics/d/n.htlm (Accessed July 15, 2007).

20. KAMEDO. The Estonia Disaster - The loss of MS Estonia in the Baltic on September 28, 1994. *KAMEDO Report 68.* Stockholm, National Board for Health and Welfare, 1997.

21. Wikipedia. Costa Concordia disaster. http://en.wikipedia.org/wiki/Costa_Concordia_disaster (Accessed June 23, 2013).

22. Wikipedia. M/V Al – Salam Boccatio 98. The sinking. http://www.en.wikipedia.org/wiki/Al'salam'Boccatio'98 (Accessed July 15, 2007).

23. Brandstrom H, Sedig K. Sinking of the MS Sleipner on 26 November, 1999. *KAMEDO Report 77.* Stockholm, National Board for Health and Welfare, 2003.

24. KAMEDO. The fire on the passenger liner Scandinavian Star April 7, 1990. *KAMEDO Report 60.* Stockholm, National Board for Health and Welfare, 1993.

25. SOLAS. International Convention for the Safety of Life at Sea (SOLAS). http://www.imo.org/Conventions/contents.asp?topic_id=257&doc_id=647 (Accessed July 15, 2007).

26. Hayward JS, Eckerson J, Collis ML. Termal balance and survival time prediction of man in cold water. *Canadian Journal of Physiology and Pharmacology* 1975; 53: 21.

27. Forsberg R. *Train Crashes – Consequences for Passengers.* Umeå, Umeå University, 2012.

28. Forsberg R, Björnstig U. One Hundred Years of Railway Disasters and Recent Trends. *Prehosp Disaster Med* 2011; 26(5): 367–373.

29. Strandberg V. Rail bound traffic – a prime target for contemporary terrorist attacks? *J Transp Secur* 2013; 6(3): 271–286.

30. Hambeck W, Pueschel, K. Death by railway accident: incidence of traumatic asphyxia. *J Trauma* 1981; 21: 28–31.

31. Robinson OJ. Moorgate tube disaster. Part 2. Clinico – pathological review. *British Medical Journal* 1975; 3: 729–731.

32. Shackelford S, Nguyen L, Noguchi T, Sathyavagiswaran L, Inaba K, Demetriades D. Fatalities of the 2008 Los Angeles train crash: autopsy findings. *Am J Disaster Med* 2011; 6(2): 127–131.

33. Nagata T, Rosborough SN, VanRooyen MJ, Kozawa S, Ukai T, Nakayama S. Express Railway Disaster in Amagasaki: A Review

of Urban Disaster Response Capacity in Japan. *Prehosp Disaster Med* 2006; 21: 345–352.

34. Lawton R, Ward NJ. A systems analysis of the Ladbroke Grove rail crash. *Accident Analysis & Prevention* 2005; 37(2): 235–244.

35. Chatterjee S. Train engineer was texting just before California crash. Reuters, October 2, 2008. http://www.reuters.com/article/ 2008/10/02/us-usa-train-crash-idUSN0152835520081002 (Accessed June 24, 2013).

36. Evans AW. Fatal train accidents on Europe's railways: 1980–2009. *Accident Analysis & Prevention* 2011; 43(1): 391–401.

37. Oestern HJ, Huels B, Quirini W, Pohlemann T. Facts About the Disaster at Eschede. *Journal of Orthopaedic Trauma* 2000; 13(4): 287–290.

38. Thurfjell K. Spricka i hjul orsaken bakom tågolyckan. [Crack in the wheels cause of train crash]. *SvD nyheter*, 2010. http://www. svd.se/nyheter/utrikes/spricka-ihjul-orsaken-bakom-tagolyckan _5437381.svd (Accessed August 28, 2015).

39. Edkins GD, Pollock CM. The influence of sustained attention on Railway accidents. *Accident Analysis & Prevention* 1997; 29(4): 533–539.

40. Shaw RB. *A history of railroad accidents, safety precautions and operating practices.* Binghamton, NY, Vail-Ballou Press Inc., 1978.

41. Semmens P. *Railway disasters of the world.* Sparkford, Patrick Stephens Limited, 1994.

42. Kichenside G. *Great Train Disasters: The World's Worst Railway Accidents.* Bath, UK, Parragon Plus Publisher, 1997.

43. Steele J. One train, more than 1700 dead. *The Guardian,* December 29, 2004. http://www.theguardian.com/world/2004/dec/29/ tsunami2004.srilanka (Accessed August 28, 2015).

44. Millegan H, Yan X, Richards S, Han L. Evaluation of Effectiveness of Stop-Sign Treatment at Highway–Railroad Grade Crossings. *Journal of Transportation Safety & Security* 2009; 1(1): 46–60.

45. Yan X, Han LD, Richards S, Millegan H. Train–Vehicle Crash Risk Comparison Between Before and After Stop Signs Installed at Highway–Rail Grade Crossings. *Traffic Injury Prevention* 2010; 11(5): 535–542.

46. Kecklund L, Ingre M, Kecklund G, et al. The TRAIN-project: railway safety and the train driver information environment and work situation – A summary of the main results. Presented at 2. Signaling Safety 2001, London, February 26–27, 2001. http://www.researchgate.net/publication/242388701_Railway_ safety_and_the_train_driver_information_environment_and_ work_situation (Accessed August 28, 2015).

47. Evans AW. Rail safety and rail privatisation in Britain. *Accident Analysis & Prevention* 2007; 39(3): 510–523.

48. Evans AW. Rail safety and rail privatisation in Japan. *Accident Analysis & Prevention* 2010; 42(4): 1296–1301.

49. Hudson S. Train fires – Special Topic Report. Railway Safety Controller, Safety Strategy & Risk, Railway Safety, London, 2001. http://archive.uktra.in/rssb/rssb-Train_fires_-_Special_Topic_ Report.pdf (Accessed August 28, 2015).

50. Gao GJ, Tian HQ. Train's crashworthiness design and collision analysis. *International Journal of Crashworthiness* 2007; 12(1): 21–28.

51. Xue X, Smith RA, Schmid F. Analysis of crush behaviours of a rail cab car and structural modifications for improved crashworthiness. *International Journal of Crashworthiness* 2005; 10(2): 125–136.

52. Forsberg R, Holgersson A, Bodén I, Björnstig U. A study of a mass casualty train crash, focusing on the cause of injuries *Journal of Transportation Safety & Security* In press.

53. CNN. Investigator: D.C. Metro crash 'a scene of real devastation.' http://edition.cnn.com/2009/US/06/23/washington .metro.crash/index.html (Accessed June 25, 2013).

54. Holgersson A, Forsberg R, Saveman B-I. Inre säkerheten i tåg eftersatt – Fallstudie efter tågkraschen i Kimstad [Interior safety in trains is neglected – a case study from the rail crash in Kimstad]. *Läkartidningen* 2012; 109(1–2): 24–26.

55. Fothergill NJ, Ebbs SR, Reese A, et al. The Purely train crash mechanism: injuries and prevention. *Archives in Emergency Medicine* 1992; 9: 125–129.

56. Ilkjaer LB, Lind T. Passengers injuries reflected carriage interior at the railway accident in Mundelsturp, Denmark *Accident Analysis and Prevention* 2001; 33: 285–288.

57. Eriksson A, Ericsson D, Lundström NG, Thorson J. Personskador vid tågurspårningar – förslag till riskbegränsande åtgärder. *Läkartidningen* 1984; 81(5): 352–354.

58. Parent D, Tyrell D, Perlman AB. Crashworthiness analysis of the Placentia, CA rail collision. *International Journal of Crashworthiness* 2004; 9(5): 527–534.

59. Braden G. Application of Commercial Aircraft Accident Investigation Techniques to a Railroad Derailment *Aero Med* 1974; 7: 772–779.

60. Cugnoni HL, Fincham C, Skinner DV. Cannon Street rail disaster – lessons to be learned. *Injury* 1994; 25: 11–13.

61. Derailment at Grayrigg, February 23, 2007. Rail Accident Investigation Branch Report, Rail Accident Investigation Branch, Government of the United Kingdom, 2014. https://www.gov.uk/ raib-reports/derailment-at-grayrigg (Accessed August 28, 2015).

62. Design flaws and poor management caused Wenzhou collision, report confirms. International Railway Gazette, January 9, 2012. http://www.railwaygazette.com/news/single-view/view/ design-flaws-and-poor-management-caused-wenzhou- collision-report-confirms.html (Accessed August 28, 2015).

63. Forsberg R, Saveman B-I. Survivors' experiences from a train crash. *Int J Qualitative Stud Health Well-being* 2011; 6: 8401. http://www.ncbi.nlm.nih.gov/pmc/articles/PMC3224231/pdf/ QHW-6-8401.pdf (Accessed August 28, 2015).

64. Englund L, Forsberg R, Saveman B-I. Survivors' Experiences of Media Coverage after Traumatic injury events. *International Emergency Nursing* 2014; 22: 25–30.

65. Weyman A, O'Hara R, Jackson A. Investigation into issues of passenger egress in Ladbroke Grove rail disaster. *Applied Ergonomics* 2005; 36(6): 739–748.

66. Iselius L. Train Accident in Germany 1998 (in Swedish with English abstract). *KAMEDO Report 79.* Stockholm, National Board for Health and Welfare, 2004.

67. Bolling R, Brändström H, Ehrlin Y, et al. The terror attacks in Madrid, Spain, 2004 (in Swedish with English summary). *KAMEDO Report 90.* Stockholm, National Board for Health and Welfare, 2007.

68. Calland V. A brief overview of personal safety at incident sites. *Emerg Med J* 2007; 23: 878–882.

69. Braden GE. Aircraft – type crash injury investigation of commuter train collision. *Aviation, Space and Environmental Medicine* 1975; 46: 1157–1160.

70. Ebbs SR, Fothergill NJ, Hashemi K. The Purely train crash: procedural difficulties. *Archives of Emergency Medicine* 1992; 9: 130–133.

71. Ukai T, Takahashi Y, Aono M. *Disaster Medicine Learned from Cases.* Tokyo, Nankodo Co., 1995.

72. Assa A, Landau DA, Barenboim E, Goldstein L. Role of airmedical evacuation in mass-casualty incidents – A train collision experience. *Prehosp Disaster Med* 2009; 24: 271–276.

73. Barry E. Villagers Rushed to Help in Frigid Russian Crash. http://www.nytimes.com/2009/11/29/world/europe/29scene .html?_r=0 (Accessed June 25, 2013).

74. Wikipedia. Road disasters. http://en.wikipedia.org/wiki/List_of_ disasters#Road_disasters (Accessed June 23, 2013).

75. Björnstig U, Albertsson P, Lundälv J, Bergh-Johannesson K, Lundin T. Major Bus Crashes in Sweden 1997–2007. *KAMEDO Report 94*. Stockholm, National Board for Health and Welfare, 2011. https://www.socialstyrelsen.se/Lists/Artikelkatalog/ Attachments/18492/2011-11-19.pdf (Accessed August 28, 2015).

76. Wikipedia. Carrollton bus disaster. http://en.wikipedia.org/ wiki/Carrollton_bus_disaster (Accessed June 17, 2007).

77. Albertsson P. Occupant casualties in bus and coach traffic. Thesis. Umeå University, 2005.

78. Petzäll J, Albertsson P, Falkmer T, Björnstig U. Wind forces and aerodynamics, contributing factors to compromise bus and coach safety? *International Journal of Crashworthiness* 2005; 10: 435–444.

79. Wikipedia. Sierre Coach Crash. http://en.wikipedia.org/wiki/ Sierre_coach_crash (Accessed June 23, 2013).

21

EMERGENCY MEDICAL SERVICES SCENE MANAGEMENT

Kenneth T. Miller

OVERVIEW

Responses to large-scale emergences in recent years have reaffirmed what has long been said about disaster response: "all disasters are local." Those jurisdictions whose plans rely primarily on outside assistance beginning with the initial stages of response are destined to fail. Stepwise, scalable incident organization is essential to meet initial goals and objectives of the response to the emergency. Large-scale multiple casualty emergencies and disasters involving large numbers of injuries or illness are complex and will initially or eventually involve many agencies at various levels of jurisdiction that may have little or no experience working together. Local planning, preparedness, interdisciplinary training, and exercises can improve familiarity with multi-agency strategic and tactical plans and improve understanding of missions, cooperation, and interoperability.

The emergency medical services (EMS) mission of triage, rapid clinical assessment, critical therapeutic interventions, medical communications, and capability- and capacity-directed transport of victims in the management of a large-scale multiple casualty emergency is part of a complex set of overlapping missions. Immediate hazard mitigation or containment for the protection of responders and protection of victims from further injury is the first priority. This may be possible quickly and the EMS mission may proceed rapidly. There may, however, be fire suppression, rescue, infectious disease, or hazardous materials concerns complicating the missions of EMS and each response component organization. Another critical early step is communication of the evolving situation to the local healthcare infrastructure to assist them with preparing to receive patients. That healthcare infrastructure will need to establish its own internal response organization to meet the needs of a potentially large number of new patients in addition to continuing to provide services to those patients already under their care and those regular patients who present for care unrelated to the disaster. This early notification may occur spontaneously through social media, the news media, or structured lines of communication.

Preparedness and planning includes local assessment of EMS and healthcare resources. A jurisdiction's decision and threshold to request mutual aid will be determined by the local depth of resources, size, scope, and anticipated duration of the multiple casualty emergency and whether the local emergency response infrastructure remains intact or is damaged or overwhelmed in the course of the evolving emergency. The need for EMS special operations may also determine the threshold for mutual aid requests. Law enforcement–EMS tactical response; technical rescue–EMS operations; water or airborne rescue–EMS platforms; infectious disease isolation; victim emergency transportation, incident victim or healthcare facility patient evacuations; clinically oriented evacuee sheltering; trauma, burn, or pediatric intensive care; anticipated long-term specialized medical care (e.g., hemodialysis for traumatic rhabdomyolysis); anticipated incident-specific pharmaceutical needs; public health surveillance; epidemiology; or laboratory support and sustained hospital outpatient and inpatient volume are among the EMS and healthcare needs that determine the timing and nature of mutual aid requests.

The scope of emergency management is mitigation, preparedness, response, and recovery. Effective EMS scene management contributes to the success of the response and mitigation phases. Because more than one jurisdiction will be involved, mutual aid resources must be requested, coordinated, and integrated at the local level with the assistance of a unified command structure. Resources may be requested through local jurisdictions; counties or regions; state, interstate, federal and, in some cases, international agencies.

CURRENT STATE OF THE ART

There are many international models for the management of multiple casualty incidents (MCIs). Some emphasize scene organization with the goal of rapid transport and limited focused prehospital medical interventions. Others emphasize more extensive field medical operations prior to transport. There are extensive variations between these models and some include those with no apparent structure whatsoever. The very nature of multiple casualty and disaster medical operations makes it difficult to conduct longitudinal prospective studies to identify, characterize, and validate optimal operational parameters and practices that maximize victim survival with practical application of available resources. The concepts discussed here are based on U.S. models of MCI management.

Dispatch, Communications, and Initial Intelligence Gathering

EMS scene management begins with the initial calls for help. The recognition of and reaction to a large-scale multiple casualty emergency may be immediate, through cellular or landline calls to a public safety answering point (PSAP), or may be delayed if the emergency concurrently damages communications or facilities. Social media has emerged as a source of rapid information. The specific location or locations of the emergency may be immediately apparent or difficult to determine if there is conflicting information from callers or widespread consequences. Emergency services access telephone numbers vary around the world and may function to allow voice communications with a public or private entity or may supply other information about the caller's location. In the United States, many communities are served by the emergency access number 911 or enhanced 911 (E-911). Other communities use a seven- or ten-digit telephone number to access emergency services. E-911 allows both voice communication of the problem or emergency and displays the address of the telephone being used to make the call. If callers are unfamiliar with the area or unable to remember the location from which they are calling or the location of the emergency, PSAP personnel will be able to assist because they will know the location of the telephone from which the call originates. E-911 also allows call backs from the PSAP to that telephone to recontact the caller for more information or clarification if necessary. The advantages of E-911 with caller address identification may be lost with calls from cellular telephones or Voice over Internet Protocol (VoIP) calls or if there are no 911 services in the affected area. GPS technologies assist responders with caller and incident scene location. Telephones that operate over the Internet, however, may send U.S.-based 911 calls to distant operators, potentially introducing delays in determining the nature and location of an emergency and in identifying the appropriate response agencies.

When consequences of the evolving emergency are widespread, the local jurisdiction may dispatch fire suppression, law enforcement, and EMS resources to conduct a "windshield survey" of their primary response areas and report back. This helps to prioritize initial responses when needs clearly exceed initially available resources. With a loss of communications infrastructure, emergency communications may need to be conducted from individual jurisdictional law enforcement, fire suppression, or EMS response stations or units.

The first point of medical decision making for EMS scene management may take place at the level of the dispatch center when a caller reports a situation and requests assistance. In the United States, emergency medical dispatchers are trained to rapidly assist the caller in characterizing the nature of the emergency by using directed systematic questioning to construct an appropriate response to the emergency. In addition, these dispatchers provide pre-arrival instructions to the caller to attempt to mitigate immediate life-threatening problems. Dispatch centers can also assist local public health authorities with surveillance for disease during a public health emergency when an actionable case definition is known by asking callers about specific epidemiological links. When emergency medical dispatchers are engaged in response unit coordination they may no longer be able to medically triage calls for help or provide pre-arrival instructions to the caller to help reduce morbidity or mortality. However, they may still be in contact with callers in immediate danger from the evolving hazards. Guided by information provided by the caller, lifesaving advice may include to shelter in place or to evacuate the hazardous area. Emergency medical dispatchers may be trained in the use of scripted protocols aimed at reducing immediate life threats at the scene for special situations.

These include sites where a perpetrator is firing a gun, a structure fire entrapment, a known or unknown evolving community infectious disease, or a chemical or radiological release. Both syndromic and dispatch call type surveillance over time coordinated with local emergency management and public health resources may provide early information in an evolving, extended operations emergency. The situation may be dynamic, requiring case-by-case decisions based on dispatcher training and experience. Sufficient and accurate actionable information is frequently lacking. The most appropriate interventions for victim and public safety personnel are often unclear prior to first responder arrival. This can be an extraordinarily high stress time for emergency medical dispatchers who are attempting to construct a picture of the emergency, structure response configurations, coordinate the response with considerable situational uncertainty, and manage calls from callers in harm's way.

Initial Response

As social media is sent out, local media report on the emergency, and local dispatch radio traffic is heard, there may be self-dispatch of local or regional responders. Agency and responder discipline and "freelancing" must be balanced with judgment to dispatch the closest, most appropriate, and available response units based on staffing, capabilities, proximity to the incident, immediate needs of the emergency, and information available to the PSAPs and dispatch centers. Emergency unit use must also be balanced with the need to maintain capacity to meet other non-incident-related community calls for help. One strategy is to dispatch mutual aid units to the incident and preserve some local and reserve units familiar with the geography, procedures, and practices to respond to concurrent emergency calls. Once an incident command structure is established, self-dispatched units can be partially managed by staging incoming responders at a designated location with a staging manager in communication with the incident command for operational assignments.

Victim location may be known or readily apparent or there may be the need for search operations. Search operations may take the form of systematic wide-area searches by air, boat, or ground. Area searches are resource intensive and often are multi-agency and multi-jurisdictional. Structural search may be initially limited by the need for structural triage for stability by structural engineers. With proper structural triage and emergency building shoring as needed, structural search may be technical, using acoustic and imaging devices, or may involve search dogs or robots. Although the objective of the search may be location of survivors, the discovery of non-survivors must be anticipated and their locations mapped.

The prioritiesTh of the initial responding resources are scene survey (within the primary response area of individual response units), critical hazard mitigation or containment (that might immediately increase mortality of survivors and include hazards such as fires, unsecured utilities, and structural instability), and assessment of the need for and requesting additional resources. In truly widespread emergencies it may be necessary to make the very difficult decision to conduct area surveys and accurately report conditions that will contribute to better resource allocation and early specific mutual aid requests without attempting hazard mitigation or addressing life safety. Such activities may ultimately reduce morbidity and mortality among those victims with the greatest potential for survival. With the nearly immediate availability of airborne television reporting in urban and suburban areas, a visual area assessment may begin with video from television news reporting. In some parts of the world, certain industries (e.g., hotels, casinos, and secured buildings and facilities) maintain extensive video or closed circuit television. Law enforcement or public safety agencies may also conduct real-time video surveillance. This is a good source of information when infrastructure is intact. This visual assessment over several local television channels or other sources combined with emergency response dispatcher and first responder information and social media feeds helps to define the scope of the emergency.

Survivors might perform initial search, light rescue, and first aid. This local citizen-based assistance may be spontaneous, structured, or a combination of the two. Businesses may have organized emergency response teams designed to meet the immediate needs of employees and trained in early mitigation of any hazards unique to that business. For example, businesses that manage secure information may have plans to care for their employees, mitigate hazards from building utilities, and maintain information security.

Industries and universities may have hazardous materials teams that are solely responsible to their facilities and serve to identify and contain any hazardous materials breaches. U.S. nuclear power plants have response, assessment, and mitigation teams for potential radiation dispersion. Communities may have organized volunteer response teams (e.g., U.S. Community Emergency Response Teams)[1] trained in light rescue, residential utilities control, first aid, sheltering, and sustainment until professional help can arrive (see Chapter 11). In larger emergencies these may be the earliest responders. Training and exercising of emergency responders should include anticipation of and coordination with spontaneous, business, or community citizen responders.

Extended Response and Incident Organization

In smaller-scope daily jurisdictional EMS incidents, the roles and responsibilities of first responders are well defined and frequently practiced. As the incident becomes larger or extends over a longer period of time, a few specific functions must quickly be established to manage the emergency. Incident organization can define success or failure of overall incident management. As resource availability and capacity allow, two initial and overlapping priorities emerge: 1) immediate hazard mitigation and 2) victim triage. To address these two priorities, two functional groups must operate simultaneously: fire suppression/rescue and EMS. The response increases in complexity as the scope of the emergency is more completely determined and new priorities emerge. An incident management system is necessary to address these complexities. Response organization can occur at many functional and jurisdictional levels. Terms that describe functions and positions can vary. To create uniformity in incident management, U.S. policymakers developed the National Incident

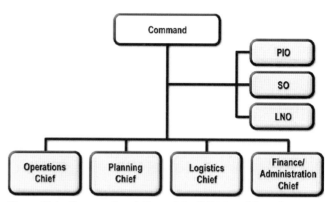

Figure 21.1. Command and General Staff (PIO: Public Information Officer; SO: Safety Officer; LNO: Liaison Officer).

Management System (NIMS).[2] The adoption and adaptation of NIMS at various jurisdictional levels is encouraged by tying its use in planning and preparedness to federal funding of eligible local jurisdictional programs.

Management of large and sustained incidents is structured around command and general staff with geographical divisions and functional branches and groups. If the incident requires greater resources and organization, the functional branches are divided into groups (Figure 21.1). If this not operationally necessary, the functional branches alone are adequate. Functional group resources can be further subdivided into task forces composed of multiple disciplines, strike teams composed of similar disciplines, or individual resources.

Command and General Staff

Command and general staff consist of an incident commander or a unified command with multiple agencies (e.g., fire, EMS, law enforcement, and public health) to manage the incident. The incident safety officer, public information officer, and any responding agency liaison officers all report to the incident commander. Also reporting to the incident commander is the general staff: operations section chief, plans section chief, logistics section chief, and finance/administration section chief.

Planning Section

The Planning Section is responsible for incident intelligence gathering, documentation, anticipation and requesting of specialized resources, coordination of technical specialists necessary to support incident operations, and the briefing of responding agency leadership throughout operational periods. During sustained operations, the Planning Section has the responsibility of writing the Incident Action Plan with the concurrence of the command and general staff and based on a standardized format.[3] The Planning Section is also responsible for organizing demobilization of resources as the incident resolves. For example, the Planning Section coordinates with local health departments and hospitals to keep the Operations Section informed about hospital and specialty care resources (e.g., burn and trauma) and ability to receive patients in an extended EMS incident. Incident EMS or medical supervisors coordinate with safety and hazardous materials officers to develop a safety plan that contributes to the Incident or Operations Action Plan and addresses occupational health hazards for remaining victims and responders. The Planning Section gathers information on agencies with the ability to transport victims greater distances to healthcare facilities remote from an emergency affecting local healthcare resources. This section also writes the plan to guide the Operations Section in accessing transportation and other resources.

Logistics Section

The Logistics Section is responsible for incident communications, acquiring and managing all equipment and materiel necessary to support incident operations, and managing and supporting a base of operations. If on-site medical care is provided to incident responders, that medical unit is also the responsibility of the Logistics Section.

Finance/Administration Section

The Finance/Administration Section is responsible for tracking incident costs and personnel time and facilitating purchases for the logistics section. This section also tracks claims for injuries to responders.

Operations Section

The Operations Section manages the various missions of the incident. It is supported by the other three general staff sections. The Operations Section may be divided into geographical divisions based on incident priorities and physical boundaries that affect those priorities. The Operations Section is further divided into functional branches and/or groups. These functional branches or groups may include multiple casualty, rescue, fire suppression, hazardous materials, or air operations branches/groups or any other function essential to the mission. Group supervisors report to branch directors, division chiefs or the Operations Section chief depending on the level of organization necessary to manage the incident (Figure 21.2).

For extended EMS operations, the Operations Section needs a multiple casualty branch (Figure 21.3). The multiple casualty branch is divided into a medical group and a transportation group. If there are multiple sites in operation, geographical divisions can be assigned to further organize incident management. The medical group has a triage unit, treatment unit, and a morgue unit.

The transportation group has a ground ambulance coordinator and a medical communications coordinator. An ambulance loading manager coordinates victim movement between the treatment unit leader and ground ambulance coordinator. If air medical transport services are in ongoing use during victim transport, the transportation group supervisor coordinates with the air operations branch/group.

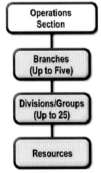

Figure 21.2. Operations Section: Geographic Divisions, Functional Branches or Groups.

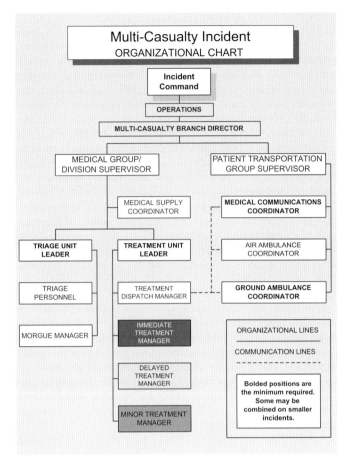

Figure 21.3. Multicasualty Incident Organization (adapted from FIRESCOPE).

Area Command

In widespread emergencies with multiple incident sites, an area command can be established to manage the response (Figure 21.4). There may be one area command with a unified command; safety officer; public information officer; agency liaison officers; and plans, logistics, and finance/administration section chiefs. Each operational site would then have an operations chief with geographical divisions or functional branches or groups.

Such extended incident organization develops over time, is structured to meet the needs of the incident, and is built from essential functions, beginning with the initial responding units. To manage a multiple casualty incident site, initial responders should establish an incident command system and appoint an incident commander and personnel to function as triage unit leader and medical communications coordinator. These essential three functions will meet the initial needs of organizing resources, assessing the incident, reporting conditions and hazards (scene safety), requesting additional resources, initiating victim triage, and establishing communications with the EMS and healthcare infrastructure.

Victim Triage and Transport

Victim triage strategies and challenges are discussed in Chapter 14. Further organization depends on the availability of additional resources to meet the needs of the incident. If sufficient ambulances are available to initiate immediate victim

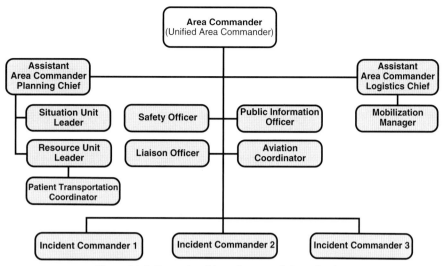

Figure 21.4. Example of Area Command Organization.

transport, a ground ambulance coordinator can be established and victims can be moved directly from triage to ambulances by triage priority. The medical communications coordinator determines the destination hospital or specialty receiving center. Management of arriving ambulances may be assigned to a staging manager reporting to the medical group supervisor, medical branch director, or operations chief, or assigned to the ground ambulance coordinator on smaller incidents. If sufficient ambulances are not immediately available or the resource needs of the MCI exceed local capacity, a treatment unit is necessary. Victims are moved to a treatment unit at a safe location by triage priority and subsequently transported in ambulances or other types of vehicles (e.g., buses or vans for minor casualties) as these resources become available. An ambulance loading manager working with the treatment unit leader and ground ambulance coordinator manages victim movement based on triage category and ambulance availability. The medical communications coordinator determines destination hospitals in consultation with healthcare infrastructure. The physical location of the medical communications coordinator is determined by many incident-specific factors. One strategy is to geographically locate the medical communications coordinator so that the ambulances loaded by triage category receive their hospital or specialty center destination assignments as they are exiting the incident. This prevents slowing down the patient loading process by allowing the ambulance loading manager and ground ambulance coordinator to load ambulances by triage category without waiting for destination decisions.

A critical concept is that components must be based on functions rather than on positions. If local responders are adequately trained and exercised on MCI management, the functions described will be accomplished without unnecessary focus on process and position titles.

Effective victim triage is essential to optimize use of limited on-scene resources and healthcare infrastructure in larger MCIs. Although many EMS systems have robust patient distribution systems, a disproportionate number of casualties may be transported to the closest hospital or a single specialty hospital such as a trauma or burn center such as during the disasters at the World Trade Center in New York City[5] and the Alfred P. Murrah Federal Building in Oklahoma City.[6] Less commonly, casualties

are indeed distributed across the system effectively according to well-rehearsed procedures, such as during the Boston Marathon bombing in the United States in 2013. Some degree of victim self-triage and self-transport can be expected (and percentages vary by country), especially before effective incident management is established and adequate resources have arrived to the incident site. The magnitude of victim self-triage and self-transport can be substantial, even in industrialized societies with highly resourced EMS systems.[6,7] Victims who have or find their own transportation can be expected to go to the closest hospitals or to those most familiar to them independent of any plan to optimally use healthcare resources. Even if scene managers use a good patient distribution system, this can result in a maldistribution of casualties to local hospitals such that one or a few facilities are overwhelmed, whereas others stand by with few casualties. Early communications about the nature and location of the incident are essential to assist the healthcare infrastructure in rapidly preparing for casualty arrival. This is particularly true if victim decontamination or infectious disease isolation is necessary. It takes time to make hospital-based decontamination systems and PPE for infectious diseases operationally ready. Hospitals may experience "reverse triage" such that self-transported victims with comparatively less severe injuries arrive before more seriously injured victims present through the EMS system.[6] Bidirectional communication between the medical communications coordinator and hospitals helps to determine whether victims of lower triage priority should be transported to more distant hospitals to avoid those that are closer and more affected by victim self-triage and self-transport. Another strategy is to designate a hospital near the incident site as a "triage facility" where patients are quickly stabilized and transferred out to other hospitals.

Communication with healthcare facilities may be direct (using radio or telephone coordination between the medical communications coordinator and hospitals) or indirect (through a dispatch or regional coordination center). Other communications modalities include web-based tracking systems of victim transport and hospital capabilities updated in real-time. Electronic victim and hospital tracking can take place via the Internet and can be backed up by microwave transmission or satellite communications. Effective hospital-based management of patients from a multiple casualty incident is dependent on establishing an internal command structure similar to the field incident management system. The Hospital Incident Command System is an example of a framework that defines positions and functions to assist hospitals with internal organization, requesting additional resources, and optimal resource use for both in-house and on-call sources.[8]

Spontaneous responders can be a management challenge during a large incident. Unplanned medical responders are unlikely to be trained, equipped, or experienced in providing medical care under hazardous conditions and are also unlikely to be familiar with EMS strategies and procedures. Informed and organized spontaneous medical responders can be an asset, however, when the size and scope of the MCI exceeds local capacity. It is essential to have a plan to manage these well-meaning volunteers; otherwise they can distract resources from their primary functions and lead to suboptimal scene management. One strategy is to attempt to collect spontaneous medical responders, brief them on the nature of the incident and assign them to the treatment unit leader. The staging area for victims in the treatment unit awaiting transportation to hospitals will likely be in a comparatively safe location and the approach to these patients' care will be somewhat familiar to spontaneous medical responders who are healthcare providers.

Medical Management

Specific treatment rendered during and after the triage process or in the treatment unit must be goal directed. Treatment depends on the capabilities and capacity of the responding resources. Because the triage process is dynamic and not complete simply when a victim arrives at the treatment unit, an important function is interval victim reassessment and re-triage if necessary. Newer triage tags are designed to display change in triage category with either improvement or deterioration. Treatment strategies likely to reduce morbidity and mortality among victims staged in the treatment unit include: maintaining an open airway, decompressing a tension pneumothorax (needle thoracostomy), controlling external exsanguinating hemorrhage (wound packing, pressure dressing, application of clot-inducing bandages, and/or arterial tourniquet) and spinal stabilization if not already accomplished. Conversely, a clinical assessment to determine whether patients need to be placed or remain in spine immobilization can be invaluable during MCIs, both to save scarce resources and to reduce discomfort and complications for patients who do not require it. Using a validated protocol, properly trained personnel can systematically judge when spinal stabilization is necessary and when it is not.[9,10] Patients without unnecessary spinal immobilization require far fewer personnel and transportation resources.

The gamut of EMS therapeutic interventions may not be available or possible depending on the number and acuity of victims, available transportation, and capacity of the EMS system. Intravascular fluid resuscitation (intravenous or intraosseous) of profound hypovolemic shock with uncontrolled hemorrhage to permissive hypotension endpoints may influence victim outcome[11,12] but little is known about outcomes-based, multiple casualty victim, clinical management strategies. Decisions on airway interventions are determined by availability of equipment and personnel, sustainment of those resources (e.g., oxygen), predicted victim survivability and the number of other victims who may survive. Goal-directed therapies for injuries or for exacerbations of underlying illnesses subsequent to those injuries should be considered on a case-by-case basis as resources allow.

Pain control can be both a humanitarian and practical intervention. Non-pharmacological pain control may take the form of effective splinting and immobilization of fractures. Pharmacological pain control depends on local scope of practice and available resources. It provides comfort to victims immobilized for long periods of time or with painful injuries who are staged in the treatment unit awaiting available transportation. Other measures to address victim comfort include providing shade or shelter for the treatment unit to reduce exposure to temperature extremes, sunlight, wind, precipitation, and the sights and sounds of the incident itself, and oral hydration when clinically appropriate.

Medical management of entrapped victims can be complex. When resources are available and the survivability of entrapped victims is judged to be sufficiently favorable to commit to extended technical rescue operations, certain medical interventions can contribute to both the stabilization of the victim and the tempo of the rescue. The treatment of easily reversible conditions and the treatment of pain may allow some downward triage (i.e., moving patients to a lower, less severe level) of selected victims and allocation of scarce medical resources to victims requiring temporary stabilizing interventions and rapid transport. Inhalation injury, blunt and penetrating trauma, traumatic rhabdomyolysis ("crush syndrome" depending on duration of entrapment and muscle mass entrapped), hypothermia, dehydration, and exacerbation of chronic illnesses are among the conditions that require field interventions. Depending on the nature of a structure's building materials and the type of event causing its failure, emergencies involving structural collapse may result in void spaces capable of supporting life. Void space ventilation, either passive by opening the void space to the atmosphere or active by using ventilation fans and a particulate respirator (e.g., disposable N95 respirator) for the victim can help reduce further risk of inhalation injury. Anticipating predictable physiologic consequences of prolonged entrapment and coordinating goal-directed medical interventions with the rescue operation are important considerations. Anticipating traumatic rhabdomyolysis, blood loss, and intravascular fluid shifts during disentanglement can reduce the risk of precipitous hemodynamic destabilization on extrication.[12] Pain management can substantially affect the tempo of a rescue effort by expediting disentanglement and extrication. Although disentanglement and extrication can involve moving the victim in ways that are unavoidably painful, pain exacerbation can be a warning that part of the rescue effort is placing the victim at risk of further injury. If victim discomfort causes the rescue effort to be repeatedly stopped and readjusted with no appreciable progress, pharmacological pain control should be used to facilitate the rescue process.

Decontamination and Special Hazards

When chemical, radiological, or biological hazards may be present or when there is concern for secondary hazardous devices such as explosives, incident organization for the purpose of victim movement remains unchanged. However, several other processes must be inserted into MCI organization and structure. The first challenge is recognition and rapid assessment of the hazard. Responders must quickly determine whether there are surviving and accessible victims and what level of responder PPE is necessary to make rapid entry and remove survivors from the immediate hazard to a safe area. The suspected nature of the hazard and initial operational decisions must be communicated to responding personnel. Triage may need to be performed in the area of safety or delayed until after initial decontamination. If triage is to be accomplished prior to emergency decontamination, triage personnel may need to work in PPE. Once the suspected hazard has been recognized, however, PPE used, initial victim rescue accomplished, and emergency decontamination performed, the process of organizing secondary triage (or primary triage if not yet performed), treatment, medical communications, resource coordination, transportation destination, and victim transport remains the same.

When there is a need for victim decontamination, there is a substantial layer of complexity and personnel requirements added to EMS scene management. First responders may need to perform emergency decontamination based on victim symptoms of known or suspected contaminant inhalation or skin contact toxicity.

In the United States, this will likely be accomplished by initial responding fire suppression personnel using handheld hose lines or elevated master streams with nozzles operated in a fog pattern. If there is believed to be a life or immediate health threat to the contaminated victims, the U.S. Environmental Protection Agency (EPA) has communicated[13,14] that water runoff can be managed (e.g., downhill from operating units on grass or gravel) but does not initially need to be contained. In the United States, runoff containment becomes a regulatory requirement after the life or health threat is mitigated and when operations transition from emergency decontamination to technical responder decontamination during hazard mitigation, deceased victim recovery, or law enforcement investigation. An attempt should be made to cohort contaminated victims to the extent possible during emergency decontamination set up. An area of safe refuge is the ideal location for this. With proper training and exercising, decontamination resources can be operationalized very rapidly (within minutes) using equipment and appliances carried on fire apparatus normally used for fire suppression. Victim contact for pre-decontamination coordination or life-threatening injury or illness intervention will likely occur with personnel wearing structural firefighting protective equipment and full-face, positive pressure, self-contained breathing apparatus (SCBA). If decontamination operations are sustained, the level of respiratory and splash protection necessary can be made based on a more objective risk assessment (see Chapter 16). Critical pre-decontamination interventions may include removal of outer clothing (which results in substantial contamination reduction), containing important personal items (e.g., personal identification) and coordinating family or companion decontamination for ambulatory victims. For non-ambulatory victims, pre-decontamination maintenance of an open airway, needle decompression of a tension pneumothorax, control of external exsanguinating hemorrhage, and spinal stabilization may be indicated. Pre-decontamination antidote administration may be impractical or medication may be unavailable. It is, however, technically feasible for providers wearing protective equipment to administer intramuscular injections (e.g., atropine and pralidoxime via auto-injectors) for critically ill victims of organophosphate/nerve agent toxicity. This intervention can stabilize the victim sufficiently to permit necessary decontamination prior to more definitive treatment. Exposure solely to gases (particularly less water-soluble gases) does not require immediate skin decontamination. Inhalation or intravenous cyanide antidote administration to critically ill victims can proceed as soon as the victim is removed from the immediate inhalation hazard and the prehospital care provider can work safely without a respirator. Similarly, radioactive particulate contamina-

tion of victims and their wounds from an explosive dispersion device is a lower priority than managing critical blunt or penetrating trauma resulting from the blast injury.[15,16] Removing the external layer of clothing, wrapping the victim to contain the radioactive contamination, critical prehospital interventions, transport to a trauma center, and initial resuscitation and damage control surgery are all priorities over radiological decontamination (see Chapter 33). Radiological decontamination can be performed at any point during medical or surgical management at which the victim is considered stabilized. Stable victims can be decontaminated prior to transport. Wound irrigation is part of the decontamination process. Because hospitals may not be sufficiently prepared to manage patients with radiological contamination, emergency planners should anticipate requests from hospitals for decontamination assistance (supplies and trained personnel), particularly if large numbers of self-transported victims arrive before hospital-based decontamination procedures are fully operational.

During a public health emergency involving an infectious disease, responder PPE may need to be enhanced for airborne or droplet transmission (e.g., SARS in 2003) or more comprehensive contact precautions (e.g., Ebola virus disease in 2014).[17] Access to sufficient protective equipment, safe donning and doffing, and recognizing when to use it can complicate field operations and limit choices of destination hospitals based on isolation capabilities and trained staff. Transport vehicles my need to be specially configured and disinfected.

Victim Tracking

Victim tracking is a challenging problem in EMS scene management of MCIs (see Chapter 28). With wireless telephone communications (including instant messaging and picture phones) widely available to victims who can communicate, their involvement in an emergency can be known by family, friends, coworkers, and the media very early in the evolution of the incident. The status and whereabouts of victims of MCIs who require custodial care and caretakers (e.g., children, elderly, or disabled) will likely be sought even before the last victim has left the scene, with some caretakers arriving to the scene in the midst of ongoing emergency operations. There is a balance between efficient victim movement from the incident to definitive medical care and documentation of important victim information at the scene. Electronic devices to connect a triage tag identifier with the identity and destination of a victim have not been rigorously and objectively compared to paper-based tracking systems in efficacy, effectiveness, protection of confidential patient information, or practicality under operational field conditions. Electronic devices can fail due to power or weather situations and would need to be immediately and widely available and operable by EMS system personnel. Any procedure or device that is used only rarely and under exceptional circumstances is at risk for failure when it may be needed most. Hospital-based patient identification and tracking is a common practice and may be augmented with the assistance of nongovernmental organizations (e.g., American Red Cross chapters) or local EMS communications infrastructure. This process, although effective, incorporates an inherent delay in victim information transmission.

Multi-Jurisdictional Coordination

Large or widespread multiple casualty emergency response by an authority having jurisdiction will likely require outside assistance. "Automatic aid" refers to public safety answering points and dispatch centers sending the closest appropriate local units independent of geopolitical boundaries. "Mutual aid" refers to interjurisdictional assistance following a specific request for that assistance, often but not exclusively with pre-event agreements defining available resources, response parameters, and administrative issues such as reimbursement procedures. Mutual aid can be between local jurisdictions, within regions of a state, from state government, between states (e.g., Emergency Management Assistance Compacts),[20] from the federal government, and between countries. Each responding mutual aid entity has its own command structure that integrates into a unified command, division, branch, or group organization of the authority having jurisdiction. Local or regional entities may request EMS mutual aid to report to the scene to assist with victim management. More distant EMS mutual aid may include ambulance strike teams[20,21] to assist with victim transport from hospitals to specialty facilities (e.g., trauma, burn, or pediatric) or from hospitals with a large number of victims to more distant hospitals. In most cases, EMS helicopters are less practical than ground transport units in MCIs because they require additional resources to operate safely and coordinate landing zones, and they can generally only carry one or possibly two victims. Additionally, many rescue helicopters do not fly at night and cannot fly in inclement weather. Air EMS resources have value if they are used to transport properly triaged victims to specialty care centers (e.g., trauma, burn, or pediatric) distant from the incident site due to geographical location or saturation of closer specialty centers during an extended incident. If extended rescue operations are necessary, specialty rescue teams or task forces with medical components may be deployed to the scene. Medical teams may be requested to support local healthcare infrastructure by expanding local or regional emergency department, critical care unit, medical-surgical unit, or public health capacity and operational sustainment, to provide free-standing treatment stations or to provide medical support to the community and shelters for special populations. Individual resources or strike teams such as specialty nurses (e.g., critical care, burn, dialysis), pharmacists, or physicians may also be requested. Disaster management systems and healthcare facility disaster management are discussed elsewhere (see Chapters 11 and 22).

RECOMMENDATIONS FOR FURTHER RESEARCH

Planning for MCI response requires more than an analysis of the organizational and technical aspects. MCI response plans must anticipate and incorporate the potential effects of victim self-triage and self-transport. Hospital and scene incident management must anticipate maldistribution of victims geographically and by acuity. In addition, response personnel must be familiar with and trained, exercised, and disciplined in the application of, their MCI plan. The plan must be adaptive to allow flexibility and deviation to meet the specific needs of an incident. Frequent exercises and scaled application of the plan to more common smaller incidents will help achieve responder familiarity and comfort and improve plan compliance. Research on victim movement and incident organization will help identify those functions that are most critical to effective patient triage and transport and allow planning, training, and exercising to address those needs.

Healthcare resources in a community can be scarce, even during daily operations. To support MCI operations, particularly for minor triage category victims, transport to free-standing emergency departments, urgent care centers, and other alternate care sites might help unload acute care facilities, allowing them to manage greater numbers of higher acuity victims. This is not common practice in the United States and will require research into the safest ways to distribute minor casualties into a broader healthcare system, as well as to address existing laws and the need for legislative relief to enable selected alternate care sites to receive victims from an incident. Development of healthcare surge capacity will assist in survivor distribution to hospitals by keeping hospitals operational as EMS destinations.

Virtually every emergency incident or disaster after-action report mentions challenges with communications. Effective and sustainable communications within jurisdictional chain of command and with outside resources are essential for command and control and optimal resource utilization. The capacity of routinely used communications systems can easily be exceeded during major incidents. Cellular telephones and local emergency radio frequencies can be saturated with communications traffic, as can handheld satellite telephones. Distance from communications centers or communications transmission equipment or terrain can compromise radio or cellular traffic. Collateral damage to communications infrastructure or power supply can render wireless telephones unusable and radio communications may be limited to line-of-sight with handheld units. Portable radio battery life, replacement, and recharging may be limited. Multi-jurisdictional radio interoperability may also be limited. Separation of law enforcement, fire suppression/rescue, and EMS radio communications may make coordination of resources difficult. Lack of redundancy in communications systems can compromise operations when one or more systems fail. Technological, political, and operational solutions are possible when combined with funding, equipment availability, familiarity, training, and exercising. As with triage strategies, communications solutions should be integrated into daily emergency services operations so that unfamiliar equipment and procedures will not be first used in times of high demand.

No triage decision scheme has been prospectively validated under large-scale MCI operational conditions. Retrospective studies on efficacy do not always translate to prospective operational effectiveness. Attempting to transport every "critical" victim to a specialty center by using advanced life support assets is not always the best use of resources or even possible to achieve. Arguably, effective triage strategies during a large multiple casualty emergency are more important to victim outcome and resource utilization than in daily single-victim trauma triage. Under- and overtriage can substantially impact the volume and acuity of victims arriving by EMS and arriving at healthcare facilities, compromising the ability of these potentially limited resources to be preserved for victims most likely to benefit and potentially ultimately compromising victim clinical outcomes.

Victim tracking from the scene, if done at all, can be as low tech as paper documentation of victim name, triage category, hospital destination, and transporting unit identifier, or as high tech as encrypted electronic scanning and wireless transmission of victim data to multiple stakeholder agencies needing this information. Such information, secured as protected patient information, would promote improvements in victim management from the incident, healthcare inter-facility transfers for specialty care, family notifications, and post-incident analysis. The more complex equipment and procedures become and the less they are used under daily operational conditions, the more likely they are to fail during a multiple casualty event. Practical, durable, affordable technological solutions or simple operational procedures should be developed.

Thoughtful, goal-directed, locally conceived and executed exercises and drills are essential to managing and coordinating the many challenges of a large MCI. Both insufficient funding and grant-driven funding for exercises can result in training that is poorly conceived with too broad or general goals and objectives and insufficient attention to local needs. The lack of sophisticated local systems, equipment, and procedures does not necessarily translate to poor MCI performance. Understanding local resources, optimizing those resources, training and exercises can result in a well-managed incident.

Continuous quality improvement studies are increasingly applied within EMS systems. Documentation of patient demographics and clinical condition may not be as thorough during MCIs as it is for incidents with few or individual patients, but post-incident analysis can provide useful data for system and response evaluation. Response intervals, staging intervals, victim transport intervals by triage category, ambulance departure-from-scene intervals, and cumulative victim transport numbers by triage acuity over time are parameters that can help characterize the timeframe of the response and of victim movement. Changes in these calculated intervals if operational changes were made on-scene during the evolution of the incident can be very instructive. These time-related data may be more readily available in an EMS system than are victim outcome data. When victim outcome data are available, hospital admission rates, duration of stay, admission diagnoses, emergency department and hospital discharge diagnoses, surgical intervention rates (e.g., trauma/general, orthopedic, and neurological surgery), critical care unit admission rates, and mortality rates can be useful to help assess triage sensitivity (false negative or undertriage rate) and specificity (false positive or overtriage rate). In well-designed MCI exercises with mock victims tagged with local triage scheme specific parameters, both "victim" movement time analysis and triage scheme sensitivity and specificity can be assessed for the purposes of adjusting future training and system deployment. Such an exercise assessment is only an approximation of operational effectiveness but can identify extremes in performance that can assist with defining future training needs. EMS systems with well-developed data management and continuous quality improvement processes may be able to capture more objective, operational data and contribute to the knowledge base for MCI management by forming MCI registries.

REFERENCES

1. Community Emergency Response Teams. https://www.citizencorps.gov/cert (Accessed June 9, 2013).
2. National Incident Management System. http://www.fema.gov/national-incident-management-system (Accessed June 9, 2013).
3. ICS Forms. http://www.firescope.org/ics-forms.htm (Accessed June 9, 2013).
4. Multi-Casualty Branch Worksheet. http://www.firescope.org/ics-multi-casual/forms/ICS-MC-305.pdf (Accessed June 9, 2013).
5. Centers for Disease Control and Prevention. Rapid assessment of injuries among survivors of the terrorist attack on the World Trade Center – New York City, September 2001. *MMWR* 2002; 51(1): 1–5.
6. Hogan DE, Waeckerle JF, Dire DJ, Lillibridge SR. Emergency department impact of the Oklahoma City terrorist bombing. *Ann Emerg Med* 1999; 34(2): 160.
7. Okumura T, Takasu N, Ishimatsu S, et al. Report on 640 victims of the Tokyo subway sarin attack. *Ann Emerg Med* 1996; 28(2): 129–135.
8. Hospital Incident Command System. http://www.emsa.ca.gov/disaster_medical_services_division_hospital_incident_command_system_resources (Accessed Dec 7, 2015).
9. Spinal Assessment Protocol, Maine EMS 2002. http://www.maine.gov/ems/documents/2011MaineEMSProtocols.pdf (Accessed June 9, 2013).
10. Domeier RM, Frederiksen SM, Welch K. Prospective performance assessment of an out-of-hospital protocol for selective spine immobilization using clinical spine clearance criteria. *Ann Emerg Med* 2005; 46(2): 123–131.
11. Dubick MA, Atkins JL. Small-volume fluid resuscitation for the far-forward combat environment: current concepts. *J Trauma* 2003; 54(5 Suppl.): S43.
12. Ashkenazi I, Isakovich B, Kluger Y, Alfici R, Kessel B, Better OS. Prehospital management of earthquake casualties buried under rubble. *Prehosp Disaster Med* 2005; 20(2): 122–133.
13. US EPA letter to US Army Soldier and Biological Chemical Command, September 1999. http://cryptome.org/runoff.htm (Accessed June 9, 2013).
14. Bushberg JT, Kroger LA, Hartman MB, et al. Nuclear/radiological terrorism: emergency department management of radiation casualties. *J Emerg Med* 2007; 32(1): 71–85.
15. Koenig KL, Hatchett RJ, Mettler FA, et al. Medical treatment of radiologic casualties: current concepts. *Ann Emerg Med* 2005; 45(6): 643–652.
16. Emergency Management Assistance Compact. http://www.emacweb.org (Accessed June 9, 2013).
17. Koenig KL, Majestic C, Burns MJ. Ebola Virus Disease: Essential Public Health Principles for Clinicians, *West-JEM*, 2014. http://www.escholarship.org/uc/item/1bh1352j#page-1 (Accessed August 8, 2015).
18. Koenig KL. Ebola Triage Screening and Public Health: The New "Vital Sign Zero". Disaster Medicine and Public Health Preparedness. http://journals.cambridge.org/action/displayAbstract?fromPage=online&aid=9587810&fulltextType=AC&fileId=S1935789314001207 (Accessed August 21, 2015).
19. Koenig KL. Identify, Isolate, Inform: A 3-pronged Approach to Management of Public Health Emergencies. Disaster Medicine and Public Health Preparedness. http://journals.cambridge.org/action/displayAbstract?fromPage=online&aid=9587816&fulltextType=RA&fileId&S1935789314001256 (Accessed August 21, 2015).
20. Ambulance Strike Team Guidelines. http://www.emsa.ca.gov/disaster/files/AST%20Manual%20and%20PTB%206-9-11.pdf (Accessed June 9, 2013).
21. U.S. Department of Homeland Security, Federal Emergency Management Agency, Ambulance Strike Teams. http://www.fema.gov/txt/emergency/nims/508_3_emergency_medica_%20services.txt (Accessed June 9, 2013).

22

HEALTHCARE FACILITY DISASTER MANAGEMENT

John D. Hoyle, Sr.

OVERVIEW

Disaster preparedness in healthcare facilities has historically been a low priority and is often viewed as a chore or unnecessary mandate. Too often it has not received the support of top management in a meaningful way. In some societies, healthcare is viewed as a right, with the expectation that the hospital be ready 24/7 to render care as needed. Lawyers may sue the unprepared hospital or healthcare professional after a disaster in some cultures. In past decades, many healthcare professional training programs, including those in the United States, have not emphasized disaster preparedness in their curricula. Even residencies in emergency medicine sometimes neglect this important subject. Since the terrorist attacks of September 11, 2001, in the United States, many healthcare training programs have begun educating students on this vital topic and its implications for their communities. Many hospitals have experienced a resurgence of interest in preparedness and have hired full-time emergency management personnel. In contrast, other institutions have only prepared minimally as required by outside entities (e.g., the local or national health authority or The Joint Commission in the United States). Hospital preparedness efforts have waxed and waned over the years, and the tempo of preparedness planning, training, and drilling has vacillated depending on national or local requirements or trends and real-world events. Preparedness efforts for hospitals, public health organizations, and long-term care facilities tend to gain momentum when a real or perceived threat is present. Because students in hospital and healthcare administration usually receive no training in emergency management, they are not fully cognizant of the possible demands that could be placed on them and their facilities during a disaster or emergency situation. An additional factor inhibiting preparedness activities is the fact that individuals could work their entire careers in a hospital and never experience a disaster. While the term "hospital" is used throughout much of this chapter, the principles discussed are meant to apply to all healthcare facilities.

History of Healthcare Disaster Planning and Preparedness

The initial efforts to formalize hospital disaster preparedness began in the United Kingdom in the days before the outbreak of World War II. As war with Germany became imminent, the British government completed planning activities started in the 1920s following the World War I bombings of London by Zeppelins. The government realized that modern airpower and munitions represented a severe threat that could produce massive numbers of casualties. Therefore, they implemented many medical preparedness measures and created the Emergency Medical Service (EMS) in the Ministry of Health to coordinate these endeavors.[1] The British EMS was unlike a twenty-first century prehospital system in the developed world; rather, it represented a planning and control agency. This group had authority over all healthcare services and had the power to regulate hospitals, designate duties for each category of hospital, create new hospitals in prefabricated huts at distant locations from target areas, and dispatch ambulance trains and buses to remove the injured to hospitals in safe areas.

The United Kingdom was divided into twelve planning regions, with the London region further subdivided into twelve sectors because of the heavy population density. Planners anticipated an initial casualty load of 35,000 victims from bombings.

Working with the military to devise estimated casualty figures, EMS quickly placed orders for 150,000 beds with linens and blankets. At the same time, EMS also ordered 226,000 litters that, with their wire mesh, could be easily cleaned or even used as decontamination stretchers. The large number of litters was also desired to reduce the frequency of transferring patients from bed to bed as they moved through multiple treatment venues. Also ordered were massive quantities of pharmaceuticals and dressings to provide for 250,000 hospital beds, 3,000 first aid posts, and 2,000 smaller first aid points.[1] Those staffing the first aid posts included physicians and nurses performing casualty clearing. Gas decontamination units were also organized and the EMS issued guidance documents.[1]

- "Structural Precautions for Hospitals Subject to Bombing Effects"
- "System for Wartime Organization of Hospitals"
- "Formation of Casualty Bureaus"
- "Medical Treatment of Gas Casualties"
- "Training and Work of First Aid Parties"

Also during this period, numerous medical faculty members published books such as *Medical Organization and Surgical Practice in Air Raids; Casualty: Training, Organization and Administration of Civil Defense Casualty Services*; and *The Treatment of Burns.*[2-4]

Before hostilities began, hospitals were reinforced with wooden beams and some constructed bed space and operating rooms in their basements. Casualty Bureaus were created to organize the medical records on patients and the deceased, and report their statistics twice daily to the EMS. An alerting system for hospitals was established. On receipt of a warning, each hospital had specified actions to take in preparation for the arrival of casualties. The British government offered reimbursement to hospitals for upgrading their facilities and providing care to casualties.

The EMS appointed a medical director for each region and sector whose responsibilities included:[1]

■ Liaise with the hospitals in the region or sector;
■ Build cooperation in planning the precise use of each hospital;
■ Distribute medical personnel between the inner and outer zone hospitals; and
■ Act on behalf of the hospital while also being an agent of the Ministry of Health.

Within the EMS headquarters, physicians were assigned as principal medical officers of EMS for each of the following services[1]

■ First aid posts
■ Ambulances
■ Medical equipment and supplies
■ Evacuation trains
■ Pathology
■ Radiology
■ Blood transfusion
■ Dental

On September 3, 1939, the United Kingdom declared war on Germany. The Ministry of Health issued orders to completely evacuate certain hospitals to make capacity available for potential war casualties. In addition, they removed civilian patients from hospitals located in areas at risk for German attack. By that evening, all such patient movements were completed. From thirty-four London hospitals, some 3,000 patients had been transferred to their previously planned destinations by using eighteen of the twenty-one improvised hospital trains. Approximately 2,000 children were evacuated to outlying hospitals by buses converted to hold ten stretchers each. The London Passenger Transport Board had fittings and hardware prepared in advance to equip 320 buses for a medical evacuation role within 12–24 hours. In other parts of the United Kingdom similar plans resulted in a total of 163,500 beds being made available for casualties. The London area contained 51,000 of these beds. In subsequent days, the number of beds made available continued to increase. Later, the EMS relaxed some of its standards and the percentage of hospital beds held in reserve for casualties was decreased. Additionally, the EMS reimbursed hospitals for empty beds.[1]

Of special concern were the cancer specialty hospitals with their stocks of radium. Authorities feared that if the hospitals were bombed, the radium might be widely dispersed and, with its long half-life, present an environmental hazard. EMS decided to assist those hospitals with protecting their therapy sources by drilling deep bore holes in which the radium containers would be lowered during air raids. For those hospitals with small quantities of radium, a specially designed steel box was created for storage. Although many hospitals suffered bomb damage, both methods were successful in protecting the therapy sources.[1]

Special centers were also established for casualties with major psychiatric illness and orthopedic, plastic, chest, head, and burn injuries. The government took over country homes and schools and established 10,000 rehabilitation and convalescent beds in these facilities.[1] All the organizational efforts by the EMS and hospitals proved to be effective when the bombing began.

The United States Prepares

The United States government sent observers to Britain from military and other agencies, including the National Fire Protection Association (NFPA), to observe the function of the UK civil defense, fire service, and EMS system. When these observers returned to the United States, they quickly began to develop systems modeled on the information obtained from the UK. On December 1, 1941, the U.S. Office of Civilian Defense (OCD) was created. On December 7, 1941, Japan attacked the U.S. naval fleet at Pearl Harbor, Hawaii. German submarines then launched torpedo attacks on freighters and tankers off the eastern seaboard of the United States.

Following these attacks, officers of the U.S. Public Health Service (PHS) were assigned to OCD to begin developing organizational schemes and medical doctrine, and determining supply requirements, while seeking the help of U.S. hospitals. The American Hospital Association, the American Medical Association, and the American Nurses Association were also instrumental in promoting medical preparedness. Guidance was developed and included publications such as those listed in Table 22.1.[5]

Hospitals developed blackout plans and formed field medical teams composed of physicians and nurses. OCD provided each team with a two-suitcase set that contained surgical instruments, pharmaceuticals, and other medical supplies. The Military Mobilization Committee of the American Psychiatric Association prepared a publication for OCD entitled, "Reactions of People Under Stress: Anxiety and its Control."

Nurses took a leadership role in preparedness, and the publication *R.N. A Journal for Nurses* carried many articles on the subject. Furthermore, the government established the U.S. Cadet Nurse Corps in 1943 to train nurses on a massive scale to meet the needs of military and civilian hospitals. Congress passed the

Table 22.1. Medical Guidance Developed for the United States during World War II

■ Equipment and Operation of Emergency Medical Field Units
■ Protection of Hospitals
■ Central Control and Administration of Emergency Medical Services
■ Guide for the Training of Volunteer Nurses' Aides
■ Field Care and Transportation of the Injured
■ Treatment of Burns and Prevention of Wound Infection
■ The Clinical Recognition and Treatment of Shock
■ First Aid in the Prevention and Treatment of Chemical Casualties

Nurse Training Act and it became Public Law 74 on July 1, 1943. Women at least 17 years of age who were high school graduates and in good health were eligible to apply. A massive recruiting campaign ensued with various Hollywood stars promoting the program. Major corporations and women's magazines ran advertisements featuring Cadet Nurses. A 10-minute film was produced with Hollywood actresses playing Cadet Nurses. This film was subsequently shown in 16,000 movie theaters before an audience of 90 million. The recruitment campaign was very successful and the yearly quota for 65,000 recruits was easily met. The last year for new admissions began in October 1945 and the final cadets were graduated in 1948. The program was administered by PHS, which had enlisted the participation of nearly all nursing schools.

PHS not only paid tuition, but also a monthly stipend for room and board. Students pledged that, in return for education, they would serve wherever needed by the government. The Cadet Nurses were also furnished uniforms specially designed for the program, bearing the insignia of PHS. The program was an immense success with 124,000 nurses graduated by its end.[6]

By 1944, the Allied Powers were prevailing in the struggle and OCD began to dissolve itself. At war's end in 1945, the United States quickly demobilized its military and the nation concentrated on the civilian economy.

The Cold War Period

In 1949, the Soviet Union exploded an atomic bomb signaling the start of the Cold War. In 1950, the U.S. Congress passed the *Civil Defense Act* and created the new Federal Civil Defense Administration (FCDA). FCDA, like its predecessor OCD, had a medical division and again enlisted the aid of hospital and medical organizations. Planning focused on the massive casualties possible from nuclear weapons. Comparing possible casualty figures from a nuclear attack against the available number of hospitals revealed that medical resources were inadequate. In 1952, FCDA developed the prototype Civil Defense Emergency Hospital, which contained 200 beds, operating room equipment, an X-ray unit, generators, a water tank, pharmaceuticals, and medical and surgical supplies. It was a complete but austere hospital, designed to be assembled in an existing building such as a school. Furthermore, the government developed First Aid Station units and created a huge medical supply stockpile that was distributed across the nation in twenty-one warehouse complexes. In addition to the portable hospitals, the supply sets in these warehouses comprised:[7]

■ First Aid Replenishment Unit – supplies to allow operation of a First Aid Station for up to 48 hours after a disaster. Weight: 1,026 kg
■ Hospital Replenishment Unit – supplies necessary for operation of a 200-bed civil defense emergency hospital, or existing hospital, for 7 days. Weight: 5,464 kg
■ Blood Collecting Replenishment Unit – supplies for collecting 1,000 U of whole blood. Weight: 1,410 kg
■ Intravenous Solutions Replenishment Unit – supplies designed to provide intravenous solutions and sets for 100 patients for 7 days. Weight 3,529 kg
■ Medical Supplies, Hospital Back-Up – supplies in original manufacturer shipping containers sufficient for 10,000 patients for 7 days. Weight 71,840 kg
■ Blood Expanders – 24 U of dextran injection. Weight 37 kg

Subsequently, FCDA created improved models of the Civil Defense Emergency Hospitals and supply quantities were increased. Later, PHS assumed operation of the improvised hospital program and produced the largest and final model in 1962. Those hospitals were named Packaged Disaster Hospitals (PDHs). The United States had a total of 2,600 PDHs, which gave the nation a medical surge capacity of 512,000 PDH beds and 7,800 PDH operating rooms. Also created was a unit named the Hospital Reserve Disaster Inventory (HRDI). This unit consisted of pharmaceuticals, medical and surgical supplies, instruments, sterile gloves, X-ray contrast media, plaster bandages, and numerous other items. HRDIs were built in 100-bed increments and civilian hospitals could apply to receive an HRDI, at no cost, based on the number of beds they had. A hospital signed an agreement that it would integrate the HRDI items into its inventory, periodically using and replacing these supplies, thus keeping the materials from expiring. In addition, FCDA distributed publications such as Health Services and Special Weapons Defense, to train healthcare personnel about nuclear, biological, and chemical weapons effects.

Fallout shelters were also created during this period to protect the occupants from radiation in the event of a nuclear attack. Fallout shelters were equipped with food, water, sanitation kits, medical kits, and radiation measurement kits to support the civilian population in these structures. The medical kits came in two sizes depending on the capacity of the shelter and contained antibiotics, sulfa drugs, and other pharmaceuticals as well as first aid supplies.

The Medical Education for National Defense (MEND) program was another notable Cold War initiative to train U.S. physicians in disaster medicine. MEND enlisted the support of all the nation's medical schools. Contracts to some universities were issued to create mass casualty curriculums. These, in turn, were distributed without charge to the medical schools to teach their students. The MEND program operated from the mid-1950s until it was cancelled in 1972.

All of the Cold War medical preparedness programs enjoyed the support of the various national and state medical and healthcare organizations. Notwithstanding this fact, funding for the PDH program and the medical warehouses ceased in 1972. These programs were cancelled despite many protests, and by the mid-1980s, most PDHs had been dismantled or given to the Agency for International Development. Parts of remaining PDHs were used to equip the first Disaster Medical Assistance Teams of the new National Disaster Medical System, which was created in 1984. The warehoused supplies were given to state surplus property programs and others were sold at auction.

The Modern Era

In the United States, various healthcare organizations and professionals made efforts to continue some of the momentum in medical preparedness that the Cold War created; however, with the demise of the Soviet Union, less attention was paid to these matters. Nevertheless, disasters continued to occur and various scientific journals reported recurring problems with emergency management systems. The 1995 sarin nerve agent attack by cultists in Tokyo caused worldwide concern and increased emphasis on both war-related and industrial chemical training, equipment, and preparedness.

In 1999, the U.S. Congress ordered PHS to assume control over the former Noble Army Community Hospital facility located at the recently closed Fort McClellan in Alabama and convert it into a mock hospital training facility. At this renamed Noble Training Center, civilian healthcare personnel, PHS officers, and other emergency responders take courses in disaster medicine, hospital preparedness, and the medical effects of weapons of mass destruction.

The U.S. Centers for Disease Control and Prevention (CDC) developed the National Pharmaceutical Stockpile, later renamed the Strategic National Stockpile (SNS). This stockpile consists of antibiotics, chemical agent antidotes, radiation treatment drugs, ventilators, vaccines, and other pharmaceuticals and supplies configured into 12-Hour Push Packages (see Chapter 18). Each package weighs 50 tons and is ready at all times for immediate air delivery to a stricken area. Conceptually, from the time the order is received to ship supplies, a Push Package can be delivered to the designated receiving point within 12 hours. However, delays can occur, and it still needs to be further distributed to the specific locality where it is needed. Even the initial 12-hour timeline varies by event. For example, although New York City received a Push Package within hours following the terrorist attack of September 11, 2001, several days elapsed before these materials arrived in New Orleans after Hurricane Katrina. Pharmaceutical manufacturers also maintain additional vendor-managed inventory (VMI) for the SNS. Governments at the local, county, and state levels have undertaken planning to receive, store, secure, and distribute the Push Package contents. The early training courses for this program were taught at the Noble Training Center. The U.S. Department of Veterans Affairs (the largest integrated healthcare system in the nation) has also developed disaster augmentation supply units for each of its approximately 152 hospitals nationwide.

As a result of the 2014 Ebola outbreak in West Africa, which included patients treated in the United States, the SNS added specialized Personnel Protective Equipment (PPE) ready to be shipped to any U.S. hospital that encounters an Ebola patient. Traditional hospital PPE is inadequate for protection from Ebola.[8] In addition to augmentation of PPE, hospital personnel in the United States and around the globe implemented many other preparedness measures related to the potential to receive an Ebola patient.

The terrorist attacks of September 11, 2001, in the United States heightened preparedness efforts worldwide. In this event, nearly 3,000 persons were killed and hundreds injured. Articles began appearing in the professional literature on mass casualty issues; universities held disaster medicine seminars; and PHS commissioned numerous studies.

The American Hospital Association (AHA), American Medical Association (AMA), American Nurses Association, and numerous other U.S. healthcare professional organizations promote preparedness to their members, to healthcare facilities, and to communities at large, and also support government preparedness programs. This includes the support offered by the AMA's Center for Public Health Preparedness and Disaster Response.[9] In a video, the organization describes the requirement for physician involvement and training in disaster medicine to include the knowledge needed for:

- How to develop rapid protocols for triaging patients;
- How to access current antidotes and vaccines;
- How to link with local community resources and local public health officials;
- How to assess and implement the local disaster plan;

- How to obtain reliable information about patients' medications without their medical records; and
- Ethics and rationing.

Other examples of preparedness efforts are illustrated in the following sample of publications.

- *Are You Prepared? Hospital Emergency Management Guidebook*, by the Joint Commission on Accreditation of Healthcare Organizations (later renamed The Joint Commission) and Dr. Christopher Farmer. 2002.
- *Emergency Preparedness, Response and Recovery Checklist: Beyond the Emergency Management Plan*, by the American Health Lawyers Association. 2004. www.healtcarelawyers .org/HLResources/PI/Pages?EmergencyPreparedness.aspx (Accessed August 22, 2013).
- *Providing Mass Medical Care with Scare Resources: A Community Planning Guide*, by the Agency for Healthcare Research and Quality. November 2006. www.Archive.AHRQ.GOV/ Research/MCE (Accessed August 22, 2013).

Likewise, AHA and their affiliated organization, the American Society for Healthcare Engineering, assist the preparedness effort with numerous activities. Many healthcare professional societies promote preparedness to their memberships with publications and seminars. Healthcare professionals contribute literature to professional journals and are serving on preparedness committees in their communities. The U.S. Agency for Healthcare Research and Quality in the Department of Health and Human Services (HHS) produces publications covering many aspects of healthcare preparedness. The Health Resources and Services Administration of HHS supervises a hospital preparedness program and awards grants for healthcare preparedness activities and equipment.

CURRENT STATE OF THE ART

Healthcare Facility Preparedness

Increased interest in addressing the need for surge capacity both in the prehospital and hospital settings emerged in the United States in 1995 with Presidential Decision Directive 39, U.S. Policy on Terrorism.[10] This directive resulted in local governments creating Metropolitan Medical Response Teams to increase their abilities to manage mass casualties. The effort was later expanded when HHS broadened the concept of the National Disaster Medical System. Originally designed to include general medical and veterinary teams, the program subsequently created burn, mental health, crush injury, mortuary, international response, and other specialty teams.

The U.S. Congress passed and allocated funding for the *Defense Against Weapons of Mass Destruction Act*, promoting surge capacity building.[11] Other federal programs brought much needed weapons of mass destruction training to healthcare personnel. Researchers published numerous articles and manuals, and policymakers developed seminars devoted to medical surge capacity building. In January 2001, The Joint Commission made significant improvements to its emergency management accreditation standards that strengthened preparedness in hospitals. The Joint Commission also defined surge capacity to include potential patient beds; available space for triage; patient management; decontamination; vaccination; available personnel of all types;

necessary pharmaceuticals, supplies and equipment; and legal capacity to deliver care under situations that exceeded licensed capacity.[12] The Joint Commission has continued to expand emergency management standards requirements each year. A central principle to these standards is the requirement that accredited hospitals have an Emergency Management Committee (EMC).

The Emergency Management Committee

Each facility's EMC should be given the charge to:[13]

■ Develop all-hazard emergency plans;
■ Perform a hazard vulnerability analysis (HVA);
■ Coordinate with other community agencies such as fire, police, EMS, public health, public works, the emergency management agency, hazardous materials unit, and ambulance dispatch center to encourage interoperability;
■ Coordinate with the medical staff and each department of the facility; and
■ Assist in training stakeholders in the plans it develops.

The EMC needs broad participation and must be multidisciplinary. Participants should include representatives from hospital administration, medical staff, nursing staff, emergency department, security department, environmental services, plant operations, materials management, pharmacy, laboratory, radiology, ancillary services, food service, volunteer services, and all other departments of the facility. Ideally, hospital leadership should appoint persons to the EMC with a known interest in disaster preparedness, or who are at least known for their enthusiastic approach to projects. The chairperson needs to be carefully selected and understand how to lead a meeting. A secretary/recorder should keep accurate minutes in a timely manner. A library of healthcare disaster materials needs to be established for all to use and each committee member should be notified as new publications become available. Members should be encouraged and funded to attend healthcare disaster seminars and to observe as many drills and exercises as possible. Plans developed should be concise, straightforward, and widely promulgated to all operating departments and nursing areas. The inclusion of disaster plan knowledge as a factor in annual employee evaluations is also an option. A good chairperson will continually challenge members to think of multiple and complex case scenarios and stress that plans must be flexible because unforeseen incidents may happen. This "process of planning" is critical as opposed to simply having a "paper plan" with which few personnel are familiar and which is sometimes written by an outside consultant who would not be participating in managing a real event. Rather than hiring an external consultant, a plan should be created by the personnel who will use it.

In today's world, EMCs need to consider the medical impact of biological, chemical, nuclear, and explosive weapons and adopt treatment protocols such as those found on the CDC website (www.bt.cdc.gov). The committee also needs to ensure that the hospital stockpiles sufficient PPE for employees and medical staff members and trains these individuals in its proper use. Additional training should include methods of decontamination, protection of the physical plant and the airflow into the hospital, obtaining supplemental supplies, and ensuring the security of utilities and the physical plant. Communications, both internal and external, can prove vulnerable and systems frequently fail. Planning for alternate methods of communication including use of amateur radio operators and messenger services are indicated. The EMC has a large task and an even greater responsibility to the hospital and community it serves. Proper executive support and funding are essential.

Familiarization with Standards for Healthcare Emergency Management

It is essential that each member of the EMC is aware of standards and guidelines that have been promulgated for healthcare emergency management. The Joint Commission standards are one example of benchmarks for accredited facilities in the United States or worldwide through the Joint Commission International program. The Joint Commission standards for hospital emergency management are contained in *The Comprehensive Accreditation Manual for Hospitals*. Comprehensive Accreditation Manuals have also been developed for

■ Ambulatory care;
■ Behavioral healthcare;
■ Healthcare networks;
■ Critical access hospitals; and
■ Long-term care facilities.

For members of the hospital EMC, the accreditation standards are found in the Environment of Care (EC) Section. Standard EC.4.11 states: "An emergency in a health care hospital or in its community can suddenly and significantly affect demand for its services or its ability to provide those services." Therefore, a hospital must have a comprehensive plan that describes its approach to emergencies in the hospital or those in its community that may affect hospital operations. *The Comprehensive Accreditation Manual for Hospitals* includes the term disaster under its definition of an emergency. The definition is somewhat long and uses some outdated terminology (e.g. "natural and manmade"; see Perspective), but is comprehensive. The manual defines an emergency as:

> A natural or man-made event that significantly disrupts the environment of care (for example, damage to the organization's building(s) and grounds due to severe winds, storms, or earthquakes); that significantly disrupts care and treatment (for example, loss of utilities such as power, water, or telephones due to floods, civil disturbances, accidents, or emergencies in the organization or its community); or that results in sudden, significantly changed or increased demands for the organization's services (for example, bioterrorist attack, building collapse, or plane crash in the organization's community).[13]

In 2009, The Joint Commission, in an early version of the chapter on Hospital Emergency Management, stated in Standard EM.02.01.01 that the Emergency Operations Plan must identify "alternate sites for care, treatment, and services that meet the needs of its patients during emergencies."[14] The numerous emergency management plan components, standards, and responsibilities of hospital leadership and medical staff are listed within EC.4.10 and EC.4.20.

In the United States, staff members who are trained for decontamination that requires them to wear PPE must be familiar with and comply with the applicable standards of the Occupational Safety and Health Administration (OSHA) of the U.S. Department of Labor. OSHA regulates the safety and health of

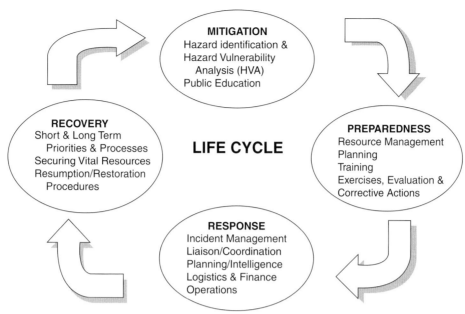

Figure 22.1. The Four Phases of Comprehensive Emergency Management.

workers by setting and enforcing standards, as well as providing training, outreach, and education. The following standards are of particular relevance to the EMC:

▪ Title 29, Code of Federal Regulations (CFR) 1910.120, Hazardous Waste Operations and Emergency Response
▪ Title 29, CFR 1910.132, Personal Protective Equipment Standard
▪ Title 29, CFR 1910.134, Respiratory Protection

OSHA has also produced a detailed publication that recommends best practices.[15] This publication discusses PPE and training for hospital first receivers. Additionally, it contains valuable references that can assist the EMC in achieving a better understanding of the issues surrounding PPE and in building a reference library. Specific recommendations regarding selection of PPE are found in Chapter 15. There are other organizations and agencies with regulatory authority, but the EMC should start with The Joint Commission and OSHA requirements.

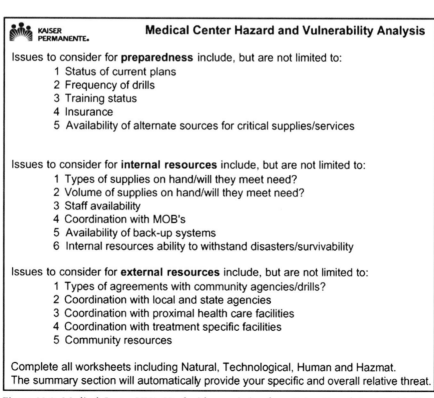

Figure 22.2. Medical Center HVA. Used with permission from Kaiser Foundation Health Plan.

Performing a Hazard Vulnerability Analysis

The Joint Commission requires accredited hospitals to have a formal document known as an HVA.[16] This process is used to identify those risks in the community that could cause an interruption or loss of a critical function or service, cause casualties, and possibly damage the hospital's physical plant. Subsequent analysis of risks identified in the HVA can then be addressed in the Emergency Management Plan.

Remembering the four phases of emergency management can aid in the preparation of an HVA.

- Mitigation – Those activities that can be undertaken, predisaster or emergency, to lessen the severity of an event. This phase also includes measures that will reduce the potential physical damage to the facility during an event.
- Preparedness – Those activities, programs, and systems that are in place before the disaster or emergency and that are used to support the response to the event. Creating inherent capacity for response to an occurrence is included.
- Response – Activities undertaken to address the immediate and short-term effects of a disaster or emergency. In the case of hospitals, it would include casualty care.
- Recovery – Activities and processes that must be undertaken to restore pre-disaster normality to the individual, facility, or community that experienced a disaster or emergency.

The U.S. Department of Veterans Affairs Emergency Management Strategic Healthcare Group has envisioned these four phases as depicted in Figure 22.1.[17]

The American Society for Healthcare Engineering of the AHA pioneered the development of hospital HVA in 2001. That same year, the Kaiser Permanente Foundation Health Plan issued their version of HVA. Both are now used extensively by U.S. hospitals. The Kaiser Permanente HVA worksheets are shown in Figures 22.2 and 22.3, and Tables 22.2–22.5.[16]

Once complete, the HVA requires a thorough review. After examination of the report, hospital emergency managers can determine the most likely threats to the community and hospital. Given this information, the institution can develop mitigation, preparedness, response, and recovery portions of the emergency management plan that address these hazards. The chair of the EMC must challenge members to think "what if" and "worst-case scenario," as well as to consider the impact of multiple events occurring simultaneously.

The hospital should collaborate with the community. The HVA should be compiled with the assistance of the local emergency management agency, fire department, EMS agency, police, hazardous materials unit, and with input from community organizations. In the United States, these entities include the American Red Cross Disaster Services, Salvation Army Disaster Services, and Voluntary Organizations Active in Disaster, as well as neighboring hospitals and the area hospital council. Similar organizations exist for other countries. If there is a major waterway or airport in the area, then HVA discussions should include additional bodies such as airport authorities, Army Corps of Engineers, Coast Guard, and state waterway police.

After generating the HVA, the next step is to rate the probability of occurrence and level of preparedness for each event. The resulting information can then be used to prepare or strengthen the facility and the emergency management plan. Nevertheless, it is possible that the HVA will not identify all potential casualty-producing incidents. The potential risks from poorly controlled nuclear weapons and radioactive material are increasing. Although the danger of all-out nuclear warfare is probably minimal, the possibility that terrorists could use one or several nuclear devices against a modern city should be addressed.

Common Factors in Disasters

To facilitate their work, the EMC should consider several factors that are common to many disasters.

1. Uncertainty – In the early stages of a disaster, it is often unclear what is transpiring, to what extent additional resources are needed, how many casualties have resulted, and the extent of the medical requirements. In addition, the exact location and magnitude of the incident may be unknown.

2. Casualty Arrival – In mass casualty incidents, especially those occurring over a wide area, the standard operating procedure of ambulance crews triaging patients and removing them in an orderly manner may not occur. In such disasters, it is common in some countries for up to 80% of the casualties to self-refer and arrive at the hospital without prehospital care on scene and en route. Casualties able to ambulate or be moved with assistance will often self-transport to area hospitals rather than waiting for arrival of EMS professionals. Well-intentioned bystanders will often transport victims in their automobiles, including those with severe injuries. Patients contaminated with hazardous materials will arrive at the hospital without having first been decontaminated at the scene. This convergence phenomenon can inundate the hospital closest to the scene with casualties, whereas other nearby facilities may receive few to none of the victims. Last, less serious cases may arrive well ahead of the most seriously injured, many of whom may be trapped in rubble.

3. Communications – Communication systems connecting the hospital to the rest of the community are vulnerable. Telephone service may fail due to overloaded circuits or physical damage. Cellular telephone communication is unreliable as the available cells can quickly become saturated. This also occurs with satellite telephones, as reported during Hurricane Katrina in the United States. Monitoring local fire, EMS, and police frequencies and having direct radio communication with first responders can greatly aid the hospital incident commander in decision making. The hospital emergency management plan should also include a provision for the use of messengers to carry information throughout the hospital in the event of telephone and computer failures. Other back-up communications options include the use of amateur radio operations and installation of emergency phones on an exchange that does not normally service the hospital.

4. Patient Care Capacity – Maintaining patient care capacity (including for those requiring hospital admission) may be problematic due to the influx of numerous casualties or a high inpatient census. The early discharge of stable patients can help the situation but the process of doing so is time-consuming, especially when family members are unable to assist. Another option includes the use of other areas in the hospital such as meeting rooms, physical therapy suites, or auditoriums for patient care to temporarily increase surge space. Hospitals must plan for supplies and staffing of these areas during the preparedness phase.

5. Staffing – Ensuring the presence of sufficient numbers of physicians, nurses, and other support personnel to staff existing patient care areas and temporarily expanded space used

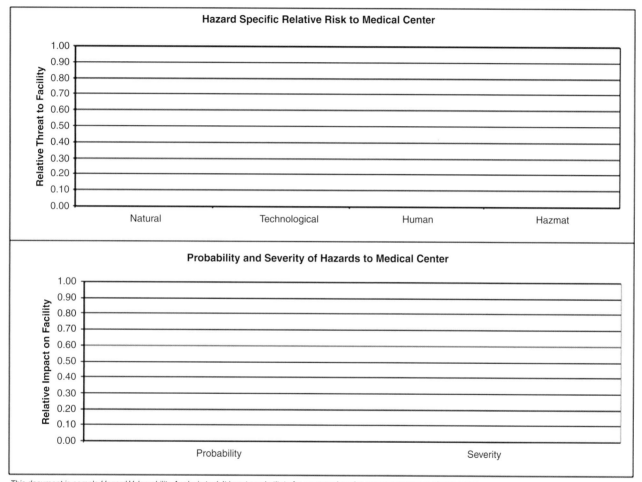

Figure 22.3. Summary of Medical Center HVA. Used with permission from Kaiser Foundation Health Plan.

for surge can be problematic, depending on the type and location of the disaster. In a severe blizzard, many individuals may have difficulty reaching the hospital. In anticipation of such circumstances, the emergency management plan should contain a list of volunteers who have four-wheel drive vehicles and are willing to transport employees and medical staff members to the hospital. In a hurricane, employees and physicians may be victims themselves, dealing with destroyed homes and offices and injured family members. In such instances, the hospital must support the staff and their family members (including pets) with sleeping accommo-

dations, shower facilities, and food service. In an infectious disease outbreak, some staff may be unwilling to report to work. Thus, the plan must account for the fact that not all staff will be willing or able to come to the hospital. The emergency management plan must provide a method for temporarily credentialing medical volunteers and a strategy for using medical personnel from country-specific volunteer medical systems such as the Medical Reserve Corps or the National Disaster Medical System in the United States.

6. Decontamination – Hospital personnel must be prepared to decontaminate victims needing such treatment prior to

Table 22.2. Hazard Vulnerability Assessment Tool for Environmental Events

EVENT	PROBABILITY	SEVERITY = (MAGNITUDE - MITIGATION)						RISK
		HUMAN IMPACT	PROPERTY IMPACT	BUSINESS IMPACT	PREPARED-NESS	INTERNAL RESPONSE	EXTERNAL RESPONSE	
	Likelihood this will occur	*Possibility of death or injury*	*Physical losses and damages*	*Interruption of services*	*Planning*	*Time, effectivness, resources*	*Community/ mutual aid staff and supplies*	*Relative threat**
SCORE	*0 = N/A* *1 = Low* *2 = Moderate* *3 = High*	*0 = N/A* *1 = Low* *2 = Moderate* *3 = High*	*0 = N/A* *1 = Low* *2 = Moderate* *3 = High*	*0 = N/A* *1 = Low* *2 = Moderate* *3 = High*	*0 = N/A* *1 = High* *2 = Moderate* *3 = Low or none*	*0 = N/A* *1 = High* *2 = Moderate* *3 = Low or none*	*0 = N/A* *1 = High* *2 = Moderate* *3 = Low or none*	*0 - 100%*
Hurricane								
Tornado								
Severe Thunderstorm								
Snowfall								
Blizzard								
Ice Storm								
Earthquake								
Tidal Wave								
Temperature Extremes								
Drought								
Flood, External								
Wild Fire								
Landslide								
Dam Inundation								
Volcano								
Epidemic								
AVERAGE SCORE								

Threat increases with percentage.

RISK = PROBABILITY × SEVERITY

Source: Used with permission from Kaiser Foundation Health Plan.

allowing them to enter the facility. Decontamination is essential not only to support patient care but also to prevent contamination of the hospital, potentially rendering it nonfunctional. The healthcare institution must maintain sufficient quantities of PPE to permit rotation of decontamination staff, taking into consideration the fatigue factor and heat load stress when wearing PPE. The selection of PPE is a complex task (see Chapter 15). Maintaining a variety of types of PPE to protect against multiple hazards and ensuring appropriate staff training is essential for worker safety.[18,19]

7. Prophylaxis – It may be necessary to offer hospital employees and the medical staff antibiotics and vaccinations as prophylaxis during an epidemic or after the terrorist release of a biological agent. A protocol is needed to ensure adequate supplies and efficient distribution methods.

8. Laboratory Support – Most hospital laboratories lack the capability to safely and definitively identify many biological weapons agents, emerging infectious diseases, or hazardous materials. The EMC must know the capabilities of the in-house laboratory and ensure that arrangements have been made with state, national, or international reference laboratories to supplement diagnostic resources within the facility in the event of an outbreak or exposure. Such diagnostic resources must be available 24/7.

9. Media Relations – Members of the media will telephone or quickly arrive at the hospital when disaster strikes. A plan must be in place to accommodate the media and also to manage them, restricting their access to patient care areas and preventing them from disrupting the hospital's response.

Often, accurate information may not be immediately available to the healthcare facility's designated public information officer. Other information may be known but disclosure may not be possible as it would violate federal privacy laws. Social media has complicated information management during disasters. The FEMA Emergency Management Institute offers disaster public information training for health department and hospital personnel.

10. Morgue – Hospitals generally have limited refrigerated space for the temporary storage of the deceased. Consideration must be given to a potentially large death toll and the subsequent need for increased storage space for remains (see Chapter 23).

11. Utilities – A disaster event could curtail some or all of the hospitals utilities. Water is especially critical for hospital operations and backup supplies must be organized in advance. Storage of water on the grounds of the facility is one option. Generators supplying emergency power may prove unreliable for extended operations. Plans should exist for renting generators and wiring them to the hospital's electrical grid. If the hospital uses fuel oil to power the generators or boilers, the EMC should calculate the number of hours or days of supply the institution has on hand under both temperate and winter conditions.

12. Supplies – With the healthcare industry relying on just-in-time inventories, supply shortages may quickly manifest. Plans are needed for emergency resupply if contracted vendors cannot respond or normal supply channels are disrupted. Community-wide planning is essential to prevent

Table 22.3. Hazard Vulnerability Assessment Tool for Technological Events

EVENT	PROBABILITY	SEVERITY = (MAGNITUDE - MITIGATION)						RISK
		HUMAN IMPACT	PROPERTY IMPACT	BUSINESS IMPACT	PREPARED-NESS	INTERNAL RESPONSE	EXTERNAL RESPONSE	
	Likelihood this will occur	*Possibility of death or injury*	*Physical losses and damages*	*Interruption of services*	*Planning*	*Time, effectivness, resources*	*Community/ mutual aid staff and supplies*	*Relative threat**
SCORE	0 = N/A 1 = Low 2 = Moderate 3 = High	0 = N/A 1 = Low 2 = Moderate 3 = High	0 = N/A 1 = Low 2 = Moderate 3 = High	0 = N/A 1 = Low 2 = Moderate 3 = High	0 = N/A 1 = High 2 = Moderate 3 = Low or none	0 = N/A 1 = High 2 = Moderate 3 = Low or none	0 = N/A 1 = High 2 = Moderate 3 = Low or none	0 - 100%
Electrical Failure								
Generator Failure								
Transportation Failure								
Fuel Shortage								
Natural Gas Failure								
Water Failure								
Sewer Failure								
Steam Failure								
Fire Alarm Failure								
Communications Failure								
Medical Gas Failure								
Medical Vacuum Failure								
HVAC Failure								
Information Systems Failure								
Fire, Internal								
Flood, Internal								
Hazmat Exposure, Internal								
Supply Shortage								
Structural Damage								
AVERAGE SCORE								

*Threat increases with percentage.

RISK = PROBABILITY × SEVERITY

Source: Used with permission from Kaiser Foundation Health Plan.

multiple hospitals depending on the same supplier if that entity has inadequate resources for the number of facilities that need them. Additionally, hospitals must include items appropriate for pediatric care in their supply inventories as they must prepare for the arrival of pediatric patients.

13. Blood Products – During a disaster, blood and blood product usage may rise above normal levels. Hospitals must anticipate this contingency and plan to address any shortfalls. Conversely, in some types of disasters, additional blood is not needed. However, well-meaning volunteers may present in large numbers wanting to donate. A system for volunteer management is important to avoid redirecting resources needed for control of the incident to handle this influx.

14. Medical Equipment – In a disaster situation, a hospital may face a shortage of beds, ventilators, respiratory therapy equipment and supplies, oxygen cylinders, intravenous infusion pumps, wheelchairs, and gurneys. Institutions must plan for supplemental delivery of these items.

15. Service Deliveries – Ensuring continuity of critical service deliveries such as medical gases, generator fuel, linens, medical and surgical supplies, foodstuffs, and waste removal is essential to continued operations. Plans must exist that maintain availability of these critically needed items.

16. Security – Plans are required for securing the facility and grounds, directing traffic, protecting human remains, and managing personal effects. During a disaster, requirements may exceed the capacity of the security department. In support of increased security demands, the emergency management plan should assign non-security personnel to provide some security duties, such as traffic direction or supervision of facility entrances. In addition, hospital security plans must permit rapid implementation of a total facility lockdown, allowing only certain supervised entrances to remain open. This is especially important when faced with contaminated casualties. Reliance on local law enforcement personnel to respond and assist is usually not an option as they will be occupied managing the disaster within the community.

17. Care of Relatives and Friends – During a disaster, family members and friends of patients may rush to a hospital, even with just the suspicion that a relative was taken there. Plans must exist for receiving and assisting family members of victims.

18. Damaged Hospitals – Hospitals are susceptible to physical damage. Tornados, hurricanes, and earthquakes have repeatedly compromised hospital function. Healthcare institutions must plan for emergent damage inspection and repair. In severe situations, hospitals must also have a strategy to

Table 22.4. Hazard Vulnerability Assessment Tool Related to Human Activity

EVENT	PROBABILITY	SEVERITY = (MAGNITUDE - MITIGATION)						RISK
		HUMAN IMPACT	PROPERTY IMPACT	BUSINESS IMPACT	PREPARED-NESS	INTERNAL RESPONSE	EXTERNAL RESPONSE	
	Likelihood this will occur	*Possibility of death or injury*	*Physical losses and damages*	*Interruption of services*	*Planning*	*Time, effectivness, resources*	*Community/ mutual aid staff and supplies*	*Relative threat**
SCORE	*0 = N/A 1 = Low 2 = Moderate 3 = High*	*0 = N/A 1 = Low 2 = Moderate 3 = High*	*0 = N/A 1 = Low 2 = Moderate 3 = High*	*0 = N/A 1 = Low 2 = Moderate 3 = High*	*0 = N/A 1 = High 2 = Moderate 3 = Low or none*	*0 = N/A 1 = High 2 = Moderate 3 = Low or none*	*0 = N/A 1 = High 2 = Moderate 3 = Low or none*	0 - 100%
Mass Casualty Incident (trauma)								
Mass Casualty Incident (medical/infectious)								
Terrorism, Biological								
VIP Situation								
Infant Abduction								
Hostage Situation								
Civil Disturbance								
Labor Action								
Forensic Admission								
Bomb Threat								
AVERAGE SCORE								

Threat increases with percentage.

RISK = PROBABILITY × SEVERITY

Source: Used with permission from Kaiser Foundation Health Plan.

Table 22.5. Hazard Vulnerability Assessment Tool Events Involving Hazardous Materials

EVENT	PROBABILITY	SEVERITY = (MAGNITUDE - MITIGATION)						RISK
		HUMAN IMPACT	PROPERTY IMPACT	BUSINESS IMPACT	PREPARED-NESS	INTERNAL RESPONSE	EXTERNAL RESPONSE	
	Likelihood this will occur	*Possibility of death or injury*	*Physical losses and damages*	*Interruption of services*	*Planning*	*Time, effectivness, resources*	*Community/ mutual aid staff and supplies*	*Relative threat**
SCORE	*0 = N/A 1 = Low 2 = Moderate 3 = High*	*0 = N/A 1 = Low 2 = Moderate 3 = High*	*0 = N/A 1 = Low 2 = Moderate 3 = High*	*0 = N/A 1 = Low 2 = Moderate 3 = High*	*0 = N/A 1 = High 2 = Moderate 3 = Low or none*	*0 = N/A 1 = High 2 = Moderate 3 = Low or none*	*0 = N/A 1 = High 2 = Moderate 3 = Low or none*	0 - 100%
Mass Casualty Hazmat Incident *(from historic events at your MC with >= 5 victims)*								
Small Casualty Hazmat Incident *(from historic events at your MC with < 5 victims)*								
Chemical Exposure, External								
Small to Medium Sized Internal Spill								
Large Internal Spill								
Terrorism, Chemical								
Radiologic Exposure, Internal								
Radiologic Exposure, External								
Terrorism, Radiologic								
AVERAGE SCORE								

Threat increases with percentage.

RISK = PROBABILITY × SEVERITY

Source: Used with permission from Kaiser Foundation Health Plan.

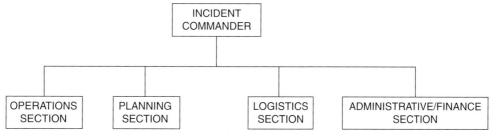

Figure 22.4. Basic Incident Command System Diagram.

evaluate hospital structural integrity and evacuate the facility if indicated.[21,22]

Health Facility Management of Disaster

When a disaster occurs, the emergency management plan must be activated and the healthcare facility must quickly mobilize its resources and key personnel, ideally before the first casualty arrives. The hospital may organize its response in a variety of ways, as long as The Joint Commission or similar requirements for coordination with community plans are met.

The Incident Command System

The Incident Command System (ICS) is a disaster management strategy that is growing in popularity among hospitals. ICS was first developed in the 1970s by California firefighters for better management of wide-scale forest and wildfires. The group who developed the ICS was known as FIRESCOPE. ICS was later adapted to the hospital setting. It offers hospitals many advantages in managing their disaster responses:[23]

- Standard organization and procedures
- Modular and scalable system for any size disaster
- Interactive management components
- Management by objectives
- Manageable span of control
- Designated incident facilities
- Comprehensive resource management
- Integrated communications
- Procedures for establishing and transferring command
- Accountability
- Easy integration with the community response
- Avoiding duplication of effort

ICS is essentially a toolbox that provides utilities for the command, control, and coordination of resources during a disaster. ICS clarifies roles and responsibilities between all persons in the system, while also organizing resources, personnel, facilities, equipment, and communications through common procedures.

The basic ICS is composed of an Incident Commander assisted by an Operations Section, Planning Section, Logistics Section, and Finance/Administration Section (see Chapter 11).

- Operations Section
  - Directly manages all incident activities and implements the Incident Action Plan.
  - Works closely with other members of the command and general staff to coordinate response tactics.
- Planning Section
  - Gathers, analyzes, and disseminates intelligence and information gleaned from available sources.
  - Manages the planning process and maintains incident documentation.
  - Compiles and develops the Incident Action Plan.
  - Tracks all incident resources.
  - Manages the activities of assigned technical specialists.
  - Develops the demobilization plan.
- Logistics Section
  - Meets the support needs for the incident, including ordering resources through appropriate procurement authorities from non-incident locations.
  - Provides facilities, transportation, supplies, equipment, maintenance support, fueling, food service, and communications.
- Finance/Administration Section
  - Establishes whether there is a specific need for financial, reimbursement, and/or administrative services to support incident activities.
  - Takes responsibility for time-keeping records and compilations of hospital costs incurred during the disaster response.

MULTIAGENCY COORDINATION SYSTEMS

In large incidents, a Multiagency Coordination System (MACS) may be established. A MACS is a combination of facilities, equipment, personnel, procedures, and communications integrated into one common system and principally relying on an Emergency Operations Center (EOC). Within the EOC, a medical operations center or joint public health command center is usually established. The hospital disaster command structure will usually report to this entity. A MACS is especially helpful in areas of high population density or where the disaster is geographically widespread. Figure 22.4 illustrates the basic incident command structure.

THE HOSPITAL INCIDENT COMMAND SYSTEM

Initially developed as the Hospital Emergency Incident Command System, in its fourth revision, the name was changed to the Hospital Incident Command System (HICS). The historical development of HICS is as follows.[23]

1987 – Hospital Council of Northern California adapts FIRESCOPE ICS to hospitals.
1991 – Hospital Emergency Incident Command System, version 1 (HEICS I) first released.
1993 – HEICS II released.
1998 – HEICS III released.
2006 – U.S. government-funded project to revise HEICS. The development of version IV creates the HICS in compliance with the National Incident Management System (NIMS).

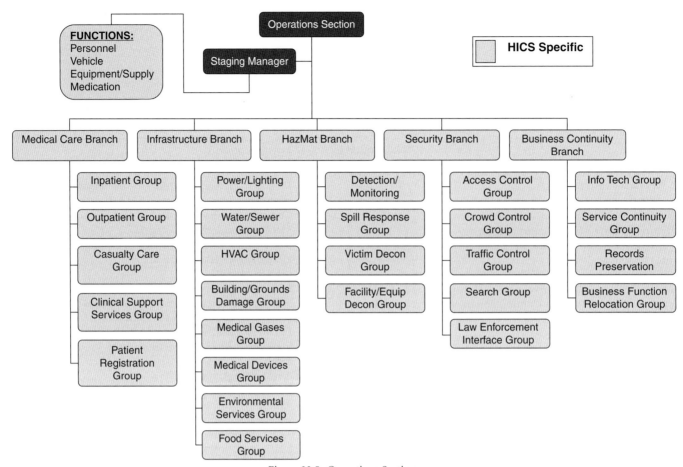

Figure 22.5. Operations Section.

2014 – HICS V released with multiple updates since the 2006 version.[24]

The HICS resources include[25]

■ Exercise scenarios;
■ Planning guides;
■ Job action sheets;
■ HICS forms; and
■ Training materials.

HICS adds healthcare-specific titles to the ICS. On the organizational chart for the command and general staff, the Incident Commander (IC) has the prerogative to add components to the chart, identifying individuals who report to the IC. An example is a medical/technical healthcare specialist needed for a response to a particular disaster. Such individuals would include:

■ Infectious disease consultants;
■ Chemical and radiological consultants;
■ Hospital administration representatives;
■ Hospital legal officers;
■ Hospital risk managers; and
■ Medical staff officers.

As previously mentioned, all ICS systems including HICS are modular and scalable according to the requirements to manage

the disaster, the hospital size, and the availability of personnel and medical staff. The EMC should decide in advance what roles will be needed and initially staff these positions with on-duty personnel. Following activation of HICS, additional personnel determined by the hospital's response needs would then be recruited to backfill these positions. The HICS chart is based on emergency functions and differs from the hospital's routine organizational or functional chart.

The command and general staff sections of Operations, Planning, Logistics, and Finance/Administration have a hierarchical structure that translates into a manageable span of control. Depending on the size and duration of the event, each section may need division into branches, with various defined groups, led by a supervisor, under the branch and reporting to the branch director. Graphically, the Operations Section could appear as shown in Figure 22.5.[23] An example of a Planning Section chart appears in Figure 22.6.[23] The Logistics Section is graphically depicted in Figure 22.7.[23]

The Finance/Administration Section of HICS includes important units for documenting costs and hospital and employee compensation during the hospital response and recovery phases. Because many hospitals have cash flow problems, this is a very significant post-disaster function. In the United States, the hospital may be eligible for reimbursement from the federal government if the president declares the event a disaster, but only if the expenses are properly documented. Also, the procurement unit within this section must keep the hospital supplied with consumable items and must arrange contracts for emergency

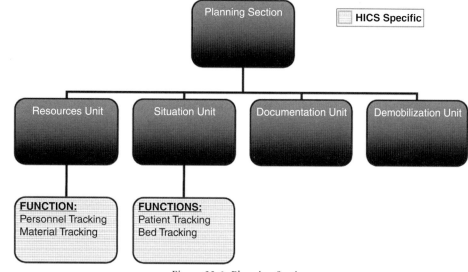

Figure 22.6. Planning Section.

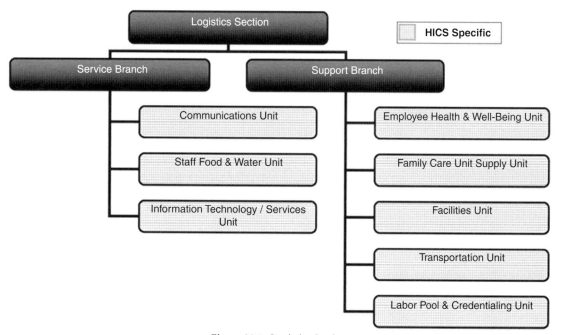

Figure 22.7. Logistics Section.

supplies. A typical Finance/Administration Section chart would be similar to that shown in Figure 22.8.[23]

While every hospital has a defined organizational chart for normal operations, the command and control system necessary to manage an emergency differs from the routine reporting structure. HICS tables of organization provide a logical framework with which to coordinate the hospital's response. Additionally, these tables allow individuals with particular strengths, not listed on the standard organizational chart for normal operations, to be used in the most effective manner. For example, the chief of surgery may request the assistance of another surgeon, perhaps with military combat medical experience, to head the medical care branch that manages mass casualties.

In smaller incidents, it may not be necessary to activate and staff the five basic HICS positions. The IC may perform all the functions alone in some cases. What is essential is that the IC

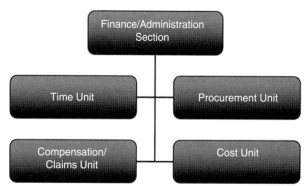

Figure 22.8. Finance/Administration Section.

has a clear picture of the incident, the estimated casualty load, and the response needed, and staffs the HICS system accordingly. HICS training is available without cost online.[24]

The National Incident Management System

ICS is an integral part of a post-September 11, 2001, U.S. initiative in managing all-hazard incidents. In 2003, the president of the United States issued Homeland Security Presidential Directive 5 (HSPD 5), directing the Secretary of Homeland Security to develop and administer NIMS. This system provides a consistent nationwide framework that enables federal, state, local, and tribal organizations to work together effectively to prepare for, respond to, and recover from all-hazard incidents regardless of cause, size, or complexity, including terrorist attacks. NIMS is built on existing concepts of incident management that have stood the test of time. NIMS represents a core set of doctrines, concepts, principles, and terminology that permit effective collaboration in incident management at all levels of governments and private organizations. HSPD 5 requires all federal departments and agencies to make adoption of NIMS by state and local organizations a condition for funding from federal preparedness grants. The components of NIMS include:[26]

- Command and Management;
- Incident Management System;
- Multiagency Coordination Systems;
- Public Information Systems;
- Preparedness;
- Planning;
- Training;
- Exercises;
- Personnel Qualifications and Certification;
- Equipment Acquisition and Certification;
- Mutual Aid;
- Publications Management;
- Resource Management;
- Communications and Information Management;
- Supporting Technology; and
- Ongoing Management and Maintenance.

NIMS was launched by then-Secretary of Homeland Security Tom Ridge on March 1, 2004. In September 2006, FEMA announced the publication of *NIMS Implementation Activities for Hospitals and Healthcare Systems*.[26] The publication outlines the seventeen elements healthcare facilities must accomplish to become NIMS compliant and eligible for federal preparedness grants:

Element 1 – Adopt NIMS at the organizational level.

Element 2 – Manage all emergency incidents, exercises, and "preplanned" events utilizing the HICS.

Element 3 – MACS: Develop connectivity capability with the area hospital command center, as used in catastrophic, wide geographical area, or smaller incidents, to the local EOC, local 911 centers, local public health, EMS, local emergency operating center, and others as appropriate.

Element 4 – Public Information System – The healthcare facility manages information with the various healthcare partners and response agencies through a Joint Information System and Joint Information Center.

Element 5 – The hospital/healthcare facility/healthcare system will track NIMS activities annually as part of the organized emergency management plan.

Element 6 – Development and coordination of a system to track local, state, and federal preparedness grants. Document that preparedness grants received meet any funding commitments.

Element 7 – Revise and update plans and procedures to incorporate NIMS components in all emergency phases and activities.

Element 8 – Participate in and promote interagency mutual aid agreements with public and private sectors.

Element 9 – Train those personnel who have emergency preparedness and response duties in NIMS by completing the free online course IS-700.a National Incident Management System: An Introduction. This online course can be found at http://training.fema.gov/IS (Accessed August 22, 2013).

Element 10 – Train those personnel who have emergency preparedness and response duties in the National Response Plan by completing the free online course IS-800.b National Response Framework: An Introduction. This course can be found at: http://training.fema.gov/IS (Accessed August 22, 2013).

Note: for both courses, it has been recommended that a phased approach would allow employees and physicians to complete the training without a time constraint burden on the hospital. Successful completion of both courses could be an element in the employee periodic performance evaluation.

Element 11 – The organization's primary emergency preparedness and response personnel complete free online courses: IS-100.HCb Introduction to the Incident Command System for Healthcare/Hospitals and IS-200.HCa Applying ICS to Healthcare Organizations. These free online courses can be found at http://training.fema.gov/IS (Accessed August 22, 2013).

Element 12 – Preparedness Exercises – The organization's emergency management program training and exercise documentation reflects the use of NIMS/ICS.

Element 13 – Participate in an all-hazard exercise program based on NIMS that involves responders from multiple disciplines, agencies, and organizations.

Element 14 – Hospitals and healthcare systems will incorporate corrective actions into preparedness and response plans/procedures.

Element 15 – Maintain a current resource inventory of medical-surgical supplies, pharmaceuticals, PPE, staffing, and so forth.

Element 16 – To the extent possible and permitted by law, the organization should work to establish common equipment and communications data interoperability with other local hospitals, EMS, public health, and emergency management agencies.

Element 17 – Apply standardized and consistent terminology, including the establishment of plain English communication standards across the public safety sector.

Hospital Physical Plant Preparedness

While the EMC is focused primarily on direct patient care capacity and capability, optimal patient outcomes depend on a functioning physical plant. Rarely do hospital personnel, even executives, think about the physical plant becoming non-operational. Hospitals and other healthcare facilities have suffered significant damage resulting from hurricanes, tornadoes, fires, and earthquakes. Therefore, the EMC must become familiar with the physical plant and its systems, and work with the plant operations leader to maximize preparedness. Ideally, the head of plant operations should be a member of the EMC. The critical hospital systems that must remain functional include

- Electrical;
- Heating, ventilating, and air conditioning (HVAC);
- Water and sewer;
- Medical equipment including vacuum and medical gases;
- Various life support and critical care systems; and
- Communications systems: pagers, public address, computers, and radios.

ELECTRICAL

In the U.S. model, there has historically been a disparity between what building codes require that emergency generators support and the hospital's electrical power requirements for patient care. The codes are designed to address life safety issues and protect occupants in the event of a power failure, fire, or other emergency. The level of electrical generator support is limited to that required to permit the occupants to safely exit the building. The code does not recognize the need to provide power for operating autoclaves, laboratory and radiology equipment, and other devices necessary for hospital function during a disaster. The members of the EMC should know what equipment and what locations receive power from emergency generators in the event of a power failure, how long the fuel supply will last when the generators are running, and how long they will run if the fuel must be shared with the boilers. Further action may be necessary to ensure these additional essential components receive emergency power. Another approach to minimize the threat of power disruption is to provide normal electrical service to the facility from two different utility substations.

Time of year can also increase the fuel consumption needs of boilers as well as pose other challenges. During a blackout in a New England winter, a small community hospital initially received emergency power from its generators. The hospital had an above-ground fuel storage tank and had forgotten to connect the immersion heater to the generator circuitry. After several hours the fuel cooled, became more viscous, and resulted in a generator shutdown.

In August 2003, a considerable portion of the northeast United States experienced a blackout, at first thought to be caused by a terrorist attack but later found to be caused by faulty equipment in Ohio. Hospitals throughout the region were forced to use emergency power – supplied by generators. As had been reported in previous disasters, several institutions experienced failure of this critical equipment and lost power. This illustrates the importance of the EMC needing to identify and maintain equipment and locations that receive emergency power from the generators.

The requirements of The Joint Commission mandating tests of the emergency generators should be considered the absolute minimum for testing the generators. Diesel engines need to be run at, or near, full load of the engine rating and not just the connected electrical load, for approximately 15% of the run time. They need a heavy load for most of the time remaining in the test. There are islands in the Caribbean that use the same type of generators as U.S. hospitals. These units may run for months without shutdown. It is what these generators are built to do if

properly exercised and maintained. U.S. hospitals do not exercise them enough and then are challenged when they cease to run. Other good practices include changing oil as recommended by the manufacturer, and changing the generator coolant at least every other year, or more frequently if recommended by the manufacturer. Only distilled water should be used to mix with the antifreeze to prevent mineral buildup and resultant loss of cooling capacity of the radiator. Batteries should be replaced every three years as a good practice, and at each oil change a sample should be sent for an independent analysis. The fuel in the tanks should be reconditioned annually by running it through a staged series of water separators and filters. Fuel should be analyzed on site until it reaches the specified clarity and quality. Further, a manual dipstick, coated with water indicator paste, should be performed weekly on each tank, rather than relying on a gauge that could be faulty.

The transfer switch that locks out commercial power and allows generated power to the hospital is a link in the chain of proper functioning. For this reason, the transfer switch needs to be periodically inspected and connections tested. If the switch fails, there will be no power to the hospital from the generators. In areas subject to earthquake, there have been instances where tremors caused emergency generators to fail. This problem can be prevented with proper mounts.[28]

An additional concern created by use of supplemental standby power is the extent to which the laboratory and radiology can operate their equipment relying on this source. Furnishing generator power to these departments is insufficient. Some devices have unique requirements relating to electrical current flow and personnel must know whether the cyclical fluctuation of the generator will cause delicate equipment to malfunction or fail completely. Such conditions must be anticipated pre-event and addressed collaboratively between EMC and plant operations representatives.

Because generators and transfer switches can malfunction even after proper maintenance, the hospital should have an ample supply of flashlights, battery-powered lights, headlamps, and batteries as a safeguard against generator failure. Illumination sources using light-emitting diodes (LED) conserve battery power and should be considered.

Natural gas is a common fuel and may power the hospital's air conditioning system, boilers, hot water, cooking ranges, ovens, and generators. Although natural gas is more reliable during storms than overhead electrical lines, it is extremely vulnerable to earthquakes and mudslides.

HEATING, VENTILATING, AND AIR CONDITIONING

In compliance with ventilation codes, a hospital in the United States can draw in more pounds of air per day than pounds of water. The typical hospital will have multiple handling units that pass the incoming air through mechanical or electronic filters, heat or cool the air, humidify or dehumidify the air, and send it to the various areas of the hospital. This air does not linger in the building and is removed by exhaust fans. Hospitals have high energy costs due to compliance with these building codes. Little recirculation is permitted as an infection control measure, and a large number of air exchanges per hour are required. If the hospital does not have adequate emergency generator capacity, there will be a shutdown of this system and also air conditioning. If the air conditioning chillers are fueled by natural gas, the loss of this supply will also shut down the units. During and after Hurricane Katrina, many hospitals in the affected area experienced temperatures of over 37°C, creating a significant hardship for patients and staff. Certain types of equipment cannot function in that temperature range. Because the applicable codes do not require emergency generator power to HVAC equipment, the prudent facility spends the extra money and purchases larger-capacity generators after a thorough analysis of emergency electrical needs. This pre-event strategy can protect the multiple services not addressed by regulatory codes that are required to operate the hospital and provide patient care. Whatever the type of disaster, planners must understand that loss of power or other utilities can severely limit patient care capacity.

The hospital's HVAC system can become a safety hazard in the event of a chemical spill. Transportation and industrial accidents can release chemicals that are carried through the air. If a hospital is downwind of a chemical plume, it will quickly draw the chemical into the building by the air-handling units, and this may in turn sicken or even kill staff and patients. The EMC, as an all-hazard planning committee, must be cognizant of this possibility and plan accordingly.

The first consideration is the location of the air intakes for the hospital. Because many chemicals are heavier than air, ground level air intakes are particularly susceptible to drawing in contamination. Some hospitals have intakes mounted on the side of the building, which is better, especially if they are 4.6 meters or more above the ground. The best location is on the roof; however, even rooftop units do not guarantee that the hospital cannot become contaminated. Due to the risk of terrorism, hospital planners must be mindful of the need for security of these air-handling intakes. Additional information about protecting the building and its occupants is found in *Guidance for Protecting Building Environments from Airborne Chemical, Biological or Radiological Attacks*.[28,29]

To protect the facility from such an event, the EMC must develop a plan to lock all external entrances to the hospital and to guard them. The engineering department must rehearse the shutdown of all air-handling units to prevent the chemical or smoke from entering into the building. Also, security officers should be taught this procedure to assist the engineer on duty or in case the engineer becomes incapacitated. If evacuation of the facility is not appropriate, using this shelter-in-place strategy to protect patients is the best option.

WATER

Water is an absolute necessity to keep the hospital functioning. The EMC should determine whether the utility company feeds water to the hospital from two directions. This is a safeguard in the event of a water main break. Another option is to have a continuous loop that surrounds the hospital property. Some hospitals have storage tanks that are constantly refreshed by a main water line. An supplementary water tank for fire protection is also a prudent investment. Additional strategies for water supply include bottled water, arrangements with water-hauling companies, and pre-event agreements with the community emergency management agency for assistance. In the case of slow-onset events such as hurricanes, the hospital can fill water bladders if they have them. These can be purchased in a variety of sizes. Bladders are also useful for on-site storage of delivered water if a means of extracting the water is available.

The EMC must also develop a water-rationing plan including alternate means of disposing of human waste. To avoid further loss of limited supplies, patient and employee commodes can be lined with plastic bags. Following use, several ounces of chlorine bleach can be added and then the contents can be double bagged. A standby contract for portable toilets can be helpful, especially for hospital personnel and visitors. Planners must determine how the facility will dispose of human waste.

Some hospitals have wells on their campuses. In these cases, the EMC must ensure the pumps are connected to the emergency generator. Wells, however, can be damaged or destroyed by earthquakes and some other types of disasters so contingency plans must be in place.

DAMAGE CONTROL

Healthcare facilities can be damaged in a disaster; however, they are expected to remain functional and remain open for patient care. For the protection of patients and personnel, the facility should have a damage control plan. The damage control plan should be developed jointly by the plant operations personnel and the EMC. The plan outlines a methodology whereby reports are received at a central point such as the hospital EOC from the various departments regarding damage their area has experienced. At the same time, management staff should dispatch employees to conduct a rapid needs assessment of every floor and department. These employees then report their findings to the EOC. A person/position designated in the Damage Control Plan then reviews the damage list and determines the emergency repair priorities in consultation with the IC and chief of the Operations Section. The work of the damage control team can be greatly facilitated if the following equipment is contained in a storage area on site: floor plans, rolls of plastic and lathing strips for covering windows, spools of wire, sprinkler plugs, hand tools, gasoline-powered rescue saws with blades for steel and concrete, dewatering pumps, portable oxy-acetylene torches, flashlights, headlamps, portable flood lights, sheets of exterior plywood, saws, pry bars, and materials for controlling chemical spills. Large-sized facilities should consider creating several such storage areas. The hospital must aim toward self-sufficiency for at least the first 72 hours and not expect external assistance from emergency response agencies because these groups are fully committed in a disaster and their capabilities are frequently exceeded.

SUPPLIES

From a preparedness standpoint, a weakness in the hospital industry is the just-in-time inventory system. Although such systems improve cash flow and are efficient during routine operations, they are unreliable in a disaster, especially one that covers a large geographical area such as Hurricane Katrina. Because a just-in-time system depends heavily on truck transportation, this can become problematic due to obstruction of transportation corridors after a disaster.

The AHA's Association for Healthcare Resource and Materials Management (AHRMM) in concert with the Health Industry Group Purchasing Association and the Health Industry Distribution Association created a preparedness document.[29] This publication consists of a core and pediatric inventory and then adds specific items needed for managing the effects of terrorist attacks with chemical, radiological, explosive, nuclear, or biological weapons. The document also contains recommendations for staff PPE. Laboratory and radiological supply needs are not included. The Minnesota Department of Health's website contains a more refined list.[30]

As previously cited in the section on History of Healthcare Disaster Planning and Preparedness, the United States no longer has the massive reserves of medical and surgical supplies of past years. In addition, reliance on the military medical service is somewhat problematic. Their first commitment is to national defense; therefore they have limited resources to participate in civilian disaster response. The reduction of combat support hospitals and other field medical units as well as diminished military medical supply inventories also limits their ability to respond.

The EMC should carefully consider the cited lists, determine desired inventory levels, and decide whether the hospital can afford to increase supply levels of frequently used items. Additionally, the materials management department can craft pre-event purchase orders, arranging contracts with suppliers for emergency shipments and mutual aid agreements with neighboring hospitals or as part of a multi-hospital system. These arrangements should part of community-wide planning to avoid multiple facilities in the region depending on the same supplier. Standby agreements should also be established with medical suppliers outside the immediate area in case local suppliers are unable to deliver the requested inventory.

COMMUNICATIONS

Communications problems are a recurring issue in most disasters. The EMC should review the stability of existing communications systems in the hospital such as the telephone, paging, and computer systems. Emergency responders increasingly rely on web-based toolboxes and social media for disaster management. If the hospital also uses these tools and the Internet fails, an auxiliary system must be available. Implementation of paper documentation and use of runners are options.

The use of cellular telephones may prove unreliable as available circuit capacity can quickly be exceeded. The same occurs with regular telephones. For any given system, the equipment is designed to handle only a certain percentage of the telephones in the area at any one time. If too many individuals attempt to place calls simultaneously, the system will not function, even if there is no physical damage. During Hurricane Katrina, even satellite telephones proved unreliable for this reason. As an alternate to the usual communication devices, the hospital should consider purchasing handheld portable radios. In addition, it is prudent to have a hospital radio system for communicating with local responders and the regional emergency management agency. The greater Cincinnati area pioneered a radio system linking all hospitals, the dispatch center, weather bureau, and three mobile units in 1965. A supervisory committee provides system quality and procedure review, and updates policies. An 800 MHz system was installed in 2011 and now all hospitals in a thirteen-county region are linked by radio. This system has proven effective over the decades. With the widespread use of social media, disaster planners should anticipate its use under disaster conditions and develop management strategies. Social media can be a useful tool but also creates a risk that inaccurate and contradictory information is rapidly disseminated to multiple sources.

The hospital EMC can also establish a relationship with an area amateur radio unit that performs disaster and emergency communications. These operators can be very helpful to the hospital for both internal and external communications. Such emergency radio teams usually belong to organizations such as the Amateur Radio Emergency Service, the Radio Amateur Civil Emergency Service, or the Salvation Army Team Emergency Radio Network.

For internal communications, the EMC should devise a plan to use messengers should other systems fail. These individuals can visit each important location within the hospital and collect and distribute the messages.

Surge Capacity for Healthcare Facilities

Background

Beginning in the early 1990s, increased attention has focused on surge capacity. The United States has suffered devastating hurricanes, earthquakes, and terrorist attacks and is concerned about mass casualties from a pandemic. Canada had a SARS outbreak that overwhelmed healthcare assets in Toronto and could have extended nationally. Many other nations have experienced significant events such as tsunamis, radiologic emergencies, catastrophic earthquakes, and terrorist attacks. There have been numerous articles and seminars on surge capacity.[32] While the concepts have been well defined, substantively little has been done to operationalize them. One reason for this is that there is little funding to hospitals to encourage development of surge capacity.

The loss of surge capacity has a variety of causes. The U.S. government cancelled the Packaged Disaster Hospital and Hospital Reserve Disaster Inventory Programs. In addition, managed care and the move to the outpatient care model have contributed to hospital closures and conversion of this space to other uses. To reverse this trend, the development of surge capacity requires new emphasis on personnel, medical supplies and equipment, and patient care space coupled with an incident management structure, frequently referred to as the 3-S System: "staff, stuff, and structure" (see Chapter 3).[33]

In 2005, the U.S. government developed a Target Capabilities List that identified priorities for Medical Surge and Medical Supplies Management and Distribution.[34] The 2007 update to the list defines medical surge as

> the capability to rapidly expand the capacity of the existing healthcare system (long-term care facilities, community health agencies, acute care facilities, alternate care facilities and public health departments) in order to provide triage and subsequent medical care. This includes providing definite care to individuals at the appropriate clinical levels of care, within sufficient time to achieve recovery and minimize medical complications. Medical surge is defined as rapid expansion of the capacity of the existing healthcare system in response to an event that results in increased need of personnel (clinical and nonclinical), support functions (laboratories and radiological), physical space (beds, alternate care facilities) and logistical support (clinical and nonclinical equipment and supplies).[34]

The document lists a variety of critical tasks in the areas of developing and maintaining plans, critical items, performance guides, and a variety of benchmarks. It is a comprehensive product that aims for high levels of preparedness, backed by exercises.[34]

U.S. hospital administrators, however, have expressed concern that little is being done at the federal level to help the nation's hospitals achieve these levels of competence in surge. They think that current initiatives fall short of the medical preparedness measures that were implemented between 1950 and 1975 as covered earlier. Yet the population of the United States continues to grow.

Table 22.6. U.S. Population, Hospitals, and Bed Statistics

Year	Population	Hospitals (All Types)	Staffed Beds
1965	194,600,000*		
1990	248,709,873	6,649	1,213,000
2000	281,421,906	5,810	984,000
2005	295,895,897	5,756	946,997
2006	298,754,819	5,747	947,412
2013	313,933,954**	5,274	924,333

* Packaged Disaster Hospital Program: 512,000 beds and 7,800 equipped operating rooms were available.
** As of July 4, 2013.
Source: U.S. Census Bureau and American Hospital Association Research Department.

In many countries, hospitals often strain under their current patient loads and would not be capable of managing an increased demand for care associated with a catastrophic event such as a pandemic or major earthquake. In the United States, there are fewer medical assets per person today than there were many years ago. As the population has grown, the number of hospitals and beds (and thereby patient care capacity) has declined (Table 22.6).

Creation of a Surge Program

The creation of surge capacity requires philosophical as well as financial support. Everyday operational requirements of hospitals and physicians' practices make this difficult. The American College of Healthcare Executives policy statement on the role of healthcare executives in emergency preparedness calls on its members to: 1) be involved in emergency preparedness; 2) ensure that their organizations develop an emergency operating plan; 3) prepare the facility to become a casualty itself from the disaster; 4) become active in interagency planning efforts and encourage adoption of an ICS; and 5) support the NIMS system among others.[35] Healthcare executives may need to delegate these responsibilities. If so, they should ensure that their designees develop robust surge capacity programs, including designation of alternate care sites. The Joint Commission also urges hospitals to create surge capacity; it produced a publication regarding surge hospitals and safe care of patients.[36]

A surge capacity plan must consider all the hazards likely to create a sudden increase in healthcare demands. A pandemic would stress the hospital with patients from their own immediate service area and be coupled by loss of staff who become ill or stay home to care for ill family members. Staff in hospitals in earthquake prone areas should anticipate receiving large numbers of victims with crush injuries, possibly at the same time they are evacuating pre-event patients. A hospital in a community with a refinery or chemical plant could expect to receive patients with toxic exposures, blast, burn, and pulmonary injuries.

Types of Surge Capacity

The hospital can expand capacity by using space within its own grounds and also in the community. This requires an inventory of available space that can potentially be used for patient care.

Examples are conference rooms, meeting rooms, physical therapy departments, solariums, and hallways.

Capacity can be acquired outside the main hospital by using auxiliary buildings on the hospital campus. Some hospitals have purchased tents to be erected on the hospital grounds. Such tents can be equipped with heating and cooling equipment. Off campus surge capacity can be planned with community leaders and local public health officials. Such external capacity is best used for less acute patients or as a step-down facility during the casualty-producing period. With owner approval, patient care capacity can be established in a variety of buildings of opportunity such as convention centers, schools, and warehouses. Pre-event planning must include an extensive review of the physical structure and environment. Sanitation and water availability are essential.[37]

Supplies

A variety of supplies are needed to support surge capacity and these include cots/litters, bedding, medical and surgical supplies, oxygen, pharmaceuticals, and sanitation supplies. Pre-event planning to acquire and store these items is necessary whether it be on the hospital grounds or held in reserve by a vendor. Some hospitals have acquired excess inventory by slowly buying the supplies over time and then rotating them into normal hospital operations. Other hospitals have stored supplies in trailers or cargo containers. It would be helpful if funds became available from third parties to permit acquisition of these supplies, such as the stockpiles and units of previous years. In the United States, the SNS has limited quantities of medical and surgical consumables and should not be counted as the only source. The Joint Commission does not mandate that hospitals maintain a specified supply level. It does require that if the local community cannot provide the resources to support the hospital's surge capacity for 96 hours, the hospital must identify response procedures for this eventuality.[38] Other standards discuss alternate care sites and requirements for the emergency operations plan to identify sites, staffing, supplies, and methods for transporting patients.[38] The Joint Commission standards are available at: www.jointcommission.org.

Staff

Adequate staffing remains a challenge because there is currently a shortage of nurses and other healthcare professionals in the United States and some other countries. Beds are frequently closed due to lack of staff. In a catastrophic situation, especially one that requires the implementation of alternate care sites, preevent plans are needed for management of medical volunteers, who in some cases are credentialed by states rather than nationally. In some cases, hospitals can implement emergency credentialing of volunteers when additional staff are required within the first few hours.[39] Inclusion of retired personnel is an option but due to possible degradation of skills, these individuals should provide care to less acutely ill patients. Local emergency medical technicians, Red Cross volunteers, and home health aides can all be used in an auxiliary role to assist regular care providers.

The Hawaii Department of Health funded a study to assess the attitudes of all state licensed physicians and nurses regarding their willingness to work in a non-hospital field medical facility. The response was highest for "natural" disasters and lowest for radiological incidents.[40] A study in Maryland of health

Table 22.7. Causes of Hospital Evacuations in the United States, 1971–1999

23% Fire within hospital	6% Fire in community
18% Hazmat within hospital	6% Flood
14% Hurricane	5% Utility failure
13% Human threat	4% Hazmat in community
9% Earthquake	

department personnel found up to 50% of public health nurses stated they would not report for duty during a pandemic.[41] Thus, even if "stuff and structure" are available, the staff may not be.

The U.S. Agency for Healthcare Research and Quality has produced many documents recommending ways to optimize existing staff and supplies during mass casualty events.[42,43] In addition to these publications, the agency has also produced an online interactive tool that estimates resources needed for such emergency responses.[44]

Evacuation

For many decades, hospitals and other healthcare facilities have included evacuation procedures in their emergency plans, but the emphasis was for use in fire events. The plans focused on moving patients from the hospital wing on fire to an adjacent area on the same floor and safely sequestering them behind fire-rated hallway doors and smoke barriers. This was the practice of "horizontal" evacuation. "Vertical" evacuation was usually included in written plans, but rarely considered or exercised. Vertical evacuation means moving patients from one floor to another or even from upper floors to outside the facility. Historically, even less effort was expended creating plans to clear the entire building and move patients to alternate treatment sites.

In a study of hospital evacuations in the United States from 1971 to 1999, Sternberg et al. found 275 reported evacuation incidents.[45] Many occurred in 1994, the year of the Northridge earthquake in southern California. The causes of these evacuations are shown in Table 22.7. A study by Schultz et al.[46] reports the findings of hospital evacuations after the Northridge earthquake. Post-event decision making and evacuation techniques are examined to inform the management of future evacuation events. A related article provides a standardized hospital evacuation data collection tool.[47]

Following the 1994 Northridge earthquake in southern California and the 2005 Hurricanes Katrina and Rita, challenges related to hospital evacuation received greater attention. Standards from The Joint Commission require both horizontal and vertical evacuation capabilities and alternate care site plans. Many hospitals have improved their evacuation plans and held evacuation drills. A notable community example is the Reno-Washoe County, Nevada, hospital evacuation project. Undertaken with a grant from FEMA through the state emergency management agency, planning began on types of evacuations, methods of evacuation, review of transportation assets, staffing requirements, patient supplies and critical medications, and locations for receipt of evacuated patients.[48] The planning group also performed a real-time exercise to assess employee reactions and the amount of time required to achieve complete hospital evacua-

tion. Analysis of the exercise findings determined the amount of time and labor needed to accomplish a total hospital evacuation. The results of the planning and exercise led to the creation of the *Multi-Casualty Incident Plan: Mutual Aid Evacuation Annex*, which was approved by the District Board of Health as policy for Washoe County.[48]

Evacuations can be partial or total depending on the situation. When an EMS helicopter crashed on the roof of a Michigan trauma center in 2008, leaking fuel flowed down an elevator shaft necessitating a partial evacuation of several floors. The associated loss of power required the use of stairwells to evacuate the patients and the injured pilot.

The following information should be considered when developing evacuation plans:

1. A facility evacuation plan must be coordinated with the local community.
2. A decision tree should be used to determine whether an evacuation order should be issued (Table 22.8). The decision to evacuate a hospital may not be a simple one and evacuation authority must be clear. An example would be the hospitals in the delayed evacuation group after the Northridge earthquake that did not initially realize they were structurally unsound.[49]
3. Variance in philosophy on the order of patient evacuation (intensive care unit patients first or ambulatory patients first) is found in hospital evacuation plans. General consensus indicates that in emergency situations, focus shifts to saving as many lives as possible rather than focusing on an individual patient. A study of hospital evacuations after the Northridge earthquake suggests that ambulatory patients should be evacuated first when time is critical. When greater time for evacuation exists, intensive care unit patients should be transferred first.[49]
4. Internal patient transportation aids may be necessary. Devices most useful for individual patient movement are wheelchairs, wheeled stretchers, backboards, and blankets. A staff member should be assigned to each to make turnaround as rapid as possible. While vendors market some specialized evacuation devices (e.g., infant carriers for multiple newborns), real-life evacuations show that these tend not to be used. Therefore, caution should be exercised to ensure practicality for a specific facility before funds as expended for such products. External patient transportation planning must account for the number of ambulances, wheelchair carriers, and commercial buses in the community, including procedures for contacting them on short notice.
5. Procedures should exist for discharging as many patients as possible, including providing follow-up care instructions, medications as needed, and transportation to domiciles if a friend or family member is unavailable.
6. A patient tracking system is needed to monitor patients, visitors, destinations, and hospital staff members who accompany patients to alternate treatment sites (Figure 22.9).
7. Coordination with the local EMS system and EOC is necessary.
8. Medical records, medications, and medical support equipment should be sent with each patient to the receiving location. Special precautions are needed for controlled pharmaceuticals and syringes.
9. Traffic patterns, both vehicular and pedestrian, must be controlled. The hospital will receive an influx of ambulances,

Table 22.8. Hospital Evacuation Checklist

PURPOSE – OVERVIEW

To provide guidance in the development or update of a hospital evacuation plan containing detailed information, instructions, and procedures that can be engaged in any emergency situation necessitating either full or partial hospital evacuation, as well as sheltering-in-place.

The expectation will be that staff may need to accompany patients and work in staging areas, in local government Alternate Care Sites (ACS) and/or at receiving facilities, subject to receiving proper emergency credentials. Drills, training, and reviews must be conducted to ensure that staff have a working knowledge of the plan and to ensure that the plan is workable.

The plan should be consistent with federal NIMS and The Joint Commission requirements

1. General Plan Requirements	
▪ Integrated with other pertinent protocols in facility's comprehensive EOP, including activation of hospital ICS	
▪ Identify backup measures for key infrastructure components/resources as appropriate	
▪ Assigned responsibilities and formal process for review and update of Evacuation Plan (Plan), including incorporation of after-action report results	
▪ Staff training including Plan overview, specific roles and responsibilities, utilization of evacuation equipment, techniques for lifting and carrying patients, and knowledge of primary/alternate evacuation routes	
▪ Uses standard terminology in common and consistent plain English language and emphasizes its use by staff during an evacuation	
2. Activation	
▪ Define criteria and authority for decision to activate the Plan	
▪ Define how the Plan is activated and how it integrates with the hospital ICS and EOP. Define the plan for communication and coordination with the MACS and/or the operational area ICS (e.g., EMS, Public Health Department Operations Center (PHDOC), or city/county EOC)	
▪ Document how shelter-in-place critical decision making has been integrated into Plan, including a determination whether state program flexibility would allow hospital to avoid full evacuation (e.g., alternate use of facilities)	
▪ Identify and/or reference public information plan (Public Information Officer (PIO), Joint Information Center (JIC) coordination as appropriate)	
▪ Identify alert and notifications to local (e.g., EMS, PHS, fire) and state agencies (e.g., Licensing and Certification (L&C)) regarding potential and/or intent to evacuate facilities and how communication will be maintained during and after evacuation	
▪ Define the type/level of evacuation that could occur (shelter-in-place, partial horizontal/vertical/external, full)	
▪ Describe the phases of implementation (i.e., staff notification, accessing available resources and equipment, preparation of patients and essential patient supplies and equipment)	
▪ Define routes and exits identified for evacuation, including area, facility, and campus diagrams	
▪ Describe the protocols for accepting and orienting staff and volunteers from other facilities to assist with evacuation	
▪ Describe the plan for the order of removal of patients and planned route of movement (prioritization) as relevant to event and evacuation type	
3. Securing Hospital Site	
▪ Define the hospital security access (e.g., lockdown) plan, including ambulance diversion	
▪ Describe the alternate sites identified for media center and labor pool, including nursing and medical staff	
▪ Define the procedures for securing the facility and perimeter	
▪ Describe procedures for security and/or management of controlled substances	
▪ Describe procedures for securing utilities, including shutting down/controlling gas, medical gases, water and electricity as appropriate to event (potentially shutting down or activating generators); consideration should be given to potential impact on equipment and systems and potential for spoilage of food and pharmaceuticals	
▪ Describe how coordination with local public safety for determination of inner and outer perimeters for hospital and staging area sites will be established	

Table 22.8. *(continued)*

4. Identification of the Alternate Site(s) – Receiving Facilities	
▪ Identify receiving facilities and government sponsored alternate care sites and contact information	
▪ Identify/reference any written documentation that confirms the commitment of these facilities (e.g., Memorandum of Understanding, contract, local emergency plans)	
▪ Define process for reaffirming/updating agreements	
▪ Define the process for contacting Operational Area Emergency Medical Services – DOC and/or facilities to:	
▪ ascertain availability at the time of the evacuation and assist with transport	
▪ notify identified facilities that patients will be evacuated to their facilities	
5. Resources/Evacuation	
▪ Identify resources/equipment available to move patients from rooms/floors and the procedure in place for inventory control	
▪ Identify the location of additional resources needed such as additional lighting sources (i.e., flashlights and batteries and portable monitors and ventilators)	
▪ Identify a clearly marked storage area available 24/7 for this equipment	
▪ Define the protocol for staff training on equipment use	
▪ Define the protocol to be utilized for ongoing assessment of the patient status for equipment and transportation needs in the event of an evacuation	
▪ Describe how communication will be maintained, and documented, for staff and outside resources	
6. Resources/Continuity of Care	
The Plan must address how continuity of care will be maintained during an evacuation for patients at all levels of clinical complexity and disability including:	
▪ How to maintain continuity of care if the usual equipment is not available during the evacuation process	
▪ How equipment identified as necessary to provide continuity of care can be moved with the patient, how to identify and track the patient's own equipment, and how to meet requirements for providing power to electrical equipment (e.g., beds, wheelchairs, ventilators, etc.)	
▪ What resources are available to maintain isolation precautions for the safety of staff and patients, including communication of need for precautions above standard precautions	
▪ How staff will be trained and drilled on the evacuation process/Plan	
▪ Identify how services that may need to continue will be provided or arranged for while repairs to facilities are being made as necessary (e.g., day treatment, dialysis)	
7. External Transportation Resources	
▪ Identify and designate areas to congregate patients according to established criteria (i.e., event, acuity, mobility levels)	
▪ List and numbers of patients by type and/or transportation resources needed (buses, vans, Advanced Life Support (ALS) and Basic Life Support (BLS) ambulances, ambulettes, trucks, wheelchair vans, etc.)	
▪ Describe the process for contacting EMS (e.g., DOC/EOC) to request and to coordinate transportation vehicle needs/resources with patient needs (i.e., patient acuity level, wheelchairs, life support, bariatric)	
▪ Identify hospital's primary and secondary/alternate transportation resources to be available if needed, including contact information	
▪ Reference documentation that confirms the commitment of required transportation resources (e.g., Memorandum of Understanding, contract, county emergency plans or protocols)	
▪ Define the process for reaffirming and updating agreements and plans	

Table 22.8. *(continued)*

8. Patient Evacuation	
▪ Specify the protocol to assure that the patient destination is compatible to patient acuity and healthcare needs, as possible	
▪ Provide evacuees with standardized visual identifiers, such as a color-coded wristband or evacuation tag, to help personnel rapidly identify special needs for high-risk conditions that, if not easily identified, could lead to injury or death of an evacuee	
▪ Establish protocols for sharing special needs information, as appropriate, with personnel participating in the evacuation, including transport agencies, receiving facilities, alternate care sites, shelters, and others involved in evacuee patient care	
▪ Identify the resources necessary to address patient needs during transport, how to access, and responsibility for acquiring and sending with the patient (e.g., "go bags," food, water, medications, etc.)	
▪ Document staff training and exercises on the traffic flow and the movement of patients to a staging area	
9. Tracking Destination/Arrival of Patients	
▪ A patient identification wristband (or equivalent identification) must be intact on all patients	
▪ Describe the process to be utilized to track the arrival of each patient at the destination	
▪ The tracking form* should contain key patient information, including the following:	
▪ Medical Record Number	
▪ Time left the facility	
▪ Name of transporting agency	
▪ Original chart sent with patient (yes/no)	
▪ Critical medical record information (orders, medications list, face sheet) (yes/no)	
▪ Meds sent with patient (list)	
▪ Equipment sent with patient (list)	
▪ Family notified of transfer (yes/no)	
▪ Private MD notified of transfer (yes/no)	
Note: Example HICS tracking forms are available	
▪ Identify protocol for linking and reuniting patients and personal possessions not taken with patients during evacuation	
10. Family/Responsible Party Notification	
▪ Describe the process for assignment of staff members to conduct and track family/responsible party notification	
▪ Define the procedure to notify patient emergency contacts/family of an evacuation and the patient's destination including protocols to communicate if initial contact attempts are not feasible or successful (e.g., hotline, Red Cross, police, etc.)	
11. Additional Governmental Agency Notification	
▪ Protocol for emergency notification to public safety for immediate response must be clearly written and communicated to staff	
▪ Protocol for emergency notification of patient evacuation to California Department of Public Health Licensing and Certification and local emergency medical services must be clearly written and communicated to staff	
▪ Define position title responsible for maintaining contact numbers in an accessible location	
12. Facility Evacuation Confirmation	
▪ Define the protocol to verify that patient care and non-patient care areas have been evacuated (i.e., orange tags, chalk on door)	
▪ Define orientation and annual staff training for room evacuation provided to all staff	
▪ Describe how the protocols will be tested during drills and/or exercises	
▪ Describe the mechanism used to communicate the evacuation confirmation protocol to the responding fire department and other facility first responders	
▪ Describe the protocol to track and account for staff, visitors and non-employees (i.e., vendors, contractors) that may be on-site during an evacuation	

Table 22.8. (continued)

13. Transport of Records, Supplies, and Equipment	
▪ Describe the procedure for transport of Medication Administration Records (MARs) patient care/medical records	
▪ Describe measures taken to protect patient confidentiality	
▪ Describe the process to transport essential patient equipment and supplies	
▪ Define protocol for transfer of patient-specific medications and records to receiving facility	
▪ Protocol for the transfer of patient-specific controlled substances sent with patients and procedure to record receipt, full count, and signature of transferring and receiving personnel	

14. Recovery, Reopening, and Repopulation of Evacuated Facilities	
▪ Criteria and responsibilities for preparing facilities for reopening and assuring resources and ability to provide appropriate patient care	
▪ Steps to be taken to ensure a safe environment (e.g., facilities, fire and safety, etc., as appropriate). See *CHA Hospital Repopulation after Evacuation Guidelines and Checklist*	
▪ Process for securing government/regulatory agency approvals (e.g., Licensing and Certification, State Pharmacy Board)	
▪ Protocols for coordination and collaboration of transportation through county ICS (e.g., EMS DOC or EOC) or directly with transport vendors	
▪ Protocols for repatriation of staff and patients back to evacuated facilities, including facility access and staff identification, communication with receiving facilities, documentation, etc.	
▪ Protocols for communication with family regarding patient status/location	
▪ Protocols for communication and coordination with EMS ICS regarding status of facilities and repatriation/repopulation.	

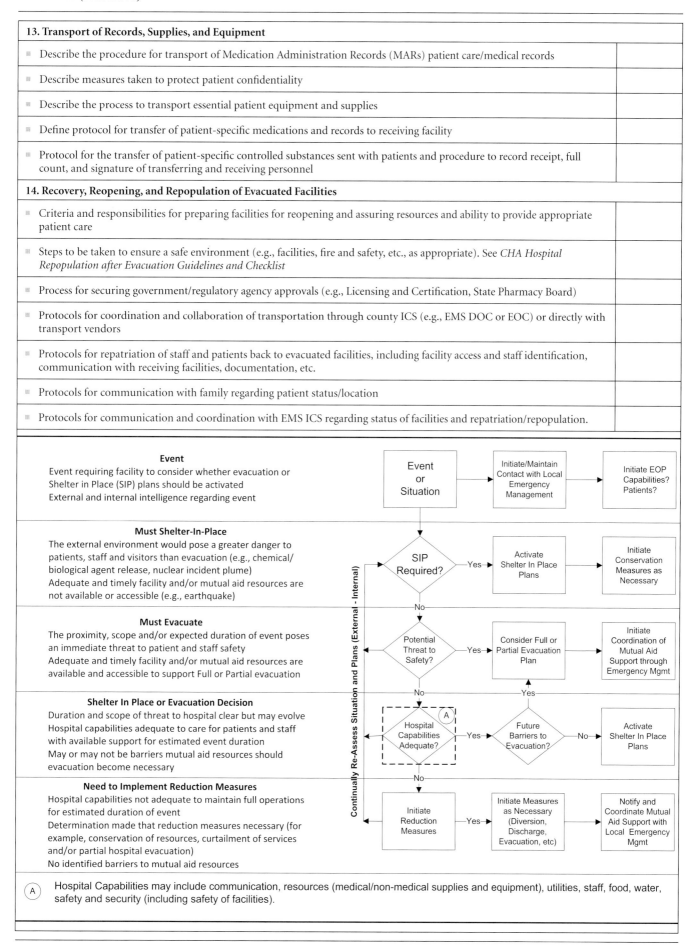

Event
Event requiring facility to consider whether evacuation or Shelter in Place (SIP) plans should be activated
External and internal intelligence regarding event

Must Shelter-In-Place
The external environment would pose a greater danger to patients, staff and visitors than evacuation (e.g., chemical/biological agent release, nuclear incident plume)
Adequate and timely facility and/or mutual aid resources are not available or accessible (e.g., earthquake)

Must Evacuate
The proximity, scope and/or expected duration of event poses an immediate threat to patient and staff safety
Adequate and timely facility and/or mutual aid resources are available and accessible to support Full or Partial evacuation

Shelter In Place or Evacuation Decision
Duration and scope of threat to hospital clear but may evolve
Hospital capabilities adequate to care for patients and staff with available support for estimated event duration
May or may not be barriers mutual aid resources should evacuation become necessary

Need to Implement Reduction Measures
Hospital capabilities not adequate to maintain full operations for estimated duration of event
Determination made that reduction measures necessary (for example, conservation of resources, curtailment of services and/or partial hospital evacuation)
No identified barriers to mutual aid resources

(A) Hospital Capabilities may include communication, resources (medical/non-medical supplies and equipment), utilities, staff, food, water, safety and security (including safety of facilities).

Source: www.calhospitalprepared.org/sites/main/files/file.attachments/hospitalevacuationplanchecklist102710.doc (Accessed August 23, 2013).

GNYHA Draft 08/20/07

Patient Critical Evacuation Information Tracking Form

NOTE: After completion of form please make THREE copies: ONE for sending facility, ONE for EMS, and ONE for receiving facility.

Sending Facility: _____

Receiving Facility: _____

Patient Name: (PRINT) _____

Date of Birth: ____ / ____ / ____   Sex: Male   Female

Transferring Facility Medical Record Number: _____

Method of Transport: Ambulatory   Wheelchair   Basic Life Support   Advanced Life Support

Emergency Contact: _____ Telephone # _____

Notified of Transfer :   YES   NO

Attending Physician: _____ Notified of Transfer: YES   NO

Primary Diagnosis: _____

Do Not Resuscitate: YES (attach copy)   NO   Advanced Directives: YES (attach copy)   NO

Healthcare Proxy: YES   (attach copy) NO

Date transferred: _____ Time of arrival at receiving facility: _____

Equipment owned by sending facility accompanying patient during transport:

_____   _____
_____   _____
_____   _____
_____   _____

COMMENTS: _____
_____
_____
_____

Prepared by GNYHA based upon documents developed by the New York State Department of Health, Continuum Health Partners, and Lourdes Hospital.

Figure 22.9. Patient Critical Evacuation Information Tracking Form.

buses, EMS personnel, and others that must be managed for maximum evacuation efficiency. For example, if sufficient elevators are available, one can be designated for ingress of EMS ambulance personnel arriving to transport patients, and another for those exiting the facility. This minimizes congestion at elevator lobbies. All unnecessary vehicles should be moved from the ambulance/bus staging area to allow optimal use of space.

10. Flashlights, headlamps, and battery-powered backup lights in corridors and stairwells are useful.

11. Staging areas are needed for patients waiting to depart the facility. This strategy prevents unnecessary exposure to outside elements. These should be under the control of an experienced fire or EMS officer, preferably equipped with a hospital frequency radio, who can supervise transportation assets in an efficient manner. Additionally, an internal triage team of physicians and nurses should be stationed in the patient staging area and in the vicinity of the loading point to perform medical assessments and render care as needed.

12. A method is needed to notify patients' family members of their alternate care destinations.

13. External security of the patient loading area is necessary to protect patients and their privacy. Additionally, the hospital facility itself must be secured.

14. Receiving facilities should develop memoranda of agreement with neighboring hospitals as well as hospitals 80–160 km away to provide mutual assistance. Joint evacuation planning that clarifies the roles and responsibilities of the evacuating hospital and the receiving hospital is necessary (Table 22.9).

Table 22.9. Receiving Hospital Evacuation Checklist

Hospital Evacuation – Receiving Hospital		
Receiving Hospital's Pre-evacuation Actions	Completed	To Do
Establish MOA with partnering facility (like organization) that addresses the sharing of staff, what is expected of the evacuating organization to bring with them, how staff will be utilized, reimbursement, liability, housing for evacuating staff, how workers compensation will be handled, continuity of patient care, location for evacuating organization's administrative staff, and so forth		
Credential healthcare providers with the partnering organization and determine level of privileging.		
Establish a location for which the evacuating organization's administration to operate.		
Provide to partnering organization a list of the types of medical specialists available to them.		
Assist in locating lodging for the evacuating hospital's staff.		
Arrange with suppliers for additional food, linens, medications, supplies, equipment, etc., and a "trigger point" for ordering and receiving them.		
Determine where incoming patients will go (both ambulatory and non-ambulatory).		
Examine possible temporary arrangements (non-traditional care sites) for patients to avoid revenue loss incurred by discharging them.		
Explain to staff the protocols that have been established with the evacuating hospital and its staff.		
Coordinate exercises prior to hurricane season where the evacuating organization practices evacuation and their partnering organization practices preparing for and receiving patients – even if it is a tabletop exercise with administrative staff.		
Visit each other's facility to gain a better understanding and appreciation of the issues each organization faces by this effort.		
Establish drop-off points so as not to interfere with day-to-day traffic.		

Source: South Carolina Hospital Association. Used with Permission.

15. For situations in which other healthcare facilities are unable to receive some or all of the evacuated patients, alternate care sites are necessary. Pre-event planning should include the identification and preparation of alternate care sites such as auditoriums, hotels/motels, and schools that could be used to house patients when hospitals are unavailable. While these sites may not be ideal for the practice of modern medicine, they should be considered as they may be the only locations for sheltering patients too ill to return home.

16. The command structure must be clearly delineated. Policies created by the Continuum Health Partner Hospitals of New York City suggest using the HICS in reverse. For example, the Logistics Chief controls the movement of patients and supplies, whereas the Planning Chief assumes responsibility for tracking patients through the evacuation process to their final destinations.[48]

Superstorm Sandy Hospital Evacuation Case Study

Superstorm Sandy wreaked destruction from the Caribbean to New Jersey, New York, and beyond. It then turned northwest, causing heavy rains, winds, and even heavy snows at higher elevations in inland states, along with power outages.

The storm was 90 nautical miles (167 km) across and by the time it reached the northeastern United States, it was measured at 945 millibars, the lowest ever in recorded history at that location. By the evening landfall on October 28, 2012, in New York City, it had weakened to a Category 1 hurricane. However, it hit at high tide and caused a massive storm surge that pushed the Hudson and East Rivers into the city, with the surge measured as high as 4.23 meters.[50]

The following seven hospitals, identified by letter to protect their anonymity, performed various evacuation activities in the wake of Superstorm Sandy.

Hospital A – This hospital lost commercial power and began using emergency generators. Subsequently, these later failed when flooding shut down the fuel pumps, which sent fuel to the generators located on upper floors. The building code called for the fuel tanks and pumps to be at ground level or below. The emergency department was flooded. Several CT and MRI units were destroyed by flood waters. Research projects were also lost. The storm surge was nearly 4.3 meters and poured water into the hospital's basement and elevator shafts to a depth of 3–3.65 meters. The telephone, email, and computer systems failed. The decision was made to evacuate over 200 remaining patients and 20 neonates, four of whom were on respirators. Some patient rooms were as high as the seventeenth floor.

Nurses, physicians, hospital personnel and first responders began the evacuation using stairwells as the elevators were inoperable. Using flashlights, teams of four to five persons transported patients on emergency evacuation devices and wheelchairs to the ground floor. Nursing staff carefully evacuated the newborns and neonates, including four on respirators. A nurse was assigned to each patient and held the baby to the chest for warmth while constantly monitoring its respirations and any other monitors or intravenous solutions.

Some required squeeze bag resuscitators. At the ground floor, area ambulances, and those from distant states, assisted the patient transfers. The nurses rode in the ambulances with the babies to the receiving hospital(s).

The operating rooms, intensive care unit and other services reopened 59 days after the storm while other services remained closed.[51]

Hospital B – This hospital also experienced loss of commercial power and went on emergency generator power. However, flooding caused the fuel pumps to shut down. Hospital personnel and National Guard members formed a line up the stairwell to pass fuel containers to the emergency generators on the thirteenth floor, but by the day after landfall, hospital management made the decision to evacuate over 700 patients. The National Guard members and first responders again helped with this massive effort using dozens of ambulances. Patients were then transported to other hospitals.

The hospital partially reopened on November 19, 2012, nearly 3 weeks after landfall, and was fully operational 99 days after its temporarily closure.

Hospital C – This hospital began to discharge patients pre-landfall owing to concerns that a nearby seawall could be breached by the storm surge. Forty ambulances, including three ambulance buses, with assistance from the National Guard, transported 130 evacuated patients.

Flood waters later entered the facility and flooded the ground floor and damaged equipment. The hospital reopened the emergency department, but diverted patients with life-threatening conditions to other hospitals until cleanup and repairs were made.

Hospital D – Four emergency generators failed at this hospital due to flooding on the night of landfall. The hospital evacuated eighty-three patients, including thirteen on life support. Local police, EMS personnel, staff from two ambulance buses operated by the State EMS Task Force, and prehospital personnel with a local private ambulance performed the evacuation. The hospital sent nurses, nurse aides, and respiratory therapists with the evacuated patients. In addition, ventilators and intravenous and feeding pumps (with their disposable supplies) were sent to the receiving hospital.

Their electronic medical record system failed. The information technology department printed copies of the patient charts prior to landfall and these were sent with the patients. Later, local first responders and public works personnel restored power using two new generators. The hospital also effectively used sandbags to hold back water; however, ground water percolated up through the floor. Despite these issues, this hospital reopened with full services in several days.

Hospital E – This long-term care hospital lost commercial power and heat, and evacuated 104 patients to a neighboring facility. The remaining patients were sheltered-in-place. Heat and hot water were restored with temporary boilers and power by temporary generators which were brought to the site.

Repairs and restoration activities required replacement of boilers, emergency generators, heating, ventilating, and air conditioning equipment, and new electric switchgear, all of which had been destroyed by flood waters.

As of November 1, 2012, they were providing all services and were reviewing available beds to determine whether they would accept new patients.[52]

Hospital F – This hospital suffered extensive flooding in its basement, which housed clinics, kitchen, central sterile supply, boilers, electrical gear (including two emergency generators), laundry, pharmacy, communications, maintenance, and engineering. Ground water continued to seep into the basement for a month after landfall.

The county executive ordered evacuation, along with the patients from its skilled nursing facility. This evacuation was completed before landfall and patients were distributed to other hospitals.

A damage assessment estimated cost of repairs and replacement of equipment to be over $30 million (USD). Several weeks after landfall, the hospital opened a temporary emergency department in heated tents and trailers. The skilled nursing facility was reopened in an off-site location. Inpatient services were planned to be reopened 6 months after landfall. However, even a year later, the hospital still remained closed, while the family practice clinic operated at an alternate location. According to the New York City Health and Hospitals corporation, resources to repair damage from Superstorm Sandy were still needed even years later.[52]

Hospital G – This hospital's leadership made the decision to begin evacuating their patients prior to landfall, owing to being in a flood zone. Approximately 130 patients were transferred, without incident, to other hospitals and most patients were escorted by their care teams.

This same hospital was evacuated a year earlier for Hurricane Irene. During Superstorm Sandy it suffered extensive flood damage and failure of all major utilities. More than 150,000 square feet (13,935 square meters) of outpatient and support areas were destroyed, as well as an MRI unit and other valuable clinical equipment.

Outpatient services were reopened 8 months after landfall.

Because Superstorm Sandy was a slow-onset disaster with advanced notice, there were several days for planning and preparations. Emergency managers arranged for additional supplies of food, medicine, and fuel oil, and prepared sandbags. Use of sandbags by some hospitals to hold back water was successful, while others found their sandbags insufficient in number or overwhelmed by the tidal surge. Percolation of ground water was also a problem. Flood waters contaminated some hospitals with bacteria, mold spores, and substances often found in flood waters such as pesticides, fuel oil, and other hazardous materials. A complete cleaning and decontamination of the affected areas, followed by culturing, was needed before re-occupancy could take place.

Hospitals often lost their computer systems and access to electronic medical records, and their off-site backup provider was only viable if it was not in or near the storm path. Cost estimates for the affected hospitals total in the several hundred million dollar (USD) range. Property damage and business interruption insurance often did not cover the costs of Superstorm Sandy losses.

Patient evacuation was labor intensive, especially with critically ill patients on life support equipment. When the elevators, or controls, were flooded, evacuation was by stairwell. Some stairwells lacked emergency battery-pack lights and were unlit. In spite of all these difficulties, evacuations were performed safely and no patient died. This is a credit to the physicians, nurses, hospital personnel, ambulance crews, and all others who assisted the effort. Of equal importance were the efforts made by other hospitals and staffs who received evacuated patients. Transferring hospitals often sent nurses and physicians to assist the receiving hospitals. The evacuation was facilitated by the New York Department of Health, which authorized hospitals to go to "Surge Capacity" status. Additionally, the influx of 350 ambulances and crews from the FEMA National Emergency Contract aided. These units were fully self-sufficient and came with their own fuel and logistic arrangements.

Unofficial numbers gleaned from media articles report that more than 7,000 patients were evacuated from hospitals, nursing homes, and adult care facilities. Of these patients, more than 1,500 had to have a second transfer to an appropriate facility to meet their needs. New York City also opened "special medical needs shelters" and had at peak greater than 1,800 patients housed in them. Additional information on New York City and Superstorm Sandy is available online.[53] The media also reported that there was only one known injury to a patient during evacuation.

The Disaster Recovery Phase

Each disaster has four phases: mitigation, preparedness, response, and recovery. Following the response phase, the hospital must recover and return to baseline operating status. If the physical plant has been damaged, the hospital can seek financial help from the U.S. Public Assistance Program of FEMA or parallel programs in other countries. Here the Finance/Administration Section of the HICS has a critical role. The Documentation Unit, Time Unit, Procurement Unit, and Compensation/Claims Unit must collect data and prepare them for presentation to FEMA. The Public Assistance Program follows the rules and regulations of the *Robert T. Stafford Act*.[54] The Finance/Administration Chief needs a financial team to tabulate the costs the hospital has incurred related to the disaster. This team also provides documentation to the hospital's insurance companies as it relates to property, liability, and business-interruption insurances. Patients' health insurance companies should also be billed as federal reimbursements are made on a last dollar basis in the United States. Unreimbursed and donated care should be carefully documented, as well as invoices for supplies and personnel wages. Such information can then be presented to the hospital's insurers and FEMA. Because of the healthcare institution's high cash demands to pay employees and vendors, the hospital may continue to incur bad debt and uncompensated care above the norm. To maintain cash flow, the hospital should discuss periodic interim payments with major health insurance companies (including the government programs Medicare and Medicaid in the United States) in advance of a disaster. The hospital's capital requirements following a cataclysmic event must be fully understood. It is imperative that the hospital have solid documentation and meet the various deadlines for filing claims. Some hospitals keep a large sum of cash on hand for purchase of needed supplies in a disaster.

RECOMMENDATIONS FOR FURTHER RESEARCH

Protecting the Hospital from Chemical and Biological Threats

The hospital physical plant should be protected from chemical, biological, or radiological plumes that could be drawn into the building by its air-handling equipment. As stated earlier, a hospital draws in more kilograms of air daily than kilograms of water to meet the infection control codes. This represents a significant vulnerability to the hospital. Incidents with tank cars carrying toxic industrial chemicals are fairly common and some have led to deaths. A hospital should avoid becoming internally contaminated, as it then becomes not only a dangerous environment for occupants, but its critical role of providing healthcare to the community is also compromised.

The U.S. Army has consistently sought better devices to detect harmful agents and has a need for real-time detection from a distance. To that end, the Army has experimented with laser beams that could reach out a few kilometers, sample the air, and sound an alarm if a harmful agent is detected. This standoff capability has also been developed into a package that can be carried by a helicopter and reach out several kilometers.

If this technology is successful, hospitals could incorporate this type of system into their overall response plans. On receiving the warning, the hospital could shut down its air-handling systems and perform a facility lockdown to protect occupants. Existing monitors are not necessarily real-time and require follow-up of samples to analyze bioparticles. Research is needed into this technology to give not only real-time warning but also to allow technology to detect the presence of harmful agents before they can reach the hospital so timely protective actions can be taken.

Improved Reserve Supply Inventory

Just-in-time inventory control systems are in use in hospitals across the United States and some other parts of the world. Therefore, a shortage of medical and surgical supplies and pharmaceuticals can be expected during a disaster. Research is needed on how to provide supply packages to equip providers to treat patients suffering from trauma, burns, respiratory injuries from chemicals, biological-induced illness, and radiation exposure. In addition, funding is needed to support the purchase, storage, rotation, and transportation of medical equipment to resupply hospitals on a timely basis. Such supply packages would contain the basic materials needed by physicians to treat the casualties from these events. This medical reserve inventory must be available at the local and regional levels to bridge the gap before supplies are available from outside sources such as the SNS.

Hospital Preparedness Funding

At the time of this writing, the U.S. Office of the Assistant Secretary for Preparedness and Response in HHS operates a bioterrorism grant program to assist hospitals with disaster preparedness. Awards to grantee hospitals are small. Preparedness costs money and health insurance companies do not consider this in their reimbursement formulas. Although communities routinely fund the operations of fire, police, and EMS through taxes, they do not share tax revenues for disaster preparedness with the first receivers of the victims – the hospitals. More funding for healthcare facilities is necessary for a comprehensive preparedness effort.

Research is needed to determine international, national, state, and local government priorities for funding hospital disaster preparedness as well as the perspective of the health insurance industry in this regard. From the research data derived, strategies can be crafted to obtain such specific funding. Hospitals must be willing to accept such funding as restricted grants and to monitor and document that the funds are being used for their designated purposes.

Radiological Training for Hospital Employees

Radiation has been stigmatized for more than 60 years with the result that most people are fearful of any amount of radiation. Research is needed on educational criteria and curriculums for each level of hospital employee, including those in service departments. This training would assist in demystifying radiation, and teach protective measures for alpha, beta and gamma radiation. In the event of a radiological/nuclear event, the goal would be to have all levels of employees know their roles for: protecting themselves; monitoring and recording radiation levels; and decontaminating casualties. Knowledge can replace fear just as it did in the 1980s when hospital personnel were first confronted with HIV. If a radiological event happens in the community or surrounding area, hospital personnel would have the knowledge to manage the incident and continue to serve their community.

Hospital Evacuation Methodology

Although evacuation of hospitals is an uncommon occurrence, there have been a number of evacuations in the past several decades. The Joint Commission requires hospitals to have plans for staged and total evacuations. Evacuations can be partial or full, can be planned before a hurricane landfall, or needed during a sudden event such as a fire, earthquake, terrorist attack, or sudden loss of utilities. Research would determine best practices for each type. While many elements in hospital evacuations are the same for both planned and sudden evacuations, all variables must be taken into account in the research, and evidence-based practices be discovered that could serve as international guidelines.

REFERENCES

1. Dunn CL. Medical History of the Second World War. *The Emergency Medical Services.* Vol. 1. London, His Majesty's Stationery Office, 1952.

2. Mitchester PH, Cowell EM. *Medical Organization and Surgical Practice in Air Raids.* London, Churchill Ltd., 1939.

3. Shirlaw GB. *Casualty: Training, Organization and Administration of Civil Defence Casualty Services.* London, Martin Secker and Warburg, 1940.

4. Wallace AB. *The Treatment of Burns.* Oxford University Press, London, 1941.

5. U.S. Government Office of Civil Defense. Author's collection.

6. U.S. Department of Health and Human Services. Office of the Public Health Service Historian. December 2006. www.uscadetnurse.org/node/4 (Accessed August 22, 2013).

7. Federal Civil Defense Administration. *Civil Defense Medical Depot.* Author's collection. n.d.

8. Koenig KL, Majestic C, Burns MJ. Ebola Virus Disease: Essential Public Health Principles for Clinicians, *WestJEM,* 2014. http://www.escholarship.org/uc/item/1bh1352j#page-1 (Accessed August 8, 2015).

9. American Medical Association. Educating Physicians on Controversies and Challenges in Health. *Disaster Preparedness: Are Physicians Ready?* http://disasterlit.nlm.nih.gov/record/1866 (Accessed August 21, 2015).

10. Presidential Decision Directive 39. U.S. Policy on Counterterrorism. June 21, 1995. http://www.au.af.mil/au/awc/awcgate/pdd39/pdd39-synopsis.htm. Also see: www.whitehouse.gov/issues/homeland-security (both accessed August 22, 2013).

11. 104th Congress. Public Law 104–201 Title XIV, Defense Against Weapons of Mass Destruction.

12. Joint Commission on Accreditation of Healthcare Organizations. Health Care at the Crossroads: Strategies for Creating and Sustaining Community-wide Emergency Preparedness Strategies. 2006. www.jointcommission.org/assets/1/18/emergency-preparedness.pdf (Accessed August 22, 2013).

13. Joint Commission. Comprehensive Accreditation Manual for Hospitals. 2006. Note: the reader should consult the latest standards and updates, available at: www.jointcommission.org.

14. The Joint Commission. Prepublication version of the 2009 Standards. The latest version of standards and updates are available at: www.jointcommission.org (Accessed August 22, 2013).

15. Occupational Safety and Health Administration (OSHA). Best Practices for Hospital-based First Receivers of Victims from Mass Casualty Incidents Involving the Release of Hazardous Substances. 2005. https://www.osha.gov/dts/osta/bestpractices/html/hospital_firstreceivers.html (Accessed August 22, 2013).

16. *Medical Center Hazard and Vulnerability Analysis.* Oakland, CA, Kaiser Foundation Health Plan, Inc., 2001. Used with permission.

17. *Disaster Life Cycle: Four Phases of Comprehensive Emergency Management,* Washington, DC, U.S. Department of Veterans Affairs, 2002.

18. Koenig KL, Boatright CJ, Hancock JA, et al. Healthcare Facility-based Decontamination of Victims Exposed to Chemical, Biological, and Radiological Material. *Am J Emerg Med* 2008; 26(1): 71–80.

19. Koenig KL, Boatright CJ, Hancock JA, et al. Health Care Facilities "War on Terrorism" A Deliberate Process for Recommending Personal Protective Equipment *Am J Emerg Med* 2007; 25(2): 185–195.

20. Gum RM, Hoyle JD. CBRNE-Chemical Warfare Mass Casualty Management. *Medscape eMedicine Reference.* 2011. http://emedicine.medscape.com/article/831375-overview (Accessed August 21, 2015.)

21. Downey EL, Andress K, Schultz CH. External Factors Impacting Hospital Evacuations Caused by Hurricane Rita: The Role of Situational Investigation. *Prehosp Disaster Med* 2013; 28(3): 257–263.

22. Downey EL, Andress K, Schultz CH. External Factors Impacting Hospital Evacuations Caused by Hurricane Rita: The Role of Situational Awareness. *Prehosp Disaster Med* 2013; 28(3): 264–271.

23. Federal Emergency Management Agency. Incident Command Resource Center. 2006. http://www.fema.gov/emergency/ims/index.shtm (Accessed August 21, 2013).

24. California Emergency Medical Services Authority. Hospital Incident Command System – Frequently Asked Questions (FAQ), http://www.emsa.ca.gov/disaster_medical_services_division_hospital_incident_command_system_faq#faq1 (Accessed August 21, 2015).

25. Federal Emergency Management Agency, Emergency Management Institute. *Fundamentals of Healthcare Emergency Management Course.* Emmitsburg, MD, FEMA, 2006.

26. Federal Emergency Management Agency. NIMS Implementation Activities for Hospitals and Healthcare Systems. 2006. http://www.fema.gov/pdf/emergency/nims/imp_act_hos-hlth.pdf (Accessed August 21, 2013).

27. Telephone Interview with John Ross, PE, former Vice President for Plant Operations, The Saint Luke Hospitals, July 2, 2013.

28. National Institute of Occupational Safety and Health. Guidance for Protecting Building Environments from Airborne, Chemical, Biological or Radiological Attacks. 2002. www.cdc.gov/niosh/docs/2002–139 (Accessed August 21, 2013).

29. Halpern P, Goldberg S, Koenig KL, Goh J. Principles of Emergency Department Facility Design for Optimal Management of Mass Casualty Incidents. *Prehosp Disaster Med* 2012; 27(2): 204–212.

30. Association of Healthcare Resource and Materials Management. Medical-Surgical Formulary by Disaster Scenario. 2002. http://www.ahrmm.org/ahrmm/news_and_issues/issues_and_initiatives/files/disaster_formularies.pdf (Accessed August 21, 2013).

31. Hick JL. Sample Medical Surgical and PPE Supplies by Disaster Type and Category of Hospital Emergency Services. 2003. http://www.health.state.mn.us/oep/healthcare/disastersupplies.pdf (Accessed August 21, 2013).

32. Koenig KL, Kelen G. Executive Summary: The Science of Surge Conference. *Acad Emerg Med* November 2006; 12(11): 1087–1088.

33. Barbisch DF, Koenig KL. Understanding Surge Capacity: Essential Elements. *Acad Emerg Med* 2006; 13(11): 1098–1102.

34. U.S. Department of Homeland Security. Target Capabilities: A Companion to the National Preparedness Guidelines. 2007. http://www.fema.gov/pdf/government/training/tcl.pdf (Accessed August 21, 2013). Note: In 2012 The Target Capabilities were consolidated and now are styled Core Capabilities. The Target Capabilities List is available at: http://www.fema.gov/PDF/government/training/TCL.pdf (Accessed Aug. 23, 2013).

35. American College of Healthcare Executives. Healthcare Executives' Role in Emergency Preparedness. 2006. Revised November 2009. www.ache.org/policy/emergency_preparedness.cfm (Accessed August 21, 2013).

36. Joint Commission. Surge Hospitals: Providing Safe Care in Emergencies. 2006. www.jointcommission.org/Surge_Hospital_Providing_Safe_Care_in_Emergencies (Accessed August 21, 2013).

37. Centers for Disease Control and Prevention. Assessment Tool for Evaluating Emergency and Disaster Shelters. 2008. http://www.bt.cdc.gov/shelterassessment (Accessed August 21, 2013).

38. Joint Commission. *History Tracking Report: 2009–2008 Requirements.* Chapter on Emergency Management EM02.01.01. Pre-publication version, Oak Brook, IL, 2008. Note: The Joint Commission now has 2013 Standards in place and has announced *New and Revised Requirements Address Emergency Management Oversight.* www.jointcommission.org/assets/1/18/JCP0713_Emergency_Management_oversight.pdf (Accessed August 21, 2013). This new requirement is effective January 1, 2014. Also see Ambulatory Buzz. In Case of Emergency Read This. http://www.jointcommissin.org/ambulatory_buzz/emergency_read_this (Accessed August 21, 2013).

39. Schultz CH, Stratton SJ. Improving Hospital Surge Capacity: A New Concept for Emergency Credentialing of Volunteers. *Annals of Emerg Med* 2007; 49: 602–609.

40. Lanzilotti SS, Galanis D, Leoni N, Craig B Hawaii Medical Personnel Assessment: A Longitudinal Study of Hawaii Doctors and Nurses, their Knowledge, Skill and Willingness to Treat Victims Related to Weapons of Mass Destruction and Naturally Caused Casualty Incidents. *Hawaii Medical Journal* 2002; 61(8): 162–173.

41. Barnett D, et al, Johns Hopkins Bloomberg School of Public Health. Study of Public Health Personnel in three Maryland Counties and Willingness to Work During a Pandemic. *BMC Public Health Journal* 2006; 6: 99. http://www.biomedcentral.com/1471-2458/6/99.

42. Phillips SJ, Knebel A, *Mass Medical Care with Scarce Resources: A Community Planning Guide.* Rockville, MD, Agency for Healthcare Research and Quality, 2007; Publication No. 05–0043; 2005. http://www.archive.ahrq.gov/research/mce (Accessed August 21, 2013).

43. Health Systems Research. *Altered Standards of Care in Mass Casualty Events: Bioterrorism and other Public Health Emergencies.* Rockville, MD, Agency for Healthcare Quality and Research, 2005; Publication No. -5-0043. http://www.archive.ahrq.gov/alstand (Accessed August 21, 2013).

44. Agency for Healthcare Research and Quality. Hospital Surge Model. 2008. http://www.archive.ahrq.gov/prep (Accessed August 21, 2013).

45. Sternberg EL, Lee, GC, Huard D. Counting Crisis: U.S. Hospital Evacuations 1971–1999. *Prehosp Disaster Med* 19(2): 150–157.

46. Schultz CH, Koenig KL, Lewis RJ. Implications of Hospital Evacuation after the Northridge California Earthquake. *N Engl J Med* 2003; 348: 1349–1355.

47. Schultz CH, Koenig KL, Auf der Heide E, Olson R. Benchmarking for Hospital Evacuation: A Critical Data Collection Tool. *Prehosp Disaster Med* July–August 2005; 20(5): 331–341.

48. Matles S. Author interview October 12, 2008; and *Multi-Casualty Incident Plan: Mutual Aid Evacuation Annex.* Washoe County, NV, District Board of Health, 2008. http://www.co.washoe.nv.us/repository/files/4/MCIPrevised1–24–08 (Accessed August 21, 2013).

49. Long R. *Required Elements for Evacuation Planning for Continuum Health Partner Hospitals.* www.gnyha.org (Accessed August 21, 2013).

50. National Oceanic and Atmospheric Agency website. www.noaa.gov.

51. Telephone interview with Doreen McSharry, MA, CIC, CHSP, June 10, 2013; www.nj.com/hudson.

52. Aviles AD. New York City Health and Hospital Corporations, Public Reports and Testimonies, March 13, 2014. http://www.nyc.gov/html/hhc/html/about/city-council-testimony-20140313.shtml (Accessed August 22, 2015).

53. NYC Office of the Mayor After Action Report on Sandy. www.nyc.gov/html/recovery/downloads/pdf/sandy_aar_5.2.13.pdf (Accessed August 25, 2013).

54. Robert T. Stafford Disaster and Emergency Assistance Act (Public Law 93–288 as amended). www.fema.gov/pdf/stafford-act.pdf (Accessed August 22, 2013).

ADDITIONAL RESOURCES

California Hospital Association. http://calhospitalprepare.org/cha-tools (Accessed August 21, 2013).

Centers for Disease Control and Prevention, Division of Environmental Hazards and Health Effects. Population Monitoring in Radiation Emergencies: A Guide for State and Local Public Health Planners. August 2007. http://emergency.cdc.gov/radiation.pdf/population-monitoring-guide.pdf (Accessed August 21, 2013).

Courses IS-100.HCb and IS-200.HCa are found at: http://www.training.fema.gov/IS/crslist.aspx?all=true.asp (Accessed August 22, 2013).

Deynes S, Kahn C, Koenig KL. Hospital Planning For Terrorist Disasters: A Community-Wide Program. *Emergency Medicine Practice* December 2009; Special Report 1–20.

FEMA Lessons Learned Information Sharing. Marathon Bombings Positive Effects of Preparedness. 2013. https://www.llis.dhs.gov/sites/default/files/BostonMarathonBombingsPositiveEffectsofPreparedness_0 (Accessed August 23, 2013).

Goralnick E, Gates J, We Fight Like We Train. *N Engl J Med* May 29, 2013; 368: 1960–1961. http://www.nejm.org/doi/full/10.1056/NJEMp1305359 (Accessed May 30, 2013).

Kaji AH, Koenig KL, Lewis RJ. Current Hospital Disaster Preparedness. *JAMA* November 14, 2007; 298(18). www.jama.jamanetwork.com/article.aspx?articleid=209407 (Accessed August 22, 2013).

Koenig KL. Preparedness for Terrorism: Managing Nuclear, Biological, Chemical (NBC) Threats. *Annals, Academy of Medicine, Singapore* December 2009; 38(12): 1026–1030.

Minnesota Department of Health. Emergency Sheltering, Relocation, and Evacuation for Healthcare Facilities, V. 4.0, April 2012. http://www.health.state.mn.us/oep/healthcare/flood.html (Accessed August 21, 2013).

National Alliance for Radiation Readiness. www.radiationready.org (Accessed August 21, 2015.)

National Security Staff. Planning Guidance for Response to a Nuclear Detonation. 2nd ed. June 2010. www.epa.gov/radiation/docs/er/planning-guidance-for-response-to-nuclear-detonation-2-edition-final.pdf (Accessed August 21, 2013).

Office of the Assistant Secretary for Preparedness and Response. U.S. Dept. of Health and Human Services. Ebola Information for Healthcare Professionals and Healthcare Settings. http://www.phe.gov/preparedness/Pages/default.aspx (Accessed December 28, 2014).

Zolla-Pazner S. Savings Specimens After Sandy. *N Engl J Med* May 8, 2013; 368(21): e27, DOI: 10.1056/NEJMp1303024.

23

MASS FATALITY MANAGEMENT

Paul S. Sledzik and Sharon W. Bryson

OVERVIEW

> For a civilization to deserve that name, all of life must be valued, including the absent life of the dead.
>
> *Mate Reyes*[1]

Caring for the sick, injured, and displaced is understandably the most important work of disaster responders. However, for the public, media, government, and society, the number of disaster fatalities often reflects the true magnitude of the tragedy. Acknowledging the effort of mass fatality managers is largely focused on the deceased; the work is actually done for the living.

The remains of those killed in disasters must be recovered, identified, and returned to families for final disposition.[2-4] Each step requires specialists in forensic science and fatality management. The processing of disaster fatalities follows legal requirements dictated by the disaster and by the jurisdiction in which the event occurred. As the primary focus of mass fatality management, victim identification involves the collection of postmortem data from the victims and antemortem information from the next of kin, and comparison of the data to establish identification. The condition of the remains also influences the process of managing the deceased. Such taphonomic factors as burning, decomposition, and fragmentation often make recovery difficult and identification complex.

Successful mass fatality management has, as its foundation, proper scientific methods and well-considered government policy guidance. Since governments work for living citizens, it is critical that the family members of the deceased and the communities in which they lived be provided information and support services to move through the culturally accepted practices of grief, mourning, and recovery.[5]

In many countries, mass fatality management has received limited attention from emergency management and disaster response agencies. Myths and uncertainty about dead bodies can be found in media reports, disaster response textbooks, and comments made by public officials. The presence of large numbers of disaster fatalities exposes fears and creates confusion among responders and government officials who lack experience in managing such events. This can lead to ineffective and misguided responses that damage two of the primary goals of mass fatality management: identification of the remains and providing factual information to family members of the deceased.

Mass fatality management is not a traditional first responder or emergency management responsibility and does not fall into typical disaster medical preparedness, training, and response models. Governments have largely overlooked funding, research, and planning for mass fatality management, despite scholarship and after-action reports detailing the short- and long-term psychological, social, and economic impact of poorly conceived management of disaster fatalities and their families. In the past decade, however, mass fatality management has become more formalized with best practice documents, research publications, and after-action reports now influencing the discipline.

This chapter examines current methods for addressing disaster fatality issues and discusses some of the complicating factors encountered during a mass fatality response. Current best practices for managing disaster fatalities are discussed. This includes exploring the unique nature of questions that mass fatality events raise, and a discussion of how to mitigate the impact of such events on families, communities, cultures, and governments.

CURRENT STATE OF THE ART

Legal and Social Concerns in Mass Fatality Management

Effective mass fatality management addresses both the legal considerations for death and the humanitarian concerns guiding respect for the deceased and their families.[3] Proper laws and procedures for mass fatality management must be in place before a disaster occurs.

Identifying human remains from a disaster is a primary objective for the medicolegal, public health, or law enforcement agency responsible for investigating deaths.[6,7] In most cultures, an official identification is required for legal reasons. Family members of the deceased require documentation of the death, usually in the form of a death certificate or similar legal instrument. Certifying death and the issuance of a death certificate allow the next of kin to legally resolve issues of insurance, wills, probate, child guardianship, and remarriage. For a typical non-disaster death, this process is usually straightforward. With large numbers of remains from a disaster, however, the process is quickly overwhelmed.

When a disaster management authority does not follow the legal requirements for death documentation and certification (e.g., by using mass graves or cremations without an attempt to identify the deceased), there are complex, long-term political, economic, psychological, and religious consequences to society.[3,8] Also, the next of kin may be unable to secure the proper legal documents to proceed with obtaining life insurance, inheritance, or government support. Jurisdictions may need to petition courts to issue documents concerning the deceased so that legal matters can be resolved.

In mass fatality events, tension may develop between individual and societal needs with regard to disposition of remains. Families' desires to proceed with funerals and other grief rites may be in conflict with medicolegal requirements for proper identification. If not kept informed about the process, family members and community leaders may begin to question the forensic efforts, particularly the time needed to complete the identification process. Providing factual and realistic information on the process allows families to understand the procedures used and reduces confusion about recovery and identification.[9,10]

Broader than the legal considerations are the humanitarian and moral obligations codified in state and national laws. These laws govern the treatment of the deceased, the need to identify decedents, and the obligation to determine the status of unidentified remains.[3] In addition to national- or state-level laws, international guidelines in the form of customary international humanitarian law guide mass fatality management. These reflect the importance of victim recovery, identification and burial of remains, and the appropriate treatment of the deceased's families.

The Geneva Conventions of 1949 and 1977 and the Law of The Hague have provisions regarding the location, identification, and disposition of human remains resulting from armed conflicts. They proscribe dignity in handling the deceased (e.g., individual burial instead of mass graves) and the importance of positive identification of remains. Signatories to these conventions consider these actions to be fundamental rights.

In 1998, the United Nations (UN) Office of High Commissioner on Human Rights issued the Guiding Principles on Internal Displacement. The guidelines, although not legally binding, comprise provisions codified by international human rights and in humanitarian law that focus on persons displaced by disasters. The principles are well regarded and promoted among UN members. Specifically, Principle 16 of the Guidelines states:

1. All internally displaced persons have the right to know the fate and whereabouts of missing relatives.
2. The authorities concerned shall endeavor to establish the fate and whereabouts of internally displaced persons reported missing, and cooperate with relevant international organizations engaged in this task. They shall inform the next of kin on the progress of the investigation and notify them of any result.

3. The authorities concerned shall endeavor to collect and identify the mortal remains of those deceased, prevent their despoliation or mutilation, and facilitate the return of those remains to the next of kin or dispose of them respectfully.

In 2005, the UN Commission on Human Rights adopted a resolution on human rights and forensic science, noting that "the practice of forensic science includes examinations and identification procedures of both dead and living persons, and underlines the importance of dignified handling of human remains, including their proper management and disposal, as well as of respect for the needs of families."

The international police organization, Interpol, published a Disaster Victim Identification (DVI) Guide to support ongoing programs in its 186 member states. In addition to antemortem and postmortem data collection forms, the guide sets forth recommendations for planning and training in DVI. Interpol's Standing Committee on DVI issues guidelines to member states for establishing DVI teams composed of forensic specialists. The committee advocates using the DVI Guide in all mass fatality events. The Interpol DVI Guide details specific procedures for mass fatality management and the process of victim identification.

In the specific area of aviation accidents, the International Civil Aviation Organization (ICAO, a specialized agency of the UN) promulgates standards and practices for international aviation operations and sets protocols for accident investigation for 191 countries. Several ICAO documents address aviation accident victim identification, including the 2013 Policy on Assistance to Aircraft Accident Victims and Their Families. This policy details the responsibilities of the State, the air operator, and others in the response to a major aviation accident.[11] The ICAO Manual of Aircraft Accident Investigation details the need for investigators to work with civil authorities in the legal identification and death certification of victims.[12]

The Pan American Health Organization (PAHO) provides a model document detailing guiding principles and procedures for states preparing for the management of human remains resulting from disasters.[3] The role of knowledgeable experts, the need for a responsible agency to coordinate efforts, the respectful handling of remains, and the importance of keeping family members and the affected community informed are integral aspects of the model law.

Public Health and Responder Safety Concerns

Despite such laws and accepted protocols, these tenets of proper treatment of the deceased are not always followed. The myth of dead bodies as disease vectors has been promulgated by the media, politicians, and misinformed disaster responders, and plays on unfounded fear of dead bodies.[13] For example, mass graves were used following the 2004 Asian tsunami and the 2010 Haiti earthquake. Comments by public officials following Hurricane Katrina in 2005 indicated a lack of scientific knowledge concerning the potential of disease epidemics spread from dead bodies.[13,14] Such actions can exacerbate the distress experienced by family members of the deceased and the community because they are unable to grieve in the culturally accepted manner.[3,15]

Although the bodies of those killed in mass disasters pose little risk of harboring diseases transmissible to the living, two areas merit consideration: the overall public health risk and the more specific risk to those handling human remains.

For those not physically handling remains, there is little risk associated with human remains. Water- and insect-borne diseases such as dysentery, cholera, plague, and typhoid fever are highly unlikely to be transmitted from human remains to the living. After death, the body temperature drops, thus killing off nearly all pathogens within the body.[3] Ebola virus disease is a notable exception as evidenced by transmission of disease to unprotected relatives of the deceased handling remains that still contain high levels of virus.[16] For those handling remains, there are risks from diseases such as hepatitis B and C, human immunodeficiency virus, tuberculosis, and other enteric pathogens;[17] however, forensic and mortuary workers take precautions against these risks during their regular work in medical examiner offices and funeral homes. Standard precautions and hygiene will typically suffice for those required to handle remains following a disaster. Forensic and mortuary workers involved in body handling and the more invasive procedures such as autopsy should use the precautions taken by forensic pathologists in their daily practices.[18] Special precautions recommended for handling of remains exposed to chemical, biological or radiologic agents are discussed later in the chapter.

The contamination of groundwater due to the leaching of body fluids from mass graves is another common misconception. No reliable evidence of groundwater contaminated by infectious diseases from corpses has been documented by public health and landfill researchers.[15] The anaerobic soil environment and the time required for any biological fluids passing through the soil to reach the groundwater would likely kill any viable pathogens.

The Role of the Event in Response Management

While disaster etiology may initially be unknown, different types of disasters require the use of specific regulations or procedures to document the scene, collect evidence, and determine the cause and manner of death. Despite problems with use of this terminology (as described in Perspective), mass fatality events have been categorized into three types based on etiology: criminal, accidental, and natural. Although similar activities occur following each of these types – search and recovery, victim identification, and disposition of remains – disasters caused by criminal intent or that are the result of an "accident" require an investigation, and thus the implementation of additional procedures. For example, the response to a criminal event requires collection of evidence for potential legal proceedings. Determining the cause of an accident requires collection of evidence so that recommendations to improve safety in the particular area of public interest can be implemented. In "natural" disasters, the cause is often known, and collecting of physical evidence is usually not required. Disease-related fatality events may require autopsy and evidence collection to determine the specific pathogen and its source. Some events initially thought to be "naturally occurring" are later determined to have illegitimate causes. Most of the evidence collected by morgue personnel for criminal and technological disasters centers around autopsy, physical evidence on the remains, identification of perpetrators (if they are killed in the event), and separation of investigative evidence that may be commingled with the remains.

In criminally-related disasters, such as the September 11, 2001, terrorist events in the United States, the terrorist bombings in Bali in 2002, the July 7, 2005, London transit bombings, and the November 2008 Mumbai terrorist attacks, collection and documentation of important forensic evidence was necessary, both at the disaster site and from the victims' remains. In these events, determining the identity of victims and the deceased perpetrators was a critical investigative avenue, as was detailing the victims' cause of death.

Following the 2002 terrorist bombing of a Bali nightclub, the Australian Interpol DVI team responded to support Balinese officials. Once local police secured the scene, techniques were used to document and collect the remains. In this event, the condition of remains helped discern the center of the blast – an important forensic determination. Analysis of the scene indicated the bomb was poorly constructed and the blast was not as powerful as it could have been. Although the number of different nationalities represented among the victims complicated the collection of antemortem information, the DVI team was able to identify all 202 victims within 4 weeks. The importance of using accepted scientific methods for identification was underscored when the DVI team positively identified nine bodies that had been previously misidentified by family members using visual recognition.[19]

In a technological disaster, such as an aircraft catastrophe, building collapse, ferry capsizing, or industrial explosion, victims must be identified and the cause of death determined. Identifying the reason for the disaster also requires collection of evidence. Once the cause is determined, investigators often make recommendations to enhance worker or passenger health and safety. For example, correlating passenger injuries with seating assignments may aid in reconstructing the sequence of events at the time of a plane crash and is useful in evaluating aircraft safety equipment.[20–22]

Assessing the cause of mortality in disasters and the resulting changes in public health codes and building requirements underscores the importance of collecting information concerning disaster fatalities and the impact of this research on the safety of the community.[23–25] Surveillance of suspicious deaths, an often-overlooked responsibility of medical examiners and coroners, can distinguish bioterrorism events from non-criminal disease outbreaks.[18]

Mass fatality events caused by chemical, biological, and radiological sources pose complications for recovery, handling, processing, and disposition of remains.[26,27] To respond effectively, the chemical or biological agent must first be identified, allowing forensic responders to plan for the level of decontamination and the level of personal protective equipment (PPE) needed. The medicolegal authority should work with the appropriate health and environmental agencies to understand the local laws regarding handling and disposition of any contaminated remains. For certain types of chemical and biological agents, there are considerations regarding burial or cremation of remains. For victims killed by anthrax, smallpox, or viral hemorrhagic fever, cremation is recommended over burial to prevent the potential spread of the disease. For victims of botulinum toxin, plague, and tularemia, experts recommend remains not be embalmed to reduce the risk to mortuary workers.[27]

Due to the high incidence of disease transmission from infected dead bodies during the 2014 Ebola outbreak in West Africa, national and international health agencies issued guidance on the safe handling of remains.[28,29] These included minimizing the handling of remains, using PPE when handling remains and proper doffing and subsequent hygiene, ensuring remains are properly wrapped in plastic or double-bagged, and thorough decontamination of surfaces that have come into contact with the victim. The guidance also suggests avoiding conducting autopsies and that remains be cremated or buried in a hermetically sealed coffin.

Radiological contamination can be internal, external, or result from shrapnel from an explosive device. Removing clothing from the deceased can reduce the risk of secondary external contamination by 90% to those recovering and processing them; most of the remaining external radiological contaminants can be removed by washing the deceased. Monitoring radiological exposure to forensic and mortuary workers and coordinating with knowledgeable experts in radiology will also help to reduce risk.[26]

Deaths from pandemic events, such as those from pandemic influenza, pose challenges because of the wide geographical area affected and long duration of time for the event. Because pandemic influenza deaths would most likely occur in homes and in hospitals in numbers exceeding the normal capacity of the local death management infrastructure, storage of remains and final disposition are important considerations.[30]

When disasters such as hurricanes, floods, and earthquakes result in fatalities, response teams must conduct search, recovery, and identification operations. The size of these responses is driven by the geographical scope of the event. Floodwaters have disinterred caskets from cemeteries, resulting in unique challenges for mass fatality managers.[30]

Mass Fatality Response and Government Agencies

While mass fatality events are infrequent, when they do occur the affected community often seeks assistance from nearby communities and municipalities, and regional and state-level government response agencies. Public and private organizations and nongovernmental organizations can provide help, ranging from offering advice to providing personnel and equipment. However, government agencies must have mass fatality plans in place in order to conduct an effective response. The complex nature of the work and the sometimes complicated nature of augmenting local or national-level resources can pose operational challenges if unplanned.

At the national level, governments usually have an agency assigned to manage disaster responses. These differ by country and state, but generally encompass emergency management, public safety, military, health ministry, homeland security, and similar agencies. Although they may not have direct responsibility for the specific requirements of mass fatality management, they often guide the overall national policy and approach to such events. Within the United States, some states have assigned mass fatality responsibilities to national-level forensic medicine institutes, local or state-level coroner offices, or other pertinent agencies with medicolegal knowledge. The capabilities of national-level governments and related state agencies differ greatly between states, based on economy and infrastructure.

Interpol DVI teams – deployable to mass fatality events in the 186 Interpol member countries – comprise experts in forensic identification such as dentists, pathologists, fingerprint analysts, and experienced support personnel. International, federal, and private deoxyribonucleic acid (DNA) laboratories are available for analysis and comparison of DNA samples. Nongovernmental agencies such as the International Committee for the Red Cross and PAHO have experts available to assist in planning mass fatality response operations. State and local funeral director or mortuary service associations can also provide assistance. Private companies specializing in disaster response operations

have also developed teams to support mass fatality management and victim identification.

Disaster Victim Identification

Positive identification of disaster victims is based on the comparison of unique biological attributes observed in the remains with concurrent evidence of these features detailed in dental and medical records, radiographs, and other reliable documents.[6] This method of comparing antemortem records with postmortem findings is routine in daily non-disaster forensic casework. Four methods are most commonly used and each method is scientifically validated using verified and accurate antemortem and postmortem documentation.

1. Comparison of dental records (e.g., radiographs and charts) with dental evidence from remains
2. Comparison of fingerprint/footprint records located in reliable repositories with friction ridge patterns from the palms, fingers, and feet of victims
3. Comparison of medical documentation of highly unique physical characteristics with similar evidence found on the remains. Such evidence includes (but is not limited to) radiographs showing healed fractures and other unique skeletal structures, implanted medical devices with serial numbers, tattoos, scars, and birthmarks
4. Comparison of DNA profiles obtained from the remains to DNA samples of the victim (direct comparison) or DNA from specific blood relatives (indirect or family comparison)

The number of victims, the composition of the victim population, and the condition of the remains influence the comparison of evidence and ultimately the timeliness of identifications. If antemortem records are available, identifications using dental, medical, and fingerprint methods can be performed quickly, usually within several days. These "conventional" methods of identification lead to the most immediate results because they involve on-site comparison of antemortem and postmortem data. The laboratory requirements to process and analyze DNA require more time than conventional methods, and DNA identifications take longer to complete.

The term "presumptive identification" is often used to refer to the process of using characteristics or items that suggest a victim's identity, but are not sufficiently unique to be definitive. A presumptive identification based on non-unique biological or portable evidence is often used as a step toward confirming an individual's identity by using some or all of the scientific methods listed previously. Jewelry, clothing, and visual recognition or facial features by next of kin are examples of methods used for presumptive identification. Personal effects such as clothing, wallets, and jewelry are portable items that are often displaced during a disaster. Visual recognition of facial features by next of kin has been shown to be inaccurate, possibly because of postmortem changes in the remains and the attendant psychological stress placed on family members involved in the process.[32,33]

Considerations in Mass Fatality Management

Before fatality management activities progress, the medicolegal authority and the primary forensic responders must begin to obtain information regarding several important concerns.

- Number of fatalities
- Potential cause of the event (e.g., criminal, accidental, natural)
- Challenges in searching for and recovering human remains (e.g., geographical area, terrain, weather)
- Type of victim population: Open (names of victims are unknown) or closed (known list of victims)
- Condition of the remains (e.g., complete, fragmented, burned, decomposed)
- Availability, types, and accuracy of the antemortem information
- Role and limitations of DNA in the identification efforts
- Concerns and expectations of society and the next of kin about the identification process

These data determine how forensic personnel will conduct their work, the amount of time the identification process will require, and the limitations to identifications.[2,34,35] They also allow mass fatality managers to determine the goals of the DVI process.

Certainly, the number of fatalities plays a role in the time required to complete the identification process, particularly when the figure rises into the thousands. However, it is the associated factors of environmental context, taphonomy, and antemortem data availability that often have a more profound effect on the identification process. As an example, consider two disasters each resulting in 100 fatalities. The first disaster leaves complete bodies recovered from level terrain, which display little taphonomic change (i.e., no burning, fragmentation, or decomposition), and for which antemortem records for the victims are easily obtainable. The second disaster causes fragmentation of remains, with nearly 5,000 fragments representing 100 victims, scattered at a depth of 3,000 meters below the ocean surface. Little is known about the victims and locating their associated antemortem information is complicated. Resolving the second event will take longer, use more resources, and require more complex fatality management decisions.

Based on the information known about a victim population at the time of the disaster, the group is categorized as either "open" or "closed." In a closed population, data about the number and identity of the victims are easily obtainable. Using personal information found on the victim or other pertinent information, authorities can contact the next of kin to obtain antemortem information. The most common example is an aircraft incident wherein a flight manifest (supported by ticket purchasing and security procedures) is the initial source for collection of antemortem information. For example, under U.S. law, passenger names and contact information are provided to federal authorities within a matter of hours following a major aviation accident, and the collection of antemortem information can begin shortly thereafter.

Conversely, an open population defines a victim group in which neither the number of victims nor their names are immediately, or in some cases ever, known. In the public response to the disaster, emergency managers and law enforcement agencies are often overwhelmed by massive numbers of inquiries regarding the missing – a common challenge with an open population disaster. Despite frequently held misconceptions, family members take actions to reunite themselves with their missing loved ones, including contacting agencies responsible for missing persons and going to the disaster site.[36] Creating an accurate list of victims and their status (i.e., alive, injured, or dead) requires a well-designed process, managed by the agency responsible for managing missing persons cases, to separate those reported missing from those actually missing. Ideally, a designated missing persons or casualty call center receives all such inquiries and develops a comprehensive list of those persons reported as missing. From this list, investigators establish a second list of those actually missing by verifying the status of a missing person, eliminating duplicate reports, clarifying misspellings, and other errors. Once a victim is known to be missing, the process of obtaining and examining antemortem data can begin.

The challenges regarding management of missing persons in open population disasters are reflected in the initial reports of the number of fatalities, which usually differ substantially from the final figures. Following the September 11, 2001, U.S. World Trade Center disaster, initial media reports indicated that as many as 10,000 people were dead or missing. Subsequent days saw the number range between 3,958 and 6,453.[37] As of November 2005, the total number reported missing due to the disaster was 2,749, of whom 1,594 had been identified.[38] More than a dozen years after the event recovery and identification operations were still ongoing. Following the Asian tsunami of 2004, the World Health Organization reported 10,000 dead and within 10 days the number expanded to 153,000.[39] The final death toll was nearly 250,000, with an understanding that the true number will never be known.[32,40] After the terrorist bombings in London on July 7, 2005, a centralized casualty call center was established (per previous planning efforts) to manage missing persons calls.[5] The center received 43,000 calls within the first hour of operation, with more than 121,000 calls received by July 25. This resulted in 12,000 missing reports being taken. This number of calls and missing persons reports, for an event that killed 56 and injured more than 700, underscores the intense public response following a disaster, and the need for authorities to implement a coordinated missing persons tracking system.

The condition of the remains also impacts the methods used for their identification and processing.[41] When related antemortem records are available, complete bodies can be identified quickly because they encompass all the unique physical characteristics needed for identification. In cases involving whole or nearly complete bodies, once the body is identified, the decedent is also identified, that is, the number of bodies equates to the number of victims. Using conventional methods, identifications are completed relatively quickly and at comparatively low cost.

Complexities arise when the bodies of multiple victims are reduced to several hundreds or thousands of body parts of varying sizes and anatomical structures. Among the fragmented remains are those containing the unique physical characteristic that will lead to a positive identification, such as a hand with ridge skin or a jaw fragment exhibiting dental work. These parts are usually identified quickly (if antemortem data are available), confirming both the victim's death and identification. Most of the fragmented remains, however, will not contain these features. These remains are examined using DNA analysis, and if identified, they can be reassociated with previously identified remains from the same individual. This ongoing process of identification presents a need for the next of kin to decide whether they wish to be notified each time a body part is identified or prefer to be notified only at the end of the identification process.

In both cases, all reasonable efforts to identify fragmentary remains are made, but there are usually remains that cannot be identified, often referred to as group remains. These remains must be managed carefully; families must be informed of their existence and must be involved with decisions regarding their final disposition.

DNA and Mass Fatality Management

DNA analysis is a powerful tool in disaster victim identification and offers a high degree of statistical confidence in its results. DNA analysis provides the ability to identify remains having no distinctive biological characteristics and the possibility of being able to identify very small fragments of hard and soft tissue. As a laboratory-based procedure, DNA analysis takes longer and is more expensive than other methods of identification. The overall DNA effort should be coordinated by the agency responsible for medicolegal DNA identification during non-disaster periods. Before DNA identification begins, several questions must be asked, the answers to which will influence the application of DNA analysis.[35] These include:

- How important is DNA to the identification effort?
- Will every person be accounted for or every fragment be identified?
- What is the minimum fragment size that will be processed for identification?
- How difficult will it be to identify everyone?
- How long will the recovery efforts last?

DNA identification requires analysis of postmortem (victim) samples, and the collection and analysis of antemortem samples, called reference samples. Reference samples include personal items of the victim that would contain DNA (direct reference samples), DNA samples from biological relatives (family reference samples), and DNA extracted from remains previously identified using conventional methods. Direct reference samples include toothbrushes, hairbrushes, personal hygiene items, and medical or pathology samples. Family reference samples are easily obtained by use of buccal swabs or blood samples. The biological relationship of the donor to the victim must be documented in order to ensure accurate results usable in the DNA comparison.

Processing of postmortem and reference samples requires DNA extraction. Once extracted, the DNA can be compared for identification. However, some samples tested will not yield DNA for analysis, because conditions such as fire, chemicals, and decomposition have destroyed or degraded DNA.[42] Very small pieces of bone can yield usable DNA for comparison, but these samples are often destroyed in the extraction process. This creates a situation in which a body fragment could be identified, but in accomplishing this, there are no physical remains to return to the family except the tube containing the extracted DNA.

Mass fatality managers must provide realistic expectations for family members, politicians, and the media about the use of DNA in the identification process. DNA analysis is a powerful tool that can be misunderstood by nonscientists. Following the World Trade Center disaster, emergency managers provided the following figures to the public on a regular basis to help manage expectations: victim samples received; victim samples analyzed; reference samples analyzed; victims identified; victims identified by DNA only; and remains reassociated with victims.[35] With this information, family members, the public, the media, and politicians could see progress and frame it within the larger context of the recovery and identification efforts.

Mass Fatality Operations

Mass fatality operations encompass several activities: location and recovery; documentation and identification; and determination of final disposition of remains and associated record-keeping. In addition, there is a need to keep family members informed during the process. Three operational locations of activity typically develop: the disaster site, the disaster morgue, and the family assistance center, where families of the deceased gather to provide and receive information. An effective response allows for continual and accurate information exchange among all three sites.

Mass fatality response teams are multidisciplinary because the nature of their participation involves both scientific analysis and cultural and religious aspects of handling human remains. Victim identification teams usually include forensic pathologists, forensic anthropologists, forensic dentists, fingerprint specialists, DNA analysts, medicolegal investigators, and forensic managers. Funeral directors, clergy, crisis mental health experts, and similarly trained personnel support both the disaster responders and the victims' families. The services and information provided to family members, often termed family assistance, are critical elements of a mass fatality response.

Search and Recovery

The search for and recovery of remains is the first part of the victim identification process. Typically, once the living and injured are treated and removed from the site, the search and rescue operations shift to search and recovery of remains.

The methods used to process a crime scene are logically applicable to the disaster scene and include locating, defining, and securing the maximum boundary of the affected area (or areas); identifying, documenting, numbering, and collecting human remains and any associated evidence; and establishing chain of custody to ensure the integrity of all evidence from the moment of recovery to final disposition. In situations where there are multiple contexts within a disaster area, each context may be managed separately; however, good communication and coordination between these operations will reduce field documentation and collection errors that can introduce confusion at the morgue and slow the identification process. Implementing a systematic approach using scientific methods ensures the scene is thoroughly documented and all evidence, including human remains, are detected, recorded and collected.[43]

The increased use of precision survey and mapping technology and geographic information systems have enhanced the ability to collect spatial data that capture the relationship between human remains, personal effects, and other physical evidence. High-resolution orthophotography and other types of remote-sensing offer responders a more accurate common operating picture that can be shared by those involved in the search and recovery efforts. These data are critical to the investigation of the accident or crime, in addition to aiding in victim identification. Where no discrete scene is present (e.g., pandemic deaths in individual homes), consideration should be given to the level of documentation needed based on the disaster, any investigation that may occur, and local laws.

Many factors influence the search and recovery process: size of the impacted area, number of fatalities, condition of the remains, chemical/biological/radiological hazards, season, terrain, and weather. For example, searching for complete bodies

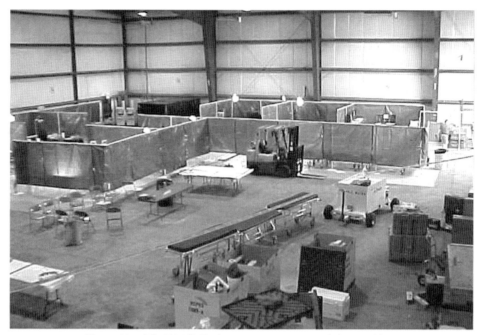

Figure 23.1. The DMORT Disaster Morgue at an Aviation Accident.

exhibiting little decomposition found in homes following a hurricane may require a period of time, but the actual documentation and recovery is relatively simple. Conversely, the fragmented and burned remains resulting from a relatively small high-speed aircraft crash caused by a terrorist attack must be carefully documented at the scene and thoroughly analyzed once in the morgue.

Disaster Morgue Selection

Selecting the location for processing remains is a critical first step in management of the disaster fatalities. Since the disaster morgue is the site of intense, stressful work, lasting weeks or months, the needs of morgue personnel should be the primary focus in determining facility location. Ideally, local authorities should identify a site before an event occurs. Health, safety, security, and adequate size are key considerations in identifying the location for the disaster morgue. Logistical considerations include adequate heating/ventilation/air conditioning, lighting, water supply, electrical capacity, telephone and high-speed Internet access, restrooms, drainage (for capturing biohazard wastes), nonporous floors, and forklift accessibility. Proximity to the disaster scene(s), adequate floor space, access for and placement of refrigerated trucks for storage of remains, and office space for workers and support personnel are additional factors. The movement of remains through the morgue facility and other areas where examinations occur should also be carefully arranged. A security plan should be implemented to preserve chain of custody and also because the morgue can become a focus of attention for family members and the media.

Disaster morgues have been successfully established in aircraft hangers, vacant warehouses, securable private buildings, and medical examiner or coroner offices when space and procedures allowed. In the latter circumstance, care is taken to separate the daily casework from disaster casework. Portable tents have also been used in situations where an existing physical facility is unavailable. Active public facilities such as schools or community centers should be avoided because of the potential psy-

chological impact on the community. Although disaster victim identification teams have worked in austere conditions, the preference is for them to conduct their work in a more comfortable environment.

Remains should be stored in refrigerated trucks or a facility cooled to a temperature that slows decomposition because this process can destroy certain soft-tissue characteristics useful for identification. Refrigerator trucks or similar storage facilities should be designated as "unprocessed" and "processed" to keep remains segregated and organized. Racking systems can be installed in refrigerated trucks or warehouse facilities to maximize storage of both complete bodies and fragmentary remains, which can be bagged and collected in bins. Careful management of remains in storage is essential so that specific body fragments can be retrieved for reexamination or release. Remains may require storage for a long period following postmortem examination, particularly if DNA analysis is being used for identification.

In the United States, the Disaster Mortuary Operational Response Team (DMORT) system has assembled Disaster Portable Morgue Units (DPMU) containing supplies and equipment for operating an incident morgue for large-scale fatality events. Some larger jurisdictions and states have also established portable morgues. DPMUs are transportable to the incident site via truck or aircraft and are supported by a team of trained responders who assemble, restock, and repack the DPMU. Equipment and supplies are stored in specialized cases and a load plan facilitates shipment. Once on site, the DPMU is usually operational in less than 24 hours. Figure 23.1 shows the DPMU established in an aircraft hangar following an aviation incident near Wilkes-Barre, Pennsylvania, in May 2000. Figure 23.2 shows the DPMU organized in an abandoned gymnasium on an inactive military base following the crash of EgyptAir 990 in October 1999. Note the walled sections denoting the workstations for the various parts of the morgue operation. Figure 23.3 depicts a schematic of morgue operations, with workstations, refrigerated trucks, and processing areas.

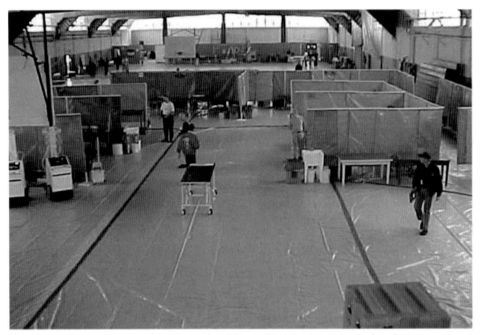

Figure 23.2. The DMORT Disaster Morgue Showing Forensic Workstations.

Incident Morgue Operations

Several standard operating guidelines for disaster victim identification and morgue operations are available from the websites of organizations such as Interpol, DMORT, the National
Association of Medical Examiners, the UK Home Office, the
U.S. National Institutes of Justice, and PAHO. These guidelines
reflect the importance of a standardized process for documen-

tation, analysis, quality assurance, and respect for the dead. The
particulars of the disaster may require modification of parts
of the morgue process, but the procedures remain largely the
same.

Figure 23.4 is a morgue operational plan that demonstrates
the typical movement of remains through the incident morgue.
Controlling the flow of the deceased into the morgue allows
for efficient processing and avoids overwhelming the morgue

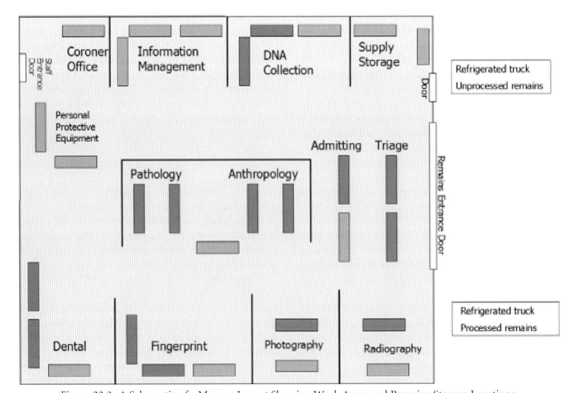

Figure 23.3. A Schematic of a Morgue Layout Showing Work Areas and Remains Storage Locations.

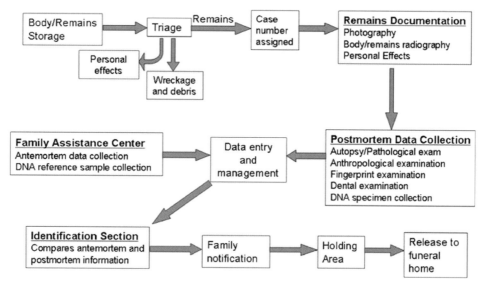

Figure 23.4. Morgue Operational Plan.

team with remains for analysis. Once brought into the morgue, remains are radiographed in their container (e.g., body bag, pouch, or transfer case). Radiographs allow for evaluation of the container's contents prior to opening. For complete bodies, radiographs can reveal explosive devices or other hazards, personal effects, forensic evidence, the extent of trauma, and potential commingling with other remains in the same container. For fragmented remains, radiographs reveal potentially identifiable body portions, evidence, personal effects, non-biological material, and the extent of commingling. Radiographs are essential for the next step, known as triage. Triage is the process of sorting human remains, first to remove any material not related to determining identity, and then to assess their potential for identification.[44,45] In the first step, four categories of materials are typically separated: 1) personal effects; 2) wreckage or other types of evidence; 3) remains with a potential for identification; and 4) remains with no or little potential for identification.

During the second step, each body or body part is assessed using a probative index that classifies remains according to their identification potential or investigative value. The probative index is incident-specific because factors such as availability and accuracy of antemortem information impact identification potential. Triage of whole bodies allows for sorting by the potential for identification, such as the presence of dental work or evidence of surgery. For fragmentary remains, triage personnel assess each body part for positive and presumptive identifying features that may lead to dental, fingerprint, medical, or DNA identification. Remains usually suitable for identification include dental specimens, large body portions, hands, feet, prosthetic devices, and bone showing healed trauma. Accordingly, remains with the greatest potential for identification are analyzed first. Small pieces of skin, fatty tissue, muscle, and similar specimens lacking characteristics usable in the identification process do not initially enter the morgue processing stream, but can be examined if the initial identification process does not account for all victims.

Following triage, remains are moved to the admitting area where a case file containing postmortem analytical paperwork

and other administrative data is created. Remains are assigned a number corresponding to the case file. A simple numbering system reduces confusion and decreases administrative errors. Remains should be assigned unique simple consecutive numbers. Letters, dashes, and similar characters should be avoided (e.g., 34/A-2, 96–0005A34). During the course of the morgue analysis, if additional remains are found commingled with a specimen, then the new body part can be brought to the admitting station and assigned the next consecutive number. Morgue personnel can preserve associated numbering systems assigned at the disaster scene if a similar logic has been applied. Data from the scene associated with the remains can be placed in the pertinent case file. After identification and reassociation of fragmented remains, the coroner or medical examiner assigns a unique victim number or case number to the remains comprising that individual.

Various technologies reduce errors in the management of large numbers of remains. For example, computer-readable barcodes and radiofrequency identification chips were used to manage remains in disaster morgue operations following the World Trade Center disaster, the 2004 Indian Ocean tsunami, and Hurricane Katrina.[46]

Once numbered, the individual remains are photographed, radiographed, and then moved through the postmortem examination stations. Forensic scientists with mass fatality experience staff these stations, which are usually referred to by the discipline conducting the work – dental, pathology, anthropology, fingerprint, and DNA. Requirements of the investigation dictate whether remains are examined at each station or just at stations that are relevant to a particular body part. At each station, information is collected according to a protocol created for the specific disaster response.

Forensic odontologists (dentists) staff the dental station, where they examine the maxilla, mandible, and any fragments thereof to document dental structures, fillings, and other unique features.[47] Fingerprint experts take prints from fingers, hands, and feet (if necessary) for comparison to existing print records. Forensic anthropologists document anatomical structures to determine sex, age, stature, and other pertinent biological attributes useful in identification, such as bone trauma or unique skeletal characteristics. Forensic pathologists examine remains for evidence of unique features, assess information relative to cause of death, and conduct autopsies if necessary. In some cases where equipment is available and the remains are complete, MRI scans can assist pathologists in this determination, thus avoiding the need for an invasive autopsy. DNA technicians take samples from soft tissue and bone, which are later analyzed in the DNA laboratory. Interaction across discipline boundaries is essential for successfully completing the process of postmortem documentation. Once finalized, postmortem data are entered into a data management system for later retrieval during the identification process.

These same forensic specialists are also involved in comparison of the postmortem data with the antemortem records – the process of positive identification. Regularly scheduled meetings between the medicolegal authority and the forensic experts allow for review of current findings and discussion of identifications. Details of each identification are documented, and the information is presented to the medicolegal authority for validation and authorization. This process usually takes place at the disaster morgue for those identifications accomplished by conventional methods. If DNA analysis is used, the identifications may take months to complete and a separate DNA identification team is established to document and validate identifications. Once a victim is identified, the next of kin is notified via the medicolegal authority's usual process for death notification. Remains may then be released to the next of kin for final disposition, or remains are maintained at the morgue awaiting reassociation based on the next of kin's decision.

Collection and Use of Antemortem Data

Collecting postmortem data is relatively simple compared with the collection of antemortem information. Locating, analyzing, and interpreting antemortem data is a more complex process because it involves work outside the morgue, reaching out to family members, medical and dental offices, government agencies, and law enforcement bureaus. The availability and usefulness of antemortem data can be affected by the disaster itself and the demographics of the victims impacted.

Antemortem data consist of three types: 1) medical, dental, and fingerprint records; 2) family interview information; and 3) DNA reference samples. Records – such as dental charts, radiographs, medical records, fingerprint cards, and photographs – detail the presence of unique biological characteristics of the victim. Because these types of records contain the most accurate and verifiable sources of information, they must be obtained through means that detail their source, that is, dental, medical, or government office. Interpol and national or state law enforcement agencies may hold fingerprint records of a victim, especially if there is a history of military service, federal or state employment, or a criminal record.

Locating the sources of antemortem records usually starts with contacting family members and friends of the deceased to conduct interviews. This process provides assistance with locating antemortem records (e.g., by providing contact information for the victim's dentist and physician), gathering information required for death certificate completion, and determining the legal next of kin. A family assistance center or similar facility is often established where specialists in funeral service and forensic identification interview family members using standardized questionnaires.

Interviewers must understand identification methods and be familiar with the antemortem data collection form. Antemortem interviews are difficult for families, and interviewers should possess the ability to work with those suffering from grief. Answers provided by family members and friends regarding the deceased's biological and medical data should be verified before use in the identification process.[48] They may, however, be the only sources of antemortem information, particularly when no medical or dental records exist and when DNA will not be used.

Antemortem data availability is affected by various factors within the victim population. For example, individuals of lower socioeconomic status may never have received dental care and thus will have no antemortem dental records. Antemortem records are also sometimes destroyed in the disaster, such as in the crash of a U.S. military chartered aircraft in Gander, Newfoundland, in 1985 and following Hurricane Katrina.[49,50]

If DNA will be used for identification, collecting direct and family reference samples requires coordination and careful documentation. For chain of custody reasons, the DNA laboratory conducting the analysis should also participate in the collection of the reference and postmortem samples. The biological relationship of the donor to the victim must be accurately documented, and sample collection kits can be tailored to ensure the reliability of family donor information.

The efforts of the missing persons call center and the antemortem data collection teams will result in the accumulation of large amounts of information. Data management software is necessary for effective data organization.[51] The nature of this large data collection effort results in errors from a variety of sources, and methods to locate and correct errors must be implemented. DNA data management is often accomplished separately, due to the unique features of the testing, but the data are cross-referenced with related antemortem and postmortem information.

The volume of antemortem information, scene documentation data, and DNA-based records generated is often dramatically underestimated. For the World Trade Center DNA identification efforts, approximately 260,000,000 pairwise comparisons were made between the nearly 20,000 remains, 6,800 family reference samples, and 4,200 direct reference samples.[52] Although the actual comparison time using computer software took only several hours, creating the data for comparison, ensuring its accuracy, and interpreting the results required many months of work.

Policy and Ethical Questions in Mass Fatality Management

The decisions and processes involved in managing and identifying disaster victims create unique policy and ethical questions arising from the interplay of three different domains: the remains of the victims, the expectations of family members and society, and the tools and technical limitations of victim identification science. These questions often concern how remains are identified, the extent of resources allocated to conduct identifications, and expectations about what is returned to the family for final disposition. Such questions include:

▪ Should the limited resources available to conduct identification be used to identify all fragmentary remains or all decedents?
▪ How large does a specimen need to be for testing?

- What should be the disposition of unidentifiable remains?
- At what point does the identification process end?
- Should remains recovered years after a disaster be processed for identification?

Answers to these questions are influenced by available resources, the characteristics of the disaster, the desires of the family members (individually and as a disaster-specific group), cultural and religious beliefs about death and final disposition of remains, societal expectations about what science can provide, and the availability of appropriate forensic identification tools and techniques.[3,35] These questions are not unique to disaster work, as forensic scientists involved in human rights investigations have raised similar concerns.[53] Additionally, the increased use of DNA testing for disaster victim identification has raised ethical questions about the use of samples for such events.[54]

DVI science has limitations that must be explained to family members and society because their expectations can be at odds with scientific capabilities. When families believe that identifications will happen quickly, scientists must convey realistic expectations to the families about the timeframe and associated complexities. This difficult but necessary readjustment helps families understand the reasons behind the answers to the aforementioned questions.[9,55]

Resolving these questions is rarely done through public dialogue, presumably because of the sensitivities of discussing the details of the event. Informed public discussion is essential, however, to answer these questions appropriately.[56,57] Family members want and deserve factual, compassionate discourse. Although the discussions may be difficult, they help families navigate the complex grief process associated with a disaster while concurrently assuring a community that their loved ones receive appropriate consideration and care.

Caring for Mass Fatality Workers

Despite their routine exposures to death, the psychological impact of disaster work on forensic responders should not be underestimated. Disaster forensic work is physically and psychologically stressful.[58-60] Even with the familiarity of working with human remains, certain tasks increase stress for most forensic responders.[61] These include the handling of personal effects, examining the remains of children, the condition of remains (particularly aspects of visual grotesqueness, odor, and tactile features), and exposure to a large number of victims. Identifying or personalizing with the victims increases emotional attachment to the remains, may reduce objectivity, and may increase vulnerability to psychological distress. Such stressors can result in normal emotional reactions, such as sadness, disgust, anger, pity, fear, and numbness. Physical reactions can include headache, sleep difficulties, intestinal problems, appetite changes, and fatigue.[62]

The most effective coping strategies involve talking with trusted coworkers, appropriate use of humor, reflecting on the larger purpose of the work, avoiding media coverage of the event (particularly information about the victims), and taking regular time off from the disaster work. Camaraderie and talking with colleagues both during and after the event has been shown to be an important source of positive feelings about a disaster response. Peer-support models, as found in fire/rescue and police agencies, are preferable for forensic responders, because outside mental health professionals typically do not understand the particular stressors of forensic work.[60] Despite the stress,

forensic responders report that disaster work is a valuable experience, provides a sense of accomplishment, and increases their appreciation of life.[58]

Assistance to Victims and Their Families of Victims

Because one of the main goals of mass fatality management is to comfort the living, it is important that appropriate support is provided to survivors and to victims' families. Issues to address include the type of help needed when a mass fatality occurs and identifying the needs of the victims and their families after the immediate emergency passes. Survivors of mass fatality events and family members of those killed often experience an "existential crisis" marked by a profound sense of emptiness and despair.[63] Family members, survivors, and others impacted in the community are likely to exist in a state of psychological shock, uncertain about the whereabouts of loved ones and about the future.[64]

Responding to the needs of those affected is complex from a logistical perspective, yet simple in determining a successful outcome. The complexities arise from the myriad of state, local, and federal agencies, private groups, and local community nonprofit organizations each attempting to provide assistance. The measure of success for those assisting family members is simple: it is determined by how effectively the needs of victims and their families are met and by the compassion demonstrated during the response.

Managing a mass fatality event requires coordination among all participants from each area of the disaster response. Prompt and precise communication about the needs of those impacted is crucial. In the chaos of the moment, however, responders can lose sight of the victims' real needs. There is a tendency to respond based on a broad generalization of what the disaster response should entail. Clearly, there are guiding general principles that influence responders when assisting victims; however, it is equally as important to stay focused on the individual impacted by the disaster. It is often best to reflect on who the victims are and what their needs may be in order to maintain the proper focus and deliver appropriate services.

Listening to victims and their families describe their needs and expectations can also help guide future responses. The U.S. Task Force on Aviation Disaster Family Assistance, formed by the passage of the Aviation Disaster Family Assistance Act of 1996, articulated a series of recommendations.[65] Family members, representatives from the commercial aviation community, government agencies, and nonprofit organizations attempted to create a more effective approach to meeting the needs of victims and their families following an aviation disaster. In the United Kingdom, the charity Disaster Action is composed of survivors and family members who provide an independent advocacy and advisory service representing the perspectives of individuals directly affected by disaster. The Fédération Nationale des Victimes d'Accidents Collectifs (FENVAC) in France comprises victims' families from various mass fatality disasters and terrorism events. In addition to supporting family members, FENVAC also serves to defend the rights of victims and to promote accountability and accident prevention.

Family members impacted by a mass fatality event describe an overwhelming sense of loss of control over their world. The loss they experience is often in the context of a larger public tragedy.[66] When individuals suffer a loss under such circumstances, they experience grief.[67] Grief is expressed in numerous ways, including physical, psychological, behavioral, and social and spiritual responses and reactions.[68] The nature of this larger public tragedy makes the grief process more difficult for victims and their families. An effective mass fatality response and recovery must carefully consider these aspects and integrate proper remedies.

The grief experienced in response to a mass fatality event is further complicated by the traumatic nature of the incident. Trauma refers to situations out of the normal range of experience and includes things such as suddenness and lack of anticipation; violence, mutilation, and destruction; preventability or randomness of the event; and the mourners' personal encounters with death. The individual experiences either a significant threat to personal survival or a shocking confrontation with the death or mutilation of others.[69] Traumatic events challenge the many assumptions people have about the world and cause them to feel they no longer control the basic facets of daily existence. An effective and responsible effort to assist victims and their family members must consider the loss experienced and the grief response in the greater context of a traumatic event.

Corr and Doka observed two main elements in ongoing responses to public tragedy: coping with loss, grief, and trauma and finding ways to adapt to a changed world.[70] Janoff-Bulman states, "In the end, it is rebuilding of this trust – the reconstruction of a viable non-threatening assumptive world – that constitutes the core coping task of victims."[71]

The path from victimization to regaining a sense of control and trust requires the individual to cope with the traumatic event and the grief resulting from the loss of a loved one. Those responding to a mass fatality must be sensitive to this emotional state and have an understanding of what is needed. A systematic approach to address the physical, psychological, social, and spiritual needs of victims and their families is vital. These approaches, which take many forms depending on the disaster, help victims and their family members begin to reestablish a sense of control. When handled properly, such interventions will also help them rebuild the shattered trust caused by the mass fatality event.

Corr describes several strategies that responders can use to aid people coping with public tragedies.[67]

- Assess the specific nature of the tragedy. Determine who is in need of help and what types of help they are seeking.
- Understand the distinct characteristics of the tragedy; each is different.
- Use available resources. Understand the contributions and limitations that exist in those providing assistance.
- Prioritize the various aspects of the response. Determine who needs help most urgently, and how and when tasks should be undertaken.
- Be flexible; needs change during the event.
- Offer assistance to the responders, both in the immediate and long term.

The lives of victims and their family members impacted by a mass fatality will be forever changed. The goal of any response should be to mitigate further trauma and help the victims reestablish a sense of control. Most individuals, with a little assistance, can use their coping skills to adapt to even the most horrific of circumstances.

RECOMMENDATIONS FOR FURTHER RESEARCH

Within the past three decades, mass fatality management has evolved from uncoordinated, unscientific interventions to interdisciplinary scientific responses involving experienced forensic professionals using well-designed and proven methods. The professionalization of mass fatality management is tied closely to technological developments, particularly the establishment of DNA identification methods and the development of emergency management as a profession. Mass fatality management will continue to benefit from technological advances, which should reduce the time required for victim identification. For example, in the area of search and recovery, the development and validation of standardized protocols to enhance capabilities in search completeness; precision mapping systems and technologies; and spatial data collection, visualization, and analysis is promising.

Emergency management and medicolegal authorities have been developing programs and guidance materials focusing specifically on mass fatality management. Several medical examiner offices in the United States employ full-time mass fatality planning and response staff and have used federal funds to purchase disaster morgues. In the United Kingdom, the Home Office established a section to manage the overall cross-government Mass Fatalities Workstream. Interpol maintains a Standing Committee on DVI that oversees their international efforts in mass fatality response. PAHO published several important documents and papers in the mid-2000s that detail approaches to fatality management.[3,4] In order to provide DVI guidelines and best practices, the United States government, through the National Institutes of Justice, funded the development of the Scientific Working Group on Disaster Victim Identification (SWGDVI) in 2010. SWGDVI brings together professionals from the international DVI community to exchange ideas regarding scientific analysis methods, protocols, training, and research related to DVI. SWGDVI is also developing consensus guidelines and best practices for DVI and conducting a gap analysis of current DVI sciences to help guide future research.[72]

Because large and complex sets of data are created during a mass fatality response, data management and quality control are critical to the victim identification process and any associated medicolegal considerations.[49,50] In the past several years, software programs have been developed that provide well-designed, effective, and user-friendly procedures for data collection and management applicable across forensic disciplines and useful in any area of the globe affected by a mass fatality event. The DVI System International, a program developed by the Interpol DVI teams, allows for entry of the postmortem and antemortem data forms, search capability, and data mining. The system is available in nine languages. The Victim Identification Profile was developed by the United States DMORTs as a data collection tool to assist in DVI. The relational database has been expanded to include a call center capability. The Unified Victim Identification System is a web-based application developed by the Office of the Chief Medical Examiner in New York City. The system comprises modules to operate missing persons call centers, provides an integrated platform to manage and collect missing persons and victim antemortem information, and serves as a case management system for the DVI process. The International Committee of the Red Cross created the Antemortem/Postmortem Database to manage, archive, and standardize data collection, and to allow for identifications to be facilitated. Given the international aspects of large-scale mass fatality events, standardizing methodologies for collecting postmortem and antemortem information will benefit all forensic responders.

Mass fatality management takes place within the context of politics and media attention. Each death in a disaster affects not only the family of that victim, but also the community and culture impacted by the event. Educating political leaders and media representatives about the complexities of a mass fatality response may help to reduce confusion for family members and the impacted community. Effective mass fatality management not only focuses on the fatalities – the most immediate need – but also on providing information for the living. Mass fatality responders must provide a standard of care reflecting both the needs of the living and the complexities of managing the deceased.

REFERENCES

1. Reyes M. El campo, lugar de la política moderna. In: *Memoria de Auschwitz*. Madrid, Editorial Trotta, 2003; 78.

2. Office of Justice Programs. *Mass Fatality Incidents: A Guide for Human Forensic Identification*. Washington, DC, United States Department of Justice, 2005.

3. Pan American Health Organization. *Management of Dead Bodies in Disaster Situations. Disaster Manuals and Guidelines.* Series No. 5. Washington, DC, PAHO, 2004.

4. Morgan O, Tidball-Binz M, van Alphen D, eds. *Management of Dead Bodies after Disasters: A Field Manual for First Responders*. Washington, DC, PAHO, 2009.

5. *Report of the 7 July Review Committee*. London, Greater London Authority, 2006. http://www.london.gov.uk/sites/default/files/archives/assembly-reports-7july-report.pdf (Accessed June 13, 2013).

6. Weedn VW. Postmortem identification of remains. *Clin Lab Med* 1998; 18: 115–137.

7. Wagner GN, Froede RC. Medico-legal investigation of mass disasters. In: Spitz WU, ed. *Spitz and Fisher's Medico-legal Investigation of Death: Guidelines for the Application of Pathology to Crime Investigation*. Springfield, IL, Charles C Thomas, 1993; 567–584.

8. Sumathipala A, Siribaddana S, Perera C. Management of dead bodies as a component of psychosocial interventions after the tsunami: a view from Sri Lanka. *Intl Rev Psychiatry* 2006; 18(3): 249–257.

9. Eyre A. Improving procedures and minimizing stress: issues in the identification of victims following disasters. *Aust J Emerg Manage* 2002; 17: 9–14.

10. Levin BGL. Coping with traumatic loss: an interview with the parents of TWA 800 crash victims and implications for disaster mental health professionals. *Intl J Emerg Mental Health* 2004; 6: 25–31.

11. International Civil Aviation Organization. *ICAO Policy on Assistance to Aircraft Accident Victims and their Families*. Doc 9998, AN/499. Montreal, International Civil Aviation Organization, 2013.

12. International Civil Aviation Organization. *Aircraft Accident and Incident Investigation*. 9th ed. ICAO Annex 13. Montreal, International Civil Aviation Organization, 2001.

13. Morgan OW, de Ville de Goyet. Dispelling disaster myths about dead bodies and disease: the role of scientific evidence and the media. *Pan Am J Public Health* 2005; 18: 33–36.

14. Arnold JL. Disaster myths and Hurricane Katrina 2005: Can public officials and the media learn to provide responsible crisis communication during disasters? *Prehosp Disaster Med* 2005; 21: 1–3.

15. Morgan OW. Infectious disease risks from dead bodies following natural disasters. *Pan Am J Public Health* 2004; 15: 307–312.

16. World Health Organization. Emergencies preparedness, response, Frequently asked questions on Ebola virus disease. http://www.who.int/csr/disease/ebola/faq-ebola/en (Accessed August 22, 2015).

17. Health concerns associated with disaster victim identification after a tsunami – Thailand, December 26, 2004–March 31, 2005. *MMWR* 2005; 54: 349–352.

18. Nolte KB, Hanzlick RL, Payne DC, et al. Medical examiner, coroners, and biologic terrorism: a guidebook for surveillance and case management. *MMWR* 2004; 53(RR08): 1–27.

19. Griffiths C, Hilton J, Lain R. Aspects of forensic responses to the Bali bombings. *ADF Health: J Aust Defense Health Serv* 2003; 4: 50–55.

20. Li G, Baker SP. Injury patterns in aviation-related fatalities. *Am J Forensic Med Pathol* 1997; 18: 265–270.

21. Lillehei KO, Robinson MN. A critical analysis of the fatal injuries resulting from the Continental flight 1713 airline disaster: evidence in favor of improved passenger restraint systems. *J Trauma* 1994; 37: 826–830.

22. Vosswinkel JA, McCormack JE, Brathwaite CEM, Geller ER. Critical analysis of injuries sustained in the TWA Flight 800 midair disaster. *J Trauma* 1999; 47: 617–621.

23. Combs DL, Quenemoen LE, Parrish RG, Davis JH. Assessing disaster-attributed mortality: development and application of a definition and classification matrix. *Intl J Epidemiol* 1999; 28: 1124–1129.

24. Logue JN. Disasters, the environment, and public health: improving our response. *Am J Public Health* 1996; 86: 1207–1210.

25. Mortality associated with Hurricane Katrina – Florida and Alabama, August–October 2005. *MMWR* 2006; 55: 239–242.

26. Wood CM, DePaolo R, Whitaker RD. *Guidelines for Handling Decedents Contaminated with Radioactive Materials*. Atlanta, GA, HHS, CDC, 2007. http://www.bt.cdc.gov/radiation/pdf/radiation-decedent-guidelines.pdf (Accessed June 13, 2013).

27. Office of Justice Programs. *Mass Fatality Management for Incidents Involving Weapons of Mass Destruction*. Washington, DC, U.S. Soldier Biological Chemical Command and U.S. Department of Justice, 2004.

28. U.S. Department of Health and Human Services, Centers for Disease Control and Prevention. Guidance for safe handling of human remains of Ebola patients in U. S. hospitals and mortuaries. 2014. http://www.cdc.gov/vhf/ebola/hcp/guidance-safe-handling-human-remains-ebola-patients-us-hospitals-mortuaries.html (Accessed December 29, 2014).

29. World Health Organization. Interim infection prevention and control guidance for care of patients with suspected or confirmed filovirus haemorrhagic fever in health-care settings, with focus on Ebola. 2014. http://www.who.int/csr/resources/publications/ebola/filovirus_infection_control/en (Accessed December 29, 2014).

30. Gursky E. A working group consensus statement on mass-fatality planning for pandemics and disasters. *J Homeland Security* July 2007.

31. Sledzik PS, Willcox AW. Corpi Aquaticus: the Hardin cemetery flood of 1993. In: Steadman DW, ed. *Hard Evidence: Case Studies in Forensic Anthropology*. Upper Saddle River, NJ, Prentice-Hall, 2003; 256–265.

32. Morgan OW, Sribanditmongkol P, Perera C, Sulasmi Y, Alphen DV, Sondorp E. Mass fatality management following the South

Asian tsunami disaster: Case studies in Thailand, Indonesia, and Sri Lanka. *PloS Med* 2006; 3(e195): 1–7.

33. Lain R, Griffiths C, Hilton JMN. Forensic dental and medical response to the Bali bombing: A personal perspective. *Med J Aust* 2003; 179: 362–365.

34. Tun K, Butcher B, Sribanditmongkol P, et al. Forensic aspects of disaster fatality management. *Prehosp Disaster Med* 2005; 20: 455–458.

35. Office of Justice Programs. *Lessons Learned from 9/11: DNA Identifications in Mass Fatality Incidents.* Washington, DC, United States Department of Justice, 2006.

36. Auf der Heide E. Common misconceptions about disasters: panic, the "Disaster Syndrome," and looting. In: O'Leary M, ed. *The First 72 Hours: A Community Approach to Disaster Preparedness.* Lincoln, NE, iUniverse, 2004; 340–380.

37. Simpson DM, Stehr S. Victim management and identification after the World Trade Center collapse. In: *Beyond September 11th: An Account of Post-Disaster Research.* Program on Environment and Behavior Special Publication #39, Institute of Behavioral Science, Natural Hazards Research and Applications Information Center. Boulder, University of Colorado, 2003; 109–120.

38. Biesecker LG, Bailey-Wilson JE, Ballantyne J, et al. DNA identifications after the 9/11 World Trade Center attack. *Science* 2005; 310: 1122–1123.

39. Fleck F. Tsunami body count is not a ghoulish numbers game. *Bull World Health Organ* 2005; 83: 88–89.

40. Thieren M. Asian tsunami: death-toll addiction and its downside. *Bull World Health Organ* 2005; 83: 82.

41. Sledzik PS, Rodriguez WC. Damnum fatale: The taphonomic fate of human remains in mass disasters. In: Haglund WD, Sorg MH, eds. *Advances in Forensic Taphonomy. Methods, Theories and Archaeological Perspectives.* Boca Raton, FL, CRC Press, 2002; 321–330.

42. Alonso A, Martín P, Albarrán C, et al. Challenges of DNA profiling in mass disaster investigations. *Croat Med J* 2005; 46: 540–548.

43. Dirkmaat DC. Forensic anthropology at the mass fatality incident (commercial airliner) crash scene. In: Dirkmaat DC, ed. *A Companion to Forensic Anthropology.* West Sussex, John Wiley & Sons, Ltd., 2012; 136–156.

44. Kontanis EJ, Sledzik PS. Resolving commingling issues during the medicolegal investigation of mass fatality incidents. In: Adams BJ, Byrd JS, eds. *Recovery, Analysis, and Identification of Commingled Human Remains.* Totowa, NJ, Humana Press, 2008; 317–337.

45. Mundorff AZ. Anthropologist-directed triage: Three distinct mass fatality events involving fragmentation of human remains. In: Adams BJ, Byrd JS, eds. *Recovery, Analysis, and Identification of Commingled Human Remains.* Totowa, NJ, Humana Press, 2008; 123–144.

46. Meyer H, Chansue N, Monticelli F. Implantation of radio frequency identification device (RFID) microchip in disaster victim identification (DVI). *Forensic Sci Int* 2006; 157: 168–171.

47. Fixott RH, Arendt D, Chrz B, Filippi J, McGivney J, Warnick A. Role of the dental team in mass fatality incidents. *Dent Clin North Am* 2001; 45: 271–292.

48. Simmons T, Skinner M. The accuracy of ante-mortem data and presumptive identification: Appropriate procedures, applications and ethics. *Proc Am Acad Forensic Sci* 2006; 12: 303–304.

49. Brannon RB Kessler HP. Problems in mass disaster dental identification: a retrospective review. *J Forensic Sci* 1999; 44: 123–127.

50. Louisiana Department of Health and Hospitals. *Reuniting the Families of Katrina and Rita: Louisiana Family Assistance Center.* Baton Rouge, Louisiana Department of Health and Hospitals, 2006.

51. Hennessey M. Data management and commingled remains at mass fatality incidents (MFIs). In: Adams BJ, Byrd JS, eds. *Recovery, Analysis, and Identification of Commingled Human Remains.* Totowa, NJ, Humana Press, 2008; 337–356.

52. Leclair B, Shaler R, Carmody GR, et al. Bioinformatics and human identification in mass fatality incidents: The World Trade Center disaster. *J Forensic Sci* 2007; 52: 806–819.

53. Williams ED, Crews JD. From dust to dust: Ethical and practical issues involved in the location, exhumation, and identification of bodies from mass graves. *Croat Med J* 2003; 44: 251–258.

54. Knoppers BM, Saginur M, Cash H. Ethical issues in secondary uses of human biological materials from mass disasters. *J Law Med Ethics* 2006; 34: 352–355.

55. Blakeney RL. *Providing Relief to Families after a Mass Fatality: Roles of the Medical Examiner's Office and the Family Assistance Center.* Washington, DC, U.S. Department of Justice, Office of Justice Programs, Office for Victims of Crime Bulletin, November 2002.

56. Keough ME, Kahn S, Andrejevic A. Disclosing the truth: Informed participation in the antemortem database project for survivors of Srebrenica. *Health Hum Rights* 2000; 5: 68–87.

57. Keough ME, Simmons T, Samuels M. Missing persons in post-conflict settings: Best practices for integrating psychosocial and scientific approaches. *J Roy Soc Health* 2004; 124: 271–275.

58. Webb DA, Sweet D, Pretty IA. The emotional and psychological impacts of mass casualty incidents on forensic odontologists. *J Forensic Sci* 2002; 47: 539–541.

59. McCarroll JE, Ursano RJ. Mental health support to operations involving death and the dead. In: Ritchey EC, ed. *Combat and Operational Behavioral Health.* Washington, DC, Department of the Army, Office of the Surgeon General, Textbook of Military Medicine Series, 2011; 717–725.

60. Brondolo E, Wellington E, Brady N, Libby D, Brondolo T. Mechanism and strategies for preventing post-traumatic stress disorder in forensic workers responding to mass fatality incidents. *J Forensic Leg Med* 2008; 15: 78–88.

61. Ursano RJ, McCarroll JE. Exposure to traumatic death: the nature of the stressor. In: Ursano RJ, McCaughery BG, Fullerton CS, eds. *Individual and Community Responses to Trauma and Disaster: The Structure of Human Chaos.* New York, Cambridge University Press, 1994; 46–71.

62. McCarroll JE, Ursano RJ, Fullerton CS, Liu X, Lundy A. Somatic symptoms in Gulf War mortuary workers. *Psychosomatic Med* 2002; 64: 29–33.

63. Thompson N. The ontology of disaster. *Death Studies* 1995; 19: 501–510.

64. Wright KM, Ursano RJ, Bartone PT, Ingraham LH. The shared experience of catastrophe: an expanded classification of the disaster community. *Am J Orthopsych* 1990; 60: 35–42.

65. Task Force on Assistance to Families of Aviation Disasters. Final Report. Washington, DC, U.S. Department of Transportation and National Transportation Safety Board, 1997.

66. Doka KJ. What makes a tragedy public? In: Lattanzi-Licht M, Doka KJ, eds. *Living With Grief: Coping With Public Tragedy.* New York, Brunner-Routledge, 2003; 3–14.

67. Corr CA. Loss, grief and trauma in public tragedy. In: Lattanzi-Licht M, Doka KJ, eds. *Living With Grief: Coping With Public Tragedy.* New York, Brunner-Routledge, 2003; 63–76.

68. Corr CA, Nabe CM, Corr DM. *Death and Dying, Life and Living.* 4th ed. Belmont, CA, Wadsworth, 2003.

69. Rando TA. *Treatment of Complicated Mourning.* Champaign, IL, Research Press, 1993.

70. Corr CA, Doka KJ. Master concepts in the field of death, dying, and bereavement: coping versus adaptive strategies. *Omega* 2001; 43: 183–199.

71. Janoff-Bulman R. *Shattered Assumptions: Towards a New Psychology of Trauma.* New York, The Free Press, 2002; 175.

72. Scientific Working Group on Disaster Victim Identification. http://www.swgdvi.org (Accessed June 13, 2013).

24

REHABILITATION OF DISASTER CASUALTIES

James E. Gosney, Jr. and Colleen O'Connell

OVERVIEW

This review primarily addresses the rehabilitation of casualties in large-scale, sudden-onset disasters. Here, the term disaster is defined as "a situation or event which overwhelms local capacity, necessitating a request to a national or international level for external assistance."[1] Providing disaster medical relief services, including rehabilitation, in developing or low-resource regions can be significantly more challenging than providing them in developed nations. Effective rehabilitation of disabling and potentially disabling traumatic injuries significantly reduces associated mortality, disability, and community burden. Typical trauma that respond to this intervention include spinal cord injury (SCI), traumatic brain injury (TBI), burn injury, and extremity injuries such as amputations, bone fractures, and peripheral nerve injury

SCI and amputation are emphasized in this chapter due to their comprehensive, long-term rehabilitation requirements and their relative importance within the emerging discipline of disaster rehabilitation. TBI and burn injury are addressed by other chapters within this reference textbook and the rehabilitation of disaster-related fractures and complex orthopedic trauma, including nerve injury, is extensively addressed in the scientific literature. Closely related disaster medicine topics are also addressed in respective chapters. These include specific types of environmental events; complex humanitarian emergencies; functional and access needs populations including persons with disabilities; mental and behavioral health; ethical issues; and international perspectives.

Rehabilitation of disaster casualties is a vital component of comprehensive disaster response. Large-scale, sudden-onset disasters often result in significant mortality and disability evidenced by the high incidence of traumatic disabling injuries as previously listed. Rehabilitation medicine manages the impaired physical and cognitive functioning of individuals through: 1) the diagnosis and treatment of musculoskeletal and neurologic injuries; 2) the prevention and treatment of related complications; 3) the reduction of physical impairments; and 4) the optimization of physical functioning. Rehabilitation can be defined as "a set of measures that assists individuals who experience or are likely to experience disability to achieve and maintain optimal functioning in interaction with their environment." Disability indicates impairment in body functions and/or structures that limit daily activities and/or restrict participation in society.[2]

Doctors qualified in rehabilitation medicine (i.e., physical medicine and rehabilitation, or PM&R) and other rehabilitation professionals provide rehabilitation services in a range of care settings. These include acute and emergency care sites, general and specialized hospitals, tertiary rehabilitation centers, outpatient and community clinics, and private dwellings. Rehabilitation professionals who may be involved include: 1) physical and occupational therapists; 2) prosthetists (P), orthotists (O), and P&O technicians; 3) rehabilitation nurses; and 4) psychologists, social workers, and counselors. Rehabilitation professionals routinely work as multidisciplinary teams and coordinate with other medical professionals and services to ensure delivery of effective rehabilitation interventions.[3] Rehabilitation services and support provided include: 1) medical and procedural interventions; 2) physical, occupational, speech-language, communication, and cognitive therapies; 3) mobility and activities of daily living training; 4) durable medical equipment and assistive technology; and 5) education, training, and counseling.

The specialty of PM&R developed significantly during WWII in response to the immediate and long-term rehabilitation needs of injured soldiers and civilians, many with SCI and amputations. The rehabilitation of persons with traumatic injuries has advanced considerably as a result of the demand created by such armed conflicts. Treatment of combat casualties has resulted in improved acute injury management practices and more effective trauma and rehabilitation systems. Whereas trauma care focuses on management of the injury, rehabilitation more holistically includes functional interventions such as mobility and activities of daily living training. Measures to facilitate emotional, mental, social, and vocational functioning are employed to facilitate full return to society.[4,5]

Disaster rehabilitation, a developing discipline within PM&R, is the rehabilitation of persons with disabling and potentially disabling traumatic injuries sustained in a disaster setting. Incidence of morbidity and mortality, absolute numbers of injuries, and relative proportions of disabling injuries vary based on the disaster type and severity as well as many other environmental and human factors. Although every disaster is unique, the injuries resulting from a particular type of disaster are qualitatively predictable. Earthquakes, for example, frequently demonstrate injury patterns related to crush mechanisms. The proximity of severe earthquake-generated ground motion to the nearest large urban center, time of occurrence, building construction, and cultural gender activity roles were reviewed for the Kashmir (Pakistan, 2004), Sichuan (China, 2008), and Haiti (2010) earthquakes. In these countries with traditional societies, temblors occurring during daytime hours when women were likely at home performing domestic duties may account for the higher incidence of females than males sustaining SCI (due to building collapse) in these earthquakes.[6,7] Earthquakes are considered the representative sudden-onset disaster due to their immediate, catastrophic impact on individual health and health systems.[8]

Rehabilitation services provided during the emergency disaster response and beyond may be insufficient, however, especially in developing regions with few resources. Local disaster management plans and policy often do not include rehabilitation. Rehabilitation infrastructure in affected regions is often inadequate and degraded further by the disaster. Moreover, responding local and foreign medical teams (FMTs) historically provide limited rehabilitative care. Rehabilitation needs of those with new injuries as well as those with existing disabilities are consequently neglected, resulting in suboptimal return of physical functioning and less socially integrated lives. The resulting increased burden of disability compromises community recovery. Increasing frequency and predominance of large-scale disasters in developing regions underscores the critical need for stronger rehabilitation systems in these areas and for appropriate rehabilitation services as part of the humanitarian medical response.[9,10]

CURRENT STATE OF THE ART

The role and benefit of rehabilitation services, including rehabilitation of people with disabling injuries, are clearly documented in large-scale, sudden-onset disasters. Recent earthquakes with written records include Armenia (1988), Bam (Iran, 2003), Kashmir, Sichuan, Haiti, and the 2011 Tōhoku Earthquake and Tsumami (2011).[11-14] Water-related disasters include the Indian Ocean Tsunami, Hurricane Katrina (United States), and Cyclone Sidr (Bangladesh).[13,15–17] Positive rehabilitation outcomes including improved physical functioning, reduced medical complications, improved quality of life, greater life satisfaction, and increased community integration are noted. Patients treated by rehabilitation physicians following the Kashmir earthquake, for example, were noted to have fewer complications, better clinical outcomes, and higher quality of life than patients in SCI centers with no specialist supervision.[18] Positive rehabilitation system outcomes include reduced length of hospital stay and demonstrated overall system effectiveness during the disaster response.[19] Cohorting earthquake SCI patients in dedicated facilities has been shown to optimize staff expertise, efficiency, and training as well as physical resource acquisition and management.[18,20]

Disaster Rehabilitation Continuum

The disaster rehabilitation continuum is similar to the comprehensive emergency management model consisting of response, recovery, mitigation, and preparation phases. Medical rehabilitation of disaster casualties based on individual clinical needs is primarily performed during the response phase, which consists of the acute and core rehabilitation stages. Longer-term rehabilitation needs are primarily addressed during the community integration stage of the disaster recovery phase that follows. Acute stage rehabilitation is generally delivered within 72 hours of the disaster. It includes initial assessment of disabling and potentially disabling injuries with triage to an appropriate level facility, perisurgical and intensive care consultation, and prevention and management of secondary complications. Core rehabilitation includes disability-specific therapy and discharge planning, and is generally performed in an inpatient facility by a rehabilitation team under the direction of a physician with rehabilitation expertise. During the community integration stage following hospital discharge, the individual may receive outpatient educational, vocational, and social rehabilitation as part of a community-based rehabilitation (CBR) program. Rehabilitation treatment plans vary based on diagnosis, available resources, and other contextual factors of the disaster. Concurrent with clinical activities focused on individual care, non-clinical operational rehabilitation activities include: 1) assessment of evolving and long-term injury patterns, rehabilitation needs, and resource requirements; 2) data collection, management, and analysis; 3) establishing systems for patient triage, discharge, referral, and tracking; 4) collaboration with other rehabilitation and healthcare service providers; and 5) coordination with the emergency management system, host health system, and government managers (Figure 24.1).

The rehabilitation recovery phase optimizes function and quality of life for injured individuals. It also develops and/or restores operation of the local rehabilitation system in alignment with the healthcare infrastructure and builds rehabilitation system capacity and sustainability. Planning for long-term rehabilitation needs is critical to community recovery and alleviates the burden of disability. Services should include accessible, ongoing rehabilitation as well as general health maintenance. Patients with SCI require regular medical follow-up to prevent complications and new amputees will need prosthesis repair and replacement.

Development of SCI infrastructure, including permanent spinal injury units, has been stimulated by the influx of local and foreign rehabilitation resources following earthquakes in Armenia (1988), Pakistan (2005), and Haiti (2010).[6,20] Prosthetic and orthotic workshops supported by the International Committee of the Red Cross (ICRC) in developing conflict-affected countries also exemplify international efforts to promote continuous post-disaster rehabilitation programming.[21] Strengthened rehabilitation systems, sometimes in countries where rehabilitation had not effectively existed, resulted in improved care for disaster casualties. It also had a similar effect on new trauma-related casualties occurring after the disaster and persons with existing disabilities. Trauma rehabilitation system improvement in disasters should align with World Health Organization (WHO) recommended standards for rehabilitation services as part of essential global trauma systems of care.[22]

Medical care, physical rehabilitation, and assistive devices including prostheses can be provided to disabled persons in developing countries through local CBR programming.[23] The relationship between CBR and the global provision of prosthetics and orthotics services is well documented.[24] In addition to universal development strategies for comprehensive rehabilitation, equalization of opportunities, and social integration of people with disabilities, CBR programs also comprise employment,

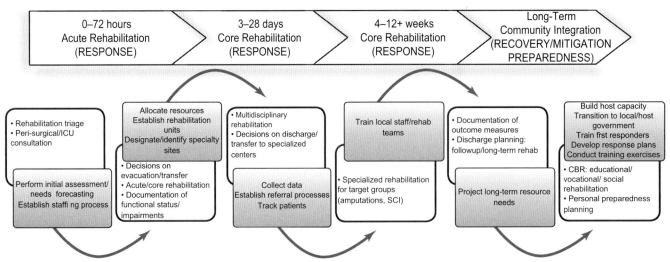

Figure 24.1. Disaster Rehabilitation Continuum by Time after a Disaster and by Stage (Phase). Key clinical activities are shown in *unshaded* boxes and key non-clinical activities are shown in *shaded* boxes. Adapted from Fig. 1. A suggested plan of rehabilitation interventions after a natural disaster in the article. "Medical Rehabilitation After Natural Disasters: Why, When, and How?" *Arch Phys Med Rehab* Vol 93, October 2012.

education, and social services. CBR programming improves individual quality of life and also raises community awareness of physical rehabilitation. CBR programming is critically important after large-scale disasters when the availability of rehabilitation services, general medical care, and public health assistance are potentially quite limited for the new and previously disabled population.[25] Displaced persons with disabilities are of special concern since they suffer isolation more frequently when displaced to a new location than when living in their home communities.[26] Studies have reported as much as a twofold increase in mortality for persons with existing physical disabilities in earthquakes.[9]

Mitigation in the context of rehabilitation for persons sustaining disaster-related injuries includes pre-disaster and emergency activities intended to limit the severity and number of casualties. Emergency planning for persons with disabilities must consider medication and equipment requirements as well as evacuation and sheltering strategy to reduce secondary casualties in a disaster. These disability measures among others are advocated in resources published by many humanitarian organizations including WHO's *Guidance Note on Disability and Emergency Risk Management for Health* and Light for the World's *Humanitarian Aid All Inclusive! How to Include People with Disabilities in Humanitarian Action.*[27,28]

Saving lives and minimizing impairment may depend on the rescue and first aid skills of first responders. Recognition of potentially disabling injuries such as suspected SCI and knowledge of proper lifting and transportation techniques can prevent further neurologic deterioration from this condition. Therefore, providing relevant pre-disaster training to the lay public and other first responders in a developing country's earthquake-prone communities may improve injury outcomes in disasters. An example of such training is found in the WHO publication Coping with Natural Disasters: The Role of Local Health Personnel and the Community Working Guide.[29] A community's emergency preparedness efforts for rehabilitation should also be prioritized in densely populated areas located near technical and nuclear industrial facilities.[30]

Preparedness within the disaster rehabilitation context focuses on strengthening the existing systems including CBR ser-

vices. Rehabilitation of disaster casualties should be addressed by local and national trauma systems and in public health disaster response plans. The absence of disaster plans and policies has been shown to compound the severity of an earthquake's impact on elements of the local healthcare system.[31] Strategic mapping of human and institutional resources is recommended. This process should include facility expansion/conversion to accommodate significant casualties as well as designating facilities for SCI, TBI, and amputation, which require specialized rehabilitation.[32] Multidisciplinary guidelines for the management of disabling injuries can be implemented in areas with high seismic activity. Examples of such guidance include those developed by Handicap International (HI) for use in earthquake-prone regions of Nepal.[33] These measures have particular importance since earthquake losses are predicted to increase in such areas due to population growth.[10] In addition, the disaster response and preparedness informational package developed from assessments of the Indian Ocean tsunami (2004) by the World Federation of Occupational Therapists (WFOT) could be modeled to assist regional community therapists.[34] Sponsorship of relevant training opportunities for rehabilitation professionals is advisable. These could include local and regional workshops, seminars at international centers, and annual society meeting attendance at international rehabilitation professional societies such as the International Spinal Cord Society (ISCoS).[35] International professional rehabilitation societies including WFOT, ISCoS, the International Society of Physical and Rehabilitation Medicine (ISPRM), and the World Confederation for Physical Therapy offer online disaster preparedness resources.[36–39] ISPRM and ISCoS also have disaster committees that address preparedness and other phases of the rehabilitation response.

Operationalizing the Disaster Rehabilitation Continuum

Operationalizing the disaster rehabilitation continuum depends to a great degree on the severity of the disaster and resource availability. A developed region with a strong rehabilitation system may require only local and domestic support, whereas a developing region may seek international assistance.

Rehabilitation systems in developing countries often have few human and physical resources. Facilities, equipment, and supplies are limited as well as trained providers and access to rehabilitation training programs and professional schools. In fact, many developing countries do not have accredited professional training programs in allied rehabilitation fields such as physical and occupational therapy, speech language pathology, and prosthetics and orthotics.[40] These countries also may lack local rehabilitation therapists, nurses, or doctors. For example, Sub-Saharan Africa has no PM&R physicians while Europe has more than 10,000 specialists who are unified by a comprehensive system of postgraduate education.[41,42] Consequently, rehabilitation practice may be entirely empirical in developing countries. Therefore, local specialized care for certain disabling injuries such as SCI and amputation may not be available in a disaster.

Societal variables in developing countries can severely affect implementation of rehabilitation services. Examples include medical, political, legal, economic, and cultural practices that limit pre-disaster acceptance of persons with disability and rehabilitation needs. Domestic physical factors such as geographical divisions, transportation corridors, and communication networks can also significantly impact disaster rehabilitation efforts. Making a positive operational impact requires effective coordination and collaboration between responding organizations, foreign and local disaster managers, and local rehabilitation services.

In a domestic disaster, rehabilitation professionals often respond to support plans by local employing institutions or government emergency managers. A rehabilitation physician may report to a local hospital and provide casualty triage assistance, for example. Providers may also deploy to another national region or internationally. International responders generally deploy as part of a civilian FMT or military unit. Others respond as employees of participating international rehabilitation NGOs such as ICRC, Christian Blind Mission, or HI. Responders provide rehabilitation in support of the sponsor's mission objectives and within their credentialed professional scope of practice. They also should receive additional pre-deployment education and training in humanitarian core competencies as well as on standards of care and how to adapt these skills to a resource-constrained environment. Sponsoring organizations and professional societies may provide this supplemental training for those functioning as a humanitarian healthcare providers.[43] Training is currently available for U.S. orthopedists, surgeons, and SCI specialists, and is being developed for rehabilitation professionals.[13,37,44,45]

The proposed WHO operational model for deploying FMTs in response to sudden-onset disasters recognizes rehabilitation as a core function of trauma care systems and recommends that FMTs provide post-disaster rehabilitation services. This model supports the WHO Humanitarian Reform process, which subsumes the WHO Emergency Response Framework, the Global Health Cluster response mechanism, and the Inter-Agency Standing Committee Transformative Agenda. This structure seeks to improve the effectiveness of humanitarian response through greater predictability, accountability, responsibility, and partnership.[46–48] A recent review of surgical care provided by FMTs in humanitarian crises also recommends that multidisciplinary surgical teams provide rehabilitation services.[49] Services should only be provided by teams with appropriate resources, however.[50] Appropriate level services are defined as Type 1 through Type 3 and would be provided by rehabilitation

care teams attached to FMTs or a national hospital. They are defined as follows. A Type 1 FMT is associated with outpatient emergency care facilities and would ideally have rehabilitation capability to help provide initial emergency care for injuries. A Type 2 FMT is associated with inpatient surgical emergency care facilities and should, at a minimum, have a rehabilitation physician or physical therapist to help manage acute general surgical trauma patients. A Type 3 FMT is part of an inpatient referral care facility and should have a rehabilitation team including a rehabilitation physician, physical and occupational therapists, and rehabilitation nurses to help manage patients with complex trauma diagnoses that include SCI, TBI, and amputation.[46]

A previous WHO guideline for rehabilitation of the physically wounded in disaster situations also proposes three levels of rehabilitation care. Level A (simple rehabilitation) would be provided in acute care general hospitals. Level B (general rehabilitation) would be provided in hospital rehabilitation departments for persons with complicated injuries affecting mobility. This involves mostly physical and occupational therapy and rehabilitation nursing. Level C (specialized rehabilitation) would be provided in rehabilitation hospitals by multidisciplinary teams for patients with complex injuries requiring comprehensive care including SCI, TBI, and amputation. This seminal consultation also considers continuity of care as well as the psychosocial and vocational implications. These guidelines were written primarily for non-rehabilitation professionals. However, other audiences who may find them useful include rehabilitation specialists supervising and training non-rehabilitation providers, primary care professionals engaged in the long-term care of the disabled, and community leaders.[51]

Role of Rehabilitation Providers

The role of the rehabilitation physician and other allied rehabilitation professional team members is determined by the FMT mission objectives, treatment care levels provided, rehabilitation team composition, resource availability, and a population's rehabilitation needs distributed over the disaster rehabilitation continuum. Roles and competencies implemented in a disaster may be adapted from those performed in standard practice settings but modified due to the austere nature of the disaster environment.[52] Rehabilitation physicians are experts in disability and trained in the diagnosis and treatment of musculoskeletal and neurological trauma and diseases. They can integrate acute rehabilitation into treatment protocols provided by FMT surgical and intensive care unit members, coordinate comprehensive inpatient rehabilitation, and facilitate discharge and referral planning. They prevent and treat secondary complications including pain and deconditioning. In addition, they prescribe medical therapies and assistive devices including prostheses and orthoses, mobility aids, and adaptive technologies. Rehabilitation physicians lead the multidisciplinary inpatient rehabilitation team and coordinate with various FMT and non-FMT providers to manage rehabilitation of patients with disabling and potentially disabling injuries.[53]

Physical and occupational therapists provide interventions to improve patient range of motion, strength, and mobility. They also diagnose and monitor musculoskeletal and neurological disease processes. Occupational therapists facilitate regaining performance of daily activities previously lost due to injury through hand function training, cognition, and environmental adaptation. Physical therapists administer lower extremity gait training

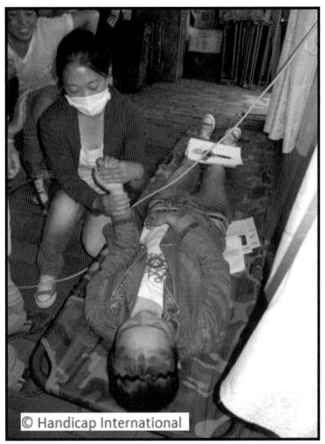

Figure 24.2. Occupational therapy is provided in a makeshift health center as part of the Handicap International disaster response to the 2008 Sichuan Earthquake. Photo courtesy of Eric Weerts, HI.

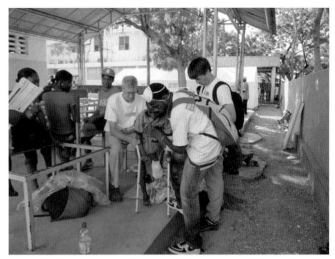

Figure 24.3. American orthotist Frank Shirley and prosthetist Al Ingersoll, as part of Handicap International France, provide therapy, data collection, and training to local non-rehabilitation staff in the days following the Haiti 2010 earthquake. Both Shirley and Ingersoll had extensive prosthetic and orthotic experience in Haiti prior to the earthquake. Photo courtesy of Colleen O'Connell.

and movement and balance exercise. All these activities facilitate early post-surgical mobilization and functional recovery, thus decreasing time to hospital discharge and increasing turnover of limited beds. Therapists coordinate patient discharge from the hospital, arrange for necessary durable medical equipment and supplies, provide CBR, and educate and train local therapy providers as well as the patient and family on the home care plan (Figure 24.2).[54,55]

Prosthetists, orthotists, and P&O technicians evaluate persons with amputations, fractures, contractures, weakness, and nerve injury. They design and fabricate prosthetic limbs and bracing in consultation with the rehabilitation team, provide training on device use, and perform modifications with replacement as needed. Prosthetists and orthotists also manage production workshops, train local service providers, and participate in CBR and long-term local rehabilitation needs planning (Figure 24.3).[56]

Rehabilitation nurses are experts in wound care. This expertise includes prevention of pressure ulcers, provision of bowel and bladder care, pain and nutritional management, and fall prevention. Nurses provide patient case management including medical documentation. They also provide essential education and training to patients, families, and caregivers to facilitate long-term recovery.[57]

Psychological distress frequently results from a severe injury and the subsequent adjustment to a new disability. This is common following amputations. Psychologists provide needed

screening for, and treatment of, post-injury mental health issues. Social workers can also provide counseling and emotional support in addition to case management services. Such services typically include coordination of necessary community resources for patients and families. Specialized rehabilitation services are especially useful in treating persons with TBI. Specialists in neuropsychology for the diagnosis and treatment of cognitive and behavioral impairment and speech-language pathology for the diagnosis and treatment of communication and swallowing disorders are particularly important.[22]

Besides the education and training of patients, families, and caregivers, rehabilitation professionals also train non-rehabilitation FMT members in rehabilitation clinical care and skills. This task-shifting provides FMTs with additional expertise to manage rehabilitation needs during the high-volume emergency response phase. Such training is critically important if FMT rehabilitation responders are understaffed.[58,59] Similarly, training can be provided by FMT rehabilitation professionals to local providers and other personnel working in regional facilities and in the community. Capacity building within the local rehabilitation system leverages service provision over the disaster rehabilitation continuum. Following the 2010 Haiti earthquake, WHO/PAHO encouraged rehabilitation experts to provide rapid training to their teams and local staff, thus maximizing integration of optimal, post-disaster rehabilitative care.[60] Current proposed FMT guidance endorses this recommendation in order to maximize the impact of consistent and continuous rehabilitation care.[46]

Based on its experiences in the Sichuan (2008) and subsequent Yushu (2010) earthquakes, HI China recognized these various training needs. It developed a technical rehabilitation training package that includes patient assessment and management tools for hospital non-rehabilitation medical staff as well as tools for patient, family, and caregiver education and training (Figure 24.4). A rehabilitation needs questionnaire is included for use by non-specialized providers to screen and refer patients to hospital rehabilitation staff for further assessment of potential

HANDICAP INTERNATIONAL *ATLAS*

EARLY PHYSICAL REHABILITATION ASSESSMENT (Version 09/2012)

TEMPORARY IMPAIRMENT ☐   or   PERMANENT IMPAIRMENT ☐

	SENSORIAL DISABILITIES	☐	SPEECH AND LANGUAGE DISABILITIES / DISORDERS	☐	INTELLECTUAL DISABILITIES	☐
	PARTIAL	COMPLETE	DETAILS / COMMENTS :			
Hearing	hard hearing ☐	deaf / mute ☐				
Visual	low vision ☐	blind ☐				

PHYSICAL IMPAIRMENT   ☐

		DETAIL / COMMENTS / THOUGHT DIAGNOSIS
Recent Fracture ☐	☐ Recent Fracture	*Loss of sensation paralysis to check*
Wound ☐	☐ Wound	
Burn ☐	☐ Burn	
Amputation ☐	☐ Amputation	
Deformity ☐	☐ Deformity	
Burn ☐	☐ Burn	
Weak Muscles ☐	☐ Weak Muscles	
Stiff Muscles ☐	☐ Stiff Muscles	

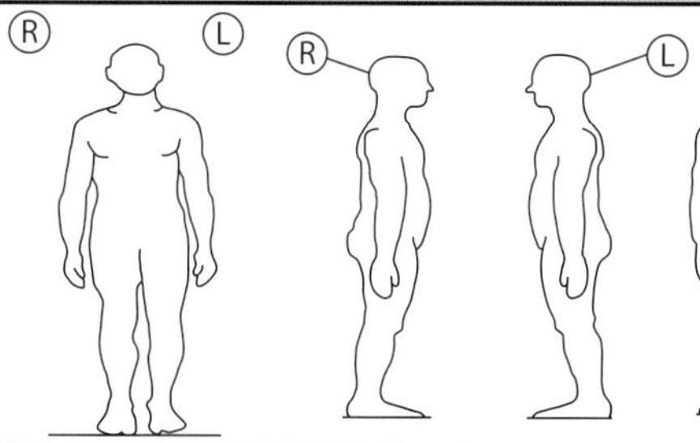

(R) (L) (R) (L)

CAUSE OF IMPAIRMENT

From birth ☐   Illness ☐ *precise* ....   Old age ☐   Accident ☐ *precise*...   From Crisis (conflict)☐ *precise*...

FIRST ASSESSMENT PHYSICAL INDEPENDANCE

DATE OF FIRST ASSESSMENT :   ASSESSOR :

DATE OF LAST ASSESSMENT :   ASSESSOR :

Is it difficult for you to do the following on your own ?	Not difficult		some difficulties		dificult		very difficult		impossible alone, need help		Comments: bladder/bowel control to define
	1st visit	Last	1st visit	Last	1st visit	Last	1st visit	Last	1st visit	Last	
Bathing	0 ☐	0 ☐	1 ☐	1 ☐	2 ☐	2 ☐	3 ☐	3 ☐	4 ☐	4 ☐	
Dressing	0 ☐	0 ☐	1 ☐	1 ☐	2 ☐	2 ☐	3 ☐	3 ☐	4 ☐	4 ☐	
Washing laundry	0 ☐	0 ☐	1 ☐	1 ☐	2 ☐	2 ☐	3 ☐	3 ☐	4 ☐	4 ☐	
Eating/Drinking	0 ☐	0 ☐	1 ☐	1 ☐	2 ☐	2 ☐	3 ☐	3 ☐	4 ☐	4 ☐	
Using toilets	0 ☐	0 ☐	1 ☐	1 ☐	2 ☐	2 ☐	3 ☐	3 ☐	4 ☐	4 ☐	
Moving in the house	0 ☐	0 ☐	1 ☐	1 ☐	2 ☐	2 ☐	3 ☐	3 ☐	4 ☐	4 ☐	
Moving long distance	0 ☐	0 ☐	1 ☐	1 ☐	2 ☐	2 ☐	3 ☐	3 ☐	4 ☐	4 ☐	
Community activities	0 ☐	0 ☐	1 ☐	1 ☐	2 ☐	2 ☐	3 ☐	3 ☐	4 ☐	4 ☐	

ICF scoring: 0= normal; 1= mild; 2= moderate; 3= severe; 4 = complete

REHABILITATION RESPONSE

REHABILITATION EXERCISE and ADVICES

Services	Date of service (dd/mm/yyyy)	Caregivers	Beneficiary	Comments	Need for Follow Up
☐ Rehabilitation........................		☐ Present ☐ Absent	☐ Present ☐ Absent		☐ Yes ☐ No Date next visit........
☐ Rehabilitation........................		☐ Present ☐ Absent	☐ Present ☐ Absent		☐ Yes ☐ No Date next visit........
☐ Rehabilitation........................		☐ Present ☐ Absent	☐ Present ☐ Absent		☐ Yes ☐ No Date next visit........
☐ Rehabilitation........................		☐ Present ☐ Absent	☐ Present ☐ Absent		☐ Yes ☐ No Date next visit........
☐ Rehabilitation........................		☐ Present ☐ Absent	☐ Present ☐ Absent		☐ Yes ☐ No Date next visit........

☐ ACTIVITY CLOSED, date:
If activity closed, ensure assessment of independance's evolution

☐ DATA ENTRY DONE date:

☐ TEAM LEADER VALIDATION, date: Signature:

WOUND CARE AND MEDICAL ADVICE

Services	Date of service (dd/mm/yyyy)	Caregivers	Comments	Need for Follow Up
☐ Wound care		☐ Present ☐ Absent		☐ Yes ☐ No Date next visit..............
☐ Wound care		☐ Present ☐ Absent		☐ Yes ☐ No Date next visit..............
☐ Wound care		☐ Present ☐ Absent		☐ Yes ☐ No Date next visit..............

☐ ACTIVITY CLOSED, date:

☐ DATA ENTRY DONE date:

☐ TEAM LEADER VALIDATION, date: Signature:

Figure 24.4. Early physical rehabilitation assessment tool for use by local rehabilitation providers and community rehabilitation health workers in areas with limited pre-disaster rehabilitation capacity. Document courtesy of Handicap International.

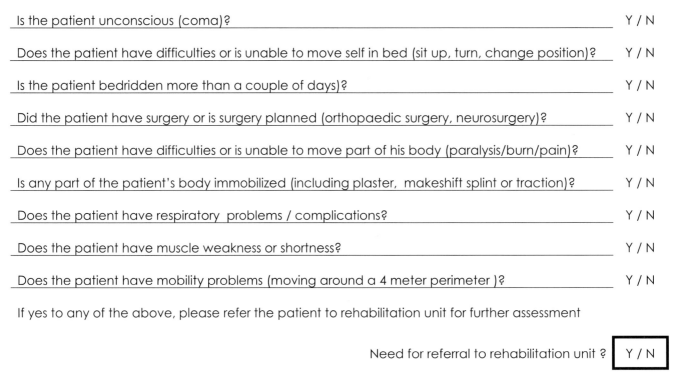

Figure 24.5. Early rehabilitation needs questionnaire for non-rehabilitation trained health workers to facilitate early identification and referral of persons with rehabilitation needs. Document courtesy of Handicap International.

needs for early intervention. An example is shown in Figure 24.5. This comprehensive collection of materials was employed during the earthquake rehabilitation response and has been integrated into standing operating procedures and emergency management plans in several hospitals within the earthquake zone.[61]

In addition to providing clinical care to individual patients and education and training to various providers, rehabilitation team members participate in non-clinical, operational rehabilitation activities. These include: 1) development and implementation of triage and referral systems for all levels of rehabilitative care; 2) comprehensive data collection and patient tracking; and 3) ongoing assessment of rehabilitation needs and resource requirements. As an example, an assessment of inpatient facilities including field hospitals in the greater Port-au-Prince area occurred immediately following the 2010 Haiti earthquake. It provided injury and resource requirement estimates as well as useful clinical management recommendations to help guide the emergency rehabilitation response.[62] Similarly, ongoing interval

assessments can inform managers regarding emerging critical requirements. These include numbers and type of rehabilitation workers, durable medical equipment, rehabilitation beds and facilities, and community rehabilitation capacity. Accurate, current assessment data and effective cooperation between the rehabilitation team and the other stakeholders facilitates rehabilitation service delivery over the disaster continuum including transition of services to local providers and systems.

Rehabilitation of Traumatic Disabling Injuries

Rehabilitation of persons with traumatic disabling injuries begins as early as possible in the disaster response and continues over the rehabilitation disaster continuum. Typical conditions are SCI, TBI, burns, and extremity injuries such as amputations, bone fractures, and peripheral nerve injury. Local and national rehabilitation professionals will emergently respond. These are in addition to foreign responders embedded on FMTs with surgical capacity, on rehabilitation FMTs, or attached to international rehabilitation NGOs. Early involvement optimizes positive rehabilitation outcomes and reduces preventable secondary complications for many disabling injuries.[63,64]

Injuries are identified, classified, diagnosed, and documented during rehabilitation triage. As an example, the International Standards for Neurologic Classification of Spinal Cord Injury (ISNCSCI) is used to classify patients with this condition.[65] Management of SCI within the critical first 72 hours after occurrence may determine outcomes, and specialized rehabilitative multidisciplinary team care is recommended.[66] Optimal management of patients with amputations also requires early rehabilitation expertise.[64] Acute rehabilitation activities can include consultation with the surgical team to determine at what level to perform the amputation. This optimizes postoperative prosthetic fitting, initiation of early mobilization protocols, and prevention and treatment of secondary medical complications. Management of complications related to SCI and amputation minimizes long-term disability and includes care for wounds, pressure ulcers, contractures, spasticity, and deconditioning. Other areas that benefit from assessment include bowel and bladder function, respiratory function, autonomic and cardiovascular function, thromboembolic risk, pain, nutrition, sexuality, and emotional health.

The surgical approach to performing a lower extremity amputation has rehabilitation implications. Ideally, the level of amputation should be below the knee and as distally as possible. Patients with a functioning knee joint will have a much better recovery. In addition, the greater the length of tibia preserved, the better will be the resulting ambulatory function. Amputations performed above the knee will significantly compromise mobility. The method of amputation used is dictated by the circumstances. The guillotine approach is indicated when attempting to free victims trapped in the rubble or when a person's life is threatened by exsanguination and an amputation must be performed quickly outside the hospital. This approach has the advantage of speed and preserving as much leg length as possible. In most other situations, however, the guillotine amputation is less desirable and should not be used.[64] Important soft tissue may be lost and this will force the surgeon to resect more bone to create soft tissue coverage of the stump during definitive closure, thus sacrificing length.

Following acute interventions, core rehabilitation therapies aim to maximize physical activity and conserve body function. Mobility restoration therapies include training in: 1) strength, balance, and range of motion; 2) ambulation and wheelchair skills; 3) sitting, standing, and transfers; and 4) bed mobility and pressure relief maneuvers. Patients receive hand function therapy and training in the performance of activities of daily living (ADL). These self-care tasks include bathing, toileting, dressing, and eating. Assessment of functional outcomes is performed using standard measures such as the Spinal Cord Independence Measure that is serially documented for interval comparison.[67] Mobility-impaired patients are evaluated and prescribed durable medical equipment such as wheelchairs and orthotic braces, which should be contextually appropriate. For example, after the Haitian earthquake, an environmentally compatible, durable wheelchair was preferred for individuals with SCI that could be easily maintained by the patient.[20]

During core rehabilitation, some patients with SCI may be transferred to a dedicated SCI center for more specialized care. Criteria for transfer will depend on injury severity and the level of rehabilitation expertise at the FMT Type 3 hospital. Persons with amputations may be discharged from a FMT Type 2 or 3 hospital to the community, depending on severity of injury. As part of the discharge process, they will receive a referral for prostheses assessment, fabrication, fitting, and functional training. Nerve injury patients who did not receive orthotic assessment in the hospital may also be referred. Most fractures can be appropriately managed at FMT Type 2 hospitals with outpatient rehabilitation referral. Patients with complex orthopedic trauma, burn injury, TBI, or multi-system trauma generally require specialized care at a FMT Type 3 hospital or a specialized center.[46,68]

Discharge planning should begin early during hospitalization, given the critical demand for hospital beds, unclear referral pathways, and disrupted patient lives. Patient families may be missing or deceased, their homes destroyed, and livelihoods lost. Therefore, location of relatives, custodianship, accessible housing, and access to medications, equipment, and referral centers must be confirmed prior to discharge. Patient tracking processes should also be established to facilitate long-term follow-up and community integration. Investigators have shown that rehabilitation follow-up is lacking in sudden-onset disasters in developing countries. The Bam (2003), Gujarat/India (2004), and Kashmir (2005) earthquakes illustrate this problem, presumably in part due to faulty discharge planning.[12,18,69] Inadequate follow-up can contribute to secondary complications in these settings.[13,20] An example of a practice to improve follow-up and prevent complications includes an SCI database employed in post-earthquake Haiti by a coalition of SCI providers.[6] Another option is establishing Disaster Vulnerability Focal Points (DVFPs). These are outpatient community and camp aid stations that are managed by HI. They provide on-site and mobile rehabilitation therapy, mobility aids, training, and psychosocial support to beneficiaries, families, and caregivers.[70] Educational training materials ensure basic continuing care for community-based rehabilitation workers, persons with disabilities, and their families and caregivers. Several model examples are worth noting. WHO offers two publications, *The Rehabilitation of People with Amputations* and *SCI India: Guidelines for Care of Persons with Spinal Cord Injury in the Community*, which are administered by the government of India's WHO Collaborative Programme.[71] *The HELP Guide For Community Based Rehabilitation Workers* is a notable training manual for non-specialized providers.[72] *Disabled Village Children: A Guide for Community Health Workers, Rehabilitation Workers, and Families* is a widely used practical tool for rehabilitating children and includes guidance on common disabling injuries, medical complications, and managing a community rehabilitation program.[73] Provision of physical rehabilitation follow-up and additional CBR activities are fundamental components of the community integration stage of recovery. Such activities should address health, education, vocation, social inclusion, and other rights of persons with disabilities. If successful, these endeavors will facilitate full participation in society over the disaster rehabilitation continuum.

Rehabilitation of persons with traumatic disabling injuries is provided based on clinical best practices and established scientific evidence in countries with developed rehabilitation and health systems. However, meeting this standard of care is often not possible in many developing countries. Here, capacity to manage complex diagnoses such as SCI and amputation is severely limited, especially in a large-scale, sudden-onset disaster. Given the lack of evidence for rehabilitation interventions in disaster, local and foreign professional rehabilitation responders are guided by a combination of clinical practice guidelines, disaster-specific protocols, sponsoring organization recommendations, personal experience, and local practice. Some standards and guidelines are not appropriate for low resource settings such as disasters. Here, best clinical judgment based on case-specific risks and benefits is required. Consequently, roles, competencies, and interventions performed by foreign and local rehabilitation professionals may be adapted from those practiced in routine care settings. They can also innovate new approaches, creating other options for implementing the standard of care in disasters. The unique disaster context thereby impacts how the standard of care is interpreted. Significant disaster rehabilitation guidelines and other reference resources are listed in Table 24.1.

Interventions, equipment, and technology are most effectively applied when they are compatible with the local disaster environment, availability of resources, and the host culture. Simple aseptic wound care technique was demonstrated to heal severe wounds, including large sacral pressure ulcers, in post-earthquake Haiti.[74] Resourceful recycling of limited materials and supplies has been effective, as shown by reuse of catheters for SCI neurogenic bladder patients in Haiti.[35] Reinforced compact civilian and military medical equipment designed for tactical use can be employed with minimal adaptation. Complementing the previous wheelchair example is the ICRC's development of high-quality, durable, and relatively low-cost polypropylene material technology for the fabrication of prosthetic and orthotic devices in low resource settings.[75] Promising examples of modern technology transfer for disaster application include: 1) an electronic patient tracking system for amputees and other vulnerable populations trialed in Haiti; and 2) an evaluation tool under development for physical functioning that is independent of language and literacy.[76,77] Resourceful and practical interventions, technologies, and equipment are required by necessity in the austere, low resource disaster environment.

RECOMMENDATIONS FOR FURTHER RESEARCH

As previously described, the scientific and gray literature affirms the value and role of rehabilitation services in large-scale, sudden-onset disasters. Although robust research exists documenting the rehabilitation of persons with traumatic disabling injuries in normal practice settings, evidence in disaster populations is extremely limited. Based on a standardized classification of evidence levels developed by the Centre for Evidence-Based Medicine, good outcomes research is scarce. Such missing investigations include Level II/III cohort studies and Level I systematic surveys with appropriate sampling and other sound epidemiological methods.[78] Level I randomized controlled trials are not feasible in the disaster setting. Level IV and V publications comprised mostly of documents published by international relief agencies predominate. This gray literature contributes minimally to the evidence base, although it remains the primary data source for humanitarian health relief workers.

The vast majority of information on disabling injury in disasters is epidemiological data derived from chart reviews of individual hospitals and similar cross-sectional studies.[9] In contrast, studies on SCI victims from the 2008 Sichuan earthquake reported functional outcomes and medical complications as well as long-term quality of life and community integration results.[79,80] The primary rehabilitation services model employed in Sichuan was shown to improve long-term physical func-

tioning in survivors.[19] The amputation literature reports functional and integration measures of lower limb amputee war victims.[81–83] The 2-year functional status of Haiti earthquake traumatic amputees has also been reported.[84]

The conduct of scientific research in disasters is extremely challenging due to numerous methodological, technical, and operational constraints.[85] Significantly, requisite baseline demographic data may not be readily available in developing regions, and data repositories may be destroyed.[86] Medical record keeping has been noted as severely lacking in large-scale, sudden-onset disasters. Host and FMT/NGO providers typically use different reporting standards and systems, complicating comparison of data.[13,49,64,87] Coordination is crucial and involves medical priorities; resource availability; study design; cooperation with local and international authorities; and mobilization of local, regional, and international staff.[88] Research partnerships in disasters are highly variable and comprise a broad range of local and foreign governments, humanitarian and disability NGOs, and institutional sponsors. Few academic institutions perform disaster research, especially in developing countries. In addition, NGOs that emphasize operational involvement in disaster response do not historically perform scientific investigations. A recent comparison of SCI research efforts from the Kashmir, Sichuan, and Haiti earthquakes highlights these issues.[6] Despite these complex challenges, the quantity and quality of disaster rehabilitation research is improving and expanding. Development of a comprehensive research agenda for the rehabilitation of disaster casualties is urgently required based on a full systematic review of the scientific and gray literature identifying existing knowledge, relevant questions, and research gaps.

Potential areas of interest for clinical research include epidemiological patterns of injury such as SCI level and completeness of deficits distal to the spinal cord lesion. Such data would help support follow-up injury and mortality studies. Timing and cause of death could be clarified with further evaluation of emergency response, rescue, extrication, and patient transfer mechanisms. Investigation of the clinical efficacy, cost effectiveness, and timing of specific rehabilitation interventions on patient functional outcomes and management of complications would better inform clinical disaster practice. Surgical approaches should be compared to non-surgical rehabilitation strategies. Additional methodologically robust studies are needed that assess long-term rehabilitation outcomes, including individual function and community vocational integration. Rehabilitation outcomes of interest also require further definition.

Rigorous scientific disaster research depends on systematic collection, reporting, and analysis of standardized data. While international data standards for specific disabling injuries in disasters do not exist, international standards and core data sets are available for some traumatic injury types, including SCI and amputation. These data sets could be adapted and extracted to standardized template forms to facilitate disaster rehabilitation data management as the global surgical community has proposed.[6,89,90] Rehabilitation data management should integrate with overall health sector efforts through coordination with international and local emergency response managers and disability stakeholders. This would accelerate incorporation of research into existing disaster management priorities and facilitate organizational data-sharing and aggregated high-quality investigations.[6]

Significant disaster rehabilitation research findings ideally become part of accepted clinical practice. The U.S. Veterans

Table 24.1. Guidelines and Resources Applicable to Delivery of Rehabilitation Services in Disasters

Guideline/Resource	Summary
Consensus Statements Regarding the Multidisciplinary Care of Limb Amputation Patients in Disasters or Humanitarian Emergencies (Harvard Humanitarian Initiative 2011)	Consensus recommendations based on extensive review of amputation guidelines and literature, with recommendations across acute care through to rehabilitation in disasters and humanitarian emergencies
Community Based Rehabilitation Guidelines (WHO 2010)	Guidelines for developing and strengthening community-based rehabilitation with focus on low- and middle-income countries
Coping with Natural Disasters: The Role of Local Health Personnel and the Community Working Guide (WHO 1989)	Collection of facts, advice, and recommended actions that can enable community leaders and health personnel to take control when disaster strikes; uses checklists, action plans, and abundant illustrations to guide community members from immediate response through recovery
Database of International Rehabilitation Research (CIRRIE)	Online searchable database of rehabilitation research conducted outside of the United States, from 1990 to current
Disability Check List for Emergency Response (HI 2004)	General protections and inclusion principles of injured persons and people with disabilities
Disabled Village Children (Werner 2009)	Practical manual of physical rehabilitation and community-based strategies, written for communities with limited resources; can be used as training resource
Early Rehabilitation Protocols for Victims of Natural Disasters (HI China 2013)	Manual of specific therapy and care instructions for disabling injuries, intended for non-specialist provision of rehabilitation services
eLearnSCI (ISCoS 2012)	Online training modules for therapists, counselors, nurses, and doctors in SCI care, appropriate for areas with limited resources; includes disasters module
Emergency Surgical Care in Disaster Situations (WHO 2005)	Guideline for emergency management of injuries including basic rehabilitation, presented in point form and accompanied by illustrations; intended for middle and low resource situations
Evidence Aid (Evidence Aid Project)	Online resource using Cochrane and other systematic reviews to provide up-to-date evidence on interventions that might be considered in the context of natural disasters and other major healthcare emergencies; includes reviews of specific injury management such as burns, fractures, TBI, and SCI.
Guidelines for Essential Trauma Care (WHO 2004)	Recommendations for achievable and affordable essential standards for injury care worldwide, including rehabilitation
Guidelines for Rehabilitation of Physically Wounded in Disaster Situations (WHO/Euro 1996)	Recommendations for facility-level team composition and specifics of therapy and care for amputations, TBI, SCI, nerve injury
Humanitarian Aid All Inclusive! (Light for the World 2013)	Guidance reader on how to include persons with disability in humanitarian action, including disaster prevention, preparedness, response, and recovery
International Perspectives on Spinal Cord Injury (WHO/ISCoS pending)	Global overview of interventions, services, health systems, and policies for people with SCI, from trauma and acute care through rehabilitation toward full participation in family and community life, education, and employment
Promoting Independence Following Spinal Cord Injury (WHO 1996)	Guide intended for mid-level rehabilitation workers, with information on SCI, including basic care, promoting independence, and community participation
Prosthetics and Orthotics Manufacturing Guidelines (ICRC 2007)	Manuals designed to promote and enhance standardization of ICRC polypropylene technology, provide support for training, and promote good practice in this field
Prosthetics and Orthotics Project and Program Guides: Supporting P&O Services in Low-Income Settings (2006)	Comprehensive resource guides to P&O programs (long-term) and projects (short-term – emergency situations) in low resources settings; collaboration of thirty-five organizations, and endorsed by the International Society for Prosthetics and Orthotics
Sphere Project Humanitarian Charter and Minimum Standards in Disaster Response (2011)	Broad standards and guidelines for the delivery of humanitarian relief
Spinal Cord Injury Clinical Practice Guidelines (Consortium for Spinal Cord Medicine)	Ten consensus and best evidence guidelines for SCI care and treatment; individual guidelines documents include acute care; bowel, bladder, and respiratory care; depression; upper extremity preservation; pressure ulcer prevention; autonomic dysreflexia; sexuality; and outcomes.
The Rehabilitation of Persons with Amputation (WHO 2004)	Manual for care and rehabilitation of persons with amputation; can be used in training healthcare personnel and as a reference for personnel working with persons with amputations.
VA/DOD Clinical Practice Guideline for Rehabilitation of Lower Limb Amputation (2008)	Guidelines with detailed peri-surgical, medical, and rehabilitation interventions for persons with lower limb amputations
Classification and Minimum Standards for Foreign Medical Teams in Sudden Onset Disasters (WHO 2013)	Recommendations for foreign medical disaster response teams including technical standards for rehabilitaton

Administration (VA) clinical practice guidelines for management of concussion (mild traumatic brain injury) and post-traumatic stress disorder (PTSD) reflect injury experience from Operation Enduring Freedom and Operation Iraqi Freedom. This knowledge has been applied to a broader beneficiary population that includes conflict veterans.[91] The challenge is to appropriately adapt existing guidelines for use in disasters as part of an evolving standard of care. The Paralyzed Veterans of America clinical practice and consumer guidelines for management of SCI and the VA clinical guidelines for the management of lower extremity amputation are examples of approaches that could serve as model guidelines for adaptation.[91,92] Additionally, disaster-specific humanitarian medical guidance can be periodically revised, such as the Harvard Humanitarian Initiative's consensus statements for the multidisciplinary surgical and rehabilitation management of patients with limb amputations after disasters. Similar guidance could also be developed for other disabling injuries such as TBI and PTSD. Finally, this expanding evidence base should be freely available online to the widest audience, including developing regions. This would be similar to the evolving Cochrane Evidence Aid repository of systematic reviews addressing humanitarian emergencies.[93] The Center for International Rehabilitation Research Information and Exchange database of international rehabilitation research is another globally accessible relevant clinical database.[94]

The clinical roles, skills, and competencies of responding multidisciplinary professional foreign and local rehabilitation providers require elaboration, as do those for non-rehabilitation staff. Related non-clinical operational rehabilitation system activities also merit relevant health services research. Novel research and development is needed in such areas as technology transfer and adaptive innovation of disaster-appropriate equipment and technological expertise. Additional research foci include: patient triage; referral and tracking systems; assessment of rehabilitation needs and resource requirements; education and training for patients, caregivers, providers, and emergency managers; and analyzing performance effectiveness. This last analysis should focus not only on the response phase of the disaster rehabilitation continuum, but also address emergency rehabilitation activities in the recovery, mitigation, and preparedness phases as well. The impact of response phase activities on rehabilitation outcomes in subsequent phases should be clarified as well as the variation in outcome performance during phase transitions. This will assist in evaluating CBR program effectiveness and sustainability. Broader analysis of local rehabilitation assets in relation to the medical and public health systems would also support long-term local rehabilitation system development and sustainability, including CBR programming. In summary, development of research endeavors examining the non-clinical operational and clinical activities of rehabilitation providers will increase the quality and impact of their efforts as part of a comprehensive research agenda for the rehabilitation of casualties after large-scale, sudden-onset disasters.

Conclusion

Rehabilitation of persons with disabling injuries in a large-scale, sudden-onset disaster significantly reduces associated mortality, disability, and community burden. Rehabilitation professionals perform a variety of clinical and non-clinical roles during the immediate emergency response and over the disaster rehabilitation continuum, facilitating optimal patient functional outcomes, quality of life, and community integration. Providing effective rehabilitation for persons with SCI, amputation, and other disabling injuries that require comprehensive, long-term rehabilitation services is especially challenging after disasters in developing, low resource countries. Effective disaster mitigation and preparedness measures are necessary to limit disability. An increase in higher quality clinical and health services research will translate into more effective rehabilitation response with greater integration of disaster rehabilitation into the overall disaster response framework. This will enhance the development of the emerging discipline of disaster rehabilitation medicine.

Acknowledgements

We sincerely thank expert reviewers from the ISPRM and ISCoS disaster committees.

REFERENCES

1. Burkle FM, Greenough PG. Impact of public health emergencies on modern disaster taxonomy, planning, and response. *Disaster Med Public Health Prep* 2008; 2: 192–199.
2. WHO International Classification of Functioning, Disability and Health (ICF). Geneva, World Health Organization. 2001. http://www.who.int/classifications/icf/en (Accessed August 8, 2013).
3. King, JC. Rehabilitation Team Function and Prescriptions, Referrals, and Order Writing. In: Frontera W, DeLisa J, eds. *DeLisa's Physical Medicine and Rehabilitation: Principles and Practice*. Philadelphia, PA, Lippincott Williams & Wilkins, 2010; 359–385.
4. Eldar R, Jelic M. The association of rehabilitation and war. *Disabil Rehabil* 2003; 25: 1019–1023.
5. Robinson L. Trauma Rehabilitation: An Introduction. In: Robinson L, ed. *Trauma Rehabilitation*. Philadelphia, PA, Lippincott, Williams & Wilkins, 2006; 1–10.
6. Gosney JE, Reinhardt JD, von Groote PM, Rathore FA, Melvin JL. Rehabilitation of spinal cord injury following earthquakes in rehabilitation resource-scarce settings: implications for disaster research. *Spinal Cord* 2013; 51(8): 603–609.
7. Priebe MM. Spinal cord injuries as a result of earthquakes: lessons from Iran and Pakistan. *J Spinal Cord Med* 2007; 30(4): 367–368.
8. Gautschi OP, Cadosch D, Rajan G, Zellweger R. Earthquakes and trauma: review of triage and injury-specific, immediate care. *Prehosp Disaster Med* March–April 2008; 23(2): 195–201.
9. Reinhardt JD, Li J, Gosney J, Rathore FA, Haig AJ, Marx M, DeLisa JA. International Society of Physical and Rehabilitation Medicine's Sub-Committee on Rehabilitation Disaster Relief. Disability and health-related rehabilitation in international disaster relief. *Glob Health Action* 2011; 4: 7191.
10. Doocy S, Daniels A, Packer C, Dick A, Kirsch TD. The human impact of earthquakes: a historical review of events 1980–2009 and systematic literature review. *PLoS Currents Disasters* April 16, 2013; 1.
11. Burke DC, Brown D, Hill V, Balian K, Araratian A, Vartanian C. The development of a spinal injuries unit in Armenia. *Paraplegia* 1993; 31: 168–171.
12. Raissi GR, Mokhtari A, Mansouri K. Reports from spinal cord injury patients eight months after the 2003 earthquake in Bam, Iran. *Am J Phys Med Rehabil* 2007; 86: 912–917.

13. Rathore FA, Gosney JE, Reinhardt JD, Haig AJ, Li J, DeLisa JA. Medical Rehabilitation after natural disasters: why, when, and how? *Arch Phys Med Rehabil* October 2012; 93(10): 1875–81.

14. Liu M, Kohzuki M, Hamamura A, et al. How did rehabilitation professionals act when faced with the Great East Japan earthquake and disaster? Descriptive epidemiology of disability and an interim report of the relief activities of the ten Rehabilitation-Related Organizations. *J Rehabil Med* May 2012; 44(5): 421–428.

15. Lancaster J. Emergency on the Subcontinent. *Harvard International Review*. August 15, 2010. http://hir.harvard.edu/emergency-on-the-subcontinent?page=0,2 (Accessed September 12, 2013).

16. Bloodworth DM, Kevorkian CG, Rumbaut E, Chiou-Tan FY. Impairment and disability in the Astrodome after hurricane Katrina: lessons learned about the needs of the disabled after large population movements. *Am J Phys Med Rehabil* September 2007; 86(9): 770–775.

17. Chiou-Tan FY, Bloodworth DM, Kass JS, Li X, Gavagan TF, Mattox K, Rintala DH. Physical medicine and rehabilitation conditions in the Astrodome clinic after hurricane Katrina. *Am J Phys Med Rehabil* September 2007; 86(9): 762–769.

18. Rathore FA, Farooq F, Muzammil S, New PW, Ahmad N, Haig AJ. Spinal cord injury management and rehabilitation: highlights and shortcomings from the 2005 earthquake in Pakistan. *Arch Phys Med Rehabil* March 2008; 89(3): 579–585.

19. Zhang X, Reinhardt JD, Gosney JE, Li J. The NHV rehabilitation services program improves long-term physical functioning in survivors of the 2008 Sichuan earthquake: a longitudinal quasi experiment. *PLoS One* 2013; 8(1): e53995.

20. Burns AS, O'Connell C. The challenge of spinal cord injury care in the developing world. *J Spinal Cord Med* January 2012; 35(1): 3–8.

21. ICRC Special Fund for the Disabled. 2013. http://www.icrc.org/fund-disabled (Accessed August 10, 2013).

22. WHO Guidelines for essential trauma care. Geneva, World Health Organization. 2004. http://whqlibdoc.who.int/publications/2004/9241546409.pdf (Accessed August 24, 2015).

23. WHO Community-based rehabilitation: CBR guidelines. Geneva, World Health Organization. 2010. http://www.who.int/disabilities/cbr/guidelines/en/index.html (Accessed August 8, 2013).

24. ISPO/WHO Statement: The Relationship Between Prosthetics and Orthotics Services and Community Based Rehabilitation (CBR). 2003. http://www.ispoint.org/resources (Accessed August, 23, 2013).

25. United Nations Enable. Disability, Natural Disasters and Emergency Situations. http://www.un.org/disabilities/default.asp?id=1546 (Accessed August 23, 2013).

26. WRC. Programs/Disabilities/Women's Refugee Commission's Work with Displaced Persons with Disabilities. New York, NY, Women's Refugee Commission. c2013. http://www.womensrefugeecommission.org/programs/disabilities (Accessed September 13, 2013).

27. *WHO Guidance Note on Disability and Emergency Risk Management for Health.* Malta, World Health Organization, 2013. http://www.who.int/hac/techguidance/preparedness/disability/en (Accessed October 14, 2013).

28. Pfeifer E, Blijkers, J, Ottacher, F, Lassmann, D, Nausner, B, Scherrer, V. *Humanitarian Aid All Inclusive! How to include people with disabilities in humanitarian action.* Vienna, Light for the World/Diakonie Katastrophenhilfe, 2013. http://www.light-for-the-world.org/uploads/media/HA_all_inclusive_web_02.pdf (Accessed August 24, 2015).

29. *Coping with Natural Disasters: The Role of Local Health Personnel and the Community Working Guide.* World Health Organization,

1989. http://helid.digicollection.org/en/d/Jwho07e (Accessed August 8, 2013).

30. Ardalan A, Mowafi H, Burkle FM, Jr. Iran's disaster risk: now is the time for community-based public health preparedness. *Prehosp Disaster Med* 2013; 28(5): 1–2.

31. Bremer R. Policy development in disaster preparedness and management: lessons learned from the January 2001 earthquake in Gujarat, India. *Prehosp Disaster Med* October–December 2003; 18(4): 372–384.

32. Eldar R. Preparedness for rehabilitation of casualties in disaster situations. *Disabil Rehabil* December 1997; 19(12): 547–551.

33. Handicap International/Nepal Red Cross Society. User friendly protocol/guidelines on post-trauma care in a large scale disaster scenario (amputation, open fracture, and spinal cord injury) ('Enhancing emergency health and rehabilitation response readiness capacity of the health system in event of high intensity earthquake' Project). European Commission Humanitarian Aid and Civil Protection (ECHO), 2013, unpublished.

34. Thomas K, Sinclair K. Disaster Preparedness and Response Information Package [CD-ROM]. Perth, Australia, World Federation of Occupational Therapists, 2006. http://www.wfot.org/Store/tabid/61/CategoryID/2/ProductID/10/Default.aspx (Accessed August 8, 2013).

35. Burns AS, O'Connell C, Rathore F. Meeting the challenges of spinal cord injury care following sudden onset disaster: lessons learned. *J Rehabil Med* May 2012; 44(5): 414–420.

36. WFOT. Disaster Preparedness and Response (DP&R). Australia, World Federation of Occupational Therapists. c2011. http://www.wfot.org/Practice/DisasterPreparednessandResponseDPR.aspx (Accessed August 23, 2013).

37. ISCoS. eLearning: www.elearnsci.org: a global educational initiative of ISCoS. UK, International Spinal Cord Society. c 2013. http://www.iscos.org.uk/resources/elearning (Accessed September 14, 2013).

38. ISPRM Rehabilitation Disaster Relief/Resources. Geneva, Kenes Associations Worldwide. c2013. http://www.isprm.org/collaborate/who-isprm/rehabilitation-disaster-relief (Accessed August, 23, 2013).

39. WCPT. Disaster Management. London, World Confederation for Physical Therapy. c2013. http://www.wcpt.org/disaster-management (Accessed August 8, 2013).

40. . WHO World Report on Disability. Geneva, World Health Organization. 2011. http://www.who.int/disabilities/world_report/2011/en/index.html (Accessed September 16, 2013).

41. Haig AJ, Im J, Adewole A, Nelson VS, Krabek B. The practice of physical medicine and rehabilitation in sub-Saharan Africa and Antarctica: a white paper or a black mark? *Disabil Rehabil* 2009; 31(13): 1031–1037.

42. Gutenbrunner C, Ward A, Chamberlain M White book on Physical and Rehabilitation Medicine in Europe (revised November 2009) *J Rehabil Med* 2007; 39(45): 1–48.

43. Burkle FM. The development of multidisciplinary core competencies: the first step in the professionalization of disaster medicine and public health preparedness on a global scale. *Disaster Med Public Health Prep* March 2012; 6(1): 10–12.

44. AAOS. Disaster Preparedness and Response Training. Rosemont, IL, American Academy of Orthopaedic Surgeons. c1995–2013. http://www.aaos.org/member/humanitarianprograms/disasterprep/dpr_trainingcourse.asp (Accessed September 14, 2013).

45. ACS. Operation Giving Back: International Disasters: Disaster Management and Emergency Preparedness (DMEP) Course. Chicago, IL, American College of Surgeons. c2004–2013. http://www.operationgivingback.facs.org/content2276.html (Accessed September 14, 2013).

46. WHO FMT Working Group. Technical criteria for classification and minimum standards for Foreign Medical Teams (FMTs). Geneva, World Health Organization, forthcoming.

47. IASC. IASC Principals Transformative Agenda. Inter Agency Standing Committee. c2013. http://www.humanitarianinfo.org/iasc/pageloader.aspx?page=content-template-default&bd=87 (Accessed September 13, 2103).

48. WHO. Humanitarian Health Action/Global Health Cluster. World Health Organization. c2013. http://www.who.int/hac/global_health_cluster/en (Accessed September 13, 2103).

49. Nickerson JW, Chackungal S, Knowlton L, McQueen K, Burkle FM. Surgical care during humanitarian crises: a systematic review of published surgical caseload data from foreign medical teams. *Prehosp Disaster Med* April2012; 27(2): 184–189.

50. Minimum Standards in Health Services. Sphere Project. *Sphere Handbook: Humanitarian Charter and Minimum Standards in Disaster Response, 2011.* Oxford, Oxfam Publishing, 2011; 331–333. http://www.spherehandbook.org (Accessed August 8, 2013).

51. Eldar R, Marincek C. WHO/EURO Consultation on Guidelines for Physical Rehabilitation of Wounded in Disaster Situations. Ljubljana Slovenia, 1996. http://www.worldcat.org/title/who-euro-consultation-on-guidelines-forrehabiliation-of-physically-wounded-in-disaster-situations-19–20-february-1996/oclc/182919614&referer=brief results (Accessed August 24, 2015).

52. Gutenbrunner C, Lemoine F, Yelnik A, Joseph PA, de Korvin G, Neumann V, Delarque A. The field of competence of the specialist in physical and rehabilitation medicine (PRM). *Ann Phys Rehabil Med* July 2011; 54(5): 298–318.

53. Gosney JE. Physical medicine and rehabilitation: critical role in disaster response. *Disaster Med Public Health Prep* June 2010; 4(2): 110–112.

54. Harrison RM. Preliminary investigation into the role of physiotherapists in disaster response. *Prehosp Disaster Med* September–October 2007; 22(5): 462–465.

55. Scaffa ME, Gerardi S, Herzberg G, McColl MA. The role of occupational therapy in disaster preparedness, response, and recovery. *Am J Occup Ther* November–December 2006; 60(6): 642–649.

56. Swiss Agency for Development & Cooperation/Landmine Survivors Network. Prosthetics and Orthotics Project Guide: Supporting P&O Services in Low-Income Settings. 2006. http://www.ispoint.org/resources (Accessed August 8, 2013).

57. Brown LM, Hickling EJ, Frahm K. Emergencies, disasters, and catastrophic events: the role of rehabilitation nurses in preparedness, response, and recovery. *Rehabil Nurs* November–December 2010; 35(6): 236–241.

58. WHO Taskshifting: global recommendations and guidelines. Geneva, World Health Organization. 2008. http://www.who.int/workforcealliance/knowledge/resources/taskshifting_guidelines/en/index.html (Accessed August 8, 2013).

59. Dawad S, Jobson G. Community-based rehabilitation programme as a model for task-shifting. *Disabil Rehabil* 2011; 33(21–22): 1997–2005.

60. De Ville de Goyet C, Pablo Sarmiento J, Grünewald F. Health response to the earthquake in Haiti January 2010: Lessons to be learned for the next massive sudden-onset disaster. Washington, DC, PAHO. 2011. http://new.paho.org/disasters/dmdocuments/HealthResponseHaitiEarthq.pdf (Accessed August 8, 2013).

61. Demey D, Nielsen S, Weerts, E. Early Rehabilitation Protocols for Victims of Natural Disaster: Capitalization Training Manual. Handicap International. 2010. Post-emergency project capitalization DVD. Handicap International. 2010. http://fr.scribd.com/doc/176227752/Early-Rehabilitation-Protocols-Eng-light (Accessed October 24, 2013).

62. O'Connell C, Shivji A, Calvot T. Preliminary findings about persons with injuries. Haiti Earthquake 12 January 2010: Handicap International Report. 2010. http://reliefweb.int/report/haiti/handicap-international-report-preliminary-findings-about-persons-injuries-ha%C3%AFti (Accessed August 8, 2013).

63. WHO International Perspectives on Spinal Cord Injury (IPSCI). Geneva, World Health Organization, forthcoming.

64. Knowlton LM, Gosney JE, Chackungal S, Altschuler E, Black L, Burkle FM Jr, et al. Consensus statements regarding the multidisciplinary care of limb amputation patients in disasters or humanitarian emergencies: Report of the 2011 Humanitarian Action Summit Surgical Working Group on amputations following disasters or conflict. *Prehosp Disaster Med* 2011; 26: 438–448.

65. Kirshblum SC, Waring W, Biering-Sorensen F, et al. Reference for the 2011 revision of the International Standards for Neurological Classification of Spinal Cord Injury. *J Spinal Cord Med* November 2011; 34(6): 547–554.

66. Consortium for Spinal Cord Medicine. Early acute management in adults with spinal cord injury: a clinical practice guideline for health-care professionals. *J Spinal Cord Med* 2008; 31(4): 403–479.

67. Catz A, Itzkovich M. Spinal Cord Independence Measure: comprehensive ability rating scale for the spinal cord lesion patient. *J Rehabil Res Dev* 2007; 44(1): 65–68.

68. Sayer NA, Chiros CE, Sigford B, Scott S, Clothier B, Pickett T, Lew HL. Characteristics and rehabilitation outcomes among patients with blast and other injuries sustained during the Global War on Terror. *Arch Phys Med Rehabil* January 2008; 89(1): 163–170.

69. Roy N, Shah H, Patel V, Bagalkote H. Surgical and psychosocial outcomes in the rural injured–a follow-up study of the 2001 earthquake victims. *Injury* August 2005; 36(8): 927–934.

70. Relief Web. Syrian crisis emergency response Lebanon – Bekaa valley: Disability and Vulnerability Focal Point project – Short project & activity report. January 30, 2013. http://reliefweb.int/report/lebanon/syrian-crisis-emergency-response-lebanon-bekaa-valley-disability-and-vulnerability (Accessed September 13, 2013).

71. Tharion G, Nagarajan G, Bhattacharji S. Guidelines for care of persons with spinal cord injury in the community. Department of Physical Medicine & Rehabilitation and Low Cost Effective Care Unit. Christian Medical College, Vellore, India. Government of India – World Health Organization Collaborative Programme 2008–2009. ftp://203.90.70.117/searoftp/WROIND/whoindia/linkfiles/NMH_Resources_Guidelines_for_care_of_persons_with_Spinal_Cord_injury_in_the_Community.pdf (Accessed August 8, 2013).

72. Loveday, M. The HELP Guide For Community Based Rehabilitation Workers: A Training Manual. Global HELP. 2006. http://www.global-help.org/publications/books/book_cbrehabilitation.html (Accessed October 14, 2013).

73. Werner D. *Disabled Village Children.* 2nd ed. 5th printing. Palo Alto, CA, Hesperian Foundation, 1999. http://www.worldforumfoundation.org/disabled-village-children-book-and-pdf (Accessed August 23, 2013).

74. Stephenson FJ. Simple wound care facilitates full healing in post-earthquake Haiti. *J Wound Care* January 2011; 20(1): 5–6, 8, 10.

75. ICRC. Prosthetics and Orthotics Manufacturing Guidelines. International Committee of the Red Cross. 2007. http://www.icrc.org/eng/resources/documents/publication/p0868.htm (Accessed August 10, 2013).

76. Haig AJ, Jayarajan S, Maslowski E, et al. Development of a language-independent functional evaluation. *Arch Phys Med Rehabil* December 2009; 90(12): 2074–2080.

77. Operational Medicine Institute. The Haiti Information Technology Rescue Project: Electronic Medical Record and Patient Tracking Assessment. 2010. http://www.opmedinstitute.org/media/upl/file_repository/OMI_HIT_RESCUE_FINAL_UN_REPORT.pdf; http://www.opmedinstitute.org/haiti (Accessed September 5, 2013).

78. OCEBM Levels of Evidence Working Group. The Oxford 2011 Levels of Evidence. Oxford Centre for Evidence-based Medicine. http://www.cebm.net/index.aspx?o=5653 (Accessed August 10, 2013).

79. Hu X, Zhang X, Gosney JE, Reinhardt JD, Chen S, Jin H, Li J. Analysis of functional status, quality of life and community integration in earthquake survivors with spinal cord injury at hospital discharge and one-year follow-up in the community. *J Rehabil Med* March 2012; 44(3): 200–205.

80. Li Y, Reinhardt JD, Gosney JE, Zhang X, Hu X, Chen S, Ding M, Li J. Evaluation of functional outcomes of physical rehabilitation and medical complications in spinal cord injury victims of the Sichuan earthquake. *J Rehabil Med* June 7, 2012; 44(7): 534–540.

81. Osmani-Vllasolli T, Hundozi H, Bytyçi C, Kalaveshi A, Krasniqi B. Rehabilitation of patients with war-related lower limb amputations. *Niger J Med* January–March 2011; 20(1): 39–43.

82. Hettiaratchy SP, Stiles PJ. Rehabilitation of lower limb traumatic amputees: the Sandy Gall Afghanistan Appeal's experience. *Injury* September 1996; 27(7): 499–501.

83. Fergason J, Keeling JJ, Bluman EM. Recent advances in lower extremity amputations and prosthetics for the combat injured patient. *Foot Ankle Clin* March 2010; 15(1): 151–174.

84. Delauche MC, Blackwell N, Le Perff H, Khallaf N, Müller J, Callens S, Allafort Duverger T. A Prospective Study of the Outcome of Patients with Limb Trauma following the Haitian Earthquake in 2010 at One- and Two- Year (The SuTra2 Study). *PLOS Currents Disasters* July 5, 2013 (last modified: July 11, 2013). Edition 1.

85. Brown V, Guerin PJ, Legros D, Paquet C, Pe´coul B, Moren A. Research in complex humanitarian emergencies: the Me´decins Sans Frontie´res/Epicentre experience. *PLoS Med* 2008; 5: e89.

86. Killian LM. An introduction to methodological problems of field studies in disasters. In: Stallings RA, ed. *Methods of disaster research.* Philadelphia, PA, Xlibris, 2002; 21–49.

87. Redmond AD, Mardel S, Taithe B, Gosney J, Duttine A, Girois S. A qualitative and quantitative study of the surgical and rehabilitation response to the earthquake in Haiti, January 2010. *Prehosp Disaster Med* 2011; 26: 449–456.

88. Abramson D, Morse S, Garrett A, Redlener I. Public health disaster research: surveying the field, defining its future. *Disaster Med Public Health Prep* 2007; 1: 57–62.

89. Burkle FM, Nickerson JW, von Schreeb J, Redmond AD, McQueen KA, Norton I et al. Emergency surgery data and documentation reporting forms for sudden-onset humanitarian crises, natural disasters and the existing burden of surgical disease. *Prehosp Disaster Med* 2012; 27: 577–582.

90. Blanchet K, Tataryn M. Evaluation of post-earthquake physical rehabilitation response in Haiti, 2010 – a systems analysis: ICED Research Report. International Centre for Evidence on Disability (ICED), London School of Hygiene and Tropical Medicine (LSHTM). 2012. http://disabilitycentre.lshtm.ac.uk/research/disaster-response-haiti (Accessed August 8, 2013).

91. U.S. Department of Veterans Affairs. VA/DOD Clinical Practice Guidelines. Washington, DC, U.S. Department of Veterans Affairs. July 10, 2013. http://www.healthquality.va.gov (Accessed September 13, 2013).

92. Paralyzed Veterans of America. Consortium for Spinal Cord Medicine. Clinical Practice and Consumer Guidelines for Management of Spinal Cord Injury. http://www.pva.org/site/c.ajIRK9NJLcJ2E/b.6431479/k.3D9E/Consortium_for_Spinal_Cord_Medicine.htm (Accessed August 8, 2013).

93. Evidence Aid/Resources: Providing resources for decision-makers before, during and after disasters and other humanitarian emergencies. Evidence Aid. c2013. http://www.evidenceaid.org/research (Accessed September 13, 2013).

94. CIRRIE. Database of International Rehabilitation Research. CIRRIE. January 3, 2013. http://www.cirrie.buffalo.edu/database/index.php (Accessed September 23, 2013).

25

CRISIS AND EMERGENCY RISK COMMUNICATION

Barbara J. Reynolds and Gilead Shenhar

OVERVIEW

Crisis and Emergency Risk Communication (CERC) is a recognized field of communication study that differs from health-risk communication and risk communication. It is used in disaster communication and combines elements of the other types of risk communication, but has emerged as a new field of communication recognized by academia. CERC is taught in universities in the United States and is being diffused internationally. In addition, the Pan American Health Organization (PAHO), World Health Organization (WHO), and North Atlantic Treaty Organization (NATO) have adopted CERC principles for their communication work. Hence, CERC is the risk communication term that will be used in this chapter.

A Case for Emergency, Crisis, and Health-Risk Communication

Health-risk communications are an important and necessary component of disaster management. While a population or community faced with a potential injury/illness-creating event (PICE) will not overcome its challenges solely through the application of appropriate communication principles, an organization can compound its problems during an emergency if it has neglected sound CERC planning. Failure to "be first," "be right," and "be credible" and deliver empathetic messages may interfere with what would otherwise be well-planned and executed response operations. Integrating CERC into the planning and early stages of disaster response will improve operations and speed recovery.[1–3]

Scenario 1. A chemical plant fire 3 km away appears to send a plume of black smoke directly over a neighborhood. A suburban parent of two preschool children calls 911 (or the equivalent emergency access number) and expects to get answers. He is told there is no evacuation information for his address. He is given no alternatives.

Scenario 2. A single mom proudly moves into her first home. Three months later, she receives an official government packet in the mail – it contains iodine tablets for her children and her to take in case of a terrorist attack on the nearby nuclear plant.

All the joy in her new home evaporates as she anguishes over the potential future radiation threat to her children. She calculates the cost of leaving this "death trap" – her new home.

Scenario 3. People in the community are suddenly dying in high numbers from an upper-respiratory disease while tests have not confirmed the infectious agent. Some in the media are speculating that it could be a new disease and possibly a bioterrorist attack. Local health officials refuse comment until their tests are completed. Community members are demanding antibiotics from their physicians while local emergency departments are overwhelmed.

Three different public health scenarios have one common denominator – people in serious need of health-risk information and officials who provided an inadequate communication response. In Scenario 1, the family was not notified to evacuate because there was no risk to them. The government officials did not recognize that they may not only need to tell people when to evacuate, but also reassure families when they do not need to evacuate, especially when they observe families in nearby communities being evacuated. In Scenario 2, government officials believed they had communicated the necessary information to the community member and that no other follow-up or reassurance was needed. In Scenario 3, the government was focused on ensuring that whatever message they communicated was complete and accurate and ignored media speculation in the interim, which left the public without guidance.

Emergency Communication Purposes

The initial objectives for public information releases from response authorities early in a crisis are to: 1) prevent further illness, injury, or death; 2) restore or maintain calm; and 3) engender confidence in the operational response.[4] During a crisis, good communication to the public is a necessity, not a luxury. For an optimal outcome, the public needs information from its leaders, and leaders need support and cooperation from the public. Many predictable, harmful individual and community behaviors can be mitigated with effective crisis and emergency risk communication. CERC tools are critical disaster resources and CERC uses sound psychological and communication research in its approach to the selection of message, messenger, and method of delivery.

What the Public Expects

The public wants to know what officials know. While this is not always possible, officials must understand the motivations behind the public's desire for information, especially early in a crisis. The public wants to accomplish the following five things with the information they obtain from public health and emergency management authorities:

1. Gain the wanted facts needed to protect them, their families, and their pets from the dangers they are facing
2. Make well-informed decisions using all available information
3. Have an active, participatory role in response and recovery
4. Act as guards over resources – both public funds and donated funds
5. Recover or preserve well-being and normalcy, including economic security

While the purpose of crisis response is to efficiently and effectively reduce and prevent illness, injury, and death, and to return individuals and communities to normal, the possibilities of harmful human behaviors combined with bad communication practices can lead to overwhelmingly negative outcomes. The following are some of the damaging situations response professionals could face:

▪ Public demand for the misallocation of limited emergency response resources
▪ Public mistrust or circumvention of public health recommendations
▪ Opportunists who play on peoples' fear or uncertainties to provide fraudulent alternate treatments
▪ Increased levels of disease and death
▪ Overreaction and wasted fiscal and medical resources during the emergency response

Executed well and early, CERC can help reduce the tendencies of detrimental human behavior and prevent negative public health outcomes.

CURRENT STATE OF THE ART

Defining Crisis and Emergency Risk Communication

Understanding how academics and practitioners define various categories of communication may be useful to inform disaster managers who face a broad and rapidly changing disaster response environment. Communication expertise, which fulfills the needs of response professionals, borrows from many areas of communication study. Professionals are increasingly calling this integrated model "crisis and emergency risk communication" as they recognize that no single communication field can fulfill the multiple and overlapping roles required of this era's complex sociopolitical environments, new technological media, and dynamic health disaster risks.[2] For a response organization to successfully communicate in a crisis, it must be fast, accurate, credible, consistent, and empathetic. To navigate the harsh realities of the information needs of the public, media, and stakeholders during an intense public-safety emergency requires more

than attaching "appendix X" to an operational plan. In a crisis, the right message at the right time is a "resource multiplier" – it helps response officials get their jobs done. Many predictable, harmful individual and community behaviors can be mitigated with effective CERC. Each crisis has its own psychological challenges; disaster response officials must anticipate what mental stresses the population will experience and apply appropriate risk communication strategies to attempt to manage these population stresses.

Crisis Communication

Crisis communication can be defined in two ways; therefore, it can cause some confusion for a practitioner seeking expert training and counsel. The term is most often used to describe an organization facing a reputational crisis and the need to communicate about that crisis to stakeholders and the public.[5] Typically, a crisis is an event that occurs unexpectedly, may not be within the organization's control, and may cause harm to the organization's good reputation or viability. An example of an organization facing a crisis is the occurrence of a mass shooting in the workplace by a disgruntled employee. In most instances, the organization faces legal or moral culpability for the crisis (unlike a disaster in which a tornado destroys the production plant), and stakeholders and the public judge the organization's response.

A second, simpler definition of crisis communication separates judgment or reputation factors in the communication and focuses primarily on factual communication by an organization to its stakeholders and the public when a disaster or emergency occurs. In this context, crisis communication could simply be the effort by community leaders to inform the public that, by law, they must evacuate in advance of a hurricane. In this definition, the organization is not being overtly judged as a possible participant in the creation of the disaster, and the information is empirically sound, so the individual can judge its veracity without the help of an expert.

The underlying thread in crisis communication is that the communicating organization is experiencing an unexpected crisis and must respond. Crisis also implies lack of control by the involved organization in the timing of the crisis event.

Communicator: Participant
Time Pressure: Urgent and unexpected
Message Purpose: Explain and persuade

Issues Management Communication

Issues management communication is similar to crisis communication; however, the organization has the luxury of foreknowledge of the impending crisis and the opportunity, to some extent, to choose the timing of its revelation to stakeholders and the public and reveal the organization's plan to resolve the issue. Again, the organization is central to the event.

Communicator: Participant
Time Pressure: Anticipated; timing somewhat in control of the communicator
Message Purpose: Persuade and explain

Health-Risk Communication

Health-risk communication is a field that has flourished in the area of environmental health. Through health-risk communication, the communicator seeks to provide the receiver with information about the expected type (good or bad) and magnitude (weak or strong) of an outcome from a behavior or exposure. Typically, the communicator provides information about an adverse outcome and the probability of that outcome occurring. In some instances, risk communication has been employed to help an individual make a choice about whether or not to undergo a medical treatment, continue to live next to a nuclear power plant, pass on genetic risks, or elect to vaccinate a healthy baby against pertussis. In some cases, risk communication is used to help individuals adjust to the knowledge that something that has already occurred, such as an exposure to harmful carcinogens, that may put them at greater risk for a future negative health outcome, such as cancer. Risk communication would prepare people for that possibility and, if warranted, give them appropriate steps to monitor for the health risk, such as regular cancer screening.

Communicator: Expert that did not participate in the event and is neutral regarding the outcome
Time Pressure: Anticipated communication with little or no time pressure
Message Purpose: Empower informed decision making

Crisis and Emergency Risk Communication

CERC balances the urgency of disaster communication with the need to rapidly communicate risks and benefits to stakeholders and the public in an evolving situation. It differs from crisis communication in that the communicator is not, at least initially, perceived as a participant in the crisis or disaster, except as an agent to resolve the crisis or emergency. CERC is a strategy used by experts to provide information to allow individuals, stakeholders, or an entire community to make the best possible decisions about their well-being within challenging time constraints. It also assists people with accepting the imperfect nature of choices during a crisis. CERC differs from risk communication in that a decision must be made within a narrow time constraint, the decision may be irreversible, the outcome of the decision may be uncertain, and the decision may need to be made with imperfect or incomplete information. This is similar to the communication that typically occurs in emergency departments, but not usually in doctors' offices. CERC represents an expert opinion provided with the goal that it benefits its receivers and advances a behavior or an action that allows for rapid and efficient recovery from the event. CERC integrates elements of all of the previously defined fields of communication and emphasizes each more or less depending on the type of disaster and the stage of the disaster response.

Communicator: Expert who is a post-event participant invested in the outcome
Time Pressure: Urgent and unexpected
Message Purpose: Explain, persuade, and empower decision making

Organizational Credibility and Trust

Research indicates that the public perceives the success of the disaster operational response by the amount and speed of relevant information they receive from emergency response officials.[6] Messages are more or less relevant as they do or do not answer important questions about actions to take to empower the receiver and reduce uncertainty.[7,8] Research also indicates that messages that are empathetic (taking the emotional perspective of the audience), appear honest and open, are relevant, and come from a trusted source are most effective in a crisis.[1,9]

In several surveys, the U.S. public was asked whom they would trust most as a spokesperson or reliable source of information if a bioterrorism event occurred in their community. Respondents trusted most the local health department or a local physician or hospital. However, respondents also trusted "quite a lot" or "a great deal" their own doctors, the fire chief, the director of the health department, the police chief, the governor, and a local religious leader.[10]

Communicating in disaster situations has become increasingly more difficult for responding organizations for a number of reasons. A complicating phenomenon is the reality that one's messages will compete with many others for credibility with the public before, during, and after the disaster. Therefore, the organization's credibility, the credibility of the spokespersons who deliver messages, and the messages' soundness from the intended audience's perspective are all critical. The explosion of alternate information channels and sources, particularly fast-paced social media, allow people to "shop around" for messengers and messages. In addition, public suspicions of scientific experts and government are increasing. The suspicions are increasing for a variety of reasons, including access to more sources of conflicting information, a reduction in the use of scientific reasoning in decision making, and political infighting.[5,9,11] Also, the media has a tendency to interview "experts" with diametrically opposed views (a point/counterpoint technique) and this can serve to confuse the public since there is no unified message. Finally, confidence in government, traditional social institutions, and industry in the United States and some other countries has severely eroded in the last 30 years.[9]

Reputational Risk Management

Organization reputational risk management is more critical than ever because of this increasing lack of confidence, shifting cultural norms, and new, faster communication technologies. Part of this is driven by the emergence of a "victim" culture that divides people into three categories: helpless victim, those who victimize, and those who rescue victims. Additional changes forcing this rethinking include the global explosion of information access, a decline in the understanding and reputation of science, and the increase of advocacy groups.[12,13]

An organization can measure its reputation through the level of stakeholder trust or mistrust. Stakeholders are people or organizations with a special connection to the organization. The Ethics Resource Council teaches that "trust is the natural consequence of promises fulfilled."[14] Mistrust is an outgrowth of the perception that promises have been broken and values violated. Trust and credibility are essential elements of persuasive communication.[15] Empathy and caring, competence, commitment, and accountability contribute to trust.[1] Three important elements – speed of response, avoiding missteps during the crisis response, and asking for forgiveness when mistakes occur – contribute significantly to maintaining and building trust during a crisis response. It is best if events that affect the organization's trust never occur, but when they do, it is not the error itself but the response to the misstep that harms the reputation. This is especially true if an organization mishandles the early phases of correcting the error. The public can forgive an organization when something goes wrong, but it will not, if the organization is perceived as uncaring. Early and empathetic action may mitigate damage. Yet, most organizations are not structured to provide rapid responses. Leaders are rarely trained for, and committed to quick, caring action. If an organization and its leaders are unwilling to build and maintain trust with their stakeholders and the general public, then executing any other elements of the communication plan is a wasted effort. Trust is foundational to CERC. There are five key elements to building trust: expressed empathy, competence, honesty, accountability, and commitment.

Empathy

Research shows that an expression of empathy should be given in the first 30 seconds of communication.[16] To do otherwise is futile, because the public will be waiting to hear whether or not you "get it." The audience is wondering whether the response official understands that they are frightened, anxious, confused, or angry. If the official neglects to articulate what the audience members are feeling in the moment, their minds will be consumed with the question "Do they get it?" and they will not hear anything the officials are saying. A sincere expression of empathy early in the communication will allow people to calm their thoughts and actually hear what the official has to say.

When someone's life is suddenly severely disrupted and something happens to them that they never believed could really happen to "me," it is important for that person to hear from the people who are there to help that they "get it." Caution: It is inappropriate to say, "I know how you feel." That phrase lacks specificity. Officials must take a moment and discern what emotion community members are feeling, such as fear, frustration, anxiety, dread, or confusion and actually name the emotion. If uncertain, say, "I can only imagine I would be feeling pretty frustrated right now," and wait to see whether the audience appears to agree.

From the time of Aristotle to today's communication and psychological research, studies continue to highlight that expressed empathy is a key component of building trust. Expressing empathy in a crisis situation is a necessity. Every credible response official that acts as a spokesperson must be prepared to sincerely and repeatedly express empathy toward those affected by the event.

Competence and Expertise

Source competence is important.[15] If an official has a title and is part of the response to a crisis, the public will assume he or she is competent until something occurs to indicate otherwise. Education, position title, or organizational roles and missions are quick ways to indicate expertise. Previous experience and demonstrated abilities in the current situation enhance the perception of competence. Another useful tool to build trust is to have an established relationship with the audience in advance of the emergency.[5] If that is not possible, a third party (who has the confidence of the audience and expresses confidence in the response organization and its officials) is useful.

Honesty

According to data from 2005, communities believe that the U.S. government routinely withholds information.[17] Before communication with a community in crisis even begins, most of the population assumes officials are withholding information. Officials should strive to treat people as they would like to be treated in a similar situation. It is inappropriate to withhold information based on a well-meaning but misguided desire to protect people or to avoid a bigger problem. The motives may be

noble, but the outcome could be the opposite. The U.S. Centers for Disease Control and Prevention (CDC) and five universities conducted a series of fifty-five focus groups in 2003. Among the findings, three themes emerged from the participants: any information is empowering; uncertainty is more difficult to accept than knowledge of something bad; and participants seek out multiple sources for information.

Holding back information as a way to "manage" the crisis in not only inappropriate, it is also impractical. With modern information technology, the public can readily find information. Assume that if more than one person knows the "facts," everyone knows the facts. Then ask, "Do you want to present the facts in context or do you want to try to clean up a mess of someone else's making?"

Bad news does not get better over time. There is consensus among professionals that the faster one delivers bad news, the better. Withholding information implies guilt and arrogance.

Do organizations choose to withhold frightening information because they do not want people to "panic?" Do they withhold information because they think it will minimize the volume of information requests from the public and media inquiries from reporters? In actuality, not knowing is worse than knowing. People can cope with bad news and the anticipation of bad things to come. Conversely, at times, there are good reasons to withhold certain information (e.g., for issues of national security). When this is the case, respectfully tell the public you are withholding information and why.

Honesty and openness in crisis communication means facing the realities of the situation and responding accordingly. It means not being paternalistic in communication but, instead, participatory – giving people choices and enough information to make appropriate decisions. In situations of great uncertainty, the public should be told why the information is not available for release.[13] To build trust, the public should be allowed to observe the process while being reminded that this method is what drives the quality of the emergency response.

Accountability and Commitment

For most people, accountability literally means "keeping the books open." If government or nonprofit money is being spent in the response to a disaster, sooner or later the public and media will demand to know to whom that money or those resources are being distributed. A savvy official would anticipate the questions and have the mechanisms in place to be as transparent as possible. One strategy would be to keep an account on a website related to the disaster with timely updates.

An organization's credibility is important at any time, but especially during a crisis. While it is relatively simple to retrospectively analyze another organization's crisis and clearly see that its leaders should have released information to the public earlier and more fully, it is much more difficult when it is "your" crisis. Achieving openness and empathy requires written policies that are practiced during exercises, have full commitment from the highest organizational leadership, and are modeled during non-crisis situations.

Crisis Communication Life Cycle

Understanding the pattern of a crisis can help communicators anticipate problems and respond effectively. For spokespersons, it is vital to know that every emergency, disaster, or crisis evolves in phases and that the communication must evolve in tandem.

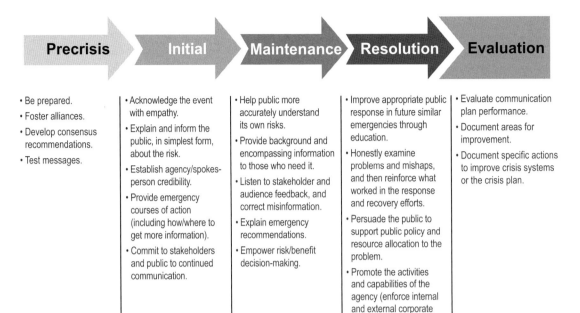

Figure 25.1. Crisis Communication Life Cycle.

By dividing the crisis into the following phases, the communicator can anticipate the information needs of the general public, stakeholders, and the media. Each phase has unique informational requirements (Figure 25.1).

Movement through the phases varies according to the triggering event. Not all crises are created equally. The degree or intensity and longevity of a crisis determine the required numbers of staff and other resources.

Pre-Crisis Phase

Communication objectives during the pre-crisis phase are:

- Be prepared
- Foster alliances
- Develop consensus recommendations
- Test messages

During this phase, all the planning and most of the work should be completed. Types of disasters that your organization may need to address can be anticipated using a hazard vulnerability analysis (see Chapter 11). Reasonable questions can be anticipated, and preliminary answers can be sought. Initial communication templates can be drafted with blanks to be completed later. Spokespersons, resources, and resource mechanisms should be identified. Training and refinements to plans and messages can be made. Alliances and partnerships can be fostered to ensure that experts are speaking with one voice.

Initial Phase

Communication objectives during the initial phase are:

- Acknowledge the event with empathy
- Explain and inform the public, in simplest terms, about the risk
- Establish and affirm organizational/spokesperson credibility
- Provide emergency courses of action (including how and where to get additional information)

- Commit to continued communication on a regular basis to stakeholders and the public

The initial phase of a crisis is characterized by confusion and intense media interest. Information is usually incomplete, and the facts are dispersed. Simplicity, credibility, verifiability, consistency, and speed are critical when communicating in the initial phases of an emergency. Information from the media, other organizations, and even within an organization may not be accurate. The communicator's role is to learn the facts about what happened, to determine the organization's response to the problem, and to verify the true magnitude of the event as quickly as possible.

In the initial phase of a crisis, there is no second chance to "get it right." An organization's reputation depends on what it does and does not say, when it says it, and the tone in which it is said. One of the best ways to limit public anxiety in a crisis is to provide useful information about the nature of the problem and what the people can do to protect themselves. During the initial phase of an event, an organization must reaffirm or establish itself as a credible source of information. Even when there is little information to offer, it can still communicate what is currently known, how the organization is investigating the event, and when more information will be available. At the very least, messages should demonstrate that the organization is addressing issues directly and that its approach is reasonable, caring, and timely.

The pressure to release information prematurely can be intense. However, all information must be approved by leadership before its release to the media. Importantly, the organization must speak with one voice and avoid giving mixed messages.

In the initial phase of a crisis or emergency, people want immediate information. They want timely and accurate facts about what happened, where it occurred, and what is being done. They will question the magnitude of the crisis, the immediacy of the threat to them, the duration of the threat, and who is going to fix the problem. Communicators should be prepared to address these concerns as quickly, accurately, and fully as possible.

Crisis Maintenance Phase

Communication objectives during the crisis maintenance phase are:

- Help people more accurately understand their own risks
- Provide background and encompassing information to those who need it. For example: How could this happen? Has this happened before? How can I prevent this from happening again? Will I be safe and secure long term? Will I recover?
- Gain understanding and support for response and recovery plans
- Listen to stakeholder and audience feedback; correct misinformation
- Explain emergency recommendations
- Empower risk-benefit decision making

As the crisis evolves, anticipate sustained media interest and scrutiny. Unexpected developments, rumors, or misinformation may place further media demands on organization communicators. Experts, professionals, and others not associated with your organization will comment publicly on the issue and sometimes contradict or misinterpret your messages. Expect to be criticized about your management of the situation.

Remaining current regarding information flow and maintaining tight coordination are essential. Processes for tracking communication activities become increasingly important as workload increases. The crisis maintenance phase includes an ongoing assessment of the event and allocation of resources.

Resolution Phase

Communication objectives for the resolution phase are:

- Improve appropriate public response in future similar emergencies through education
- Honestly examine problems and mishaps, and then reinforce what worked in the recovery and response efforts
- Persuade the public to support public policy and resource allocation
- Promote activities and capabilities of the organization both internally and externally

As the crisis resolves, there is a return to baseline operations, with increased understanding about the event as complete recovery systems are implemented.[5] This phase is characterized by a reduction in public and media interest. Once the crisis is resolved, an organization may need to respond to intense media scrutiny of how the event was managed. It may have an opportunity to reinforce public health messages while the issue is still current. A public education campaign or changes to a website may be necessary. Research has shown that a community is usually most responsive to risk avoidance and mitigation education directly after a disaster has occurred.[1]

Evaluation

When the crisis is over, evaluate communication plan performance and determine specific actions to improve crisis systems or the crisis plan.

Communication in a Crisis Is Different

Communicating in a crisis is different than during normal conditions. In a serious crisis, affected people may process and act on information differently. During crisis situations, individuals are often unable to collect and process information in a timely manner and, thus, rely on established routines for situations that are, by definition, novel.[5] Since people absorb information they receive during an emergency in a manner different from non-emergency situations,[7] the potential for miscommunication increases. The way people assimilate information, process it, and act on it can change when they or their loved ones are under the threat of illness or death.[16] Importantly, people will simplify complex information, attempt to force new information into previous constructs, and cling to current beliefs.[18] Therefore, if the emergency message requires asking people to do something that seems counterintuitive, they may hesitate to act. Because people tend not to seek out contrary evidence and are adept at maintaining their beliefs, conflicting or contrary information may be misconstrued to conform to established beliefs.[12] They may reject new information.

Use of imagery in decision making and persuasion may cause people to be influenced by irrelevant factors.[14] Scientists report that people's brains are hard-wired to engage in sensory-emotive logic. Messages created with the belief that people are linear thinkers who make logical decisions may fall short of their expectations.[19] Hill contends that the old way of thinking is that individuals proceed through steps in decision making from cognitive to affective, and then to behavioral. However, scientific results based on tracing the brain's circuitry show that long before learning through the logical basis of the message, people are influenced on a largely unconscious, emotive level, particularly when they feel threatened and anxious.[1,19] Therefore, it is important that response officials consider what images are being presented to people and show people what they should be doing, not just tell them. Spokespersons should "model" the behavior they want from the public. Non-verbal behavior is of great importance when the audience feels threatened.

An "action message" can provide people with the feeling that they can take steps to improve a situation and not become passive victims of the threat. Physical and mental preparation relieves anxiety, despite the expectation of potential injury or death. Therefore, to reduce the likelihood of victimization and fear, the public must feel empowered to take action. Show them the positive actions to take; avoid focusing on negative images.

Other aspects of decision making are affected during a crisis. The following behaviors are commonly exhibited:

Simplify

Under intense stress and possible information overload, people overlook the nuances of messages or avoid the effort to juggle multiple facts by simplifying what they have heard.[18] To cope, people may not attempt an analytical and reasoned approach to decision making. Instead, they may rely on habit, long-held traditions, following the lead of others, and such stereotyping as classifying participants as "good" and "bad" guys.

Maintain Current Beliefs

It may be difficult to change peoples' beliefs during a crisis or emergency, especially if one's communication requires asking them to do something that seems counterintuitive (e.g., getting out of a "safe" car and lying in a ditch instead of outrunning a tornado).[15] People are adept at maintaining faith in their current beliefs and tend not to seek out contrary evidence. They also exploit conflicting or contradictory information about a subject by interpreting it as consistent with existing beliefs. For example:

"I believe that chocolate is good. Some studies say chocolate is bad for your health. Some studies say chocolate is good for your health. I choose to believe that no one knows for sure, and I'll continue to eat chocolate."

People may remember what they see and may believe incorrect or conflicting information. They tend to believe what they have experienced in their own lives. Faced with new risks in an emergency, people rely on experts. However, supposedly reputable experts may disagree regarding the level of threat, risks, and appropriate recommendations. Furthermore, recommendations from the same expert may change over time as more is understood about the nature of the threat. The evolving nature of emergencies and the natural give and take among experts and their tendency to enjoy the peer process could leave the general public with increased uncertainty and fear. The media often fosters point/counterpoint discussions, regardless of the validity of the differing views. Research indicates that, often, the first message to reach the listener is the accepted message, even though more accurate information may follow.

With this in mind, CERC principles stress that simplicity, credibility, verifiability, consistency, and speed are critical when communicating in an emergency. An effective message must be repeated, come from a legitimate source, be specific to the emergency being experienced, and offer a positive course of action.

During a Disaster, What Are People Feeling?

People experience a wide range of emotions. While there is variability between people, patterns emerge in a crisis. Response officials need to understand this diversity and why communicating in a crisis is different.

There are a number of psychological barriers that could interfere with the cooperation and response from the public. Many of them can be mitigated through the work of a leader with an empathetic and honest health-risk communication style.

Fear, Anxiety, Confusion, and Dread

Chaos theory related to crises emphasizes that disasters that take a toll on human life are inherently characterized by change, high levels of uncertainty, and interactive complexity.[5] The majority of people in the United States will experience at least one traumatic event "outside the range of normal human experience,"[21] sometime within their lifetimes. How well someone may cope with those traumatic events depends on personal resilience (see Chapter 6). Personal resilience is a person's ability to maintain equilibrium in the face of trauma and loss. Resilience is often described as the protective factors that foster positive outcomes and help humans to thrive after extreme disasters.[21] The following psychological resources protect victims of disaster: coping efforts, self-efficacy, mastery, perceived control, self-esteem, hope, and optimism.[22] In disaster situations, some people feel a sense of dissociation and that the familiar normal world they knew is gone. These feelings may be mitigated with quick, firm directions for action.[23] Survivors' fear, anxiety, and despondency can be reduced to manageable levels by reducing situational uncertainty with information, by giving individuals or communities actions to take that restore a sense of control, and by modeling optimistic behaviors.[1,15,23] These are all activities that can be achieved through mass communication. However, the messages must be crafted carefully and acknowledge the emotional toll.

In a crisis, one can expect that people in the community are feeling fear, anxiety, confusion, and, possibly, dread. The spokesperson in a crisis should not attempt to eliminate these feelings. If that were the goal, failure would be a certainty. Instead, these are the emotions that one should acknowledge in a statement of empathy. "We've never faced anything like this before in our community and it can be frightening."

Hopelessness and Helplessness

If the community, its families, or individuals let their feelings of fear, anxiety, confusion, and dread grow unchecked during a crisis, psychologists predict they will begin to feel hopeless or helpless.[24] A reasonable amount of fear is acceptable. Instead of striving to "stop the panic" and eliminate fear, help the community manage its fears and lead it to productive actions. Action helps overcome feelings of hopelessness and helplessness. Give people things to do. As much as possible, give them relevant things to do – things that are constructive and relate to the crisis they are facing. Anxiety is reduced by action and a restored sense of control. This should be the primary objective for risk communication in a crisis.

The actions may be symbolic (e.g., put up the flag) or preparatory (e.g., donate blood or create a family check-in plan). Some actions need to be put into context. Be careful about telling people things they should do without telling them when to do them. Phrase these preparatory actions in an "if–then" format. For example: "Go buy duct tape and plastic sheeting to have on hand, and if (fill in the blank) occurs, then seal one interior space in your house and shelter-in-place."

The public must feel empowered and in control of at least some parts of their lives if officials want to reduce fear and feelings of victimization.[24,25] Plan ahead and think of actions for people to perform. Deliver instructions in action messages, even if the instruction is as simple as "check on an elderly neighbor."

The Myth of Panic

Contrary to what is seen in the movies, people seldom act completely irrationally or panic during a crisis.[7] Certainly there are anecdotal reports of people running into burning buildings, remaining in a car stuck on the tracks with a train speeding toward them, and becoming emotionally paralyzed to the point of helplessness. However, the overwhelming majority of people can and do act reasonably during an emergency. Behavior during a crisis described by the media as "panic" often represents reasonable, self-protective actions.

How people absorb or act on information they receive during an emergency may be different from non-emergency situations. In other words, the primitive part of the brain that supports survival of the human species is activated (i.e., the "fight or flight" mechanism). One cannot predict whether someone will choose fight or flight. However, everyone's behavior will fall at some point on the continuum. Extreme "fighters" may resist taking most actions to keep themselves safe until the very last moment. And extreme "fleers" may overreact and take extraordinary additional steps to make themselves extra safe, well in advance of the threat. These normal reactions to a crisis, particularly when at the extreme ends, are often reflected back in the media and described erroneously as "panic." In actuality, panic behavior is defined as behavior counter to survival. While officials responsible for getting a recommended response from the community may have the impression that people are engaging in extreme behavior, in reality, the overwhelming majority of people do not.[26] The condition most conducive to panic is not bad news; it is conflicting messages from those in authority. People are the most likely to panic (although still not all that likely) when they feel that they cannot trust what those in authority are telling them or when they feel misled or abandoned in dangerous territory. When authorities start hedging or hiding bad news in order to prevent panic, they are likely to exacerbate the risk of panic.

During the fall 2001 U.S. anthrax incident, for example, media reported local shortages of the antibiotic known as ciprofloxacin (Cipro) because people began to seek prescriptions, anticipating the threat of anthrax. If individuals request a prescription for Cipro, even though they live on the other side of the country from where the exposures occurred, is that really a panic behavior or counter to their survival? No; it is their survival instinct leading to a behavior they believe will be self-protective. If a person hears a community leader saying "don't panic," the individual may believe that the message only applies to others. While securing a Cipro prescription, he thinks he is rationally taking steps to ensure his survival, and someone else must be panicking. If response officials describe individual survival behaviors as "panic," they will alienate their audience and render them unable to receive the public health message. Instead, officials should acknowledge people's desire to take protective steps, redirect them to actions they can take, and explain why the unwanted behavior is potentially harmful to them or the community. Officials can appeal to people's sense of community to help them resist maladaptive actions aimed at individual protection.[27]

When people overwhelm emergency hotlines with calls, they are not panicking. They want the information they believe they need and officials should have. As long as people are seeking information, they may be fearful, but they are not acting helpless, nor are they panicking. Seeking information is appropriate during a crisis. Share available data and explain that there is a process in place to gain more information. Do not be pedantic or paternalistic – be honest and humble about what is and is not known in the situation. Empower people to draw solid health conclusions for themselves and their loved ones.

Uncertainty

Uncertainty increases anxiety if there is a perception of danger or threat.[13] To reduce anxiety, people gather and process information and seek options that confirm or discredit their beliefs. The information used in this process does not have to be accurate. In fact, to improve coherence and reduce anxiety, people choose sources selectively and discount information that is distressing or overwhelming. People who are seeking information to reduce anxiety from dangerous uncertainty are particularly attentive to behaviors and language styles of persons in power.[13] They may choose a familiar source of information over a less familiar source, regardless of the accuracy of the information. People less certain of their ability to process information involving complex situations may choose an advocate to collect and interpret information for them, especially if the information is not provided in their native language or a medium familiar to them (e.g., social networking).

Early in a crisis, there are typically more questions than answers. The cause of the disaster and full magnitude of the situation may be uncertain. Even the actions people can take to protect themselves may be unclear. A danger early in a crisis, especially if one is responsible for fixing the problem, is to promise an outcome outside one's control. One should never utter a promise, no matter how heartfelt, unless it is in one's absolute power to deliver. Officials can hope for certain outcomes, but most cannot be promised. New York Mayor Rudy Giuliani cautioned, "Promise only when you're positive. This rule sounds so obvious that I wouldn't mention it unless I saw leaders break it on a regular basis."[28]

People can manage the anxiety of the uncertainty if officials share the process the organization is using to get the answers.[7,27] "I can't tell you today what's causing people in our town to die so suddenly, but I can tell you what we're doing to find out. Here's the first step," or "It's too early to declare that this is the pandemic we've been predicting – but this is still a serious health concern because the virus is transmitting between humans. Here are the steps we're taking next."

In a crisis, people believe any information is empowering. Tell them what is known now and most importantly tell them what is not known and explain the process being used to get answers.

If people are not panicking, why is there sometimes confusion during a crisis, especially in the early stages? Just because an individual action is driven by survival instincts, it is not necessarily the best behavior for the community as a whole. There are a number of troublesome expected behaviors that can and do occur in major catastrophes. For example, a person interested in survival may seek out special relationships for favors or another may start a rumor based on faulty information-seeking. A leader should be aware of these behaviors and be prepared to confront them in communications to the public.

Acknowledge People's Fears

When people are afraid, the worst thing to do is pretend that they are not. The second worst message is to tell them they should not be afraid.[1] Both actions leave people feeling alone with their fears. Mishandling people's fears is related to improper reassurance, but conceptually different, for example, "Everything is under control" versus "Don't worry."

Even when the fear is totally unjustified, people do not respond well to it being ignored – nor do they respond well to criticism, mockery, or statistics. These approaches are marginally effective even when the fear is warranted. Instead, acknowledge fears while concurrently providing people the information they need, thereby placing their fears into context. Giving people permission to be excessively alarmed about a bioterrorist threat (but still telling them why they need not be overly worried) makes it far more likely that they will actually be reassured.

Stigmatization

In some instances, victims may be stigmatized by their communities and refused services or public access.[29] Fear and isolation of a group perceived to be contaminated or risky to close contacts will hamper community recovery and impede evacuation and relocation efforts. In a disease outbreak, a community is more likely to separate from those perceived to be infected.

During the 2002–2003 SARS outbreak, believed to have originated in China, cities worldwide reported that the public avoided visiting Chinatown sections of their cities. The governor of Hawaii publicly ate dinner in the Chinatown section of Honolulu to help counter this stigmatization. This is a good example of leadership modeling behavior desired by the public.

Response officials must be sensitive to the possibility that, although unintentional and unwarranted, segments of their community could be shunned because they become "identified" with the problem. This could have both economic and psychological effects on the well-being of community members and should be challenged immediately. This stigmatization can occur absent any scientific basis and could come not only from individuals but entire nations. During the avian influenza outbreak in Hong Kong in 1997–1998 and during the West Nile virus outbreak in New York City in 1999, policies of other nations banned the movement of people or animals, absent clear science calling for those measures.

Perception of Risk

The perception of risk is also vitally important in emergency communication. Risks have variable acceptance.[1,6] A wide body of research exists on issues surrounding risk communication. The following emphasize that the public accepts some risks more than others.

- Voluntary versus involuntary: Voluntary risks are more readily accepted than imposed risks.
- Personally controlled versus controlled by others: Risks controlled by the individual or community are more readily accepted than risks outside the individual's or community's control.
- Familiar versus exotic: Familiar risks are more readily accepted than unfamiliar risks. Risks perceived as relatively unknown are perceived to be greater than risks that are well understood.
- Origin: While crisis etiology is not always initially known, risks perceived to be generated by nature are better tolerated than risks thought to be caused by human actions.
- Reversible versus permanent: Reversible risk is better tolerated than risk perceived to be irreversible.
- Statistical versus anecdotal: Statistical risks for populations are better tolerated than risks represented by individuals. An anecdote presented to a person or community (i.e., "one in a million") can be more damaging than a statistical risk of 1 in 10,000 presented as a number.
- Endemic versus epidemic (catastrophic): Illnesses, injuries, and deaths spread over time at a predictable rate are better tolerated than illnesses, injuries, and deaths grouped by time and location (e.g., annual motor vehicle collision deaths versus individual airplane crashes).
- Fairly distributed versus unfairly distributed: Risks that are not directed at a group, population, or individual are better tolerated than risks that are perceived to be targeted.
- Generated by trusted institution versus mistrusted institution: Risks generated by a trusted institution are better tolerated than risks that are generated by a mistrusted institution. Risks generated by a mistrusted institution will be perceived as greater than risks generated by a trusted institution.
- Adults versus children: Risks that affect adults are better tolerated than risks that affect children.
- Understood benefit versus questionable benefit: Risks with well-understood potential benefit and harm reduction are better tolerated than risks with little or no perceived benefit or reduction of harm.

In any discussion of risk, the scientist may perceive 1 risk in 10,000 as an acceptable risk, while the listener may anecdotally be familiar with that one adverse outcome and believe that the risk is personally much greater. Perception of risk involves more than numbers alone.

Response officials must carefully assess event magnitude. Typically the magnitude of the event is measured by the number of people injured, ill, or dead, and/or the dollar amount and geographic spread of property damage. The causative agent is also important. The principles of risk communication are vital when developing messages during an emergency. If it is the first emergency of its type – irrespective of etiology or magnitude – communication challenges will increase, even if the severity of the crisis is not as great as previous events. Officials should measure the magnitude of a crisis based on three things: 1) the degree of physical and mental impact on people (i.e., how many are ill, sick, or dead); 2) the degree of property damage; and 3) the emotional toll the crisis takes on the population, based on attributes related to crisis etiology.

Role of the Spokesperson

The right spokesperson at the right time with the right message can save lives. The following emergency risk communication principles should be incorporated into messages:

- Acknowledge fears. Do not tell people they should not be afraid. Fear may be a reasonable reaction. One effective technique for calming fears is for spokespersons to share a reason why they are not afraid (based on expert knowledge) and let people conclude for themselves why these experts are less concerned. Never follow with "so don't be afraid."
- Express wishes. "I wish we knew more." "I wish our answers were more definitive." An "I wish" phrase expresses empathy.
- Give people things to do. Offer a range of responses – a minimum response, a maximum response, and a recommended middle response. For example: "Don't drink the tap water; buy bottled water or boil the tap water."
- Acknowledge the shared misery. Some people will be less frightened than they are miserable, feeling hopeless and defeated. Acknowledge the misery of a catastrophic event, then help move people toward hope for the future through the actions of the organization and through actions that they can also take.
- Give anticipatory guidance. If officials are aware of future negative outcomes, they should let people know what to expect (e.g., side effects of antibiotics). If it is going to be bad, tell them.
- At some point, be willing to address the "what if" questions. These are the questions everyone is thinking about and wants answered by experts. Although it is often impractical to encourage "what ifs" when the crisis is contained and not likely to affect large numbers of people, it is reasonable to answer these hypothetical questions as people need to prepare emotionally. If officials do not answer the "what if" questions, someone with much less at risk regarding the response's outcome will likely answer them. If spokespersons are not prepared to tackle "what ifs," they may lose credibility and the opportunity to address the "what if" questions with reasonable and valid recommendations.
- Be a role model and ask more of people. Many trauma experts agree that the psychological outcome of a community as a whole depends on resilience (see Chapter 6). A critical role of spokespersons is to ask people to bear the risk with them. People can tolerate considerable risk. If spokespersons

acknowledge the risk, its severity, and complexity, and acknowledge fears, they can then ask people to accept the risk during the emergency and work toward solutions.

Five Communication Failures that Inhibit Operational Success

Communication experts and leaders with real-life disaster experiences have determined that certain approaches should be avoided as they will cripple or even destroy disaster response operational success.[8,29] Tactics to avoid include:

■ Mixed messages from multiple experts
■ Information released late
■ Paternalistic attitudes
■ Not countering rumors and myths in real-time
■ Public power struggles and confusion

Mixed Messages

The public needs a unified message rather than a selection of options for action. During the mid-1990s, the Midwestern United States experienced a spring of great floods. Response officials determined that the water treatment facilities in some communities were compromised and that a "boil water" directive should be issued. A problem developed when multiple response organizations, governmental and nongovernmental, issued directions for boiling water and each of them was different. Compounding this issue is the fact that, in the United States, people turn on the faucet and clean water comes out. Few people know the "recipe" to boil water because they have never needed it. Examples of people who might be unable to choose the correct option for sterilizing water include: a young mother who needs to mix her infant son's cereal with water, a middle-aged son caring for his immunocompromised mother receiving chemotherapy, or a sister living down the street from her HIV-positive brother whose T-cell count is low. Even healthy people are risk-adverse to the consequences of not choosing the right boil-water instructions.

When faced with a new threat, people want a consistent and simple recommendation. They want to hear absolute agreement about what they should do and they want to hear it from multiple experts, through multiple sources. Even correct messages can be damaging if delivered improperly. If messages are inconsistent, the public will lose trust in the response officials and begin to question every recommendation.[1,8,29] Local, state, regional, and national response officials and their partners must work together to ensure messages are consistent, especially when the information is new to the public.

Information Released Late

Following the September 11, 2001, U.S. terrorist attacks, many people wanted advice on whether or not to buy a gas mask and requested information from CDC. Three weeks after the attack, CDC had an answer on its website. During the 3 weeks that CDC took to develop and vet its answer, a number of experts were willing to give an answer; however, it was not the correct one. When CDC issued advice to the public not to buy gas masks, the gas mask aisles at local Army-Navy Surplus stores were already empty. While few could contemplate the consequences of a September 11–type attack, officials must anticipate and create a process to quickly react to the information needs of the public. If authorities cannot give people what they need when they need

it, others will. And those "others" may not have the best interests of the public in mind when they offer advice.

If the public expects an answer from an organization on something that is answerable and it does not provide it or direct them to someone who can, people will be vulnerable to receiving bad advice from unscrupulous or fraudulent opportunists.

Paternalistic Attitudes

Putting on the American film actor John Wayne's swagger and ostensibly answering the public's concerns with a "don't worry little lady, we got ya covered" is ineffective in the information age. People want and expect to be provided information that allows them to come to their own conclusions.[30] As a response official, it is insufficient to satisfy one's own worries with copious bits of information and then state a bottom line message that is unsupported by the currently known facts. As difficult as it may be, spokespersons must help the public to reach the same conclusion by sharing the knowledge with them that led to it. Response officials should determine what they learned that made them believe the situation was not worrisome and then share this information.

Treat the public like intelligent adults and they will act like intelligent adults.[7,24,32] Treated any other way, they will either turn on officials or behave in ways that seem illogical. Officials are leaders, not parents, for the public. Never tell people "don't worry." Tell people what they need to know and allow them to reach the conclusion that they do not need to worry. Engage the public in the process and they will follow.[22,31]

Not Countering Rumors in Real Time

During a pneumonic plague outbreak, how successful will an organization's drug distribution program be if a rumor starts that there are not enough drugs for everyone? What system is in place to monitor what is being said by the public and the media? How will officials react to false information?

Do not spread rumors by holding press conferences every time a rumor surfaces, but be aware that a press conference may be necessary if a rumor has been widely published. If the rumor is circulating on the Internet, post a response on the Internet and have a telephone information service ready to manage the rumor. The media will report rumors or hoaxes unless officials rapidly explain why they are false. Have an open, quick channel to communicate to the media for use when monitoring systems detect a troublesome rumor. Do not think, "this is preposterous, and no one will believe it." In a crisis, the improbable seems more possible. Deflect rumors quickly, with facts.

Public Power Struggles or Confusion

In an actual event, one U.S. governor held a press conference about a public safety crisis at the same time the mayor of the city was holding one on the other side of town. This set the tone for speculation about who was in charge and what was or was not true.

In the information age, it is easy to see how this could happen. Sometimes there may be a power struggle over jurisdictions or other issues. These issues should be resolved quickly and confidentially. It is disconcerting to the public to think that the people responsible for helping them are not getting along. All partners need to have clearly defined roles and responsibilities. When they overlap, and they do, make sure officials can settle concerns without causing headlines about power struggles or, worse, confused response officials. When all else fails, stay in the scope of one's responsibility and refrain from declaring "I'm in charge" without being certain that you are.

Even if everyone participates in the same press conference, officials could send the wrong message to the public. If people are jockeying for the microphone or looking back and forth at each other hoping someone will answer a reporter's question, the public will be left with the impression that there is confusion and power struggles among the leadership.

Early in the sniper shooting incident in metropolitan Washington, DC, Montgomery County Police Chief Charles Moose formally requested involvement by the U.S. Federal Bureau of Investigation (FBI). Although there were concerns about what that might mean to local law enforcement, the chief chose to involve the FBI and did it quietly and apparently seamlessly, at least to the public. At no time did the public perceive a power struggle among the response agencies. This, however, was a community that had previously experienced a terrorist attack at the Pentagon and an anthrax attack at the Capitol. It had learned the value of a united front with multiple jurisdictions working cooperatively for the good of the community. Turf wars need to end the moment a crisis begins. A good plan can help avoid turf wars from the start.

The Message – Content Is Critical in an Emergency

Identify Your Audiences and Their Concerns

The receiver of communication will judge the content of the message, the messenger, and the method of delivery. Each of these aspects must be considered in planning for CERC. The public's awareness of government is heightened during a crisis. A lack of continuity, control, adequate resources, or full knowledge of the event can invoke fear and threaten social unity.[31] The public's needs can be judged three ways: 1) their relationship to the incident; 2) their psychological differences (e.g., "fight or flight" response and emotional versus adaptive coping); and 3) their demographic differences.

Possible audiences for CERC include:

- Public within the circle of disaster or emergency for whom action messages are intended
  - Concerns: Personal safety, family safety, pet safety, stigmatization, property protection
- Public immediately outside circle of disaster or emergency for whom action messages are not intended
  - Concerns: Personal safety, family safety, pet safety, interruption of normal life activities
- Emergency response and recovery workers, law enforcement involved in the response
  - Concerns: Resources to accomplish response and recovery, personal safety, family safety, pet safety, public image
- Public health and medical professionals involved in the disaster response
  - Concerns: Resources adequate to respond, personal safety, family safety, pet safety, public image
- Family members of victims and response workers
  - Concerns: Personal safety, safety of victims and response workers
- Healthcare professionals outside the response effort
  - Concerns: The public mentally "trying on" and then prematurely acting on or rejecting treatment recommendations; ability to respond to patients with appropriate information; access to treatment supplies if

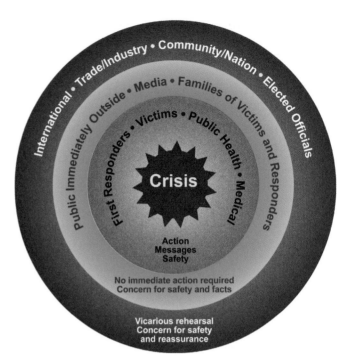

Figure 25.2. Audience Relationship to the Event.

needed/wanted; and how to volunteer to respond to the disaster area
- Civic leaders at local, state, and national levels
  - Concerns: Response and recovery resources, liability, leadership, quality of response and recovery planning and implementation; opportunities for expressions of concern; trade and international diplomatic relations
- Legislative bodies (e.g., U.S. Congress)
  - Concerns: Protecting and informing constituents, review of statutes and laws for adequacy and adjustment needs, opportunities for expressions of concern by public officials to their constituents
- Trade and industry
  - Concerns: Business issues (loss of revenue, liability, business interruption), protection of employees
- National community
  - Concerns: Public mentally rehearsing treatment and then rejecting recommended treatments (vicarious rehearsal), risks to self, readiness efforts
- International neighbors
  - Concerns: Vicarious rehearsal, risk to self, readiness efforts
- International community
  - Concerns: Vicarious rehearsal, risk to self, exploration of readiness
- Stakeholders and partners specific to the emergency
  - Concerns: Inclusion in decision making, access to information
- Media
  - Concerns: Personal safety, access to information and spokespersons, fact-checking, deadlines

Each audience desires a specific message (Figure 25.2). Prioritize the development of messages for listeners based on their involvement.

Remember the basics when creating messages. Audience segmentation and demographics remain relevant during a crisis. Consider the following:

- Education
- Current subject knowledge and experience
- Age
- Disability (hearing or sight impaired)
- Language spoken/read
- Cultural norms
- Geographic location

How Audiences Judge Messages in a Crisis

Expect an audience to immediately judge the content of a message in the following ways.

SPEED OF COMMUNICATION

Was the message timely? Research indicates that the first message received on a subject sets the stage for comparison of all future messages on that subject. If the public hears that the world is flat, and then someone comes along and says "the world is round," that message may face resistance because of inflexible beliefs. Also, the speed with which one responds to the public can be an indicator of how prepared one is to respond to the emergency. More rapid speeds suggest that there is a system in place and that needed action is being taken. If the public is not aware that officials are responding to the crisis, it is the same as a non-response. The public may then lose confidence in the organization's ability to effectively manage an incident, and the organization will need to reallocate needed resources to convincing the public that the response system is working.

First impressions are lasting impressions. If an organization fails to gain public confidence early, it will be nearly impossible to recover the public trust. This does not necessarily mean having all the answers; it means having an early presence so the public knows that officials are aware of the emergency and that there is a system in place to respond. A great message delivered after the audience has moved on to other issues is a message not delivered at all.

There are two important reasons to strive to be the first source of information in a crisis. The public uses the speed of information flow in a crisis as a marker for judging preparedness.[6] A perfect operational response may be irrelevant without concurrent health-risk communication. Even when a hazardous materials team in the U.S. city of Atlanta responded within 2 minutes of a chemical plant fire, immediately evacuated the scene, and determined that the fire should be allowed to burn instead of being extinguished with water that could spread hazardous chemicals into the water table, the local news coverage was filled with sound bites from angry families. People saw the black smoke and wanted to know if they should evacuate, but were unable to receive rapid, practical information. Parents, gripping the hands of their small children, castigated the people who knew but did not tell them that they were safe. Living in the information age means being expected to not only save lives, but also to tell people that lives are being saved concurrent with an unfolding event.

The second reason is a psychological principle. When people seek information about something they do not know, the first message they receive carries the most weight.[23] There is a tendency for people to accept the information and then, if they hear a second message that conflicts with the first, weigh the messages against each other. This is especially dangerous if the first message is incorrect but sounds logical.

For example, the news media reports that health officials are swabbing the noses of congressional staffers for anthrax spores to see if they need to take antibiotics. A member of the lay public is exposed to a white substance in the break room of his factory, and he thinks he should get a nose swab too. In fact, a positive or negative nose swab for anthrax spores is not a reliable way to determine if someone should be given antibiotics. That determination is made with other data such as proximity to the exposure site and ventilation systems. Even so, reasonable people who were misinformed that nasal swabs were useful in making medical treatment decisions will expect to receive the same care as people in the news who they may perceive to be more privileged. It is better to use resources to distribute an early correct message, rather than wasting them later to correct a faulty first impression.

FACTUAL CONTENT OF THE MESSAGE

The public will listen for factual information, and some will be expecting to hear a recommendation for action. Get the facts right, repeat them consistently, avoid sketchy details early on, and ensure that all credible sources deliver the same facts. Speak with one voice. Preparation is critical. Consistent messages are vital. Inconsistent messages increase anxiety and quickly damage experts' credibility.

Crafting the Best Messages

Consider the following when creating an initial communication to an audience:

- For the general public, present a short, concise, and focused message (sixth-grade level). It is difficult in a heightened state of anxiety or fear to internalize copious amounts of information. Get the bottom line out first. In time, the public will want more information.
- Cut to the chase. Initially provide only relevant information. Avoid starting with a lot of background information. Do not spend time establishing the identity of the spokesperson or the organization. One sentence should be sufficient.
- Give action steps in positives, not negatives (e.g., "In case of fire, use stairs" and "stay calm" are positive messages; negative messages include "do not use elevator" and "don't panic.")
- Repeat the message. Repetition reflects credibility and durability. Correct information is correct each time it is repeated. Reach and frequency, common advertising concepts, teach that the message is more apt to be received and acted on as the number of people exposed to the message (i.e., reach) and the number of times each person hears the message (i.e., frequency) increase.
- Create action steps in threes or rhyme, or create an acronym. These are ways to make basic information easier to remember, such as "stop/drop and roll" or "KISS – keep it simple, stupid." Three is not a magic number, but in an emergency, it is likely that the public can absorb three simple directions. Research indicates that somewhere between three and seven bits of information is the limit for people to

memorize and recall.[26] For example: "Anthrax is a bacterium that is treated with antibiotics. Anthrax is not transmitted from person-to-person. Seek medical care if exhibiting the symptoms of anthrax: fever, body aches, and breathing problems."

■ Use personal pronouns for the organization. "We are committed to (fill in the blank)" or "We understand the need for (fill in the blank)."

Avoid:

■ Technical jargon and medical terminology
  ■ Instead of saying "people may suffer morbidity and mortality," say, "people exposed may become sick or die."
  ■ Instead of "epidemic" or "pandemic," say "outbreak" or "widespread outbreak."
  ■ Instead of "deployed," say "sent" or "put in place."
  ■ Instead of "correlation," say "relationship" (avoid using "cause").
■ Unnecessary filler – background information (save for other outlets/times)
■ Condescending or judgmental phrases (e.g., "You would have to be an idiot to try to outrun a tornado" or "Only hypochondriacs would need to walk around with a prescription for Cipro.") Most people are neither idiots nor hypochondriacs, and both ideas have crossed their minds. Do not insult the audience by word or tone. That does not mean condoning the behavior; instead, validate the impulse but offer a better alternate and then explain the reasons why it is better.
■ Attacks. Attack the problem, not the person or organization.
■ Promises/guarantees. Guarantee only what you can deliver; otherwise, promise to remain committed throughout the emergency response.
■ Discussion of money. During the initial phase, discussion of the magnitude of the problem should be in the context of the health and safety of the public or environment. Loss of property is secondary. Also, a discussion of the amount of money spent is not a surrogate for the level of concern and response from an organization (what does that money provide?).
■ Humor. Seldom is humor a good idea. People seldom "get the joke" when they are feeling desperate. Humor is a great stress-reliever behind closed doors. While inappropriate humor is sometimes used as a coping mechanism, be careful not to offend others responding to an emergency, even behind closed doors. Be especially sensitive when speaking to the public.

Know the Needs of Stakeholders

Stakeholders are identifiable groups of people or organizations who can be reached in more ways than through the media. They self-identify as stakeholders. Response organizations do not determine whether these groups have something at stake in the crisis – the stakeholders do. They believe the organizations are beholden to them in some way and these groups expect to communicate with the organization directly and not only via the news media.

The highest level of respect toward a stakeholder group is for the organization's leader to meet face to face with them.

Organizations need to determine who, in a crisis, should be invited to meet with its leaders, or be called by its leaders or receive a handwritten note or personalized email from its leaders. The organization's leaders cannot do all of these things for all stakeholders, so they must delegate some of these activities. For example, Mayor Giuliani attended as many funerals as possible for the firefighters, police, and government workers who died on September 11, 2001, in New York City. By not delegating that task, he chose his stakeholder priorities wisely.

Stakeholders are people or groups with a special connection to an organization and its involvement in the emergency.[24] Anticipate and assess the incident from the stakeholders' perspective. They will be most interested in how the incident will affect them. Stakeholders are expecting something from the organization. It could be as simple as information released through a website and email or as complex as in-person meetings with key organization officials.

In crisis communication planning, the first step in responding to stakeholders is to identify them. Stakeholders vary according to the emergency, but core stakeholders will be common to every emergency and will expect communication with the organization.

Not all stakeholders are supporters of the organization; nonetheless, it is critical to identify unsupportive stakeholders and be prepared to respond to them appropriately. Generally, stakeholders fall into three categories based on their responses in a crisis: advocates, adversaries, and ambivalents. The response to stakeholders depends on the category. The key is to anticipate stakeholders' reactions based on their affinity for the organization and the way that similar groups have reacted in the past when this type of crisis has occurred.

An emergency or crisis may be an opportunity to strengthen an organization's partner and stakeholder relationships as stakeholders see the organization in action. A positive response will enhance the organization's credibility. Do not forget to consider existing stakeholder controversies or concerns and how the ongoing relationship will color their attitudes during this incident.

By planning ahead and identifying as many stakeholders as possible before the event occurs, and the means for communication with them, an organization will be prepared to show stakeholders respect by attending to their needs for communication with the organization.

Expending energy on stakeholder communication during a crisis is valuable for at least two reasons. First, they may have information of value to the organization. They have viewpoints outside the organization. Few stakeholders will be shy about pointing out deficiencies. It is preferable for the organization to hear these criticisms directly rather than indirectly through the media. Second, stakeholders may be able to help communicate messages for the organization. They may have credibility in circles the organization does not. If an organization is forthcoming with them, it may face fewer problems during the crisis recovery.

Research has shown that leaders and their organizations make five errors during a crisis according to stakeholders.[15,25,30] They include the following: 1) inadequate access; 2) lack of clarity; 3) no energy for response to stakeholders; 4) too little too late, and 5) perceptions of arrogance. Most of these represent a lack of resources and planning directed at stakeholder communication.

The Town Hall Meeting

Facing a community in a town hall meeting or citizen's forum during a crisis may be the most difficult communication task asked of a response official. Nevertheless, this is an important responsibility. It is essential for response officials to allow the community the opportunity to meet and discuss aspects of the response, and for officials to be held accountable.

Do not convene a town hall meeting without preparation and practice. A poorly managed meeting can lead to lack of community support. Be aware that the people who come to a town hall meeting are not representative of the entire community. They are usually the most angry or frightened. The basic principles for a successful meeting are:

- Let people talk. Do not allow experts to lecture. The more people talk, the more successful they will judge the meeting.
- Solicit questions. Listen to questions before offering solutions. Officials may be surprised to find out that what they think are the issues are in fact not the community's issues. The key is not to offer solutions to problems; rather, empower the audience to discover solutions.
- Be respectful of people's input. Praise them for being willing to offer ideas. Encourage participation.
- Tell the truth. Organizers should admit when they do not know something and follow up to get people the information they are seeking.
- Do not lose your temper. Meeting participants may have been emotionally hurt, feel threatened by risks out of their control, feel they are not respected, or have had their fundamental beliefs challenged. Set aside your anger. Instead, strive to understand.

Sometimes people appear angry because they are advocates for a particular position on an issue. These people become "angry" when the cameras are focused on them. Sometimes people appear angry because they hope to litigate. Set ground rules and remind people that, in *this* town hall meeting, everyone must behave respectfully if they want to be heard. Do not allow hecklers to gain control. Remain calm and take a little more abuse than most people would expect. In so doing, the legitimately angry community members will soon come to the rescue, demanding that the hecklers behave.

Despite all the risks officials face in holding a town hall meeting, they work for the people and, therefore, should hold these meetings. Set realistic goals for the meeting. It is not the responsibility of organizing officials to have everyone leave the meeting happy. Sometimes, the goal should be to listen, simply listen. Never promise what cannot be delivered, no matter how easy it would be to do so in the moment. Under-promise and over-deliver.

While delivering a lecture may be easier than facilitating an interactive discussion, it is much less likely to change beliefs or behavior. The lecturer can express opinions and emotions, and does not have to take others' points of view into account. A lecture does not engage the audience. If people are upset, they want to be heard. Officials should limit opening remarks to 5 minutes or less, because the audience will likely be thinking about what they want to say, rather than listening to someone else. Let them say it.

Telling is easier; asking is more difficult. Asking questions is a deliberate action. It forces the process to slow down and compels people to stop and think before replying. Instead of attempting to persuade individuals or community groups to take an action, allow them to convince themselves through a self-discovery process. The key is not to provide the solution, but to help the audience discover its own solution.

How does one help an audience discover its own answers? This is accomplished by asking the right questions. Using feedback as a tool, ask the audience questions that will create awareness about the situation in such a way as to empower them to make difficult choices. As many therapists will attest, a person who comes up with his own answer and says something in his own voice will take ownership of that idea. It is better to ask a leading, open-ended question than to make an interpretation. The right questions can help an audience to make the necessary connections between the information provided by experts and the best possible choices for them in the specific situation. This strengthens the audience's tendency to claim ownership for the insights.

For example, if a severe communicable disease outbreak were to occur, a challenge for emergency response and public health officials is the possibility that civil rights may need to be temporarily suspended to control the spread of disease. An extreme case would be the need to quarantine individuals or communities (see Chapter 17). A population that understands the need for quarantine will be more likely to comply with public health instructions.

Questions to Assist the Lay Public with Taking Ownership of Protective Public Health Measures

- Start with broad, open-ended questions.
  - Examples: What challenges have (you or your community) faced that required consensus building to solve the problem? How did it go? What did you learn from those experiences? Were there difficult choices to make?
- Then, ask questions to discover the explicit wants, needs, and desires of the audience.
  - Examples: What is most important to (you or your community) when faced with a problem to solve? Consensus building? Putting the greater good for the greater number first? Avoiding conflict? That the solution is fair and equitably distributed? Ensuring that everyone has a voice and is heard? That reasonable alternatives are fully explored?
- Follow with questions that are more specific to the current situation.
  - Examples: What are the ramifications to (you, your family, your community, the nation) when faced with this current problem? What consequences are you hoping to avoid? What do you see as the worst outcome for (you or your community)? What courses of action do you believe could lessen this outcome?
- Then, ask questions that encourage audience members to state the benefits they would like to see result from a course of action.
  - Examples: What benefits would you or your community expect if this disease did not spread further? Since you've brought up quarantine, what benefits

would (you or your community) expect if you accepted quarantine as a course of action to reduce spread of disease?

▪ Once the audience sees and expresses the benefits, it will be much easier to demonstrate how a particular strategy can solve the problem.

    ▪ Examples: From what I understand, you are looking for a way to protect (yourself, your family, your community) from more illness or death? If I can explain how quarantine will meet those needs, are you open to implementing it? If you think quarantine would work in this effort, how do you see the quarantine being explained and implemented for the entire community?

Allowing people to persuade themselves is not an easy process. Done poorly, it can seem condescending or manipulative. It takes practice and a great deal of empathy. However, it is worth the effort, because it is the most effective way to gain acceptance in thought and behavior.

RECOMMENDATIONS FOR FURTHER RESEARCH

Following the anthrax events in 2001 in the United States and the struggles CDC experienced with communication at that time, it developed key principles for use in CERC for future potential injury creating events. CDC successfully applied these principles in response to Hurricane Katrina and in preparation for pandemic influenza. However, there are vital areas of emergency risk communication that require urgent consideration and research such as those related to vicarious rehearsal (described next) and outreach to special populations.

Vicarious Rehearsal and Risk Communication

In an emergency, some recovery and specific health recommendations are directed at victims and those exposed or who have the immediate potential to be exposed. However, information technology allows people to vicariously participate in a crisis that is not an immediate danger to them. These people will mentally rehearse the crisis as if they are experiencing it and "try on" the courses of action presented, which, in reality are being presented to the directly affected victims of the crisis. Because these "armchair" victims have the luxury of time to decide their chosen course of action, they may be much more critical about its value to them. In some cases, these people may reject the proposed course of action and choose another or insist that they too are at risk and deserve the recommended remedy (e.g., an emergency department visit or a vaccination). These concerned, but unexposed, persons may place an undue burden on already thin response and recovery resources. Research is needed to help determine the best way to manage the anxiety created by those who are vicariously involved in a crisis event and who then believe they also should be taking a mediating action. Alternate "action" messages may be needed for people who are not really threatened but are vicariously feeling threatened and may be primed to take an action they should not take. In addition, how should treatment messages be communicated to ensure that those who should act on them do, and those who should not, will not?

Emergency Messages in Multicultural Settings

Can emergency communication that may only reflect a nation's dominant-culture's perspectives appropriately influence behaviors of persons from non-dominant groups? Research related to culture and crisis is inconsistent.[13] In crisis situations, event-specific messages may need to be rapidly developed. However, efforts to tailor messages could slow information flow, thereby creating additional challenges to credibility and trust. In addition, if messages were culturally tailored in some crises, there may be potential for messages to be misinterpreted as "selective" or culturally biased, which could increase mistrust or create a perception of stigmatization. For example, because historically most cases of H5N1 occurred in Asia, if health officials tailored messages specific to Asian Americans, it might be perceived by some in the population that the messages focused on their differences and separateness, thus stigmatizing them.

If cultural differences in messaging are neglected during a public safety emergency, will this result in increased levels of illness or death among non-dominant groups, or are people's information needs essentially the same when reacting to serious threats, thus obliterating cultural differences and rendering culturally attuned messaging unnecessary? When the entities communicating to these diverse populations are authoritative governments (i.e., local, state, and federal) that have the power to suspend civil rights, ration scarce pharmaceutical resources, and control information flow, will the absence of culturally appropriate messages complicate disaster operations? These questions should form the basis of crisis communication research to ensure equitable support to all members of the community.

In an international setting, differing cultural norms (e.g., collectivist versus individualistic societies), political structures, media practices, and aversions to risk make the application of CERC principles more challenging. An important area of future research is to determine to what extent these principles are universally accepted across cultures and which must be adapted based on national and cultural differences. Zaltman's research emphasizes the commonalities among all human cultures and suggests that people are more alike than different.[34] However, can health-risk communication mitigate inherently harmful behavior among a population? For example, can it prevent the tendency for people to go to the seaside to watch for a tsunami or to gather as a group to discuss whether to exit a burning building? Is there a difference between cultural adaptation for pre-event messaging versus communications during the event?

The initial objectives for public information releases early in a crisis are to: prevent further illness, injury, or death; restore or maintain calm; and engender confidence in the operational response. With looming crises such as pandemic influenza, which will involve many national and cultural groups, additional research on these issues is urgent.

Summary

Crisis and emergency risk communication is an essential tool to achieve preparedness during routine times, but an even more important tool during emergencies. The case study of the Israeli experience provides useful information, but this knowledge must be evaluated and adapted to other systems before implementation. Clear, effective, and coordinated CERC before, during, and after an event is challenging, but effective.

Case Study 1 – The Israeli Risk Communication Experience

In recent history, Israel has experienced several large-scale events that necessitated a robust risk communication program in order to prepare the Israeli population to best protect themselves, and to save lives during the events. CERC is one of the most important tools used in Israel for disaster management.

The homeland defense is based on several layers that include early warning, active and passive defense. An example of active defense is the use of an anti-missile system. Passive defense is based on several elements, with CERC being one of the most important components. It also includes other elements such as: bomb shelters, medical support, alert systems, and search and rescue.

Major events include:

1. War against Terror

    Terror events (mostly suicide bombers) targeting the civilian population killed more than 785 persons and injured more than 5,600, especially during the years 2000–2004.

2. Second Iraqi War (Operation Iraqi Freedom)

    Israel had only a few months to prepare the population and to provide protection in case of a conventional or unconventional attack (2002–2003). Iraq fired thirty-nine Scud missiles at Israel during the first Gulf War, all armed with conventional explosives. It was known that they possessed weapons of mass destruction.

3. Second Lebanon War (2006)

    a. During the second Lebanon war, Hezbollah (an extremist Shiite Muslim organization in Lebanon) attacked the northern part of Israel with more than 4,000 rocket missile launches. This resulted in more than 4,300 civilian casualties (half of them who developed mental illnesses) and an additional 42 civilian deaths.

    b. The war started precipitously (without any warning time to prepare the population) and lasted 33 days.

4. Cast Lead Operation (2008)

    a. The goal of this operation was to stop rocket fire into Israel from the Gaza strip. During the 24 days of the operation, more than 1 million people in Israel were under immediate threat of rockets.

    b. During the operation, the public remained on imminent alert to enter protective zones. Overall, 3 civilians were killed, 183 were injured and 548 developed acute stress reactions.

5. Mount Carmel forest Fire (2010)

    a. The fire claimed 44 lives. The dead were mostly Israel Prison Service officer cadets in a bus trapped by the fire. More than 17,000 people were evacuated, and the area sustained massive property and environmental damage.

    b. During the event, Israel requested international assistance.

6. Pillar of Defense (2012)

    a. During the 8-day operation, 1,506 rockets were fired at Israel from the Gaza Strip, aimed to strike the civilian population.

    b. The areas most highly targeted had more than 1 million inhabitants, mainly in the southern part of the country.

    c. In order to protect the country's population, an active defense system with "Iron Dome" rocket interceptor

systems was installed. During the operation, 3 Israeli civilians were killed and 202 were wounded.

Understanding the basic infrastructure of Israel is critical in order to put the information that follows into context (Table 25.1).

Table 25.1. Basic Infrastructure of Israel

- 8 million inhabitants, many are new immigrants (e.g., from 1989 to 1996, about 670,000 people emigrated from Russia). In comparison, in 1948, Israel had 806,000 inhabitants.
- Area – 21,643 square kilometers
- Gross domestic product (GDP) per capita – $32,200 USD (2012)
- Religion: 75% Jewish; 17% Muslim; 2% Christian; 1.6% Druses; 4% other
- The only democracy in the Middle East
- Israel is a single state with a single command structure (single police force, single fire department, single emergency medical system)
- Multi-lingual – Hebrew, Arabic, English, Russian, Amharic
- High percentage of population with military service background
- Population is well-educated
- Majority of hospitals are public (not private)
- Has a huge civil protection organization "Home Front Command," established in 1992; It is a military organization, civilian-oriented, based mainly on reserve duty personnel. One of its main goals (by law) is to prepare the Israeli population and to educate and train them on civil protection issues.

Insights and Observations

OBSERVATION #1

Preparing a country – and especially the population – requires extensive time and effort, willing and engaged decision-makers, and a sizeable budget.

It takes a substantial amount of time to prepare a country for the essential threats. Preparations must be coordinated with all relevant organizations, should begin in advance, and should be revised during and after the event.

OBSERVATION #2

A country must identify and prepare for legitimate threats. Using cost-benefit analyses, decision-makers must set priorities since limited resources (including the public's time and attention) make it impossible to prepare for all hazards concurrently. As an example, in preparing for Operation Iraqi Freedom, Israel focused on mitigating a conventional or unconventional missile attack through public education on the use of gas masks and how to prepare a shelter (Figure 25.3). Subsequently, during Operation Pillar of Defense, education and training focused on mitigating a conventional rocket attack.

OBSERVATION #3

The plan must be developed, tested, and evaluated in advance and be continuously updated. It should include roles for all relevant organizations and the media. Periodic exercises, some of which include the population, must be conducted to test the plan (Figure 25.4).

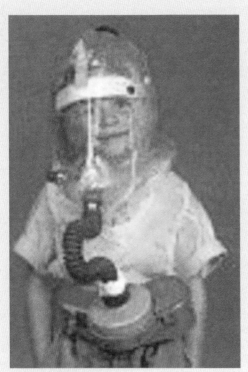

Figure 25.3. A Child's Gas Hood.

The plan should include:

- Instructions for protective behaviors
- Emergency announcements
- Videos that provide guidance to the public (these are labor-intensive to prepare)

- Expert analysis and explanation via interviews. Simply having information is inadequate. Experts must also be able to clearly and honestly communicate their knowledge to the public.
- Information through use of social media tools such as Facebook and Twitter
- Information via smartphone applications
- Information centers
- Informational websites
- Information sheets (e.g., within phone books and via leaflets)

The plan must be continuously reassessed. The situation is dynamic and therefore the plan must be modified to adjust to the changing environment.

OBSERVATION #4

Work with the media. The media is the key source of information for the public before and especially during events. Therefore, positive collaboration is essential. In Israel, the media are considered to be first responders. Therefore, they must be educated and take part in exercises. They need to understand the threats and the needs of the population. For example, they must understand that a terror event is a double-edged sword (i.e., when the media brings publicity to a terror event, it assists the terrorists in achieving their goals). In today's information age, there are many opportunities for bystanders to transmit video or pictures from the event. For example, during Operation Pillar of Defense or Cast Lead, national and international television studios broadcast real-time footage generated from smartphones.

To develop an effective relationship with the media, it is useful to understand their goals:

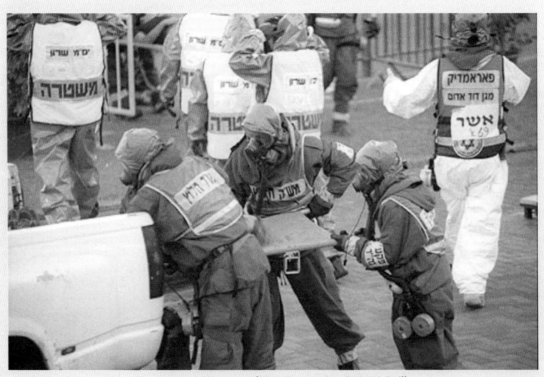

Figure 25.4. A Weapons of Mass Destruction (WMD) Drill.

- Timely news coverage, 24/7
- Up-to-date information
- Relevant material
- Newsworthy events
- Both breaking news and smaller stories with emotional appeal

During events, spokespersons should deliver the known information as soon as possible. The goal is to be first, be right, and, above all, be credible. If appropriate officials do not provide information directly to the public, someone else might do so (and it might be the wrong information and also lead to rumor reporting). Once rumors are spread, it will be very difficult to change the public's mind and convince them to trust authorities again.

The media also provides critical information to emergency managers from the scene of an event, at times even before the traditional first responders arrive.

An effective strategy for the successful implementation of a crisis communication plan is the use of "national spokespersons." The method links each spokesperson to one of the major television channels in various languages. National spokespersons provide a standardized message to the public with instructions, information on vital services, guidelines, tools, knowledge and skills to empower them to protect themselves, thus saving lives. They became the known faces within the public and have a huge positive influence on protective human behavior.

OBSERVATION #5

Continuously reassess the public's needs. To be effective, public officials must assess the status of the public in real-time. Providing guidelines is necessary, but not sufficient. In addition, the public needs instruction and support. Several methods are useful to assess the public's needs:

- Surveys: During crises times, daily surveys should be conducted. Ask the population the key questions that allow assessment of the effectiveness of preparedness or response actions. For example, in the War against Terror, officials learned that the public fully understands instructions and implements protective actions.

- Focus groups: Conduct focus groups in order to evaluate the effectiveness of plans. For example, focus group participants gave feedback on educational films or evaluated experts and spokespersons.
- Special officers trained in the psychosocial effects of war serve as observers throughout the country.
- Media: It is important to monitor and evaluate how the media presents information to the public. Media monitoring also assists officials with assessment of the public mindset regarding the crisis.
- Call centers: Officials have established call centers where the public can receive information. During times of crises, the volume of calls increases dramatically. For example, during the 33 days of the second Lebanon war, the Home Front Command received and processed 161,380 phone calls from the public. In addition to having the ability to rapidly expand capacity to manage increased inquiries, it is critical to provide a uniform message and standardized information between the various call centers.
- Interviews: Direct interviews with the public can provide useful feedback.

OBSERVATION #6

Public interest and awareness varies depending on the stage of event preparation. During non-emergent times, the public is occupied with day-to-day problems and concerns. Therefore, it is nearly impossible to persuade them to prepare for something that "might happen." However, when the situation is rapidly changing, the public immediately wants all available relevant information. Since it requires significant time to prepare this information, officials should create it in advance to the extent possible and use it at the relevant time.

Officials also use special methods to deliver important information in routine time. For example, beginning in 2007, the Israeli government conducts an annual nationwide exercise from the level of the cabinet to the level of the population. The exercise includes local authorities, government ministries, schools, first responder organizations, the private sector and nongovernmental organizations. The exercises typically follow a national preparedness campaign, as "Google trends" have shown an elevation in public awareness during this time (Figure 25.5).

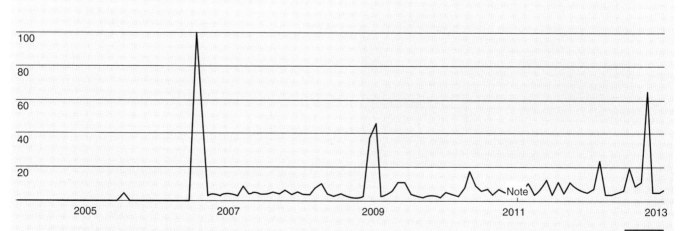

Figure 25.5. Graph Using Google Trends Tool Showing Heightened Israeli Public Awareness during War Times or Operations and during National Exercises.

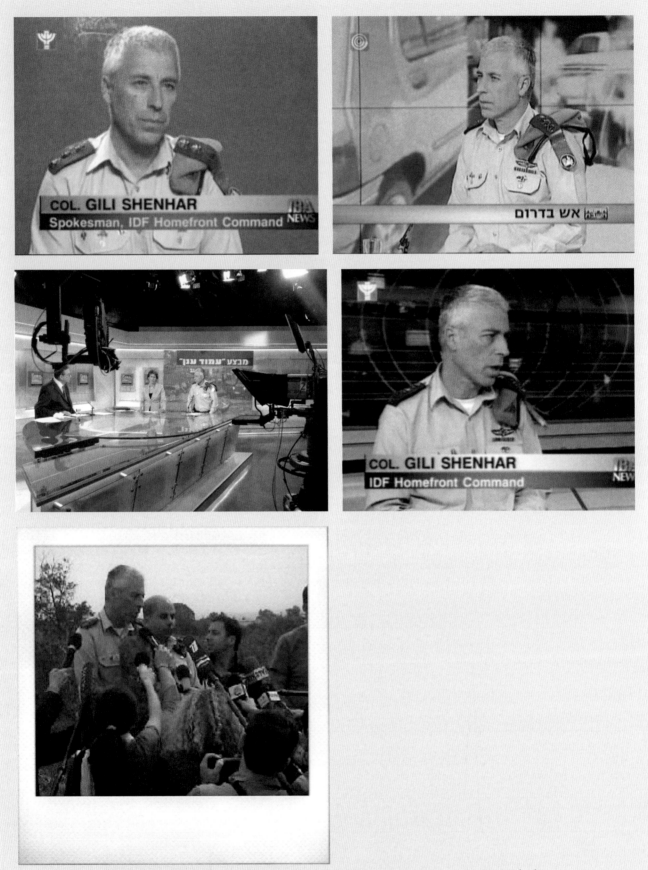

Figure 25.6. Sample Photos of Public Officials Engaging in Various Communication Methods.

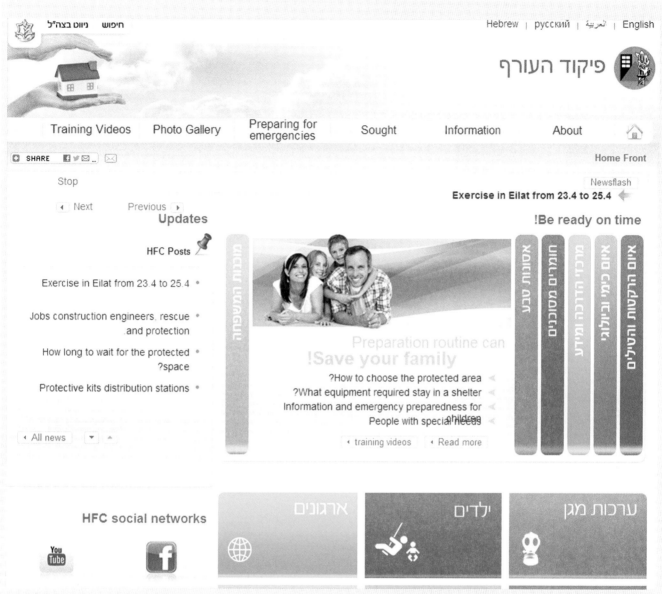

Figure 25.7. Written Materials Available Online and in Multiple Languages.

During the 2006 war and other operations, the level of awareness for emergency was very high, as expected. While lower in comparison to wartime, there are spikes during national exercise times as well.

OBSERVATION #7

Leaders must deliver an answer that satisfies the majority of the population. In the words of Pareto, "20% of people consume 80% of your time." The Israeli approach, however, is to provide information to the entire public and not only to the majority. Children, the elderly, and people with disabilities have special needs. For example, when an alert is being announced, the same alert is sent to deaf people via a pager that was given to them in advance of the event.

OBSERVATION #8

A key principle is "achieving resilience" (see Chapter 6). Life must go on as close as possible to "normal," even during days that the homeland is under terrorist or missile attacks.

Those opposed to the State of Israel (both countries and terror organizations) believe it would be much easier to achieve their goals by fighting against the civilian population than by fighting directly against military forces. The Israeli population has been educated about this concept. For example, Israeli citizens understand the goal of terror – "to kill one and to frighten thousands." To show resilience, the Israeli population continues its normal life, even after a terror attack (keep going to the cinema, eating at restaurants, using public transportation and so forth, even minutes after a terror event). This is a good example of resilience, and risk communication is an important tool to achieve it.

The same concepts apply to wartime scenarios. The goal is for the population to continue their normal lives as soon as possible and as close as possible to baseline. Therefore, it is critical to provide the public with timely information. While information about the threat can cause a rise in anxiety, when it is accompanied by guidance for feasible actions, it leads to preparedness, self-sufficiency, and lower fear levels. For example, during Operation Pillar of Defense, when the public understood that civil protection guidelines save lives, it raised their level of resilience.

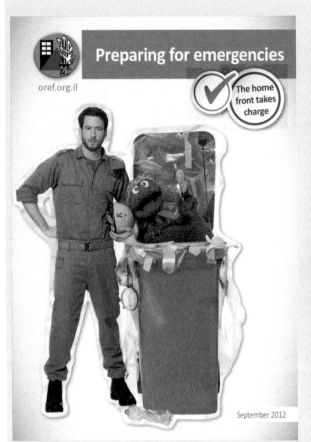
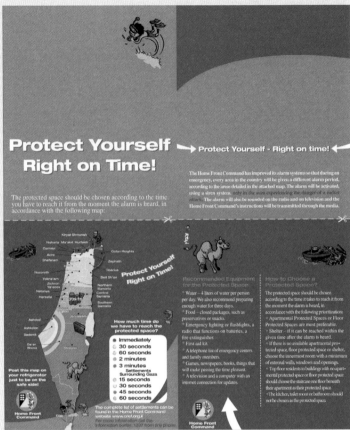

Figure 25.8. Leaflets Distributed to the Public during a National Campaign before a National Exercise.

OBSERVATION #9

Different people learn and are affected in different ways. Officials should use a wide array of methods to communicate with the public. The following are some of the techniques used:

■ Public training and exercises.
■ Media: National television channels remain the principle way to address the public, with main radio channels being the second most frequent (Figure 25.6).
■ Internet: Public officials should prepare and present important information in several languages and include pamphlets that the population can download from the Internet (www.oref.org.il and Figure 25.7).
■ Written materials: During national campaigns and especially during crisis time, special information pamphlets were distributed through several methods (mail, newspaper delivery, at major food stores). These pamphlets provided key information regarding what a family should do and how they should do it, before, during, and after an attack (Figure 25.8).
■ School and workplaces: These are important sites for information distribution.
■ Cell phones: Major security announcements can be sent via instant messaging to mobile phones. Newer systems selectively send automatic security messages only to the population in a designated area, simultaneously in several languages (Figure 25.9).

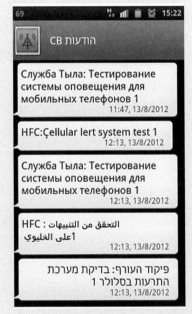

Figure 25.9. Sample Automated Text Messages in Multiple Languages.

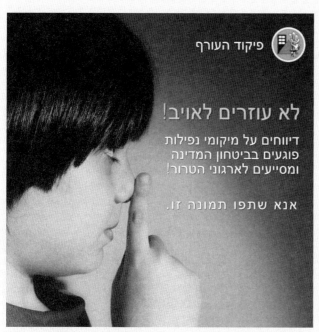

Figure 25.10. Example of a Public Message: Don't Let an Enemy Know Where the Rockets Hit, Please Share the Picture.

■ Call centers: A national call center provides standardized answers to the public's questions. This call center manages all issues regarding civil defense. At every local authority, there is also a call center. Coordination of the national and local call centers is critical to ensure that callers receive a single, uniform message.

■ Social media: Messages via social media are rapidly spread to the public via the Internet (Figure 25.10).

OBSERVATION #10

Israel is a multilingual society because it is a new immigrant country. Therefore, risk communication messages must be prepared and delivered in several languages. It is essential to be able to deliver a comprehensive message in Hebrew, Arabic, English, Russian, and Amharic. In addition, tourists and foreign laborers may need information in other languages. Messages must be culturally appropriate – a protective action that may be acceptable in one culture may be unacceptable or forbidden to another group of people. For example, different pictures must be used for orthodox and less religious audiences (Figure 25.11).

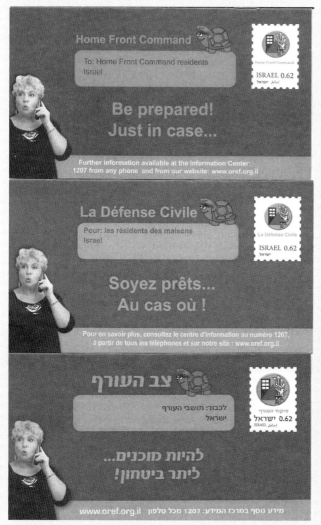

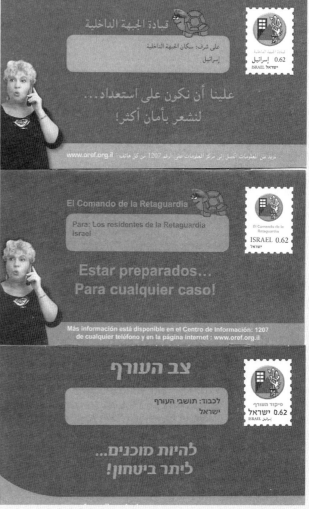

Figure 25.11. Leaflet in Several Languages (Hebrew has two configurations, one for orthodox Jews without a photo of a woman).

Case Study 2: Pandemics and Social Media: The U.S. CDC Builds Trust

By April 2009, CDC had been anticipating the next pandemic influenza virus for nearly half a century. Following the terrorist attacks in 2001, in addition to standard disease detection and laboratory skills, CDC started a new emphasis on its emergency public risk communication skills.

In 2002, CDC first adopted its CERC framework, with the goal to provide rapid, credible information to the public. CERC strived to break down the bureaucratic, paternalistic, and one-way communication historically used in crisis response. Instead, CERC championed meeting the needs of the public with simple, relevant and credible communication during a crisis. The following are the six basic principles of CERC:

1. **Be First:** If the information is yours to provide by organizational authority, do so as soon as possible. If you can't, then explain why you can't (e.g., it's classified) or the process you are using to get needed information to those involved.
2. **Be Right:** Give facts in increments. Tell people what you know when you know it, tell them what you don't know, and tell them *if* you will know relevant information later.
3. **Be Credible:** Tell the truth. Do not withhold information to avoid embarrassment or the possible "panic," which seldom happens. Uncertainty is worse than not knowing and rumors are more damaging than difficult truths.
4. **Express Empathy:** Acknowledge in words what people are feeling; it builds trust. "We understand this is worrisome."
5. **Promote Action:** Give people things to do. It calms anxiety and helps restore order.
6. **Show Respect:** Listen. Treat people the way you want to be treated, the way you want your loved ones treated – always – even when hard decisions must be communicated.

The first three of the six CERC principles focus on organizational responsibilities. The final three highlight psychological stressors and perceptions of the audience that influence meaningful communication.

These principles guided decisions about the use of social media in CDC's response to the 2009 H1N1 influenza pandemic. Social media – seen as interactive communities and hosted services meant to increase collaboration and sharing of information – provided rich choices to support CDC's desire to communicate with, not to, the public in a more personal and targeted way. What was uncertain was whether the use of social media during the H1N1 outbreak would increase or decrease the public's trust in CDC's recommendations and response.

The purpose of public health is to efficiently and effectively prevent or reduce illness, injury, and death across the lifespan. CDC must have the public's trust to achieve these goals. For example, without a trusted reputation, the public could: ignore important health recommendations, resulting in increased disease and death; make demands for the misallocation of limited resources; circumvent public health policies; and succumb to opportunists who offer fraudulent alternate treatments.

Before social media tools were widely available, CDC relied primarily on a 24/7 national call center (1–800-CDC-Info) in English and Spanish to answer calls from the public. In addition, CDC regularly posted the answers to "frequently asked questions" on its website.

CDC made the conscious decision to maintain scientific integrity in its messaging through these new media (e.g., it used simple, but formal language rather than jargon) and also to respect the norms of the social networks it joined. For example, Facebook is a self-correcting environment and CDC understood that individuals should be free to post their beliefs and concerns, some of which were counter to CDC's science and recommendations. As is the custom, individuals on Facebook offered corrective information, not the agency.

FACEBOOK

Here are excerpts from CDC's Facebook H1N1 discussions regarding the value and safety of influenza vaccination.

Male: Never had any flu vaccination for 10 years and never had any problem … UNTIL last month I give it a try … BIG mistake, first time feeling sick like a dog … tsk tsk … talking about conspiracy theory

Female 1: baaaa baaaaa Amazing how many of you are clueless. I would swear that you are being paid to post your nonsense here. By whom? I can think of a few possibilities. hmmmm Oh and my uncle just got his h1n1 shot and got sick with the flu within 1 weeks' time. Go ahead baaaaaaaaaaa get that shot.

Female 2: what flu did he get sick with? was it confirmed h1n1? If he got sick within a week his inoculation was too late, it takes 2 weeks before the antibodies make you immune to the virus. Makes me sick how many people think the flu vaccines are killing so many people and causing autism. Now there is the conspiracy. Go take a microbiology class, and an anatomy and physiology class. Stop reading junk science articles.

Within a short time, an individual in the community helped dispel a recurring misperception – that the flu shot can cause the flu – and explained why someone might become ill with the flu after having received the vaccine.

TWITTER

Twitter allowed for some public self-correction, and was also a helpful tool to distribute information and address "issues of the day" by providing simple health facts (Figure 25.12). The following are examples of tweets during the outbreak:

RT @FluGov Be Advised of New Spam Myth in Circulation. CDC has NOT implemented a vaccination program requiring registration.

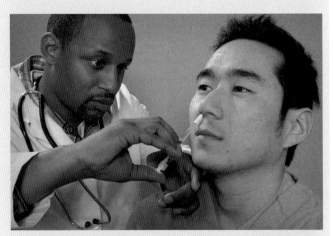

Figure 25.12. Sample Tweet Regarding H1N1 Vaccination.

RT @CDCFlu H1N1 Flu Vaccine – Why the Delay? Watch a new CDC video to find out how flu vaccines are made: http://is .gd/4OVFq

RT @CDCFlu Anyone with asthma is at higher risk for flu-related complications. Learn more: http://is.gd/3jwfB

Did using social media have any impact on the public's perception of CDC's trustworthiness during the H1N1 response? The American Customer Satisfaction Index documents CDC's quarterly score jumped from 74 to 82 (out of 100). Research further indicated that people who used social media gave CDC higher satisfaction ratings than those who did not, were more likely to return and recommend the site to others, and rated CDC as more trustworthy than those who did not use CDC's social media tools (Figure 25.13). In a pilot study, compared to a sampling of other federal agencies, CDC scored highest for online participation, collaboration, and trust. While these preliminary findings are encouraging, more research is needed.

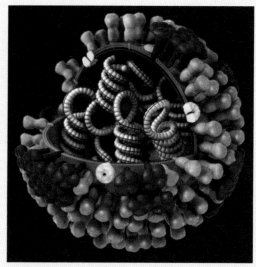

Figure 25.13. A 3-D Graphical Interpretation of an Influenza Virus. Social media helped dispel myths about how this virus harms people.

REFERENCES

1. Reynolds B, Galdo J, Sokler L. *Crisis and emergency risk communication.* Atlanta, GA, Centers for Disease Control and Prevention, 2002.

2. Reynolds B, Seeger M. Crisis and emergency risk communication as an integrative model. *J Health Commun* 2005; 10(1): 43–55.

3. Seeger MW, Reynolds B. Crisis Communication and the Public Health: Integrative Approaches and New Imperatives. In: Seeger M, Sellnow T, Ulmer RR, eds. *Crisis communication and the public health.* Cresskill, NJ, Hampton, in press.

4. National Response Plan. Emergency Planning: National Response Plan. 2005. http://www.dhs.gov/dhspublic/interapp/editorial/editorial_0566.xml (Accessed August 16, 2005).

5. Seeger MW, Sellnow TL, Ulmer RR. *Communication and organizational crisis.* Westport, CT, Praeger, 2003.

6. Fischer HW III. *Response to Disaster.* Lanham, MD, University Press of America, 1998.

7. Clarke, L. The problem of panic in disaster response. 2003. http://www.upmc-biosecurity.org/pages/events/peoplesrole/clarke/clarke.html (Accessed September 1, 2005.)

8. Seeger MW. Best Practices in Crisis and Emergency Risk Communication. *J Appl Commun Res* 2006; 34: 232–244.

9. Peters RG, Covello VT, McCallum DB. The determinants of trust and credibility in environmental risk communication: An empirical study. *Risk Analysis* 1997; 17(1): 43–54.

10. Pollard WE. Public Perceptions of Information Sources Concerning Bioterrorism Before and After Anthrax Attacks: An Analysis of National Survey Data. *Journal of Health Communication* 2003; 8(1)93-103.

11. Tomes N. The making of a germ panic, then and now. *Am J Public Health* 2000; 90(2): 191–198.

12. Andreasen AR. *Marketing social change: Changing behavior to promote health, social development, and the environment.* San Francisco, CA, Jossey- Bass Publishers, 1995.

13. Brashers DE. Communication and uncertainty management. *Journal of Communications* 2001; 51(3): 477–497.

14. Navran FJ, "If 'Trust Leads to Loyalty' What Leads to Trust?" Ethics Resource Center, 1996, http://www.ethics.org/resources (Accessed August 22, 2015).

15. Brehm SS, Kassin S, Fein S. *Social Psychology.* 6th ed. Boston, Houghton Mifflin Company, 2005.

16. Reynolds B. *Crisis and emergency risk communication: By leaders for leaders.* Atlanta, GA, Centers for Disease Control and Prevention, 2004.

17. CDC, unpublished survey data. Personal conversation CDC and Red Cross Liaison. August 2005.

18. DiGiovanni C. Domestic terrorism with chemical or biologic agents: psychiatric aspects. *Am J Psychiatry* 1999; 156: 1500–1505.

19. Novac A. Traumatic stress and human behavior. *Psychiatric Times.* 2001. http://www.mhsource.com (Accessed July 22, 2005).

20. Hill D. Why they buy. *Across the Board* 2003; 40(6): 27–33.

21. Bonanno GA. Loss, trauma, and human resilience: Have we underestimated the human capacity to thrive after extremely aversive events? *Am Psychol* 2004; 59(1): 20–28.

22. Norris F. *50,000 disaster victims speak: An empirical review of the empirical literature, 1981–2001.* Atlanta, Georgia State University, 2001.

23. Young BH, Ford J, Ruzek JI, Friedman MJ, Gusman FD. Disaster mental health services a guidebook for administrators and clinicians. n.d. http://www.ncptsd.org/publications/cq/v4/n2/masterdm.html (Accessed August 19, 2005).

24. Tierney KJ. *The public as an asset, not a problem: A summit on leadership during bioterrorism.* Center for Biosecurity, University of Pittsburgh Medical Center. 2003. http://www.upmc-biosecurity.org/pages/events/peoplesrole/tierney/tierney_trans.html (Accessed September 7, 2004).

25. Izard CE. Translating emotion theory and research into preventive interventions. *Psychol Bull* 2002; 128(5): 796–824.

26. Solso RL. *Cognitive Psychology.* 6th ed. Boston, Allyn and Bacon, 2001.

27. Hesselbein, F. Crisis management: A leadership imperative. *Leader to Leader* 2002; 26(Fall): 4–5.

28. Giuliani R. *Leadership.* New York, Miramax, 2002.

29. Reynolds B, Deitch S, Schreiber R. *Crisis and Emergency Risk Communication: Pandemic Influenza.* Atlanta, GA, Centers for Disease Control and Prevention, 2006.

30. Reynolds B. Response to best practices. *Journal of Applied Communication Research* 2006; 34(3): 249–252.

31. Hecht TD, Allen NJ, Klammer JD, Kelly EC. Group beliefs, ability and performance: The potency of group potency. *Group Dynamics: Theory, Research, and Practice* 2002; 6(2): 143–152.

32. Crocker J, Nuer N. Do people need self-esteem? Comment on Pyszynski, et al. *Psychol Bull* 2004; 130(3): 469–472.

33. Sturmer S, Snyder M, Omoto AM. Prosocial emotions and helping: The moderating role of group membership. *J Pers Soc Psychol* 2005; 88(3): 532–546.

34. Zaltman G. *How customers think: Essential insights into the mind of the market.* Boston, Harvard Business School Press, 2003.

ADDITIONAL RESOURCES

Reynolds BJ, Earley E. Principles to enable leaders to navigate the harsh realities of crisis and risk communication. *Journal of Business Continuity & Emergency Planning* 2010; 4(3): 262–273.

Reynolds BJ. Building trust through social media. CDC's experience during the H1N1 influenza response. *Mark Health Serv* 2010; 30(2): 18–21.

26

TELEMEDICINE AND TELEHEALTH: ROLE IN DISASTER AND PUBLIC HEALTH EMERGENCIES

Adam W. Darkins

OVERVIEW

Telemedicine and Telehealth

Electronic information and telecommunications technologies are routinely delivering clinical services at a distance. Telephones, pagers, and fax machines are longstanding examples of using technology in this way. Telehealth describes how these existing and newly emerging digital technologies are incorporated into clinical practice in support of patient/provider interactions, when the parties involved are separated by distance and/or time.[1,2] The suggested value for using telehealth in routine clinical practice is that it increases access to care and improves the quality of care.[3,4] Telehealth enables healthcare providers typically located in clinics and hospitals within cities or towns to virtually consult with their patients in urban, rural, or remote areas. The scope of services provided via telehealth is quite diverse: it can vary from direct consultation with patients in their homes by video using their own computers, laptops, or cell phones to remotely supporting critical care patients in intensive care units (Tele-ICU).[5,6] Increasingly, people worldwide are digitally interconnected on a range of information technology devices such as cell phones and telecommunication networks. Ever-increasing telecommunications functionality, along with innovation in the devices supported by such functionality, means that opportunities are burgeoning for providing healthcare services virtually. This is true for both the delivery of routine healthcare services and support for emergency medicine. A vision for leveraging these assets in ways that can revolutionize the management of public health emergencies is relatively easy to outline, and not new.[7] The major challenge in making this a reality is not creation and/or dissemination of the vision. It is in aligning policy, legislation, regulation, and clinical operations to assure safe, robust, secure, and sustainable services. Redundancy is necessary to ensure that the emergency and disaster response provided by telehealth does not, itself, become a casualty of an incident it is deployed to relieve.

Visions of using telehealth to support emergency and disaster management have existed for many decades. Over this period of time, the promise of what telehealth can contribute has been revisited and frequently extolled in multiple projects. So far, the rhetoric of using telehealth in emergency care and disaster relief has not translated into an operational reality of improved care delivery. However, there are good reasons to suppose that the field is currently on the cusp of a revolution, one that will meld physical and virtual assets into an integrated response to public health emergencies. Such an integrated effort, based on analyses performed using big data, will increase responsiveness and flexibility, decrease mortality and morbidity, and lower costs by reducing travel and optimizing effective use of telehealth.[8]

There is a sense that war represents a series of consecutive public health emergencies. This makes the military a fertile environment for exploring future uses of technologies in emergency and disaster response.[9] To this end, telehealth was deployed in Bosnia in the early 1990s, and has subsequently been used in the in the Iraq and Afghanistan conflicts.[10,11] An example of this technology transfer from warfare to peacetime is demonstrated by technologies that monitor vital signs to help triage and prioritize the management of battlefield casualties.[12] These devices are being adopted for civilian applications such as use in sports medicine and home telehealth.

Despite the increasing availability of wireless connectivity, and established proof of concept for many areas of telehealth, it still remains a niche activity in terms of its overall impact on healthcare delivery worldwide.[13] Within emergency medicine and the management of public health emergencies, the use of telehealth is the exception rather than the rule, other than for one telehealth technology that is ubiquitous – the telephone. When the telephone was first introduced into healthcare, it was viewed with the same trepidation as telehealth receives now. Societal trends in technology acceptance suggest that it is inevitable that a range of new digital information technologies will follow the telephone, pager, and fax machine into routine operational use throughout healthcare. When this transformation is complete and these technologies are fully socialized into routine care delivery, including disaster medical care and public health emergencies, it is likely that the term telehealth will become redundant. By then, care supported by telehealth will be deemed usual care. In the meantime, the concept of telehealth provides a useful framework on which to envision, plan, and manage current projects. The concept can also help evaluate how various clinical, technological, and business processes are integrated to establish robust systems for delivering care virtually and ensuring networks are safe, efficacious, and cost-effective.

Role of Telemedicine and Telehealth in Public Health Emergencies

A hallmark of a public health emergency response is an urgent need to bring a range of assets, including healthcare services, to bear at an incident site in order to control, contain, and mitigate the situation. Typically, local healthcare assets at the incident site are insufficient, depleted, or otherwise inadequate. Additional generalist and specialist healthcare provider expertise is required for the immediate triage, treatment, and follow-up of the acutely affected population. The specific nature of a public health emergency dictates the major sources of casualties requiring triage and care, such as burns, blast injuries, crush injuries, chemical exposure, or release of an infectious agent. Frequently, the exact nature of the problem is initially unknown. Consequently, there is a clear role for telehealth in the initial acute phase of a public health event to remotely assess, triage, and monitor those affected.[14] Once the initial phase of an emergency abates, the healthcare assets deployed need to evolve. The emphasis of medical intervention should transition toward providing long-term primary care and assessing the immediate and prolonged effects of the event on the remaining at-risk population. As part of this rapid process of evolution, healthcare providers need to refocus from delivering acute care to assessing the more protracted changes in physical and mental health status of the affected population. This change will provide an accurate prognosis on specific health risks to individual patients and their family caregivers, as well as communicating public health data to relief organizations and to the population at large.

In the immediate aftermath of a public health emergency, the scope of healthcare needs is not clearly apparent. A traditional emergency response is based on anticipating various scenarios and usually provides pre-event planned generic responses. Such generic responses operate until more precise information about the size and scope of the incident is identified as it unfolds, so the response can be tailored to the incident. Effectively managing the various assets deployed depends on assessing the risk to both individuals and population subsets. Assessment of the specific healthcare needs has traditionally depended on the sequential physical review of casualties, and their ongoing treatment and monitoring. Widespread availability of smartphones now offers a potential means of identifying the site and severity of casualties using global positioning systems (GPS), vital sign monitoring, and voice/text communication.[15,16,17]

But for now, successful management of a public health emergency still depends on having the necessary healthcare assets already on-site, deploying resources to the disaster zone from distant locations, or transporting individuals elsewhere for care. Therefore, a self-evident rationale exists for using telehealth in public health emergencies. It functions as a decision support tool for those at the event site who, by the nature of public health emergencies, may not have the skills to deal with everything that confronts them.

A vision for the role telehealth can play in public health emergencies is as follows: *Telehealth is a vital decision support tool to assist all public health emergency responders in saving lives, reducing avoidable morbidity, and managing the care of patients with medically unexplained symptoms.*

During a disaster, large numbers of people are concerned about potential threats to their health from the event, even if they have minimal symptoms. This significant subset of the population is particularly challenging for first responders to assess, and telehealth can play a major role in managing their care. This group often places as great a demand on the emergency response as those with immediately apparent major injuries or illnesses. Among the group with medical concerns or unclear symptoms are those whose health status may dramatically deteriorate some time later, such as from an emergency that may or may not be attributable to the concurrent event. A typical example of this is a patient with preexisting heart disease who suffers an acute myocardial infarction precipitated by the stress of a major disaster even though the person is not at any risk from the event. Also in this group are people with psychological trauma following the event, which if not recognized, may suffer long-lasting sequelae (Case Study 26.1), but if recognized early are amenable to treatment.[18]

In this scenario, telehealth can be particularly beneficial in providing guidance to healthcare personnel in remote facilities as well as first responders regarding the management of large patient populations who present with "medically unexplained symptoms." Telehealth can provide access to a specialist's advice that will help distinguish between patients concerned about an exposure but who are actually well versus those who are truly ill and require observation or treatment. There are currently three main modalities of telehealth that are mature, in routine use, and readily available for deployment in emergency and disaster management. They are: 1) telehealth via real-time clinical videoconferencing;[19] 2) tele-monitoring of vital signs;[20] and 3) store-and-forwards telehealth.[21]

The functionality to support real-time video, vital sign monitoring, and digital image exchange is becoming more available for mobile devices. However, this capability has not yet

---

CASE STUDY 26.1[18]

During the morning rush hour on March 20, 1995, a cult terrorist group known as the Aum Shinrikyo placed containers of the nerve agent sarin in five of the carriages on three of Tokyo's underground railway lines. The release of this material resulted in alarms from fifteen subway stations as people arrived with breathing difficulties, muscle weakness, and altered levels of consciousness.

Approximately 6,000 people were exposed to the chemical agent. Of these, 3,227 went to the hospital. There were 493 hospital admissions to forty-one hospitals. Those seen in the hospital manifested classic cholinergic symptoms with nicotinic effects predominating. Twelve people died as a result of the incident and several developed permanent neurological sequelae. However, the vast majority of the victims were acute psychological casualties – people who feared they might have been exposed to sarin vapor, but had no real contamination. For at least 5 years after the attack, many of those exposed continued to manifest symptoms of post-traumatic stress disorder, a condition that may have been mitigated if there had been earlier recognition and treatment.

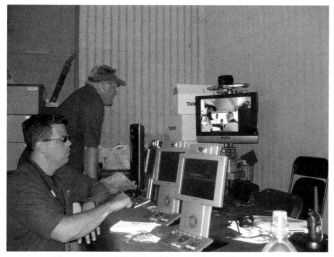

Figure 26.1. Clinical Video Conferencing System.

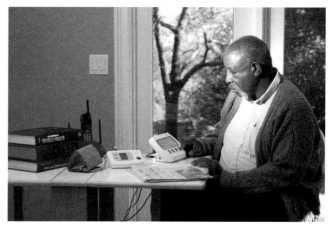

Figure 26.2. Home Telehealth Device.

translated into the widespread use of telehealth at the population level, even though there are anecdotes of how individual patients have benefited. Privacy concerns, the logistics of matching supply and demand for healthcare resources, and inadequate payment systems are delaying the broad use of telehealth on consumer devices.[22] As a result, no system is currently providing routine telehealth-based support for clinical care on consumer devices in a manner suitable to facilitate a coordinated and systematic response to public health emergencies. Intuitively, it is only a question of time before this is possible. Technologies described herein are ones currently available to provide formal healthcare services via telehealth. One can expect these functionalities to become generally available on consumer electronic devices as clinical, technical, business, and regulatory barriers to this transition are overcome.

Practical Technologies to Provide Telehealth-Based Services

Clinical videoconferencing systems such as that illustrated in Figure 26.1, together with the requisite telecommunications connectivity to link patients and providers, enable real-time videoconferencing to provide consultation and advice on clinical care. Although it is not currently possible to directly perform a physical examination on a patient when using these systems, there are emerging telehealth technologies that suggest this will be possible in the future.

Real-time videoconferencing for clinical purposes, also known as synchronous telehealth, allows an expert clinician from any specialty to help manage patients who are in geographically distant locations (from as close as several miles to as far as thousands of miles away). Clinicians providing synchronous telehealth can:

▪ Diagnose
▪ Triage
▪ Make treatment recommendations such as advise antibiotics and analgesic medications
▪ Supervise procedures such as wound debridement and fracture reduction
▪ Mentor and train
▪ Manage and monitor staff at a distance

Synchronous telehealth services can supplement or provide otherwise unavailable on-site specialist expertise in the immediate aftermath of a public health emergency. Examples include:

1. Management of burn patients requiring urgent access to plastic surgical specialty care
2. Provision of access to specialist assets such as infectious disease consultants to identify and manage an infectious disease outbreak and proactively assist in disease prevention throughout all phases of the emergency
3. Provision of counseling and therapy services to both the affected population and emergency responders who have mental health needs secondary to traumatic events they have witnessed
4. Protection of specialist emergency response healthcare personnel assets in a bioterrorism event by enabling clinicians to render advice from a distant location that does not expose them to contagious agents
5. Provision of direct videoconferencing and real-time symptom monitoring technologies to support quarantine or ongoing surveillance in the home

Routine monitoring of vital signs and health status using commercial off the shelf (COTS) home telehealth devices (such as illustrated in Figure 26.2) are in everyday clinical use. Such devices enable the monitoring of patients with chronic diseases such as diabetes and congestive heart failure in their own homes and local communities. The telecommunications connectivity needed to support these technologies includes regular telephone lines, cellular technology, broadband Internet, and satellite.

Routine recording of vital signs and patient's responses to interactive disease management protocols administered on home telehealth devices can rapidly alert a remotely located clinician to a patient's deteriorating condition. Once this health risk is identified, healthcare personnel can initiate an appropriate response. The intervention may include: 1) providing health information; 2) supporting patient self-management through providing advice; 3) prescribing new drugs; 4) adjusting existing medications; 5) initiating an emergency in-home visit; or 6) prompting a preemptive hospital admission. If the clinician monitoring the patient needs further expert assistance, they can rapidly seek guidance from other colleagues if the telehealth devices are part of a larger telehealth network. Once it is in place, the infrastructure of a home telehealth network readily lends itself for deployment to assist in a public health emergency. Examples include:

1. Quarantine of an exposed population (and isolation of an infected population) in the event of pandemic influenza or a bioterrorism event with a contagious agent such as pneumonic plague or smallpox
2. Monitoring the definitely exposed and those at risk from possible exposure to a pathogen after a bioterrorism incident
3. Direct videoconferencing into the home

There are many scenarios in which the response to a public health emergency or disaster cannot cope with the sheer numbers of people it faces. These victims threaten to overwhelm a limited healthcare response capacity and require management in ways that limit the spread of a contagious pathogen. Home telehealth offers a surge capacity that may otherwise be much more costly, or even impossible to provide.[23]

The acquisition, storage, retrieval, and forwarding of digital, clinical, and radiological images, known as store-and-forward or asynchronous telehealth, provides a simple mechanism for obtaining remote advice from expert clinicians who can report on digital images, radiographs, EKGs, and ultrasound studies. This resource makes it possible to deploy general and lesser skilled personnel to the site of the public health emergency, improving the effectiveness of limited specialist resources. These deployed first responders can receive advice on triage, immediate care, and ongoing management of those they are assessing at a distance.

It is now possible to obtain digital images, video, and special investigations from readily available consumer devices such as cell phones and computer tablets, and send these for expert review. Smartphones are in development that can perform auscultation, slit lamp views of the eye, view eardrums, obtain ultrasound, and take EKGs.[24–28] However, their status with medical device regulatory bodies remains in question in many instances.[29] The potential is rapidly emerging for front line emergency responders to have convenient access to telehealth-enabled devices that can provide diagnoses and objectively triage injured victims at an incident site. Store-and-forward technologies are converging with both clinical videoconferencing and home telehealth technologies to provide comprehensive telehealth solutions that will transition onto these mobile platforms.

Despite compelling reasons for the use of telehealth in the management of public health emergencies that have been recognized for over a decade, it remains an underutilized resource. Lack of adoption by mainstream emergency and disaster management teams is likely attributable to the following challenges:

1. Poor understanding of the potential for telehealth in emergency and disaster management
2. Lack of standardized clinical pathways
3. Non-interoperability of information technology and telecommunications networks
4. Immaturity of the vital business and management processes that are required to support and sustain telehealth-based services
5. Conservatism of those currently providing emergency services in the absence of compelling evidence on the clinical effectiveness and efficacy of telehealth as compared to traditional practice
6. A focus on developing customized point-to-point telehealth systems that offer limited emergency management tools,

instead of creating telehealth networks that deliver routine care across the spectrum of need. Such comprehensive systems would be readily transferable to provide accessible and verifiable clinical expertise to support a public health emergency response
7. The absence of a clear vision among policymakers and senior managers who are wedded to legacy systems that rely on physical resources

One expert in the field has summarized these challenges. This individual states that widespread adoption of a networked telehealth response in emergency and disaster management is being unnecessarily held back, despite a compelling vision of telehealth as a means of saving life and reducing avoidable morbidity associated with public health emergencies. This compelling vision is not being translated into clear strategies for technology deployment, marshaling clinical services, and integration into the overall emergency and disaster response. Efforts are needed to move this vision into operational reality by investment in technology and creating clinical operations guides that deliver robust, easily accessible, and flexible models of care to deliver the just in time services this revolutionary new approach promises.

Operations guides for implementing telehealth into the emergency response have been developed.[30] However, silos in the traditional organization and management of healthcare restrict development of the clinical, technical, management, and business frameworks needed to provide the foundation for large-scale telehealth networks. To date, approaches in this area have focused on developing a framework supporting exceptional emergency situations, not creating integrated solutions that link to routine delivery systems for emergency care. An important first step to improve this situation is bringing together multidisciplinary groups of subject matter experts to create operations guides for using telehealth in emergency care and disaster management. Ultimately, however, professional organizations, technology panels, standard setting bodies, legal/regulatory bodies, and government must be fully engaged in this process. Until this wider collaborative approach is embraced for standardizing the role of telehealth, these electronic networks cannot reach the critical mass necessary to realize their promise of transforming public health emergency management. Elements of the information and telecommunication technologies needed for the healthcare component of emergency and disaster management are already used in other aspects of the emergency response. One example is the remote assessment of physical damage and ongoing risk profiles after disasters.[3] The implementation gap that occurs when introducing telehealth in many situations primarily relates to human behavior, and not necessarily to an unfulfilled need for the "right" technology infrastructure.

The seven challenges to delivering services via telehealth in public health emergencies mirror those limiting telehealth growth in routine healthcare delivery. Six are related to human nature, and one is based on technology. Early adopters who advocate the use of the telehealth response in public health emergencies often suggest developing customized telehealth solutions that are used exclusively for this purpose and not used in routine healthcare operations.[32] However, a pioneering application of telehealth to provide support in a disaster suggests an alternate strategy (Case Study 26.2), that of building on existing systems that are used in non-emergency situations.[33,34]

Despite this compelling demonstration of telehealth's value, the knowledge gained from Spacebridge is repeatedly forgotten

CASE STUDY 26.2[33,34]

On December 7, 1988, an earthquake measuring 7.2 on the Richter scale struck Spitak, Armenia, killing 50,000 people. The Soviet Union took an unprecedented step in allowing international relief workers to provide aid to the homeless and injured. With town and surrounding community hospitals destroyed, there was an urgent need for medical services. One element of this response was an offer from the U.S. National Aeronautics and Space Administration (NASA) to the Soviet government to provide telehealth support. This project was called "Spacebridge" because it was established under the auspices of an existing 1987 agreement between the United States and the Soviet Union that allowed for the joint exploration of space for peaceful purposes. The aims of Spacebridge were to provide consultations to a hospital in Yerevan in the Soviet Union from U.S. medical centers in Utah, Texas, Maryland, and the Uniformed Services University of the Health Sciences in the specialty areas of rehabilitation, plastic surgery, mental health, public health, and epidemiology.

Technical issues that needed resolution before implementing the project were:

■ Establishing terrestrial and satellite-based telecommunications links
■ Harmonizing technology protocols and procedures to enable video, voice and fax communications to support remote consultations
■ Agreeing on common telehealth and staff training procedures
■ Finding suitable translation services to accommodate different languages
■ Ensuring patient privacy for telehealth consultations.

The outcomes of the project were that 400 clinicians from the Soviet Union and the United States provided expert consultations to 253 of the injured. The Spacebridge was deployed again on two further occasions with similar success. The first was following a train collision outside Ufa, Russia, when 300 people were killed and many burned following a gas explosion. The second was to help trauma victims following the political uprising in Moscow in October 2003.

technologies and associated models of care delivery have been previously validated by an existing pool of clinicians with readily available appropriate skill sets. Routine operations guides ensure that these clinicians are comfortable with telehealth and familiar with the practicalities of using it to deliver care. The following nine issues must be addressed to achieve success in moving from proof of concepts to established and accepted network systems:

1. Clarifying the health needs the system must address
2. Identifying and verifying a pool of clinicians who can address these needs virtually
3. Standardizing clinical processes
4. Creating a means of contact and communication between first responders and remote clinicians
5. Using reliable, user-friendly, robust, and interoperable technology
6. Ensuring adequate primary and backup telecommunications bandwidth
7. Managing legal and regulatory issues such as patient privacy
8. Addressing business and management aspects
9. Considering psychosocial issues

Telehealth and Systems Reengineering

To address these issues, there has to be an associated business case that justifies embarking on a telehealth implementation. For telehealth to be a serious proposition as a standard part of the emergency response, it must have clear clinical and economic justifications. Supplementing existing routine and emergency healthcare delivery systems with telehealth is a sophisticated process. It requires major reengineering of current healthcare delivery systems. Redesigning a system involves more than merely adding telehealth technologies and their supportive information platforms to deliver essentially a duplicate version of current services. A "provide the technology and they will use it" approach to telehealth implementation without an accompanying change in management's agenda is likely to fail. Rather, fundamental changes in clinical and business processes are necessary to reengineer healthcare services to develop and sustain telehealth networks.

Creating telehealth networks that can provide support in public health emergencies will radically transform emergency preparedness in both developed and developing parts of the world. This endeavor requires investment in technology, clinical change management, and associated organizational development. Although simulations and pilot projects exist, the widespread investment necessary to implement these changes and maintain the ongoing clinical, technology, and business processes for telehealth networks has not yet been made. Decision-makers should carefully consider this investment before implementing telehealth programs. Once such changes are made to incorporate telehealth into standard practice, there is no easy method for reverting back to implementing the previous technologies. For example hospitals that have adopted picture archiving and communication systems to replace the use of X-ray film in routine radiology services do not anticipate reversing the process.[3] Resources to reverse implementation of this system would include recreating X-ray film archives, reemploying staff, reinstituting radiology storage rooms, and then investing in additional equipment and staff training. This brief description of the business process reengineering that accompanies the implementation of picture archiving illustrates how telehealth application

and rediscovered. It still must be translated into routine telehealth deployment.[35] In retrospect, a major reason for Spacebridge's success was undoubtedly the long-standing expertise of both NASA and the Soviet Space Agency in the remote monitoring and managing of people (astronauts and cosmonauts) as part of their respective space programs. A recurring theme in after-action discussions following limited use of telehealth in disasters is recognition of its value in individual anecdotal cases and frustration that it is not more widely deployable. Intuitive sense and experience, such as the use of Spacebridge, illustrate the value of deploying an existing telehealth network that provides routine care and repurposing it to deliver emergency medical capacity in support of a disaster response. In this manner, the requires a systems approach, one that usually creates multiple interdependencies. Risk management strategies associated with telehealth require the clinical, technology, and business components of the new system to be documented, managed, maintained, and updated. Creating an initial telehealth project or program is complex, and its long-term support and maintenance is infinitely more so. Such support processes for a new program include staff training, quality management, systems maintenance, ongoing contracting, and a continuity of operations plan (COOP). The vital roles of training and maintenance/support are often neglected when considering implementing a telehealth system.

The benefit of connecting local hospitals and their associated clinicians with the site of a public health emergency is well described.[37] This chapter assumes general familiarity with such point-to-point approaches to telehealth in disasters and will therefore concentrate on the systems approach to create interoperable telehealth networks.[38] The magnitude of public health emergencies, and the challenges they present, require that telehealth provide a sizable and reliable resource that deals with the associated substantive problems in an efficient, effective, and consistent manner.

The will, financing, and focus involved in undertaking a widespread systems reorganization to implement a telehealth program requires that decision-makers embrace change. Which of these drivers is the eventual vehicle of change will vary according to circumstances. In the case of implementing technology-based telehealth solutions, the pace of change typically depends on the baseline level of technology sophistication within the organization.[39] In regard to telehealth's role in supporting emergency preparedness, there are currently some innovators and early adopters, but a preponderance of traditionalists remain resistant to these programs. Given this general resistance to organizational change, and a comfort with the traditional emergency response, there is currently no overarching driver at the operational, policy, or political levels that supports the changes involved in creating and then sustaining telehealth networks. Understanding how these systems will eventually evolve and implementing the clinical, technological, and business systems to support telehealth is neither a conceptual exercise nor a question of fashionable technologies. It must be based on pragmatic considerations of underlying patient care needs in population terms coupled with appropriate support systems. This needs-driven approach to shape systems that support care requires a service-oriented architecture in an organization, something that will be discussed later.[40]

Health Needs as Drivers of Telehealth Implementation for Emergency and Disaster Management

Developing telehealth networks to support public health emergencies requires a clear understanding of population-level patient needs whether voluntarily adopted in the short term or imposed out of necessity in the future. Telehealth must function to: 1) manage these needs more effectively than can be done by the elements of the traditional emergency response; 2) offer solutions at lower cost; and 3) protect healthcare workers. Meeting these stipulations raises the following questions:

1. What are the challenges confronting traditional management in responding to public health emergencies that telehealth can resolve?

2. In practical terms, can telehealth provide a viable solution to these deficiencies?

A case for creating telehealth networks to systematically support emergency services requires more than a commitment to embracing new technology. The successful creation of telehealth networks depends on ensuring they support clinical processes that management personnel can readily apply at the scene in real-time situations. The system must provide a useful adjunct for management and treatment of the acutely ill and injured population. It is the ability of a technology to resolve a clinical need in this way that ultimately drives its adoption into mainstream healthcare usage. What are the needs of patients and staff associated with public health emergencies that telehealth can fill?

By their very nature, public health emergencies and disasters are unpredictable in terms of their causation, timing, occurrence, location, and the damage and disruption they produce. The RAND Corporation defines public health emergency preparedness as:

> The capability of the public health and healthcare systems, communities, and individuals to prevent, protect against, quickly respond to, and recover from health emergencies, particularly those whose scale, timing, or unpredictability threatens to overwhelm routine capabilities. Preparedness involves a coordinated and continuous process of planning and implementation that relies on measuring performance and taking corrective action.[41,42]

The main mission for public health emergency preparedness is, therefore, to provide an anticipatory response to unpredictable events. Conceptually, this response prevents, proactively manages, and adapts to the changing way in which most disasters unfold. The traditional emergency preparedness approach has been based on managing this unpredictability by creating systems that seek to impose elements of certainty. Such elements include:

▪ The range of possible eventualities that an emergency preparedness response team might face has been fully determined.

▪ Clear procedures and processes have been formulated to deal with these situations.

▪ The logistics in terms of required people, equipment, supplies, communications, and transport to manage likely eventualities have all been determined.

▪ The command and control structures are in place to manage the initial response and subsequent activities.

This traditional approach to preparedness of defining certainty in relation to public health emergencies is essentially an exercise in Newtonian physics. This classical physics theory takes a linear view of systems, one in which knowledge of the constituent parts allows its behavior to be accurately predicted. The reality of public health emergencies is that they are anything but certain. The only thing that is predictable is that the disaster response will not be implemented precisely according to the plan. Yet, if responders use a basic command and control infrastructure, the event can be managed well. The emergency response attempts to bring order, predictability, and ultimately levels of control to disaster management. Information technologies have fostered new approaches to the logistics and management of situations from industrial production to military conflict by enabling the operations of just-in-time systems. This creates a more flexible and adaptable response, one that replaces the Newtonian view of events with one that views situations as part of a complex adaptive system. This changed approach is relevant to the role of telehealth networks in providing flexibility and adaptability to healthcare services in an unfolding public health emergency.

Telehealth offers ways in which population needs for healthcare services can be addressed dynamically. The traditional Newtonian approach has its merits in that it is necessary to have an armamentarium of services. The complexity of a public health emergency does not result from unidentified healthcare needs. The appropriate resources to meet these needs have been considered and are potentially accessible. It is the logistics of ensuring the right care is available at the right time in the right place that is the main challenge. Telehealth offers this just-in-time flexibility to supplement the traditional physical response to a disaster or to provide urgent support in areas of neglected healthcare delivery. As with the delivery of routine healthcare services, the main benefit of telehealth in emergency and disaster management is that it allows for the reengineering of clinical processes and a flexible response to changing circumstances.

Since 2010, the horizon for telehealth has radically shifted and continues to evolve. The advent of smartphones will significantly change the complex adaptive response that telehealth can offer. Before the smartphone, use of telehealth in emergency and a disaster management response usually required deployment of telehealth assets that were expensive, inflexible, and largely in the hands of emergency responders. Connecting disaster victims to emergency responders required the victims' physical co-location with the telehealth technologies. However, with the advent of the smartphone, its potential new role in telehealth may facilitate a quantum change in emergency and disaster management. This device could effectively place telehealth technologies in the hands of the affected population and enable a personalized response aimed at these affected individuals. Such changes could replace the current stylized logistic response that is frequently mismatched in size, scope, and specificity for the event to which it is deployed. Apps on smartphones have the potential for:

∎ Storing and exchanging health-related information
∎ Transmitting vital sign data
∎ Videoconferencing
∎ Making telephone calls
∎ Text messaging
∎ Downloading emergency management instructions
∎ Locating and tracking individuals via GPS

There are a myriad of challenges that require resolution to reliably use smartphones as part of an emergency response. Apart from creating the necessary apps, data exchange systems, and associated communication policies, telehealth programs must adhere to regulatory privacy and jurisdictional requirements. Although using smartphones in this way may be piloted at the city or state level, it will ultimately require national government coordination and involvement. Standards and regulation will be critical in achieving this result.

A typical emergency response encompasses a wide spectrum of primary, secondary, and tertiary healthcare needs. Such a response usually involves governments at the local, state, and federal levels. It necessitates these bodies working collaboratively with nongovernmental organizations (NGOs) and volunteers. A range of professional and allied staff may be involved at various stages including engineers, aid workers, volunteers, law enforcement, water and sanitation workers, transportation and healthcare professionals, and public health representatives. The public health emergency response includes much more than healthcare services alone. Such services, whether delivered physically or via telehealth, must be considered within the context of the wider response. The information technologies, videoconferencing capabilities, and telecommunications bandwidth necessary to support telehealth is equally applicable for non-healthcare professionals' use in other aspects of assessing and managing the emergency response. The current discussion will be limited to the healthcare services response to public health emergencies, but recognizes that this is only one component of a broader system.

The effectiveness of the public health emergency response depends on the adequacy of logistics and communications. Detailed plans must provide sound and effective strategies for managing the variety of situations that may be encountered during the phases of a disaster, including allowances for unexpected contingencies. Embedding telehealth within current healthcare services systems can be accomplished by introducing it directly into existing strategies and programs. For example, the breakdown of routine transportation services during a disaster can be mitigated by implementing a telehealth program.

The example of using telehealth in situations where there are transportation difficulties is one of many possible scenarios. There are endless combinations and permutations whereby telehealth can be incorporated into an emergency response. In August 2005, Hurricane Katrina illustrated how a sudden loss of critical infrastructure could rapidly render inadequate the ability to deliver healthcare to the population. Telehealth was deployed during Hurricane Katrina, but without a coordinated approach for incorporation into the traditional emergency response.[43] Telehealth can assist with the provision of basic emergency response elements as shown in Table 26.1.

Mounting an effective emergency response with telehealth is dependent on attention to detail. Assessments of the disaster response to Hurricane Katrina, the Indonesian tsunami, and Hurricane Sandy in 2012 are prototypical of all such responses.[44] They suggest there could better coordination of agencies and assessment of needs in the local community to ensure the resources deployed are appropriate, efficacious, and cost-effective. A glimpse of how smartphones can assist in these complex tasks as a telehealth modality was shown in Hurricane Sandy. During this storm, one of the top application (app) downloads was the Red Cross Hurricane App, which combines a storm tracker with emergency functions such as a flashlight and alarm.[45] The app also features a first aid database and a notification system for quickly and easily informing loved ones of a person's safety.

As with non-emergency healthcare, progress is being made to standardize the response elements to a public health emergency.[46,47] Since the destruction of the World Trade Center in New York on September 11, 2001, and the anthrax attacks in its aftermath, the need for an effective response to disasters in the United States has received increased scrutiny by politicians and the general public. As a result, new funding opportunities have arisen, and with them have come enhanced expectations of safety and security for the public. With increasing accountability for a return on investment in emergency preparedness, the issues of dealing with unpredictability and uncertainty receive greater

Table 26.1. Basic Management Elements for the Public Health Emergency and Disaster Response

1. Persistent surveillance/monitoring to detect a threat to the public health
2. Verifying the existence, identifying the associated location(s), and determining the extent and causation of a public health emergency
3. Mobilizing the appropriate voluntary, local, state, federal, and nongovernmental organization responses to the public health emergency
4. Ascertaining the legal milieu and enforcing laws and regulations to protect health and ensure public safety
5. Instituting existing policies and plans that verify, manage, and contain the emergency
6. Informing the public about the emergency and the appropriate actions they need to take
7. Providing the appropriate triage, preventative, curative, palliative, and investigative services to protect and treat individuals and animals affected by the emergency
8. Depending on risk and exposure related to the emergency, personnel must evacuate, quarantine, or shelter-in-place the affected/exposed population
9. Transitioning from the initial emergency response to routine operational management in the aftermath of the immediate emergency situation
10. Reviewing the outcomes, opportunities for improvement, and need for revision of laws, regulations, policies, and procedures

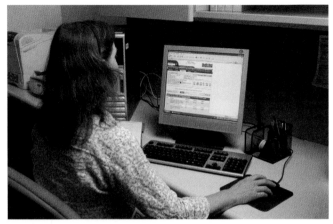

Figure 26.3. Population Management via Home Telehealth.

attention.[48] For example, the elusive search for a solution to containing the threat of pandemic influenza has sharpened the attention of governments on the financial accountability of emergency preparedness systems.[49] As the following telehealth emergency response scenario shows, managing the consequences of pandemic influenza exemplifies how telehealth should be applied within this framework of financial awareness.

Telehealth Emergency Response Scenario

In the event of a high virulence pandemic, there will likely be widespread contagion and loss of life without an effective vaccine for protection. In the evolving public health emergency, engagement of national governments and international collaboration will be necessary to mount a humanitarian response of unprecedented complexity. From a practical perspective, there will be insufficient hospital capacity to care for infected patients and it would be better to manage many of the victims in outpatient locations. Home and community settings (e.g., community centers and hotels) could be used to house those affected and segregate those who have been exposed but have not yet become ill. Home telehealth devices offer one option for monitoring people and helping to manage their treatments remotely, such as via telephone. By employing telehealth, fewer healthcare professionals would be needed to monitor and manage a population of patients (100 or more patients can be managed by each nurse). In the event of a pandemic, healthcare professionals will also become infected, thereby reducing the workforce. Home telehealth-based quarantine systems, if adequately designed and appropriately engineered, offer a solution to the lack of surge capacity. Figure 26.3 depicts a healthcare professional managing a population of patients who are being monitored on home telehealth systems. The monitor provides population-level data that

are viewable on a simple Internet browser-based application that enables expanded viewing to the level of individual patients.

The most significant benefit that telehealth brings to healthcare delivery, whether providing routine care or emergency care, is that patients can receive care at their location, and don't need transportation to a specialist. Healthcare decision making often takes place in hospitals. Telehealth makes it possible to move the locus of healthcare decision making from the hospital to home or a local community setting. When the physical locations of patient and practitioner are changed through the use of telehealth, it is particularly important to pay close attention to the continuum of care. The purpose of monitoring a patient at home in the routine delivery of care is to facilitate treatment in the home or arrange for care in a more appropriate setting. Logically, such monitoring activities can provide supportive care during public health emergencies.

Individuals who are being treated for injuries sustained in a disaster may have existing medical histories that impact how, where, when, and even if they should continue to receive care. After the initial patient assessment is performed at the disaster site and health-related problems are detected, patients begin receiving treatment. They may need ongoing monitoring, and if so, it is important to have medical information available for clinicians to compare any change in patient status with a prior baseline. If the patient requires evacuation and subsequent care is undertaken at a different location by another clinician, information about the preceding treatment regimen, such as medications or surgeries, should be available. Telehealth enables the virtual management of patients across the continuum of care. Telehealth is a safe and effective addition to the delivery of care, provided that the necessary processes are in place to coordinate patient management. If these processes are not in place, telehealth can result in further fragmentation of care and make it less safe. Although aspects of a written patient record can be verbally communicated, sent by fax, or physically attached to the patient, the optimal way to support medical management across the continuum of care using telehealth is to implement an electronic health record (EHR). In the absence of an EHR, there are major limitations to how widely telehealth can be used.

It is difficult to build a viable business case for telehealth in the absence of an EHR.[50] Many telehealth applications have rudimentary EHR systems that can support continuity of care but fall short of a comprehensive EHR. These limited software packages lack the advantages of well-developed systems with modules for pharmacy and applications that link with laboratories, operating rooms, and emergency departments. The creation and implementation of EHRs into healthcare systems is a major socioeconomic issue for any nation and has implications for payment systems as well as privacy and confidentiality of personal healthcare information. Implementation of EHRs is proceeding to varying degrees, at variable paces, and with differing success rates in healthcare systems worldwide. The EHR is vital to creation of telehealth networks; the two systems are synergistic in public health emergencies. An EHR provides more than just a tool for the management of individual patients. Aggregated information from an EHR can offer valuable data for assessing needs, planning services, and patient monitoring and evaluation. If data were available from those who are triaged and assessed, this would transform the management of public health emergencies. Real-time data on a population's needs would allow a dynamic response with coordination of healthcare services within a wider emergency management context at the local, national, and international level. This would help manage the logistics of evacuating casualties to outside regional medical facilities. The EHR also could facilitate consistent epidemiological surveillance of those affected by a public health emergency. If an EHR had existed to assist with patient management during the sarin incident in Tokyo, for example, it would have been much easier to understand how long-term symptoms related to initial exposure.

The Electronic Health Record and Telehealth

In the routine delivery of healthcare services, the use of information technology to coordinate care has been recognized at the policy level.[51] A health information system is a clear prerequisite to providing safe and effective consultations via telehealth. The success of organizations such as the U.S. Department of Veterans Affairs (VA) in implementing telehealth is, in part, attributable to the presence of its EHR. The EHR facilitates the ability to change the location of care. In public health emergencies, there is a critical health information need to support: 1) monitoring, surveillance, and planning; 2) managing the care of those with health problems resulting from the emergency situation; and 3) caring for patients with existing health problems that may have been exacerbated or compounded by the emergency situation.

The EHR offers tools to manage patients across the continuum of care associated with an emergency and disaster response, just as it does in routine healthcare delivery. It facilitates changing the location of care because it allows the process of healthcare decision making to move closer to the patient. It removes the necessity for the patient to visit traditional hospitals in order to receive expert assessment and care. EHRs and telehealth enable a much more flexible approach to the delivery of care. Major changes in healthcare, emergency, and disaster management often follow what occurs on the battlefield. The Korean War introduced the concepts of rapid evacuation and the mobile army surgical hospital that persisted as standard operating procedures throughout the Vietnam War and until the end of the First Gulf War. The acute management of wounded soldiers totally changed with Operations Enduring Freedom and Iraqi Freedom. Initial triage and stabilization now take place closer to the site at which the injury occurred, and definitive treatment may happen in another country or even on another continent. Patients need only be "stabilized" prior to transport rather than "stable."

The value of an EHR in a public health emergency was exemplified by the evacuation process for patients in the New Orleans VA Medical Center who were relocated to other VA centers in advance of Hurricane Katrina in 2005. The EHRs for these evacuated VA patients were available nationally within 48 hours.[52] Impressive examples such as this show the value of the EHR when used for routine care delivery in emergency situations, both for patients affected by the acute event as well as those who require chronic care for existing health conditions. In a population that is aging and suffering from an increasing burden of chronic disease, public health emergencies affect the daily care of these patients in ways that can be life-threatening, such as the separation of diabetic patients from their insulin supply. Many other areas of human activity, such as commerce and industry, already use information technology systems to communicate, coordinate, and evaluate complex undertakings. These systems resolve logistical problems in analogous ways to the emerging use of the EHR and telehealth in healthcare.

Although an EHR is of particular importance to telehealth, it must be kept in perspective, and viewed cautiously to avoid overzealous and uncoordinated efforts to introduce such systems. It is a considerable challenge to implement the hardware and software components of an EHR. Implementing an EHR with the associated training, information technology support, cyber security, interoperability, and other modular components it requires (such as laboratory and blood transfusion packages) is a colossal undertaking. To succeed, an EHR project must be well planned, particularly in developing countries. Key principles are listed in Table 26.2 for the implementation of information technology systems in developing countries to support routine operations.[53] These same principles apply to projects in developed nations and to telehealth systems.

Basic requirements for an EHR are even more complex than for other systems. Therefore, even if unanimous support existed for an international EHR system to coordinate emergency responses, the challenges of implementing an integrated system offering a public health benefit would severely impede its development, even in developed countries. However, nascent elements of a future solution can be seen in projects like the common alerting protocol that is an attempt to standardize alerts in the event of disasters.[54] The rudimentary nature of the information systems that can be deployed widely in a developed country was shown by the experience with Katrina Health in the United States.[55]

Table 26.2. Recommendations for Implementing Information Systems Nationally and Internationally

Ensure the information technology system can support the individual, organizational, and institutional needs of users

Avoid simultaneous implementation in an entire large country of one overarching project

Avoid implementing state of the art technology with unskilled professionals

Limit the number of project components

Ensure clear ownership of the project and acceptance by users

Ensure compatibility of systems and collaboration among participants

Telehealth logically builds on health information systems for two reasons. First, the EHR provides necessary information that is needed for continuity of care and assists both the referring practitioner and the teleconsulting practitioner in making appropriate treatment decisions. Second, the telecommunications infrastructure required for distributing an EHR helps provide the business case and routine operational telecommunications backbone for a telehealth network. The routine exchange of an EHR on local area networks and wide area networks (WANs) of healthcare organizations sustains the network and ensures basic interoperability, cyber security, and privacy requirements. These same items apply directly to other systems on the network, such as telehealth. If the organization's information technology infrastructure is not sophisticated enough to implement the requirements of an EHR, it will restrict the development of a telehealth network. An adequate telecommunications infrastructure is as important to the development of telehealth services as water is to a hydroelectric power generation project.

Telecommunications Technology Support of Telehealth

Telecommunications technologies are changing the lives of people worldwide. Developing nations that lack impediments to innovation from vast legacy systems, such as public telephones that use copper wire, are leapfrogging over developed countries in their use of new technologies for commercial, leisure, and entertainment purposes. The inflexibility that protecting legacy telecommunications systems impose on developed countries mean that developing states may assume a leadership role ahead of wealthy nations in creating the preeminent technology-based healthcare delivery systems of the future. These governments may also demonstrate how such systems will integrate with the emergency response to public health emergencies.

The availability of traditional telephone service and integrated services digital networks (ISDN), as well as broadband, cellular, radio, and satellite communications, are the basic building blocks for data exchange that can support telehealth services. The ability to use telephone service, ISDN, broadband, or satellite communications to connect a patient at one point with a clinician at another site is known as point-to-point telehealth. This will be described in more detail later. Given access to the necessary finances and political willpower, it is possible purchase the equipment and telecommunications bandwidth to establish a telehealth project that can support routine healthcare delivery almost anywhere in the world. The step-by-step addition of new participants on point-to-point telehealth networks is unlikely to create networks of the size and complexity needed to assist in routine healthcare delivery, much less support services needed during disasters. The reason for this relates to the nature of telecommunications networks and fundamental systems requirements that can be traced back to the development of the telephone.

After its invention, the telephone was of limited use to the general population because the connections were all point-to-point. The worldwide network of telephone services that is now supported by standard telephone systems, wireless networks, satellites, and the Internet was initially made possible by the development of telephone exchanges that allowed direct dialing. These same key developments are needed for a telecommunications infrastructure that can support telehealth, and depend on similar technology solutions, standards, and logistics to ensure they are interoperable. It is outside the scope of the current discussion to describe international efforts associated with telecommunications standardization. However, there are efforts underway to standardize the emergency response to public health emergencies. Although telecommunications needs have been recognized, telehealth is not yet a supported application.

Telehealth and the Standardization of Support Services for the Emergency Response to Public Health Emergencies

The Sphere Project is an attempt to define a Humanitarian Charter and Minimum Standards for Emergency Response.[56] It lists contingencies to consider when managing disaster situations, from monitoring clinical conditions to logistical issues such as burials. However, it only references telecommunications and does not mention telehealth. Telecommunications are a vital part of disaster relief. By their very nature, telehealth services are based on a telecommunications infrastructure. A robust interoperable telecommunications network is a prerequisite for telehealth. The need to develop this telecommunications network for emergency and disaster relief has long been recognized at the international level, but has been slow to evolve. The Tampere Convention was unanimously adopted on June 18, 1998, by delegates from seventy-five countries and updated in 2012.[57] Its elements require countries to facilitate provision of prompt telecommunication assistance in the event of a disaster. The convention covers the deployment of reliable, flexible telecommunication services. Regulatory barriers that impede the use of telecommunication resources for disasters are waived during such events. This waiver includes licensing requirements for allocated frequencies, restrictions on the import of telecommunication equipment, and mobilization of humanitarian teams. The Tampere Convention also eased restrictions for the use of life-saving telecommunication equipment but did not aid its standardization. The relative inertia in attempts to harmonize telecommunications platforms globally is due to commercial and political considerations coupled with the relative inflexibility of large legacy systems. These issues lie outside the current discussion of the role of telehealth in public health emergencies. However, as a consequence of this lack of standardization, there are problems with interoperability of communication systems, including telehealth. The functional continuity of telecommunications systems is vital if they are to support the delivery of health and other services in public health emergencies, as illustrated in Case Study 26.3.

The vulnerability of telecommunications networks to disasters was exemplified by Hurricane Katrina.[58] Rescue attempts

---

CASE STUDY 26.3

On August 29, 2005, Hurricane Katrina made landfall in southeast Louisiana and Mississippi. As a consequence of the hurricane and subsequent flooding, 1,577 people died in Louisiana, Mississippi, and Alabama. Hundreds of thousands of people were left homeless and a massive humanitarian relief effort mounted. The event was a severe test of emergency preparedness in terms of logistics and readiness. It took 48 hours to restore even the most basic telecommunications services on a widespread scale.

during Katrina were plagued by problems with inoperability of telecommunications systems. To help rectify this deficiency in the United States, part of the telecommunications spectrum has been dedicated to emergency and disaster management services.[59] Considerable work remains to secure land-based telecommunications infrastructure and standardize it in ways that are necessary to support the safe and robust networking services needed for widespread telehealth expansion.

Satellite-based services provide the most reliable and consistently available telecommunications systems in the event of a public health emergency. A disaster such as an earthquake, hurricane, flood, or cyber terrorist attack can disrupt land-based telecommunications systems. Despite the theoretical back-up and redundancy of telecommunications fiber in WAN systems, there are often situations where critical points of failure can occur with damage at a single site. Any design for telecommunications systems that support telehealth should contain back-up arrangements that involve a contingent WAN based on satellite communications.

The need to have a contingent WAN applies to both the routine delivery of healthcare and to telehealth networks that support a disaster response. The value of using telehealth to provide services at a distance is that existing care delivery systems are redesigned to make medical interventions more accessible. Usually the physical provision of certain services can either be reduced or completely curtailed because telehealth offers care more economically and effectively. The end result is that information technology-mediated services replace interventions that were once delivered directly and offer care in situations where the ability to physically deliver services may not be possible. This makes it vital to ensure that telecommunications back-up and redundancy plans exist in the event of failure of the primary technology. Telehealth-based services will never replace the need to provide direct care during a public health emergency, but telehealth should be considered as part of the emergency response armamentarium, with the aim of providing a flexible and adaptive response. In mounting this flexible and adaptive telehealth response, a critical issue is determining how clinicians and responders at the scene will be connected via telehealth networks. This will require the development of a common telecommunications "dial plan" for telehealth services, whether limited to the emergency response or applied to telehealth provision generally.[60]

Telephone and cell phone networks have a standardized system to assign numbers and support connections between individuals on the basis of dialing the requisite numbers. This organized system of interconnectivity is known as a "dial plan." A dial plan to connect telehealth clinicians over telecommunications networks must have a standardized structure and must link remote healthcare responders into a prioritized telecommunications infrastructure. It would be pointless to have a widespread network of clinicians available for an urgent disaster response and then rely on a publicly available telecommunications system to support them. Questions related to the dial plan and access issues emphasize the need for improvement in the human aspects of telehealth networks and how they are organized.

Telecommunications standards for video functions that connect clinical workstations are rapidly changing as point-to-point services are evolving toward multi-point services. The H.320 video protocol for point-to-point communication over ISDN is evolving to the H.323 protocol that allows simultaneous multi-point connections.[61,62] Video services over large telecommunications networks are now increasingly Internet Protocol (IP) based.[63] There are constraints on the expansion of web-based services to support IP video on the scale that large telehealth networks will require. These should be resolved with the newest version of IP, IPv6. The use of IP as the basis for telecommunications connections raises the possibility that large telehealth networks may assemble from smaller existing systems as a network of networks and not as a separate undertaking. Informal networks such as Skype are available but not encrypted.

Clinical Care Networks to Support a Telehealth Response to Public Health Emergencies

A single provider who personally knows the on-site clinician and is linked by satellite-based videophone can improve care and decrease mortality. A relationship-based initiative like this illustrates a benefit of telehealth, but it is not readily scalable beyond a certain size. A systems approach to telecommunications networks is necessary to support large-scale public health emergencies. Emergency managers must assemble and connect the various components of the clinical care network that provide such support. This network is likely to constitute a core of practitioners that have competencies in:

◼ Trauma and orthopedics
◼ Emergency and critical care
◼ Neurosurgery
◼ Plastic surgery
◼ Infectious disease
◼ Public health
◼ Pediatrics
◼ Psychiatry
◼ Burn care

In the event that such a network must be assembled rapidly, it might be possible to use spontaneous volunteers. However, the planning and processes necessary to construct a reliable telehealth network requires that the appropriate systems are already in place to:

◼ Verify that staff (volunteer or otherwise) are trained and fit to practice
◼ Establish a registry of staff that identifies their appropriate credentials, clinical specialties, and contact details
◼ Ensure that staff have access to equipment that is compatible and interoperable and can link via the necessary telecommunications bandwidth
◼ Develop operations guides for staff that focus on explicit processes and communication
◼ Train staff in the use of telehealth systems, ensure they are aware of its limitations, and that they know the level of support on which they can rely at the patient site
◼ Develop and implement quality assurance and outcomes measures as well as the systems to monitor them post-event
◼ Construct the necessary systems within emergency response teams to manage and coordinate telehealth-supported healthcare interventions

Of the seven processes just listed, numbers the first six all currently exist in healthcare but must be adapted to the emergency response. To support the clinical and technology arrangements that make telehealth possible, associated business processes are needed.

Business Processes That Support Telehealth Networks

Healthcare systems vary worldwide in terms of management style, reimbursement, and funding allocation strategies for care. Telehealth facilitates the provision of healthcare irrespective of how it is delivered. The two main approaches to the provision of care are dedicated services and service lines.

Dedicated services are implemented through traditional hierarchies that are professionally based and represent distinct silos Examples include orthopedic surgery, emergency medicine, physical therapy, and occupational therapy. This construct bases the delivery of care on the expertise of those providing it rather than on the patients who receive it. Telehealth can readily fit into this arrangement, assuming the clinical activity can be coded on associated information systems and the workload captured by an individual professional discipline and sub-specialty.

A service line arrangement is one in which the services provided dictate the managerial arrangement. An example is mental health services. Telehealth itself can be managed as a separate service line. This pattern of service delivery is more reflective of the care given to patients. In this arrangement of services, telehealth can be coded for workload purposes as its own entity.

The workload supported by telehealth services is accurately captured, whether delivered as a dedicated service or a service line. Telehealth is distinctly different from other healthcare practice in that there are two separate episodes of care associated with each telehealth encounter. The first is the support of the patient at the site and the second is the consultation services of the clinician who is providing advice from a distance. This duplicative coding requirement can present challenges in some healthcare systems in which the concept of two separate episodes of care occurring simultaneously at two separate sites is anathema.

The arrangements for reimbursement or supplemental funding after a disaster is complex and variable within and between nations. The ability to systematically code for telehealth activity means that it is possible to accurately capture workload data and thereby ensure that an accurate reckoning is made for the costs of providing services. Telehealth relies on electronic technologies and it is possible to automate the process of capturing workload activity by using standard codes. One example is the use of Health Level 7 (HL-7) codes generated by the technologies instead of relying on manual coding of information by clinicians. The ability to track clinical activity and associated costs of telehealth encounters is a vital part of developing telehealth-based services. The nature of large networks that rely on electronic technologies is that they need a stream of high-volume, low-cost applications to sustain them. Telehealth networks are sustainable up to a certain size by the variable types of grant funding and barter that often typifies the development of innovative new services in healthcare. However, to achieve a critical mass of permanently sustainable funding, the processes of workload capture, clinical coding, and financial recompense should be as clear and explicit as the clinical and technology processes associated with telehealth. Data from good financial and accounting systems provide a basis on which to conduct routine clinical outcomes studies for effectiveness and continuous quality management.

CURRENT STATE OF THE ART

Introduction

The current state of the art with respect to the use of telehealth in public health emergencies is varied and somewhat rudimentary.

Within the wider healthcare arena, telehealth is an innovation that is emerging but lacks the information systems necessary to support it in ways that will transform it into a fully-fledged healthcare activity. In many situations, telehealth activities are fragmented and it is difficult to gauge its effectiveness. It is typically a separate endeavor undertaken within an existing clinical service in an informal way, not supported and coordinated at the enterprise level.

Although the current role of telehealth in public health emergencies is limited and variable, there are several modalities of telehealth in use including:

- Real-time clinical videoconferencing
- Home telehealth
- Store-and-forward
- Public telephone systems
- Amateur radio
- Web-based information

State of the Art for Real-Time Videoconferencing Applications

The World Health Organization provides information on telehealth activity worldwide with sections on: Africa; Americas; South-East Asia; Europe; Eastern Mediterranean; and Western Pacific.[64] Expertise from within and between these regions is potentially available to assist in the event of a public health emergency. The current status of telehealth deployment in emergency preparedness situations is largely that of a single or small group of clinicians providing variable support. There are organizations seeking to develop a clinical network of physicians who can offer humanitarian assistance via telehealth. Humanitarian Emergency Logistics & Preparedness is one such organization.[65] It maintains a website through which it strives to mediate ISDN and IP-based video consultations.[66] This initiative and others like it are works in progress. These are grassroots efforts that are attempting to develop an international network of telehealth providers. There is a tremendous willingness and enthusiasm amongst individual clinicians to participate in humanitarian assistance via telehealth. Despite this enthusiasm, there are logistical issues that limit implementation. The goal of voluntary, governmental, and international agencies is to harness the volunteerism of clinicians into telehealth networks. Progress by such agencies toward achieving this goal is hampered by the lack of interoperable registries to certify the credentials of these volunteers and the cost of satellite communications, which provide the only current assurance of telecommunications operations continuity.

Satellite Communications for Synchronous Telehealth in Emergency and Disaster Management

In 2006, there were upwards of 150 communication satellites that could be used for telehealth.[67] While this number is growing, the cost of satellite communications remains prohibitively expensive and so many third world countries are unable to use this technology. Despite these cost constraints, when the United Nations Scientific and Technical Subcommittee of the Committee on the Peaceful Uses of Outer Space met in 2007, it identified the programs that were contributing to the increasing availability and use of space-based solutions to support disaster management.[68] These included:

- Italian-Argentine Satellite System for Emergency Management (SIASGE)
- RADARSAT-2 (Launched in December 2007; Canada's next generation commercial radar satellite) to reinforce the ability to detect potential disasters
- Use of Indian Remote Satellite (IRS) images
- Indian National Satellite System (INSAT)-based communications and telemedicine services for post-disaster relief operations
- Advanced Land Observing Satellite ("Daichi") of Japan
- Indian Space Research Organization (ISRO) satellite-based search and rescue network (this helped save thirty crew members on board the ship *Glory Moon* in 2006)
- International Satellite System for Search and Rescue (COSPAS-SARSAT) mission control center of Nigeria, which had been supporting search and rescue operations in aviation-related disasters

Although the U.S. military is similarly bound by cost considerations regarding satellite usage, it participated in the Pakistan earthquake relief effort in 2005. The military demonstrated that a robust consultation service for infectious disease, trauma, pediatrics, and dermatology could be established via satellite communications.[69]

Recent satellite deployments that promise to support telehealth include a system that will provide broadband satellite services to New England.[70] The system is supported by one fixed location site and several mobile healthcare units composed of three trucks and one vessel. This network will support delivery of medical care to migrant farm workers in Maine, New Hampshire, and Vermont. This manner of mobile telehealth deployment mirrors the functional requirements of systems needed for public health emergencies.

Another promising innovation that may impact telehealth is the Google Loon project.[71] This network of balloons floats in the stratosphere, approximately 20 km above the earth's surface. It provides Internet coverage connecting people in rural and remote areas and resolves coverage gaps. This system could permit online access after disasters and offer crucial connectivity to support telehealth.

Land-Based Communications for Synchronous Telehealth in Emergency and Disaster Management

The PROACT system (Preparedness & Response On Advanced Communications Technology) is a synchronous telehealth project based at the University of Kentucky in the United States.[72] It was established to bring public health, medical, and other experts together from anywhere within the United States via interactive videoconferencing. Its aim is to supplement other elements of the emergency response by:

- Bringing the regional coordinators together on a regular basis;
- Delivering disaster preparedness and response educational programming to communities;
- Engaging communities in statewide planning and response efforts;
- Reaching out across state lines to other PROACT-like networks for regional and national disaster response; and
- Providing a channel to connect victims of disasters with specialists from anywhere in the world, including the U.S. Centers for Disease Control and Prevention in Atlanta.

The activities of PROACT mirror those outlined by the Southern Governors Association. This group called for the inclusion of telehealth in emergency preparedness and seeks to develop a network of networks to evolve telehealth capacity for emergency preparedness.[73]

Bandwidth, logistics, regulations, and other constraints mean that the status of real-time clinical videoconferencing (and store-and-forward telehealth) has been relatively unchanged since the Telemedicine Spacebridge to Armenia.[10] During operations between March and July 1989, the use of Spacebridge resulted in more appropriate diagnoses being made in 26% of the patients seen. Anecdotal experience repeatedly shows similarly improved outcomes when telehealth is used in this sporadic way. Proponents of telehealth see its value in public health emergencies and call for the development of the telehealth networks that are necessary to support its widespread operational deployment. Opposition to creating these telehealth networks stems from the lack of scientific evidence to support them. Telehealth use in disasters is, therefore, in the classic dilemma that besets many new innovations in healthcare. Delays in creating the networks that will demonstrate the widespread benefits of telehealth are the norm until scientific evidence for improved outcome can be shown.

Real-Time Simulations Using Synchronous Telehealth

To show the benefits of telehealth and provide evidence of effectiveness, telehealth network simulations have been developed.

- **Operation Strong Angel.**[74] The United States Navy Third Fleet organized this simulated humanitarian response in Hawaii in June 2000. It took place within the umbrella of the concurrently occurring Rim of the Pacific Exercise.[75]
- **North Carolina Domestic Training Exercise.**[76] This training exercise took place in June 2002 at Camp Lejeune Marine Corps Base in Jacksonville, North Carolina. It used existing telehealth networks supplemented by rapidly deployable systems like satellites to show how telehealth could enhance the traditional emergency response to a disaster.
- **Shadow Bowl.**[77] In January 2003, the U.S. Super Bowl sporting event was used as the backdrop to a simulated homeland security exercise that examined community readiness and medical response. Telehealth was used as part of this medical response.

There is a commonality of findings from all these simulations. The first and most important is that it is possible to mount an effective telehealth response within the wider emergency response. Even with the advantages of forewarning and planning, it is a complex undertaking to develop the telecommunications infrastructure to support telehealth. Integrating the telehealth response and the use of information technologies into the existing emergency response is challenging. Operational details that reflect the clinical, technical, and business considerations highlighted in the Overview section can be problematic. Telehealth networks should be based on realistic simulations.

State of the Art of Home Telehealth Applications

Patient monitoring and telemetry has been featured in simulation exercises but the use of home telehealth technologies to manage disasters has not occurred in real events. Home telehealth technologies have the potential to provide surge capacity, such as during pandemic influenza. The current development of home telehealth services and networks is at an early stage and needs to evolve. Relevant issues for the development of home telehealth networks and the provision of surge capacity are:

- The home telehealth industry is emerging and rapidly increasing in sophistication and interoperability of technology, although still in its infancy;
- Creation of a strategy for technology distribution;
- The telecommunications capacity needed to support such networks;
- The location for the necessary clinicians;
- Identification of the protocols and procedures these clinicians would use;
- The method used to interface home telehealth with other services;
- Approaches to training and retraining staff; and
- Development of the necessary patient self-management and family/community caregiver tools.

Without resolution of these issues, the use of home telehealth will likely remain sporadic and show limited benefits. In the aftermath of Hurricane Katrina, the care provided to veterans via telehealth in areas not devastated by the hurricane continued uninterrupted. The only exception was the need to transfer support for this remote care from clinicians at hospital sites that were destroyed to other hospital locations.

State of the Art for Store-and-Forward Applications

The Swinfen Charitable Trust, a United Kingdom-based charitable organization, has provided routine medical services to third world countries and shown the great value of store-and-forward technologies.[78] However, such initiatives are limited in size with respect to the "people networks" on which they depend. They rely on relationships that are not easy to expand in a complex disaster unless the necessary practices, processes, and procedures have been detailed in advance and embedded in the emergency response.

There is increasing use of informal telehealth modalities to provide support in emergency and disaster situations. Examples include the use of email and transfer of digital images over a variety of telecommunications platforms, including cameras in cell phones. These activities are usually ad hoc, poorly documented, and use the general public telecommunications systems. They are, therefore, vulnerable to failure if these networks cease to function. Instead, they need to become part of dedicated networks to support emergency and disaster management. As such, the current status of store-and-foreword technologies:

- Is sporadic and mostly informal;
- When formalized, is part of a real-time videoconferencing response;
- Is subject to the vagaries of telecommunications support;
- Lacks access to accompanying health record systems; and
- Has major privacy and cyber security deficiencies in its informal usage.

State of the Art for Public Telephone Systems

By definition, there is ubiquitous use of telehealth in both routine healthcare and emergency and disaster operations when the public telephone system is accessed. However, this resource is subject to disruptions from network damage and to inadequate capacity due to sheer call volume during a disaster. Despite its limitations, the public telephone system is a mainstay in healthcare delivery. Its use is routine and understood and cell phone technology makes it mobile. It does not lock individuals to set locations in the way that the old copper-wired systems did. The telephone system is often the way in which telehealth systems are deployed that involve clinical videoconferencing. Important initiatives in relation to an expanded role for the telephone in providing healthcare are: 1) to work toward prioritization of users on public telephone systems to ensure that emergency responders are guaranteed immediate access; and 2) to use the telephone and telephone call centers as sources of public information and epidemiological surveillance.[79]

The Current Role of Amateur Radio Networks in Providing Telehealth

There is a danger with telehealth, as with all new innovations, of not recognizing existing capabilities. An invaluable part of the telecommunications support during disasters has been amateur radio.[80] Users of amateur radio are often trained and skilled communicators. The emergency management community recognizes these competencies when discussing the Amateur Radio Service. Amateur radio users are a resource that can act as a conduit to help agencies exchange information. They may not understand the medical and health terminology, but the ability to transmit the information accurately makes them an invaluable communications bridge.

The Current Role of Web-Based Information

The use of the Internet to provide web-based information and resources is a worldwide phenomenon. The volume of health-related information on the Internet that may be pertinent in the event of a public health emergency is so great that it could not all be synthesized and verified.

The Internet itself may be a target of terrorist or hacker-related actions. The effect of this activity could be local, national, or conceivably worldwide. If a patient's EHR were purposely altered, this could lead to a well-meaning telehealth provider inadvertently administering a fatal treatment. In addition, continuous access to the Internet requires electricity services that can be finite despite generators, batteries, and solar energy. Furthermore, bandwidth capacity might be inadequate to accommodate large numbers of users simultaneously. Thus, a total reliance on posting information on the Internet is unwise and printed or published written materials are needed as a backup.

The veracity of Internet information is a critical issue. There have been large purchases or liquidations of stock and other financial instruments triggered by false rumors published on the Internet. The propagation of misinformation in the form of urban legends is well known. Web-based information sources must be credible, authoritative, accessible, and usable by those with disabilities, such as visual impairment.

Examples of credible information sources valuable to emergency responders and the public are the sites for the U.S. Joint Pathology Center and Center for Disaster and Humanitarian Assistance Medicine. The pathology center Is the federal government's premier pathology reference center supporting the

Military Health System, Department of Defense, and other federal agencies.[81] The Center for Disaster and Humanitarian Assistance Medicine is supported by the Uniformed Services University of the Health Sciences in Bethesda, Maryland. Its website is a resource that provides information about chemical and biological warfare and terrorism.[82] Information contained on the site is derived from the organization's 25 years of instruction on management of events related to weapons of mass destruction use.

Using the web to distribute information requires resources and expertise to maintain the data and keep it scientifically correct and valid. There is also concern that by publicly posting information about the emergency response on the Internet, one may be providing information to terrorists as well as the intended audience.

Web-based resources that provide information to the general public at the local, national, and international levels are currently grossly inadequate with regards to content and quality. Web-based training modules are increasingly providing information for emergency responders. However, this information is often applicable only to the individual sponsoring organization, and not linked with common standards and the operational policies and procedures of other groups.

RECOMMENDATIONS FOR FURTHER RESEARCH

In the previous sections of this chapter, it has been stressed that the use of telehealth in disasters is at a rudimentary and formative stage. To move forward and use telehealth as a tool to transform elements of the healthcare response, it is critical that investigator pursue the following areas of research and development:

1. Policy considerations
2. Organizational strategic considerations
3. Network of networks
4. The clinical effectiveness of telehealth in disasters and public health emergencies
5. Robustness, standardization and interoperability of technology
6. Understanding that telehealth is a complex adaptive system[83]

Policy Considerations

The role of telehealth is not yet formalized into policy in terms of its impact on the routine delivery of healthcare services, let alone for public health emergencies. Governments and health services are notoriously reactive when it comes to policy development in healthcare. The EHR and telehealth are simultaneously transformative and disruptive technologies and organizations. Healthcare professionals worldwide are reluctant to embrace the EHR and telehealth for these reasons. The crisis that affects the delivery of both routine and emergency healthcare services in terms of access equity requires a focus on the patient. Telehealth is a technology that benefits patients by transferring services from healthcare facilities to the home and local community. Lack of support from hospitals and existing healthcare infrastructure is a powerful barrier to change.

Recommendation 1: Central governments and healthcare services should consider telehealth in formal policy terms.

Organizational Strategic Considerations

Similar reservations exist in healthcare and emergency response organizations to adopting telehealth in their approach to managing disasters. In part, this is because healthcare organizations do not plan ahead in a strategic manner and consider the impact of new technologies. This strategic approach should be incorporated into the broader consideration of health informatics and telecommunications implementation, and mandates innovative new methods for reimbursement.

Recommendation 2: Telehealth should be part of the emergency and disaster management strategies for all healthcare organizations.

Networks of Networks

Healthcare organizations develop their own Intranets based on evolving information and communication technologies. Business, technical, and privacy/confidentiality/cyber security considerations make these Intranets self-contained, offering limited access to the Internet and connectivity with other healthcare entities. Access to the breadth and volume of healthcare services needed in a public health emergency requires that networks of networks aggregate and self-assemble in an organized and cohesive manner to offer integrated and interoperable services.

Recommendation 3: International agencies, central governments, and healthcare organizations should link telecommunications networks and clinical services that provide both routine medical care and emergency and disaster management.

Research on the Clinical Effectiveness of Telehealth

Global demographic trends identify that more people are living in areas where an increase in natural disasters are predicted, particularly due to climate change.[84] The use of telehealth in disasters must be based on scientific evidence that it is clinically efficacious and cost-effective. Although evidence is accumulating for the effectiveness of telehealth in certain areas, such evidence is currently lacking for its application in public health emergencies.[85] A research agenda should be developed and include ethical dilemmas faced by disaster medicine investigators. There are special research considerations in a fast moving technological area like telehealth.[86] For example, the approach of the traditional randomized controlled trial is rarely appropriate.

Recommendation 4: A comprehensive research agenda should be developed and funded at the international and national levels to generate the evidence necessary to support the use of telehealth networks for emergency and disaster management.

Robustness, Standardization, and Interoperability of Technology

Telehealth in general, and the home telehealth industry in particular, is an emerging enterprise. The future use of telehealth depends on creating robust technologies that are standardized and interoperable. The experience of cellular technologies in public health emergencies shows the dangers of inoperability. The electronic components required to support telehealth must be engineered to exacting specifications and developed under the necessary standards for interoperability. Wherever possible, these new assets should be compatible with existing technologies to maximize the function of older systems (backwards compatibility).

Recommendation 5: Governmental bodies and international/national technology standardization agencies must develop robust and interoperable telehealth technologies that enable the widespread deployment of these assets in disasters.

Telehealth Requires a Complex Adaptive System

The implementation of telehealth by emergency and disaster management should occur in ways that can improve the response to contemporary threats and address risk.[87] A successful approach must embrace rather than deny uncertainty. Telehealth should be developed within the context of building networks of organizations committed to a process of continual inquiry, informed action, and adaptive learning. This approach is one that recognizes complexity and is different from the traditional linear anticipatory response from emergency and disaster management. The emergency response to a disaster is, above all, a logistical one. Using a scientific approach to logistics management, investigators are beginning to examine the emergency and disaster response.[88] The similarities between business logistics and those of disaster relief are substantial, and each can learn from the other. Information systems are important to both.

Recommendation 6: Organizational development should encompass both linear and complex adaptive approaches as appropriate in developing and implementing telehealth networks.

Conclusion

Telehealth has many advantages in the management of disasters and public health emergencies. It offers the potential for enhancing patient care, improving efficiency in allocation of scarce resources, and protecting emergency responders, all in a cost-effective manner. With improvements in technology and enhanced research efforts that demonstrate evidence for efficacy, telehealth will become an increasingly important tool for the emergency managers of the future.

REFERENCES

1. Health Care Resources and Services Administration. Telehealth. http://www.hrsa.gov/ruralhealth/about/telehealth (Accessed August 22, 2013).
2. Darkins A, Cary M. *Telemedicine and Telehealth: Principles, Practice, Performance and Pitfalls*. New York, Springer, 2000.
3. Access Morland LA, Raab M, Mackintosh MA, et al. Telemedicine: A Cost-Reducing Means of Delivering Psychotherapy to Rural Combat Veterans with PTSD. *Telemed J E Health* 2013; 19(10): 754–759.
4. Müller-Barna P, Schwamm LH, Haberl RL. Telestroke increases use of acute stroke therapy. *Curr Opin Neurol* February 2012; 25(1): 5–10.
5. Darkins A, Ryan P, Kobb R, et al. Care Coordination/Home Telehealth: the systematic implementation of health informatics, home telehealth, and disease management to support the care of veteran patients with chronic conditions. *Telemed J E Health* December 2008; 14(10): 1118–1126.
6. Lilley E. Tele-ICU: Experience to Date. *Journal of Intensive Care Medicine* September 13, 2009; 1–7.
7. Grossmann ZR, Sorondo B, Holmberg R, Bjorn P. Telemedicine consultation for emergency trauma: the 130 million square foot trauma. *Bull Am Coll Surg* June 2011; 96(6): 12–19.
8. de Lissovoy G. Big data meets the electronic medical record: a commentary on "identifying patients at increased risk for unplanned readmission." *Med Care* September 2013; 51(9): 759–760.
9. Butler FK, Jr., Blackbourne LH. Battlefield trauma care then and now: a decade of Tactical Combat Casualty Care. *J Trauma Acute Care Surg* December 2012; 73(6 Suppl. 5): S395–S402.
10. Calcagni DE, Clyburn CA, Tomkins G, et al. Operation Joint Endeavor in Bosnia: telemedicine systems and case reports. *Telemed J* Fall 1996; 2(3): 211–224.
11. Blank E, Lappan C, Belmont PJ, Jr., et al. Early analysis of the United States Army's telemedicine orthopaedic consultation program. *J Surg Orthop Adv* Spring 2011; 20(1): 50–55.
12. Khitrov MY, Rutishauser M, Montgomery K, et al. A platform for testing and comparing of real-time decision-support algorithms in mobile environments. *Conf Proc IEEE Eng Med Biol Soc* 2009: 3417–3420.
13. Zanaboni P, Wootton R. Adoption of telemedicine: from pilot stage to routine delivery. *BMC Med Inform Decis Mak* January 4, 2012; 12: 1.
14. Case T, Morrison C, Vuylsteke A. The clinical application of mobile technology to disaster medicine. *Prehosp Disaster Med* October 2012; 27(5): 473–480.
15. Thompson C, White J, Dougherty B, et al. Using Smartphones to Detect Car Accidents and Provide Situational Awareness to Emergency Responders. *Lecture Notes of the Institute for Computer Sciences, Social Informatics and Telecommunications Engineering* 2010; 48: 29–42.
16. Lee YG, Jeong WS, Yoon G. Smartphone-based mobile health monitoring. *Telemed J E Health* October 2012; 18(8): 585–590.
17. Hee Hwang J, Mun GH. An evolution of communication in postoperative free flap monitoring: using a smartphone and mobile messenger application. *Plast Reconstr Surg* July 2012; 130(1): 125–129.
18. Kulling P. *The Terrorist Attack with Sarin in Tokyo on 20th March 1995*. Kamedo Report 71. Stockholm, 1995.
19. Wade V, Karnon J, Elshaug A, Hiller J. A systematic review of economic analyses of telehealth services using real time video communication. *BMC Health Services Research* 2010; 10: 233.
20. DelliFraine JL, Dansky KH. Home-based telehealth: a review and meta-analysis. *J Telemed Telecare* March 2008; 14(2): 62–66.
21. Bonnardot L, Rainis R. Store-and-forward telemedicine for doctors working in remote areas. *J Telemed Telecare* January 2009; 15(1): 1–6.
22. Istepanian RSH, Jovanov E, Zhang Y. Guest editorial introduction to the special section on m-health: Beyond seamless mobility and global wireless healthcare connectivity. *IEEE Transactions on Information Technology in Biomedicine* 2004; 8(4): 405–414.
23. Boaz T, McManus J, Koenig K. The Art and Science of Surge: Experience from Israel and the U.S. Military. *Acad Emerg Med* 2006; 13(11): 1130–1134.
24. Hawes C. Get rid of your stethoscope! *Pract Neurol* December 2010; 10(6): 344–346.

25. Lee W. Slit Lamp Adapters turn Smartphones into Clinical Cameras. http://www.ophthalmologyweb.com/Featured-Articles/136817-Slit-Lamp-Adapters-turn-Smartphones-into-Clinical-Cameras (Accessed August 25, 2015)

26. Hill D. Now Your Smartphone Can Be Used to Diagnose Ear Infections at Home. http://singularityhub.com/2012/07/15/now-your-smartphone-can-be-used-to-diagnose-ear-infections-at-home (Accessed August 25, 2013).

27. Wojtczak J, Bonadonna P. Pocket mobile smartphone system for the point-of-care submandibular ultrasonography. *Am J Emerg Med* March 2013; 31(3): 573–577.

28. Sinatra S. Is Your Smartphone the Latest ECG Machine? http://www.drsinatra.com/is-your-smartphone-the-latest-ecg-machine (Accessed August 25, 2013).

29. US Food and Drug Administration. Mobile Medical Applications. http://www.fda.gov/MedicalDevices/ProductsandMedicalProcedures/ConnectedHealth/MobileMedicalApplications/default.htm (Accessed August 25, 2013).

30. Balch B. Developing a National Inventory of Telehealth Resources for Rapid and Effective Emergency Care: a white paper developed by the American Telemedicine Association Emergency Preparedness Response Special Interest Group. *Telemed J E Health* August 2008; 14(6): 606–610.

31. Adams BJ, Arn Womble J, Ghosh S, Friedland C. Deployment of Remote Sensing Technology for Multi-hazard Post-Katrina Damage Assessment within a Spatially-Tiered Reconnaissance Framework. The 2nd International Conference on Urban Disaster Reduction, Taipei, Taiwan, November 27–29, 2007. http://www.researchgate.net/publication/267833599_Deployment_of_Remote_Sensing_Technology_for_Multi-Hazard_Post-Katrina_Damage_Assessment (Accessed September 1, 2015).

32. Garshnek V, Burkle FJ. Applications of Telemedicine and Telecommunications to Disaster Medicine. *J Am Med Inform Assoc* 1999; 6: 26–37.

33. Merrell RC, Doarn CR. Disasters-How Can Telemedicine Help? *Telemed J E Health* 2005; 11(2): 511–512.

34. United States–USSR. Telemedicine Consultation Spacebridge to Armenia and Ufa. Presented at the Third U.S.–USSR Joint Working Group on Space Biology and Medicine. Moscow and Kislovodsk, USSR, December 1–9, 1989. http://www.quasar.org/21698/nasa/spacebridgeq.htm (Accessed August 25, 2013).

35. Doarn C, Merrell R. Spacebridge to Armenia: a look back at its impact on telemedicine in disaster response. *Telemed J E Health* September 2011; 17(7): 546–552.

36. Siegel E. Psychological factors affecting the *adoption of PACS*. Appl Radiol 2002; 31: 19.

37. Simmons SC, Murphy TA, Blanarovich A, et al. Telehealth technologies and applications for terrorism response: a report of the 2002 coastal North Carolina domestic preparedness training exercise. *J Am Med Inform Assoc* March–April 2003; 10(2): 166–176.

38. Garshnek V, Burkle F. Applications of telemedicine and telecommunications to disaster medicine – Historical and future perspectives. *J Am Med Inform Assoc* 1999; 6: 125–127.

39. Moore G. Crossing the Chasm and Inside the Tornado. *Harper Business* 1991.

40. Natis YV, Schulte WR. *Introduction to Service-Oriented Architecture.* Gartner Research, 2003. https://www.gartner.com/doc/391377?ref=ddisp (Accessed September 1, 2015).

41. RAND Center for Domestic and International Health Security. http://www.rand.org/news/press/2007/04/05.html (Accessed August 25, 2013).

42. Nelson C, Lurie N, Wasserman J, Zakowski S Conceptualizing and Defining Public Health Emergency Preparedness. *American Journal of Public Health* December 2006; 8(4): 449–471.

43. Federal Telemedicine Update. September 19, 2005. http://www.federaltelemedicine.com/n091905.htm (Accessed August 25, 2013).

44. Raymond C. Offenheiser, President, Oxfam America. Testimony before the U.S. Senate Foreign Relations Committee. February 10, 2005.

45. American Red Cross. Red Cross Hurricane App. http://www.redcross.org/news/article/Its-Officially-Hurricane-Season–Are-You-Prepared (Accessed August 25, 2013).

46. http://www.sphereproject.org/handbook/pages/navbook.htm?param1=0 (Accessed July 27, 2007).

47. Homeland Security Presidential Directive 21. 2007. http://www.whitehouse.gov/administration/eop/ostp/nstc/biosecurity (Accessed August 25, 2013).

48. Nelson N, Lurie N, Wasserman J, Zakouski S. Conceptualizing and Defining Public Health Emergency Preparedness. *American Journal of Public Health* 2007; 97 (Suppl. 1): S9–S11.

49. Pandemic and All-Hazards Preparedness Act (S.3678). July 18, 2006.

50. Telemedicine & Health IT. American Telemedicine Association. Http://www.Americantelemed.Org/News/Policy_Issues/Hit_Paper.Pdf (Accessed December 7, 2007).

51. Institute of Medicine. *Crossing the Quality Chasm: A New Health System for the 21st Century.* Washington, DC, National Academy Press, 2001.

52. Hurricane Katrina's Veteran Victims in the Nation's Capital. http://www.washingtondc.va.gov/news/katrina.asp (Accessed September 1, 2015).

53. Ceesay I. Public Financial Accountability In Pakistan. The Impact of PIFRA on Capacity. World Bank. Pakistan Country Financial Accountability Assessment. Report Number 27551-PAK. December 2003.

54. http://xml.coverpages.org/CAPv11–12649.pdf (Accessed July 23, 2007).

55. Lessons From Katrina Health. http://www.markle.org/downloadable_assets/katrinahealth.final.pdf (Accessed July 29, 2007).

56. http://www.sphereproject.org/handbook/pages/navbook.htm?param1=0 (Accessed July 6, 2007).

57. http://www.itu.int/ITU-D/emergencytelecoms/tampere.html (Accessed July 6, 2007).

58. Written Testimony of Vincent D. Kelly, President and Chief Executive Officer, USA Mobility before the FCC's Independent Panel Reviewing the Impact of Hurricane Katrina. March 6, 2006. http://www.fcc.gov/eb/hkip/GSpeakers060306/ACT1010.pdf (Accessed July 6, 2007).

59. http://www.fcc.gov/pshs/spectrum/700mhz (Accessed July 7, 2007).

60. Cisco. http://www.cisco.com/en/US/docs/voice_ip_comm/pgw/9/dial_plan/guide/DP_Pref.html (Accessed September 1, 2015).

61. H.323 Protocol Definition. http://www.pcmag.com/encyclopedia_term/0,2542,t=H320&i=44036,00.asp (Accessed August 7, 2007).

62. http://www.h323forum.org (Accessed August 25, 2013).

63. Cisco Systems. Internet Protocols. http://www.cisco.com/univercd/cc/td/doc/cisintwk/ito_doc/ip.htm (Accessed August 7, 2007).

64. http://www.who.int/goe/publications/goe_telemedicine_2010.pdf (Accessed August 25, 2013).

65. Humanitarian Emergency Logistics & Preparedness. http://www.disasterlogistics.org (Accessed August 25, 2013).

66. http://www.disasterlogistics.org (Accessed August 25, 2013).

67. Conference Report. Satellite Applications for Telehealth in the Developing World. *Journal of Telemedicine and Telecare* 2006; 12: 321–324.

68. United Nations Scientific and Technical Subcommittee of the Committee on the Peaceful Uses of Outer Space http://www.oosa.unvienna.org (Accessed August 25, 2013).

69. Meade KM, Lam D. A deployable Telemedicine Capability in Support of Humanitarian Operations. *Telemedicine and e-Health* 2007; 13: 331–340.

70. http://c3otelemedicine.com/2013/01/what-about-satellite-based-telemedicine (Accessed August 25, 2013).

71. http://www.google.com/loon (Accessed August 25, 2013).

72. PROACT – Preparedness & Response On Advanced Communications Technology. http://www.mc.uky.edu/kytelecare/proact.asp (Accessed August 25, 2013).

73. Southern Governors Homeland Security/Telemedicine Project. http://www.stateline.org/live/ViewPage.action?siteNodeId=136&languageId=1&contentId=15759 (Accessed August 25, 2013).

74. Balch D, West V. Telemedicine used in a simulated disaster response. *Stud Health Technol Inform* 2001; 81: 41–45.

75. Rim of the Pacific Exercise (RIMPAC). http://www.globalsecurity.org/military/ops/rimpac.htm (Accessed August 25, 2013).

76. Simmons SC, Murphy TA, Blanarovich A, et al. Telehealth technologies and applications for terrorism response: a report of the 2002 coastal North Carolina domestic preparedness training exercise. *J Am Med Inform Assoc* March–April 2003; 10(2): 166–176.

77. Balch D, Taylor C, Rosenthal D, et al. Shadow Bowl 2003: a collaborative exercise in community readiness, agency cooperation, and medical response. *Telemed J E Health* Fall 2004; 10(3): 330–342.

78. Swinfen Charitable Trust. http://www.swinfencharitabletrust.org (Accessed August 25, 2013).

79. Rolland E, Moore K, Robinson V, McGuinness D. Using Ontario's "Telehealth" health telephone helpline as an early-warning system: a study protocol. *BMC Health Serv Res* 2006; 6: 10. Published online February 15, 2006. http://www.pubmedcentral.nih.gov/articlerender.fcgi?artid=1431529 (Accessed August 25, 2013).

80. The Amateur Radio Emergency Service (ARES). http://www.arrl.org/FandES/field/pscm/sec1-ch1.html (Accessed August 10, 2007).

81. The U.S. Joint Pathology Center. http://www.jpc.capmed.mil (Accessed September 16, 2014).

82. Center for Disaster and Humanitarian Assistance Medicine (CDHAM). http://www.cdham.org (Accessed August 25, 2013).

83. Kovacs G, Spens S. Humanitarian logistics in disaster relief operations. *International Journal of Physical Distribution & Logistics Management* 2007; 37(2): 99.

84. Brookings. Trends in Natural Disaster Response and the Role of Regional Organizations. Http://Www.Brookings.Edu/Events/2013/04/22-Natural-Disaster-Trends (Accessed September 15, 2013).

85. Agency for Healthcare Research and Quality (AHRQ) – Telemedicine for the Medicare Population – Update. http://www.ncbi.nlm.nih.gov/books/NBK37953 (Accessed August 25, 2013).

86. Grigsby J, Bennett RE. Alternatives to randomized controlled trials in telemedicine. *J Telemed Telecare* 2006; 12 (Suppl. 2): S77–S84.

87. Comfort K. Risk, Security, and Disaster Management. *Annual Review of Political Science* 2005; 8: 335–356.

88. Kovacs G, Spens S. Humanitarian logistics in disaster relief operations. *International Journal of Physical Distribution & Logistics Management* 2007; 37(2): 99.

27

COMPLEX PUBLIC HEALTH EMERGENCIES

Frederick M. Burkle, Jr.

OVERVIEW

Public Health Emergencies

The term "public health emergencies" denotes disasters that adversely impact the public health system and its protective infrastructure (water, sanitation, shelter, food, energy, and health) thus resulting in both direct and indirect consequences to the overall health of a population. When this protective threshold is destroyed; overwhelmed; not recovered or maintained; or denied to populations through political violence, war, conflict, or other disasters, classic consequences, all preventable, emerge. Outbreaks of communicable disease and food shortages leading to undernutrition and eventual malnutrition inevitably result in worsening vulnerability and insecurity, population displacement, loss of livelihoods, and poverty.

Public health emergencies occur more often in developing countries where public health infrastructure, adequate numbers of health sector workers, and basic medications and equipment are lacking or nonexistent. An exception occurs in developed countries when urban environments become more populous and dense, commonly with migrants experiencing low socioeconomic status and increased vulnerability. Rapid unsustainable urbanization occurs when the population numbers exceed the capacity of the public health infrastructure to service and protect the people, especially the poor. This increases, within the urban boundaries, the gap between the have and have-not populations. Urban occupancy for the disadvantaged is often limited to unfavorable disaster-prone areas with poor or absent infrastructure. Such a combination of factors results in high risk for a major public health emergency to occur if additional essential infrastructure loss were to occur, for example, with an earthquake or tsunami. Similar public health emergencies happen whenever the protective public health cover is breached in large-scale disasters such as was the case with Hurricane Katrina and the 2004 Indian Ocean tsunami. Two years after Hurricane Katrina, a 47% increase in mortality was reported in New Orleans.[1] This negative outcome of the public health impact of the disaster results from system resources and infrastructure deficiencies that are similar to the familiar and prolonged adverse conditions common to countries at war in Asia and Africa. Additionally, large-scale epidemics, pandemics, and other biological, chemical, or radiation disasters have the potential to cause unprecedented public health catastrophes. By definition, public health emergencies result in dire health consequences and share similar health indices such as increased mortality and morbidity, which remain the most sensitive indices of short- and long-term impact and outcome.

Complex Humanitarian Emergencies

The focus of this chapter is the prototypical public health emergency commonly referred to collectively as complex humanitarian emergencies (CHEs). Descriptively, "complex" is added to define a worsening or absent political, economic, governance, security, and social system that either catapults or accelerates a deteriorating public health environment and severely curtails its recovery.[2] The political violence and warfare commonly grows so severe that it requires international humanitarian assistance and United Nations (UN) peacekeeping or peace enforcement assets to protect the civilian population. CHEs have also been called "complex political emergencies," a term favored by some to emphasize the pervasive political violence that is at the core of these tragedies.[3]

Additional public health emergencies are covered elsewhere, and although they may differ in cause, all are conceptually linked by similar consequences brought about by the disruption in the protective cover that public health provides to a population. CHEs have been defined by the U.S. Centers for Disease Control and Prevention (CDC) as "situations affecting large civilian populations which usually involve a combination of factors including war or civil strife, food shortages, and population displacement, resulting in significant excess mortality."[4] The twentieth century is known for cross-border wars such as WWI and WWII, the Korean War, and the 1991 Persian Gulf War, yet few understand that during that time more people were killed by war, conflict, and its consequences within their own countries rather than in foreign lands.

CHEs represent the most common human-generated disasters of the past three decades. Internal crises are often catalyzed by longstanding social and gender inequities, poverty, judicial injustices, cultural incompatibilities, ignorance, racism, oppression, tribalism, and religious fundamentalism, all of which adversely influence public health and access to it.[2] In the past three decades, the agricultural and protective public health infrastructure has declined while hunger in the world (defined as without food for basic health) has climbed to over 1 billion.[5] The chronic, smoldering political violence adversely affects access to and availability of health facilities and services, leading to increasing mortality and morbidity rates among the most vulnerable populations (e.g., women, children, elderly, and disabled). Such data go uncounted, unnoticed, and without political attention from the outside world. While the number of CHEs has declined over the last decade, the few that remain are more complex, longer lasting and more insecure. Despite the lower number of reported wars, the number of crisis-affected countries and territories across four continents at risk for conflict remains essentially unchanged. Politically, these are commonly referred to as "failed" or "fragile" states.

CURRENT STATE OF THE ART

Measuring the Human Cost of CHEs

Characteristically, CHEs are initially confined within nation-state borders and result in massive numbers of internally displaced persons/populations (IDPs) who stay within their country's borders. Political violence and its direct effects on individuals occur first, resulting in death and injury.[3] In time, IDPs begin to experience the consequences of being separated from essential public health services, and mortality and morbidity from indirect causes begin to escalate. Most CHEs risk affecting neighboring countries with escaping refugees (defined as persons or populations crossing into a neighboring country) and risk in spreading, over time, the political turmoil and the conflict itself across borders.

Without epidemiological studies, the short- and long-term impact of various forms of political violence would remain elusive. Studies performed in the early 1990s highlighted the dominance of public health consequences and the preponderance of civilian victims. Epidemiological studies detect and verify continued health problems, confirm whether victims are benefiting from aid operations, and often catalyze major alterations in the direction and strategies of the international relief community and governmental donors. The additional lack of local and nation-state capacities in governance, economics, public safety, communications, and transportation work against an efficient and effective recovery and normalization to pre-disaster health indices.

Data analysis suggests that CHEs have changed substantially over the last three decades, especially in the overall levels of insecurity.[6] Security assessments and relief strategies have not yet evolved effectively to deal with worsening security, especially as it impacts civilians and the relief community. The humanitarian community relies on use of specific direct and indirect indices to: 1) assess consequences including severity of the conflict; 2) measure the impact or outcome of interventions in declining mortality and morbidity; and 3) identify the most vulnerable of populations requiring care. The most common baseline health indices followed are:

- Mortality or death rates;
- Morbidity rates;

- Nutritional status;
- Aid program indicators to ensure predicted impact and outcome;
- Age and sex-specific mortality and morbidity rates critical to determine population vulnerability; and
- Attack rates and case fatality rates crucial during outbreaks and epidemics.

Direct Indices

Direct effects of political violence result in death, injury, and disabilities, including psychological, as well as the direct consequences resulting from a lack of protection from, and respect for, international humanitarian law. Direct effects are quantitative in nature and subject to organized attempts to measure, i.e., population-based cluster sampling. They are more readily detectable and it is easier to hold people accountable for them than for indirect effects.

Intervention from outside agencies and organizations is initially driven by reports of battlefield and civilian deaths. Assessment teams use both direct observation and rapid assessment tools to measure the consequences of the conflict on essential public health parameters such as access to and availability of food, water, sanitation, shelter, health, and fuel. Initial assessments focus on measurements for crude mortality rates and younger than age 5 mortality rates. As the humanitarian community becomes more established, follow-on surveys include population-based cluster samplings and studies that further disaggregate the crude mortality rates to determine age and sex vulnerability (i.e., infant and maternal mortality and morbidity rates). Ongoing surveys and surveillance ensure that management responses meet Sphere (Humanitarian Charter and Minimum Standards in Disaster Response) and other essential public health standards.[7]

The assumption is that low-cost humanitarian aid, if properly administered and managed, will reduce the direct indicator rates to prewar conflict levels or better within 4–6 months.[6] As the direct effect mortality rates decline however, so does outside interest and relief aid from donor agencies and governments, often giving a false assurance of success.

Indirect Indicators

It is the indirect collateral damage effects of conflict resulting from population displacement, disruption of food supplies, destroyed health facilities and public health infrastructure, and consequences, such as poverty and destroyed livelihoods that will ultimately account for 90% or more of overall mortality and morbidity (Figure 27.1). Women and children are the most common victims, as are the elderly and those with disabilities. No existing data sets, however, measure indirect death tolls. This issue proved to be highly contentious in the 2003 war with Iraq, and numbers of indirect deaths among civilians, even today, remain in dispute. Except for a few countries, the humanitarian community has no idea how to gauge the worldwide extent of indirect deaths.

In contrast to direct indices, indirect deaths are rarely measured, are more functional and abstract in nature, frequently require qualitative or semi-quantitative measures, and their accuracy is difficult to confirm. In CHEs, the health system and public health infrastructure is the first to be destroyed and last to recover or be rehabilitated. In the post-conflict phase, the risk of continuing death and disability from environmental, communicable, and noncommunicable diseases related to the lack of this

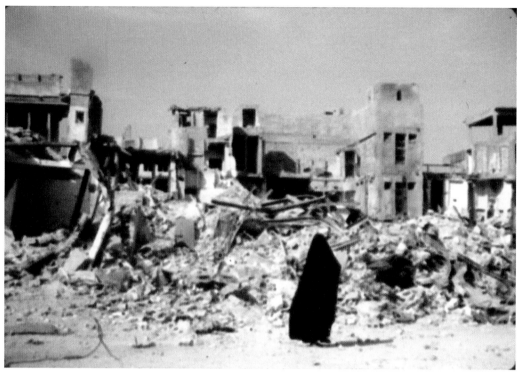

Figure 27.1. "Collateral damage" goes beyond injury and death. The fragile and superficially placed piping seen in the foreground was the main water artery to this village in Iraq. Public health infrastructure may be different than the normal standard for civilian contractors, the military, and aid workers. Public health "indirect" deaths are more prevalent than direct deaths from weaponry and violence. Photo by Frederick M. Burkle, Jr. – used with permission.

recovery may continue to decay up to 10 years post-conflict and the effects may far exceed the immediate loses from the war itself.[8,9] Similar consequences are found in countries contiguous to the conflict.

Despite the cessation of hostilities, subtle and rarely counted mortality and morbidity result from those now out of work and despondent, demobilized soldiers, and IDPs who are more likely to suffer suicide, depression, and alcohol and drug use. A sensitive marker of the continued community decay and economic and physical insecurity is an increase in sex-based violence among intimate partners.[10] In developing countries experiencing residual post-conflict insecurity, families struggling to recover economically will frequently delay reenrollment of their children to school, usually females – a factor that subtly correlates with high child mortality rates. Over the past decade, humanitarian assistance has moved from insecure rural Africa and Asia to overcrowded urban areas.[11]

Urban aid is predominantly focused on protecting single or widowed mothers with young children seeking some semblance of security, education, and essential public health and social services after their rural economies are destroyed. Many have been forced to resort to prostitution to avoid abject poverty, and then commonly contract sexually transmitted diseases. The increased density of urban populations has rapidly outstripped the fragile and poorly maintained public health infrastructure. Few urban conclaves have safe water and sanitation. More than 2.5 billion people, almost one of every two people in the developing world, do not have adequate water and sanitation.[11] Globally, nearly 4,000 children die each day from unsafe water and lack of basic sanitation facilities.[11] In areas where the vector exists, outbreaks

of dengue fever serve as a marker of economic decay and worsening governmental services resulting from increased breeding of mosquitoes in the stagnant water of failed public rubbish collection systems.[12]

Achievement Indicators

Achievement indicators refer to the completion of certain humanitarian-related missions, such as emergency delivery of military rations and rebuilding of clinics and hospitals. Coalition military and private contractors prefer to use achievement indicators rather than outcome indicators in measuring effectiveness of their interventions. Achievement indicators do not necessarily result in improved outcomes or guarantee the functional return of the health and public health infrastructure. Whereas these functions are critical to the relief process, claims of success in humanitarian aid and reconstruction must be viewed with caution when achievement indicators alone are used.

Epidemiology of CHEs

CHEs can be divided into developing, smoldering or chronic country, and developed models, all with differing data presentations.[2,4] Models are valuable in predicting priorities for immediate aid, even before confirming field level assessments. There are overlaps in these three models, especially when developed country conflicts persist with failed public health infrastructure, resulting in failing indices similar to those seen in developing countries. Iraq once enjoyed stable health indices indicative of a developed country. In 2007, after 4 years of war and a worsening public health infrastructure, the infant mortality rate equaled

Table 27.1. Developing Country Health Profile

- 90% of deaths are preventable
- Outbreaks of communicable diseases
- Malnutrition and micronutrient diseases
- Absent protective public health infrastructure
- Major deficiencies in WHO childhood vaccine protection
- Mental health consequences most often unmeasured and untreated
- Internally displaced and refugee populations
- Weaponry, usually small arms and machetes, accounts for 4–11% of deaths
- High crude mortality rates range from 7–70 times normal baseline
- Higher mortality rates in orphaned and unaccompanied children
- High case fatality rates

Table 27.2. Smoldering or Chronic Country Model Health Profile

- Many years of chronic violence
- Social and political unrest
- Poor maintenance of basic public health infrastructure
- High environmental degradation
- Little or no access to and availability of health and education
- Below-sustenance-level economy
- Chronic malnutrition and stunted growth
- Children grow up knowing only a culture of violence
- Few indigenous healthcare providers
- Lack of basic reproductive health services
- Organized mental health services generally nonexistent
- Incidents of violent surges, resulting in peaks in death rates from direct violence and sudden-onset consequences of chronic conditions (i.e., acute malnutrition and dehydration in children with chronic malnutrition)
- Primarily small arms deaths and wounds, advanced weaponry increasing
- Violent surges increase internally displaced and refugee populations

that of Afghanistan and Sierra Leone.[13] Reported acts of genocide, ethnic cleansing, and torture are a common element of all models of CHEs.

Developing Country Model

Developing country CHEs primarily occur in central Asia and Africa and are characterized by a health profile that exacerbates preventable diseases, such as infectious diseases and malnutrition, resulting from lack of protective levels of food, water, sanitation, shelter, and healthcare (Table 27.1).[14] This results in high crude mortality rates, the majority coming from deaths of children younger than 5. Seventy-five percent of the world's epidemics occur during CHEs.[2] Outbreaks typically occur from unprotected endemic diseases. The major causes of mortality and morbidity are diarrhea and dehydration; malnutrition and micronutrient diseases such as vitamin A, C, and B6 deficiencies; complications from childhood vaccine-preventable diseases such as measles and tetanus; complications from acute respiratory infections; and malaria (Figures 27.2, 27.3–27.5, 27.6–27.7, 27.8, 27.9, 27.10, 27.11, 27.12, 27.13).

CHEs result in people attempting to flee the war and conflict. If they flee their homes but are unable or unwilling to cross the country's border they are termed IDPs. With international

law they remain under the authority of the host country, even though national forces may be attempting to find and kill them. This contradiction remains a dilemma for the international community, a well-known illustration being the forced abandonment of fleeing Tutsi civilians by UN peacekeeping forces in Rwanda. Characteristically, IDP mortality and morbidity rates are among the highest. Nongovernmental organizations (NGOs) have difficulties gaining access to IDPs and, in their attempts, often face danger from national or rebel forces. Populations who cross borders to flee death and prosecution are given refugee status under international law and the protective UN agency benefits, both physical and political, that these provisions provide. Once international programs are in place in refugee camps, the health indices begin to improve and in time may prove better than the neighboring country housing the camps. Crucially, similar aid programs must benefit the surrounding countryside to prevent resentment and new hostilities from erupting.

Primary care, public health and preventive medicine, infectious disease, obstetrical, and emergency medicine, all adapted to a resource poor environment, are the skills required of expatriate healthcare assets.[15] The World Health Organization (WHO) provides immediate assistance in the form of Emergency Health Kits that provide basic health supplies for a population of 10,000 for 3 months. Additional surgical and safe birthing kits are available.

Smoldering or Chronic Country Model

Countries such as Sudan, Haiti, and Gaza have experienced high levels of conflict for many decades, resulting in a suboptimal health profile (Table 27.2) with characteristics of a country suffering both developmental failure and ongoing requirements for all basic public health services (food, water, sanitation, shelter, health, and fuel) essential for survival. Absent or poorly maintained public health infrastructure results in chronic and untreated survivors of preventable diseases. Expatriate health workers and NGOs frequently serve as the rudimentary public health system for the country, but are often prevented by insecurity from providing care to persecuted and minority groups. Communicable diseases within these countries, other than HIV/AIDS, are similar to those seen in the developed world in the early 1900s.

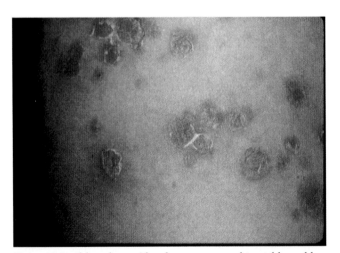

Figure 27.2. Although considered a common and treatable problem in the western world, impetigo patients are triaged as urgent in refugee camps and among internally displaced populations, especially if the victims are malnourished. Impetigo can progress rapidly from a minor skin infection to septicemia when micronutrient deficiencies and severe malnutrition exist. Photo by Frederick M. Burkle, Jr. – used with permission.

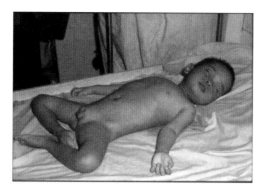

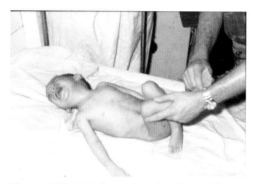

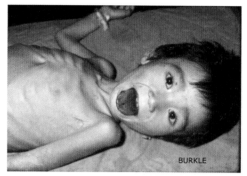

Figures 27.3–27.5. Scurvy, or vitamin C deficiency and other micronutrient deficiencies (especially A and B1) must be suspected in prolonged war where malnutrition exists. These cases, seen in Vietnam in the 1960s presented as minor bruising, severe pain when the limbs were moved, and fragile tongue lesions that easily bled. Similar cases were seen in East African camps in the 1990s when the waste diet given to refugees lacked micronutrient supplements. Vitamin C serves as a coenzyme in the metabolic reaction of clotting. Once parenteral vitamin C was administered, the pain from bleeding under the periosteum rapidly ceased. Photo by Frederick M. Burkle, Jr. – used with permission.

Because of chronic high vulnerability, these countries are more prone to adverse consequences of disasters. Haiti has suffered from increased deforestation and lack of tree-root structures that serve to protect other countries from worsening floodwaters. In recent years, uncontained floodwaters resulted in between several hundred to more than 3,000 preventable deaths from mudslides and drowning. A dilemma for the international community has been the frustration of responding to an emergency situation within a country that chronically suffers smoldering environmental decay. The environment suffers incrementally

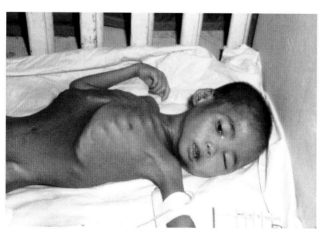

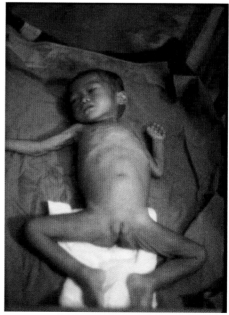

Figures 27.6–27.7. Severely dehydrated children exhibiting extreme loss of skin turgor. Examples of dehydration and malnutrition are common in complex emergencies, especially in Africa and Asia. Photo by Frederick M. Burkle, Jr. – used with permission.

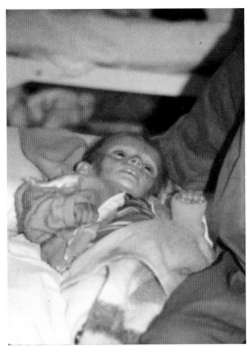

Figure 27.8. A Kurdish child with severe dehydration from diarrhea. The diagnostic "old man facies" occurs with severe loss of body water and electrolytes. Further examination was not allowed. Confirmatory laboratory tests are rarely available. These cases are usually field-managed as isotonic losses with oral rehydration. With clinical improvement the family trusted the physician to complete the physical examination. Photo by Frederick M. Burkle, Jr. – used with permission.

with each added conflict or environmental insult (e.g., drought, famine, post-hurricane flooding). Current disaster terminology may not accurately describe the problems that exist. As with Haiti and Sudan, it is unclear whether to describe these events as emergencies or as more as developmental crises. A category is needed to connote the situation of an inability of the international community, mainly restricted by existing international sovereignty laws, to intervene on the behalf of innocent civilians who may never see a sustainable lifestyle.

This model results in a chronic excess of younger than age 5 death rates. Rebel force violent surges result in an increase in adult direct death rates that often represent ethnic cleansing. A return to the chronic epidemiological picture occurs when the fleeing IDPs and refugees again succumb to preventable deaths and increased morbidity from an environment of barren desert conclaves and hastily built refugee camps (Figures 27.14–27.16).

Required professional expatriate assets are similar to that following an acute emergency in a developing country.[15] Without emphasis placed on stable governance and long-term nation-state development, including education and training of indigenous healthcare workers, these countries risk repeating similar emergency crises over and over again.

Developed Country Model

Prior to recent warfare, the former Yugoslavia, Chechnya, and Iraq enjoyed health profiles similar to that of Western industrialized countries (Table 27.3). As with the previous two

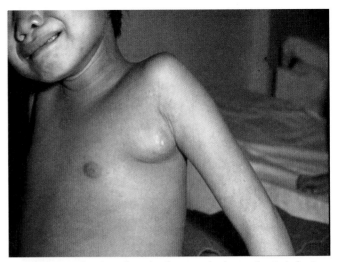

Figure 27.9. Bubonic and septic plague and other endemic infectious diseases are common when the public health infrastructure is destroyed by war and conflict. This figure illustrates an axillary bubo. Gram stain confirmed Gram negative bipolar rods. Photo by Frederick M. Burkle, Jr. – used with permission.

models, worsening political violence results in IDPs and also refugees seeking permanent asylum in willing countries. The dominance of advanced weapon–related deaths is characteristic of this model. When these weapons are fired in an indiscriminate manner, the resulting deaths by the age and sex epidemiology should reflect their representation within the baseline population demographics; however, epidemiological studies in Kosovo

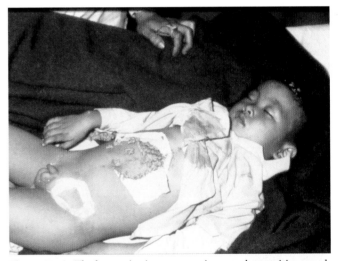

Figure 27.10. The humanitarian community must be sensitive to cultural beliefs that are not dismissed as modern medical care is added. In this toxic and comatose child, an inguinal bubo was surrounded with a lime substance believed to prevent spread. A paste material was placed over the umbilicus with "Chinese medical writings" as petitions to the "evil spirits" that caused disease. Onion flakes were placed in the hair for fever. The child had a febrile seizure immediately after this photo was taken. The mother, thinking that I had provoked an evil spirit within her child with the foreign instrument (camera) I held in my hand, fled with her child. The mother only agreed to return the child for treatment if I was removed as the healthcare provider. This being impossible, I managed the case from a distance through locally trained assistants. Photo by Frederick M. Burkle, Jr. – used with permission.

Table 27.3. Developed Country Model Health Profile

- Occur in baseline populations who are relatively healthy
- Demographic and disease profiles similar to western industrialized countries
- Excess trauma deaths from war-related advance weaponry and small arms
- Excess age and gender related deaths increase during times of ethnic cleansing
- Few epidemics
- Excess mortality from untreated chronic diseases
- Significant rates of elderly with undernutrition
- Rape, abductions, and psychological traumatic exposures common

showed excess death rates in patriarchal males and young adult males of military age. This study became pivotal in Hague war crime trials as evidence of targeted ethnic cleansing.[16]

In the former Yugoslavia, the elderly population resisted displacement and often showed rapid decline in health due to undernutrition, stress-related mental health conditions, and exacerbation of chronic diseases such as diabetes, hypertension, and cardiac disease as violence separated them from sources of their medications. Ethnic cleansing methods resulted in rape, abductions, and assassinations. Interestingly, epidemics are uncommon in this model, in part because the educated population is aware, even in the worst of conditions, of the need for some semblance of basic hygiene including hand washing.

With worsening security, attacks against civilian and military targets include increasingly lethal improvised explosive device attacks and landmine detonations. Victims exhibit unprecedented multi-organ high-velocity blast effects. Fragile civilian health systems lack the capacity to manage complicated resuscitations for multiple organ failure, multiple limb loss, acute respiratory distress syndrome, and traumatic brain injury and the specialized care required for prolonged recovery and rehabilitation.

With the emphasis on traumatic casualties, the international requirements for aid include emergency medicine, surgical, and anesthesia specialties (Figures 27.17 and 27.18).[15] Such

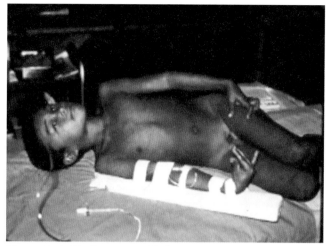

Figure 27.12. Vaccine preventable diseases are common. Tetanus arising from a foot lesion caused severe lockjaw in this 10-year old male. Hyperventilation with nasal flaring resulted in secondary tetany. This child survived with parenteral penicillin and antitoxin. Photo by Frederick M. Burkle, Jr. – used with permission.

services and resources rarely arrive from outside the country before 3 days' time. The best programs are those that use previously educated and trained indigenous healthcare providers. These local personnel assume augmented responsibilities for emergency healthcare and stabilization during and immediately after the traumatic event, with delayed surgery, intensive care,

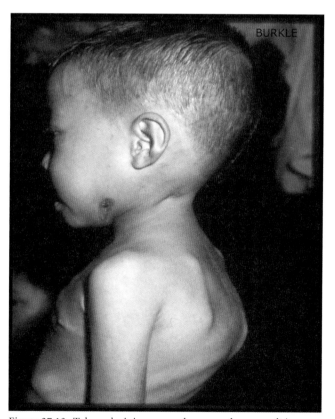

Figure 27.13. Tuberculosis is commonly seen and may result in many secondary cases in crowded camps. This child exhibits both Pott's disease and a scrofula lesion of the neck. Photo by Frederick M. Burkle, Jr. – used with permission.

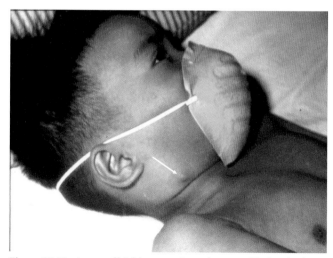

Figure 27.11. A case of highly contagious pharyngeal bubonic plague stemming from a cervical bubo with visible flea bite site. Photo by Frederick M. Burkle, Jr. – used with permission.

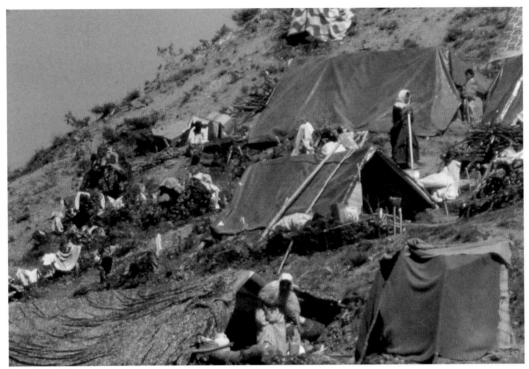

Figure 27.14. Refugee Camp Conditions in Northern Iraq, 1992. Camp demographics are critical in determining requirements and vulnerability. As Kurdish men were killed by Saddam's Iraqi forces, or were fighting to keep their own territory safe, the fleeing Iraqi Kurds were primarily children (50%), women (30%), and the elderly (20%). Logistics and healthcare in the precarious camp tents placed on the side of mountains had to adapt to unique needs. Photo by Frederick M. Burkle, Jr. – used with permission.

evacuation, and other interventions provided by the international community. It is essential that international responders provide necessary skill training to local healthcare providers so that the level of competency remains improved even after the international "experts" leave.

Communicable Diseases in CHEs

Connolly and colleagues found that communicable diseases, alone or in combination with malnutrition, account for most deaths in CHEs.[17] Disease transmission is promoted by poor and dense population conditions common to refugee camps (Figures 27.14, 27.15, and 27.16). Refugees fleeing the slaughter from small arms and machetes in Rwanda rapidly crowded makeshift camps across nation-state borders. A camp at Goma, in the former Zaire, surged to a population of more than 300,000 in 5 days. Crowding contributed to outbreaks of dysentery and cholera that killed thousands more. Whereas effective interventions are often possible in camp settings, populations covering large and poorly accessed geographical areas or entire countries pose a greater challenge. Health workers, at a minimum, must have an operational understanding of communicable diseases and the management in austere environments of diarrheal disease (watery, bloody, and non-bloody) and dehydration, acute respiratory infections, measles, tetanus, malaria, meningitis, tuberculosis, HIV/AIDS, viral hemorrhagic fevers, cholera and dysentery, and trypanosomiasis and leishmaniasis.

Standard case definitions for these diseases are critical to reduce variability in reporting. Epidemiological studies confirm, for example, that control of diarrheal diseases occurs through provision of clean water, simple hygiene practices, and sanitation systems; distribution of soap; training of clinical staff and indigenous health workers in aggressive rehydration therapies; and improved basic health services and disease detection. Western medical and nursing personnel generally lack education and training in tropical disease diagnosis and management, and lack experience with the manner in which HIV/AIDS, tuberculosis, and malaria first present with advanced complications in a resource poor environment. Management of region-specific pharmaceutical resistance must be researched before deployment, with special attention to malaria resistance and to the less frequent clinical presentations of tropical diseases such as dengue fever and Japanese B Encephalitis (Southeast Asia), and leprosy (Sudanese refugees).

There are three key elements to humanitarian interventions in communicable disease.[17]

1. Prevention and control of communicable disease
   a. Adequate campsite planning and shelter
   b. Water and sanitation
   c. Immunization
   d. Vector control
   e. Epidemic preparedness and response
2. Case management
   a. Use of standard treatment protocols
   b. Simplified and efficient drug regimens
   c. Syndromic management protocols for acute respiratory diseases and sexually transmitted diseases are often necessary where diagnostic facilities are lacking
3. Assessment, surveys, and surveillance
   a. Rapid health assessments and an initial overview of immediate consequences and needs

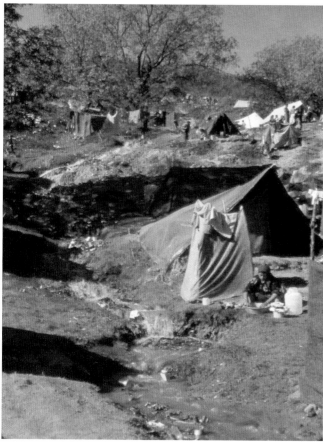

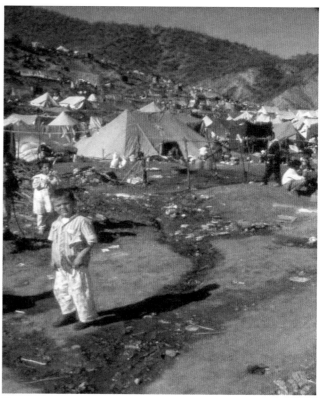

Figure 27.16. Mountain streams ended up as stagnant and polluted pools at the base of the camp where children played. Simple and easily corrected public health solutions must be sought to prevent outbreaks. Photo by Frederick M. Burkle, Jr. – used with permission.

Figure 27.15. This figure illustrates camp conditions that contributed to 80% of childhood deaths resulting from diarrhea and dehydration secondary to common waterborne bacteria and viruses. Water from melting snow that ran through the camp was polluted by makeshift toilet facility runoff and the washing of soiled laundry. Photo by Frederick M. Burkle, Jr. – used with permission.

preventable childhood disease, such as measles, highlight the inherent threat to the immune system that results from malnutrition and micronutrient disease. Micronutrient diseases such as vitamin A deficiency, even without other

  b. Surveys consisting of intermittent, focused assessments that gather population-based health data
  c. Surveillance consisting of ongoing, systematic gathering, analysis, and interpretation of health data

Trends and baseline epidemiological information are critical for program and mission interpretation and as measures of long-term effectiveness and post-conflict recovery and rehabilitation.

Malnutrition and Micronutrient Diseases in CHEs

Food shortages may be generalized across the entire population, limited to the most politically and economically vulnerable within certain ethnic, religious, or minority groups, or found only in IDPs and refugees. A challenge for proper nutrition is that the cost of basic foods such as rice, maize, sugar, and wheat has skyrocketed in many countries. The most vulnerable in these populations are children, especially infants and children younger than 5 years of age and those unaccompanied or orphaned, women both pregnant and lactating, the elderly, and the disabled. Mortality and morbidity are most often the result of communicable diseases and malnutrition or a combination of the two (Figures 27.2–27.8). Death due to measles is rare in a non-malnourished population.[18] In CHEs, deaths from the complications of a simple and

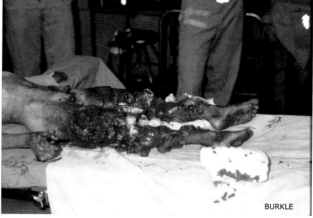

Figure 27.17. A preadolescent male who built a mine to kill "occupying forces" and accidentally triggered the device, sustaining these severe injuries. More visible hemorrhage was prevented by massive vasoconstriction physiologically available as a last measure before death in children. With anesthesia, this hormonal protection ceased and he rapidly lost what remained of his meager blood volume. In this case, the surgical team was aware of this risk and instituted protective blood, fluids, and venous access before anesthesia was begun. Decoding of vital signs, looking for fragile stroke volume losses, is a required skill when western monitoring technologies are unavailable. Photo by Frederick M. Burkle, Jr. – used with permission.

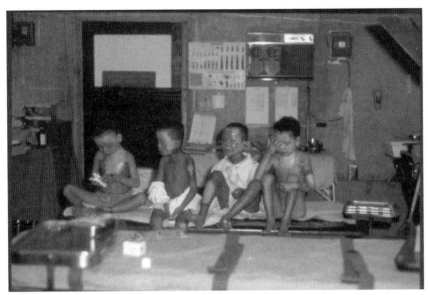

Figure 27.18. All resources are scarce and must be efficiently used without wastefulness. In this figure, multiple burn patients received care using the contents of a single surgical pack. This pack was also aged and contained World War II–era sulfa powder. Photo by Frederick M. Burkle, Jr. – used with permission.

manifestations of malnutrition, inhibit biochemical and cellular protective processes essential to infectivity and pathogenicity of an infectious agent.

Malnutrition is best appreciated as a combined threat of protein, energy, and micronutrient deficiencies referred to as protein-energy malnutrition. It is characterized by four therapeutic elements, all of which must be addressed in every malnourished victim.

1. Overall nutritional status is rapidly assessed first by mid-upper arm circumference in both children and adults, followed by surveys using more specific weight-for-height measures, and then long term through surveillance-based Z-scores.
2. Micronutrient deficiencies, especially vitamins A, C, and B6, are common and assumed to be present in severe malnutrition, but additional deficiencies should be assessed based on known regional and geographical deficiencies such as iron and iodine. If disorders such as scurvy, beriberi, pellagra, and xerophthalmia are prevalent in the population, all those with severe malnutrition should be assumed to have deficits in the micronutrients that lead to these diseases until proven otherwise.
3. Assume all those who are malnourished are either harboring an infectious disease or are susceptible to one and its complications. Severely malnourished are often unable to mount fever, positive skin tests (tuberculosis), or leukocytosis as indications of an occult infectious disease. Even when skin tests are positive, it is frequently unclear whether this is the result of prior Bacille Calmette-Guérin (BCG) immunization rather than acute tuberculosis infection. This is especially challenging since WHO recommends BCG vaccine be administered at birth in the developing world.
4. Assume all malnourished children to be dehydrated. Hydration must be addressed immediately with determination of whether dietary supplementation alone or hospital-based

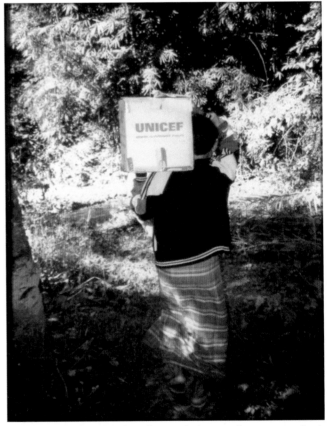

Figure 27.19. The majority of resupply in complex emergencies is through local logistical networks such as these rehydration salts, from the United Nations Children's Fund (UNICEF), being trekked through jungle trails along the Burmese border to a refugee camp run by the International Rescue Committee. Photo by Frederick M. Burkle, Jr. – used with permission.

therapies are required. The international community rarely provides parenteral rehydration, even in cases of cholera. Studies suggest, and clinical experience confirms, that oral rehydration is as effective as or better than parenteral rehydration, even in the most severe cases.[19] Oral rehydration is also much cheaper, logistically easier to use, and less labor intensive (Figure 27.19). International workers must gain experience and confidence in oral rehydration techniques and rehydration salts designed for austere environments.

Children entering a camp setting are assumed to be vitamin A deficient with no immunity to measles. Effective humanitarian assistance requires immediate measles immunization, vitamin A supplementation, and possibly prophylactic antibiotic coverage. Humanitarian relief efforts in developing countries are directed toward support of breast-feeding with extra rations and micronutrient supplementation to mothers, identifying those infants and children requiring wet nurse supplementation, and supplementary and therapeutic feedings (with hospitalization) for those most severely ill and malnourished. Women in developed countries at war (e.g., former Yugoslavia) more often than not have adopted many developed country habits such as bottle-feeding while working outside the home. Rates of breast milk substitute use of 60% or more provoke a crisis when outside supplies cease as the war escalates. The humanitarian community in the former Yugoslavia and other developed countries in crisis had no option but to rapidly reorganize the logistics system to supply and distribute breast milk substitute and weaning foods.

Psychosocial and Mental Health Problems

Assessment instruments and interventions developed in western countries are medically focused (emphasizing diagnosis and treatment of selected individuals) and rarely assess their cross-cultural impact or accuracy. Individuals suffering from psychosocial and mental health problems often present differently depending on their environments (Figure 27.20). They require interventions adapted to their situations and culture. Many interventions promoted over the last three decades are not based on sound scientific evidence or best practices, and they have not been evaluated for their feasibility or effectiveness in the contexts in which they are being used, especially among multicultural populations.[20]

Current thinking recommends interventions that promote unity of psychosocial, mental health, and public health approaches while equally emphasizing community and medically based programs along with traditional multicultural and family-centered structures. This approach helps in clarifying that extreme human rights abuses, so prevalent in humanitarian crises, will no longer be simply medicalized. It forces an appreciation that a broader psychosocial, mental health, and public health services approach is necessary to address the variety of cultural, religious, and political factors that threaten well-being among these populations (Figure 27.21).

Culture can be considered, in part, to be a collection of coping mechanisms or behaviors shared by a group of people. These behaviors are learned ways of navigating the world safely, and having been developed and refined over centuries, these behaviors are often recognized as defining a culture and its strengths. CHEs, especially those resulting in displacement, involve upheaval to the extent that many of these behaviors are

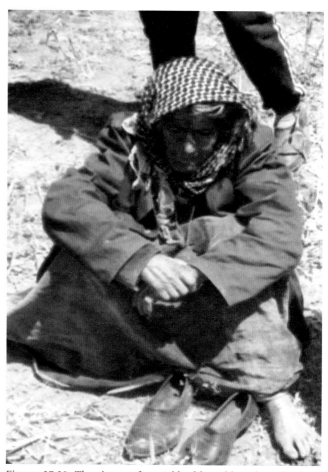

Figures 27.20. The picture of mental health problems brought about by war depicts an elderly and overtly psychotic woman abandoned by her family to U.S. military forces believing that the United States held magical powers to cure her mental illness. Photo by Frederick M. Burkle, Jr. – used with permission.

no longer appropriate or possible. Psychosocial programming in the immediate period after a crisis should include approaches aimed at making as many of these behaviors as possible appropriate and possible once more.[21,22] This consists of reestablishing many of the physical and social structures that existed prior to the disaster.

- Reconnecting families
- Reconnecting communities
- Reestablishing security

Risk Factors

CHEs produce risk factors that increase both individual and population propensity for developing psychosocial and mental health problems and for compounding the severity of disease in persons with existing psychological conditions.[22–24] Behavior of neglected and abused mentally ill in a refugee camp setting can lead to an erosive impact on the fragile social fabric of displaced communities. Additional factors include, but are not limited to:

- Poor health and nutrition;
- Separation from family and caregivers (Figure 27.22);
- Suboptimum perinatal care, neglect, and under-stimulation of children;

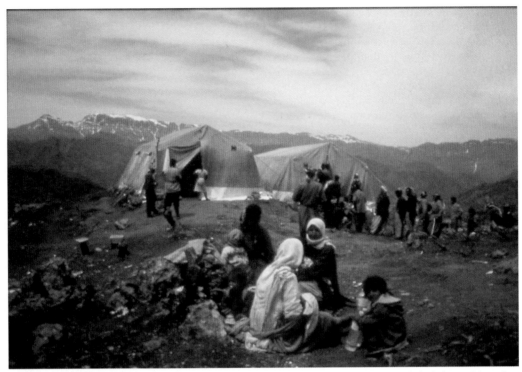

Figure 27.21. Makeshift Tents for Women on the Left and Infants on the Right. Kurdish fathers objected to the resuscitative measures taken on their ill infants, claiming that death was dictated by religious beliefs. The humanitarian community must recognize cultural, religious, and ethnic restrictions and develop a dialogue that both addresses and balances health requirements and local values. Photo by Frederick M. Burkle, Jr. – used with permission.

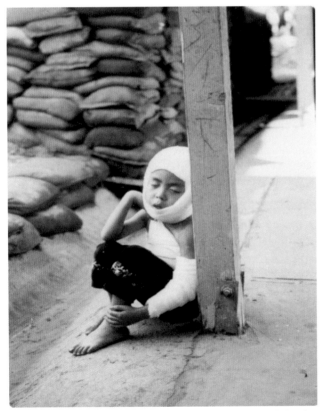

Figure 27.22. The last remaining survivor when her family's bunker was destroyed in an air raid, this child was mute and refused to be held or receive care within the hospital wards. Photo by Frederick M. Burkle, Jr. – used with permission.

- Exposure to chronic communicable diseases that affect the brain;
- Risk of traumatic epilepsy; and
- Exposure to extreme and repeated stress and sleep deprivation.

War, conflict, and camp conditions often place those with existing conditions at greater risk for:

- Abuse, including gross dereliction, stigma, ostracism, and sexual violence;
- Child abduction, youth violence/death;
- Family separation and displacement;
- Neglect or abandonment by family and caretakers;
- Exploitation (Figure 27.23);
- Destruction of supportive institutions and services, including psychiatric facilities and medications;
- Life-threatening physical illnesses;
- Suicide;
- Conditions that foment hatred and revenge; and
- Unremitting conditions that lead to worsening disability and premature death, especially among the elderly.

Interventions

Common guiding principles and strategies for the humanitarian community in developing interventions for populations exposed to extreme stressors include:[22–25]

- Contingency planning before the acute emergency;
- Assessment before intervention;
- Inclusion of long-term development perspectives;

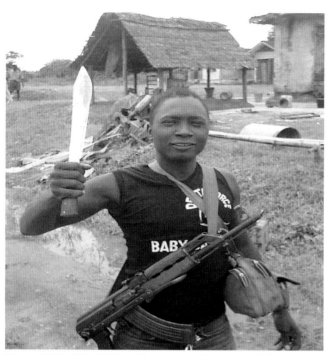

Figure 27.23. This child soldier was a self-designated "general" in the rebellion against the Taylor regime in Liberia. Threatening and unpredictable, he also demonstrated childlike behaviors and needs. Originally from Sierra Leone, he was abducted at the age of 8 and knew nothing but war and killing. Photo by Frederick M. Burkle, Jr. – used with permission.

- Collaboration between agencies;
- Provision of treatment in primary care and community settings;
- Access to services for all in need;
- Training and supervision; and
- Monitoring indicators, including project impact.

Immediate psychosocial interventions should focus on supporting public health activities aimed at reducing mortality and morbidity, mitigating the burden on the community of managing the seriously mentally ill who need specialized psychiatric care, and mobilizing community-based resiliency and adaptation to new circumstances affecting people during the emergency. These immediate interventions may mitigate more serious mental illness in a large portion of the affected population.

The challenge for the humanitarian community is to support the population in the displacement camp. Humanitarian agencies and UN agency organizations usually have limited resources and are faced with displaced populations with overwhelming needs. Experience has shown that projects imported to manage behavioral and mental health problems frequently lack cross-cultural sensitivities or benefits and may prove detrimental. Such programs and their inexperienced personnel have no place in these critical situations. Indigenous and expatriate mental health professionals with specific skills should be properly identified and vetted to provide the best value-added expertise to a community-based approach. In doing so, they will provide care where most needed. Psychiatric, psychological, and social work practitioners trained in developed countries may play a critical role in training; providing consultation, supervision, and specialized care to the most seriously mentally ill; and providing assess-

ments and evidence-based investigations, preferably through a culturally sensitive partnership with the local population, indigenous healers, and caregivers. Limited resources must be directed to improve capacity of family basic survival needs through a community-oriented approach.

Psychosocial and mental health services need to be provided through both primary healthcare and community settings. Presentations tend to fall into three categories:[25]

1. Severe psychological reactions to trauma
2. Significant behavioral signs and symptoms in individuals who may be able to cope and adapt once peace and order are restored (this subgroup generally represents the majority of the population)
3. Disabling psychiatric illnesses (new or exacerbation of existing illnesses)

THOSE SUFFERING FROM SEVERE PSYCHOLOGICAL REACTIONS TO TRAUMA

Displacement from home and familiar cultural and religious surroundings may cause cognitive and emotional disorganization in the displaced population. This is often catalyzed by some degree of "experienced brutality" (e.g., rape, physical and mental torture, witnessing of killings of family and friends), which because of fear of possible reprisal and stigma may not be easily or readily revealed to healthcare workers. Beyond the physical suffering that occurs, displaced people are often deprived of their livelihoods and suffer a loss of identity, purpose, and community. Displacement camps are frequently crowded, poorly designed, and inadequately serviced. When war and conflict damage traditional ways of life, cultural bereavement, along with individual bereavement, can be key determinants of psychological distress. It is not uncommon that once the displaced population witnesses success in the ethnically relevant community programs for the severely mentally ill, the same programs may see increased numbers presenting with acute trauma-related symptoms. This suggests that the initial barriers of stigma and suspicion tend to decrease with time.

Options for programming include both population-based interventions and conventional, "western-oriented," one-on-one therapies. Mental health disorders common to displaced populations without a history of mental illness but with history of trauma exposure (including manifestations in children and adolescents), include several of the psychiatric diagnoses defined in the *Diagnostic and Statistical Manual of Mental Disorders* (DSM-5).

- Situational depression and major depressive disorder;
- Drug and alcohol use;
- Somatization;
- Anxiety;
- Post-traumatic stress disorder (PTSD); and
- Comorbidity of depression and PTSD.

Claims of large populations experiencing PTSD have limited evidence; research suggests that only a minority of those exposed to mass violence suffer from this disorder, with numbers varying from 4–20%.[23–25] A purely medical model of intervention that focuses on PTSD to the exclusion of other diagnoses is problematic in that it may fail to address other issues that present in the population; however, epidemiological evidence indicates that symptoms commonly associated with both PTSD and depression are identified in most cultures. Ethnographic assessments that recognize culturally determined language for relevant symptoms may help identify individuals suffering from these disorders.

THOSE PRESENTING WITH SIGNIFICANT PSYCHOSOCIAL AND/OR BEHAVIORAL PROBLEMS WHO MAY BE ABLE TO ADAPT AND COPE ONCE STABILITY IS RESTORED

Complaints presenting in this group generally differ in degree and these persons often demonstrate a greater ability to cope and adapt. Culture and community cohesiveness determines, to a large extent, how war, trauma, and displacement are experienced and what coping mechanisms are used. Programmatic emphasis can be placed on community-based initiatives that focus on strengthening family and kinship ties; promoting indigenous healing methods; facilitating community participation in decision making; fostering leadership structures; and reestablishing spiritual, religious, social, and cultural institutions and practices that restore a framework of cohesion and purpose for the whole community. The goal is to encourage and strengthen pre-event coping and adaptive capacities of the population. Program strategies are developed to reduce stress and encourage normal activities and active participation of those displaced.[25] Examples include:

- Establishing cultural and religious events, including funeral ceremonies and grieving rituals involving spiritual and religious practitioners;
- Restarting formal or informal schooling and recreational activities;
- Promoting adult and adolescent participation in relief activities, especially those that facilitate the inclusion of social networks of people without families;
- Organizing community-based self-help support groups, especially focused on problem-sharing, brainstorming for solutions and effective ways of coping, and mutual emotional support and community-level initiatives; and
- Economic redevelopment initiatives such as microcredit or income-generating activities.

The psychosocial and mental health response in the immediate post-disaster period often emphasizes this type of approach. In addition, a program commonly called Psychological First Aid can be introduced.[26] It is an assessment strategy and an intervention that entails basic, nonintrusive pragmatic care. The focus is on listening but not forcing talk, assessing needs and ensuring that basic needs are met, encouraging but not forcing company from significant others, and protecting people from further harm. With this approach many of the "symptoms" of mental health disorders may resolve, increasing the likelihood that those who continue to have symptoms have specific disorders requiring specific treatment.

THOSE SUFFERING FROM DISABLING PSYCHIATRIC ILLNESSES

Psychoses and severe mood disorders (including DSM-5–defined diagnoses of major depression and bipolar disease) cause considerable disability in every culture worldwide. How these disorders are conceptualized, recognized, and managed across cultures and in a conflict or post-conflict situation may differ considerably. Although it may be possible to diagnose psychotic disorders that were present prior to the event after a crisis occurs, providing sustained and effective treatment may be diffi-

cult. This places considerable stress on the families of those with severe illness and may exacerbate the ongoing stress to the camp population especially if their behaviors are disruptive or even dangerous. For anxiety and mood disorders that existed before the disaster, it is often impossible to distinguish the symptoms of these disorders from normal responses to an overwhelming crisis event.

Although emergency health services are usually void of mental health personnel, including psychiatrists, some promise has been found among programs that use local psychiatric nurses and community volunteers to provide services. Whenever possible, psychiatric interventions should be included as part of the established primary healthcare system, but even these resources may be severely lacking.

For the severely mentally ill, the impact of treatment is frequently dramatic, with reintroduction of antipsychotic medications and supportive community follow-up that can include rehabilitation in traditional family structures. In camps, community volunteers can provide outreach services, family education and support, and links to other agencies that can assist with rehabilitation. Basic needs of patients in custodial psychiatric hospitals must be addressed if the crisis becomes protracted.

Newer psychotropic medications, often those familiar to foreign aid workers with experience in psychiatric treatment, are both scarce and prohibitively expensive. Aid workers must advocate for what is best for the populations they are attempting to serve and coordinate these requirements with the ability of local healthcare workers to sustain any medications from outside resources.[21]

Measuring and Monitoring Effectiveness

In general, the key psychological and psychiatric functional indicators based on Sphere standards for interventions are:[7]

- Individuals experiencing acute mental health distress after exposure to traumatic stressors have access to psychological first aid at health services facilities and in the community.
- Care for urgent psychiatric complaints is available through the primary healthcare system.
- Individuals with known psychiatric disorders continue to receive relevant treatment; harmful, sudden discontinuation of medications is avoided.

The International Response to CHEs and the Changing Face of Humanitarian Assistance

The UN Charter was launched at the end of World War II in 1945 to handle declared cross-border wars that resulted in large numbers of refugees. The Geneva Convention and International Humanitarian Law guided aid interventions. Much effort was placed on ensuring that the practice of humanitarian care was steered by the "humanitarian principles" of neutrality, impartiality, universality, and independence. By the 1990s and the end of the Cold War, unconventional, intrastate, prolonged conflict and warfare began to dominate international crises. The Geneva Convention, written to protect populations from the influence of cross-border wars, became less relevant. By the turn of the century, non-declared unconventional wars became the norm along with the rise of non-state actors and social media–driven nation-state revolts (e.g., Arab Spring), and the inclusion of private groups and militaries all claiming a humanitarian role. In addition, conflicts are complicated by the ominous influences of climate change extremes that drive out populations, especially IDPs seeking security in urban conclaves, and increasing numbers of distributional conflicts related to scarcity of water, food, and energy resources. Many in the humanitarian community are no longer working in war zones but in crime scenes (e.g., Democratic Republic of Congo) where organized armed violence is not fought on ideological principles but due to greed over natural resources such as petroleum, gold, diamonds, uranium, copper, silver, phosphate, and plutonium just to name a few. Today, over half of UN peacekeeping forces are deployed to locations where these natural resources play an active role in the armed conflict.

Western-dominated aid is changing rapidly. Security for humanitarian workers depends on the perception that workers are independent, neutral, and impartial. Humanitarian aid, especially since the Iraq and Afghanistan wars, is seen as a pretext for occupation or an alibi for western domination and where aid workers are targeted not for their assets and resources but rather as unwelcome outsiders. Violence against aid workers increased steadily since 2004, although between 2011 and 2012 began to drop. Still, over 187 incidents of aid worker deliberate violence were recorded in 2012, with 46 workers killed, 54 injured, and 87 kidnapped.[27] More aid workers have been killed than UN peacekeepers, making aid work one of the deadliest occupations from increasing targeted killings, hostage taking, kidnapping, armed raids, ambushes, carjacking, illicit taxing, and prevention of access to beneficiaries. This has led to the doubling of closures or yearly suspensions of critical aid projects. Western-based aid agencies rely more on remote administration and programming and depend on unsupervised indigenous workers. In the second decade of the twenty-first century, half of the world's beneficiaries of aid are Muslim. New Muslim NGOs and non-state organizations increasingly provide humanitarian aid, but international oversight is lacking, especially in the guarantee that humanitarian principles are being practiced (e.g., Syrian War).

The UN Charter language inadequately addresses internal conflict and the genocidal actions that dominate modern-day emergencies. Sovereignty of individual nation states is steadfastly protected under the present Charter and severely limits the UN from entering any sovereign country to protect a minority population from ethnic cleansing and outright genocidal acts. Article II, Part 7, right of sovereignty reads: "Nothing contained in the present Charter shall authorize the United Nations to intervene in matters which are essentially within the domestic jurisdiction of any state."[28]

Only the UN Security Council has legal authority to respond militarily. The peacekeeping and peace enforcement actions permitted under Security Council Resolutions to cease internal nation-state conflicts are often too little and too late in protecting these populations. Operational successes occurred in the Kurdish crisis of Northern Iraq, the Balkans, and East Timor, but little changed the overall course of conflicts in the poverty-stricken, remote, and austere environments of Rwanda and the Democratic Republic of the Congo or during the prolonged debacles in the Sudan, Somalia, and later Syria.

The UN-led humanitarian response community – made up of NGOs; the Red Cross Movement (resources from both the International Committee of the Red Cross and the Federation of Red Cross and Red Crescent National Societies); UN agencies such as UNICEF, WHO, the UN High Commissioner for Refugees; and others – has worked to protect civilian populations both within conflicted countries and on their borders. Over the last three decades, however, this traditional UN-led multi-national response system has been criticized for being ad hoc, unprepared, under-resourced, and overwhelmed by legal restrictions of an ill-equipped UN system. Without a major reform of the UN Charter that would favor human rights over exclusive sovereignty and include a standing UN task force of their own, the role of the UN in addressing any internal conflicts will remain limited in the future.

With increasing insecurity in places such as Iraq and Afghanistan, the political preference by western-led coalitions has been to bypass the UN-led system and traditional humanitarian community in favor of a non-UN military force. Humanitarian relief and reconstruction operations have been led by military resources and private contractors. Claims that these partnerships have succeeded when the UN-led humanitarian community has failed are in doubt.

Globalization has strengthened many Asian countries that have become economically interdependent with western industrialized countries. When the 2004 Indian Ocean tsunami occurred, a Western-led consortium of military assets (from the United States, India, Australia, Japan, Canada, and others), the World Bank, like-minded NGOs, and private contractors responded with the goal of ensuring rapid economic recovery. The consortium referred to the tsunami disaster as a CHE because two affected countries, Aceh Province in Indonesia and Sri Lanka, have ongoing rebel insurgencies. Less economically developed areas of the world remain dependent on the conventional, underfunded, and under-resourced UN-led humanitarian community that is driven by rights-based humanitarianism. Whether either of these models will persist in the midst of donor country and international organization political change remains to be seen.[29,30]

Judt suggests that future coalitions of the willing will be powerless to respond appropriately to large-scale "natural disasters, famine, droughts, floods, resource wars, population movements, economic crises, and regional pandemics" and "will have to act through others in collaboration, cooperation, and with little reference to separate national interests or boundaries."[30] The UN and its agencies, such as WHO, UNICEF, and the UN High Commission for Refugees, have mature and tested "inter-national early-warning, assessment, response, and coordination mechanisms for when states fray and collapse." The UN works best in handling crises "when everyone acknowledges the legitimacy of its role."[31] Major power political interference and influence impedes the opportunity for the UN to fulfill leadership in a consistent and predictable manner. In the meantime, it is not known how the world will manage future complex humanitarian and other large-scale public health emergencies.

RECOMMENDATIONS FOR FURTHER RESEARCH

As stated, even though the absolute number of CHEs has declined, the list of countries in crisis remains long with little information on the impact of these crises available for monitoring and evaluation. The world community must find new ways to prevent instability in fragile countries and apply resources that emphasize political and economic sustainability. Furthermore, a professional civil–military approach is desirable to many of these crises, but political competition, relevant education and training, funding, and lack of a modern-day UN Charter, among many other factors, have severely limited progress toward these good intentions.

Research critical to conflict studies remains unattended, especially in topic areas concerned with: vulnerable populations, advances in international law that address access and protection, public health priorities, and sustainability. Awareness driven by globalization, especially Internet access to information, has led the world's population to expect equity, transparency, and accountability in global health and humanitarian assistance. Populations have little tolerance for responses that are imperfect, ad hoc, and politically motivated. There are concerns that disaster management issues, especially those resulting from public health emergencies, if not fully addressed, will further complicate the widening rift between the world's haves and have-nots. Recent events suggest that disasters occurring in countries economically interdependent with economic powers will receive robust relief that is directed at rapidly recovering the economy. In contrast, disasters in economically poor countries will be left to depend on fragile UN–, UN agency–, and Red Cross/Red Crescent Movement–led responses that have limited funding and resources. Such inequities are apt to foment additional political unrest. Furthermore, a previously unrecognized public health overlap between conventional disasters and CHEs has been described. Conventional disasters and CHEs can occur during or following either event, and epidemics commonly occur during CHEs. Unlike the findings in CHEs, the data do not support the often-repeated assertion that "epidemics, especially large-scale epidemics, commonly occur following large-scale conventional disasters." This emphasizes that training and tools are needed to help bridge the gap between the different types of organizations and professionals who respond to conventional disasters and CHEs to ensure an integrated and coordinated response.[32] Similarly, researchers have suggested that climate change induced drought and water scarcity have also increased the risk for conflict, presumably as populations compete over diminishing availability and access to food products. However, the link between climate change and war is unclear and has forced researchers to recognize the multidisciplinary possibilities, both physical and social (quantitative and qualitative) that might build the connections leading to conflict.[33]

Public health is no longer relegated only to issues of healthcare and prevention. Rather, public health is being redefined to include transportation, communications, public safety, judiciary, good governance, and many other critical entities that are necessary for a village, a nation, and the global community to function. Public health and health indices have and will always be one of the most sensitive measures of the recovery process and its ultimate success or failure. Indeed, despite all the attention and resources that CHEs have received over the last three decades, the state of health of women and children, especially in disaster prone areas, has declined. Public health and agricultural infrastructure in both developing and developed countries have not expanded to meet population and maintenance demands. CHEs, which were first considered "water wars" in some resource areas of the world, must now be seen as public health (infrastructure and system) wars in deprived areas that lack the buffer capacity to respond to the insults that disasters provoke. Public health must take precedence over politics and must not be driven by political motives. Disasters keep nation states and the global community honest by revealing vulnerabilities in the public health system and infrastructure. Through immediate recognition that public health systems and infrastructure play a monumental role in the consequences and recovery of large-scale disasters, public health will be seen in a new light. This involves focusing on strategic and security issues that deserve heightened attention, including an international monitoring system and international law protections. If this does not become a priority, public health emergencies will continue to increase as a pivotal challenge for future disaster managers and the global community.

REFERENCES

1. Stephens KU, Grew D, Chin K, et al. Excess mortality in the aftermath of Hurricane Katrina: A preliminary report. *Disaster Med Public Health Prepare* 2007; 1(1): 16–20.
2. Burkle FM. Complex humanitarian emergencies: A review of epidemiological and response models. *J Postgrad Med* 2006; 52(2): 109–114.
3. Zwi A, Ugalde A. Towards an epidemiology of political violence in the Third World. *Soc Sci Med* 1989; 28(7): 633–642.
4. Burkholder BT, Toole MJ. Evolution of complex disasters. *Lancet* 1995; 346: 1012–1015.
5. Clapp J. Hunger and the Post-2015 Development Agenda. Triple Crisis: Global Perspectives on Finance, Development, and Environment. http://triplecrisis.com/hunger-and-the-post-2015-development-agenda (Accessed June 22, 2013).
6. Human Security Report 2005: War and Peace in the 21st Century. Human Security Centre, University of British Columbia, Canada. Oxford, Oxford University Press, 2005; 123–144.
7. *Humanitarian Charter and Minimum Standards in Disaster Response.* Geneva, The Sphere Project/Oxfam, UK, 2004 (Revised).
8. Ghobarth H, Huth P, Russett B. The long-term consequences of civil war on public health. *Soc Sci Med* 2004; 59: 869–884.
9. Ghobarth H, Huth P, Russett B. Civil wars kill and maim people long after the shooting stops. *Am Pol Sci Rev* 2003; 97(2): 189–202.
10. UN Office for the Coordinator of Humanitarian Affairs. Gender-based violence: a silent, vicious epidemic. IRIN In-Depth. www.irinnews.org/IndepthMain.aspx?IndepthId=20&ReportId=62814 (Accessed November 20, 2008).
11. UNICEF. Water and Sanitation. http://www.unicefusa.org/work/water (Accessed June 22, 2013).
12. Dengue fever, a man-made disease. *The Economist.* May 2, 1998; 21(U.S. print edition).
13. Save the Children. State of the world's mothers: 2006. Saving the lives of mothers and newborns. http://www.savethe children.org/publications/mothers/2006/SOWM_2006_final.pdf (Accessed November 20, 2008).
14. Roberts L, Hoffman CA. Assessing the impact of humanitarian assistance in the health sector. *Emerg Themes Epidemiol* 2004; 1: 3.
15. VanRooyen MJ, Eliades MJ, Grabowski JG, et al. Medical relief personnel in complex emergencies: Perceptions of effectiveness in the former Yugoslavia. *Prehosp Disaster Med* 2001; 16(3): 145–149.
16. Spiegel PB, Salama P. War and mortality in Kosovo, 1998–99: an epidemiological testimony. *Lancet* 2000; 355(9222): 2204–2209.
17. Connolly MA, Gayer M, Ryan MJ, et al. Communicable diseases in complex emergencies: Impact and challenges. *Lancet* 2004; 364(9449): 1974–1983.
18. Koenig KL, Burns MJ, Alassaf W. Identify-Isolate-Inform: A Tool for Initial Detection and Management of Measles Patients in the Emergency Department. *WestJEM* 2015. http://escholarship.org/uc/item/0sz9b7kp (Accessed August 8, 2015).

19. Curioso WH, Miranda JJ, Kimball AM. Learning from low income countries: What are the lessons? Community oral rehydration units can contain cholera epidemics. *Br Med J* 2004; 329(7475): 1183–1184.

20. Van Ommeren M, Saxena S, Saraceno B. Mental and social health during and after acute emergencies: emerging consensus? *Bull World Health Organ* 2005; 83: 71–76.

21. Silove D, Ekblad S, Mollica R. The rights of the severely mentally ill in post-conflict societies. *Lancet* 2000; 355: 1548–1549.

22. Silove D. The psychological effects of torture, mass human rights violations, and refugee trauma: Toward an integrated conceptual framework. *J Nerv Mental Dis* 1999; 187: 200–207.

23. Mollica RF, Lopes-Cardoza B, Osofsky HJ, et al. Mental health in complex emergencies. *Lancet* 2004; 364: 2058–2067.

24. Mental health in emergencies: Psychological and social aspects of health of populations exposed to extreme stressors. Geneva, World Health Organization. 2003. www.who.int/_mental_health/media/en/640.pdf (Accessed November 20, 2008).

25. Burkle FM, Chatterjee P, Bass J, Bolton P. Guidelines for the psycho-social and mental health assessment and management of displaced populations in humanitarian crises. In: *Public Health Guide for Emergencies*. Geneva and Baltimore, International Federation of Red Cross and Red Crescent Societies and Johns Hopkins University Medical Institutions, 2008.

26. United States Department of Veterans Affairs. Psychological First Aid: Field Operations Guide. www.medicalreservecorps.gov/file/mrc_resources/mrc_pfa.doc (Accessed December 2, 2008).

27. Aid Worker Security Database. 2012. https://aidworkersecurity.org (Accessed June 22, 2013).

28. Charter of the United Nations. www.un.org/aboutun/charter/unflag.htm (Accessed November 20, 2008).

29. Burkle FM. Globalization and disaster management: public health, state capacity and political action. *J Intl Affairs* 2006; 59(2): 241–265.

30. Bello W. The rise of the relief-and-reconstruction complex. *J Intl Affairs* 2006; 59(2): 281–297.

31. Judt T. Is the UN Doomed? *The New York Review of Books*. February 15, 2007; 54(2). www.nybooks.com/articles/article-preview?article_id=19876 (Accessed November 20, 2008).

32. Spiegel PB, Le P, Ververs MT, Salama P. Occurrence and overlap of natural disasters, complex emergencies and epidemics during the past decade (1995–2004). *Confl Health* 2007; 1(1): 2.

33. Solow AR. A call for peace on climate and conflict. Comment. *Nature* May 9, 2013; 497: 179–180.

28

PATIENT IDENTIFICATION AND TRACKING

Andreas Ziegler

OVERVIEW

Patient identification and tracking is one of the greatest challenges in disaster management. The difficulty in tracking disaster victims has been highlighted not only for disasters affecting developing countries as in the 2004 Indian Ocean tsunami or the Haiti earthquake,[1] but also for disasters in high income industrialized countries as illustrated by Hurricane Katrina in the United States[2,3] or the 2011 Tōhoku Earthquake and Tsunami.[4]

Events of all sizes present challenges for patient tracking. This includes time-limited multiple casualty incidents (MCIs). Reports document logistical challenges for emergency services personnel,[7] including difficulties in determining where patients are transported,[5,6] even in situations where the initial number of patients is known.[8,9]

MCI management doctrines contribute to the patient tracking challenges. These principles include that patients are categorized according to their treatment and transport priorities and, to avoid overburdening a single facility, conveyed to multiple hospitals and by various types of vehicles and agencies (sometimes using mutual aid). Hospitals in turn may initiate secondary transfers of patients to other facilities with appropriate treatment capabilities. In addition, depending on the country and system, many patients spontaneously leave the scene and present to hospitals without evaluation and treatment by prehospital personnel.

Even in events with an intact transportation and communication infrastructure, the environment can be challenging[10,11] since responders will converge from multiple jurisdictions and rapidly engage in non-routine activities.[12] This scenario will also affect the quality of record keeping. While each entity involved will likely attempt to document the care provided, there may not be a single body that amasses all patient encounter data quickly enough to facilitate situational overview.

Small-scale events without infrastructure disruptions also commonly result in communications disruptions (e.g., use of radios on different channels). Communications may completely fail (e.g., breakdown of mobile phone networks due to overload).

Situations with infrastructure destruction will create even greater hurdles for effective response.[1] The influx of responders will be larger[12,13] and will require additional layers of coordination.[10]

In addition to tracking patients requiring medical care, disaster managers must track evacuees[2,14] who left their homes either because of destruction or due to imminent hazards (e.g., those present after the 2011 Tōhoku Earthquake and Tsunami).

A large number of shelter sites[14] or repeated relocation will make tracking of evacuees even more difficult. After Hurricane Katrina, researchers reported that families were relocated an average of 3.5 times, with a maximum of 9 times.[2] Families can also be separated during complex or prolonged disasters. Children are particularly vulnerable to separation from their families. Chung et al. reported that 7% of parents did not recognize their child in a photograph.[15] Consequently family reunification has been identified as a major issue in disaster management. All of these issues are magnified in conflict situations.

Importance of Patient Tracking

Although difficult, proper identification and tracking of patients and evacuees is an indispensable component of any effective response to MCIs and disasters. Several themes illustrate this need.

Proper Allocation of Resources by a Common Operational Picture

Real-time information and the ability to effectively communicate it are essential elements of disaster management.[7,16] Situational awareness[10] is critical to inform real-time decision making during rapidly evolving events. It is of particular importance in medical responses, where the effective use of limited resources has direct implications on the management and survival of casualties.[17,18]

Examples of limited resources include specialized transportation means and unique hospital capabilities.[4] Investigators have described segmentation of response (various agencies from multiple jurisdictions) as a main obstacle to sufficient information sharing.[19]

Psychological Impact of Uncertainty

Not knowing about the fate of family members, relatives, and friends can be unbearable and create as much, or more, anxiety than actual destruction and loss of property.[2] Uninjured relatives enter the "victimization cycle" as soon as they grasp the possibility that their family members belong to the victims.[20] Effects of the disaster rapidly spread beyond the actual disaster site or sites and may cause public distress.[5]

Experts suggest that uncertainty may be worse than receiving confirmation of death.[2,20] Immediate provision of information – which must be based on proper identification and tracking – is vital to enable effective family support and alleviate public distress.[21]

Workload for Healthcare Facilities

Healthcare facilities may have increased workload if uninjured relatives seek information about their potentially involved family members either in person or via phone or other means of communication; this may overwhelm the hospitals and detract needed resources from managing acute casualties.[21]

Experts describe intra-hospital patient tracking as an area in need of improvement. Techniques used in disciplines such as aviation or supply chain management might prove useful.[19,22,23] For example, the Mass Casualty Tracking Application (MCTA) uses air traffic control paper strips sorted into strip holder bays to provide situational overview about in-hospital patient flows.[22]

Family Reunification

The World Health Organization (WHO) stated that, even during disasters, "all children have a right to a family and families have a right to care for their children. Unaccompanied and separated children should be provided with services aimed at reuniting them with their parents or customary caregivers as quickly as possible. Interim care should be consistent with the aim of family reunification, and should ensure children's protection and well-being."[24]

Historically, this goal has often been unachievable. After Hurricane Katrina,[25] researchers used mathematical simulation to show that delayed family reunification slightly increased mortality and also increased the costs for inpatient care.[26] Following the Katrina experience, attention to the unique needs of children in disaster situations intensified.[27,28,29]

Restoration of Healthcare Services

After the immediate hazard has been addressed, emergency managers should shift focus to restoration of pre-disaster level healthcare services. While a return to baseline operations may not be possible in a catastrophic event, if obtainable, it will mitigate a second surge of patients with untreated and undertreated chronic medical problems. These patients along with those with incipient mental health issues may overwhelm the healthcare system.[25]

Appropriate identification and tracking information is necessary to allow access to old medical records and to insurance files in order to give survivors and evacuees access to appropriate medical care, including mental health care.

Hazard Management

Knowing the identity and location of patients, or of persons who came in contact with them, may become a national or even international priority, such as in containment of an outbreak.[2] Patient identification and tracking can facilitate successful epidemiologic investigations.[30]

Defining Patient Identification and Tracking

Despite the importance of patient identification and tracking, there is no universally accepted definition of this term. As is common in the emerging field of disaster medicine, the literature contains inhomogeneous nomenclature; many terms are used besides "tracking," including "documentation," "labeling," "recording," "registration," "tracing" and "information management."

Authors have criticized the shortage of evidence-based literature and stated that the science of patient tracking is in its infancy.[2] Several prototypes have been developed and some solutions are commercially available, but there is a lack of standardization and consolidation or even basic terminology consensus (e.g., on an essential data set). Hence the need to find a more efficient method for tagging and tracking disaster victims is frequently listed as an unresolved issue requiring further research.[16,31]

Part of the challenge in codifying a consistent nomenclature for patient tracking is that it is not a "one size fits all" issue. Events may be small- or large-scale; with or without intact infrastructure; with or without a scene or multiple scenes; sudden-onset or with warning; and time-limited or evolving. Patient identification and tracking may be needed in multiple settings such as the field, the hospital, or a medical shelter. Literature may be difficult to identify due to lack of standardized search terms.

Articles on tracking might be identified by searching the keyword "triage," since the concepts of "triage," "tagging," and "tracking" are difficult to separate. While an important component of identification and tracking, technology by itself (e.g., barcodes or Radio Frequency Identification [RFID]) does not constitute a tracking system.

For purposes of this chapter, the following definition of patient identification and tracking will be used: application of a dedicated system to detect victims and monitor their locations (including casualties, deceased, evacuees, or otherwise affected persons).

Patient identification and tracking comprises the whole "chain of rescue" and is applicable in all phases of MCI or disaster management from onset through recovery.[7] Keeping track of patients includes knowledge of:

▪ total numbers;
▪ current location;
▪ destinations; and
▪ basic information on health status, including current triage categories.

A system of patient identification and tracking does not replace standard medical records.

CURRENT STATE OF THE ART

Defining a state of the art for patient identification and tracking is challenging for several reasons. The literature is not consolidated within a single specialty or even language; the definition is variable; and the technology is progressing rapidly and not well tested or studied.

Due to these limitations, a single recommendation for a patient identification and tracking system is not possible. Instead,

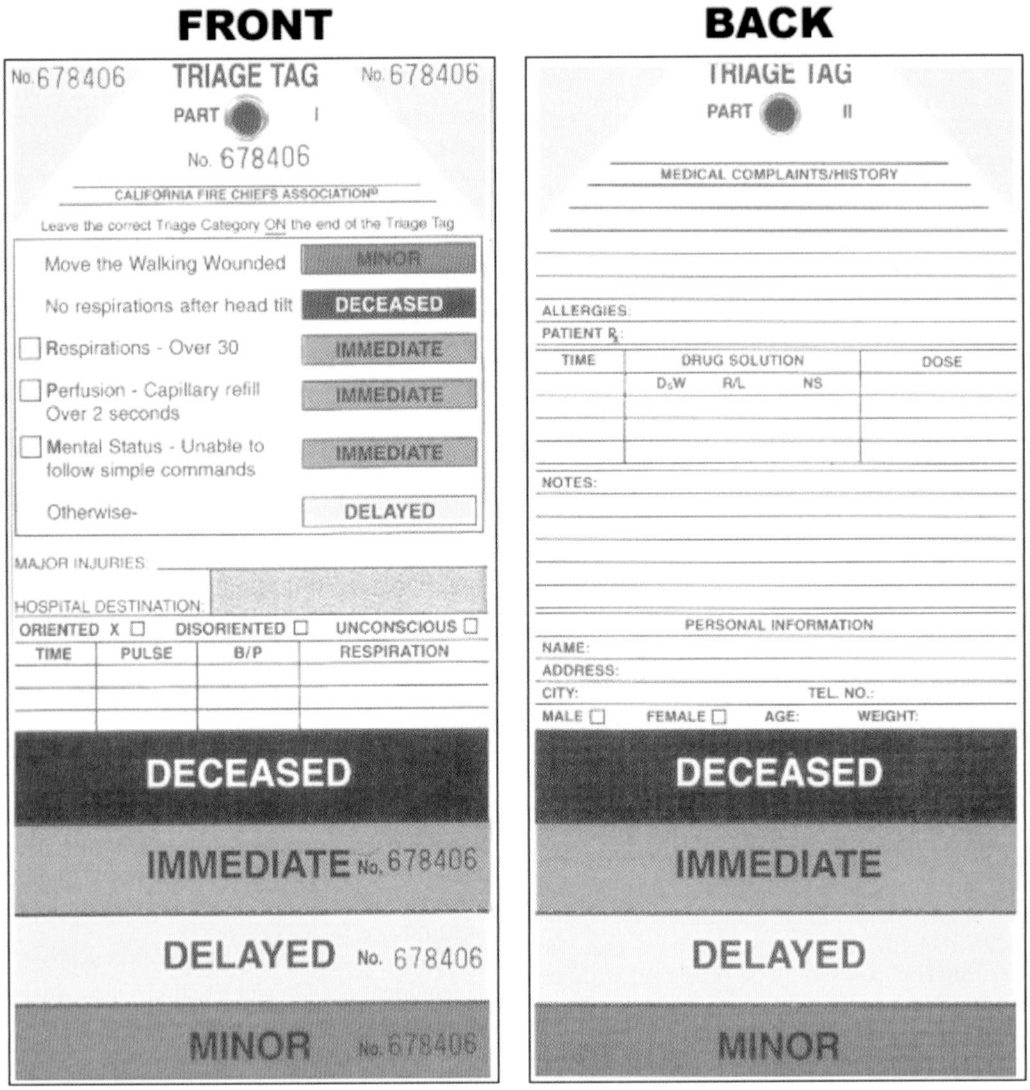

FRONT

BACK

Figure 28.1. Original Triage Tag, with Unique Numeric Identifier but No Barcode. Copyright © California Fire Chiefs Association. Reprinted with permission.

this chapter will provide a general discussion of underlying principles coupled with examples of patient tracking systems described in the literature.

The first part is a literature overview giving a comparison of paper-based and electronic patient tracking systems (ePTS). Available guidance about patient identification and tracking is cited. After that, basic considerations for tagging are presented, followed by a discussion of data issues and desirable data management functions of an ePTS. The chapter closes with a discussion of possible or probable technical elements of an ePTS and of organizational issues related to system development and implementation.

Paper-Based Patient Tracking Systems

In the digital age it is logical to explore and use techniques to improve ergonomics, safety, reliability, traceability, and quality in patient care.[32] Nevertheless the predominant systems currently used for triage as well as for tracking rely on use of paper triage tags.[33] Figures 28.1 and 28.2 illustrate an original paper

triage tag and a newer revision of the tag that includes barcoding and also the possibility to indicate that the patient is contaminated.

While paper triage tags and clipboards of notes have the undisputable advantage not to malfunction or require batteries or electricity, paper-based methods are time-consuming, labor intensive, and prone to human error.[34,35] Disadvantages of paper tags compared to ePTS include:

■ Bad weather conditions and illegible handwriting can diminish the usefulness of paper systems.[13,36,37]

■ The amount of information that can be recorded is limited due to lack of space.[8,13,37] The recorded information is often ill-structured.[32]

■ A manual count of triaged and tagged patients is necessary to provide a situational overview.[8]

■ Paper triage tags do not provide information about the dynamic location of the patient.[8,11]

■ Some triage tag systems do not easily allow changes to the triage category, particularly improvements.[8,13] As triage is a

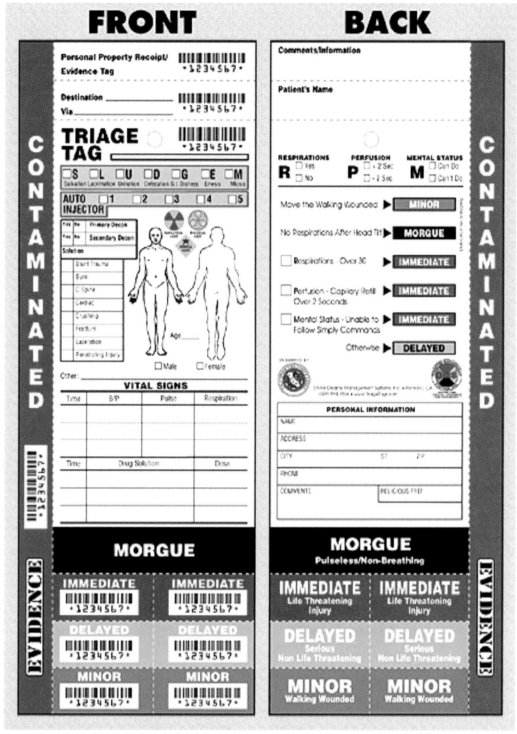

Figure 28.2. Medical All Risk Triage Tag. Note the "1-d" barcode on the front. Copyright © California Fire Chiefs Association. Reprinted with permission.

continuous process, a system to document reassessments is necessary.[38]

▪ Prioritization of multiple patients within a single triage category is not provided by triage tags.[8]

▪ Monitoring of vital signs requires additional actions or equipment.

▪ Although paper tags are relatively inexpensive, it is costly to maintain updated versions; in addition, triage tags vary widely in manufacture design and are not standardized, making training and interoperability difficult.[37]

▪ Data may be lost during transport of the victim.[37]

▪ Information on the tags is not secure and may be unintentionally disclosed, thereby violating patient privacy protection rights.[37]

▪ Paper tags are problematic in chemical, biological, radiological, and nuclear (CBRN) situations; it is difficult to complete tags while wearing personal protective equipment (PPE), and they are generally not sufficiently durable to withstand wet decontamination.[39]

These weaknesses of paper-based triage and documentation systems are further aggravated by the inherent unreliability of communication systems,[37] as observed previously.

As expected, direct comparisons between paper and electronic systems – mainly by means of exercises – usually find advantages of ePTS in regards to tracking and localization. ePTS data capture and safety features are generally described as at least as good and reliable as those for traditional paper-based systems. Researchers published such findings for the following ePTS prototypes:

▪ WIISARD (Wireless Internet Information System for Medical Response in Disasters);[30,37,40]
▪ DIORAMA (Dynamic Information Collection and Resource Tracking Architecture) – where an average reduction of 30% in evacuation time was found;[41] and
▪ AID-N (Advanced Health and Disaster Aid Network) – where the system was shown to triple the number patients that could be triaged over a given time period.[11]

A properly designed computerized system can improve data capture and reduce inaccuracies.[19] ePTS were shown to reduce missing and duplicated patient identifiers. Rapid access to information regarding numbers and status or triage classification of casualties facilitated decision making.[30,17] When applied in exercises, ePTS improves evaluation opportunities by providing more objective data and better comprehensive event reconstruction as compared with paper tags.[42]

Several groups have developed systems designed to improve victim tracking and the management of medical information in mass casualty events by instant access to identity and location information. Lenert[30] and Pate[2] provide excellent overviews.

The technologies applied comprise barcode readers, RFID, global positioning system (GPS), and miniaturized vital signs monitors; all of which are linked by wireless network technologies. These solutions will be highlighted during the discussion of technical issues.

Smartphones have become ubiquitous. At times, they have led to the design of real-time, ad hoc medical information management systems. After the Haiti earthquake, such an improvised system succeeded in improving disaster victim tracking, triage, patient care, facility management, and theater-wide decision making.[1]

Governmental Guidance

Guidance documents from the United States are the most readily available and will be used as examples. In a discussion about Hurricane Katrina, Pate notes that the "failure of the nation to adequately track victims ... has been identified as a major weakness of national and local disaster preparedness plans" and prompted government and private industries to "acknowledge that existing paper-based tracking systems are incapable of managing information during a large-scale disaster."[2]

The detailed U.S. National Response Framework of 2008 only briefly mentions "registration and tracking of evacuees" as a capability necessary to fulfill Emergency Support Function 6 (ESF 6), Mass Care, Emergency Assistance, Housing, and Human Services. While not explicitly described in ESF 8, Public Health and Medical Services, the list of functions implies that tracking is an essential capability for this area as well.

In 2009, the Agency for Healthcare Research and Quality within the U.S. federal government published "Recommendations for a National Mass Patient and Evacuee Movement, Regulating, and Tracking System."[3] This document recommended the creation of a national system for use during a multi-jurisdictional mass casualty or evacuation incident. The goal of the system would be for "locating, tracking, and regulating patients and evacuees"[3] (with "regulating" meaning to ensure transport on an appropriate vehicle to an appropriate location), as well as to improve decision making regarding transportation, resource allocation, and incident management, and to facilitate family reunification. The authors asserted that the number of jurisdictions using patient tracking systems was unknown at that time (but certainly a small percentage), as there were few compelling reasons for using these systems on a daily basis.

Tracking people between any pair of locations or monitoring movements of patients from an incident scene to a receiving hospital was regarded as "not unlike the processes employed by package delivery companies,"[3] where each package must be uniquely identified and tagged (e.g., barcoded), and its whereabouts reported into a central database. Policymakers proposed using the same processes to transmit a unique identifier and the triage category for people being evacuated from a disaster zone. The system must account for the fact that, unlike packages, people can also move of their own volition.[3] Figures 28.3 and 28.4 provide examples of two such systems.

Authorized users could access tracking data for a variety of purposes. For example, to assist with casualty distribution, emergency operations center personnel can monitor and track casualties and the number of patients transported to each hospital. Hospital personnel can track incoming casualties and prepare for specific casualty types. An open website can be established so that the public can query the database to determine the location of loved ones.[3]

Similar considerations for patient tracking were published after the events of September 11, 2001, in the United States.[43] These defined the following goals:

▪ Ability to monitor a person's progress through the system in order to keep track of patient locations and treatment updates;
▪ Capability of linking into a common operational picture to assist with deployment of emergency responders;
▪ Ability to attach to patients;
▪ Capability of identifying triage priority, clinical status and personal information, and remotely transmitting it in real-time to a common operational picture available to commanders and command centers, hospitals, and other key personnel; and
▪ Ability to provide command centers with an operational picture containing real-time information about the local system's resource status and patient care capabilities.

Solutions for Patient Tagging

Unique Identifiers

A unique identifier needs to be assigned for every registered person. Developers have proposed creation of such identifiers based on patient-specific data (e.g., date of birth, name, and sex),

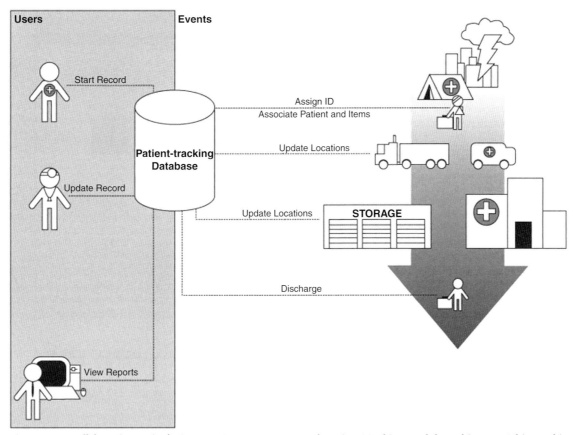

Figure 28.3. Collaborative Fusion's Community Response System's Patient Tracking Module Architecture. This graphic details one potential patient information path through the patient-tracking system. The beginning point of the patient's journey may vary. A patient may present to the hospital independently and the ID would be assigned there, or the patient may be transported from one hospital to another and have multiple record updates. Copyright © 2007, Collaborative Fusion, Inc., reprinted with permission.

but most systems use location-specific alphanumeric numbering similar to the numbers assigned to paper triage tags.[5,19]

The numbering used within the tracking system should be compatible with hospital registration systems. At a minimum, the system should be capable of linking the identification number with other numbering systems used in healthcare (e.g., HL-7 identification numbers) or administration (e.g., social security or insurance numbers). Standardized tagging would simplify and facilitate efficiency for inter-hospital transfers.[16] Attempts to capture information directly from patients or their personal documents (e.g., driver's license) and use this as an identifier have not been successful.

Barcodes

One of the simplest ways to upgrade paper triage tags to ePTS would be

1. to amend the tags with a barcode;
2. to supply responders with handheld devices for barcode scanning and data entry; and
3. to connect these devices via a wireless network to a central data storage and viewing unit.[36]

Utrecht Emergency Hospital personnel developed such a system.[19,23] The decision to use barcodes as an interactive non-keyboard method was the result of the proven reliability of barcodes, their cost-effectiveness, and the prior use of similar technology in the hospital.

Between 2002 and 2004, researchers developed the Victim Tracking and Tracing System (ViTTS) in the Netherlands. ViTTS uses injury cards (triage tags) with a barcode that links to a unique identification number. Emergency workers scan the barcode with a handheld device linked to a local network at the scene. The first responding ambulance personnel create a wireless network equipped with a mobile access router that establishes a secure, high-capacity data system. As soon as data are entered, they are viewable by all authorized users. Once the victim's identity becomes known, the barcode number can be coupled with the social insurance number.[5]

The emergency tracking system implemented in the St. Louis area of Missouri uses similar barcoded bracelets scanned by Wi-Fi or cellular-enabled devices.[44] Data are also shared with the American Red Cross as a designated disaster relief organization.

Some authors suggested that barcoded, pre-event printed wristbands could aid in triage and treatment and in reporting victim information to command centers; and that the universal implementation of such a system would augment surge capacity.[16]

Another model proposed the use of barcode stickers, which are printed by using field devices and are resistant to harsh environmental conditions. These stickers could be attached not only to the triage tag, but also to the patient's body and

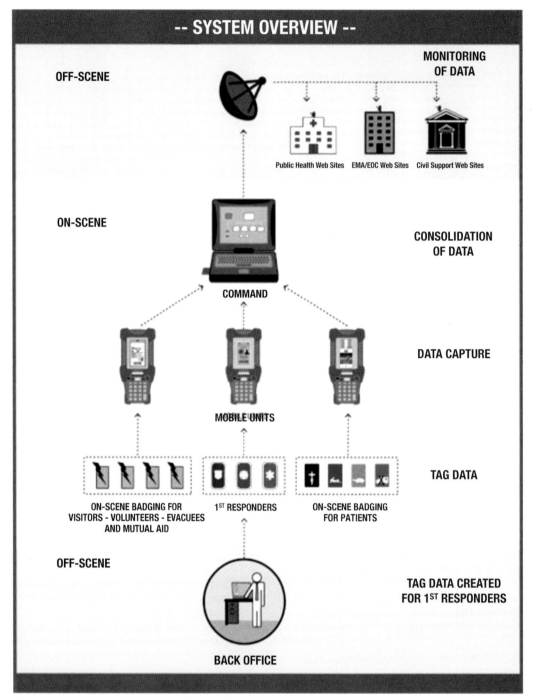

Figure 28.4. Data capture is performed via handheld units capable of scanning triage tags; these units then upload data to a local laptop, where data are consolidated, viewed, and sent to off-scene users (including hospitals and command centers). Reprinted with permission.

belongings.[32] Attaching stickers to triage tags before an incident occurs is another option.[36]

Radio-Frequency Identification (RFID)

RFID technology is not new to the medical sector. It has been used for many purposes to enhance patient safety (including patient identification, medication safety, or surgical process management) and hospital efficiency (by tracking supplies and equipment).[45]

An RFID system typically consists of a tag, a reader, and some sort of data processing equipment, such as a computer. Passive RFID tags store only a tiny amount of data and are powered by the energy emitted from the reader; their range is limited to about a meter. Active RFID tags have a battery and continuously transmit and receive signals. They can store vast amounts of data, have a lifespan of several years, and can be read over distances up to 100 meters.[46]

One ePTS prototype using RFID technology is the Dynamic Information Collection and Resource Tracking Architecture or DIORAMA. Every patient in the disaster scene is tagged with a DIORAMA electronic tag (D-tag) showing the severity of the patient's injury (red, yellow, green, and black) in the same way as paper tags. Moreover, each emergency responder (e.g., paramedic, firefighter, police officer) and resource is also equipped with a DIORAMA tag.[41] All these active wristband RFID tags transmit information to a server via a wireless network. For patients, this time-stamped information includes the severity of injury and current location. This information transfer operates automatically without victim or staff intervention.

Responders can carry readers or position them at set locations such as casualty collection points. They have a range of up to 100 meters.[47] While these devices have proven successful in exercises, the authors concede that the expense, size, and complexity of the wristband devices may make them impractical to distribute in adequate numbers to monitor all victims of a large-scale disaster.[41]

Other RFID-based prototype systems include SOGRO (Sofortrettung Großunfall) in Germany[48] and the Wireless Internet Information System for Medical Response in Disasters or WIISARD in the United States.[30,40] The developers of WIISARD adopted RFID technology rather than barcodes because barcode reader performance can be significantly impaired if lighting is inadequate.[37] In the Nordic countries, investigators developed another RFID-based ePTS prototype that uses mobile phones with integrated RFID readers as field terminals.[17]

The U.S. military developed an integrated software-hardware system called MASCAL to enhance management of resources at a hospital during a mass casualty situation. MASCAL uses active RFID tags to track patients, equipment and staff.[18]

Intelligent Tags

In addition to signal transmission for tracking and location, the WIISARD RFID system displays the victim's triage status in an easily visible way by use of signal lights. These devices were primarily designed to be usable in CBRN environments and are therefore water resistant so that they will continue to function if the patient undergoes decontamination.[30] These intelligent triage tags automatically record selected vital parameters like oxygen saturation;[49] the tag also serves as an electronic medical record.

The Trauma Patient Tracking System (TPTS), also a prototype, supplies all patients with a device that continuously reports their locations. They are connected to a base station via a wireless network. When out of range, the tag is capable of logging its own positional history and later uploading these data to the server once connectivity is restored.[50]

Wearable Sensors

Another initiative is the combination of ePTS (with the localization or tracking function) with wearable vital sign sensors. This strategy should alert responders to any deterioration of patient status so that reassessment can be performed.[9,13]

Several groups have explored the option of using "motes" (a type of low-power and low-cost computer for sensor networks) for application in disaster management.[30,51,52] In the CodeBlue project, a wireless pulse oximeter and a wireless two-lead electrocardiogram (EKG) were combined to a sensor mote collecting heart rate (HR), oxygen saturation (SpO2), and EKG data and transmitting those data over a short-range (100 meter) wireless network.[52]

Researchers developed prototype electronic triage tags for the Advanced Health and Disaster Aid Network (AID-N). These tags provide the following functionalities: triage status display (with colored lights), vital sign monitoring, location tracking, and alarm signaling.[8,9]

None of the mentioned prototypes have been introduced into routine practice. Cost to implement such a system, with hundreds or thousands of wearable sensors, can be prohibitive. Automatic display of triage status based on measured parameters is also non-trivial.

ePTS Functions and Limiting Conditions

Data Entry

The first-time patient data can be entered into the system is at the initial contact with medical care. Irrespective of the technology used to assign the unique patient identifier (paper tags, barcode wristbands, or any ePTS), manual data entry is necessary, either on the tag itself or into the handheld device connected to the ePTS network. Data entry is labor intensive and time-consuming; therefore, adequate human resources must be allocated. This can be challenging, as emergency responders have been shown to prefer to care for patients rather than take time to enter data.[1] Responders should consider unconventional solutions such as use of scribes, volunteers, or members of organizations uninvolved in initial patient assessment.

Multiple Locations for Data Entry

Data entry requirements to register a new patient should be kept as simple as possible. The system should allow amending data at a later point of time, when more resources become available.[3] ePTS should have capacity to include patients lacking identifying information (e.g., "unknown male, about 40 years old").

Efficient ePTS must allow data entry at multiple points and from multiple users. While historical data should be preserved as new information is added, the system should be designed to automatically limit duplication of data that would unnecessarily enlarge the database. There should be a clear and simple method for data reconciliation for conflicting data set entries. Furthermore, there should be an effective process for finding and merging multiple entries if patients have been registered with different identifier numbers at different locations.

Amount of Data vs. Essential Data Set

Several recommendations for a minimal data set for ePTS have been published, usually differentiating between mandatory basic data fields and desirable additional information elements.[53]

Mandatory or essential data typically consist of elements like triage tag number or name (if available), sex, date of birth or age, current location and transfer destination, triage category, and initial condition/chief complaint.[3] The system should be designed to capture the initial location and also track sequential locations by having multiple time-stamped data fields.

The "additional information" data field may include such elements as: more detailed medical and treatment information, additional personal information (including full name, contact information or telephone number, most current address or home zip code, social security number or equivalent), and patient permission for information sharing. Some authors suggest including distinguishing characteristics of the individual like eye color, birthmarks, tattoos, and scars.[54]

As technological possibilities expand, it is important to keep data entry requirements as simple as possible so that personnel can perform the task with little or no training and in a minimal amount of time.

Whether using high-tech or low-tech solutions, it is prudent to reduce the amount of information being collected. The more data collection is requested from responders, the less compliant responders will be, and the more data quality will decrease and propensity for errors will increase. In addition, the more data fields required, the slower the data will be transmitted via the networks.

Tracking systems should collect only the data necessary to reconstruct the events surrounding the incident and document medical histories sufficient to facilitate patient care and protect against malpractice claims. It would be a waste of time and resources to collect excessive data that will have no future use. ePTS have a specific purpose and are not intended to replace routine medical records.

The type of incident determines the needed frequency of data updates. For example, family assistance centers receiving requests for information might require frequent data updates every 30 or 60 minutes.[20,21] Conversely, policymakers at a national level might only require daily updates. For conflict situations with a search for missing persons, such as by the Red Cross Tracing Services, much longer update intervals may be acceptable.[55]

Inclusion Criteria

Planners should clarify whether ePTS should include only patients transported by prehospital providers or also self-evacuees.[7] Ideally, any person involved in a multi-jurisdictional incident who seeks medical attention or otherwise needs assistance (e.g., with evacuation) should be registered in the database.[3] A registry should include all patients:

- transported via the prehospital system to a hospital or other medical treatment site;
- admitted to a hospital with illnesses/injuries/medical conditions that were a direct or indirect result of the disaster;
- receiving care at a field treatment site;
- evacuated (by self or with assistance) or transferred to another healthcare facility; and
- who died.

Ideally, patients seeking care at a clinic or physician's office should also be included.

Flags for Special Conditions

Even registries specifically designed to assist in family reunification have been shown to be of limited use for unaccompanied minors; children may be either afraid or unable to report themselves to such registries.[15]

ePTS should include provisions to highlight special conditions related to high vulnerability – for example, a check box for "unaccompanied minor" for children separated from their families. Inclusion of database flags to highlight special needs related to medical care or support is recommended.

Data Viewing and Presentation

The purpose of data gathering and transmission is to present an appropriate format at the appropriate location. Data must be made available to authorized persons both at the individual level (e.g., for admitting hospitals) and at the aggregate level (e.g., for command centers).[3,5] An ideal data presentation portal allows:

- Simultaneous tracking of multiple patients at multiple locations for multiple incidents in real or near real time;
- creation of searches with multiple parameters;
- regulation of access for authorized persons only;
- exportation of data in all formats required by other authorized organizations or institutions; and
- provision of appropriate input into decision support systems used in command centers.

Data Security

Data security refers to measures to prevent unauthorized access to computers, databases, and websites and to protect data from loss or corruption. ePTS must ensure patient and evacuee confidentiality against stalkers or other predators.[3]

In addition to protection for central servers and data access portals, the following issues should be considered:

- network security (for Wi-Fi or Terrestrial Trunked Radios (TETRA) or similar);
- protection for other data transmission technologies (like RFID);[45]
- data protection in case of loss or theft of handheld devices;[37]
- data protection against corruption (to include austere environments); and
- legal compliance (e.g., with patient privacy regulations).[53]

Security requirements need to be balanced with ease-of-use – for example, it should not be necessary to reenter a password after each short time of non-use.

System Reliability and Redundancy

Over-reliance on technical solutions is precarious as disasters frequently involve infrastructure disruptions. Nonstructural damage and interruption of lifelines (like water or electricity) are a frequent cause of hospital evacuations after earthquakes.[14] These same conditions can threaten the viability of ePTS. The following are recommended:

- Regular use and charging of handheld devices;
- Adequate spare batteries; and
- Availability of a paper-based backup plan.

System Usability in Hazardous Environments

For use during CBRN incidents, patient tags and handheld registration devices need to be encapsulated such that they are water-and explosion-proof. It must be possible to use any device (and to hear any alarm) while wearing PPE.

Some electronic tracking systems have been specifically developed for such conditions (e.g., WIISARD).[30] Alternate approaches, such as using colored clothing pegs to designate patient priorities during events involving chemical exposures, are also described.[39]

Technical Components of ePTS

Primary requirements for ePTS are:

1. to collect data (either at the incident site or at the healthcare facility or both), enter them into a device and transmit them to a central server; and
2. to display, aggregate, and disseminate these data via a web portal.

The peripheral components of the patient tracking systems described in the literature comprise:

1. A tag with a unique identifier attached to the patient; either the identifier is machine readable (e.g., a barcode)[5,23,44] or the tag transmits data to a reader (e.g., by RFID);[17,30] the tag can have additional functions (e.g., display, recording) or even monitor vital signs.
2. A field data tool to interface between tagging technology and a database that allows time-stamped data entry and connects to the central server. The devices used for this purpose include: handheld devices,[5,9,30] rugged laptop and/or tablet personal computers,[17,32] and handheld terminals used by delivery services.
3. The communication technology by which the field data tools transmit information to a central database.

Many systems and prototypes rely on the availability of public infrastructures like Wi-Fi networks, although such wireless access is not ubiquitous and is prone to interruption in disasters. To mitigate this potential cause of failure, some workgroups have created their own network standards[30] or used multiple transmission technologies including satellite phones,[50] TETRA,[17] or General Packet Radio Service (GPRS).[5,50]

The central application for data display and dissemination typically consists of:

1. The "back end" – usually a standard relational database coupled with conventional web interfaces (use of an industrial-strength database from an established vendor is recommended).
2. The "front end" – some form of user interface viewable in many locations. This is mostly a web-based interface. It should be contemporary and incorporate industry standard metaphors and conventions.
3. A network to link viewers of the data (typically the public Internet).

   Any Internet-dependent application is only as robust and reliable as the network (and the public power grid).

Any chosen data system should be as easy to use as a standard web portal. Small-scale systems may be cheaper than products from market leaders; however, they may require special knowledge to use, may trigger pop-up blockers and anti-spamware, and may not have been tested in-depth for usability and stability.

While it is unnecessary for patient tracking systems to have the structure described here, these are the approaches most frequently described in the literature.

The "Adam system" from Israel does not include any prehospital components. Adam interfaces online with hospitals' patient registration systems to locate and identify casualties (Figure 28.5). The goal is to provide family support centers with information on patient location. Casualties not carrying any identification are photographed for that purpose.[20,21]

MCTA, developed and evaluated at the Uniformed Services University of the Health Sciences in the United States, avoids

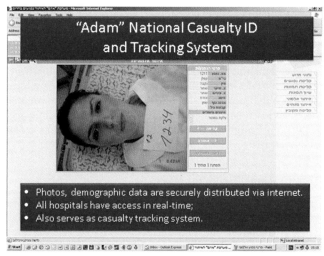

Figure 28.5. "Adam" National Casualty ID and Tracking System. Developed by Prof. Pinchas (Pinny) Halpern, MD. Chair, Emergency Department, Tel Aviv Medical Center.

the use of high technology. MCTA uses paper strips which are placed into strip holder bays like they are in air traffic control applications (Figure 28.6). This system allows efficient intra-hospital patient tracking without any dependence on high-tech devices or uninterrupted energy supply.[22,56]

Localization Technologies

Researchers have begun to develop localization technologies for use in tracking systems. Whereas Lenert assumed in 2011 that "most devices on the network would not have built in geolocation capabilities,"[30] this statement is generally outdated for outdoor areas, as any modern device has built-in GPS.[37] Localization within buildings, however, remains a challenge;[13] some approaches combine GPS with other systems for indoor tracking.[11,51] In RFID-based systems, localization information can be derived from signal triangulation using the received signal strength of RFID tags.[18,41,47] However the frequently asserted

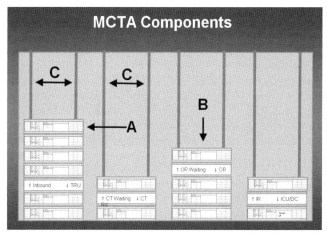

Figure 28.6. MCTA Components. Developed by Dr. Les Folio, National Institutes of Health; Dr. Jason Hoskins, Captain, U.S. Air Force; Rick Hansen, President, APS Global LLC & Professor of Practice at Capitol College; Dr. Justin Woodson, Lt. Colonel, U.S. Army; Dr. Cliff Lutz, Colonel, U.S. Army.

rationale that real-time location of victims and responders is essential when there is a disaster scene[52] is not always valid.

The goal of patient tracking must be carefully considered, rather than allowing technology to dictate what systems are put in place. It might be sufficient to attach an inexpensive machine-readable bracelet to every patient and to deduce the patient location from that position in the rescue chain where the bracelet was most recently scanned (e.g., at the ambulance loading area or the target hospital). Localization technologies are an area for future research.

Organizational Issues for ePTS

Developers of ePTS must consider several organizational issues. As noted previously, there is no standard definition of patient tracking. Therefore, the first consideration is to define the main purpose of the ePTS.

▪ Is it incident management, triage documentation, patient tracking, evacuee tracking, family reunification, or a combination of more than one of these?

▪ Is the system intended for use in all kinds of disasters and MCIs or only for special threats like CBRN?

▪ What is the intended organizational level of information sharing? Will the system be used on the municipal, district/county, province/state, or national level, or even for supranational information exchange?

▪ Who is intended to provide the data? Results may be better if data are collected from emergency responders and the system can be used in everyday operations.[3,7] Ease of use will facilitate the opportunity to assign the task of data entry to volunteers or untrained personnel.

▪ Who is intended to use the collected and aggregated data? The data access portal should be as easy to use as any ordinary (but well-designed) website. The amount of information collected needs to be balanced with use-specific data update interval needs.

▪ Which interfaces are necessary to connect the new ePTS to existing registration systems or administrative databases?[3,54]

▪ What are the legislative and regulatory requirements (e.g., patient privacy rules)?[16,54]

▪ What are the budgetary constraints?

Another challenge is that technology is advancing so rapidly that any system will likely be outdated as soon as it is fully developed or introduced into practice. However, the main barriers to the development of patient identification and tracking systems are the organizational issues delineated in this chapter, rather than technological or scientific constraints.

RECOMMENDATIONS FOR FURTHER RESEARCH

While it is tempting to believe that patient identification and tracking should be as simple or streamlined as tracking packages by delivery companies, this is not the case. Communication and information management, including patient tracking, is likely to remain a challenge for disaster management well into the future. Of particular concern is the durability and reliability of advanced technologies in disaster situations. The following are important research questions:

1. What are the essential data elements? Are current systems attempting to collect too much data?

2. How can compliance and quality of data entry be improved? Would better ease of use of a system improve accurate and complete data collection?

3. How can system stability, reliability, and usability be assessed in catastrophic disaster situations?

4. Can patient tracking systems be created with the capability to transition to baseline operations? How long are tracking systems needed?

5. How much location information is necessary for effective disaster management and what would be the best and most cost-effective way to provide this information?

6. Could a wearable sensor be developed that displays patient status based on measured parameters in a simple and reliable way?

Much work remains to be done to improve the current state of the art of patient identification and tracking.

REFERENCES

1. Callaway DW, Peabody CR, Hoffman A, Cote E, Moulton S, Baez AA, Nathanson L. Disaster mobile health technology: lessons from Haiti. *Prehosp Disaster Med* 2012; 27(2): 148–152.

2. Pate BL, Identifying and Tracking Disaster Victims, State-of-the-Art Technology Review. *Fam Community Health* 2008; 31(1): 23–34.

3. Agency for Healthcare Research and Quality. *Recommendations for a National Mass Patient and Evacuee Movement, Regulating, and Tracking System*. Rockville, MD, Agency for Healthcare Research and Quality, January 2009. http://archive.ahrq .gov/prep/natlsystem (Accessed July 7, 2014).

4. Matsumoto H, Motomura T, Hara Y, Masuda Y, Mashiko K, Yokota H, Koido Y. Lessons learned from the aeromedical disaster relief activities during the Great East Japan Earthquake. *Prehosp Disaster Med* 2013; 28(2): 166–169.

5. Marres GMH, Taal L, Bemelman M, Bouman J, Leenen LPH. Online Victim Tracking and Tracing System (ViTTS) for major incident casualties. *Prehosp Disaster Med* 2013; 28(5): 445–453.

6. Juffermans J, Bierens JJLM: Recurrent medical response problems during five recent disasters in the Netherlands. *Prehosp Disaster Med* 2010; 25(2): 127–136.

7. Hamilton J. Automated MCI Patient Tracking: Managing Mass Casualty Chaos Via the Internet. *JEMS* 2003; 28(4): 52–56.

8. Massey T, Gao T, Welsh M. The Design of a Decentralized Electronic Triage System. *AMIA 2006 Symposium Proceedings*; 544.

9. Gao T, White D. A Next Generation Electronic Triage to Aid Mass Casualty Emergency Medical Response. *Proceedings of the 28th IEEE* 2006; 6501.

10. Howitt AM, Leonard HB. Beyond Katrina: improving disaster response capabilities Working papers. http://www.ksg .harvard.edu/taubmancenter/emergencyprep/downloads/ beyondkatrina.pdf (Accessed July 7, 2014).

11. Gao T, Massey T, Selavo L, et al. The advanced health and disaster aid network: a light-weight wireless medical system for triage. *IEEE Trans Biomed Circuits Syst* September 2007; 1(3): 203–216.

12. Howitt AM, Leonard HB. Improving response capabilities. *Crisis Response Journal* 2006; 2(4): 1–4.

13. Chan TC, Killeen J, Griswold W, Lenert L. Information technology and emergency medical care during disasters. *Acad Emerg Med* November 2004; 11(11): 1229–1236.

14. Ukai T. The Great Hanshin-Awaji Earthquake and the problems with emergency medical care. *Ren Fail* September 1997; 19(5): 633–645.

15. Chung S, Mario Christoudias C, Darrell T, Ziniel SI, Kalish LA. A novel image-based tool to reunite children with their families after disasters. *Acad Emerg Med* November 2012; 19(11): 1227–1234.

16. Carlton M. Surge Capacity Management and Patient Identification in Disaster Preparedness. *Access Management Journal.*

17. Jokela J, Rådestad M, Gryth D, et al. Increased situation awareness in major incidents-radio frequency identification (RFID) technique: a promising tool. *Prehosp Disaster Med* February 2012; 27(1): 81–87.

18. Fry EA, Lenert LA. MASCAL: RFID Tracking of Patients, Staff and Equipment to Enhance Hospital Response to Mass Casualty Events. *AMIA 2005 Symposium Proceedings*; 261.

19. Noordergraaf GJ, Bouman JH, van den Brink EJ, van de Pompe C, Savelkoul TJ. Development of computer-assisted patient control for use in the hospital setting during mass casualty incidents. *Am J Emerg Med* 1996; 14(3): 257–261.

20. Gagin R, Cohen M, Peled-Avram M. Family support and victim identification in mass casualty terrorist attacks: An integrative approach. *International Journal of Emergency Mental Health* 2005; 7(2): 125–131.

21. Adini B, Peleg K, Cohen R, Laor D. A national system for disseminating information on victims during mass casualty incidents. *Disasters* 2010; 34(2): 542–551.

22. Hoskins JD, Graham RF, Robinson DR, Lutz CC, Folio LR. Mass casualty tracking with air traffic control methodologies. *J Am Coll Surg* June 2009; 208(6): 1001–1008.

23. Bouman J, Schouwerwou R, Van der Eijk K, van Leusden A, Savelkoul T. Computerization of Patient Tracking and Tracing During Mass Casualty Incidents. *Eur J Emerg Med* 2000; 7(3): 211–216.

24. World Health Organization. Unaccompanied and Separated Children in the Tsunami-Affected Countries – Guiding Principles. 2005. http://www.unicef.org/protection/Separated-20Children-20Guiding-20Principles-20Tsunami%281%29.pdf (Accessed August 23, 2015).

25. Abramson D, Garfield R. On the Edge: Children and Families Displaced by Hurricanes Katrina and Rita Face a Looming Medical and Mental Health Crisis. National Center for Disaster Preparedness & Operation Assist. 2006. http://www.preventionweb.net/english/professional/publications/v.php?id=2958 (Accessed July 7, 2014).

26. Barthel ER, Pierce JR, Speer AL, et al. Delayed family reunification of pediatric disaster survivors increases mortality and inpatient hospital costs: a simulation study. *J Surg Res* September 2013; 184(1): 430–437.

27. National Commission on Children and Disasters. Report to the President and Congress. 2010. http://archive.ahrq.gov/prep/nccdreport/nccdreport.pdf (Accessed July 7, 2014).

28. Markenson D, Redlener I. Pediatric terrorism preparedness national guidelines and recommendations: findings of an evidenced-based consensus process. *Biosecur Bioterror* 2004; 2(4): 301–319.

29. National Advisory Committee on Children and Terrorism. Recommendations to the Secretary. June 12, 2003. http://health.mo.gov/emergencies/pediatrictoolkit/CommunityPlanningforChildren/NationalAdvisoryCommitteeonChildrenandTerrorismRecomm.pdf (Accessed July 7, 2014).

30. Lenert LA, Kirsh D, Griswold WG, Buono C, Lyon J, Rao R, Chan TC. Design and evaluation of a wireless electronic health records system for field care in mass casualty settings. *J Am Med Inform Assoc* November–December 2011; 18(6): 842–852.

31. Mackway-Jones K, Carley S. An international expert Delphi study to determine research needs in major incident management. *Prehosp Disaster Med* 2012; 27(4): 351–358.

32. Lauraent C, Beaucourt L. Instant Electronic Patient Data Input During Emergency Response in Major Disaster Setting. *Stud Health Technol Inform* 2005; 111: 290–293.

33. Cole SL, Siddiqui J, Harry DJ, Sandrock CE. WiFi RFID demonstration for resource tracking in a statewide disaster drill. *Am J Disaster Med* May–June 2011; 6(3): 155–162.

34. Branas CC, Sing RF, Perron AD: A case series analysis of mass casualty incidents. *Prehosp Emerg Care* 2000; 4: 299–304.

35. Morris G. Common errors in mass casualty management. *JEMS* 1986; 11(2): 34.

36. Plischke M, Wolf KH, Lison T, Pretschner DP. Telemedical support of prehospital emergency care in mass casualty incidents. *Eur J Med Res* September 9, 1999; 4(9): 394–398.

37. Demers G, Kahn C, Johansson P, Buono C, Chipara O, Griswold W, Chan T. Secure scalable disaster electronic medical record and tracking system. *Prehosp Disaster Med* October 2013; 28(5): 498–501.

38. Briggs S. Triage in mass casualty incidents challenges and controversies. *Am J Disaster Med* March–April 2007; 2(2): 57.

39. Okumura T, Kondo H, Nagayama H, Makino T, Yoshioka T, Yamamoto Y. Simple triage and rapid decontamination of mass casualties with colored clothes pegs (STARDOM-CCP) system against chemical releases. *Prehosp Disaster Med* May–June 2007; 22(3): 233–236.

40. Buono CJ, Chan TC, Killeen J, Huang R, Brown S, Liu F, Palmer D, Griswold W, Lenert L. Comparison of the effectiveness of wireless electronic tracking devices versus traditional paper systems to track victims in a large scale disaster. *AMIA Annu Symp Proc* October 2007; 11: 886.

41. Ganz A, Yu X, Schafer J, D'Hauwe S, Nathanson LA, Burstein J, Ciottone GR, Lord G. DIORAMA: Dynamic Information Collection and Resource Tracking Architecture. *Conf Proc IEEE Eng Med Biol Soc* 2010: 386–389.

42. Ingrassia PL, Carenzo L, Barra FL, et al. Data collection in a live mass casualty incident simulation: automated RFID technology versus manually recorded system. *Eur J Emerg Med* February 2012; 19(1): 35–39.

43. MIPT (National Memorial Institute for the Prevention of Terrorism) und DHS. National Technology Plan for Emergency Response to Catastrophic Terrorism. 2004. www.riskintel.com/library/34 (Accessed July 7, 2014).

44. Hamilton J. Automated MCI Patient Tracking: Managing Mass Casualty Chaos Via the Internet. *JEMS* 2003; 28(4): 52–56.

45. Zhang Z, Qi Q. An Efficient RFID Authentication Protocol to Enhance Patient Medication Safety Using Elliptic Curve Cryptography. *J Med Syst* May 2014; 38(5): 47.

46. Davis S. Tagging along. RFID helps hospitals track assets and people. *Health Facil Manag* 2004; 17(12): 20–24.

47. Ganz A, Yu X. Scalable Patients Tracking Framework for Mass Casualty Incidents. *33rd Annual International Conference of the IEEE EMBS.*

48. Red Cross Germany. SOGRO (SOfortrettung bei GROßunfall) [Immediate Rescue in MCIs]. 2014. http://www.sogro.de (Accessed July 7, 2014).

49. Lenert L, Palmer DA, Chan TC, Rao R. An Intelligent 802.11 Triage Tag For Medical Response to Disasters. *AMIA 2005 Symposium Proceedings*; 440.

50. Maltz J, Ng TC, Li D, Wang J, Wang K, Bergeron W, Martin R, Budinger T. The Trauma Patient Tracking System: implementing

a wireless monitoring infrastructure for emergency response. *Conf Proc IEEE Eng Med Biol Soc* 2005; 3: 2441–2446.

51. Tollefsen W, Pepe M, Myung D, Gaynor M, Welsh M, Moulton S. iRevive, a Pre-hospital Mobile Database for Emergency Medical Services. *IJHTM* Summer 2004.

52. Lorincz K, Malan DJ, Fulford-Jones TRF, et al. Sensor networks for emergency response: challenges and opportunities. *Pervasive Computing IEEE* 2004; 3: 16–23.

53. U. S. Department of Health and Human Services. Summary of the HIPAA Privacy Rule. 2005. http://www.hhs.gov/ocr/privacy/hipaa/understanding/summary (Accessed July 7, 2014).

54. Blake N, Stevenson K. Reunification: keeping families together in crisis. *J Trauma* August 2009; 67(2 Suppl.): S147–S151.

55. Federal Emergency Management Agency. Attachment F: mass care. In: *Guide for All-hazard Emergency Operations Planning.* 1996. http://www.fema.gov/pdf/plan/slg101.pdf (Accessed July 7, 2014).

56. Graham RF, Hoskins JD, Cortijo MP, Barbee GA, Folio LR, Lutz CC. A Casualty Tracking System Modeled After Air Traffic Control Methodology Employed in a Combat Support Hospital in Iraq. *Military Medicine* 2011; 176(3): 244.

EXPLOSIVE EVENTS

Glenn D. Burns and John M. Wightman

The opinions and assertions herein are the private views of the authors, and are not to be construed as official or as reflecting the views of the U.S. government, Department of Defense, or Department of the Air Force. This is in part a U.S. government work. There are no restrictions on its use.

OVERVIEW

Explosive events occur in many settings. They can have a variety of etiologies, which can be accidental or intentional. Many blasts damage only property, but every explosion can be classified as a potential injury/illness-creating event (PICE). It is the human impact with which this chapter is mostly concerned. Injuries may occur to individuals or groups. Massive and multiple explosions may affect entire communities or larger regions, resulting in a disaster, commonly defined as an event that results in a demand that exceeds the supply of existing resources.

Most explosive events are unlikely to result in major catastrophes, as defined by Lumley and Ryan, "where the social fabric of a society is disrupted and the medical infrastructure fails."[1] However, some important exceptions exist. A single bombing of the only hospital in a region may cause temporary failure of the local healthcare system, until external resources are mobilized. Multiple, intentional explosions specifically targeting critical services may impact a larger population to a greater degree. A nuclear detonation would likely disable much of a city's infrastructure. Volcanic eruptions have, and will again, create devastation on local, regional, national, and global levels.

Individual Impact

Blast injuries to persons encompass the full spectrum of polytrauma. Individual physical injuries range from minor abrasions to "total body disruption" associated with wide scattering of multiple body parts. These are detailed under sections on pathophysiology and clinical care. Short- and long-term effects on survivors and their families can be devastating.

The focus of healthcare attention is often only on resuscitation, stabilization, and definitive medical and surgical care. Victims requiring hospitalization may also need prolonged rehabilitation, physical therapy, and occupational therapy before returning, to some degree, to their pre-injury lives. Even those blast-exposed individuals who did not access the healthcare system through emergency medical services (EMS) or a hospital may be in need of identification and follow-up services, particularly as regards to their mental health.

Not all blast-injured casualties require hospitalization. Many minimally injured victims may be discharged from the emergency department (ED) if they have appropriate social support and adequate access to follow-up within the healthcare system. At the other end of the spectrum, some casualties will require intensive initial resuscitation and stabilization, multiple surgical procedures, ongoing physiological support, and management of complications that develop. Hospitalization at a regional referral center is frequently necessary to coordinate the many services essential for management of complex, multidisciplinary issues seen in victims surviving severe blast injuries.

Epidemiology

Intentional bombings are common throughout the world. Most are relatively small in scale, but frequent in occurrence. However, large-scale attacks have occurred in many countries over the last few decades. Numerous reports of individual incidents have appeared in the medical literature. Many of these were referenced or discussed in the first edition of this textbook.[2] More recent events include the terrorist bombings at the 2013 Boston Marathon. The detonation of two improvised explosive devices (IEDs) with added shrapnel in crowds near the finish line resulted in 3 immediate deaths, and 173 other victims who either self-evacuated or were transported to one of several local EDs: 17 (9.8%) in critical condition, 25 (14.5%) in serious condition, and the remaining 131 (75.7%) classified as less-serious. An additional 109 persons presented to a variety of locations for care over the subsequent week, mostly for minor wounds or persistent hearing symptoms. Although epidemiological research is still pending at the time of this writing, initial perspectives on the incident are available.

Over the last few decades, prospective trauma registries have captured larger groups of casualties in low-intensity conflicts, primarily from Northern Ireland and Israel, and war, primarily in Afghanistan and Iraq. However, comparison of data regarding injuries from IEDs shows little change from the 1970s. The majority of casualties can be discharged from the ED and only a small fraction will die of wounds after reaching the hospital. Soft-tissue injuries, minor fractures, and hearing problems dominate in minor cases. Penetrating trauma to various body parts, traumatic amputations and other open fractures, open or closed traumatic brain injury (TBI), and burns comprise the majority of injuries in patients requiring admission.

Hamid published a comprehensive review of accidental explosions between 1906 and 1964 that included analysis of more than 100 fatalities.[3] Most reports, however, are less comprehensive and describe only single events. Two days after the 2013 Boston Marathon bombings, an accidental explosion occurred at a fertilizer plant in Texas. Fourteen people were killed, most of them emergency responders, and another 200 victims were injured.[4] Unlike Boston, this event occurred in a small town in east-central Texas without a robust healthcare infrastructure to locally manage hundreds of casualties. Researchers report the outcome of a similar explosion at a petroleum plant in another small town in Texas in 1989. Victims included 22 killed, 131 injured on-site, and 3 other people injured from 3–5 km away.[5]

Accidental industrial blasts also occur in the manufacture and recreational use of explosives. The use of fireworks, especially by non-professionals, has resulted in many injuries throughout the world every year. In an American study, boys 10–14 years old were found to be the population at highest risk, though 60% of all victims were older than 14 years.[6] Injuries affected the hands, face, and eyes in order of descending frequency. Seven percent of patients were hospitalized.

A report from Finland described all accidental and intentional blast injuries over a 5-year period from 1991–1995.[7] Fireworks were the cause in 29%, explosive materials in 25%, and rupture of pressurized containers in 13%. Soft-tissue injuries and burns were the most common injuries, but traumatic amputations and crushing injuries also occurred. Two victims for every 100,000 persons in the general population were admitted every year for an average of 11 days.

There is a paucity of data on the epidemiology of natural explosions. A computerized search of the medical literature regarding the Mount St. Helens volcanic blast of 1980 – the largest in the United States in the last century – revealed less than a dozen clinical articles describing medical and mental health consequences. Even as massive as this explosion was, only fifty-seven people were reported dead or missing, likely due to a short but adequate warning time. Volcanic eruptions and explosions are discussed in more detail in Chapter 43.

Societal Impact

The cited non-accidental events represent terrorist actions. They do not include blast injuries from landmines and other conventional warfare, which are certainly PICEs, but are beyond the scope of this chapter, as is the societal impact of war itself. Some data, however, are available. From the beginning of the Global War on Terrorism in October 2001 through July 2013, there were 3,349 (2,249 American, 444 British, and 656 other Coalition) deaths plus 17,674 injuries from IEDs and conven-

tional explosive munitions in Operation Enduring Freedom. In Operation Iraqi Freedom, casualties included 2,787 killed and 22,979 injured due to explosive blasts. In both conflicts, these numbers report only Coalition military service members; they exclude enemy combatants and civilians.

Unrelated to conventional warfare, intentional bombings remain common throughout the world. Over a 20-year period in the United States from 1983–2002, there were 21,237 explosive bombings, 6,185 incendiary bombings, 7,581 attempted bombings, and 1,107 bombs that exploded prematurely during manufacture or before proximity of intended targets.[8] However, the U.S. Department of Justice's extensive database does not allow for much clinical analysis.

The societal impact of one or more sudden traumatic events is difficult to measure. One useful investigation of the clinical epidemiology of a large explosion is from the April 1995 bombing of the Murrah Federal Building in Oklahoma City.[9] This event created a paradigm shift in the conduct of disaster research.[10] It was estimated that over 400,000 people in the metropolitan area were affected in one manner or another.[11] There were documented adverse effects on the mental health of portions of the exposed population: injured survivors, families and acquaintances of those killed and injured, and people whose level of fear and stress were heightened by the event. Long-term epidemiological studies following the events of September 11, 2001, have been appearing gradually in the medical literature. The impacts of explosive events on local healthcare systems have been more frequently reported, and will be detailed in this chapter.

CURRENT STATE OF THE ART

Research into the mechanisms of blast injuries, and their clinical evaluation and management has proceeded steadily over the last century, with accelerations in periods of wartime. Some information gained during World War II is just as relevant today, while more recent biochemical and imaging technologies with enhanced computing power and sophisticated mathematical modeling have allowed keener insights into pathophysiological mechanisms applicable to the world's most recent wars. Kluger described four areas of essential knowledge for medical personnel: blast physics, injury patterns, triage, and "treating multiple patients with multidimensional injuries."[12]

Blast Physics

Understanding the physics of explosions enables anticipation of trauma in blast-exposed individuals, some of whom will have no immediate symptoms or external signs of injury. Basic comprehension of the mechanistic forces involved will aid healthcare workers in identifying the full spectrum of blast injuries, especially those that may initially be clinically occult.

Blast Waves

Natural explosions and some industrial accidents occur when gasses confined under high pressure are suddenly released. Most intentional blasts are created by high-order or low-order explosives, both of which involve the rapid chemical conversion of a liquid or solid material into a gas of essentially equal numbers of molecules in an equal volume. Low-order explosives burn rapidly to generate gas, whereas high-order explosives detonate to create gas in nanoseconds. As a consequence, this newly formed gas with highly compacted molecules is under extreme pressure. The initial pressure generated by detonation of the high-order explosive cyclotrimethylene trinitramine, the primary ingredient in Composition C4, is typically greater than 30 GPa. The power of an explosive is customarily normalized to an equivalent weight of trinitrotoluene (TNT) because it is mathematically related to its mass; however, it may be different depending on the substance.[13]

Molecules composing the newly formed high-pressure gas are forced away from each other at supersonic speeds. They push against and compress molecules in the surrounding atmosphere faster than baseline thermal motion can disperse them. This "stacking" generates a dense band of greatly compacted air or water, depending on the surrounding milieu. The energy of this band is propagated spherically away from the epicenter of the explosion as an impulse blast wave. Its leading edge, which is typically only a few millimeters thick, is called the blast front. As a blast wave passes a fixed location, a sudden rise in atmospheric pressure occurs, and force is transmitted to objects.[14] The positive-phase impulse represents the initial spike of overpressure as the blast front speeds past the reference point. Because explosive gasses continue to expand from their origin, a negative-phase impulse of relative vacuum follows. As its energy dissipates, a blast wave eventually deteriorates into a high-magnitude acoustic wave.

High-order explosive detonations cause such a rapid increase in pressures at their blast fronts – and, hence, force generation from high pressure to low pressure – that their blast waves are also referred to as shock waves. Low-order explosives generally do not release sufficient energy fast enough to demonstrate the shattering effects of shock waves. Thermobaric and volumetric weapons, fuel-air explosives, and nuclear detonations create prolonged blast waves, but these are unlikely to be acquired or delivered by non-military groups. Nonetheless, some industrial accident scenarios may mimic this effect, with blast wave characteristics between those of nuclear devices and conventional high-order explosives. These thicker blast waves tend to envelope objects after the initial shock effect of the blast front.

Pressure differentials between the blast front and the surrounding atmosphere also create net movement of molecules that generate a blast wind. Detonation of a high-order explosive causing a peak static overpressure of 35 kPa (strong enough to rupture half of exposed eardrums) may also generate a dynamic pressure sufficient to create wind speeds of 70 m/s.[15] Although they only exist briefly, blast winds can propel objects and people considerable distances. The wind created by a one-ton truck bomb may exceed 400 m/s.[14]

Internal Force Propagation

When a blast front contacts an object, the band of high pressure exerts a force on the object. This is called blast loading. This briefly applied but high-magnitude force creates an acceleration of the object's surface to a peak velocity and maximal displacement, until the elasticity of the surface overcomes its inertia. This rapid surface acceleration induces an internal stress wave propagated into the object roughly parallel to the direction of the incident wave. Solid objects, such as building surfaces, tend to shatter under this stress. More compliant surfaces, such as those of the human body, tend to compress under the force then rebound to their former shape once the blast wave passes. The magnitude of the stress wave in animal tissues is proportional to the peak surface velocity. Figure 29.1 shows the relationships of body wall acceleration, peak velocity, and internal pressure

generation. Compression also creates tangential shear waves proportional to the degree of displacement as surfaces are stretched inward. When this rapid compression occurs at the chest wall, it develops too fast to allow internally increased air pressure to decompress through tracheal venting.[15–17]

Pathophysiology

Mechanisms of internal organ injury following blast exposure are multifactorial, but stress and shear on biological tissues may result from overwhelming the elasticity of the tissue, thus causing damage in some ways similar to blunt trauma. An illustrative analogy is found in the *Textbook of Military Medicine*:

> An aluminum beverage container that is pushed in only slightly will pop back to its original shape when the force is removed (and any work done by that force is recovered). The onset of damage occurs when the stress equals the tensile strength of the material. As the stress increases beyond the tensile strength, the work done by the excess external force will not be recovered.[15]

The primary effects of blast overpressure tend to more severely affect air-containing structures of the body. Differential velocities of stress waves traveling through water-density tissues and through air-density lumina create additional internal shear waves that can tear parenchyma at air-tissue interfaces. This can also occur at any location where a density transition is present.[15–17]

The Northern Ireland Hostile Action Casualty System was devised in an effort to quantify blast loading and its effects on various organ systems. The system estimates injury severity though use of five nonparametric groupings of charge-weight against three groupings of intervening distances.[18] Investigators calculated overpressures in psi (1 psi = 6.895 kPa) then grouped them into descriptors of blast loading: < 20 psi = minor; 20–50 psi = moderate; 51–80 psi = severe; and > 80 psi = very severe. Of the 828 casualties registered into this database between 1970 and 1984, there were roughly equivalent numbers in each of the four groups (Table 29.1). No casualty in the first three groups died of "severe chest injury alone . . . with no serious external injury," whereas 17% of those with very severe blast loading were in this category and presumably died of blast lung injury (BLI). Of the forty-two patients who died in a hospital, twelve did so during the initial ED resuscitation and fourteen during or shortly after an initial surgery. Half of the delayed deaths were due to severe head injury, and half were due to respiratory failure – whether from BLI, acute respiratory distress syndrome (ARDS), or a combination of both could not be established with certainty.

Injury Classification

The trauma caused by explosive detonations has traditionally been categorized by mechanism. Primary blast injury (PBI) is caused by the effects of the blast wave transmitting forces into the body. Secondary blast injuries are ballistic injuries from fragments, shrapnel, and debris energized by the explosion or associated blast wind. Tertiary blast injuries occur when people are displaced by forces of the blast front and blast wind – and are thrown through the air, tumble along the ground, and impact objects.

Further categorization is less standardized. The taxonomy described by Stuhmiller is useful in the description of quaternary blast injury and other trauma not directly related to the explosion. He depicted quaternary injuries as those resulting directly

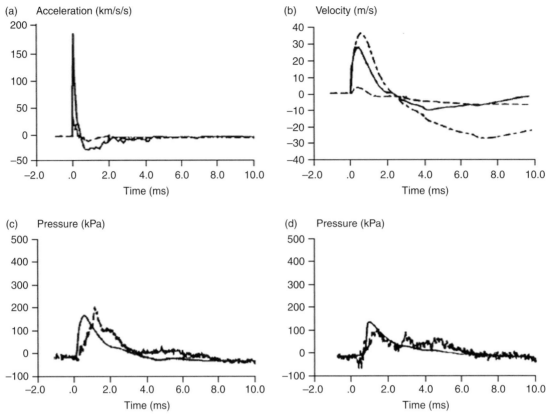

Figure 29.1. Mathematically predicted (solid lines) and experimentally measured (dashed lines) thoracic dynamics caused by blast loading after detonation of 2.2 kg of Composition C4 to the right side of a sheep: (A) acceleration of the right rib cage peaked near 200 km/s²; (B) velocity of the right rib cage peaked near 40 m/s; (C) pleural pressure under the right rib cage peaked at more than 210 kPa (30 psi); and (D) airway pressure in the right lung exceeded 100 kPa (14 psi). This figure is in the public domain as published by the Office of the Surgeon General of the United States Army, Falls Church, Virginia, USA. Reproduced from the *Textbook of Military Medicine*, 1991: 266.

Table 29.1. Relationship of blast loading to severity of injury in 828 casualties from terrorist bombings in Northern Ireland 1970–1984. Adapted with permission from the *British Journal of Surgery* 1989; 76(10): 1006–1010. The article did not specify whether the number of dead represented only those who did not reach medical care, or all deaths in non-disrupted casualties. Major, moderate, and minor injuries were not rigorously defined.

	Blast Loading Overpressure Categorization			
	Minor *<20 psi*	*Moderate* *20–50 psi*	*Severe* *51–80 psi*	*Very Severe* *>80 psi*
Number of cases	255	135	200	238
Total body disruption	0.0%	3.0%	2.0%	9.7%
Dead	2.0%	17.8%	17.0%	51.3%
Major injury	5.5%	9.6%	19.0%	11.3%
Moderate injury	9.0%	11.9%	17.5%	6.3%
Minor injury	83.5%	57.8%	44.5%	21.4%

1 psi = 6.895 kPa

from "all explosion-mediated injuries not associated with pressure or wind effects," most notably thermal, toxic, and asphyxiant mechanisms.[17] Collateral injuries – such as crush from building collapse, fall from a height, or a motor-vehicle crash – would then encompass all other outcomes. Other authors have hypothesized a quinary category of a "hyperinflammatory state" that can lead to hemodynamic instability.[18] Although the exact pathophysiology is uncertain, a toxicological response to the materials contained in many explosives has been suggested, which would move this cellular mechanism out of the quaternary blast injuries described by Stuhmiller.[17]

Obtaining a description of potential mechanisms of injury is important in the management of trauma victims, but these categorizations are more useful when devising equipment and tactics related to injury prevention. Those caring for these patients after an explosion need to know that presentations include a constellation of thermal, penetrating, blunt, crush, toxic, and other injuries, in some cases similar to those from non-blast mechanisms.

INJURY PATTERNS AND INITIAL MANAGEMENT

Because non-PBI mechanisms result in conventional trauma familiar to most healthcare providers, this section focuses on injury patterns primarily resulting from the blast wave itself.

Brain

Severe open and closed head injury is the most common cause of death in blast-injured casualties.[9,14,19] Evaluation and management of blast-induced TBI is generally similar to that of blunt and penetrating trauma from other mechanisms. Computed tomography (CT) is commonly employed, but should not be used for every patient. Rather, history and physical examination should guide clinicians. Mild cases of TBI are often missed, unless patients are properly screened for subtle functional impairments. In a 10-year study of accidental explosions, more than one-third of patients seen at the Maryland Institute for Emergency Medical Services Systems with a normal Glasgow Coma Score had some element of TBI that went undetected on the initial evaluation.[20]

The role of imaging has not been well-defined for TBI solely due to primary or quaternary mechanisms. During mass casualty situations, some authorities have recommended that CT be reserved for diagnosing intracranial mass lesions during the initial management phase – the period when casualties are arriving.[21] Otherwise, CT or magnetic resonance imaging (MRI) can be deferred based on symptoms developed during observation while more immediately serious casualties are being managed.

Blast-induced TBI, which may be distinct from classic blunt or penetrating trauma mechanisms, ranges from mild to severe. The pathophysiology of damage is not well understood and often not apparent using conventional imaging techniques.[22] Putative mechanisms of primary TBI are likely a combination of gross acceleration, skull deformation and rebound, surge of blood and cerebrospinal fluid from the blast-loaded thorax, air emboli from blast-injured lungs, micro-implosions in the brain substance, dysfunction of the blood-brain barrier, superoxide and toxicological effects, and electromagnetic pulse injury from superheated gases. Local biochemical and systemic metabolic derangements contribute to the injury patterns.[23,24] A trial published in 2013 suggests that N-acetylcysteine administered within 24 hours of injury decreases immediate sequelae of mild TBI such as dizziness, hearing loss, headache, memory loss, sleep disturbances, and neurocognitive dysfunction.[25]

All blast-exposed individuals must be screened for TBI. Neurological deficits found on examination of blast victims range from subtle dysfunction to complete unresponsiveness. Key screening questions for potential neurological injury include: Do you have headache, vertigo, unsteadiness, or nausea?[2] This may help identify patients at risk for mild TBI and allow early initiation of casualty protection and medical management. No specific assessment methodology for subtle neurocognitive deficits has proved superior in all settings, though one successful screening tool is the Military Acute Concussion Evaluation (MACE).[26] Even patients believed not to have TBI should be provided detailed instructions regarding post-concussion syndrome and post-traumatic stress disorder (PTSD), which may be more closely related than previously suspected.

Eyes, Ears, Sinuses, and Throat

Auditory and ocular injuries were the most frequently missed in one Israeli report of mass casualty incidents.[21] Healthcare providers should ask questions focused on visual and auditory symptoms:[2]

Do you have pain or problems with your eyes or ears? Any decreased vision represents a penetrating foreign body or intraocular hemorrhage until proven otherwise. Ringing, roaring, or decreased hearing is common, but determination of the long-term effect on hearing requires detailed audiometric testing on serial follow-up evaluations.

What does your pain feel like? Eye pain is typically severe, and blepharospasm may make thorough examination difficult. Ear pain caused by a ruptured tympanic membrane (TM) is often sharp initially, but wanes over time.

Foreign material and penetrating eye injuries are common after explosions. Hyphema[14] and a variety of macular abnormalities,[17] without obvious blunt or penetrating mechanisms, have been postulated as forms of PBI. The management of penetrating and non-penetrating eye injuries is beyond the scope of this chapter; however, ultrasound has been suggested as a screening tool for ocular damage in blast-injured casualties.[28]

Temporary hearing loss and tinnitus are common, the severity of which typically decreases at greater distances from the explosion. This can make communications challenging. Rupture of the TM also occurs frequently. Permanent hearing loss can result from irreparable damage to structures of the inner ear.[29,30] Transient, intermittent, and/or permanent blast-induced vestibulopathy and dysequilibrium can also occur, most commonly due to tearing of microstructures within the cochlea. Symptoms can also manifest remotely after the injury, and should be considered in patients with vertigo and a history of exposure to blast overpressure. CT imaging of the temporal bones can be diagnostic for this injury.

Blast auditory injury (BAI) is not life-threatening, but should be considered after patients are stabilized. Practitioners should examine the ears using direct otoscopy. TM perforation, disruption of the ossicular chain, and gross contamination should be noted. Rupture and blood together could be indicative of concomitant TBI. In the absence of multiple casualties, an otolaryngologist should be consulted and the patient should be seen within 1 day if there is significant debris in the ear or the torn edges of the TM require realignment.

TM rupture may be a marker for TBI.[31] It indicates exposure to blast overpressure, thus prompting mental-status and neurological examinations. On the other hand, contrary to previous expert opinions, the presence of TM rupture in patients without pulmonary manifestations in the first hour after injury does not appear to be a surrogate marker of sufficient blast overpressure to produce delayed-onset BLI.[32] Absence of TM rupture makes BLI less likely, but does not completely eliminate the possibility.[33]

Chest

Blast waves that gain access to the upper respiratory tract can cause pharyngeal, laryngeal, and tracheal petechiae and ecchymoses.[16,34,35] These findings may indicate sufficient blast loading to also cause BLI. However, blast waves do not cause BLI via an air pulse down the respiratory tract. Rather, BLI is caused by forces applied to the chest wall.

A variety of injuries may occur in the lungs due to tissue tearing. Blood can leak into the parenchyma, into the pleural space, or into the airways. Air can leak into the tissues, into the pleural cavity, or into the circulatory system. Box 29.1 summarizes the conditions resulting from air-tissue interfaces in the chest.

The prototypical BLI is hemorrhage into the pulmonary tissues and small airways. This can range from subpleural petechiae to contusions of various shapes and sizes.[34,35] The degree of damage is proportional to the peak chest-wall velocity.[36] Figure 29.2

Box 29.1. Conditions resulting from disruption of tissue interfaces in air-containing structures of the torso. This information is in the public domain as published by the Center for Total Access, Fort Gordon, Georgia, USA. It was adapted from the *Special Operations Forces Medical Handbook,* 1st ed., 2001, pp. 7–23.

Chest

Escape of air
    into lung parenchyma results in traumatic
        pseudocyst
    into pleural space results in pneumothorax
    into vasculature results in systemic air
        embolism

Escape of blood
    into lung parenchyma results in pulmonary
        contusion
    into pleural space results in hemothorax
    into airways results in hemoptysis

Abdomen

Escape of air
    into bowel parenchyma results in
        pneumointestinalis
    into peritoneal space results in
        pneumoperitoneum
    into vasculature results in portal air embolism

Escape of blood
    into bowel parenchyma results in bowel-wall
        hematoma
    into peritoneal space results in hemoperitoneum
    into bowel lumen results in GI hemorrhage

GI = gastrointestinal

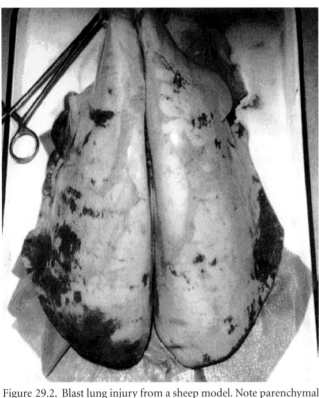

Figure 29.2. Blast lung injury from a sheep model. Note parenchymal contusions, the most severe of which are found in areas of the lung between reflecting surfaces such as the chest wall and diaphragm. Also note some hemorrhages located under the intercostal spaces. This photograph is in the public domain as published by the Office of the Surgeon General of the United States Army in Falls Church, Virginia, USA. It was reproduced from the *Textbook of Military Medicine,* 2012, p. 275.[17]

shows pulmonary contusions of various severities in different locations in a sheep model. Pulmonary lacerations can result in alveolar-venous fistulae; traumatic emphysema, if contained within the lung parenchyma; and hemopneumothoraces and bronchopleural fistulae, if involving the visceral pleura.

Alveolar-venous communications can allow air to enter the pulmonary venous circuit, travel to the left heart, and be ejected as systemic air emboli. Organ infarction and death can occur within minutes. Air embolism can also occur following blunt or penetrating trauma.[37] Bronchopleural fistulae can lead to unilateral or bilateral tension pneumothoraces.[38] Both of these conditions can be rapidly and significantly exacerbated by positive-pressure ventilation (PPV).[14,37] Some experts suggest that the commencement of PPV can accelerate death in initial survivors.

Medical personnel should ask targeted questions of casualties who can speak:[2]

"Are you short of breath?" Dyspnea may indicate tension pneumothorax, hemopneumothorax, pulmonary contusion, or shock from hypoxia, hemorrhage, or systemic air embolism.

"Do you have any chest discomfort?" Penetrating or blunt trauma, pneumothorax, and myocardial ischemia due to coronary air embolism can all cause chest pain.

"What does your pain feel like?" Pain associated with pneumothorax is typically sharp and focal, lateral or central, and aggravated by breathing until the lung is completely collapsed. Pain of pulmonary contusion is often described as dull and diffuse. Discomfort may wax and wane with respirations. Bronchospasm or difficulty expanding the chest may be described as tightness. Chest pain that seems consistent with an acute coronary syndrome may be due to air embolism to one or more coronary arteries.

"How much effort is required to breathe?" Dyspnea at rest may indicate shock due to external or internal hemorrhage; hypoxia due to airway obstruction or pneumothorax; or severe pulmonary contusion. Increased severity of dyspnea on exertion suggests the presence of BLI or pulmonary damage by another non-PBI mechanism.

Physical examination findings consistent with BLI include tachypnea; difficulty completing sentences in one breath; dry cough, with or without wheezing; hemoptysis of varying degrees; diminished breath sounds indicative of pulmonary contusion,

Table 29.2. Severity categories for BLI reported by Pizov et al., which may help predict the necessity for use of PPV and PEEP. This table is in the public domain as a U.S. government work. It was adopted from the *Annals of Emergency Medicine* 2001; 37(6): 664–678. Assumptions are: ambient air has an F_IO_2 of 0.21, a non-rebreather mask delivers F_IO_2 in the range 0.50–0.70, and bag-valve-mask delivers F_IO_2 in the range of 90–96%.

	BLI Categorization		
	Mild	*Moderate*	*Severe*
Bronchopleural fistulae	Absent	Possible	Present
Infiltrates on plain chest radiography	Unilateral	Bilateral but asymmetrical	Bilateral and diffuse
p_aO_2-to-F_IO_2 ratio examples	>200 torr $p_aO_2 > 42$ torr on $F_IO_2 = 0.21$ $S_PO_2 > 75\%$ on $F_IO_2 = 0.21$	60–200 torr p_aO_2 36–120 torr on $F_IO_2 = 0.60$ $S_PO_2 = 75$–90% on $F_IO_2 = 0.60$	<60 torr $p_aO_2 < 56$ torr on $F_IO_2 = 0.93$ $S_PO_2 < 90\%$ on $F_IO_2 = 0.93$
PPV requirement	Unlikely for a respiratory problem	Highly likely but conventional methods usually effective	Universal and unconventional methods often necessary
PEEP requirement	<5 cmH_2O if PPV required	5–10 cmH_2O usually necessary	>10 cmH_2O if volume-controlled PPV still used

F_IO_2 = fraction of inspired oxygen; p_aO_2 = arterial dissolved oxygen; S_PO_2 = arterial oxygen saturation as measured by pulse oximetry

pneumothorax, or hemothorax; inspiratory rales or dullness to percussion caused by interstitial edema, parenchymal hemorrhage, or hemothorax; and poor chest-wall expansion caused by decreased lung compliance. Rapid, shallow respirations are characteristic of BLI casualties.

Pizov et al. published a report on their observations regarding BLI severity of victims from bombings on commuter buses in Israel.[38] They were able to classify injuries into mild, moderate, and severe based on plain chest radiography, arterial blood-gas (ABG) analysis, and the presence of bronchopleural fistulae. Contusion densities on chest radiographs ranged from localized unilateral to massive bilateral, whereas the p_aO_2 to F_IO_2 ratio (PFR) was a marker of lung injury impairing oxygen diffusion.

Wightman and Gladish combined this classification with information from other studies to create the correlates of clinical information with the need for PPV (Table 29.2).[14] Mild BLI, defined as one lung focally injured and a p_aO_2 maintained over 5.6 kPa on an ambient F_IO_2 of 0.21, may require supplemental oxygen administration, but generally will not require PPV for respiratory compromise. Moderate BLI, defined as most of one lung or both lungs involved asymmetrically and an inability to maintain a p_aO_2 of 17.4 kPa with an F_IO_2 of 0.60 using a non-rebreather mask (NRBM), normally requires some period of volume-controlled ventilation using reasonable levels of positive end-expiratory pressure (PEEP) or pressure support. Severe BLI, defined as the inability to achieve a p_aO_2 of 8.1 kPa with an F_IO_2 of 0.93 using a bag-valve-mask (BVM) system, often requires pressure-controlled ventilation, inverse inspiratory-to-expiratory ratios, and permissive hypercapnia.

Wightman used the oxygen-hemoglobin dissociation curve to estimate pulse oximetry (S_PO_2) measurements corresponding to PFR categorizations for use in the out-of-hospital setting.

These recommendations assumed no major left or right curve shifts, no significant elevations in altitude, and no hemoglobin or mitochondrial toxins.[2] Mild BLI is defined as any S_PO_2 reading at or above 75% hemoglobin saturation on ambient air. Moderate BLI exists with any reading at or above 75% on a NRBM. Severe BLI is diagnosed by a reading less than 90% when using a BVM.

BLI is uncommon from terrorist bombings in open-air civilian settings.[39] Most victims close enough to high-order detonations to sustain BLI are killed by other blast mechanisms. One notable exception is the terrorist bombing event behind the U.S. Embassy in Nairobi, where BLI was a significant finding in victims. This was likely due to the charge detonating in a space surrounded by three multistory buildings that reflected the blast wave multiple times.[40] In distinction, explosions in confined spaces create casualty populations with much higher proportions of survivors manifesting BLI – especially when devices did not generate many fragments or shrapnel, or victims were protected from significant secondary ballistic objects.[41,42]

Katz and colleagues described the connection between confined spaces and increased incidence of PBI in initial survivors.[41] They reported on fifty-five casualties transported to two major medical centers in Jerusalem following detonation of a 6-kg device placed under a seat inside a commuter bus. Close to half of the casualties were evaluated and discharged from the EDs. All twenty-nine admitted patients had PBI of the ears, lungs, or bowel. For victims less severely injured but still admitted, there was a 29% (5/21) incidence of BLI and a 10% (2/21) incidence of "nonperforating bowel injury," that is, presumptive blast intestinal injury (BII). In casualties with more severe injuries, 75% (6/8) had BLI and 25% (2/8) had BII.

Pizov and colleagues pooled data from two similar explosions in commuter buses to report on their experiences with managing

BLI.[38] Forty-seven victims were found dead at the scenes and one more died on ED arrival. Of the seventeen survivors, fifteen (88%) had BLI. Nine (60%) had pneumothoraces, which were bilateral in seven. Five had clinically significant bronchopleural fistulae.

Patients with tension pneumothorax require needle thoracentesis followed by tube thoracostomy. Unilaterally decreased breath sounds and evidence of clinical shock should prompt immediate pleural decompression. Air escape without clinical improvement should raise suspicion for bronchopleural fistula, which may require one or more chest tubes, independent lung ventilation by preferential intubation of the unaffected lung or use of a dual-lumen endotracheal tube, or interventional surgery. In mass casualty scenarios, chest tubes before radiography have been recommended for any serious thoracic injury. If bilateral tension pneumothoraces have been ruled out in patients with cardiac arrest, resuscitative thoracotomy should not be performed, because these casualties most often have non-survivable pulmonary contusions.[21]

Spontaneous, negative-pressure ventilation is preferred over PPV whenever possible.[14] In a study of BLI patients admitted to the ICU at one Israeli medical center, 61% were intubated in the field or on arrival to the ED and 14% were intubated within 2 hours for progressive respiratory distress. The other 25% did not require mechanical ventilation.[42] Noninvasive PPV has been used successfully to avoid endotracheal intubation in some patients.[43] When invasive PPV becomes necessary, the initial use of PEEP up to 10 cmH$_2$O is acceptable early in management.[38] The need for more PEEP to maintain oxygenation should prompt a reassessment of ventilator mode, with consideration of pressure-control ventilation rather than the more commonly employed volume-control method.[2]

Systemic arterial air embolism should be considered any time a communication between the airways and the pulmonary venous circuit is suspected, such as with hemoptysis.[44] Embolic infarction syndromes related to one or more vascular distributions may be noted on clinical examination.[14,44] Semi-left-lateral decubitus or prone positioning have theoretical but unproven benefits.[14] Otherwise unexplained cardiac arrest might also suggest systemic air embolism. When managing individual cases (i.e., not in a resource-constrained setting), if the side of injury can be determined, resuscitative thoracotomy with hilar twist may be lifesaving.

Optimal fluid management in patients with BLI is controversial, just as it is for pulmonary contusions due to blunt chest trauma. Colloids have been recommended over crystalloids for BLI, but outcome data are lacking. Following blunt trauma, neither the amount nor type of fluid seems to make a significant difference.[45,46] Similar issues exist for blast and blunt TBI.[14]

ABG analysis is useful for stratifying patients into mild, moderate, and severe lung injury, regardless of etiology – for example, due to BLI (Table 29.2), blunt contusion, or ARDS (Table 2).[14,38] The presenting PFR is predictive of outcome in blunt pulmonary contusion.[45,46] Most other laboratory tests are unlikely to be helpful in early identification or management of PBI.[47] During mass casualty situations, individual facilities will need to assess current resources and surge capacity to define specific laboratory protocols for blunt, penetrating, and thermal trauma.

A plain chest radiograph is essential in victims with any traumatic torso-related complaint. This may also be used to confirm endotracheal, thoracostomy, and gastric tube placements. The cardiac silhouette may be enlarged as a result of right heart overload from increased pulmonary vascular resistance due to significant BLI.[48] Although almost any radiographic finding might have a conventional traumatic cause, manifestations of BLI include interstitial or alveolar fluid, hemothorax, pneumothorax, or pulmonary pseudocyst.[45,49] Infiltrates consistent with pulmonary contusions are the most common parenchymal findings. Pulmonary injury severity can also be categorized radiographically (Table 29.2).[38]

Additionally, as more emergency medical providers are trained in the use of ultrasound, this will likely become a useful tool in the rapid assessment of pulmonary and intra-thoracic injury. Ultrasonography is a relatively inexpensive method to screen large numbers of patients rapidly at the point of care, and also allows for out-of-hospital evaluation in ways not possible with traditional radiographs. This is especially true in the evaluation for pericardial effusion, pneumothorax, and hemothorax. There are currently no accepted standards for the use of ultrasound in the evaluation of blast chest trauma, however this is an emerging area of study.

Chest CT is an imaging option to quantify interstitial and alveolar fluid, and relate findings to ventilatory requirements of mild and severe categories, similar to those of Pizov et al.[38] In one report of patients with non-blast trauma, all those with more than 28% airspace filling required ventilatory assistance; none with 0% to 18% filling did.[50] Transthoracic and transesophageal echocardiography have been used to image air bubbles transiting cardiac chambers.

Abdomen

Box 29.1 summarizes conditions resulting from disruption of air-tissue interfaces in the abdomen. When stress-induced pressure differentials cause tissue tearing of air-containing structures in the gastrointestinal (GI) tract, these organs can bleed into the mesentery, bowel wall, or lumen. Figure 29.3 shows contusions

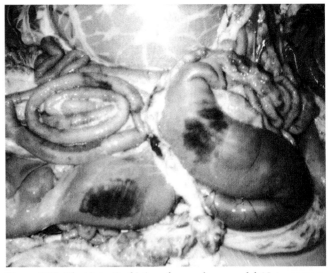

Figure 29.3. Blast intestinal injury from a sheep model. Note segmental parenchymal contusion in areas against the body surface. Also note intraluminal blood visible through other areas of relatively intact bowel wall. This photograph is in the public domain as published by the Office of the Surgeon General of the United States Army in Falls Church, Virginia, USA. It was reproduced from the *Textbook of Military Medicine*, 2012, p. 274.[17]

of the bowel wall and intraluminal hemorrhage in a sheep model. Weakened parenchyma can rupture, releasing air and GI contents into intrathoracic, intraperitoneal, or extraperitoneal spaces. The colon is the organ most commonly affected, likely because of its larger gas content.[48,51,52] Tension pneumoperitoneum has been reported.[53]

Overall, the incidence of BII in initial survivors ranges from 1–33% depending on explosive energy, distance from the epicenter, wearing of body armor, air versus water medium, closed versus open airspace, and multiple other factors.[52] Based on literature from World War II and Israeli Naval battles, BII is more common in victims exposed to underwater blasts.[48] Fragments do not travel very far in water, but blast waves are propagated much greater distances than they are in air. Individuals treading water or buoyed upright by a flotation device have no TM exposure, only partial thoracic exposure, and full abdominal exposure to underwater blast fronts. Hence, the abdomen receives proportionally greater blast loading.[15]

Targeted questions to ask casualties are similar to those for blunt abdominal trauma:[2]

"Do you have abdominal or testicular pain, nausea, urge to defecate, or blood in your stools?" BII may cause visceral, parietal, or referred pain. Tenesmus and hematochezia are relatively common presenting complaints.

"What does your pain feel like?" Stretched bowel wall feels like a persistent gas bubble with possibly sharp and crampy waves as it is affected by peristalsis. Once the bowel ruptures, pain often decreases until peritonitis begins. The pain of peritonitis is commonly diffuse and severe, and may be associated with fever.

The abdominal, flank, back, genital, perineal, and rectal examinations are the same as for any other polytrauma patient, though the probability of bowel rupture is comparatively higher. Moreover, pathology can evolve over time as bowel-wall weakening can be delayed by several days following BII without immediate rupture.[54–56] Blast-injured casualties with any abdominal signs or symptoms require serial examinations over several days.

Ancillary evaluation protocols for individual patients should be similar to those for blunt abdominal trauma, except clinicians must realize that the pretest probability of bowel rupture is higher, especially following closed-space explosions.[14] Routine plain chest radiographs should be scrutinized for free intraperitoneal air. Focused assessment with sonography for trauma (FAST) or CT may be employed to visualize free intraperitoneal fluid. FAST may also be used as a rapid screening tool for intraperitoneal hemorrhage, whether or not combined with a specific triage methodology. However, a detectable amount of hemorrhage is an uncommon finding in intestinal perforation from any cause. CT, especially without GI contrast material, is also not particularly sensitive in detecting bowel rupture.[52]

Other Primary Blast Injuries

A syndrome of bradycardia and hypotension without blood loss has been described in blast-injured soldiers.[34] Blast loads directed only toward the chest in animal models cause a unique, vagal nerve-mediated form of cardiogenic shock without compensatory vasoconstriction.[57] This phenomenon occurs within seconds of exposure, and partially resolves over 1 to 2 hours. Pressure-sensitive pulmonary C-fiber receptors may be the initiating afferent limb of this reflex.[58]

Blast loading can also damage solid organs through displacement of body surfaces, shear-wave stretch, and acceleration at organ attachments. The heart and intra-abdominal solid organs may sustain petechiae, contusions, lacerations, or rupture. Mesenteric, retroperitoneal, and scrotal hemorrhages have also been reported.[35]

The combination of stress-wave induced shattering of bone and subsequent blast wind can tear off all or portions of the extremities and the head. Isolated torsos were all that were found of many victims exposed to the 1998 detonation of one metric ton of TNT-equivalent explosives behind the U.S. Embassy in Nairobi. Multiple traumatic limb amputations, with or without genital and intrapelvic injury, has become the signature IED injury in the Afghanistan conflict.[59,60] Nonetheless, survival to reach definitive medical care is now common. Fourteen amputations occurred in survivors of the 2013 bombings at the Boston Marathon.

Local Medical Responders

Destruction of structures and associated debris resulting from explosive blasts hampers initial rescue efforts of first responders. The threats of accidental or intentional secondary blasts; evolving hazards such as fire, smoke, toxic substances, and building collapse; and potential follow-up attacks with ballistic weapons can restrict local responders' abilities to reach victims. Even when victims are located, single or combined threats can affect the speed and accuracy of clinical assessment prior to movement of patients out of these hazardous environments.

No matter how clinically contraindicated the rapid movement of blast victims may seem, the risks of lingering in an area of recent explosive activity to more adequately stabilize victims may be greater than any risk associated with early rescue or transportation. Organizations tasked with first response should anticipate the unique challenges of rapid evaluation, triage, initial treatment, and evacuation of individual or multiple blast victims.

Stein and Hirschberg described four out-of-hospital management phases based on their experiences with terrorist bombings in Israel.[21] The "chaotic phase" is characterized by ambulatory victims self-evacuating or being transported from the scene by well-meaning bystanders. No professional responders have arrived, and no Incident Commander has assumed control of the situation. The "reorganization phase" begins with the arrival of law-enforcement, fire/rescue, and EMS assets. Triage is performed and resources are allocated for the most seriously injured casualties. The "site-clearing phase" involves evacuation of known patients and thorough searches for missed victims. In urban settings in Israel, scenes are typically cleared in less than 3 hours. The "late phase" encompasses the time required for all victims suffering from blast-related injuries to present for care. Minimally injured casualties and those with medical or emotional complaints usually seek care within 1–2 days of the event.

Einav and coauthors suggested three phases: rapid on-scene triage with a minimum of medical interventions; urgent evacuation of critically injured casualties to the nearest hospital for resuscitation and stabilization; and transportation of all other casualties to more distant and presumably less-burdened facilities, so as not to overwhelm those closest to the scene.[61] A fourth phase might be the redistribution of casualties from less-capable hospitals to regional trauma or medical centers.

Singer and colleagues detailed the Israeli experience in out-of-hospital responses to terrorist attacks.[62] The first medical team that arrives does not provide care. Its primary function is scene assessment and communication to Incident Command. Key transmission elements include: 1) type of event; 2) estimated casualty numbers; 3) location(s) of casualties; 4) safe approach and evacuation routes; and 5) estimated time of first casualty arrival at the closest hospital. As the next wave of medical teams arrive, they evaluate and manage casualties as they find them. Larger responses would allow additional medical teams to be assigned to different geographical regions.

Access

The potentially unstable environment associated with explosive blasts may limit search and rescue efforts. There is a dearth of best-practice recommendations for out-of-hospital responders. However, a few observations can be stated.

Significant rescue and response efforts require coordination among public safety agencies, including emergency management, fire/rescue, law enforcement, and public health. As such, emergency management partners should use the Incident Command System (ICS). Coordination with utility companies allows rapid response to situations that put rescuers at risk, such as ruptured pipelines or damaged power lines. Bomb squads or military explosive ordnance disposal teams may be required, if unexploded devices are discovered.

Explosions can cause collapse of buildings and other structures. Access to trapped victims falls under the discipline of urban search and rescue (US&R). Delayed access may result in natural progression of pathophysiological processes, with more complications from blast manifesting before medical personnel can make initial contact with victims or prior to extrication to medical teams at a casualty collection point (CCP). Conditions unfamiliar to EMS providers may exist. Some examples include confined-space hypoxia and hypercarbia; restriction of chest-wall expansion; dust, smoke, or toxic inhalations; prolonged, and possibly irreversible, hemorrhagic shock; compartment and crush syndromes; dehydration; and advanced wound infections and sepsis in delayed rescues. Delays in evacuation can similarly result in abnormally prolonged medical-responder patient-contact time prior to extrication and evacuation for stabilization or definitive care at a hospital or alternate site.

Collapse of smaller structures may result in larger proportions of victims surviving to hospital admission. With the collapse of larger structures, outcomes are less favorable, as was observed in those victims trapped inside the Murrah Federal Building in Oklahoma City. In that event, the relative risk of dying was over sixteen times greater in the collapsed portion than it was in other areas of the structure.[9] The only fatality that did not occur as a direct result of the explosion was a rescuer with inadequate PPE who sustained a head injury caused by a falling object.

A "direct-threat environment" exists when responders are exposed to an active hazard. In some situations, scene security becomes a higher priority than casualty care, in order to prevent responders from becoming casualties themselves. When responders could be actively threatened by approaching the victim, it may not be appropriate to attempt immediate rescue. Casualties who can move under their own power should be directed to a safer location if possible. During a military-style attack, they should be told to either move to cover or remain still, so as not to attract attention and become a target again.

If a responder proceeds to a casualty and encounters a hazardous situation, most medical interventions would be inappropriate until both patient and provider are in a safe location. On the battlefield, care under fire is usually confined to control of rapidly exsanguinating external hemorrhage. Immediate airway issues from blast injuries are rare. Basic remedial maneuvers require a constant position, and adjunctive interventions can be dangerously time-consuming in a direct-threat situation. If the responder subsequently moves to a position of safety, more interventions could be undertaken and the casualty could be moved using field-expedient lifts, carries, or other available methods.

An "indirect-threat environment" occurs when rescuers are not experiencing an active threat, but are at risk because of proximity to a hazard. Potential risks and benefits must be weighed before any decisions on access and rescue are made. Safety is a prime function of the ICS. Evolving sensor technologies may facilitate locating victims, and even assessing their physiological statuses. This information will better inform decisions regarding responder risk versus patient benefit.

Out-of-Hospital Triage

Although triage is usually discussed in the context of a disaster or mass casualty scenario where inadequate resources exist to meet medical needs, triage occurs daily in medical settings around the world. It can be applied to any decision related to allocation of resources.

Undertriage refers to categorizing victims into a lower acuity category than their conditions warrant and risks excessive morbidity and mortality from delays in care. On the other hand, overtriage categorizes victims into higher acuity categories than necessary and commits resources that might be needed elsewhere. Whereas undertriage mostly affects individual casualties, the overtriage rate has been postulated to have a linear relationship to mortality in the overall population of critical casualties.[63] However, no evidence is available demonstrating this assertion. All publications to date on the subject describe only associations. It is equally valid to postulate that the strain of working at mass casualty events with higher mortality rates results in more overtriage. Since no studies currently exist demonstrating a cause and effect relationship, either interpretation is equally valid (see Chapter 14). Nonetheless, during resource-constrained responses, incorrect triage decisions have far-reaching consequences on the community affected by the disaster.[64]

Three general domains for the application of field triage have been suggested: targeting, treatment, and transportation.[2] Each must also be viewed in the context of potential hazards for the responders. For instance, care provided to a bleeding victim might be different in a structure partially on fire than it would be on a street with traffic blocked.

"Triage for targeting" refers to locating and accessing victims of an explosive blast. Reconnaissance by aircraft may be helpful in assessing the affected area, but there are limited best practices or technological solutions to support the process of victim location beyond rescuers conducting thorough on-the-ground searches. This may be hampered by debris or hazardous materials dispersed by the energy of the explosion and the blast wind; lack of technical expertise to enter collapsed structures or buildings on fire; or inadequate security to neutralize the threat of additional armed attacks.

Assigning personnel assets to geographical areas with the highest probability of containing salvageable victims should be coordinated through the ICS. External assistance in the form of specialized search-and-rescue teams and equipment may be necessary.

"Triage for treatment" in the out-of-hospital setting involves sorting casualties based on required medical interventions. This presumes that patients requiring the most immediate lifesaving interventions are the ones who will be triaged to the highest priority category, if adequate resources are available to treat everyone.

There are a number of triage systems available for use in mass casualty settings (see Chapter 14). Simple Triage and Rapid Treatment (START) and Secondary Assessment of Victim Endpoint (SAVE)[65] encompass one such system, which has been commonly employed in the United States for many years. However, the SALT (Sort, Assess, perform Lifesaving interventions, and Treatment and Transportation) methodology[66] has received considerable attention in recent years. Internationally, there are other triage systems commonly in use, such as Triage Sieve and Sort in the United Kingdom and an algorithm created by CareFlight in Australia. There are no prospective studies of the performance of any triage system during an actual disaster. Most published articles examined medical records retrospectively, which has led to any conclusions being severely hampered by missing data and small numbers of critically injured patients, the group that would presumably most benefit from rapid and accurate triage.

Most field triage systems divide casualties into some combination of five categories (listed in order of priority): immediate, delayed, minimal, expectant, and dead. However, the Magen David Adom (MDA) Israeli National EMS system uses three categories: urgent, non-urgent, and dead. MDA has the advantage of being a nationwide network with centralized organization in a relatively small geographical area, but many response systems in other communities could adopt a similar approach.

Immediate or urgent casualties are those for whom immediate lifesaving intervention is required. However, the resources needed to save the life of any given casualty in this category are as variable as the conditions that cause the life-threatening problems. When immediately available, and not anticipated to be needed elsewhere, most communities and cultures have an expectation that the necessary resources will be committed. However, if these resources are not available in the timeframe required, cannot be obligated to a single patient, or must be redistributed to many patients (e.g., the time a medical provider can spend with a single patient, or the need for large amounts of resuscitative fluids or blood), casualties in the immediate category might be reclassified into the expectant category.

Other victims would be non-urgent in the Israeli system. Delayed casualties are categorized based on the triage officer's brief assessment as those not needing immediate lifesaving intervention, but without a potentially life-threatening condition excluded. Minimal casualties are those believed to have conditions not requiring intervention during the mass casualty situation in order to prevent undue mortality, morbidity, or suffering.

Although the expectant category derives from medically austere military settings with typically longer evacuation times, it may be necessary to use this designation in civilian settings when needs outstrip resources. Many EMS educators teach an approach to expectant casualties as if they are "expected" to die,

or are otherwise labeled as "unsalvageable." A better approach (for these casualties, who would have otherwise been categorized as immediate) would be to "expect" reevaluation, and initiate more aggressive management once sufficient resources become available.

Whichever methodology is applied, two dynamics are critical: the responders must be intimately familiar with the chosen technique; and they must reassess patients and reassign categories dynamically to optimize victim benefit and allocation of resources. Casualty receivers must also be aware of the system or systems used in their communities, so they are prepared for the types of casualties presenting in each triage category. One caveat to this is that excessive retriaging can also create bottlenecks in patient flow, leading to delays in definitive care.

"Triage for transportation" is less understood outside of the military. It should be self-evident that patients incapable of moving themselves to treatment facilities will ultimately require evacuation. Most of the world's military organizations use triage to sort patients into categories for allocation of scarce transportation resources. In the U.S. Army and Marine Corps, for example, "urgent" patients are those requiring a higher level of treatment within the next 2 hours. "Priority" patients are those who require additional treatment within 4 hours. "Routine" patients require movement to a higher level of care setting within 24 hours, so this would rarely apply to a civilian disaster setting in the developed world. Nonetheless, significant constraints on the availability of evacuation assets, long distances, and lack of suitable destinations may force consideration of this category. Civilian agencies also have the option of changing the expected time frame, for example to 6 or 12 hours, instead of 24 hours.

Some casualties can be placed in a "convenience" category when their conditions would not be expected to deteriorate if care could not be rendered for longer than 24 hours. If this category is employed, these patients would be placed on a medical conveyance only when extra space is available, and no medical attention is required during transportation (e.g., a patient with an uncomplicated pregnancy who requires management in a non-combat zone setting). Because this classification is used by the military for individuals with a medical condition who need only physical movement out a given location, it would likely have limited utility in civilian disaster settings.

The Israeli MDA uses only "urgent" and "non-urgent" triage categories for making treatment and transportation decisions. In a paper that defined mass casualty incidents as those of "large enough scale to recruit most of the rescue teams…within a defined region, regardless of the actual number of casualties," Einav and colleagues examined evacuations from urban and rural scenes of terrorist bombings over a 2-year period.[61] Approximately one in every five victims were deemed to be urgent, although a few incidents were not related to explosions, and those that did result in blast-injured casualties encompassed both open-air and closed-space detonations. However, even in large urban areas, less than half of these critical casualties were evacuated to trauma centers, although most of the remainder were transported to other medical centers as opposed to smaller hospitals. The vast majority of patients arrived at the closest facility, whether self-evacuated or transported by ambulance.

Ideally, critically injured blast casualties should be managed at trauma centers, when available.[67] Children should be transported to hospitals with pediatric capabilities.[68] Consideration should be made for the reintegration of injured children and parents, as separation may lead to social disruption and impediments to care. Less critical casualties should be dispersed to less-burdened facilities farther away from the incident.[62] Use of helicopters, which represent high-value, low-density assets in any disaster response, must be carefully considered. Effective transportation systems for critical casualties require significant community and regional preparedness before an event, but evacuation processes are made even more complex by ongoing threats following initial explosions. Difficult on-the-spot decisions must be made in determining the best mode of transportation (e.g., ambulance or nonmedical vehicle of convenience, ground or air) and best destination for casualties who did not self-evacuate, based on triage category and specific injury types.

Out-of-Hospital Care

Once patients are adequately assessed in a relatively safe environment, the individual out-of-hospital care each victim receives should not be affected by the specifics of post-blast settings. This is true as long as due consideration is given to the potential for exceeding available time, personnel, equipment, and supply resources. Civilians responding to a threatening environment should be aware of the tactical emergency casualty care (TECC) recommendations.[69] These guidelines discuss appropriate care in direct and indirect threat, time-constrained, and resource-limited situations.

Mass casualty out-of-hospital care may require EMS providers to employ techniques with which they are less familiar. Examples include use of methods other than direct pressure to control hemorrhage, since this action consumes medically trained personnel resources that may be more effective elsewhere. Exsanguinating extremity hemorrhage may necessitate control with a proximal tourniquet, either by applying a prefabricated or field-expedient device or inflating a sphygmomanometer to a pressure higher than systolic blood pressure. The use of tourniquets in modern wartime has shown that correctly placed extremity tourniquets improve survival.[70,71] They may also have applications in disaster medicine, but specific use criteria are needed in the civilian setting.[72] Clot enhancing agents such as kaolin, microporous polysaccharide microsphere, mineral zeolite, or poly-N-acetylglucosamine (chitosan) may be useful adjuncts, or applied primarily for truncal or proximal extremity wounds where tourniquets cannot be used.[73]

Although rarely reported in the literature, massive hemoptysis from severe BLI may compromise a victim's airway. If simply allowing patients to attain their own best position for oxygenation and ventilation is ineffective, one lifesaving intervention is to selectively intubate the least injured lung, if sufficient time and resources are available.[14] This can be accomplished blindly as depicted in Figure 29.4.[74] In 99% of cases, a standard endotracheal tube passed orally to its full depth will cause the tip and balloon to sit in the right mainstem bronchus. After cuff inflation and a few ventilations, unilateral isolation should be assessed. If more blood passes around the tube than through the tube, then the right lung is protected from left-sided hemorrhage. If more blood passes through the tube, the right lung is likely the origin, and the left lung must be selectively intubated.[2]

Increased airway pressure or decreased venous pressure exacerbates the risk of air entering the pulmonary venous circuit.[44] Rescuers should permit victims to breathe spontaneously whenever possible.[14] The head should be kept at the level of the heart. When other injuries allow, casualties with unilateral blunt or penetrating chest trauma can be positioned on the side of injury; this will increase venous pressures. Victims with BLI might benefit from semi-left-lateral decubitus or prone positioning, but no studies have demonstrated efficacy. The semi-left-lateral position (i.e., halfway between left-lateral and prone positions) places the coronary artery ostia in their lowest positions, thereby decreasing the likelihood of air entering these vessels. Prone positioning places the left atrium at its highest point to potentially prevent air from passing through the mitral valve into the left ventricle and being ejected into the systemic circulation.

Tension pneumothorax is common in BLI patients, and may be bilateral.[38] Rescuers must be taught to rapidly recognize the presentation of this condition and act quickly to prevent continued hemodynamic compromise. The three potential indications for emergent needle thoracentesis in the field are: 1) unilaterally decreased breath sounds and any clinical evidence of shock; 2) unilateral penetrating chest trauma and severe or rapidly progressive respiratory distress; or 3) bilaterally decreased breath sounds in a moribund patient who is still attempting to breathe.

Intravenous access is indicated in most trauma patients. However, fluid administration may not be required in all situations, especially when resources are relatively scarce. If external bleeding is controlled and ongoing internal hemorrhage is not suspected, volume expansion is unnecessary in casualties who are not hemodynamically compromised, in shock, or unstable. Hypovolemic deterioration would not be expected without continued bleeding. Patients without ongoing hemorrhage, but clinically determined to be in shock, should be resuscitated with isotonic crystalloid fluids or other volume expanders (e.g., Hextend™) to the point of shock reversal. Healthcare providers can administer fluids in 5-ml/kg boluses, thus theoretically minimizing the impact on potentially damaged lungs. Vital signs should improve, but attaining normal values is not necessary. If external or internal bleeding cannot be expeditiously controlled, there is no point in administering exogenous fluids. It is unlikely to be beneficial and may, in fact, be harmful.[75]

Permissive hypotension is a well-established tenet of damage-control resuscitation in the absence of significant head injury. A clinical practice guideline for surgical facilities managing trauma in Afghanistan was made available by the Joint Theater Trauma System in February 2013.[76] However, no substantial evidence for its utility in the out-of-hospital setting has been published since Bickell and colleagues showed improved mortality following penetrating torso trauma in the early 1990s.[77] A consensus was published in the UK in 2000 that intravenous fluids should not be administered in the out-of-hospital setting if a radial pulse is palpable.[78] More recent guidelines for TECC[69] and tactical combat casualty care (TCCC)[79] echo this recommendation.

Evacuation

While local and regional protocols as well as existing disaster plans are the primary determinants of transportation modes and patient destinations, the post-blast environment creates additional considerations. Experience has shown that many, if not most, disaster victims self-evacuate before the arrival of rescuers. This was true following the 1995 sarin incident in Tokyo.[80] This phenomenon was also described after several accidental and intentional explosions.[67,81,82] On the other hand, following the almost-simultaneous detonations of high-order explosives in four commuter trains in Madrid in 2004, "the vast majority of survivors" were evacuated by ambulance.[83] Walking times to area hospitals were not provided.

The intent of scene control and incident command with regard to evacuation is to determine the best destination for

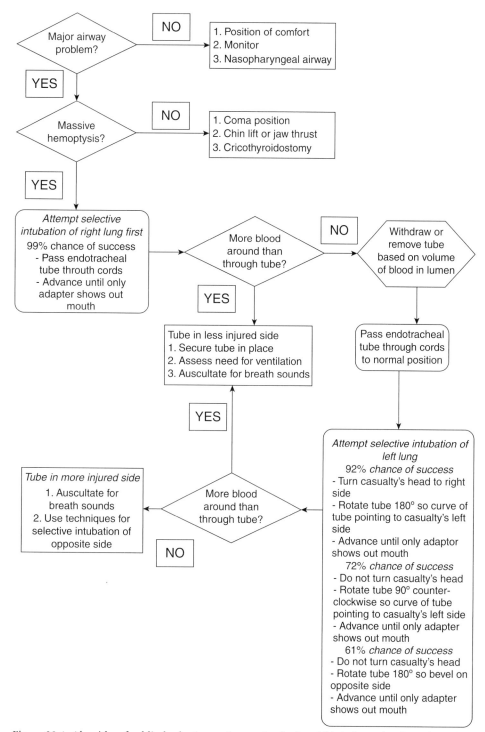

Figure 29.4. Algorithm for blind selective-mainstem intubation. This information is in the public domain as published by the Center for Total Access in Fort Gordon, Georgia, USA. It was adapted from the *Special Operations Forces Medical Handbook*, 2nd ed., 2008, pp. 7–24.

casualties, based on moment-to-moment clinical parameters matched to ever-changing capabilities and capacities of receiving facilities. In a 2-year analysis of evacuations from terrorism-related mass casualty incidents, one Israeli study found that most casualties were transported to the closest ED, despite centralized control of their EMS system.[61]

Unsecured scenes after an attack, or the threat of accidental or intentional secondary explosions may preclude or seriously delay the use of civilian evacuation assets. Nonmedical vehicles of opportunity in the area of the explosion are sometimes used to transport victims to a safer nearby CCP or all the way to a hospital.

Factors that can prevent airborne evacuation of patients include scene safety considerations, natural explosions (e.g., volcanic eruption), or even poor weather conditions unrelated to the disastrous event. In additional, some helicopters do not fly at night. Waterborne evacuation is not often considered, but, in certain locations, may be an option. Aeromedical evacuation requires pilots and medical personnel to consider the effects of altitude on conditions such as hypoxemia, air emboli, pneumocephalus, ocular air after penetrating trauma, pulmonary pseudocyst, pneumothorax, pneumoperitoneum, and bowel injury. All of these can be worsened by decreased partial pressure of oxygen and reduced atmospheric pressure, the latter of which enables existing trapped air to expand.

Receiving medical facilities may be primarily affected by the event, or their capacity secondarily degraded by inaccessibility, utility failures, or staff absenteeism. They may also be overwhelmed by unusual patient volumes and severities in a disaster's aftermath. This may be especially true for any specialty referral centers.

Specialized Responses

Some explosive events pose additional challenges for local responders. Specialized teams with subject-matter expertise and problem-specific training exist in many countries to assist local authorities and respond when requested. Incident managers must be aware of these external assets so they can request, coordinate, and oversee deployment of such resources within their jurisdictions.

Urban Search and Rescue

Many victims injured in collapsed structures are rescued by well-meaning bystanders. Nonetheless, it remains important for the lay public, public safety professionals, and out-of-hospital medical personnel to understand the significant dangers involved in attempting to rescue victims trapped in collapsed structures. One of the first principles taught to first responders is scene safety. Untrained approaches to victim extrication run the risk of additional harm to existing casualties and turning would-be rescuers into additional casualties, thereby increasing the demand for rescue resources, while simultaneously decreasing the supply.

Professional US&R teams exist in many countries; however, they are usually not plentiful, and are often controlled by governmental organizations higher than the community level. For instance, U.S. federal US&R teams are unlikely to be available to assist local rescuers in the first 3–4 days after an incident, unless positioned in the region in advance of an anticipated event. On the other hand, many fire/rescue personnel around the world have been cross-trained in some of these specialized rescue techniques. Individuals may even serve on federal US&R teams in a reserve capacity. Some local fire departments or regional coalitions of organizations have pooled resources to formalize their own US&R capabilities, which can be dispatched by local authorities.

Dirty Bombs

Dirty bombs are any explosive device that intentionally releases a secondary agent (e.g., chemical, biological, radiological). Most people associate this term with radiological dispersion devices (RDDs), but blast energy can be used to disseminate many hazardous or infectious materials. Triage and treatment of biological and chemical casualties are discussed elsewhere (see Chapters 31 and 32).

RDDs, if constructed properly and employed effectively, have the potential to pose a significant risk to an exposed population. Most plausible terrorism scenarios involve acquisition of open-source isotopes. These can either be disseminated with an explosion or delivered in manners similar to biological and chemicals (e.g., contamination of food, distribution through ventilation systems). Radioactive sources simply carried near or placed in the vicinity of people are called radiological exposure devices (REDs). These emanate ionizing radiation, but generally do not cause radiological contamination. Internal contamination via inhalation or ingestion poses the greatest health threat.

Detection of an occult isotope release or covert attack is beyond the scope of this chapter. However, once identified, treatment of radiological casualties is possible (see Chapter 33). The U.S. Department of Health and Human Services hosts a comprehensive website on the medical management of radiation-exposed patients (http://www.remm.nlm.gov). More public domain information is available from the U.S. Armed Forces Radiobiology Research Institute's *Medical Management of Radiological Casualties* handbook (free download available at: http://www.usuhs.mil/afrri/outreach/pdf/3edmmrchand book.pdf). For expert assistance, the U.S. Department of Energy maintains a worldwide 24/7 consultation capability in its Radiation Emergency Assistance Center/Training Site (REAC/TS) (contact information is available at http://orise.orau.gov/reacts).

Nuclear Detonations

Accidental or intentional nuclear detonation is a particularly devastating disaster, because it creates a combination of thermal, blast, and radiological injuries in a massive number of casualties in addition to major infrastructure destruction over a wide area. Blast-wave overpressures from nuclear detonations may be orders of magnitude greater in amplitude than conventional high-order explosives and several meters thick with positive-phase impulses lasting seconds instead of milliseconds. These are expected to crush objects and people. Combined with an intense blast wind, disintegration or total body disruption usually occurs. Casualties of nuclear PBI are usually unsalvageable, even if found intact. Secondary, tertiary, quaternary, and collateral blast injuries are the more likely mechanisms seen in initial survivors of nuclear detonations, because the extreme overpressures typically result in fatal PBI.

As many as 80% of casualties directly injured by a nuclear detonation might have thermal trauma of various degrees either alone or in combination with blast or radiation injury.[84] Mass burn care is by itself a daunting consideration for medical planners and responders, even in the absence of a nuclear event (see Chapter 30). The medical and surgical management of serious burn injury requires significant resources, even for a few individual victims. Irrespective of concomitant radiation injury, no validated triage guidelines exist for such an event, and it has been suggested that organizations follow their routine mass casualty protocols with transfer to burn centers when feasible.[85]

Local Medical Receivers

The most significant challenges for receiving hospitals relate to degraded capacity when victim needs exceed available resources. Staffing shortfalls and infrastructure failure must also be considered when facilities are directly affected by the event. Although Israel has had some success in redirecting patients seeking care for problems unrelated to the disaster, patients in most countries continue to seek care for a variety of medical and surgical conditions. The ability of hospitals to rapidly and accurately screen patients for such problems and refer them to other sources of care may enhance disaster operations at the receiving facility. Hospitals should have a disaster management plan, which evaluates baseline capabilities and surge capacity for handling any type of PICE. While difficult to assess ahead of an event, projecting numbers and types of personnel that would respond when their own lives, families, or homes have been affected helps to determine realistic capability.

Primary Triage

The ED is usually a hospital's primary site for receiving patients requesting unscheduled care. Thus, it is often designated as the place where primary (initial) triage occurs following an off-site mass casualty event. As on any day, all presenting patients must be effectively screened for emergency conditions, in addition to those due to the blast or explosion. Therefore, the ED staff or other designated team performing triage must assess for specific blast-related complaints and physical examination findings. This will facilitate early identification of less obvious injuries that may otherwise be missed. Targeted questions are listed in the injury patterns and initial management section of this chapter.

Part of primary triage's function might be to relieve bottlenecks in the ED by dispersing casualties not requiring ED management directly to other services within the hospital. For example, some immediate casualties, who may have had temporizing interventions in the field or at the primary triage location, could be sent directly to operating theaters or intensive care units (ICUs). Delayed casualties can be diverted to large receiving areas or sent directly to general medical wards for assessment by physicians and nurses stationed there. Although these healthcare providers may be less experienced with trauma management, they should have training in the evaluation of blast-injured casualties for specific life-threatening problems that may develop over time. Minor casualties could be seen at hospital or community clinics. One Israeli study reported that patients admitted directly from triage were sent to the following locations: 28% to an operating theater, 10% to an ICU, and 58% to a hospital ward.[86]

One of the major bottlenecks in mass casualty management of trauma victims is the need for radiological services. One process used in Israel is to send all casualties with non-immediate soft-tissue wounds to general medical wards for histories and physical examinations. If potentially serious delayed injuries are discovered, blood typing and possibly ABG analysis are generally the only laboratory studies necessary. Portable plain chest radiographs could be obtained on the wards, if equipment and technicians are not needed more urgently in the ED, ICU, and operating theater.

After all immediate patients are cleared from the ED, delayed patients can be brought back to the ED for expert reevaluation and any additional ancillary studies. Non-contrast CT has been used to screen all body areas of concern for blast, blunt, and penetrating trauma. Both plain radiographs and CTs are used to identify and localize foreign bodies from debris, shrapnel, and bone fragments from a suicide bomber or other victim.[87] Surgical decision-making and ED dispositions can then be based on clinical examination and imaging results.

Emergency Care

Injuries from explosions include penetrating, thermal, and blunt mechanisms. Clinicians experienced in trauma management should be familiar with all of these. Initial management of various conditions associated with PBI were discussed in the sec-

tion on injury patterns. Permissive hypercapnia[88] and permissive hypotension[76,78,79] should be considered in blast-injured casualties who do not have significant head injuries requiring maintenance of more normal carbon dioxide pressures and higher cerebral perfusion pressures.

Causes of persistent shock include unrecognized hemorrhage, tension pneumothorax, or cardiac tamponade; other cardiogenic causes such as myocardial contusion and air-embolism-induced myocardial infarction; or neurogenic causes such as blunt, penetrating, or air-embolism-induced damage to spinal sympathetic nerves.

Causes of persistent altered mental status or seizures include conventional blunt or penetrating head injury; stroke from cerebral air embolism; hypoxemia from lung injury; or shock from etiologies just described. Intracranial lesions resulting in focal deficits are typically due to cerebral or extra-axial hemorrhage.

Visualization of air in retinal vessels, mottling of nondependent areas of skin, or demarcated tongue blanching are insensitive, but specific indicators of systemic air embolism.

Anesthesia and Surgery

Older journal articles have suggested that patients with BLI have worse outcomes when operative procedures were required within a day after injury. This was presumed to result from PPV and inhalational anesthesia causing unrecognized pneumothoraces and bronchopleural fistulae to create tension pneumothoraces, or forcing air into the pulmonary vasculature to create systemic air emboli. Some experienced authors recommended prophylactic chest tubes for any BLI patient undergoing surgery. Local, regional, or spinal anesthesia were the preferred methods. These complications seem less likely with modern monitoring equipment, and might be further mitigated by an understanding of the risks and benefits of PPV.[14,89] Thousands of surgeries have been performed on blast-injured casualties under general anesthesia during recent conflicts without known complications directly attributable to PPV.

Stein and Hirschberg recommend dividing hospital-based surgical care into initial and definitive phases.[21] The "initial phase" is the interval when casualties continue to arrive and the final number of patients remains unknown. They recommend that only the minimum acceptable level of care should be practiced during this period. Casualties categorized as immediate/urgent should be screened in the ED by personnel familiar with trauma management. Hemodynamically unstable patients should be taken emergently to an operating theater, if one is available. Facility-wide blood use should be controlled by a senior surgeon. The "definitive phase" allows a more conventional approach to surgical management, once the total patient load is known and the operational status of current and surge resources assessed. Non-exsanguinating torso injuries should take precedence over fracture management, wound cleansing, debridement, and other minor procedures. Investigators published a comprehensive review of the surgical management of blast-induced abdominal trauma in 2011.[52]

Healing after planned surgical procedures can be significantly complicated by radiation exposure.[84,90,91] Major surgical interventions must be performed within the first 2 days, or be delayed months until later in the "convalescent phase" of acute radiation syndromes (see Chapter 33). Therefore, damage control, irrigation, and debridement of significant conventional wounds are normally conducted in this time window. A "second look" procedure may be indicated, if performed within the next day or so. However, any attempt at fracture repair or wound closure beyond this period is likely to result in nonunion and dehiscence, respectively.

Intensive Care

Victims of terrorist bombings who need critical care often have high Injury Severity Scores.[87,92] In a study from Israel published in 2006, 26.6% of casualties from suicide bombers required ICU management compared to 6.7% of other trauma patients.[86] In the detailed study by Pizov et al., examination of fifteen BLI patients in ICUs found that only one could be managed without PPV, and eight (53%) required pressure-controlled ventilation or high-frequency jet ventilation.[38] A subsequent study by Avidan et al. from a different institution reported that seven of twenty-eight (25%) of BLI patients were managed without intubation.[43] Permissive hypercapnia has been recommended to keep transalveolar pressures less than 35–40 cmH$_2$O, while still facilitating adequate oxygenation.[38,88] Nitric oxide inhalation has also been used.[38,43] Extracorporeal membrane oxygenation (ECMO) has been suggested for extreme cases.

Arterial air embolism is a rare but serious complication of BLI. It was suspected in only two cases of BLI patients admitted to Israeli ICUs over a 10-year period in one study.[43] One patient developed an acute electrocardiographic injury pattern and suffered cardiac arrest. The other developed a left hemiparesis without CT or MRI abnormalities. Both cases resolved with medical management. However, details of treatment were absent, particularly with regard to hyperbaric oxygen therapy, which is the definitive treatment for air embolism after temporarily placing the patient on 100% oxygen to wash out dissolved nitrogen. Transferring potentially unstable patients out of the ED or ICU to a hyperbaric chamber, or secondary transportation to another facility that offers this resource, can be logistically difficult.

Mass casualty situations may severely challenge ICUs with patients being sent directly from the ED, and post-operative patients requiring intensive care. According to a report by the American College of Chest Physicians' Task Force for Mass Critical Care:

> Most countries have insufficient critical care staff, medical equipment, and ICU space to provide timely, usual critical care to a surge of critically ill and injured victims.... [M]any people with clinical conditions that are survivable under usual healthcare system conditions might have to forgo life-sustaining interventions. Failure to provide critical care will likely result in high mortality rates.[93]

In situations of overwhelming casualty numbers, scarce resources must be justly allocated to provide only "essential care" for the greatest number of critical patients, rather than attempting to stretch existing or surge resources to deliver customary or "usual" treatment to all ICU patients.

One model recommends that hospitals with ICU capabilities be prepared to manage three times their normal capacity for a minimum of 10 days, in order to be as prepared as reasonably possible for any of several disaster scenarios.[94] The Sequential Organ Failure Assessment (SOFA) score may be a useful tool to estimate prognosis in ICU patients. It can assist triage decisions when allocating critical care resources after initial surge capacity has been maximized and patients have been secondarily redistributed between regional hospitals, but prior to the arrival of significant external assets.[95]

Additional Triage

Secondary, tertiary, and subsequent triage decisions occur at any point after primary triage. The first decision is where to send patients after initial evaluation and management in the ED or other location. Additional triage decisions could also involve transfer to regional centers. In non-disaster settings, specific criteria have been studied to determine the need for interfacility transportation to a trauma center.[96] Many countries have established regional referral centers to provide specialty services, which may not be offered at all hospitals (e.g., burn care, hyperbarics, neurosurgery, traumatology). Established transfer patterns may require revision under surge or crisis conditions at both sending and receiving facilities. When resource availability is exceeded, overwhelmed local hospitals will need to perform triage of patients to facilities designated by an Emergency Operations Center (EOC) overseeing total community or regional resources. Depending on the capacity of those included in "normal" referral patterns, transfer out of the affected area may be necessary. In the United States, this can be coordinated through the National Disaster Medical System (NDMS) for federally declared disasters (see Chapter 11).

Knowing the length of time required to establish this level of coordination and how many patients can be managed prior to realistic activation of these resources is essential, and should also be considered in organizations' disaster response plans. A realistic assessment of capabilities is essential to the ability to appropriately triage patients. Undertriage is a risk if the system has not appropriately assessed capabilities prior to actual contingencies and can lead to exceeding the capacity of the medical system.

Disposition

Many patients with open wounds do not require hospital admission. Tetanus immunization status must be assessed and updated if necessary; prophylactic antibiotic administration is often provided; and interventions for body-substance exposures from a suicide bomber or other victims are considered. Blood, bone, and other biological tissues can contact or penetrate casualties – and these substances may be contaminated with infectious agents.[97,98] The U.S. Centers for Disease Control and Prevention (CDC) has recommended stratifying casualties into three risk groups: 1) penetrating injuries or exposures to "nonintact" skin; 2) mucous-membrane exposures; and 3) superficial exposure to intact skin.[99] Within each of these risk categories, guidelines are discussed for hepatitis B and C viruses, human immunodeficiency virus, and *Clostridium tetani*. Post-exposure prophylaxis for hepatitis B virus is recommended for individuals presenting from the scene of an explosive event with nonintact skin or mucous membrane exposure to body fluids or parts.[100] Conversely, HIV prophylaxis is not routinely recommended, and only if exposure is to a known or highly likely HIV-infected source.[101]

All open wounds should be irrigated, yet few can be debrided due to personnel constraints in mass casualty situations. If, for example, ten casualties had ten wounds each, then 100 wounds would require debridement. More casualties with more wounds per casualty – like those depicted in Figure 29.5 – would exponentially increase the workload. This could require allocation of surgical resources that might be better employed in the operating theater for intracavitary injuries and open fractures,

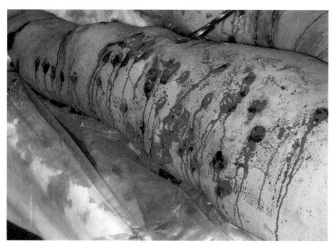

Figure 29.5. Multiple penetrating wounds of the lower extremities from ballistic projectiles following a suicide bombing. Photograph reprinted with permission of Lippincott Williams & Wilkins from Almogy et al. Suicide bombing attacks: update and modifications to the protocol. *Ann Surg* 2004; 239(3): 295–303.

managing post-operative patients in ICUs and on wards, or arranging patient transfers to other facilities.

Discharge planning at ED and hospital levels requires coordination in the setting of disasters. Patients displaced by events may find it difficult to return home. Several issues must be considered when discharging such patients: 1) security; 2) physical structure of the patient's home or extended-care facility; 3) status of utilities and food services in that area; 4) accessibility to emergency services (e.g., no telecommunications, EMS overwhelmed) and outpatient healthcare (e.g., portable oxygen, pharmaceuticals, in-home nursing care); and 5) ability to return for in-hospital treatments of chronic conditions (e.g., chemotherapy, dialysis).

Although it might be possible for patients to remain in the hospital, this could further limit the admission and treatment capacity of the facility as well as increase risk of nosocomial infections and other complications for individual patients. Patient transfer to less-crowded facilities is another option, but one that would require systematic employment of validated protocols guiding "rapid discharge." This process is predicated on a triage methodology for assessing which admitted patients can be discharged safely from a medical facility to ensure adequate resources to treat an incoming surge of casualties.

From a pulmonary standpoint, patients without chest complaints who have normal chest radiographs and arterial oxygenation should be considered for ED discharge. Missed pulmonary contusions will likely develop relatively slowly, enabling patients to return to the ED, provided they have rapid access to an EMS system or adequate social support and available transportation. Any patient with an abdominal complaint or objective finding should have a surgical consult and be observed in the hospital. Such patients should not be discharged until BII has been excluded or sufficient time has passed to significantly reduce the possibility of late bowel perforation.[14]

Patients with isolated TM rupture may be discharged home with instructions to protect their ear canals from foreign material, including water. Antibiotics are not indicated unless there is established infection with myringitis or otitis following a delayed presentation. Most perforations will heal spontaneously, especially those involving less than 80% of the TM surface.

Follow-up

Most blast-exposed and blast-injured casualties require follow-up evaluation for medical concerns, psychological assessments, forensic investigations, and research data. If managed appropriately, BLI mortality and lasting morbidity is not the norm. Follow-up pulmonary examinations of eleven BLI patients admitted to ICUs, who had an average hospital length-of-stay of more than 1 month, found that none had respiratory complaints, and most had normal chest radiographs and pulmonary function tests 1 year later.[102] In a retrospective study of short- and long-term outcomes of ICU patients following terrorist bombings, only 24% of survivors contacted had some degree of respiratory sequelae 6 months to 21 years after injury.[40] Care of discharged patients with BII should follow standard surgical practices.[14] Patients with TM rupture must be followed for assessment for cholesteatoma formation.[103]

Healthcare Systems

During mass casualty situations, the goal of care may need modification, so that the most good can be done for the most people. Optimal care cannot be provided to all when resources are constrained. The concepts of "essential care" or "minimum acceptable care" may require consideration. There are no widely accepted definitions for what constitutes these situation-specific alterations in care. In some circumstances, identifying those who will benefit most from "optimal care" may be possible, in which case such individuals would receive high priority for resource allocation.[104] Acceptability will likely vary regarding how each event impacts a given community's culture of expectations. Conflicts between the healthcare system and the community served may arise when differences in expectations are not adequately communicated in advance.

Permanent Facilities

Hospitals can be directly and adversely affected by explosive blasts, regardless of the cause. Direct explosive damage to healthcare facilities may limit the capacity of casualty-receivers to manage those patients who either find their own transportation or are transported by others to surrounding EDs. The most critical challenges for operations of healthcare systems are:

- Fire;
- Structural integrity;
- Staff, patient, and visitor injuries;
- Personnel's ability to access the facility or specific work areas;
- Access to or replenishment of supplies and equipment;
- Functioning utilities and internal and external communications;
- Adequacy of supervisory and managerial support; and
- Transportation of patients into (or out of, if evacuating patients) and within the facility.

Power loss may disrupt lighting, medical equipment, and safety systems. Disruption of water supplies may affect the adequacy of clean drinking water, and water for personal hygiene and infection control. Sewage outflow may also be affected. Widely scattered debris or direct damage to roads may make it difficult for personnel to report for work. Those already on duty at a facility may need to work extended shifts, or additional days, without relief. Supplies may not be replenished, or malfunctioning medical equipment repaired. Additional information is available in Chapter 22.

In a 1991 event, bombers specifically targeted the military wing of an orthopedic specialty hospital in Belfast.[105] Attackers placed a device of unknown size in a basement fire-exit tunnel near a location where personnel would be watching a major sporting event while off-duty. Two floors above collapsed into the basement room injuring nine people. Two victims died immediately; three seriously injured individuals sustained fragment injuries, burns, and smoke inhalation; and four casualties with minor injuries were able to self-extricate.

Only a resident physician, junior surgeon, and anesthetist were on duty at the time, since no ED existed in this particular facility and the detonation occurred during off-hours. The resident became the Incident Commander until the local fire department arrived. PPE was not available. Although two wards in the wing were evacuated to other areas of the same facility, there were no casualties elsewhere. In this example of an intentional attack against a hospital, sufficient external resources were rapidly available to manage the situation.[106]

However, a device the size of the one used in Nairobi or Oklahoma City employed against a city's multistory hospital would likely result in thousands of casualties. Many victims, some already inpatients with a wide variety of resource needs, would require evacuation to other area hospitals, since the targeted building would likely sustain significant damage and be partially or totally unusable. Hospitals do not commonly practice complete evacuations, although the events surrounding the 1994 Northridge earthquake and 2005 Hurricanes Katrina and Rita revealed that catastrophic circumstances can make such a drastic and extremely difficult action necessary.

The availability of medical personnel to respond should be considered in these situations. Reunification of healthcare providers with their families and loved ones may interfere with their performance or whether they remain at the scene if involved, report to their assigned duty locations, or depart for home. On September 11, 2001, one of the physicians responding to the terrorist attack on the Pentagon was married to one of the victims in the building itself. This provider was of limited value due to her understandable distress while searching for her husband.

Surge Capacity

Surge capacity is a concept that can be intuitively grasped yet remains difficult to define in specific terms. A broad-scope approach to defining a community's surge capacity must include the following areas: out-of-hospital care (e.g., fire/rescue and EMS), in-hospital care, community and extended care (e.g., freestanding same-day surgery centers, medical clinics, and nursing homes), and medical (e.g., pharmacies, outpatient imaging centers) and nonmedical (e.g., electricity, telecommunications, water and sewer) assets supporting healthcare delivery.[107] Addressing surge capacity must include each of the aforementioned component areas if a community intends to accurately assess its true overall capacity and to improve its surge response. The United States and Israeli military experiences suggest that those providing leadership must understand the art and science of surge capacity to successfully manage real-world contingencies. Such issues include risk communication, comprehensive training, creative use of resources, command and control, communications, and effective use of technology.[108] Additional

information, including a description of the 3-S System for surge capacity, is available in Chapter 3.

Temporary Facilities

A variety of temporary facilities might be established by governmental and nongovernmental organizations to mitigate the human impact of an overwhelmed healthcare system. In the context of a community's emergency operations plan, the likelihood of complete infrastructure disruption by a single nonnuclear explosive event is low. The media could use public service announcements to direct persons in need of medical, surgical, psychological, and other services to locations designated by a functioning EOC. Shelter considerations are discussed in Chapters 10 and 11.

In disaster situations requiring additional healthcare capacity, consideration should also be given to employing resources developed for other purposes. An example of this dual-use approach is the U.S.-based Modular Emergency Medical System created primarily for a response to biological terrorism. If prepared and integrated into a community's disaster plans prior to an event, the concept provides a framework for expanding community healthcare capacity as required. One or more high-volume reception and triage facilities can be established directly within affected areas by employing the Neighborhood Emergency Help Center concept. This strategy provides initial community healthcare that is more accessible when victims do not have ready access to transportation, roads are impassible or unsecured, ED capacities are overwhelmed, or there are no post-event functioning healthcare institutions. When hospitals are full, the Acute Care Center concept establishes one or more off-site inpatient facilities. These entities are equipped to manage large volumes of patients with less serious conditions, thus allowing hospitals to focus on more seriously ill and injured victims. However, initial staffing depends on local medical assets.

Rapid Needs Assessments

The rapid determination of infrastructure dysfunction and initial resource needs is critical to providing an effective management, and beginning the process of recovery from an explosive event. One or more rapid assessments are necessary to determine the level of response required. Aerial surveys of the affected area are the preferred approach for determining damage extent.

On-the-ground needs assessments can also identify victims with injuries and illnesses, whether event-related or not. Illnesses may be new or exacerbations of chronic conditions, either from inability to access customary care or exposure to dust, smoke, or other dispersed materials. Healthcare access, in the forms of EMS availability or capabilities of individuals and families to travel to medical facilities, can also be surveyed.

External Response

Major disasters disrupt and overwhelm local response capacity to a degree that outside assistance may be required to help mitigate the human impact of the event. Higher levels of government may control regional resources. Responses are coordinated through an EOC capable of coordinating all necessary resources.

In some countries, federal healthcare assistance to a region may be in the form of a Disaster Medical Assistance Team (DMAT). In the United States, a DMAT is a community-based asset of NDMS under the operational control of the Federal

Emergency Management Agency (FEMA), which is activated by the local Federal Coordinating Center. DMAT personnel provide medical care during a disaster or other local, regional, or state event necessitating expansion of surge capacity. DMATs are composed of fifty or more physicians, physician assistants, nurses, pharmacists, respiratory therapists, paramedics, emergency medical technicians, and a variety of healthcare, logistical, and administrative personnel. They function as rapid-response elements, which are self-sufficient for 72 hours, and supplement local medical care by providing capability to treat up to 250 patients per day in a fixed or temporary site. Roles and responsibilities of DMATs may include triage, provision of acceptable care in medically austere settings, and preparation for evacuation to more appropriate healthcare facilities. DMAT personnel may also be deployed to more distant facilities to assist in receiving large numbers of patients from affected areas. Chapter 11 provides additional information.

Public Information

The ultimate goal of any public educational effort is to prevent problems before they occur. In the United States, CDC advocates for standardization of public health messages issued for a variety of events (see Chapter 25). Medically-related information disseminated to the public and to healthcare personnel should be based on evidence where it exists. Messages should focus on immediate and delayed signs and symptoms of injuries and mental health problems incurred following an explosive blast. Representatives of local, regional, or state public health departments and hospital coalitions can facilitate crisis and emergency risk communication via the media, as well as real-time needs assessments via ongoing monitoring of the situation. Public health assets can further support the medical community in these scenarios by developing surveillance instruments to enhance early identification of TBI and the need for psychological first aid (see Chapter 9).

RECOMMENDATIONS FOR FURTHER RESEARCH

As with many research questions in public health, it is difficult to measure the results of interventions designed to prevent an outcome. Particularly in the field of disaster medicine, comparisons can usually only be made to similar events that were analyzed in the past. Any research beyond that of observation is hampered by the fact that explosive events are extremely heterogeneous. Exposure time, place, and population are difficult to predict, and the number of exposed individuals is usually relatively small without a valid cohort or control group. For these and other reasons, true meta-analyses have not been possible, although some authors have examined multiple individual incidents to determine whether any knowledge can be identified. There are no prospective, double-blinded, randomized, controlled, clinical trials of blast-injury management on humans.

Natural explosions are rare, but their power ranges from sudden steam releases that shower debris in the immediate area to volcanic eruptions that explode with forces exceeding those of military-grade nuclear weapons. Accidental explosions related to human activity range from destruction of single houses following ignition of concentrated natural gas to massive industrial explosions, which might also include dispersion of hazardous materials. Bombings and other intentional blasts also vary significantly, ranging from devices rupturing small compressed-gas cylinders to detonation of truckloads of high-order explosives.

Ideally, disaster research should be multidisciplinary and collaborative, with defined data-collection instruments created before the event occurs.[10,109] Uniform data sets must be created, vetted, and validated for explosive events; universally collected during training exercises and real-world responses; and shared between agencies and the medical community for analysis and future applications. Specific areas of interest would include risk mitigation; system preparedness; out-of-hospital access, triage, medical care, and evacuation; hospital primary triage, resource allocation, and patient redistribution; medical, surgical, and psychological evaluation and management; and medical and non-medical infrastructure recovery. A myriad of governmental and nongovernmental organizations have promulgated best practices. These agencies have codified the knowledge to be gained and applied to the next event. However, little high-quality outcomes research on the response process has been published in open sources.

Response System Preparedness

Security, public safety, protection of critical infrastructure, and preservation of medical capacity must be immediate considerations following an explosive event. Therefore, they must also be dominant topics for readiness research. Many organizations have received large amounts of funding for preparedness, mitigation, response, and recovery activities. However, decisions on how to spend those funds are often formed from anecdotal reports and personal opinion, not on evidence-based research. Even the concept of all-hazard preparedness – presumably a more efficient method for planning, equipping, and training for a variety of predictable and unpredictable scenarios – has not been rigorously demonstrated to be the best approach for responses to heterogeneous PICEs. The same could be said about the U.S. National Response Framework and National Incident Management System (NIMS).

On the other hand, explosive events are a common problem, with which response organizations must contend, whether or not there are evidence-based recommendations for best practices. Standardization, currently through the NIMS structure in the United States, seems like a good first step toward quality research into all phases of the disaster cycle, assuming that useful data are being collected and appropriately analyzed. After-action reports can be useful, but they do not constitute research.

One report took a paradigm for approach to disaster response – promulgated by the American Medical Association – and applied it to several recent bombings in order to determine common findings.[109] Population-based measures of effectiveness must be created for domestic emergency management in all countries, just as they have been for humanitarian responses to disasters and complex emergencies in the developing world. Healthcare system surge capacity is another area that deserves increased attention, although it has been a focus for many professional groups, including the Society for Academic Emergency Medicine, American College of Surgeons, and World Association for Disaster and Emergency Medicine.

Hazard Determination

Determining the likelihood of natural or accidental explosions, or detecting the first or additional intentionally planted explosive devices, is a key function of operational risk management. Excessive concern for responder safety could delay care for casualties with immediate needs, but overwhelming desire to help victims could lead to responder injury, worsening the overall situation. Significant research is being conducted by the U.S. Department of Defense and related agencies to detect IEDs in military scenarios. Knowledge translation and technology transfer should aid the public safety sector as new tactics, techniques, and procedures are developed.

Depending on the type of explosive event, any one of many active or passive sensing methodologies could be layered to assist in risk determination. Acoustic and seismic; chemical; and electromagnetic, infrared, and visual technologies all exist – but research into their best application, employment tactics, and analysis for decision-making is needed or remains classified to governments and militaries. Determining the best platforms for these sensors is another question that must be answered. Animals have been used effectively to detect chemical signatures in the air, but several electronic devices have been designed for similar purposes. Visual and X-ray techniques, either directly by humans or remotely through ground-based robots, are already used by bomb squads and explosive ordnance disposal teams throughout the world. Manned and unmanned aerial systems – from military aircraft to remotely controlled microvehicles – are on the cutting edge of hazard detection.

Personal Protective Equipment

Secondary devices, the possibility of additional natural or accidental explosions, release or threat of hazardous materials release, potential structural collapse or water-vessel sinking, and many other scenarios require protection of responders. Decontamination of hazardous materials and PPE for healthcare providers in these situations is addressed in Chapters 16 and 15, respectively. With regard to blast injuries, ballistic protection is the most important deliberation.

Bomb fragments released after detonation have the potential to cause injury at the greatest distance from the blast site and penetrating trauma is the mechanism that kills or injures the majority of victims in the absence of structural collapse. Intervening barriers protect against secondary blast injury, but not PBI.[16] Helmets and body armor are crucial in preventing penetrating injury to critical organs, but the latter can increase coupling of the blast wave to the body surface, and may magnify its translation into internal stress waves.[110] Research and reviews on improved armor designs have been published, but more work would be beneficial. Research into hearing protection that remains functional in the out-of-hospital environment is also needed.

Clinical Care

Many more questions than evidence-based answers exist in the research agenda for blast injuries. Triage, for instance, requires substantial additional scientific investigation. Even the ability to conduct triage effectively in situations with significant ongoing threats has been questioned. Several authors have retrospectively applied mass casualty triage systems to patients in existing databases in an attempt to answer some of these questions.[111] However, no significant prospective research has been published.

From the field, what is the best destination for casualties in each of the four most common triage categories? Should those with minimal injuries be primarily directed or sent to hospitals out of the affected region? In rural settings, should victims be transported to a closer hospital for stabilization, or evacuated over longer distances to a regional trauma center?

In the field or in the hospital, how much medical evaluation is required for a blast-exposed individual without significant external injury? Does categorization into mild, moderate, and severe BLI based on imaging and PFR assist in subsequent clinical decision-making? Do interventions based on any categorization method have a significant impact on outcome? Designing research investigations to answer these questions is difficult given the complex environments involving different overpressures, body positions relative to the blast front, intervening barriers and armor, and quarternary effects on fixed structures and moving vehicles. Specific injury types and their severities occur over a wide range of blast overpressures.

Do seemingly minor head injuries have long-term consequences requiring early detection to enable preventative treatments? No specific risk factors for BLI sequelae have been found other than those related to ARDS. However, the brain may be different. Further research on TBI is needed and is a high priority topic, but the degrees to which ultrastructural and functional changes contribute are largely unknown. If inflammatory and neurohumoral mechanisms are pathophysiologically important, can they be modulated to improve outcome?

Does specific early management of non-life-threatening injuries change long-term outcome? In military theaters of operation, there is a significant effort being made to identify blast-exposed persons at risk for TBI. Unlike most civilian populations, military populations are expected to be at risk for blast trauma. Therefore, pre- and post-exposure MACE scores can be obtained and compared after any event.

How do primary blast injuries obscure the management of other trauma during and after initial resuscitation? Massive hemoptysis can complicate airway management. Tension pneumothoraces are often bilateral and involve bronchopleural fistulae. Systemic air embolism is difficult to diagnose and treat during initial trauma resuscitations.

Should "standard" resuscitation measures be adjusted for blast-exposed casualties? Is it beneficial to place a blast victim in a different body position other than supine? Can left-lateral, semi-left-lateral, or prone position improve oxygenation or decrease the risk of systemic air embolism? Does delay of intubation and PPV until absolutely necessary improve or worsen outcomes? Higher airway pressure may be required to oxygenate, but excessive airway pressure may increase risk of pneumothorax and systemic air embolism. Shock must be avoided or reversed and inadequate fluid resuscitation may perpetuate lower pulmonary pressure, thus increasing the risk of systemic air embolism. However, is there any difference between standard 20-ml/kg crystalloid fluid boluses compared to smaller, more-frequent aliquots of fluid with regard to improving perfusion without causing secondary lung or brain injury? Is there a best fluid type? What is the optimal ratio of fluids to blood products and ratios of various types of blood products when indicated?

Potential complications related to standard operative and critical care also deserve research attention. What are the risks of tension pneumothorax and tension pneumoperitoneum? Are prophylactic chest tubes necessary and safe for PPV, inhalational anesthesia, or air transport as advocated by some experienced authorities? Can ventilator-associated complications be prevented by assessing specific risk factors or taking prophylactic measures? Could early independent lung ventilation decrease complications and improve outcome?

Longitudinal Studies

Blast-injured casualties should be followed long-term for the emergence of medical and neuropsychiatric sequelae. In addition, researchers should examine the impact of blast exposure on the lives of victims in general, as well as their families and society as a whole. Most longitudinal studies on primary and secondary blast injuries have evaluated eye and ear trauma. Two studies suggested that late sequelae from BLI is unusual.[40,102] No longitudinal studies of BII could be found in the literature.

Although many longitudinal mental health studies have examined survivors from the 1995 Oklahoma City bombing, research into the neuropsychiatric ramifications of sudden and unexpected trauma following explosions is in the early stages. In 2008, the U.S. Department of Defense announced a $300 million (USD) effort to fund research in the epidemiology, clinical care, and long-term effects of TBI and PTSD. The U.S. Congress also appropriated nearly as much to study battlefield injuries. While a good start, more emphasis and funding for research surrounding explosive events is needed to increase the world's ability to care for blast victims.

REFERENCES

1. Lumley J, Ryan JM. Disasters and catastrophes. In: Lumley JSP et al. eds. *Handbook of the Medical Care of Catastrophes.* London, Royal Society of Medicine, 1996; 1–8.

2. Wightman JM, Kharod CU. Explosive events. In Koenig KA, Schultz CH, eds. *Koenig & Schultz's Disaster Medicine: Comprehensive Principles and Practices.* 1st ed. Cambridge, Cambridge University Press, 2010; 393–422.

3. Hamit HF. Primary blast injuries. *Ind Med Surg* 1973; 42: 14–21.

4. Fertilizer plant explosion: pre-planning makes the difference in facilitating for hundreds of injured victims. *ED Manag* 2013; 25: 78–80.

5. Zane DF, Preece MJ. Study of the Phillips tragedy gives insights into etiologies of plant blast injuries. *Occup Health Saf* 1992; 61: 34, 36, 38–40.

6. Centers for Disease Control and Prevention. Fireworks injuries in the United States. *Morb Mortal Wkly Rep* 2000; 49: 545–546.

7. Makitie I, Paloneva H, Tikka S. Explosion injuries in Finland 1991–1995. *Ann Chir Gynaecol* 1997; 86: 209–213.

8. Kapur GB, Hutson HR, Davis MA, Rice PL. The United States twenty-year experience with bombing incidents: implications for terrorism preparedness and medical response. *J Trauma* 2005; 59: 1436–1444.

9. Mallonee S, Shariat S, Stennies G, et al. Physical injuries and fatalities resulting from the Oklahoma City bombing. *JAMA* 1996; 276: 382–387.

10. Quick G. A paradigm for multidisciplinary disaster research: the Oklahoma City experience. *J Emerg Med* 1998; 16: 621–630.

11. Smith DW, Christiansen EH, Vincent R, Hann NE. Population effects of the bombing of Oklahoma City. *J Okla State Med Assoc* 1999; 92: 193–198.

12. Kluger Y. Bomb explosions in acts of terrorism – detonation, wound ballistics, triage and medical concerns. *Isr Med Assn J* 2003; 5: 235–240.

13. Bailey A, Murray SG. *Explosives, Propellants, and Pyrotechnics.* London, Brassey, 1989.

14. Wightman JM, Gladish SL. Explosions and blast injuries. *Ann Emerg Med* 2001; 37: 664–678.

15. Stuhmiller JH, Phillips YY, Richmond, DR. The physics and mechanisms of primary blast injury. In: Bellamy RF, Zajtchuk R, eds. *Conventional Warfare: Ballistic, Blast, and Burn Injuries.* Falls Church, VA, Office of the Surgeon General of the United States Army, 1991; 241–270.

16. Yelverton JT. Blast biology. In: Cooper GJ, Dudley HAF, Gann DS, et al., eds. *Scientific Foundations of Trauma.* Oxford, Butterworth-Heinemann, 1997; 200–213.

17. Stuhmiller JH. Blast injury: translating research into operational medicine. In: Lenhart MH, Friedl KE, Santee WR, eds. *Military Quantitative Physiology: Problems and Concepts in Operational Medicine.* Falls Church, VA, Office of the Surgeon General of the United States Army, 2012; 267–302.

18. Kluger Y, Nimrod A, Biderman P, Mayo A, Sorkin P. The quinary pattern of blast injury. *Am J Disaster Med* 2007; 2: 21–25.

19. Mellor SG, Cooper GJ. Analysis of 828 servicemen killed or injured by explosion in Northern Ireland 1970–84: the Hostile Action Casualty System. *Br J Surg* 1989; 76: 1006–1010.

20. Bochichio GV, Lumpkins K, O'Connor J, et al. Blast injury in a civilian trauma setting is associated with a delay in diagnosis of traumatic brain injury. *Am Surg* 2008; 74: 267–270.

21. Stein M, Hirschberg A. Medical consequences of terrorism: the conventional weapon threat. *Surg Clin North Am* 1999; 79: 1537–1552.

22. Mac Donald CL, Johnson AM, Cooper D, et al. Detection of blast-related traumatic brain injury in U.S. military personnel. *N Engl J Med* 2011; 364: 2091–2100.

23. Desmoulin GT, Dionne J-P. Blast-induced neurotrauma: surrogate use, loading mechanisms, and cellular responses. *J Trauma* 2009; 67: 1113–1122.

24. Rosenfeld JV, McFarlane AC, Bragge P, Armonda RA, Grimes JB, Ling GS. Blast-related traumatic brain injury. *Lancet Neurol* 2013; 12: 882–893.

25. Hoffer ME, Balaban C, Slade MD, Tsao JW, Hoffer B. Amelioration of acute sequelae of blast induced mild traumatic brain injury by N-acetylcysteine: a double-blind, placebo controlled study [abstract]. *PLoS One* 2013; 8(1): e54163.

26. French L, McCrea M, Baggett M. The Military Acute Concussion Evaluation (MACE). *J Spec Op Med* 2008; 8(1): 68–77.

27. Phillips BN, Chun DW, Colyer M. Closed globe macular injuries after blasts in combat. *Retina* 2013; 33: 371–379.

28. Ritchie JV, Horne ST, Perry J, Gay D. Ultrasound triage of ocular blast injury in the military emergency department. *Mil Med* 2012; 177: 174–178.

29. Singh D, Ahluwalia KJS. Blast injuries of the ear. *J Laryngol Otol* 1968; 82: 1017–1028.

30. Okpala N. Management of blast ear injuries in mass casualty environments. *Mil Med* 2011; 176: 1306–1310.

31. Xydakis MS, Bebarta VS, Harrison CD, et al. Tympanic membrane perforation as a marker of concussive brain injury in Iraq [letter]. *N Engl J Med* 2007; 357: 830–831.

32. Leibovici D, Gofrit ON, Shapira SC. Eardrum perforation in explosion survivors: is it a marker of pulmonary blast injury? *Ann Emerg Med* 1999; 34: 168–172.

33. Peters P. Primary blast injury: an intact tympanic membrane does not indicate the lack of a pulmonary blast injury. *Mil Med* 2011; 176: 110–114.

34. Desaga H. Blast injuries. In: *German Aviation Medicine: World War II.* Washington, DC, Office of the Surgeon General of the United States Air Force, 1950; 1274–1293.

35. Sharpnack DD, Johnson AJ, Phillips YY. The pathology of primary blast injury. In: *Conventional Warfare: Ballistic, Blast, and Burn Injuries*; 271–294.

36. Axelsson H, Yelverton JT. Chest wall velocity as a predictor of nonauditory blast injury in a complex wave environment. *J Trauma* 1996; 40(3 suppl.): S31–S37.

37. Yee ES, Verrier ED, Thomas AN. Management of air embolism in blunt and penetrating thoracic trauma. *J Thorac Cardiovasc Surg* 1983; 85: 661–667, discussion 667–668.

38. Pizov R, Oppenheim-Eden A, Matot I, et al. Blast lung injury from an explosion on a civilian bus. *Chest* 1999; 115: 165–172.

39. Cooper GJ, Maynard RL, Cross NL, Hill JF. Casualties from terrorist bombings. *J Trauma* 1983; 23: 955–967.

40. Kalebi AY, Olumbe AK. Forensic findings from the Nairobi U.S. Embassy terrorist bombing. *East Afr Med J* 2006; 83: 380–388.

41. Katz E, Ofek B, Adler J, et al. Primary blast injury after a bomb explosion in a civilian bus. *Ann Surg* 1989; 209: 484–488.

42. Leibovici D, Gofrit ON, Stein M, et al. Blast injuries: bus versus open-air bombings – a comparative study of injuries in survivors of open-air versus confined-space explosions. *J Trauma* 1996; 41: 1030–1035.

43. Avidan V, Hersch M, Armon Y, et al. Blast lung injury: clinical manifestations, treatment, and outcome. *Am J Surg* 2005; 190: 927–931.

44. Ho AM-H, Ling E. Systemic air embolism after lung trauma. *Anesthesiology* 1999; 90: 564–575.

45. Richardson JD, Franz JL, Grover FL, Trinkle JK. Pulmonary contusion and hemorrhage: crystalloid versus colloid replacement. *J Surg Res* 1974; 16: 330–336.

46. Bongard FS, Lewis FR. Crystalloid resuscitation of patients with pulmonary contusion. *Am J Surg* 1984; 148: 145–151.

47. Harmon JW, Sampson JA, Graeber GM, et al. Readily available serum chemical markers fail to aid in diagnosis of blast injury. *J Trauma* 1988; 28(1 suppl.): S153–S159.

48. Huller T, Bazini Y. Blast injuries of the chest and abdomen. *Arch Surg* 1970; 100: 24–30.

49. Adler OB, Rosenberger A. Blast injuries. *Acta Radiol* 1988; 29: 1–5.

50. Wagner RB, Jamieson PM. Pulmonary contusion: evaluation and classification by computed tomography. *Surg Clin North Am* 1989; 69: 31–40.

51. Wani I, Parray FQ, Sheikh T, et al. Spectrum of abdominal organ injury in a primary blast type. *World J Emerg Surg* 2009; 4: 46.

52. Owers C, Morgan JL, Garner JP. Abdominal trauma in primary blast injury. *Br J Surg* 2011; 98: 168–179.

53. Oppenheim A, Pizov R, Pikarsky A, et al. Tension pneumoperitoneum after blast injury: dramatic improvement in ventilatory and hemodynamic parameters after surgical decompression. *J Trauma* 1998; 44: 915–917.

54. Para H, Neufeld D, Schwartz I, et al. Perforation of the terminal ileum induced by blast injury: delayed diagnosis or delayed perforation? *J Trauma* 1996; 40: 472–475.

55. Tatić V, Ignjatović D, Jevtić M, et al. Morphological characteristics of primary nonperforative intestinal blast injuries in rats and their evolution to secondary perforations. *J Trauma* 1996; 40(3 suppl.): S94–S99.

56. Cripps NPJ, Cooper GJ. Risk of late perforation in intestinal contusions caused by explosive blast. *Br J Surg* 1997; 84: 1298–1303.

57. Irwin RJ, Lerner MR, Bealer JF, et al. Cardiopulmonary physiology of primary blast injury. *J Trauma* 1997; 43: 650–655.

58. Irwin RJ, Lerner MR, Bealer JF, et al. Shock after blast wave injury is caused by a vagally mediated reflex. *J Trauma* 1999; 47: 105–110.

59. Mamczak CN, Elster EA. Complex dismounted IED blast injuries: the initial management of bilateral lower extremity amputations with and without pelvic and perineal involvement. *J Surg Orthop Adv* 2012; 21: 8–14.

60. Mossadegh S, Tai N, Midwinter M, Parker P. Improvised explosive device related pelvi-perineal trauma: anatomic injuries and surgical management. *J Trauma Acute Care Surg* 2012; 73(2 Suppl. 1): S24–S31.

61. Einav S, Feigenberg Z, Weissman C, et al. Evacuation priorities in mass casualty terror-related events: implications for contingency planning. *Ann Surg* 2007; 239: 304–310.

62. Singer AJ, Singer AH, Halpern P, et al. Medical lessons from terror attacks in Israel. *J Emerg Med* 2007; 32: 87–92.

63. Frykberg ER, Medical management of disaster and mass casualties from terrorist bombings: how can we cope? *J Trauma* 2002; 53: 201–212.

64. Kennedy K, Aghababian RV, Gans L, Lewis CP. Triage: techniques and applications in decision making. *Ann Emerg Med* 1996; 28: 136–144.

65. Benson M, Koenig KL, Schultz CH. Disaster triage: START, then SAVE – a new method of dynamic triage for victims of a catastrophic earthquake. *Prehosp Disast Med* 1996; 11: 117–124.

66. Lerner EB, Schwartz RB, Coule PL, et al. Mass casualty triage: an evaluation of the data and development of a proposed national guideline. *Disast Med Public Health Prep* 2008; 2(Suppl 1.): S25–S34.

67. Leiba A, Halpern P, Kotler D, et al. Case study of the terrorist bombing in Tel Aviv market – putting all the eggs in one basket might save lives. *Int J Disast Med* 2005; 2: 157–160.

68. Waisman Y, Amir L, Mor M, et al. Prehospital response and field triage in pediatric mass casualty incidents: the Israeli experience. *Clin Pediatr Emerg Med* 2006; 7: 52–58.

69. Committee on Tactical Emergency Casualty Care. Tactical emergency casualty care guidelines. http://c-tecc.org/tactical-emergency-casualty-care-guidelines (Accessed June 22, 2013).

70. Beekley AC, Sebesta JA, Blackbourne LH, et al. Prehospital tourniquet use in Operation Iraqi Freedom: effect on hemorrhage control and outcomes. *J Trauma* 2008; 64(Suppl. 2): S28–S37.

71. Kragh JF, Walters TJ, Baer DG, et al. Practical use of emergency tourniquets to stop bleeding in major limb trauma. *J Trauma* 2008; 64(Suppl. 2): S38–S50.

72. Doyle GS, Taillac PP. Tourniquets: A review of current use with proposals for expanded prehospital use. *Prehosp Emerg Care* 2008; 12: 241–256.

73. Neuffer MC, McDivitt J, Rose D, et al. Hemostatic dressings for the first responder: a review. *Mil Med* 2004; 169: 716–720.

74. Kubota H, Kubota Y, Toyoda Y, et al. Selective blind endobronchial intubation in children and adults. *Anesthesiology* 1987; 67: 587–589.

75. Cloonan CC. Immediate Care of the Wounded: Circulation. http://www.operationalmedicine.org/TextbookFiles/Cloonan/Circulation.pdf (Accessed June 1, 2013).

76. United States Army Institute for Surgical Research. Joint Theater Trauma System clinical practice guideline: damage control resuscitation at level IIb/III treatment facilities. http://www.usaisr.amedd.army.mil/assets/cpgs/Damage%20Control%20Resuscitation%20-%201%20Feb%202013.pdf (Accessed November 7, 2013).

77. Bickell WH, Wall MJ, Pepe PE, et al. Immediate versus delayed fluid resuscitation for hypotensive patients with penetrating torso injuries. *N Engl J Med* 1994; 331: 1105–1109.

78. Morrison CA, Carrick MM, Norman MA, et al. Hypotensive resuscitation strategy reduces transfusion requirements and severe postoperative coagulopathy in trauma patients with hemorrhagic shock. *J Trauma* 2011; 70: 652–663.

79. Committee on Tactical Combat Casualty Care. Tactical combat casualty care guidelines. http://www.health.mil/Libraries/120917_TCCC_Course_Materials/TCCC-Guidelines-120917.pdf (Accessed June 22, 2013).

80. Okumura T, Takasu N, Ishimatsu S, et al. Report on 640 victims of the Tokyo subway sarin attack. *Ann Emerg Med* 1996; 28: 129–135.

81. Hogan DE, Waeckerle JF, Dire DJ, et al. Emergency department impact of the Oklahoma City terrorist bombing. *Ann Emerg Med* 1999; 34: 160–167.

82. Rodoplu U, Arnold JL, Tokyay R, et al. Mass-casualty terrorist bombings in Istanbul, Turkey, November 2003: report of the events and the prehospital emergency response. *Prehosp Disaster Med* 2004; 19: 133–145.

83. Peral-Gutierrez de Ceballos J, Turégano-Fuentes F, Pérez-Diaz D., et al. 11 March 2004: The terrorist bomb explosions in Madrid, Spain – an analysis of the logistics, injuries sustained and clinical management of casualties treated at the closest hospital. *Crit Care* 2005; 9: 104–111.

84. Lenhart MK, Mickelson AB, eds. *Medical Consequences of Radiological and Nuclear Warfare.* Falls Church, VA, Office of the Surgeon General of the United States Army, 2013.

85. Saffle JR, Gibran N, Jordan M. Defining the ratio of outcomes to resources for triage of burn patients in mass casualties. *J Burn Care Rehabil* 2005; 26: 478–482.

86. Aharonson-Daniel L, Klein Y, Peleg K. Suicide bombers form a new injury profile. *Ann Surg* 2006; 244: 1018–1023.

87. Singer P, Cohen JD, Stein M. Conventional terrorism and critical care. *Crit Care Med* 2005; 33(1 Suppl.): S61–S65.

88. Sorkine P, Szold O, Kluger Y, et al. Permissive hypercapnia ventilation in patients with severe pulmonary blast injury. *J Trauma* 1998; 45: 35–38.

89. Leissner KB, Ortega R, Beattie WS. Anesthesia implications of blast injury. *J Cardiothorac Vasc Anesth* 2006; 20: 872–880.

90. Flynn DF, Goans RE. Nuclear terrorism: triage and medical management of radiation and combined-Injury casualties. *Surg Clin N Am* 2006; 86: 601–636.

91. Williams G, O'Malley M. Surgical considerations in the management of combined radiation blast injury casualties caused by a radiological dirty bomb. *Injury* 2010; 41: 943–947.

92. Adler J, Golan E, Golan J, et al. Terrorist bombing experience during 1975–79: casualties admitted to the Shaare Zedek Medical Center. *Isr J Med Sci* 1983; 19: 189–193.

93. Christian MD, Devereaux AV, Dichter JR, et al. Definitive care for the critically ill during a disaster: current capabilities and limitations. *Chest* 2008; 133(5 Suppl.): S8–S17.

94. Rubinson L, Hick JL, Hanfling DG, et al. Definitive care for the critically ill during a disaster: a framework for optimizing critical care surge capacity. *Chest* 2008; 133(5 Suppl.): S18–S31.

95. Devereaux AV, Dichter JR, Christian MD, et al. Definitive care for the critically ill during a disaster: a framework for allocation of scarce resources in mass critical care. *Chest* 2008; 133(5 Suppl.): S51–S66.

96. Newgard CD, Hedges JR, Adams A, Mullins RJ. Secondary triage: early identification of high-risk trauma patients presenting to non-tertiary hospitals. *Prehosp Emerg Care* 2007; 11: 154–163.

97. Braverman I, Wexler D, Oren M. A novel mode of infection with hepatitis B: penetrating bone fragments due to the explosion of a suicide bomber. *Isr Med Assoc J* 2002; 4: 528–529.

98. Wong JM, Marsh D, Abu-Sitta G, et al. Biological foreign body implanted in victims of the London July 7th suicide bombings. *J Trauma* 2006; 60: 402–404.

99. Chapman LE, Sullivent EE, Grohskopf LA, et al. Postexposure interventions to prevent infection with HBV, HCV, or HIV, and tetanus in people wounded during bombings and other mass casualty events – United States, 2008. *Disast Med Public Health Prep* 2008; 2: 150–165.

100. Centers for Disease Control and Prevention. Blast injuries: post-exposure prophylaxis for bloodborne pathogens. http://emergency.cdc.gov/masscasualties/blastinjury-postexposure.asp (Accessed November 6, 2013).

101. CDC National Center for Injury Prevention and Control, Division or Injury Response; Blast Injuries: Fact Sheets for Professionals, pg. 25. http://www.nasemso.org/Projects/Domestic Preparedness/documents/CDC-Blast-Injury-Fact-Sheet.pdf (Accessed August 24, 2015).

102. Hirschberg B, Oppenheim-Eden A, Pizov R, et al. Recovery from blast lung injury: one-year follow-up. *Chest* 1999; 116: 1683–1688.

103. Kronenberg J, Ben-Shoshan J, Modan M, et al. Blast injury and cholesteatoma. *Am J Otol* 1988; 9: 127–130.

104. Hirschberg A, Holcomb JB, Mattox KL. Hospital trauma care in multiple-casualty incidents: a critical review. *Ann Emerg Med* 2001; 37: 647–652.

105. Hodgets TJ. Lessons from the Musgrave Park Hospital bombing. *Injury* 1993; 24: 219–221.

106. Barbisch DF, Koenig KL. Understanding surge capacity: essential elements. *Acad Emerg Med* 2006; 13: 1098–1102.

107. Tadmor B, McManus J, Koenig KL. The art and science of surge: experience from Israel and the U.S. military. *Acad Emerg Med* 2006; 13: 1130–1134.

108. Jenkins JL, McCarthy ML, Sauer LM, et al. Mass-casualty triage: time for an evidence-based approach. *Prehosp Disast Med* 2008; 23: 3–8.

109. Lerner EB, O'Connor RE, Schwartz R, et al. Blast-related injuries from terrorism: an international perspective. *Prehosp Emerg Care* 2007; 11: 137–153.

110. Cripps NPJ, Cooper GJ. The influence of personal blast protection on the distribution and severity of primary blast gut injury. *J Trauma* 1996; 40(3 Suppl.): S206–S211.

111. Cone DC, MacMillan DS. Mass-casualty triage systems: a hint of science [editorial]. *Acad Emerg Med* 2005; 12: 739–741.

PART III
CLINICAL MANAGEMENT

Subpart IIIA: CBRNE and HAZMAT

30

Burn Disaster Management: Planning and Resource Needs

Tina L. Palmieri, Ariel Tessone, and Joseph Haik

OVERVIEW

Disasters are becoming an unfortunate fact of life. As such, planning for disasters is important to mitigate damage, accelerate recovery, and facilitate reconstruction. Fundamentals of disaster planning including surge, triage, and resource utilization should be components of all plans. However, certain types of disasters merit special consideration due to their frequency, impact, or overlap with other scenarios. Burn mass casualty disasters are among the categories that adhere to an overall disaster planning algorithm but require specific alterations to the plan due to the nature and treatment of burn injuries. Burns disasters can occur in conjunction with natural phenomena (such as an earthquake or volcanic eruption), military actions, terrorist attacks (bombings), or accidents (factory explosions, chemical spills). Burn care after such events poses several challenges. First, due to fiscal constraints and optimization of burn outcomes, burn care is provided in a relatively small number of centers with limited capacity to accommodate increases in patient volume. Second, provider knowledge of burn care has been limited to a small number of highly trained individuals, which limits locations where care can be provided. Finally, burn injuries have significant resource requirements in terms of physical facilities, personnel, and supplies not only for the first few days after an incident, but for weeks thereafter. As such, separate consideration for burn disaster planning is prudent. The purpose of the chapter is to first describe an overall strategy for burn surge disaster planning and triage, followed by specific considerations for resources and personnel in a burn mass casualty event.

CURRENT STATE OF THE ART

Burn Surge

Although surge capacity for burn casualties is a subset of overall surge systems, creating such capacity for these victims has some unique features and deserves special attention. A review of the detailed planning in burn surge can assist in defining critical points of failure in surge planning. Developing burn surge capacity has historically been a challenge. Table 30.1 describes

Table 30.1. Burn-Related Disasters

- Café fire, Volendam, January 2001
  - 245 casualties, mean TBSA 12%
  - 182 admitted, 112 in ICU
  - 10 died, 78 transported abroad
- Night club fire, Rhode Island, February 2003
  - 215 victims, 96 died at scene, 4 later
  - 64 sent to trauma center
  - 151 transported to 15 other facilities
- Matsa typhoon, August 2005
  - 118 chemical burn casualties

the number of burn patients resulting from several large events. Burns generally fall into the high complexity/low numbers spectrum of surge scenarios but victim numbers can escalate rapidly depending on the incident. Resources for the management of burn casualties are unique and limited. In many countries, management of these victims relies on a system of regional burn centers. Specially trained personnel, burn-specific supplies, and specialized units are necessary to optimize outcomes for burn patients. In addition, a management system to distribute mass burn casualties is essential. This reflects the basic surge requirements of "staff, stuff, and structure" identified in Chapter 3.

The first step in preparing for a burn surge event is to identify potential threats (such as geographical proximity to industrial or military facilities, low socioeconomic conditions, and a lack of compliance with safety recommendations) and define different scenarios by probability. Not every incident can be predicted; however, a small number of scenarios can represent their respective groups. For instance, the July 2010 fire that swept through a village in the eastern Democratic Republic of Congo presents different challenges than those presented by the 2002 Bali bombings, but maybe similar to the 2001 fireworks disaster in Lima, Peru.[1-3] These scenario groups should be identified and ordered by probability. Knowledge gained in similar locations after previous events can be applied in future events (e.g., the Democratic Republic of Congo health authorities could utilize knowledge acquired in Peru).

The second step in preparing for a burn surge event should be identification of resources available for reallocation from traditional uses. These include: 1) non-burn-specialized staff that can take part in the management of burn patients (general surgeons, anesthesiologists, intensivists, general surgery nurses, intensive care nurses, and post-operative unit nurses); 2) hospitalization capability in departments other than burn units (plastic and general surgery wards, intensive care units, and post-operative recovery units); and 3) medical equipment, supplies and medications (in particular, large volumes of intravenous fluids and airway equipment).

The third step should be to define the systems component that will indicate which of these resources should be used in each phase of event management. Burn surge, as in other trauma, has three management phases. The first is the management at the scene or scenes of the incident, the second is hospital or alternate care facility management (such as further resuscitation and surgical interventions as indicated), and the third is the rehabilitation phase. During the planning phase, it is critical to define outcomes-based triage criteria by which patients would be distributed to nontraditional burn treatment areas. The first patients to be assessed are not always the ones that require hospitalization in a burn unit.

Kelen and McCarthy state that "staffing for maximum known demand is not economically sound, because the physician or provider would be idle for considerable periods during lower demand times."[4] In addition, even if there were no fiscal constraints, it would likely be difficult to provide adequate training to an unlimited number of staff until new learning techniques such as virtual reality are perfected. In resource-constrained environments, a number of small interventions can be reserved for the highest skilled providers, in this case, the burn surgeon if available. In the initial phases, estimation of burn size and initiation of fluid resuscitation, escharotomies where indicated, and the decision regarding admission to a burn unit or other care location should be conducted by an experienced burn provider. Ideally, a burn surgeon should be involved in daily wound evaluations, decisions regarding the need for surgery, and the surgery itself. However, these responsibilities can be delegated to an experienced burn nurse or physician assistant (PA). The final decision on the need for surgery should be made by a burn surgeon but this can be done remotely. In situations where the burn surgeon is in the operating room while a burn unit patient's wounds are available for inspection during dressing changes, decisions can be made with the aid of digital photography and oral briefing by the relevant staff member (nurse, PA). In the rehabilitation phase, a different type of specialist can provide services in consultation with a burn surgeon. In general, other physicians (general surgeons, emergency physicians, and anesthesiologists) can perform other medical interventions. Thus, non-burn specialists with basic surgical skills can create surge capacity for burn patients by augmenting personnel resources.

If resources are sufficient, the following guidelines are useful in the hospital or definitive alternate care site setting:

1. Burn triage should be carried out by a team of one burn surgeon and two nurses, one of which should be a burn nurse. Adherence to American Burn Association (ABA) guidelines for admission and discharge is desirable. A reasonable approach would be to use one such team per inflow of approximately twenty patients per hour.

2. Initial resuscitative care should include general trauma evaluation, initial laboratory and imaging studies, emergent procedures as indicated (such as hemorrhage control and evacuation of a pneumo/hemothorax), escharotomies, and initiation of fluid resuscitation. If staff are available, each patient should be managed by one physician (emergency physician, general surgeon, or trauma physician) and one nurse. Every three such teams should have two rotating nurses or one rotating nurse and one nursing assistant (can be a trained volunteer). There should be at least one burn surgeon and one anesthesiologist for every ten such teams.

3. In the acute care phase, patients should be divided into major burn patients and minor burn patients. Since every patient with more than 20% total body surface area (TBSA) burns requires fluid resuscitation, and since escharotomies can be mandatory even in small deep burns restricted to one location, these are not optimal criteria for determining whether patients are in the "major" burn category. Rather, the criteria for a major burn patient should be: 1) need for mechanical ventilation or impending respiratory failure; 2) inhalation injury; 3) hemodynamic, septic, or other shock states; 4) special body areas burned (genitalia or deep facial burns); 5) greater than 30% TBSA; 6) major accompanying trauma (head trauma or visceral injury); 7) single or multi organ failure; 8) underlying medical conditions that indicate major systemic diseases (ischemic heart disease, diabetes, or malignancy); and 10) disability (paraplegia or loss of hearing). All other patients are designated as minor burn patients.

4. Minor burn patients can be managed with the resources of general and plastic surgery departments by the department staff (physicians and nurses) with regular patient to caregiver ratios. Ideally, a burn specialist should perform daily patient assessments (a ratio of up to one burn physician to thirty patients is the goal).

5. Major burn patients should be managed in a burn unit or in an intensive care unit. Post-operative units are an alternate if burn unit capacity has been exceeded.

6. The ideal burn nurse to patient ratio for major burn patients is 1:1. Nurses trained in intensive care, general surgery, and plastic surgery can care for burn patients if staff surge capacity is needed. In this case, one out of three nurses should be a burn nurse (daily dressing changes are usually performed in teams of three; therefore, a team of three nurses can treat three patients). Taking all that into account, optimally each patient requires 4.2 full time nursing equivalents, 1.4 of which are specialized burn nurses. Another requirement should be that in each shift there will be at least one burn nurse per three patients. This requirement does not change the number of full-time nurses needed; however, it does require that patients are grouped into threes.

7. The physician to patient ratio for major burn patients should ideally be 1:4 at most. A burn surgeon should perform daily assessments of each patient. Therefore, each patient requires 0.7 full time physician equivalents, 0.35 of which should be burn surgeons. The other physician positions can be filled by general surgeons, anesthesiologists, and intensivists. Most major burn patients will require surgical care. Each medical facility should have at least three burn surgeons dedicated to surgery (two surgeons per procedure, working 16 hours a day, 7 days a week for a limited duration). If PAs are available, the physician to patient ratio can be increased to 1:6 with two PAs

working with each physician. The ratio of burn physicians to other physicians stays at 1:2.

8. Other caregivers and personnel needed include:
   a. Nursing assistants – one for every three patients (1.4 full-time positions)
   b. Medical clerks – one (two if more than ten patients)
   c. Respiratory, physical, and occupational therapists – one of each for every ten to fifteen patients
   d. Social worker – one
   e. Respiratory technician – one
   f. Psychologist – one
   g. Qualified volunteers (such as retired trained personnel) – as many as possible

9. Exact guidelines for the rehabilitation phase are difficult to establish. Almost all major burn patients will require rehabilitation before discharge (and all will require rehabilitation after discharge). Since most major burn patients will be hospitalized for acute care for a few weeks, healthcare providers have time to coordinate rehabilitation services.

Other Considerations

STAFF

Augmentation of staff with expertise in burn care is a critical element for creating surge capacity. Planning should account for the fact some personnel will be unable (due to injury, death, or lack of transportation infrastructure) or unwilling to report to work during a disaster. To prepare non-burn specialists (such as plastic surgery and general surgery nurses) to assist in a burn disaster, basic burn training coupled with a rotation in a burn unit rotation at least every 2 years is desirable. Nurses from other departments who have experience in treating ventilated patients should also be considered for pre-event training in burn management. Surge plans should specify staff members who can be allocated to assist during a burn disaster. These staff members should be aware of their responsibilities and trained prior to the event. Just-in-time training after an event occurs may be a useful adjunct if additional personnel are required.

OUTPATIENTS

Most patients with injuries limited to burns can be managed as outpatients. Professional triage that complies with ABA guidelines can identify patients who do not need acute care services, thereby preserving staff, equipment, and patient care space for more severely injured patients. Community medical services should be capable of treating patients with burns of up to 15–20% of TBSA in noncritical body regions.

TRANSFER

Since burn events fall under the "low numbers/high complexity" end of the spectrum, highly specialized multidisciplinary teams will be needed to manage patients from these types of disasters. If possible, patients should be transferred to an appropriate facility from the scene. In some cases, however, severely burned patients may require rapid transfer to a tertiary medical center after initial stabilization at a non-burn facility.

In addition to transferring patients to other facilities, resources can be brought in to augment capacity at a burn center. Local, regional, national, and even international resources may be needed in mass burn disasters. Local resources are most easily allocated and should be used first. A regional system should be in place for resource sharing. Physicians and nurses can be allocated for short periods of time based on a daily assessment of

patient needs. National disaster management plans should state which backup resources are available and detail logistics for their movement to a burn center.

Patient length of stay in a burn center must be considered. Burn patients usually remain hospitalized well into the recovery phase of a disaster, especially when combined injuries are present. For example, in Israel, 25.6% of terror-related burn casualties are still hospitalized 1 month after their admission.[5] Two major effects of this prolonged length of stay are:

1. Continuous demand for resources including personnel, hospitalization facilities, medical equipment, and medications; and
2. Shifts in management strategies (such as increased referrals or outpatient treatment) must be initiated to maintain capacity to care for non-event related patients.

After the Surge: Triage and Burn Management

Planning for a burn surge event requires consideration of multiple variables. One of the key elements of burn surge involves the ability to triage patients to assure that existing resources benefit the greatest number of people. Burn injury triage has a major advantage over other types of disaster-related triage: burn survival probability can be objectively estimated at the time of injury. Burn extent and patient age are directly related to survival after burn injury. As such, burn triage tables have been developed based on national burn data sets (Table 30.2).[6] These triage tables assist in optimizing resource utilization to provide the best outcome for the greatest number of patients. Patients with high mortality/high resource utilization or patients with non-survivable burns can be identified at the scene. Resources can be focused on patients with high likelihood of survival. Burn triage tables have been incorporated into many disaster plans and can assist first responders in decision-making. Given the limited number of centers capable of treating major burn injury, triage will need to take a tiered approach and consider the following: 1) initial available transportation assets may not be capable of transferring patients long distances to a major burn center; 2) major burn centers will not have the capacity to accommodate massive numbers of patients with burn injury; and 3) supplies and trained personnel will become progressively limited over time. As such, trauma centers or other facilities capable of handling high acuity patients with major wounds may need to provide initial patient care. Determining the resources needed for surge capacity in a burn mass casualty incident necessitates an understanding of basic burn pathophysiology as well as the different potential etiologies of burn mass casualty incidents.

Basic Burn Pathophysiology

Burn injury results in a series of physiologic responses that impact treatment and resource needs after a disaster. Burn injury severity is described based on both depth and extent of burn injury. Burn depth is related to several factors: how long the skin is exposed to a heat source, the temperature of the heat source, skin thickness, and skin perfusion.[7] In general, the greater the duration of exposure, the higher the temperature, and the thinner the skin, the deeper the resultant burn injury. The thickest skin is on the soles of the feet and palms of the hand; the thinnest is on the inner wrist and eyelids. First-degree burns involve

Table 30.2. Triage tables developed from ABA National Burn Repository. Probability of survival based on age, burn size, and presence or absence of inhalational injury

Triage Table Non-Inhalation Injury

Age	Burn Size Group, % TBSA WITHOUT Inhalation Injury									
	0–9.9	10–19.9	20–29.9	30–39.9	40–49.9	50–59.9	60–69.9	70–79.9	80–89.9	≥ 90
0–1.99	Very High	Very High	High	High	High	High	Medium	Medium	Medium	Medium
2–4.99	Outpatient	Very High	High	High	High	High	High	Medium	Medium	Medium
5–19.99	Outpatient	Very High	High	High	High	High	High	Medium	Medium	Low
20–29.99	Outpatient	Very High	High	High	High	Medium	Medium	Medium	Medium	Low
30–39.99	Outpatient	Very High	High	High	Medium	Medium	Medium	Low	Low	Expectant
40–49.99	Outpatient	Very High	High	High	Medium	Medium	Medium	Low	Low	Expectant
50–59.99	Outpatient	Very High	High	Medium	Medium	Low	Low	Expectant	Expectant	Expectant
60–69.99	Very High	High	Medium	Medium	Low	Low	Expectant	Expectant	Expectant	Expectant
≥ 70	High	Medium	Medium	Low	Low	Expectant	Expectant	Expectant	Expectant	Expectant

Triage Table Inhalation Injury

Age	Burn Size Group, % TBSA WITH Inhalation Injury									
	0–9.9	10–19.9	20–29.9	30–39.9	40–49.9	50–59.9	60–69.9	70–79.9	80–89.9	≥ 90
0–1.99	High	Medium	Medium	Medium	Medium	Medium	Low	Low	Expectant	Expectant
2–4.99	High	High	High	High	High	Medium	Medium	Medium	Low	Low
5–19.99	High	High	High	High	Medium	Medium	Medium	Medium	Low	Low
20–29.99	Very High	High	High	Medium	Medium	Medium	Medium	Low	Low	Expectant
30–39.99	Very High	High	High	Medium	Medium	Medium	Medium	Low	Low	Expectant
40–49.99	Very High	High	Medium	Medium	Medium	Low	Low	Low	Low	Expectant
50–59.99	High	Medium	Medium	Medium	Medium	Low	Low	Expectant	Expectant	Expectant
60–69.99	Medium	Medium	Medium	Low	Low	Low	Expectant	Expectant	Expectant	Expectant
≥ 70	Medium	Medium	Low	Low	Expectant	Expectant	Expectant	Expectant	Expectant	Expectant

Outpatient: No admission required, survival ≥ 95%
Very High: Survival ≥ 90%; length of stay ≤ 14–21 days, 1–2 operations
High: Survival ≥ 90%; length of stay 14–21 days, multiple operations
Medium: Survival > 50% and < 90% (mortality 10–50%)
Low: Survival > 10% and < 50% (mortality 50–90%)
Expectant: Survival ≤ 10% (mortality ≥ 90%)

only the epidermis; as such, they are painful but require no additional treatment other than providing analgesia. Second-degree burns extend into the dermis and result in a blister formation. Although second-degree burns will heal within 2 weeks, they will require some form of wound care during that time.[8]

Third-degree burns extend through the dermis and result in full thickness destruction of the skin. In general, third-degree burns will require surgical excision or grafting if extensive; if small, they will require prolonged wound care for more than 2 weeks. Hence, third-degree burns will have higher resource utilization

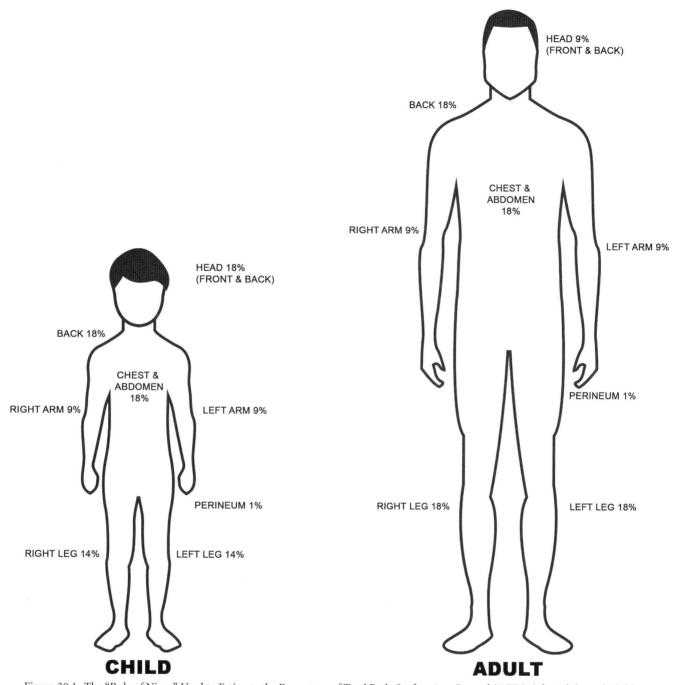

Figure 30.1. The "Rule of Nines" Used to Estimate the Percentage of Total Body Surface Area Burned (%TBSA) for Adults and Children.

for an extended period of time compared to other forms of injury.

The second factor determining burn treatment is extent of burn injury. Burn extent is categorized based on the percent of the body surface area burned. In normal circumstances, the "rule of nines" is used to estimate body surface area involvement. This system identifies the percentage of body surface area represented by various anatomic regions as a multiple of the number nine (Figure 30.1).[9] The numbers are modified slightly for children due to the relative increase in head size and decrease in leg surface area. Only regions that have a second- or third-degree burn (i.e., have at least blistering) are used in the total burn size estimation. Unfortunately, early estimates

of burn size, even without the presence of a disaster, either over- or underestimate by an average of 20%.[10–12] This could be a major limitation in a disaster response; for example, a 25% burn needs resuscitation, while a 5% burn does not. A second, easier way to estimate burn size is to use the patient's palm, which represents 1% of the patient's total body surface area. This can be done expediently by a rescuer by holding up the victim's palm to his own, estimating the size, and then using that dimension to estimate burn size. This has the theoretical advantage of being able to calculate burn size in non-circumferential and irregular wounds, but there is limited prospective data directly comparing the palm estimation with the "rule of nine" technique.

Table 30.3. Toxic Elements in House Fires

Gas	Source	Effect
Hydrogen cyanide	Wool, silk, nylon	Headache, coma, respiratory failure
Carbon monoxide	Organic matter	Tissue hypoxia
Benzene	Petroleum plastics	Mucosal irritation, coma
Ammonia	Nylon	Mucosal irritation
Hydrogen chloride	Plastics	Severe mucosal irritation
Aldehydes	Wood, cotton, paper	Severe mucosal, pulmonary damage
Nitrogen dioxide	Wallpaper, wood	Pulmonary edema, dizziness

A major magnifier of burn injury severity is the concomitant presence of inhalation injury. In general, inhalation injury increases both hospital length-of-stay, need for mechanical ventilation, fluid requirements, and mortality (Table 30.2).[13] It will also raise the level of triage acuity for any patient at a given age and percent TBSA burn. The three types of inhalation injury include: exposure to toxic gases/hypoxia, upper airway edema, and chemical injury to lung parenchyma due to smoke exposure. Exposure to toxic gases (other than vesicants) is greatest in enclosed spaces and leads to a high mortality at the scene (50% of mortalities in a house fire). Such exposure may result in mechanical ventilation and/or medical management for toxic chemical products of smoke. The most notable gases include carbon monoxide and cyanide. A table of toxic chemicals released when common household goods burn is included in Table 30.3. Upper airway edema is due to mucous membrane injury above the glottis and usually occurs in the setting of prolonged exposure to heated smoke in a confined space. Other potential scenarios that could cause injury and/or edema above the glottis include massive burns with resultant anasarca, inhalation of hot steam, vesicants, trauma, or chemicals. Intubation is required to prevent asphyxia from an edematous airway. Disasters causing upper airway edema will result in a high need for mechanical ventilation within hours of an incident, but duration of support needed is generally limited to 24–72 hours. Finally, the third type of inhalation injury, injury to lungs due to exposure to smoke or particles, can result in prolonged need for mechanical ventilation due to lung injury. Lung parenchymal injury magnifies the impact of burn injury, increases the risk of pneumonia and death, and increases hospital length-of-stay. The combination of inhalation injury and burn injury will result in high ICU resource utilization for a prolonged period of time.

If the patient has circumferential burns of either the extremities or the chest, these two areas should be monitored closely to detect the need for escharotomy and for the development of compartment syndrome. Burn eschar on the chest may interfere with ventilation and if this is the case, chest escharotomy should be performed without delay. For the extremities, eschar will act as constricting bands first occluding the venous return, then the arterial inflow. If available, Doppler signals should be followed hourly. Diminution of the signal or a change in its character is an indication for escharotomy. This procedure is performed with a scalpel or with electrocautery. If performed properly, minimal bleeding results because the incision remains just below the burn within the subcutaneous tissues. If much bleeding is encountered, the incision is too deep. Patients receiving massive amounts of fluid may also develop compartment syndrome. This results from an increase in the tissue pressure within a nonexpansible compartment of the body. The compartment may be within the skull, the chest, the abdomen, or the extremities. If compartment syndrome is suspected in the extremities, compartment pressures should be measured unless escharotomy has been performed and compartments are decompressed. The pressures are measured with an 18-gauge needle connected to an arterial pressure transducer. The absolute intramuscular pressure is measured in each compartment. A difference between diastolic blood pressure and intramuscular pressure of less than 10–20 mmHg in any one compartment is suggestive of compartment syndrome. In addition, the muscles in the compartment being measured should be squeezed. A sluggish rise in the pressure tracing with this maneuver is nearly pathognomonic of compartment hypertension. In all cases, to prevent tissue death and systemic crush syndrome, the key treatment principle if compartment syndrome develops is to decompress the involved compartments immediately.

The body's response to a burn wound also impacts resource requirements. One of the hallmarks of burn injury is fluid loss through the damaged skin. Prior to the initiation of aggressive fluid resuscitation in the management of burn victims, the burn size that resulted in a 50% mortality was ~30% TBSA. Outcomes improved significantly after this practice changed and large fluid volume administration became the norm. Major burn wounds, defined as greater than 20% TBSA, will require significant fluid administration, most pronounced in the first 24 hours, but continuing until wound closure. Initial fluid requirements can be estimated by the Parkland formula: 4 ml/kg/% burn over 24 hours, half in the first 8 hours and the remainder in the next 16 hours.[14] This can result in enormous intravenous fluid requirements. For example, a 70-kg male with a 40% TBSA burn will require approximately 11,200 ml of fluid in 24 hours. Intravenous fluids and/or supplies needed for intravenous fluid administration could easily be completely consumed. Fluid losses continue until wounds are closed. The daily maintenance intravenous fluid needed after the first 24 hours is the sum of basal requirements plus evaporative losses. Basal adult fluid needs are derived from the formula 1,500 ml × body surface area. For children less than 20 kg, the calculation is 2,000 ml × body surface area. The infusion rate in milliliters per hour to replace daily adult evaporative losses is estimated by the formula (25 + %TBSA burn) x body surface area. For children less than 20 kg, the formula estimating infusion rates in milliliters per hour to replace evaporative loss is (35 + %TBSA burn) x body surface area. Hence, the need for large volumes of intravenous fluid for weeks after burn injury is a real possibility in a major burn disaster. The role of oral fluid resuscitation for major burn injury requires further investigation, as intravenous fluid supplies (fluids, IV catheters, tubing, etc.) are likely to become limited.

Major burn wounds increase the body's overall metabolic state.[15–18] As a result, patients have a higher baseline temperature, heart rate, respiratory rate, and metabolic rate throughout the acute phase (even up to 6 months) after injury. Particular attention should be paid to temperature control, as patients lose heat through their wounds and have a limited ability to generate heat by shivering. Enteral nutrition is administered via naso-enteral feeding tubes due to the patients' inability to eat the number of calories required to maintain body weight. In a major disaster, enteral nutrition supplies are likely to become limited due to the prolonged need for high-volume feedings. Medications often used to ameliorate the hypermetabolic response, including oxandrolone and propranolol, may not be available. In addition, burn patients are immunocompromised. Major burn patients initially have a dramatic increase in white blood cell (WBC) count due to demargination of WBC after injury. However, at days 2–5, the WBC count plummets, and patients develop decreased T-cell and B-cell responsiveness. This immunosuppression, combined with the loss of skin, amplifies the risk of infection from not just the wounds, but from bacteria in the lungs (pneumonia), urine (urinary tract infection), and blood (sepsis). Traditional markers of an evolving septic process, such as elevated temperature and WBC count, are less useful in detecting infection after burn injury due to the systemic inflammatory response syndrome (SIRS) ubiquitously present in major burn injury. Judicious use of antibiotics in a disaster will be important to maintain availability for documented infection.[19] Widespread prophylaxis will likely result in a critical shortage of antibiotics and accelerate antibiotic resistance.

The most obvious supply needs after a major burn incident will be products associated with wound care. Initial cleaning of the burn wound is vital early after injury to minimize the bacterial load and infection risk. Hence, soap and water as well as a place to wash wounds are needed. There are a vast array of burn care products available ranging from creams, ointments, and gels to silver impregnated dressings. The ideal product is one that is easy to apply, effective in minimizing bacterial invasion, and has a long half-life (i.e., can be left on the patient for an extended period of time). The most frequently used antimicrobial cream is silver sulfadiazine. The advantages of silver sulfadiazine include effectiveness against a broad range of flora, easy application, low incidence of adverse response, physician/nurse familiarity with the product, and relatively abundant supply. The disadvantages of silver sulfadiazine include twice daily or daily reapplication (with concomitant wound cleaning and redressing), induction of leukopenia, and formation of a film on the wound, making it difficult to evaluate for inexperienced practitioners. Silver impregnated dressings, which can be left on for up to 1 week, may have a role in disaster management, but practitioner inexperience, lack of stockpiles, and dressing coordination can be issues.[20]

Other Burn Care Supply Needs

Burn patients also require other resources in large amounts. First, burn injuries are painful, and patients may require large amounts of narcotics and analgesics.[21] Although the pain is generally greatest immediately after burn injury, severe pain occurs with dressing changes, movement, therapy, and manipulation of vascular devices for months after injury. Second, the surgical treatment of burn wounds has intense resource requirements. Definitive treatment of burn wounds often requires multiple operative interventions. Having access to a fully equipped operating room with trained personnel may be a rate-limiting step in burn patient treatment. First, the burn wound is excised using specialized equipment. Next, a skin graft obtained from an unburned area on the patient or a temporary allograft/xenograft/skin substitute is placed over the excised wound. Blood loss during these procedures, even with the use of a tourniquet, is prodigious. Two percent of total blood volume is lost per percent burn excised on the trunk, arms, legs, and perineum; 5% of total blood volume is lost per percent burn excised on the face.[22] For example, a burn excision of the anterior and posterior trunk (approximately 36% TBSA) will result in a loss of 72% of the patient's blood volume. The need for blood products extends throughout hospital stay, as patients with burn injuries have both decreased production and increased destruction of red blood cells. Delays in excision result in greater blood loss. Hence, in a major disaster when definitive care is delayed, healthcare providers can anticipate that blood product requirements will be higher than in normal case scenarios. As a consequence, blood and blood products must be used judiciously.

Burn Care Resource Needs: People

As mentioned in the surge section, burn care requires a team of people for a prolonged period of time. Although the highest volume of work occurs in the first 24–48 hours after burn injury, burn patients have ongoing wound care and physiologic needs for months after the onset of injury. Wound care, in particular, can be problematic, as the therapy for burns has been concentrated, on the whole, in burn centers. In a major burn event, a shortage will exist of nursing personnel who are familiar with complex burn wound care. Burn wound care is both physically and emotionally draining for burn care providers, as patients often cannot cooperate with dressing changes due to fatigue and/or sedation. The patient's room is hot due to the patient propensity to develop hypothermia, limbs are edematous and heavy, wounds can be malodorous, and patient responses may impede dressing change activity. These conditions will persist for months after the initial incident in patients with major burn injury. Plans for provision of appropriate numbers of adequately trained personnel (as described in the surge capacity section) must address short-term commitments (lasting days) and well as long-term needs (lasting months). These requirements should be incorporated into disaster planning scenarios. Other paraprofessionals, including respiratory therapists, occupational and physical therapists, dieticians, and pharmacists will all be important to optimize care, enable patient healing, and increase patient throughput. Complete operating teams experienced in massive transfusion and trauma must be available during grafting periods.

Other Considerations

Not all burns are created equal. Although burn disaster planning adheres to the basic tenets of surge capacity and triage, it is important to remember that the cause of a burn disaster influences not only surge capacity, but resource utilization, personnel and equipment requirements, and structural requirements. For example, although flame burn injuries appear to present a uniform insult, several factors have been demonstrated to increase resource utilization in flame burn injury. These include: 1) concomitant traumatic injury; 2) delay in seeking care; 3) inhalation injury; 4) exposure to other chemicals; 5) recreational drug use; 6) compartment syndrome (circumferential burns); and 7) anatomic location of the burn. Additional traumatic injury, in particular, is a formidable challenge, and makes it difficult to both triage and predict resource utilization.[23] The treatment of the majority of chemical burns is irrigation with water until the substance is completely washed away. Hence, areas set aside for decontamination and access to copious amounts of water should be available. The prognosis of cutaneous radiation burns differs from traditional burn wound care.[24] Burn or trauma in combination with radiation injury markedly increases mortality, primarily due to infection. In general, excision and grafting of radiation burns needs to occur either within the first 24–48 hours or be delayed for at least a month due to the effects of radiation exposure on wound healing. Patients with cutaneous burns who are not successfully grafted early will have prolonged open wounds with frequent episodes of breakdown and may ultimately require complex surgical tissue flaps to achieve wound closure.

RECOMMENDATIONS FOR FURTHER RESEARCH

Although much is known about burn treatment and burn care, this knowledge is centralized. Virtually every burn triage algorithm relies on determination of burn size, yet this important variable may be estimated inaccurately by untrained providers. A fundamental research priority in burn mass casualty preparation is development of protocols or methods to increase accuracy and minimize variability in initial burn size estimates during the triage phase. Burn wound depth also drives both triage and treatment. A noninvasive, easy to use method that provides accurate depth assessment, such as Doppler studies, thermal imaging, and other modalities could help to streamline burn wound care.

Providing effective wound care is the major source for resource utilization in a burn scenario. Development of the "ideal" wound dressing that is easy to apply, provides optimal healing environment, decreases pain, can be left in place for prolonged periods of time, and is readily available would mitigate the complications of delayed triage to definitive care. Finally, the "holy grail" of burn treatment is the development of a skin substitute or cultured skin that can be used to definitively close a burn wound within days of injury. As mentioned previously, oral resuscitation regimens are needed to augment and provide adequate hydration to large numbers of individuals in a burn mass casualty. Burn mass casualty planning is indeed rife with opportunities for meaningful high-impact research.

Planning for a burn mass casualty event is challenging due to the extent and duration of facility, personnel, and supply needs. Understanding the fundamentals of burn care and utilizing characteristics of burn injury to develop triage and surge protocols is essential in the development of actionable burn mass casualty plans. Although burn mass casualty plans should follow established algorithms, those algorithms should be modified based on evolving situations. Special consideration should be given to requirements impacting patient flow, resource utilization, personnel, and structure (bed availability). Collaboration between mass casualty planners and trained burn providers will be needed to optimize burn mass casualty protocols. Such interaction will foster development of much needed research that can improve overall survival and quality of life after a burn mass casualty event.

Acknowledgment

The authors wish to thank Dr. John McManus and Dr. Ruben Gomez for their work on the first edition of this chapter. Some of that material has been included in this version.

REFERENCES

1. DRC Burn Survivors Suffering. News 24. http://www.news24.com/Africa/News/Congo-Burn-survivors-suffering-20100704 (Accessed September 27, 2014.)
2. 2002 Bali Bombings. Wikipedia. http://en.wikipedia.org/wiki/2002_Bali_bombings (Accessed September 27, 2014).
3. 291 dead in Lima: the social roots of Peru's tragic fire. World Socialist Website. http://www.wsws.org/en/articles/2002/01/peru-j28.html (Accessed September 27, 2014).
4. Kelen GD, McCarthy ML. The Science of Surge. *Acad Emerg Med* 2006; 13(11): 1089–1094.
5. The Israeli National Trauma Registry (ITR). The Israel National Center for Trauma and Emergency Medicine Research, Gertner Institute for Epidemiology and Health Policy Research, Sheba Medical Center, Ministry of Health, Tel-Hashomer, Israel.
6. Taylor S, Jeng J, Saffle JR, Sen S, Greenhalgh DG, Palmieri TL. Redefining the outcomes to resources ratio for burn patient triage in a mass casualty. *J Burn Care Res*, 2014; 35(1): 41–45.
7. Moritz AR, Henriques FC. Studies of thermal injury II: The relative importance of time and surface temperature in the causation of cutaneous burns. *Am J Pathol* 1947; 23: 695–720.
8. Zawacki BE. The natural history of reversible burn injury. *Surg Gynecol Obstet* 1974; 139: 867–872.
9. Hettiaratchy S, Papini R. Initial management of a major burn: II – assessment and resuscitation. *BMJ* July 10, 2004; 329: 101–103.
10. Collis N, Smith G, Fenton OM. Accuracy of burn size estimation and subsequent fluid resuscitation prior to arrival at the Yorkshire Regional Burns Unit. A three year retrospective study. *Burns June* 1999; 25(4): 345–351.
11. Hammond JS, Ward CG. Transfers from emergency room to burn center: errors in burn size estimate. *J Trauma* October 1987; 27(10): 1161–1165.
12. Giretzlehner M, Dirnberger J, Owen R, Haller HL, Lumenta DB, Kamolz LP. The determination of total burn surface area: How much difference? *Burns* 2013; 39(6): 1107–1113.
13. Colohan SM. Predicting prognosis in thermal burns with associated inhalational injury: a systematic review of prognostic factors in adult burn victims. *J Burn Care Res* July–August 2010; 31(4): 529–539.
14. Baxter CR. Guidelines for fluid resuscitation. *J Trauma* 1981; 21: 687–690.
15. Wilmore D, Aulick L. Metabolic changes in burned patients. *Surg Clin N Amer* 1978; 58: 1173–1187.
16. Jaboor F, Desai M, Herndon D, Wolfe R. Dynamics of the protein metabolism response to burn injury. *Metabolism* 1988; 37: 330–337.
17. Bessey P, Jiang Z, Wilmore D. Post-traumatic skeletal muscle proteolysis: the role of the hormonal environment. *World J Surg* 1989; 13: 465–471.
18. Newsome T, Mason A, Pruitt B. Weight loss following thermal injury. *Ann. Surg* 1973; 178: 215–217.
19. Greenhalgh DG, Saffle JR, Holmes JH 4th, Gamelli RL, Palmieri TL, et al. American Burn Association consensus conference to define sepsis and infection in burns. *J Burn Care Res* 2007; 28: 776–790.
20. Wasiak J, Cleland H, Campbell F, Spinks A. Dressings for superficial and partial thickness burns. *Cochrane Database Syst Rev* March 28, 2013; 3: CD002106.
21. Gregoretti C, Decaroli D, Piacevoli Q, Mistretta A, Barzaghi N, et al. Analgo-sedation of patients with burns outside the operating room. *Drugs* 2008; 68: 2427–2443.

22. Housinger TA, Lang D, Warden GD. A prospective study of blood loss with excisional therapy in pediatric burn patients. *J Trauma* 1993; 34: 262–263.

23. Atiyeh B, Gunn S, William A, Dibo S. Primary triage of mass burn casualties with associated severe traumatic injuries. *Annals of Burn and Fire Disasters* 2013; 26: 48–52.

24. DiCarlo AL, Maher C, Hick JL, Hanfling D, Dainiak N, et al. Radiation injury after a nuclear detonation: medical consequences and the need for scarce resources allocation. *Disaster Med Public Health Prep* 2011; 5(Suppl. 1): S32–S34.

31

CLINICAL ASPECTS OF LARGE-SCALE CHEMICAL EVENTS

Jonathan Newmark

OVERVIEW

Since the dawn of civilization, chemical materials have been a part of human life. Nearly 100,000 different commercial chemicals are known, and several thousand new chemicals are developed yearly. Of these new chemicals, nearly a thousand reach the commercial market. Annual worldwide chemical production is estimated at 363 million metric tons (400 million short tons). Of this production, most is bulk stored and bulk transported. Thus, there is a risk of large-scale release with resulting environmental and health effects. In the past century, specific chemicals have also been developed to use as weapons with the intention to harm or kill humans.

Human toxicity from chemical exposure has been well recorded since the beginning of the industrial age. Recognition and investigation of those effects have allowed the development of therapeutic interventions. Toxic effects of chemicals may result from exposures to small amounts such as present in foods or medications, or larger amounts resulting from accidental or intentional releases from storage or transportation facilities. But the actual toxicities of each compound are not always well understood because of the huge number of possible interactions with thousands of chemicals and individual patient variability.

The human toxic effects of smaller chemical exposure events have generally been well managed because there are rarely more than one or two patients requiring care at a time. Large-scale exposures vastly complicate the medical response to a toxic chemical event, principally because of overwhelming logistical difficulties.

Interactions between chemicals and people depend on pharmacokinetics (absorption, distribution, metabolism, and elimination) and specific toxicities or modes of action. Much of the clinical information about toxic (warfare) chemical effects has been collected from studies of young, healthy military men. Extrapolation of those data to other subsets of the population (children, the elderly, females, persons with complicating medical illnesses, immunocompromised patients, patients on medications, and the mentally ill) can be difficult. Additionally, research findings in nonhuman systems may correlate poorly with human systems.

Immediate and near-term lethal sequelae of chemical events, even those intentionally orchestrated, rarely occur in more than 3–5% of exposed individuals. But longer-term sequelae are often poorly understood and may not develop for many years. This has, in many cases, given rise to claims of causation which result in years of litigation.

Large-scale chemical events trigger public anxiety and fear to a degree that is strikingly disproportionate to the number of deaths. The media appears to be a primary contributor to this public anxiety, largely as a result of its presentation format. The medical community must assist the media with both its presentation of content and methods.

The mode of death in most chemical exposures results from respiratory failure, so attention to pulmonary function is always a major part of chemical preparedness. But many chemicals cause protean, multi-organ effects, some of which can be delayed. A good example is the delayed keratopathy seen years after sulfur mustard exposure. Programs to address the chemical threat must be multifaceted and span multiple medical disciplines.

During the time period termed "recovery," the medical community has unique responsibilities. Critical assessment of the long-term clinical aspects of the event should include both medical and psychological sequelae. Careful long-term evaluations of all the victims from an exposure should be undertaken in a fashion similar to the follow-up programs after the September 11, 2001, U.S. terrorist attacks in New York City. Carefully documented clinical and laboratory victim data should be collected in a medically accessible database for future review and use. This long-term clinical/medical review should be undertaken independent of legal, political, or commercial interests in the event. Critical assessment must also be made of the medical aspects of mitigation, preparedness, and response in the event. This assessment must be compiled and produced as a reference document, available for immediate and later review. This is a disaster preparedness review with a medical focus and should also be produced independent of legal, political, or commercial interest in the event. These two types of review should begin as soon as possible after a chemical release.

CURRENT STATE OF THE ART

Chemical History

Since at least 1000 BC, chemicals in some form have been used as weapons. Initially those chemicals were found as natural materials that could be used to produce a particular desired effect when extracted from geological deposits. Recent archaeological discoveries in Dura-Europos, in present-day Syria, the site of a battle between the Persians and Romans in 276 AD, seem to indicate that the defending Persians used bitumen and sulfur to asphyxiate their enemies attempting to take the fortress by tunneling into it.[1]

In approximately 670 AD, the Byzantine Greeks developed a combination of materials that, when ignited, became an effective weapon. So-called Greek fire was a combination of uncertain composition that probably contained naphtha, sulfur, saltpeter, and pitch. When used against enemy ships, this "wet, dark, sticky fire" would float on water, stick to ships, and even continue to burn underwater. It was almost impossible to extinguish and hence was particularly effective against enemy wooden ships. Greek fire not only produced substantial physical damage, but also, perhaps much more importantly, spread extraordinary fear among the enemy. That fear was the result of failures to anticipate the use of the material as a weapon, develop adequate weapon protection, control the immediate effects of the weapon, and learn the method of manufacture of Greek fire and develop plans for its future use.

Substantial effort was expended in attempting to educate sailors about the methods of use and effects of Greek fire. Fear that this was a weapon "of the devil" was mollified. Training in methods of flame control helped ease anxiety as well. These early forms of "disaster preparedness" helped overcome the advantage of fear that Greek fire carried.

By the eighteenth century, the discovery of unique chemicals such as cyanide and chlorine was quickly followed by recognition of their harmful effects. Shortly thereafter, various military forces around the world proposed use of these materials, specifically for their toxic properties. Although no army had yet weaponized chemicals, this concern was sufficient to merit specific mention in the Geneva Protocols, ratified in 1899. During World War I, large-scale production and use of chemical agents as toxic weapons became common.

French riot control agents were perhaps the first chemical weapons of WWI. They had previously been deployed by the Paris police. Riot control agents were relatively ineffective, however, because highly motivated soldiers could easily tolerate their irritant effects.

On April 22, 1915, after extensive preliminary preparation and some false starts, the Germans released approximately 136 metric tons (150 short tons) of chlorine from approximately 6,000 cylinders over a 7-km front line near Ypres, Belgium. Large clouds of a yellow-green, intensely irritating gas spread in the direction of the opposing French. Chlorine gas is heavier than air. As a result, the clouds settled into the very trenches that the soldiers thought would protect them. Choking and gasping, those soldiers ran from an unknown substance, perhaps inhaling greater quantities simply as a result of their physical activity. The effects of that first attack, by some accounts, included 2,000 deaths and up to 20,000 wounded.[2]

The Allies quickly identified the chemical agent used and shortly retaliated in kind. Within months, chlorine, and later phosgene, diphosgene, and chloropicrin, were produced, weaponized, and used in large quantities by both the Germans and the Allies. These agents are primarily toxic by inhalation. Accordingly, the development of increasingly effective gas masks diminished the "value" of these agents. Of course, gas masks were useful only if the soldiers had adequate education and training and were highly motivated. Use of the gas mask for any period of time was exceptionally uncomfortable. As a result, the soldiers often used them only when their noses provided an alarm. Chlorine, with its intensely irritating aroma, prompted immediate mask use and thus could be avoided. Phosgene, a later weapon development, had a more pleasant smell, likened to newly mown hay. As a result, inhalation of toxic amounts of phosgene easily occurred prior to donning of the mask. A delayed physiological effect, with frequently lethal pulmonary edema, occurred in 4–12 hours. Victims, appearing and feeling normal during the first few hours after exposure, would often continue full military activities. Later, it was learned that exercise during the "latent period" prior to development of pulmonary edema resulted in more rapid onset of more intense disease. This delayed onset of a sometimes-lethal respiratory failure was commonly seen in an individual who initially appeared and felt well. Extreme fear and anxiety resulted among the troops who never knew where or when they would become affected. Intensive efforts to provide the soldiers with a better understanding of chemical weapons and the circumstances/likelihood of their use were combined with improved mask protection. There was a resulting decrease in medical aid station visits for both real and imagined gas exposures.

Because improved Allied education, training, and equipment, especially gas masks, led to a decrease of effectiveness of the German chemical attacks, the Germans introduced a novel chemical material. On December 17, 1917, sulfur mustard, active either as a liquid (below 14°C) or as a vapor, was first released. Sulfur mustard damaged any topical/epithelial surface of contact. Unprotected eyes, skin, and respiratory tracts suffered inflammatory damage to a degree related to the "dose" to which the individual was exposed. Sulfur mustard had a unique aroma, often characterized as similar to garlic or horseradish; however, severe exposure, particularly to the liquid, could occur with a minimal warning aroma. The primary molecular effect of the chemical agent, alkylation of nucleic acids, occurred within the first few minutes of contact. An intense, irritating, inflammatory biological response to that contact would typically occur after a latent period of some hours to days depending on the exposure dose. As a direct result, soldiers would often develop clinical symptoms distant in time and place from their original exposure. There was no available technology to permit identification of sulfur mustard–contaminated areas. As a result, soldiers were unable to identify contaminated places or even people. Fear of cross-contamination seriously compromised their daily activities. Blindness, painful skin blisters, and respiratory symptoms including cough, wheezing, and substantial shortness of breath occurred in soldiers without obvious sulfur mustard contact. An overwhelming sense of fear of chemicals resulted. Soldiers would avoid any areas that had unusual smells, suspecting that mustard might be present. Certainly this fear was one of the most important effects of the use of chemical weapons.

By the end of the war more than half of all shells fired were filled with a chemical agent, often sulfur mustard. Estimates suggest that approximately 25% of all WWI casualties were chemically related, of which 70% or more were caused by sulfur mustard. The ease of chemical weapon manufacture attracted the attention of many countries after WWI. This resulted in substantial research, manufacture, weaponization, and stockpiling of chemical agents, particularly including mustard, in anticipation of possible future needs.

Since the discovery of mustard in 1850 by Guthrie, the intense inflammatory effects of mustard have been recognized. There has been substantial research regarding its cellular and systemic toxicity; however, no specific antidote has been identified to date. Each instance of its use subsequent to WWI has been associated with production of large numbers of debilitated and disabled individuals. Medical statistical assessment of these injuries during WWI has documented the frequency, distribution, and duration of illness of each of the bodily systems involved. Of perhaps greatest interest is the documentation of a 3–5% death rate, largely respiratory. An important comparison is the WWI Allies' 25% death rate from conventional weapons. This statistically and perhaps surprisingly low death rate appears consistently throughout records of subsequent large-scale chemical events, whether accidental or terrorist-related.[2]

The organophosphate nerve agents were originally developed by the IG Farben chemical company in Germany in 1938–1940 as possible insecticides. They are now considered the most toxic and significant chemical weapons with respect to military and civilian planning. Although the first two nerve agents, tabun and sarin, were weaponized and stockpiled by Nazi Germany during World War II, they were never used on the battlefield. American and Soviet forces discovered German rounds filled with these agents, as well as soman, which was developed too late in the war to be weaponized, and immediately began production of munitions containing nerve agents. The first attested battlefield use of these weapons was by Iraq during the Iran–Iraq War from 1984–1987. Sarin was also used by the Japanese cult Aum Shinrikyo in the famous Tokyo subway attack of 1995.

Despite the (relatively) low death rate that has historically occurred from chemical events, both military and public perception is that chemical events, whether accidental or intentional, are to be greatly feared. The degree of fear surrounding chemical events appears to be disproportionate to the degree of actual illness and death. Similar degrees of seemingly excessive public fear are evident in nearly every report of a chemical event. Fear of a chemical event, in fact, seems to create much more public distress than the actual morbidity and mortality created by the release itself. For this reason, disaster preparedness professionals have expressed concern about possible terrorist use of easily available toxic industrial chemicals (TICs).[3] In theory, the difficulty of acquiring or manufacturing a military-style agent could be bypassed and an equally large-scale public effect could be achieved by making use of commercially available chemicals. In the public mind, chemicals are "all cut from the same cloth" and hence reports of any release are likely to provoke substantial public reaction: fear and terror. It appears that even the threat of TIC use may be enough to trigger intense public anxiety and terror.

Chemical Warfare and Terrorism Agents: Clinical Considerations and Treatment Recommendations

Healthcare personnel should suspect an exogenous chemical attack whenever there are multiple patients with similar acute symptoms, especially after exposure to air with an odd smell or color. Chemical agents likely to be used in a large-scale terrorist attack overwhelmingly fall into four categories of compounds:

pulmonary intoxicants, cyanides (mislabeled "blood agents"), vesicants, and nerve agents. Two categories, cyanides and nerve agents, have specific antidotes that must be administered in a time-sensitive manner. For the other two categories of agents, only supportive care is available.

Of the four categories, pulmonary intoxicants and vesicants tend to produce delayed effects. Unlike biological agents with incubation periods typically lasting days, the latent period for these chemical agents tends to be on the order of hours to a day. For cyanides and nerve agents, symptoms are more likely to be immediate or to appear with a latent period of only seconds to minutes.

Certain general principles apply for any suspected mass casualty event involving chemical agents. Decontamination is the most important. Although decontamination of patients exposed to chemical agents may be useful for the patients, it is even more important in order to avoid contamination of other patients, healthcare providers, and treatment facilities. During the Tokyo sarin attack in 1995, an estimated 10% of the emergency department staff developed miosis, the first sign of sarin vapor poisoning. This was because they failed to remove patients' clothes before the exposed victims entered the emergency department. Sarin vapor, trapped in air cells of clothing, caused symptoms in the healthcare workers. A useful concept for chemical agent exposures is to consider patients as contagious without being infectious. This concept will remind properly trained emergency staffs to remove clothing and do at least a brief decontamination of patients suspected of chemical exposure before they enter the facility.

The specific physical state of the agent is an important consideration in determining efficacious decontamination procedures. True vapors or gases require much less attention to full-body decontamination, since clothing removal will eliminate 90% or more of the risk to healthcare workers. Cyanides and pulmonary intoxicants are likely to be only vapor or gas hazards because they are all vapors at standard temperature and pressure. Mustards and nerve agents, on the other hand, are liquids at standard temperature and pressure. Liquid chemical agents require full-body decontamination. Thus, it is critical to obtain the exposure history. Even though mustards and nerve agents are liquids at standard temperature and pressure, in many likely scenarios, exposure to patients will only be in the vapor phase. Agents such as the nerve agent sarin, which evaporates rapidly from the liquid phase at standard temperatures, can overwhelmingly cause vapor hazards rather than liquid hazards. In the Tokyo subway attack, 30% sarin solution was spilled out onto the floor and seats of subway cars. Although the agent causing intoxication was liquid, essentially none of the roughly 5,500 people who presented for care were directly touched by the liquid. Instead, they inhaled sarin vapor, which evaporated from the floor of the subway car and was carried throughout the subway system by the movement of the train.

Physical removal of contaminants is superior to all known catalytic or chemical methods of decontamination. Water or soap and water, if applied quickly and in sufficient quantities, is an appropriate decontaminant for a liquid chemical agent on the skin. The U.S. military developed doctrine for tactical situations in which water was not available in sufficient quantities, and has relied on 0.5% bleach for decades. This solution is a tenfold dilution from the commercially available product, which is 5% bleach (a concentration that is damaging to normal skin). Reactive Skin Decontamination Lotion (RSDL) has been licensed by the U.S.

Table 31.1. Recognizing Health Effects of Chemical Agents by Category

Agent	Agent Name	Unique Characteristics	Initial Effects
Nerve	Cyclohexyl sarin	Miosis (pinpoint pupils)	Miosis (pinpoint pupils)
	Sarin	Copious secretions	Blurred/dim vision
	Soman	Muscle twitching/fasciculations	Headache
	Tabun		Nausea, vomiting, diarrhea
	VX		Copious secretions/sweating
			Muscle twitching/fasciculations
			Breathing difficulty
			Seizures
Asphyxiant ("blood agents")	Arsine	Possible cherry red skin	Confusion
	Cyanogen chloride	Possible cyanosis	Nausea
	Hydrogen cyanide	Possible frostbite*	Patients may gasp for air, similar to asphyxiation but more abrupt onset
			Seizures prior to death
Choking/pulmonary-damaging	Chlorine	Chlorine is a greenish-yellow gas with pungent odor	Eye and skin irritation
	Hydrogen chloride		Airway irritation
	Nitrogen oxides	Phosgene gas smells like newly mown hay or grass	Dyspnea, cough
	Phosgene		Sore throat
		Possible frostbite*	Chest tightness
Blistering/vesicant	Mustard/Sulfur mustard (HD, H)	Mustard (HD) has an odor like burning garlic or horseradish	Severe irritation
	Mustard gas (H)		Redness and blisters of the skin
	Nitrogen mustard (HN-1, HN-2, HN-3)	Lewisite (L) has an odor like penetrating geranium	Tearing, conjunctivitis, corneal damage
	Lewisite (L)	Phosgene oxime (CX) has a peppery or pungent odor	Mild respiratory distress to marked airway damage
	Phosgene oxime (CX)		May cause death
Incapacitating/behavior-altering	3-Quinuclidinyl benzilate (Agent BZ)	May appear as mass drug intoxication with erratic behaviors, shared realistic and distinct hallucinations, disrobing and confusion	Dry mouth and skin
			Initial tachycardia
		Hyperthermia	Altered consciousness, delusions, denial of illness, belligerence
		Mydriasis (dilated pupils)	Hyperthermia
			Ataxia (lack of coordination)
			Hallucinations
			Mydriasis (dilated pupils)

* Frostbite may occur from skin contact with liquid arsine, cyanogen chloride, or phosgene.
Source: Modified from State of New York, Department of Health.

Food and Drug Administration (FDA) as a skin decontaminant for all chemical agents. It is not approved in wounds. Therefore, if the skin is broken, providers should use sterile saline or sterile water as a rinse. Work done in the 1950s in the Netherlands, however, shows that many household products including corn oil are equally as effective decontaminants as 0.5% bleach. The key concept is to decontaminate as quickly as possible, using some physical agent that will wash the patient's skin. Verification of decontamination in a large civilian attack involves confirmation that the patient has been washed. In military settings, detector papers (M8 and M9 paper) that turn specific colors if a liquid chemical agent is still present have been applied to patients' skin.

Another general principle revolves around logistics. For pulmonary intoxicants and mustards, which have no specific anti-dotes, proper management to improve survival requires that severely exposed patients be transported to intensive care settings. In these cases, evacuation to a higher level of care may be more valuable than actual emergency treatment. By contrast, for the more rapidly acting cyanides and nerve agents, immediate care may be necessary even before the patient is properly decontaminated, possibly even in the "hot zone."

Pulmonary intoxicants and cyanides have the potential to result in casualties after industrial accidents in many communities. The vesicants and nerve agents do not generally cause casualties outside of military or terrorist scenarios. Table 31.1 summarizes the initial health effects of the various chemical agent categories. Table 31.2 lists initial decontamination and treatment recommendations for these agent categories. A useful

Table 31.2. Decontamination and Initial Treatment Recommendations for Chemical Agent Categories

Agent	Decontamination	First Aid	Other Patient Considerations
Nerve	Remove clothing immediately Gently wash skin with soap and water Do not abrade skin For eyes, flush with plenty of water or normal saline	Decontaminate skin Atropine before other measures 2-PAM Cl Repeat as needed Diazepam or midazolam if severe exposure and/or if clinically seizing	Onset of symptoms from dermal contact with liquid forms may be delayed Repeated antidote administration may be necessary
Cyanide	Remove clothing immediately if no frostbite[a] Gently wash skin with soap and water Do not abrade skin For eyes, flush with plenty of water or normal saline	Rapid treatment with oxygen Specific IV cyanide antidotes (sodium nitrite and then sodium thiosulfate, or hydroxocobalamin)	Arsine and cyanogen chloride may cause delayed pulmonary edema
Pulmonary intoxicants	Remove clothing immediately if no frostbite[a] Gently wash skin with soap and water Do not abrade skin For eyes, flush with plenty of water or normal saline	Fresh air, forced rest Semi-upright position If signs of respiratory distress are present, oxygen with or without positive airway pressure may be needed Other supportive therapy, as needed; in severe cases may require intubation	May cause delayed pulmonary edema, even following a symptom-free period that varies in duration with the amount inhaled
Blistering/vesicant	Immediate decontamination is essential to minimize damage Remove clothing immediately Gently wash skin with soap and water Do not abrade skin For eyes, flush with plenty of water or normal saline	Immediately decontaminate skin Flush eyes with water or normal saline for 10–15 minutes If breathing difficulty, give oxygen Supportive care: may require intubation in severe cases	Mustard has an asymptomatic latent period There is no antidote or treatment for mustard Lewisite has immediate burning pain, blisters later Specific antidote British Anti-Lewisite (BAL) may decrease systemic effects of Lewisite; only available IM in small quantities Phosgene oxime causes immediate pain Possible pulmonary edema
Incapacitating/behavior-altering	Remove clothing immediately Gently wash skin with water or soap and water Do not abrade skin	Remove heavy clothing Evaluate mental status Use restraints as needed Monitor core temperature carefully Supportive care	Hyperthermia and self-injury are largest risks Hard to detect because it is an odorless and non-irritating substance Possible serious arrhythmias Specific antidote for cholinergic agents such as BZ (physostigmine) may be available

pocket-sized summary reference for the following discussions is the Medical Management of Chemical Casualties Handbook published by the U.S. Army Medical Research Institute of Chemical Defense.[4]

Pulmonary Intoxicants

A large variety of agents cause pulmonary toxicity by the inhalation route. Many of these are toxic industrial chemicals or materials. A few have been used in warfare or in terrorist attacks. Space does not permit detailed discussion of the entire list.

Most pulmonary intoxicants primarily affect only the respiratory tree and do not cause systemic or multi-organ toxic-

ity. With this generalization in mind, further categorization is useful. Highly reactive or water-soluble pulmonary intoxicants cause toxicity in the central compartment of the respiratory tract: the trachea, large bronchi, and larynx. Typical examples of these include hydrochloric acid and ammonia. Among the weaponized agents, sulfur mustard is another good example of intoxicants affecting these structures, although its primary use in terrorism or warfare is as a vesicant. By contrast, pulmonary intoxicants that are less reactive or water-soluble do not react with the structures of the central component, and thus are able to reach the alveoli. They exert primary effects on this peripheral pulmonary compartment. Classic examples of this category include phosgene, oxides of nitrogen (the major component of photochemical smog), and perfluoroisobutylene, the combustion product of Teflon®. Central agents cause irritation, local edema, and, in severe cases, pseudomembrane formation through sloughing in large airways. Peripheral agents tend to disrupt the alveolar-capillary membrane, causing transudation of fluid and producing non-cardiogenic, toxic pulmonary edema. In phosgene intoxication, this probably occurs due to acylation at the alveolar-capillary membrane. Certain agents, such as chlorine, have mixed effects.[5]

The distinction between central and peripheral pulmonary toxicants is a matter of degree and is not absolute. Large exposures to peripheral agents can also affect the central structures, and vice versa. But it is a useful distinction in conceptualizing the primary damage caused by the two categories of pulmonary toxicants.

The common industrial and military pulmonary agents are gases at standard temperatures and pressures. While they may be mucous membrane irritants (chlorine is a good example) and thus cause transient tearing and salivation, only their pulmonary effects are life-threatening. Because they are gases, decontamination is a relatively minor issue. Clothing removal and a quick wash-down of the patient should suffice to protect both provider and emergency treatment facilities.

While all pulmonary intoxicants can produce shortness of breath, the peripheral and central syndromes clinically differ. Central pulmonary agent toxicity manifests as stridor, laryngospasm, and dyspnea. These symptoms are often associated with a latent period that varies according to the specific intoxicant and the amount inhaled, but which is typically on the order of several hours. A severe toxic exposure to a centrally acting agent can cause sudden complete airway obstruction either from edema or by the sloughing of pseudomembranes; these patients can deteriorate rapidly.

By contrast, peripheral pulmonary agent toxicity manifests first as dyspnea, with or without chest tightness. These symptoms occur in the absence of coughing or any signs of pulmonary compromise, either on direct auscultation or even on X-ray. This is because the initial phase of pulmonary edema involves leakage of fluid from the capillaries only into the interstitial space. Until fluid has penetrated into the alveoli themselves, there will only be symptoms without signs. After that point, rales and crackles develop with clear signs of edema on X-ray. As the syndrome intensifies, arterial blood gases will show hypoxemia, and sequestration of up to 1 L/h of fluid in the lungs may lead to hypovolemia and hypotension. This clinical picture is very atypical for cardiogenic pulmonary edema. Patients die of respiratory failure due to hypoxia, hypovolemia, or both. WWI data clearly show that exertion during the latent period of peripheral pulmonary toxicity can exacerbate the situation and turn a minor illness into a life-threatening emergency.

At the time this chapter is being written, no biomarker exists that can discriminate between potentially exposed patients who may be at high risk for the development of non-cardiogenic pulmonary edema within hours. Such a biomarker would be of great help to those in charge of the disaster response because it could identify individuals having the highest need for evacuation to an intensive care unit level of pulmonary support.

Although the latent period may be sufficiently long to insure the patient is no longer being exposed at the time of medical evaluation, it is important to confirm that the patient has been removed from the agent's source. The development of symptoms and signs of pulmonary toxicity within four hours of exposure is a poor prognostic sign regardless of therapy. This is true for both the central and peripheral syndromes. There is no specific therapy for pulmonary agent toxicity. Therapy is entirely supportive.

For central pulmonary toxicity, the key principle is to maintain the integrity of the airway. In severe cases, where pseudomembranes can form and obstruct the airway, endotracheal intubation or even emergency tracheostomy may be required. For primarily peripheral toxicity, intubation with positive end expiratory pressure may be needed. Fluid management should be judicious. These patients, unlike those experiencing cardiogenic edema, are actually hypovolemic. Thus, diuretics are relatively contraindicated and intravenous fluids may be required in multi-liter quantities. Treat hypoxia directly as warranted by monitoring blood gas results in expectation that supportive care will allow the respiratory system to recover.

There are no specific antidotes for pulmonary damage from any of the pulmonary toxicants.[6] More modern forms of respiratory support, including positive end-expiratory pressure (PEEP), are not specific for these syndromes.[7] Antibiotics are not generally advocated prophylactically and are given only when cultures prove infection is present. Animal studies have not yet shown value in the use of agents such as N-acetylcysteine. The use of steroids is not supported by animal or clinical experience.[8]

Most patients with isolated toxicity from inhaled pulmonary intoxicants recover if supportive care is provided in a timely manner. A few peripheral pulmonary intoxicants are associated with interstitial fibrosis post-crisis, including oxides of nitrogen. Phosgene and chlorine, the two most common agents in terrorist scenarios, cause acute syndromes from which patients recover with no apparent lasting structural damage on subsequent pathological examination. This implies that management of patients with these intoxications may become more of a logistical challenge than a medical one.

Cyanides

Cyanides are not considered to be useful battlefield agents, but are high threats for use as a terrorist weapon due to their rapid action. The commonly cited cyanide products, hydrogen cyanide and cyanogen chloride, are close to their boiling points at standard temperatures and pressures. They are occasionally used in criminal scenarios for small-scale attacks, usually against specific individuals, to poison water and food supplies close to the point of consumption.

As a method of large-scale attack against a population, cyanides are not well adapted because the gaseous phase of cyanide ion is lighter than air. Hence, in an outdoor attack, cyanide dissipates rapidly. The reason for the high interest in cyanides as terrorist weapons lies in the possibility of using them in an indoor environment against a large crowd, such as in a sports arena, religious structure, government building, railroad station, or airport terminal.

Cyanide ion, is a normal part of the environment. There is even a normal human cyanide level, based on dietary intake of cyanogenic plants. It is present in all organic media. Smokers of tobacco, for example, average three times the normal human baseline cyanide level in blood. Cyanide ion is also a required cofactor for many human enzymes, including vitamin B12. Because humans evolved in an environment containing cyanide, unlike any of the other chemical agent classes, people also evolved a mechanism to detoxify small quantities of this ion, based on the hepatic enzyme rhodanese. This mechanism underpins antidotal therapy for cyanide poisoning.

Cyanide's mode of action is to inhibit the electron transport chain in mitochondria, at the level of the last enzyme in the chain, cytochrome oxidase or cytochrome a^3. Cyanide ion has a high binding affinity for various metals, including iron, which is the central atom in this enzyme. Once cyanide binds to the iron in this enzyme, aerobic metabolism ceases; cells can only continue metabolism by switching to the inefficient anaerobic metabolic pathway. With nonfunctional electron transport chains, cells cannot utilize oxygen to make glucose and carry out other metabolic functions. As a consequence, venous blood no longer appears blue, and this explains the classic "cherry red" appearance associated with cyanide victims. As a result, cyanide victims are *not* cyanotic. The term "cyanide" (Greek for blue) originates from Prussian blue (not cyanosis), the compound from which Von Scheele originally isolated the molecule in 1782.

Cyanide causes a primary histotoxic anoxia. It affects cells in direct proportion to their metabolic rate. Cyanide crosses the alveolar-capillary barrier and circulates via the blood, giving rise to the old misnomer "blood agent" for cyanide. This term is still in use despite the fact that the blood is only a passive carrier for cyanide. Blood is essentially unaffected by the passage of cyanide, since most blood cells have very few mitochondria. In humans, the most actively metabolic cells are those in the carotid bodies, which serve as baroreceptors. Thus, inhalation of a sizable cyanide challenge causes initial hyperpnea, hypotension, and syncope. The second most highly metabolic cells are those of the brain. Therefore, the next symptom of cyanide poisoning, which in large exposures occurs almost instantaneously, is loss of consciousness followed shortly by seizures, probably caused by hypoxia. Within seconds to minutes, central apnea affects the medullary breathing centers. Cardiac tissue will become affected next, causing vascular instability leading to cardiopulmonary arrest and death within about 8 minutes if there is no treatment.

Via the inhalation route, cyanide is one of two chemical agent classes that can cause a virtually instantaneous loss of consciousness and seizures. The other is the nerve agents. Key concepts for the differential diagnosis are detailed later.

Removal of the patient from the source of contamination is crucial and may be lifesaving. Because the body has its own detoxification mechanism, humans can metabolize a small amount of cyanide. Clinical experience has shown that simple removal from the source of cyanide can revive mild cases of poisoning.[9]

Although the mechanism is not well understood, nasal or mask oxygen therapy is helpful acutely in cyanide poisoning. While theoretically implausible since mitochondrial electron transport chains are inhibited, rendering cells unable to use oxygen, oxygen therapy should be instituted rapidly as it has been proven clinically effective. In addition to oxygen, specific antidotal therapy is valuable for acute cyanide poisoning, but only if it can be instituted in a timely manner. There are two major forms of antidotal therapy, the multi-component cyanide antidote kit and hydroxocobalamin.

The cyanide antidote kit is based on beagle dog experiments performed in the 1930s that showed the components of the kit were capable of saving animals exposed to up to twenty lethal doses of cyanide gas. Conceptually, it consists of two antidotes used sequentially. The first antidote, a nitrite (not nitrate), induces methemoglobin formation. Methemoglobin, with its iron in the Fe^{+3} (ferric) state rather than the Fe^{+2} (ferrous) state of normal hemoglobin, binds to cyanide ions with even greater affinity than does cytochrome a^3. Hence, creation of a methemoglobin pool, which results from therapy with nitrite,

will extract cyanide from cytochrome a^3 and rapidly restore normal cell function. Nitrite is given either via inhalation of an amyl nitrite ampoule or via intravenous administration of sodium nitrite. The inhaled ampoules have never been approved by the FDA but are available in the United States in a state of "regulatory discretion." The dose for sodium nitrite from the vial provided in the cyanide antidote kit is 10 ml. If a repeat dose is required, half of the second vial (5 ml) should be administered. For children, the U.S. military recommends 0.33 ml/kg of the standard 3% nitrite solution given slowly over 5–10 minutes. Nitrite will cause hypotension, and so patients should be lying down when they receive it, whether inhaled amyl nitrite or intravenous sodium nitrite. The use of nitrite alone, however, will create a pool of cyanmethemoglobin in the blood. This is unstable, and unless the second antidote is given, cyanide will eventually dissociate from methemoglobin and cause subsequent toxicity.

The second antidote, sodium thiosulfate, is necessary because the body cannot tolerate a large pool of cyanmethemoglobin indefinitely. In order to permanently eliminate the cyanide ion from the body, sodium thiosulfate, a sulfur donor, is administered as a cofactor to activate the liver stores of rhodanese. The result of this reaction is that rhodanese forms sodium thiocyanate, which is excreted harmlessly in the urine. Sodium thiosulfate is administered via the intravenous route only. The kit contains two 50-ml vials; if the patient requires more than one dose, half of the second vial (25 ml) should be administered. The U.S. military recommends a pediatric dose of 1.65 ml/kg of the standard 25% solution. In fire victims, whose oxygen carrying capacity may have been reduced by exposure to carbon monoxide, it has been standard practice for many years to avoid the methemoglobin former (nitrite) and proceed directly to sodium thiosulfate.

Hydroxocobalamin is commonly used in Europe, and in 2007 was licensed by the FDA as an alternate cyanide antidote (Cyanokit©). It binds stoichiometrically (1:1) to circulating cyanide and forms cyanocobalamin (vitamin B12) which the body tolerates well. One disadvantage is that hydroxocobalamin is a huge molecule and 1:1 binding means that large volumes of hydroxocobalamin must be used via the intravenous route. Additionally, unlike the nitrite and thiosulfate solutions in the antidote kit, hydroxocobalamin must be reconstituted from powder. It also tends to induce an orange color to the skin. Extensive clinical experience from the Paris Fire Brigade has demonstrated that hydroxocobalamin can be used as on-scene treatment by trained first responders. The adult dose is two 2.5-g vials administered intravenously over 15 minutes after reconstitution, with a second dose of two 2.5-g vials given as needed. The most common side effect of hydroxocobalamin is chromaturia (urine tends to turn purple), although this in itself is harmless. In many of the published cases in which hydroxocobalamin has been used, sodium thiosulfate was also given; these treatments are, therefore, not mutually exclusive. Hydroxocobalamin has advantages over nitrite. It does not cause methemoglobinemia (diminishing oxygen carrying capacity) or hypotension, and is safe in pregnancy. However, it takes longer to administer and requires the infusion of large volumes.[10,11] Cyanide antidotal recommendations are summarized in Table 31.3.

Vesicants

Sulfur mustard, the prototypical vesicant agent, has been a military threat since it first appeared on the battlefield in Belgium

Table 31.3. Antidotal Recommendations for Cyanide Poisoning

Patient	Mild (Conscious)	Severe (Unconscious)	Other Treatment
Child	If patient is conscious and has no other signs or symptoms, antidotes may not be necessary.	Sodium nitrite: 0.12–0.33 ml/kg, not to exceed 10 ml of 3% solution slow IV over no less than 5 minutes, or slower if hypotension develops *and* Sodium thiosulfate: 1.65 ml/kg of 25% solution IV over 10–20 minutes Consider IO administration (off-label) if IV access cannot be obtained quickly	For sodium nitrite–induced orthostatic hypotension, normal saline infusion and supine position are recommended. If still apneic after antidote administration, consider sodium bicarbonate for severe acidosis.
Adult	If patient is conscious and has no other signs or symptoms, antidotes may not be necessary.	Sodium nitrite: 10–20 ml of 3% solution slow IV over no less than 5 minutes, or slower if hypotension develops *and* Sodium thiosulfate: 50 ml of 25% solution IV over 10–20 minutes Hydroxocobalamin (Cyanokit©), one vial reconstituted at scene, administered IV, an effective alternate; given over 15 minutes and repeated as needed	

during World War I. In modern times it retains its military potential as well as posing a terrorist threat because of manufacturing simplicity and extreme effectiveness. Sulfur mustard accounted for 70% of the 1.3 million chemical casualties in WWI and an estimated 45,000 Iranian casualties during the Iran–Iraq War. Other vesicants of lesser importance include nitrogen mustard (still used in cancer chemotherapy), Lewisite, and phosgene oxime, which will not be discussed in detail.

Sulfur mustard constitutes both a vapor and a liquid threat to all exposed epithelial surfaces. Like peripheral pulmonary agents, mustard's effects are delayed, appearing hours after exposure. Organs most commonly affected are the skin (erythema and vesicles), eyes (ranging from mild conjunctivitis to severe eye damage), and airways (ranging from mild upper airway irritation to severe bronchiolar damage). Following exposure to large quantities of mustard, precursor cells of the bone marrow are damaged, leading to pancytopenia and secondary infection. The gastrointestinal mucosa may be damaged, and there are sometimes central nervous system (CNS) signs of unknown mechanism. No specific antidotes exist; management is entirely supportive.[12]

Mustard dissolves slowly in aqueous media, such as sweat. Once dissolved, however, it rapidly forms extremely reactive cyclic ethylene sulfonium ions, which react with cell proteins, cell membranes, and especially DNA in rapidly dividing cells. Mustard's ability to react with and alkylate DNA gives rise to the effects characterized as "radiomimetic" (i.e., similar to radiation injury). Mustard has many biological effects, but the actual mechanism of action is largely unknown. Mustard reacts with tissue within minutes of entering the body. Its circulating half-life in unaltered form is extremely brief.

Topical effects of mustard occur in the eyes, airways, and skin, in that order of sensitivity. Absorbed mustard may produce effects in the bone marrow, gastrointestinal tract, and CNS. Direct injury to the gastrointestinal tract may also occur following ingestion of the compound through contamination of water or food.

Erythema is the mildest and earliest form of mustard skin injury. It resembles sunburn and is associated with pruritus, burning, or stinging pain. Erythema begins to appear within 2 hours to 2 days after vapor exposure. Time of onset depends

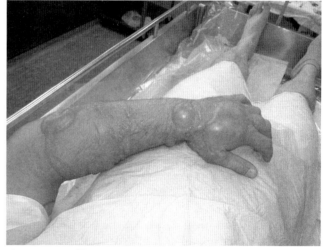

Figure 31.1. Sulfur mustard casualty. This explosive ordnance technician came in contact with liquid sulfur mustard while disabling an old World War I U.S. Army round. Photo by Newmark, with permission of the patient and the staff of the Temple University Hospital burn unit, Philadelphia, Pennsylvania.

on the severity of exposure, ambient temperature and humidity, and type of skin. The most sensitive sites are the warm moist locations and thin delicate skin, such as the perineum, external genitalia, axillae, antecubital fossae, and neck.

Within erythematous areas, small vesicles can develop, which may later coalesce to form bullae. The typical bulla is large, dome-shaped, flaccid, thin-walled, translucent, and surrounded by erythema. The blister fluid is a transudate with a clear to straw-color. It becomes yellow over time and tends to coagulate. The fluid does not contain mustard and is not itself a vesicant. Lesions from high-dose liquid exposure may develop a central zone of coagulation necrosis with blister formation at the periphery. These lesions take longer to heal and are more prone to secondary infection than the uncomplicated lesions seen at lower exposure levels. Severe lesions may require skin grafting (Figure 31.1).

Sulfur mustard vapor is a centrally acting pulmonary intoxicant. The primary airway lesion is necrosis of the mucosa with possible damage to underlying smooth muscle. The damage begins in the upper airways and descends to the lower airways in a dose-dependent manner. Usually, the terminal airways and alveoli are affected when death is imminent.

Necrosis of airway mucosa causes exfoliation of epithelial debris, sloughing, or "pseudomembrane" formation, as with any centrally acting pulmonary agent. These membranes may cause obstruction of the bronchi. During World War I, high-dose mustard exposure caused acute death via this mechanism in a small minority of cases.

The eyes are the organs most sensitive to mustard vapor injury. The latent period is shorter for eye injury than for skin injury and is also exposure concentration–dependent. After low-dose vapor exposure, irritation evidenced by reddening of the eyes may be the only effect. As the dose increases, the injury includes progressively more severe conjunctivitis, photophobia, blepharospasm, pain, and corneal damage, which may lead to severe visual impairment.

Ninety percent of eye casualties heal in 2 weeks to 2 months without sequelae. Scarring between the iris and lens may follow severe exposure; this scarring may restrict pupillary movements and may predispose victims to glaucoma. The most severe damage is caused by liquid mustard. After extensive eye exposure, severe corneal damage with possible perforation of the cornea and loss of the eye can occur. In some individuals, chronic eye irritation, sometimes associated with corneal ulcerations, has been described 10–20 years after exposure.

A few Iranian casualties from the Iran–Iraq War have developed a delayed neovascularization of their corneas that caused late-onset blindness. The relationship of this to an animal model finding known as mustard gas keratopathy is an area of active research.[13]

The mucosa of the gastrointestinal tract is susceptible to mustard damage, either from systemic absorption or ingestion of the agent. Mustard exposure in small amounts will cause nausea and possible vomiting lasting up to 24 hours. The mechanism for the nausea and vomiting is not understood, but mustard does have a cholinergic-like effect. The CNS effects of mustard remain poorly defined as well. Large exposures can cause seizures in animals. Reports from WWI and Iran described the behavior of persons exposed to small amounts of mustard as sluggish, apathetic, and lethargic. These reports suggest that minor psychological problems could linger for a year or longer.

The causes of death in the majority of cases with mustard toxicity are sepsis and respiratory failure. Mechanical obstruction via pseudomembrane formation and agent-induced laryngospasm is important in the first 24 hours, but only in cases of severe exposure. From the third through the fifth day after exposure, a secondary bacterial pneumonia can be expected due to invasion of denuded necrotic mucosa. The third wave of death is caused by agent-induced bone marrow suppression, which peaks 7–21 days after exposure and causes death via sepsis. Early warning of impending marrow suppression is a drop in the lymphocyte count beginning as early as 24 hours. Polymorphonuclear cells may actually rise at first and then begin falling at 3–5 days.

A patient severely ill from mustard toxicity requires the general supportive care provided to any critical patient as well as the specific care given to a burn patient. Liberal use of systemic analgesics, maintenance of fluid and electrolyte balance, nutritional support, use of appropriate antibiotics, and other general measures are necessary. As stated previously, no specific antidote for mustard exposure exists. This may need to await a better understanding of the underlying pathophysiology, which has eluded researchers for over a century.

The management of a patient exposed to mustard may vary from simple treatments, such as the provision of symptomatic care for a sunburn-like erythema, to complex interventions, such as the provision of sophisticated critical care to an individual with burns, immunosuppression, and multisystem involvement. Before raw denuded areas of skin develop, especially with less severe exposures, topical cortisone creams or lotions may be beneficial. Some basic research data suggest benefit from the early use of anti-inflammatory preparations. Small blisters (< 1–2 cm) should be left intact. Because larger bullae will eventually break, they should be carefully unroofed. Denuded areas should be irrigated three to four times daily with saline, other sterile solutions, or soapy water, and then liberally covered with a topical antibiotic, such as silver sulfadiazine or mafenide acetate, to a thickness of 1–2 mm. Some experts advocate sterile needle drainage of large blisters, collapsing the blister roof to form a sterile dressing. Mustard blister fluid does not contain sulfur mustard, only sterile tissue fluid. Healthcare staff should not fear contamination.

Systemic analgesics should be used liberally, particularly before patient manipulation. Monitoring of fluids and electrolytes is important in any sick patient. However, fluid loss after mustard exposure is not of the magnitude seen with deeper thermal burns. Overly rigorous hydration seems to have precipitated pulmonary edema in a few Iranian casualties sent to European hospitals.

Conjunctival irritation from a low vapor exposure will respond to any of a number of available ophthalmic solutions after the eyes are thoroughly irrigated. A topical antibiotic applied several times a day will reduce the incidence and severity of infection. Animal laboratory data have shown remarkable results with commercially available topical antibiotic/glucocorticoid ophthalmologic ointments applied early. Topical glucocorticoids alone are not of proven value, but their use during the first few hours or days may significantly reduce inflammation and subsequent damage. Ophthalmologic consultation is indicated and further use of glucocorticoids should be at the specialist's discretion. Vaseline or a similar substance should be applied regularly to the edges of the lids to prevent them from adhering together.

A productive cough and dyspnea accompanied by fever and leukocytosis occurring within 12–24 hours of exposure is indicative of a chemical pneumonitis. The clinician must avoid use of prophylactic antibiotics to manage this process. Infection often occurs on the third to fifth day and is signaled by fever, pulmonary infiltrates, and an increase in sputum production with a change in color. Initial antibiotic therapy should await evidence of infection from sputum Gram stain; regimens can then be tailored according to the results of sputum culture and sensitivity. Studies suggest that Iran–Iraq War veterans may develop a chemical pneumonitis responsive to treatment with erythromycin 400–600 mg/day, but antibiotic therapy must continue for 6 months following mustard exposure.

Intubation may be necessary for laryngeal spasm or edema, facilitating better ventilation and suctioning of the necrotic inflammatory debris. Early use of PEEP or continuous positive airway pressure (CPAP) may be beneficial. Pseudomembrane formation may require fiber-optic bronchoscopy for removal of the necrotic debris. Bronchodilators are effective for treatment of bronchospasm. If additional relief of bronchospasm is needed, glucocorticoids should be added. Otherwise, there is little evidence that the routine use of glucocorticoids is beneficial.

Leukopenia begins approximately 3 days after major systemic absorption of mustard. Marrow suppression peaks at 7–14 days. In the Iran–Iraq War, a white blood count of ≤ 200 cells/μL usually resulted in death of the patient. This value is not apparently a property of mustard toxicity per se, but is a marker of general immune system failure as a whole. AIDS patients who reach such low white counts also have a high risk of death. Sterilization of the gut by non-absorbable antibiotics should be considered to reduce the possibility of sepsis from enteric organisms. Cellular replacement (bone marrow transplants or transfusions) may be successful. In one study, granulocyte colony-stimulating factor produced a 50% reduction in the time for the bone marrow to recover in nonhuman primates exposed to sulfur mustard and should be considered in human exposure.[14] Antiemetics may be necessary for gastrointestinal side effects. Mustard has the potential for multi-organ chronic sequelae, including delayed corneal neovascularization causing blindness, chronic pneumonitis or "mustard lung," permanent skin dysfunction in affected areas, and a probable increased incidence of cancers, particularly pulmonary. A recent review summarizes experience from Iranian casualties.[15]

Lewisite, a chemically unrelated compound, causes a remarkably similar syndrome to sulfur mustard. There are two important clinical differences between Lewisite and sulfur mustard, however. Lewisite is a direct skin irritant, so early detection of exposure is more likely. This means that decontamination may be more effective in preventing systemic damage, thus reducing the probability of use for either a military or civilian terrorist attack. The other difference is that Lewisite is an arsenical compound so it can be treated with a chelating agent that binds arsenic. The antidote, British anti-Lewisite or dimercaprol, was developed in the 1930s and remains available as a chelating agent. The only U.S. FDA-approved formulation is an intramuscular (IM) injection dissolved in peanut oil, to which some patients are allergic.

Nerve Agents

The organophosphorus nerve agents are the deadliest of the chemical warfare agents. They work by inhibition of tissue synaptic acetylcholinesterase, creating an acute cholinergic crisis. Death ensues because of respiratory depression and can occur within seconds to minutes.[16]

The classic nerve agents include tabun (GA), sarin (GB), soman (GD), cyclosarin (GF), and VX. VR, similar to VX, was manufactured in the former Soviet Union. The two-letter codes are a NATO international convention and convey no clinical implications. All of the nerve agents are organophosphorus compounds, which are liquids at standard temperatures and pressures. The "G" agents evaporate at about the rate of water, except for cyclosarin, which is oily, usually evaporating within 24 hours after deposition on the ground. Their high volatility makes a spill of any amount a serious vapor hazard. In the Tokyo subway attack, 100% of the symptomatic patients inhaled sarin vapor that spilled out on the floor of the subway cars. VX, an oily liquid, is the exception. Its low vapor pressure makes it much less of a vapor hazard but potentially a greater environmental hazard. The nerve agents tabun and sarin were first used on the battlefield by Iraq against Iran during the first Persian Gulf

War (1984–1987). Estimates of casualties from these agents range from 20,000 to 100,000.

Acetylcholinesterase inhibition accounts for the major life-threatening effects of nerve agent poisoning. Reversal of this inhibition by antidotal therapy is effective, proving that this is the primary toxic action of these poisons. At cholinergic synapses, acetylcholinesterase, bound to the postsynaptic membrane, functions to terminate neuron stimulation and thus regulate cholinergic transmission. Inhibition of acetylcholinesterases causes the released neurotransmitter acetylcholine to accumulate abnormally. End-organ overstimulation, manifesting as cholinergic crisis, ensues. Clinical effects of nerve agent exposure are identical for vapor and liquid exposure routes if the dose is sufficiently large. The speed and order of symptom onset however, will differ.

Contact with nerve agent vapor is overwhelmingly the most likely exposure route in both battlefield and terrorist scenarios. Vapor exposure will cause cholinergic symptoms in the order that the toxin encounters cholinergic synapses. The most exposed synapses on the human integument are in the pupillary muscles. Nerve agent vapor easily crosses the cornea, interacts with these synapses, and produces miosis, described by Tokyo subway victims as "the world going black."[23] Rarely, this can also cause eye pain and nausea. Exocrine glands located in the eyes, nose, mouth, and pharynx are exposed to the vapor next, and cholinergic overload here causes increased secretions manifesting as lacrimation, rhinorrhea, and excess salivation. Finally, toxin interacts with exocrine glands in the upper airway and bronchial smooth muscle causing bronchorrhea and bronchospasm, the combination of which can result in hypoxia.

Once the victim has inhaled the vapor, it passively crosses the alveolar-capillary membrane, enters the bloodstream, and inhibits circulating cholinesterases, particularly free butyrylcholinesterase and erythrocyte acetylcholinesterase. Both enzymes can be assayed but measurement may not be easily interpreted without a baseline, since cholinesterase levels vary enormously between persons and over time in an individual healthy patient.

The gastrointestinal tract is usually the first organ system to become symptomatic from blood-borne nerve agent exposure. Cholinergic overload causes abdominal cramping and pain, nausea, vomiting, and diarrhea. After the gastrointestinal tract is involved, nerve agents affect the heart, distant exocrine glands, muscles, and brain. Because there are cholinergic synapses on both the vagal (parasympathetic) and sympathetic sides of the autonomic input to the heart, changes in heart rate and blood pressure are unpredictable. As discussed earlier, remote exocrine activity will include over-secretion in the salivary, nasal, respiratory, and sweat glands – the patient will be "wet all over." Blood-borne nerve agents overstimulate neuromuscular junctions in skeletal muscles, causing fasciculations followed by frank twitching. If the process continues, adenosine triphosphate in muscle cells will eventually be depleted and flaccid paralysis will ensue. Overstimulation at the post synaptic membrane also causes prolonged depolarization of these structures, resulting in eventual blockade of neurotransmission and enhancement of flaccid paralysis.

Due to the wide distribution of the cholinergic system in the brain, sufficient doses of blood-borne nerve agents cause rapid loss of consciousness, seizures, and central apnea, leading to death within minutes. If respiration is supported, status epilepticus may ensue. If status persists, neuronal death and permanent brain dysfunction may occur. In a few cases of mild nerve agent intoxication, patients recovered, but reported weeks of irritability, sleep disturbances, and other nonspecific neurobehavioral symptoms. These may reflect posttraumatic stress or direct nerve agent toxicity that is not well understood.

The time from exposure to development of full-blown cholinergic crisis after nerve agent vapor inhalation can be minutes or even seconds; however, there is no depot effect. Therefore, symptoms do not continually progress over hours and the maximal toxic effects are achieved fairly quickly. Since nerve agents have a short circulating half-life, improvement should be rapid with no subsequent deterioration if the patient is treated with antidotes and supportive care.

Exposure to liquid nerve agents differs in speed and order of symptom onset. A nerve agent on intact skin will partially evaporate and partially be absorbed, causing localized sweating and then localized fasciculations when it encounters neuromuscular junctions. Once in muscle, it will cross into the circulation and cause gastrointestinal discomfort, respiratory distress, heart rate changes, generalized fasciculations and twitching, loss of consciousness, seizures, and central apnea. The time course will be much longer than with vapor inhalation; even a large, lethal droplet can take up to 30 minutes to have an effect, and a small, sublethal dose might require up to 18 hours before toxicity is detected. Clinical deterioration that occurs hours after initiating treatment is far more likely with liquid than with vapor exposure. Additionally, miosis, practically unavoidable with vapor exposure, is not always evident with liquid exposure and may be the last symptom to present. This is due to the relative insulation of the pupillary muscle from the systemic circulation.

Unless a nerve agent is removed by specific therapy (oximes), its binding to cholinesterase is essentially irreversible. Erythrocyte acetylcholinesterase activity recovers at about 1% per day. Plasma butyrylcholinesterase recovers more quickly and is a better guide to recovery of tissue enzyme activity.

Acute nerve agent poisoning is treated by decontamination, respiratory support, and three antidotes – an anticholinergic, an oxime, and an anticonvulsant. In acute cases, all of these forms of therapy may be given simultaneously. Death from nerve agent poisoning is almost always due to respiratory failure. Ventilation will be complicated by increased resistance and secretions. Atropine should be given before ventilation or as it begins, as it will facilitate this intervention.

In theory, any anticholinergic could be used to treat nerve agent poisoning, but worldwide the choice is invariably atropine because of its wide temperature stability and rapid effectiveness. Atropine can be administered either intramuscularly or intravenously. It rapidly reverses cholinergic overload at muscarinic synapses but has little effect at nicotinic synapses. Therefore, atropine can quickly treat the life-threatening respiratory effects of nerve agents but will probably not reverse neuromuscular and possibly sympathetic effects. In the field, military personnel in some countries are given MARK I kits, which contain 2 mg atropine in auto-injector form for intramuscular use (Figure 31.2). In addition, some civilian agencies are now stockpiling this product (FDA-approved in the United States). One can only give a full auto-injector dose; dividing the drug between more than one individual is not possible. The initial loading dose is 2, 4, or 6 mg, with retreatment every 5–10 minutes until the patient's breathing and secretions improve. The Iranians initially used larger doses during the Iran–Iraq War where oximes were in short supply.[17] Pediatric auto-injectors are now available at

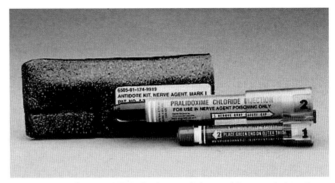

Figure 31.2. The MARK I dual auto-injector kit containing 2 mg atropine and 600 mg 2-pralidoxime chloride. This is being replaced by the ATNAA, first for military and then for civilian use. Photo courtesy of U.S. Army Medical Research Institute of Chemical Defense, Aberdeen Proving Ground, Maryland.

dosages of 0.5 and 1.0 mg for rapid IM administration; however, the intravenous route is preferred when this is logistically feasible, especially in small children. There is no upper bound to atropine therapy in a patient either intramuscularly or intravenously. A total average adult dose for a severely toxic patient usually ranges from 20–30 mg.

In a mildly symptomatic patient with miosis only and no other systemic toxicity, atropine or homatropine eye drops may suffice for therapy. This will produce roughly 24 hours of mydriasis. Frank miosis or imperfect accommodation may persist for weeks or even months after all other signs and symptoms have resolved.

Oximes are nucleophiles that reactivate a cholinesterase enzyme whose active site has been bound to a nerve agent. Therapy with oximes disassociates the enzyme from the nerve agent, restoring normal enzyme function. These antidotes are indicated primarily for the reversal of muscle paralysis and target nicotinic receptors. They have little impact on secretions or bronchospasm. Oxime therapy is limited by a chemical process referred to as aging. Oximes require the presence of a side chain molecule on nerve agents to be effective. This side chain is removed from the nerve agent by biologic processes at a characteristic time-dependent rate. The nerve agent-enzyme complex has "aged" when the side chain is removed. Aged complexes are negatively charged, and oximes cannot reactivate negatively charged molecules. Therefore, oximes cannot reactivate cholinesterase enzymes once the nerve agent to which they are bound has aged. The practical effect of this differs from one nerve agent to another, since each ages at a characteristically unique rate. VX essentially never ages, sarin ages in 3–5 hours, and tabun ages over a longer period. All of these rates are so much longer than the patient's expected lifespan after untreated acute nerve agent exposure that they may be ignored from a clinical standpoint. Soman, on the other hand, ages in 2 minutes. Thus, after only a few minutes following exposure, oximes are useless in treating soman poisoning. The oxime used varies by country; the United States has approved and fielded 2-pralidoxime chloride (2-PAM Cl). MARK I kits contain auto-injectors of 600 mg of 2-PAM Cl. Initial loading doses are 600, 1,200, or 1,800 mg. Since blood pressure elevation may occur after administration of 45 mg/kg in adults, field use of 2-PAM Cl is restricted to 1,800 mg/hour intramuscularly. During the time when more oxime cannot be given, atropine alone is recommended. In the hospital setting, 2.5–25 mg/kg of 2-PAM Cl intravenously has

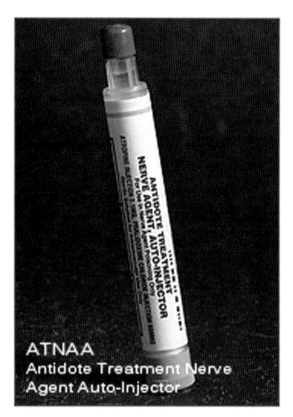

Figure 31.3. Antidote Treatment Nerve Agent Auto-injector, containing 2.3 mg atropine and 600 mg 2-pralidoxime chloride. This is the military dual-chamber autoinjector; the civilian version is called DuoDote. Photo courtesy US Army Medical Research Institute of Chemical Defense, Aberdeen Proving Ground, Maryland.

been found to reactivate 50% of inhibited cholinesterase. The usual recommendation is 1,000 mg through slow intravenous drip over 20–30 minutes, with no more than 2,500 mg over a period of 1–1.5 hours.

Dosage recommendations for children are less certain than for adults and are based on extrapolations from adults; further studies are needed in children.[18] In small children weighing less than 10–12 kg(< 25 pounds), auto-injectors, even the pediatric doses, may not be practical. Additionally, the clinical syndromes in children may be harder to recognize; in particular, seizures in children often manifest without tonic-clonic movements and may be missed. The U.S. FDA has approved a single cartridge auto-injector, ATNAA (Antidote Treatment Nerve Agent Auto-injector), which contains both 2.1 mg atropine and 600 mg 2-PAM Cl (Figure 31.3). This was shown bioequivalent to the MARK I kit, but requires only half as long to administer (requires only one injection, not two). In civilian practice, the trade name for this item is DuoDote©. DuoDote© is gradually replacing the MARK I kit in the Strategic National Stockpile (SNS) CHEMPACK kits forward-deployed for civilian emergencies.

Some studies of patients exposed to organophosphate pesticides have shown oxime therapy to be ineffective in that setting. This limitation does not appear to apply to nerve agent poisoning, at least in commonly used animal models. At present, the prudent recommendation appears to be to treat with an oxime if actual nerve agent exposure is suspected or confirmed.

Nerve agent–induced seizures do not respond to the usual anticonvulsants used for status epilepticus. The only class of anticonvulsants that has been shown to stop this form of status is the benzodiazepines. Diazepam is the only benzodiazepine approved for seizures in the United States in humans, although other benzodiazepines, especially midazolam, work well against nerve agent–induced seizures in animal models. Diazepam is manufactured in 10-mg injectors for intramuscular use and given to U.S. military forces for this purpose. Civilian agencies stockpile this product, convulsive antidote for nerve agent (CANA), which is not generally used in hospital practice. Extrapolation from animal studies indicates that adults will probably require 30–40 mg of diazepam, intramuscularly, to stop nerve agent–induced status epilepticus. In the hospital, or in a child too small to tolerate the auto-injector, intravenous diazepam may be used at similar doses. The clinician may confuse seizures with the neuromuscular signs of nerve agent poisoning. In the hospital, early electroencephalography is recommended in order to distinguish between non-convulsive status epilepticus, actual seizures, and postictal paralysis. Intravenous lorazepam is also effective. Antidotal recommendations for the treatment of acute nerve agent poisoning are found in Table 31.4.

Extensive animal work carried out by the U.S. Army has shown that midazolam is superior to diazepam and all other tested benzodiazepines in stopping nerve agent–induced seizures. Midazolam does not carry FDA approval as an anticonvulsant at the time of writing this chapter, despite being used off-label for this purpose for many years. A New Drug Application for midazolam for this purpose has been accepted by the FDA and it is hoped that approval will be forthcoming. Once this milestone is achieved, both military and civilian authorities plan to recommend IM midazolam as the anticonvulsant of choice. An important milestone in this effort was the completion of a large NIH-funded clinical study in 2012, which demonstrated that IM midazolam was superior to IV lorazepam in stopping status epilepticus of any cause in a community setting. The improved results with midazolam were largely derived from the shorter time to administer IM drugs via auto-injector. This study opened the door to general use of IM auto-injectors in civilian practice for the first time.[19]

The major differential diagnosis for acute nerve agent poisoning is acute cyanide poisoning, particularly in a mass casualty event involving multiple patients presenting similarly. Both can develop acutely and involve loss of consciousness, seizures, and respiratory depression. Cyanide poisoned patients tend to remain non-cyanotic acutely because their venous blood remains red and oxygenated. Cyanide poisoned patients do not show the prominent miosis and increased secretions typical of nerve agent poisoned patients.

Incapacitating Agents

During the 1960s there was much interest on the part of U.S. intelligence agencies and military planners in developing an agent which would incapacitate, rather than kill, opposing forces. The only product that ever emerged from this program was 3-Quinuclidinyl benzilate, later termed Agent BZ, a weaponized anticholinergic. The mechanism of action of this compound is the exact opposite of nerve agents; it blocks acetylcholine from interacting with post-synaptic cholinergic receptors. It causes profound, but unpredictable, behavioral and psychiatric syndromes which gradually resolve without treatment. Because of

Table 31.4. Antidote Recommendations Following Exposure to Nerve Agents

Patient Age	Antidotes Mild/Moderate Effects	Severe Effects	Other Treatment
Infants (0–2 yrs)	Atropine: 0.05 mg/kg IM, or 0.02 mg/kg IV; and 2-PAM Cl: 15 mg/kg IM or IV slowly	Atropine: 0.1 mg/kg IM, or 0.02 mg/kg IV; and 2-PAM Cl: 25 mg/kg IM, or 15 mg/kg IV slowly	Assisted ventilation after antidotes for severe exposure
Child (2–10 yrs)	Atropine: 1 mg IM, or 0.02 mg/kg IV; and 2-PAM Cl: 15 mg/kg IM or IV slowly	Atropine: 2 mg IM, or 0.02 mg/kg IV; and 2-PAM Cl: 25 mg/kg IM, or 15 mg/kg IV slowly	Repeat atropine (2 mg IM, or 1 mg IM for infants) at 5- to 10-min intervals until secretions have diminished and breathing is comfortable or airway resistance has returned to near normal.
Adolescent (>10 yrs)	Atropine: 2 mg IM, or 0.02 mg/kg IV; and 2-PAM Cl: 15 mg/kg IM or IV slowly	Atropine: 4 mg IM, or 0.02 mg/kg IV; and 2-PAM Cl: 25 mg/kg IM, or 15 mg/kg IV slowly	
Adult	Atropine: 2–4 mg IM or IV; and 2-PAM Cl: 600 mg IM, or 15 mg/kg IV slowly	Atropine: 6 mg IM; and 2-PAM Cl: 1,800 mg IM, or 15 mg/kg IV slowly	Phentolamine for 2-PAM Cl-induced hypertension: (5 mg IV for adults; 1 mg IV for children). Diazepam for convulsions: (0.2–0.5 mg IV for infants < 5 years: 1 mg IV for children > 5 years; 5 mg IV for adults), or bioequivalent doses of midazolam.
Elderly, frail	Atropine: 1 mg IM; and 2-PAM Cl: 10 mg/kg IM, or 5–10 mg/kg IV slowly	Atropine: 2–4 mg IM; and 2-PAM Cl: 25 mg/kg IM, or 5–10 mg/kg IV slowly	

the unpredictability of Agent BZ, the U.S. military cancelled its incapacitating agents program in the 1980s and all of the stocks of BZ were destroyed. Since then there have been allegations of use of either BZ or related compounds by Serbian forces in the Yugoslav civil war in 1995 and in alleged chemical attacks in Syria in 2013.

In the Moscow theater siege of 2002, Russian security forces attempted to gain control of an establishment that had been taken over by Chechen terrorists who were holding hundreds of occupants hostage. They exposed the captors and hostages to a chemical agent later identified as a derivative of the common anesthetic fentanyl. Unfortunately, the authorities failed to let emergency personnel, especially hospital personnel, know to what category this agent belonged. Additionally, the agent proved to have a low safety factor, and over a hundred of the theater's occupants succumbed to respiratory failure. Knowledge that the agent was a narcotic would have assisted emergency physicians in choosing naloxone as an antidote. This was the first known application of a fentanyl derivative in a law enforcement scenario. Fentanyl derivatives have never been developed for military use, and have never been used by law enforcement outside of Russia. They, like cyanides, probably are most likely to be used in confined spaces such as the theater.

Chemical versus Biological Emergencies

Because all-hazards preparedness often groups chemical and biological hazards together, it is worthwhile making the differences explicit. Although person-to-person transmission of chemical toxins, such as sulfur mustard, is a real concern, actual person-to-person infection common in plague and smallpox does not occur with chemical agents. This would suggest that preparation

for a chemical attack is somewhat easier than for an attack using an infectious agent. But this apparent advantage is largely offset by the speed with which most chemical agents cause illness. In an attack using cyanide or nerve agents, one will have only minutes to administer antidotes to reverse toxicity and prevent death in severely poisoned individuals. The response structure built within the U.S. government for an infectious disease outbreak or biological attack, including distribution of antibiotics and vaccines, is much too slow to be useful in a chemical attack. This is the major reason why those responsible for the SNS in the United States have deployed CHEMPACKs, caches of nerve agent and cyanide antidotes, within 1 hour's reach of 90% of the U.S. population.

Besides speed of symptom development, the biggest difference between chemical and biological attacks lies in the necessity for decontamination. Decontamination is often unnecessary in biological attacks, since the incubation period of most weaponized agents is on the order of days, and people will have generally bathed and changed clothes before the attack has been identified. In chemical attacks, decontamination plays a more prominent role. Exposed individuals remain potential victims until they have been decontaminated. In addition, those experiencing toxicity are a danger to others, most importantly first responders and medical personnel, until they have been decontaminated. While a detailed discussion of decontamination can be found elsewhere (see Chapter 16), it is worth noting that this has become the rate-limiting step in many civilian exercises; many people are unwilling to disrobe and be decontaminated in a mass casualty setting. At the time of writing this chapter, the U.S. Department of Health and Human Services (HHS) is funding work in several U.S. cities to measure the actual value of decontamination by various methods in a mass casualty setting. It is undeniable, however, that in the Tokyo subway attack, 10% of emergency room personnel developed miosis, a sign of poisoning, because their patients had not been decontaminated. Healthcare workers developed mild symptoms from exposure to the vaporized sarin in patients' clothing. Decontamination will remain a major issue in chemical preparedness for the foreseeable future.

Lastly, for planning purposes, one major difference between chemical and biological hazards is the presence of a robust chemical industry and supply chain in industrialized countries. Boxcars and trucks loaded with toxic chemicals such as chlorine move up and down the railways and highways of countries every day. Chemical facilities are present throughout most regions. This contrasts greatly with the lack of an equivalent risk from biological hazards. A chemical truck or railcar can become a weapon by the simple application of a conventional explosive. Thus, chemicals may be attractive to those seeking to do harm because of their availability.

Examples of Chemical Events: Implications for Disaster Preparedness

Intentional (Non-State-Sponsored) Chemical Events

CYANIDE POISONING OF WATER SUPPLY IN 1985 – THE COVENANT, THE SWORD, AND THE ARM OF THE LORD

The Covenant, the Sword, and the Arm of the Lord (CSA) was a survivalist group primarily interested in large-scale murder to "hasten the return of the Messiah by carrying out God's judgments."[20] The group was conceived in 1971 by a fundamentalist preacher, James Ellison. The group planned and prepared for Armageddon, which would result in the destruction of the American economic system. On April 22, 1985, an FBI raid of the CSA compound revealed a stockpile of machine guns, ammunition, an antitank rocket, and an armored car. The FBI found 114 liters of potassium cyanide. CSA initially explained that the cyanide was to be used for pest poisoning. Further FBI analysis revealed there had been extensive discussions and planning with intent to use the cyanide to poison water supplies in New York, Chicago, and Washington.[20]

General Commentary

The toxicity of a chemical agent is principally dependent on the quantity delivered. Therefore, cyanide, or other toxic materials such as organophosphates, would be sufficiently diluted if placed in a large community water supply, rendering the biological effect negligible.

To poison a population intentionally by contaminating its drinking water requires either extraordinary quantities of agent or delivering the agent within the water pipeline closer to the victims. Small quantities of cyanide have often been used in criminal tampering with drugs and food products. The Chicago Tylenol® contamination event in 1982 was the first documented U.S. incident of food tampering with cyanide. Seven deaths resulted from distribution of the poisoned capsules to six stores in the city. A number of subsequent "copycat" events occurred over the next several years with additional deaths. Despite a $100,000 reward offered by Tylenol® manufacturer Johnson & Johnson, the perpetrator has not been caught. Prior to 1982, tamper-proof capsules and packaging were virtually unknown. Subsequent to the tampering events, public anxiety mushroomed. Manufacturers of packaged foods and medicines promptly responded with development and application of an extraordinary variety

of complex and protective packaging. It appears that this extra level of "public protection" consumes many millions of dollars yearly. The cost/benefit of the extra packaging has yet to be measured. On such occasions, public anxiety, often fueled by media speculation, may present a far greater problem than the medical issues.

Mitigation

Communities with public water suppliers routinely participate in a risk assessment and vulnerability analysis concerning possible compromise of their water supplies. Normally, problems of environmental disaster or drought are a primary focus. As a result of such notorious industrial poisonings as the Minamata mercury-poisoning event in Japan (resulting in ~400 deaths and 1,000 permanent injuries), many cities have also become concerned about environmental "pollutant" contamination. Risk assessment and vulnerability studies for possible environmental pollution are, in fact, just the type of action that would be useful for mitigation of possible chemical, biological, or radiation contamination.

Preparedness

Specific medical preparations for possible water supply contamination have long been an accepted part of military preparedness. Civilian medical systems, however, rarely have adequate detection equipment or response technology to counter intentional contamination of the water supply. By federal regulation, U.S. communities have developed an interactive disaster preparedness committee, the Local Emergency Planning Committee. Primarily through this type of community-wide organizational structure, such issues as water supply risks can be addressed in a cooperative fashion with appropriate assistance requested from organizations such as the Environmental Protection Agency (EPA) at the state and federal levels.

Response

Despite threats by many organizations and individuals, at the time of this writing, no such large-scale intentional water supply contamination has occurred. EPA has undertaken an extensive public information, planning, and preparation effort to assist the general population in understanding the scope of this concern. This is a fine example of national governmental mitigation and preparedness for a perceived risk.

NERVE AGENT USE IN 1995 – AUM SHINRIKYO

On June 27, 1994, a successful chemical attack was undertaken in Matsumoto, a city (population 200,000) situated in the northern Japanese Alps, 201 km northwest of Tokyo. The Aum Shinrikyo, a 40,000 member, well-funded "doomsday" cult perpetrated the attack. The use of sarin, a military organophosphate poison, resulted in seven deaths among nearly 600 victims. Five victims were found dead, two were transported to the hospital in full cardiac arrest, dying within 4 hours, and one victim survived in a vegetative state due to (presumed) hypoxic encephalopathy. This individual ultimately died of respiratory failure in August 2008. There were fifty-six hospitalizations distributed among six hospitals. Several victims required intubation and mechanical ventilation. Generalized seizures were noted in many of the severely affected victims. There were 208 additional outpatient clinic medical evaluations and 277 symptomatic victims who did not seek medical care. The first report of the event came as a telephoned request for an ambulance 2 hours after the exposure. Eight of the fifty-two rescuers and one doctor providing care showed symptoms of poisoning as a result of (presumed) cross-contamination. One rescuer required hospitalization. Ten years later, a long-term questionnaire-based survey of local residents showed 73% of exposed and 44% of unexposed residents reporting psychological problems. [21] The intent of the attack, prevention of a legal decision in a local civil suit, was achieved by poisoning the three judges involved. Sarin was specifically identified as the toxic agent in a sample taken from a local pond on July 4, 1994. Those data and other related law enforcement concerns provided sufficient evidence for a police raid of the principal Aum Shinrikyo facilities, planned for March 1995. The Tokyo subway sarin attack, however, occurred first.[22]

On March 20, 1995, Aum Shinrikyo cult members released approximately 24 liters of a sarin solution estimated to be 30% pure. The perpetrators may have had atropine sulfate injections available for personal use if necessary.[23] Sarin was distributed into eleven polyethylene bags, although probably fewer bags were actually opened. Five different subway trains were involved, all of which were scheduled to arrive within 4 minutes of each other between 8:00 and 8:10 AM at the Kasumigaseki Station. The station was selected for its proximity to Tokyo's National Police Agency and Finance Ministry as part of the cult's plan to signal the beginning of Armageddon and to specifically attack members of a chemically trained police squad. The first notification of a medical emergency was directed to the city fire department within minutes of the attack. Some fifteen subway stations called within the next several minutes. Area hospitals were notified at 8:16 AM, but the initial report was of a gas explosion. Therefore, the hospitals prepared to receive patients with burns and carbon monoxide poisoning. It was more than an hour before emergency dispatch recognized the disaster as a single event. Ultimately 131 ambulances and 1,364 emergency medical technicians (EMTs) were dispatched to the affected subway stations. Poor communication with the Emergency Operations Center resulted in EMT transport of all nearby victims directly to St. Luke's International Hospital (SLIH). Even though SLIH had a mutual aid agreement with another nearby hospital to take less ill patients, this agreement could not be implemented because all available transportation was otherwise occupied. SLIH saw 649 victims within the first 24 hours. The EMTs attempted triage at the scene of the release and some medical support; however, there was no on-scene clothing removal, decontamination, antidote administration, or intubation of victims with severe respiratory distress. The EMTs had no personal protective equipment. Of the 1,364 EMTs who worked to transport victims to hospitals, 135 developed clinical evidence of sarin poisoning requiring some medical therapy, including at least twenty-five hospitalizations. SLIH had three entrances, each of which remained open, allowing full access to patients, relatives, television crews, and various bystanders. Not all victims arriving at the hospital were directed to disrobe or shower. As a result, 110 hospital staff members at SLIH (23% of the staff) themselves experienced some symptoms of sarin exposure due to cross-contamination.

There were twelve deaths as a result of the attack. Six deaths occurred within 2 hours of the event and the remaining six deaths occurred from 20–80 days later. Some deaths were among the subway station personnel, who apparently cleared sarin-contaminated waste with bare hands and no respiratory protection. From available medical reports at SLIH, it appears that the

two deaths (of 1,000 patient seen) resulted from cardiac arrest. One ultimate survivor arrived in full arrest and was immediately intubated and provided ventilatory support. She recovered and was discharged 5 days later. Of particular interest, this 21-year-old woman apparently received no specific antidote until approximately 90 minutes after her exposure. Notification that sarin was the offending agent did not occur until approximately 10:30 AM, 2.5 hours after the event. Reportedly, a military physician recognized the clinical signs and symptoms as indicative of a nerve agent exposure. Beginning at that time, oxime therapy was provided for those severely affected. SLIH quickly devised a treatment protocol that enabled the victims to be more rapidly treated. An official prosecutor's report puts the number of injuries at 3,938. Of a total of 4,973 people reportedly seen at Tokyo hospitals within the first 24 hours, approximately 1,100 were hospitalized. Of all patients reporting to Tokyo hospitals complaining of chemical agent exposure, some 74% showed no clinical signs or symptoms. These patients apparently presented largely because of media announcements reporting the event and suggesting that civilians who "felt unwell" should immediately go to the hospital. SLIH conducted a post-event questionnaire-based evaluation of 610 victims. At 1 month after the event, nearly 60% reported symptoms interpreted as indicative of post-traumatic stress disorder (PTSD). Repeated studies at 3 and 6 months showed similar percentages of individuals with such symptoms. People reported flashbacks, insomnia, depression, and nightmares. Some individuals' very high anxiety prevented their subsequent use of the subway. Long-term (10 years) follow-up has been reported and shows persistence of long-lasting psychological problems and PTSD in some victims.[21,24]

Despite legal and political action and subsequent intense investigation of the Aum cult, there is evidence of more recent Aum activity in the Ukraine, Belarus, Kazakhstan, and Russia. In March 1998, a reported Aum member telephoned the Russian newspaper *Itar-Tass* with a threatened plan to spread a toxic gas throughout the Moscow subway system.[25]

General Commentary

Aum Shinrikyo has produced the greatest number of non-state-sponsored chemical (and biological) attacks on record. Between April 1990 and March 1995, Aum undertook ten biological attacks. There were no recorded casualties. Between November 1993 and July 4, 1995, Aum undertook a total of twelve chemical attacks (one phosgene, two cyanide, five VX, and four sarin) with 20 deaths and approximately 1,300 injured.[26] Reports from various medical facilities in Tokyo have expanded knowledge of the time course and clinical response to sarin vapor. Inhalation of sarin vapor produces clinical effects very rapidly, within seconds to minutes. Individuals contaminated by sarin typically demonstrate peak disease symptomatology within the first 30 minutes after contact with the agent, provided further exposure ceases (i.e., removal from the site).[27]

Individuals who reach a medical care facility alive will likely survive even without specific antidotal therapy unless other complications supervene. At SLIH, one individual arrived in full cardiac arrest. Specific antidotal therapy (atropine and pralidoxime chloride) was not provided until more than 90 minutes after exposure. The victim nevertheless survived without complications. Two other victims suffered respiratory arrest in the setting of seizures after hospital arrival. Immediate provision of diazepam and mechanical ventilation were effective in preventing their deaths.

Of the more than 5,500 individuals reportedly involved in the Tokyo event, some 1,100 were hospitalized, mostly with recognized nerve agent–related signs and symptoms. Assuming that this cohort of 1,100 was "truly" exposed, the death of "only" 12 individuals among this group represents an important detail in terms of disaster preparedness for this and many other chemical events. In a large-scale chemical event, sizeable numbers of patients may be transported or self-present to nearby facilities. As was seen in the Tokyo event, only a very small number of these individuals will likely suffer immediately life-threatening illness. Importantly, the illness in Tokyo primarily presented as respiratory distress. In all cases, immediate identification of severely affected victims with immediate application of respiratory support was sufficient to stabilize the victims even without immediate use of antidote. Certainly, later provision of atropine and oxime appeared to ameliorate the degree and shorten the time of the illness. The rapid application of basic and advanced life support principles appears to have been of critical importance. This observation further suggests that first responders and first receivers should be fully qualified and prepared to provide respiratory support, including ventilation and intubation, possibly even at the scene of the event.

A minority of Tokyo subway sarin attack survivors reported longer-term (months, occasionally years) symptoms of diminished mental acuity, headaches, nightmares, and sleep disorders. One patient was found to have a delayed neuropathy. The relationship of this deficit to his sarin exposure remains unclear.[21,23]

Mitigation

The medical system in Tokyo supported a complex, well-organized, and well-trained disaster preparedness organization that was in place prior to the nerve agent attacks. The principal threat to the city was considered to be an earthquake. Therefore, much of the planning and training was focused on the medical care for large numbers of trauma victims. As is often the case, the nerve agent event was unexpected in size and scope. There had been no education or training for a large-scale chemical contamination event outside of the military structure. Despite the experiences of World War II, there was no repository of medical knowledge or experience in dealing with large events on which civilian disaster planners could draw. Therefore, a hazard analysis or vulnerability assessment did not exist.

Preparedness

Equipment designed for deployment in a contaminated environment was scarce and first responders were not well trained in its use. Contamination of a very large percentage of the first responders emphasized the importance of such preparation.

Response

The local hospitals managed a very large number of individuals within a short period of time. There was little attention paid to patient decontamination or to health professional self-protection, presumably due to lack of training and complicated by an overwhelming influx of vapor-contaminated patients. Consequently, in some areas of the hospitals, up to 25% of the hospital staff suffered clinical effects of cross-contamination. Nevertheless, the most severely ill victims were identified expeditiously and treated with appropriate focus on critical components of their illness. Respiratory failure and seizures were the principal life-threatening illnesses. These were handled very competently. Of note was the absence of early specific antidotal

therapy. Although the victims presented with evidence of cholinergic excess, the possibility of organophosphate toxicity was not considered for about 2 hours. When the etiology was finally identified, individuals with severe illness had either already expired or were significantly improved, having been intubated and ventilated.

Recovery

In the years after the event, the medical authorities in Tokyo have carefully reviewed the medical response, found associated challenges, and enacted realistic improvements in the city's disaster preparedness plans. Yanagisawa makes a particularly valuable recommendation for organized medical evaluation and follow-up of such a large-scale event by using an integrated team including epidemiological, neurological, and psychiatric disciplines.[21] Perhaps the most important result of the event has been the development of a National Disaster Center in Tokyo. This facility is a day-to-day resource and training facility for disaster preparedness. In the event of a large-scale disaster, the facility can be converted to provide medical care for disaster victims.

IMPROVISED EXPLOSIVE DEVICES AS CHEMICAL WEAPONS IN IRAQ FROM 2004–2007

In 2007, improvised explosive devices (IEDs) in various forms became the single greatest cause of death among U.S. troops in Iraq. Nearly 57% of the 327 U.S. deaths during the first 6 months of 2007 were the result of IEDs. The increasing complexity of IEDs has been associated with greater difficulty in detecting and defending against them, resulting in an increasing mortality rate. This has continued to be the case as American involvement in Iraq ended and attention shifted to Afghanistan. Recent escalation of their complexity has resulted from incorporation of chemicals into the device. Both military (sarin and mustard) and industrial (chlorine) chemicals have been added to the devices, resulting in substantially increased anxiety regarding their danger.

In May 2004, an IED constructed from a 155-mm artillery round, possibly left over from a Saddam Hussein-era stockpile, was found to contain the military nerve agent sarin. Two U.S. soldiers who rendered the IED safe received a vapor challenge of sarin, and required treatment for "minor exposure." Neither individual required antidotes, and both returned to duty after convalescence for 3 weeks and completed their tours of duty in Iraq. But 1 year later, one of the two soldiers developed complaints of memory loss for sequences, crucial to his job as an explosive ordnance soldier, and had abnormal neuropsychological testing results. His status gradually improved over the next 2 years. He remained on active duty and was promoted in a competitive field. It is not possible to say definitively whether his mild and temporary psychological abnormality was due to post-traumatic stress or to some delayed or chronic sarin toxicity.[28] During that same month, an IED containing military mustard agent was also found.[29]

In early February 2007, some vehicle-borne IEDs were found to contain liquefied chlorine canisters. Explosion of these devices resulted in chemical exposure for some victims and associated illness. The addition of chemicals to the IEDs in effect produced a weapon similar to the chemical weapons of World War I. Most of the injuries related to the IEDs were from associated physical trauma, however. The effects of the chemical component achieved in World War I resulted from much larger quantities of chemicals delivered by munitions specially designed for that purpose. IEDs "accompanied" by chemicals are unlikely to achieve a World War I–equivalent toxic effect. The military/public reaction and associated psychological distress from use of a "chemical warfare agent" may have as much effect as the physical damage itself.[30] As has been noted before, the best defense against such public (and medical responder) anxiety derives from education and training. Accordingly, concerns regarding a chemical release associated with IEDs have prompted training responses within the United States. Of note is the annual Golden Guardian Exercise undertaken in the State of California. There, focus on the traumatic/explosive effects of an IED has been broadened to incorporate concern about the appropriate response to other materials (e.g., nerve agents), which might possibly be incorporated with the IED.[31] The military response to incorporation of chemical (and possibly biological and radiological/nuclear) materials with an IED has led to development of various remotely operated robotic devices with detectors capable of identifying chemical, biological, and radiological/nuclear materials (e.g., Talon® Robots).

Examples of Unintentional Chemical Events

Ammonia Release in 2002 in Minot, North Dakota

At 1:37 AM on January 18, 2002, 31 railroad cars (out of 112) derailed in an incident 0.8 km west of Minot (population 36,567), a city in the U.S. state of North Dakota. Five cars carrying anhydrous ammonia suddenly ruptured, releasing an estimated 555,300 liters of the chemical. This vaporized immediately into a large plume. An estimated 11,600 people were residing in the plume-involved area. There were twelve serious injuries, including one traumatic death, and 320 additional individuals sustained minor injuries.

The derailment damaged local power lines at the site. Electricity supplied to 2,820 residences was disrupted. The conductor notified the central emergency dispatch number (911) in Minot by personal cell phone. The violent rupture of the tank cars caused some sections to be propelled as far as 356 meters from the site. Temperature was −21°C and winds were 10–12 km/h from the west. Very low ambient temperature and slow winds kept the plume from rising. Deleterious health and medical effects were minimized because most residents were indoors asleep at the time. The plume that formed was an estimated 91 meters high and 4 km wide as it ultimately drifted downwind to cover 8 km of the valley containing Minot. The local fire department chief, responding to notification by the 911 emergency dispatch operator, arrived on scene within 10 minutes and established a command post.

In the involved area, one couple attempted to flee their home in a truck. Their vehicle crashed into a house across the street from their residence. The female passenger returned to their house but the 38-year-old male driver collapsed outside. Ammonia vapors were described as so intense as to severely limit visibility in the immediate area. The Incident Commander prohibited first responders from entering the site due to a substantial risk to personal safety. Approximately 3 hours after the event occurred, first responders were allowed entry to begin rescue of victims in the immediate area; 60–65 persons were ultimately evacuated. An attempted rescue of the collapsed truck driver failed due to responders not wearing self-contained breathing apparatus (SCBA). All other residents were instructed to shelter-in-place with notification provided by warning siren, cable television interrupts, and radio notification. Many residents did not

hear the siren due to its location, and residents without power did not receive the media notification. The collapsed driver was ultimately rescued approximately 3.5 hours after the event and found to be unresponsive. The 911 system handled over 2,800 calls, and instructed people to remain in their homes, shut down their furnaces and air handling systems, shelter in their bathrooms and turn on their showers, and breathe through wet clothes. Residents with wells, whose power was interrupted, were unable to operate their showers. At 4:15 AM the plume reached the nearest (Trinity) hospital. The hospital was not evacuated. Closing down the heating, ventilation, and air-conditioning system was effective in preventing infiltration of much of the ammonia.

Seven minor injuries requiring hospital evaluation occurred in the 122 firefighters and 11 police personnel who responded, including several dispatchers. These injuries were mostly eye irritation, chest discomfort, respiratory distress, and headaches.

At 2:15 AM, the first casualty reached Trinity Hospital. The hospital disaster plan was activated at 2:30 AM. Ultimately more than 370 persons were evaluated. Eleven individuals required hospitalization, three as the direct result of chemical burns to the eyes and face. Two individuals required mechanical ventilation. The Minnesota National Guard Civil Support Team arrived later that day. The railroad corporation quickly established a claims and assistance center. The rapidity of this action may have reduced much of the public distress after the event.[32,33]

The National Transportation Safety Board (NTSB) began its activities early that morning, with inspection personnel fully active the same day. Town public meetings were conducted to assure residents that recovery efforts were fully underway. Much of the public commentary, however, focused on the belief that the 911 system as well as other components of the emergency response plan appeared to have failed the community. An informal review of public perception was undertaken in September 2004 during a Department of Justice Disaster Preparedness Program in North Dakota. Many residents spontaneously reported their continued dissatisfaction with the Minot emergency response, reflecting that they felt abandoned by on-scene personnel. The NTSB report noted that Minot had undertaken a disaster preparedness drill the prior September that had enhanced the effectiveness of the emergency response and that a 3-hour restriction of emergency responders from the involved area was appropriate to their personal safety.[34]

General Commentary

An evaluation of this event, conducted per federal regulation by NTSB, was completed and reported on March 9, 2004.[35] This was a comprehensive evaluation that also included a brief assessment of disaster preparedness within the first responder and medical community. Although the authors of this particular section of the report were not identified, and so their medical review qualifications are therefore uncertain, there is no other publicly available comprehensive evaluation of the medical (hospital and first responders) response to the event. Public anxiety is typically very difficult to control during a large-scale event. In this case, post-event efforts to explain the sheltering-in-place process and address other public concerns regarding feelings of abandonment were not entirely effective. Two years later, there was persistent public perception of inadequate emergency response. Such perceptions can continue to erode necessary public confidence in the emergency response systems of the community. This is an important public relations issue.

Mitigation

Minot has, for a number of years, performed high-quality hazard analysis and risk assessment in regards to dangers associated with rail transportation of toxic materials.

Preparedness

A citywide exercise involving all emergency responders was conducted 4 months prior to the event. Details of the after-action report for that exercise are not readily accessible; hence specific identified weaknesses are not available for comment. It does appear that first responder equipment and training issues may have contributed to some limitations of movement and work activities for individuals within the ammonia cloud.

Response

Specific response details for the emergency medical system, fire department, and hospital are not readily available. However, the NTSB report provides some insight into the disaster response activities of the prehospital and medical system. Although a more complete first response/medical review would be highly desirable, the NTSB report stands as an example of an available document that allows some degree of retrospective analysis of the event.

Recovery

The city review of the event reportedly identified several problems with communications. These seem to have been addressed; however, important issues of public confidence in Minot's emergency response system apparently remain.

METHYL ISOCYANATE RELEASE IN 1984 IN BHOPAL, INDIA

On the night of December 2, 1984, an approximately 24 metric ton (27 short tons) leak of methyl isocyanate (MIC) occurred at a Union Carbide of India industrial plant in Bhopal (population 900,000). Atmospheric conditions included a relatively low wind speed and a nocturnal temperature inversion. These conditions resulted in a gas cloud that moved slowly, primarily close to the ground, ultimately covering approximately 40 km^2 of the surrounding city. The cloud rapidly engulfed the homes of a large number of primarily poor and uneducated residents. The cloud may have contained additional contaminants and decomposition byproducts such as phosgene, mono methylamine, hydrogen cyanide, various oxides of nitrogen, and carbon monoxide, although specific data are unavailable. An estimated 500,000 people were exposed and approximately 3,000–15,000 deaths occurred. Accurate statistics are unavailable for a variety of reasons, but a 2–3% death rate seems consistent with available information.

Most immediate and near-term MIC deaths appear to have occurred due to respiratory effects of the chemical. MIC produces airway inflammatory changes, contributing to airway obstruction. MIC also appears to produce a delayed pulmonary edema, much like phosgene. This effect may have contributed to the impression that phosgene was also released during the event. Additional concern was expressed about the possibility of cyanide or various decomposition products of MIC acting as contributing factors. There was no direct evidence to support that concern.

On the evening of the event, an estimated 400,000 people fled the city in an uncontrolled evacuation. Nearly half of those who lived more than 10 km away from the event site left, reacting out of fear. Approximately 2 weeks later, during attempts to neutralize the remaining MIC at the Union Carbide plant, public fear resulted in a second wave of mass evacuation involving approximately 200,000 people. The local medical system, which consisted of approximately 300 doctors and 1,800 hospital beds, was entirely overwhelmed. An estimated additional 1,500 people are reported to have died in subsequent months due to injuries caused by the release.[36]

Insofar as possible, near-term medical care was provided by local facilities that were later assisted by Indian government aid. Additional support was provided by a number of non-governmental organizations. Long-term evaluation of medical and health consequences of exposure have been conducted by a variety of individuals and organizations, both private and public. Their data suggest multiple possible long-term MIC effects that will require further investigation, although such data are somewhat compromised by both ongoing legal/political difficulties and substantial challenges associated with establishing and following a cohort of exposed individuals.

General Commentary

The Bhopal event occurred in a country with limited and poorly developed resources. The sudden release of a large toxic vapor cloud, whether accidental or (as suggested by Union Carbide) intentional, resulted in the world's single most catastrophic chemical event at the time of this publication. A more careful analysis of the event from a perspective of disaster preparedness is warranted.

Mitigation

The city of Bhopal had a population of 900,000 people at the time of the release. Nearly 200,000 lived within 10 km of the Union Carbide plant. The majority of these individuals were poor, living in housing that often consisted of no more than tin shacks. Recognizing the risks associated with living close to a chemical plant, the provincial government attempted to encourage residents to move away. It appeared, however, that individuals actually preferred to live close to a business that might offer many new, well-paying jobs to the local residents. The local government maintained few records of the identities or even the numbers of these individuals. There was no record maintained of any individuals with special needs. No governmental or local political organization existed that collectively represented these individuals. The few city organizations responsible for the health or safety of the local population received no effective citizen input. In the absence of a specific citizen action group, there was no organization able to collect information regarding the potential risks of a disaster in the neighborhood of the chemical plant. Thus, no hazard assessment or vulnerability analysis was performed. The nearby first responder community (fire and police) had little awareness or understanding of the possibility of a large toxic leak. Accordingly, there was little education, training, or equipment acquired for that possibility. The local medical facilities and personnel were equally limited in their awareness or understanding of the possibility of a large toxic leak.

Preparedness

The nearby residents were unaware of the risks posed to their community by industrial facilities in the area (specifically the Union Carbide plant). In the absence of an organization like the Local Emergency Planning Committees found in the United States, there was no clear effort directed toward preparing for an industrial chemical event. No evidence exists that local hospitals had become aware of the dangers or risks of the industrial plants in their immediate area or had made efforts to understand and prepare for those risks. Union Carbide had established a small clinic at the entrance to the facility. A physician was hired 8 months prior to the event to act as an occupational physician for the facility. Evidence is lacking that the physician either initially had or subsequently acquired particular expertise with respect to MIC. Furthermore, there is no evidence that the company physician was active in preparing either the local medical or civilian community for possible chemical exposures.

Response

Immediately after the incident, notification of the surrounding population was ineffective. There had been no community education or training identifying appropriate responses to the alarm sirens. Accordingly, the neighboring residents did not react to the emergency alarm. Arrival of irritating fumes drove many individuals to escape on foot. Running resulted in the need for deeper respirations – likely causing inhalation of greater amounts of MIC with each labored breath. Some individuals, unable or unwilling to run away, effectively sheltered-in-place and survived the toxic event. Emergency communications between the Union Carbide Plant, local government, first responders, and local medical facilities and personnel were poor or nonexistent. Confusion with respect to what particular substance was released appeared to play a major role in complicating both medical and logistical response to the event. There was much criticism regarding the lack of "correct" medical information, training, and appropriate equipment. Although no specific antidote existed, such criticism reflects the deeper problem of failure to educate and train the population. While MIC is now recognized as an irritating substance with pulmonary edema effects similar to phosgene, this information was not available to the local medical community at the time. Accordingly, lifesaving efforts were directed toward immediate symptomatic therapy – principally the control of obvious respiratory failure. Most near-term deaths clearly resulted from respiratory failure. The actual number of deaths can only be estimated. With the data available, it is not possible to determine the relative importance of the following factors in relationship to those deaths:

1. Inadequate/insufficient medical equipment – there is no evidence that specific preparations had been made for large numbers of individuals with respiratory compromise. Even had hundreds of ventilators been available, appropriately trained personnel to manage them were lacking.
2. Inadequate medical knowledge/experience – basic education and training of local medical personnel did not occur. Plant operator could have easily provided details of the risks/toxic effects of MIC and other large-quantity chemicals stored at the Union Carbide facility. This should have been the responsibility of the occupational physician at the facility. As noted, however, the number of victims with respiratory failure would have exceeded even the best preparation with large numbers of ventilators, given the absence of personnel to manage them.
3. Inadequate numbers of medical practitioners – additional numbers of trained medical personnel were needed, but not immediately available. In some countries such as the United States, chemical facilities have trained groups of their on-site industrial workers in basic life support. In case of a chemical event, these on-site workers can act as immediately available first responders.

Recovery

Subsequent to the event, both the Bhopal government and various private organizations have maintained a roster of exposed individuals. Some of these victims have received compensation. Several private and university medical groups have undertaken cohort follow-up assessment of the victims. These group studies have revealed some very important medical observations regarding the long-term effects of MIC exposure; however, there appears to be no centralized repository for this accumulated medical information. There is little evidence that information gleaned from such cohort studies has been incorporated into routine medical practice in the local area.

Decontamination of the exposed area is a concern to local medical facilities. Plant operators have not completed site cleanup, and a variety of toxic materials remain in residual solid wastes. Local medical personnel and hospitals have received little if any information regarding the medical aspects of these materials.

The Bhopal event has prompted international discussion that may ultimately lead to an improved nationally coordinated medical recovery response in India. Similar to the practices of NTSB, the following thoughts are proposed. Shortly after the incident, as part of the recovery, a data collection team (best sponsored by the national government) should undertake responsibility for:

1. Victim demographics – immediate recording (names/identifiers) of deaths, injuries, and individuals residing in the area of exposure.
2. Clinical demographics – the capturing of any clinical information established for the individuals noted.
3. Establish epidemiological studies for near- and long-term follow-up of victims.
4. Establish specialty treatment centers for both medical and psychiatric aspects of near- and long-term victim illness.
5. Prepare a report evaluating the quality of pre-event mitigation and preparedness within the local (and perhaps provincial) medical community. The quality of the response should also be benchmarked to adherence by the medical system to previously established local emergency plans.

Medical Response to Large-Scale Chemical Events

In circumstances of large-scale chemical events, early knowledge of the specific materials involved is an ideal medical goal. This is, however, an illusory target. Specific antidotes are available for only two significant types of toxic chemical exposures: organophosphates and cyanide. Commercial/industrial formulations of cyanide and organophosphates typically present as dermal or ingestion exposures. There is a slower onset and progression of the clinical illness, often affording ample time to deliver appropriate antidotal therapy. Military/chemical warfare organophosphates and cyanide, when presenting as inhaled agents, act very rapidly, often within seconds to minutes. Consequently, antidotal therapy of both organophosphate and cyanide inhalational exposures must be delivered immediately on-site. This implies the necessity of establishing stockpiles of antidote as "far forward" or as close to the location of care as possible, in areas of actual or suspected risk.

The U.S. government recognized this requirement for deployment of antidote near the location of patient care when it augmented the SNS. The U.S. Centers for Disease Control and Prevention (CDC) maintains this cache of drugs and equipment, and now has modified it to include a "far forward" CHEMPACK component. CHEMPACKs are positioned pre-event at locations all over the United States within 1 hour of 90% of the U.S. population. CHEMPACK stocks contain nerve agent antidotes and cyanide antidotes, and CHEMPACK sites include hospitals, police stations, EMS headquarters, and even a few county jails. CDC pays for the maintenance of these stockpiles and the rotation of expired antidotes. First responders train to break open CHEMPACKs in case of a suspected chemical attack.

Aside from antidotal therapy, medical management of a large-scale chemical event is generally accomplished by symptomatic assessment. Many have recommended that responders should try to group casualties by syndrome characteristics into exposure from one of the four types of chemical agents discussed previously (syndromic assessment). An extensive medical literature has been produced on the subject of rapid assessment of injured individuals. A large number of medical responders has been educated and trained in a systematic approach to the rapid assessment and categorization of exposed individuals. The Simple Triage and Rapid Treatment (START) system allows very rapid identification of those victims needing immediate, lifesaving care. Assessment of three major bodily systems (airway/respiration, circulation, and neurological) can be quickly and consistently accomplished even by nonmedical personnel with minimal training. Cone and Koenig have proposed a modification of this triage system for use for mass casualties exposed to a chemical agent.[30] A pediatric format (JumpSTART) has been developed as well, however, none of these systems have been adequately validated (see Chapter 14).

As suggested by the examples herein, the majority of immediate and near-term chemical event–related illness results in respiratory compromise. Immediate and near-term toxic respiratory illness caused by a chemical event is very amenable to intervention with relatively simple and inexpensive technology. Thus rapid identification and intervention in these respiratory "immediates" is of the highest value.

The National Library of Medicine's CHEMM website (see Useful Websites section) was developed to provide just-in-time, government-validated information on possible chemical exposures that could be used in real-time by first responders, regardless of medical background. One feature intended to help with initial assessment is the Chemical Intelligent Syndromes Tool (CHEMM-IST) algorithm, which uses syndromic patterns to categorize the event into one of the four major exposures: pulmonary intoxicants, cyanides, organophosphate/cholinesterase inhibitor, and vesicant/mustard.

The federal response to events in the United States is dictated by the NRF. Many federal agencies play roles in dealing with a chemical event, ranging from the FBI (law enforcement) to the Coast Guard (National Spills Center) to the EPA (cleanup). Information on the NRF, including its founding documents, can be found on FEMA's website.[37]

RECOMMENDATIONS FOR FURTHER RESEARCH

General Comments

The funding for new research into large-scale chemical events is almost entirely derived from government agencies because there is very little industrial or pharmaceutical market for products that will emerge from such investigations. The two major funding streams in the United States are from the Department of Defense, through its Chemical and Biological Defense Program, and from HHS. These two programs regularly coordinate on multiple levels to ensure that the two departments will synergize and not duplicate efforts. Certain specific areas, such as pulmonary agents and cyanides, which are considered to represent a greater threat to civilians than the military, are of particular interest to HHS. At the time of this writing, the department's biggest investments are in improved countermeasures against cyanides, which are no longer seen as a major battlefield threat by the military.

Most of the original work on response to chemical agents was carried out by the military, and the treatment protocols that resulted are intended primarily for young, prescreened, healthy adults ages 18–65. Very little work has been done on any of the countermeasures discussed in this chapter in children, the elderly, pregnant women, or immunosuppressed patients. Every suggestion made here should be read as applying to these populations as well, perhaps with greater urgency than the original military population.

The original focus of most research done on chemical agents was only with the acute effects of poisoning. A more general emphasis is needed on the long-term effects. These include a wide spectrum of issues, many of which are still controversial. Examples include: pulmonary fibrosis seen after recovery from poisoning with oxides of nitrogen; delayed neovascularization and blindness seen in Iranian war veterans poisoned with sulfur mustard; possible carcinogenesis seen after sulfur mustard poisoning, particularly in the lung; and questions of chronic neurologic dysfunction alleged in survivors of nerve agent poisoning.

Animal models are a specific research issue. We have imperfect animal models for most of the agents listed. Not only are better animal models urgently needed for research, but they will be crucial in future years for obtaining licensure in the United States from the FDA for any developed countermeasures. None of the standard animal models used for work with sulfur mustard (pig skin, mouse ear) or nerve agents (rats, guinea pigs) exactly replicates the toxidrome seen in humans.

Research Priorities in Specific Categories of Chemical Agents

Pulmonary Agents

After over a century of research, we are still woefully ignorant of the molecular mechanisms of action associated with many pulmonary agents, particularly those that cause delayed peripheral non-cardiogenic pulmonary edema. Phosgene is emblematic of these agents. Presumably, mechanisms of damage are similar across a large number of pulmonary toxicants, including many toxic industrial chemicals. Mixed peripheral-centrally acting pulmonary toxicants, such as chlorine, may pose different problems on the molecular level.

In poisoning by toxicants causing delayed-onset non-cardiogenic pulmonary edema, such as phosgene, we have no reliable way to identify those among the exposed population who are at high risk for the development of pulmonary edema. Since this condition will require intensive care, it should be a priority to develop a diagnostic test, perhaps a biomarker, that can predict which patients are likely to develop edema. Some work has been done with plethysmography; however, this has not proven sufficiently reliable. Development of a predictive marker would have great impact not only on the management of specific patients, but of mass casualty events generally.

Once pulmonary edema develops, management presently consists of intensive care with intubation and pulmonary support. ICU care for pulmonary edema is primarily designed for cardiogenic cases, including dieresis and strict fluid management. Pulmonary edema caused by peripherally acting pulmonary toxicants, by contrast, involves massive fluid displacement from the circulation into the lungs, and these patients are actually fluid-depleted. We need better protocols to manage this unusual form of pulmonary edema.

Cyanides

Administration of all currently available cyanide antidotes require intravenous line placement. This is time-consuming, very difficult in children, and ill-suited to rapid treatment of large numbers of casualties. We urgently need a non-intravenous antidote, ideally administrable through an IM auto-injector similar to nerve agent antidotes. HHS is funding work on three promising candidates: cobinamide, sulfanegen, and dimethyl trisulfide. An IM cyanide antidote could make a huge difference in a mass casualty event involving cyanide.

Study of individual cyanide poisoning cases demonstrates that many patients recover without the use of antidotes at all.[9] Available antidotes have significant side effects, notably hypotension from nitrites. In an individual case this may not matter, but in a mass casualty event from cyanide poisoning, a method to identify that minority of cases who absolutely require antidotes would improve scene management and triage.

Mustard and Other Vesicants

As with pulmonary toxicants, the cellular and molecular mode of action for sulfur mustard remains elusive after 110 years of research. Much experimental work in animals has demonstrated that sulfur mustard works via multiple pathways, including inflammation and bone marrow suppression. We still need better understanding of the critical pathways in the development of mustard injury, both acute and chronic.

It would greatly assist both those caring for individual patients and those responsible for scene management and triage if there was a method to identify individuals exposed to sulfur mustard who will subsequently develop severe injury. Such injuries include pulmonary and upper airway compromise as well as the development of systemic problems such as bone marrow suppression. At present, the only rough guide available is the percentage of body surface area exposed to liquid; this is not helpful in the case of a vapor challenge and is only very approximate for those exposed to liquid. Biomarkers for exposed victims who will require higher levels of care would be extremely helpful in management.

Mustard-induced neutropenia has not been well-studied in the military research program. However, one investigation demonstrated that granulocyte colony stimulating factor (originally developed as a method to protect the bone marrow from cancer chemotherapy) can lessen the impact of sulfur mustard on hematopoietic cells.[14] Data are needed that would support a more robust recommendation for ideal management of patients exposed to unknown levels of sulfur mustard, particularly those who may already be immunosuppressed.

Nerve Agents

Midazolam is more rapidly effective against nerve agent–induced seizures than any other benzodiazepine, including diazepam. It also prevents seizures from recurring with greater efficacy than any other drug in this class. At the time of this writing, the military chemical defense program is pursuing FDA approval of midazolam for the indication of nerve agent–induced seizures in adults, while the civilian program is pursuing broader indications. This will probably result in significant near-term improvement in nerve agent poisoning management.

For many years, the military chemical defense program has pursued a bioscavenger. This circulating compound would detoxify a nerve agent before it travels through the bloodstream, interacts with cholinergic synapses, and causes the toxic effects that threaten the patient's life. In theory, warfighters protected by a circulating bioscavenger could be deployed unencumbered by protective equipment. Human butyrylcholinesterase can function as a circulating bioscavenger in animals and is safe in humans. However, it is only effective stoichiometrically (i.e., one molecule of butyrylcholinesterase detoxifies one molecule of nerve agent). Consequently, the effective dose is quite large, and because butyrylcholinesterase has to be isolated from human plasma, the expense of this product will be in excess of $10,000 per dose. Efforts are underway to identify a catalytic bioscavenger that would detoxify the nerve agent but require only a fraction of the dose of a stoichiometric bioscavenger. Unfortunately, animal experiments to date demonstrate that the only way to achieve this outcome is probably to develop a cocktail of scavengers, some of which detoxify only the G-series nerve agents and others that detoxify only the V-series.

A better oxime is needed that effectively targets rapidly aging nerve agents such as soman. The military chemical defense program is working on several possible replacements for 2-PAM Cl that will have greater efficacy against such nerve agents.

The U.S. military program is also investigating scopolamine, a well-known anticholinergic drug, as an addition to the present nerve agent treatment regimen. Unlike atropine, it crosses the blood-brain barrier and treats CNS nerve agent poisoning. Its ultimate role in the management of nerve agent victims is not yet clear and much developmental work remains.

Defining the long-term negative clinical effects from nerve agent exposure is crucial, particularly those impacting neurobehavioral functions. We do not yet have a clear understanding of how many of the alleged chronic effects seen after nerve agent poisoning are due to actual chemical toxicity and how much is potentially due to psychological trauma (PTSD), to hypoxia, or to the postictal state.[38,39] Improved understanding of this pathophysiology has been hampered by failure to develop good animal models.

Efforts have been underway for several years to develop a neuro-protectant for the central nervous system. This product would insure improved neurologic function after nerve agent exposure. Several compounds are being studied in both the military and civilian programs, including the centrally acting cholinesterase galantamine and several experimental drugs. One hurdle for this program is reliably defining animal behavioral abnormalities to facilitate research.

Incapacitating Agents

It remains unclear how much research should be devoted to incapacitating agents. No investigations are presently underway in any western country examining anticholinergics such as Agent BZ, which is no longer stockpiled by any government. Efforts are underway to better understand the toxicity of many different fentanyl derivatives.

Research Priorities in Response to Chemical Attacks

Perhaps the most urgent need in response research is validation and optimization of best practices for mass casualty decontamination. Decontamination doctrine is a mixture of old principles inherited from World War I practice and animal studies. A large workshop held in 2012 by the U.S. Department of Homeland Security demonstrated that we still lack a clear understanding of how effective various methods of decontamination are at reducing hazards, both to patients and to caregivers. At the time of this writing, HHS has funded its first grant in this area. Evidence-based guidelines are needed specifically for the civilian setting that optimize the process of decontamination. These guidelines should take into account such issues as age diversity, current medical conditions, and the challenge of disrobing during an incident. Military doctrine does not deal with these issues.[40,41]

In a chemical incident, the speed of response is much more crucial than it is for biological incident. However, the response system, particularly on the federal level, is really designed for the slower pace of a biological event. Exercises utilizing both moulaged victims and tabletop instruction at local, state, and federal levels are important in developing a response system robust and flexible enough to address a rapidly evolving chemical incident.

Part of the response to a chemical incident is the development of a tiered system of medical care. For victims exposed to pulmonary and vesicant agents, the highest priority for care will be evacuation to a location where ICU-type interventions are available. Immediate on-scene treatment is less critical. This is fundamentally different from the usual approach to triage in mass casualty events. Practicing triage strategies that incorporate evacuation is an essential part of exercises held at all levels, with modifications for each locality's specific needs.

Another aspect of the local response is the proper use of media to disseminate important messages. This could include broadcasts requesting that exposed but asymptomatic individuals shower at home and then present for evaluation at an out-of-hospital treatment center. Without advanced planning and exercises, local, state, and federal authorities will not have established relationships with media outlets that could be extremely helpful in alerting the public. Media relations should be part of plans and should be exercised and practiced along with other aspects of the response.

Even the possibility that one has been exposed to a toxic chemical can be a severely stressful experience. No consensus exists on the best way to manage acute or subacute/chronic psychological stress among those who either were exposed or who think they were exposed to an agent. The scale of this problem is huge. In the 1995 Tokyo attack, 80% of patients presenting for care had no signs or symptoms of poisoning. Research on the most expeditious way to deal with the fears of large numbers of people would be very helpful to planners and responders.

At present, the disaster medicine community lacks a robust, standardized medical review process. CDC carries out epidemiologic studies, but has never formalized a full-scale process of review. This assessment should include not only traditional epidemiology, but review of first responder and hospital professional actions as well. One model for this in the United States is the Chemical Security Emergency Preparedness Program (CSEPP), which took a comprehensive review of care in the communities where the Army's eight former chemical stockpile sites were located. CSEPP still operates at the two sites where demilitarization has not yet concluded. This could serve as a national model.

Useful Websites

In the United States, the National Library of Medicine, part of the National Institutes of Health (NIH), has created a Chemical Hazards Emergency Medical Management website, open to anyone without pre-registration. It is specifically intended for the civilian first responder. It includes a quick syndromic differential diagnosis, CHEMM-IST, to aid the civilian first responder in categorizing a chemical mass casualty event by toxidrome. The tool is intended to facilitate rapid field diagnosis. It is updated by NIH and other government experts on an ongoing basis.

For more detailed information on specific agents, the reader is directed to the Medical Aspects of Chemical Warfare portion of the *Textbook of Military Medicine*, published by the Borden Institute and Walter Reed Army Medical Center.[42] This volume, as well as the shorter treatment handbook published by the Chemical Casualty Care Division of the U.S. Army Medical Research Institute of Chemical Defense, is available on the division's website.[43] Non-military organizations must register for the website in advance, a process that usually takes 2–3 business days. Emergency personnel who may need to care for chemical casualties should therefore register their organizations during the planning phase so that they can access current data during an event.

Acknowledgments

This chapter incorporates material written for a previous edition of this textbook by John S. Urbanetti, MD. The opinions herein expressed are solely those of the author and not necessarily those of the Joint Program Executive Office for Chemical/Biological Defense, the Department of the Army, or the Department of Defense.

REFERENCES

1. Patel SS. Earliest Chemical Warfare – Dura-Europos, Syria. *Archaeology Magazine* 2010; 63(1).

2. Hilmas CJ, Smart JK, Hill BA. History of chemical warfare. In: Tuorinsky SD, ed. *Textbook of Military Medicine: Medical Aspects of Chemical Warfare.* Washington, DC, Office of the Surgeon General and Borden Institute, Walter Reed Army Medical Center, 2008.

3. Robinson JPP. Chemical Weapons and International Cooperation (Revision 1) in Public Discussion Meeting. *Elimination of Weapons of Mass Destruction.* British PugwashGroup. September 8, 2004. British Association 2004 Festival of Science, University of Exeter, UK, 2005; 1–9.

4. Chemical Casualty Care Division. *Medical Management of Chemical Casualties Handbook* 4th ed. Aberdeen Proving Ground, MD, U.S. Army Medical Research Institute of Chemical Defense, 2007.

5. Grainge C, Rice P. Management of phosgene-induced acute lung injury. *Clin Toxicol* (Phila) 2010; 48(6): 497–508.

6. Sciuto AM, Hurt HH. Therapeutic treatments of phosgene-induced lung injury. *Inhal Toxicol* 2004; 16(8): 565–580.

7. Parkhouse DA, Brown RF, Jugg BJ, et al. Protective ventilation strategies in the management of phosgene-induced acute lung injury. *Mil Med* 2007; 172(3): 295–300.

8. deLange DW, Meulenbelt J. Do corticosteroids have a role in preventing or reducing acute toxic lung injury caused by inhalation of chemical agents? *Clin Toxicol* (Phila) 2011; 49(2): 61–71.

9. Wurzburg H. Treatment of cyanide poisoning in an industrial setting. *Vet Hum Toxicol* 1996; 38(1): 44–47.

10. Thompson JP, Marrs TC. Hydroxocobalamin in cyanide poisoning. *Clin Toxicol* (Phila) 2012; 50(10): 875–885.

11. Bebarta VS, Tanen DA, Lairet J, Dixon PS, Valtier S, Bush A. Hydroxocobalamin and sodium thiosulfate versus sodium nitrite and sodium thiosulfate in the treatment of acute cyanide toxicity in a swine (Sus scrofa) model. *Ann Emerg Med* 2010; 55(4): 345–351.

12. Hurst CG, Patrali JP, Barillo DJ, Graham JS, Smith WJ, Urbanetti JS, Sidell FR. Vesicants. In: Tuorinsky SD, ed. *Textbook of Military Medicine: Medical Aspects of Chemical Warfare.* Washington, DC, Office of the Surgeon General and Borden Institute, Walter Reed Army Medical Center, 2008.

13. Ghasemi H, Ghazanfari T, Ghassemi-Broumand M, et al. Long-term ocular consequences of sulfur mustard in seriously eye-injured war veterans. *Cutan Ocul Toxicol* 2009; 28(2): 71–77.

14. Anderson DR, Holmes WW, Lee RB, et al. Sulfur mustard-induced neutropenia: treatment with granulocyte colony-stimulating factor. *Mil Med* 2006; 171(5): 448–453.

15. Mansour RS, Salamati P, Saghafinia M, Abdollahi M. A review on delayed toxic effect of sulfur mustard in Iranian veterans. *Daru* October 2012; 20(1): 51. Entire article available in English translation at www.pubmed.com (Accessed May 1, 2013).

16. Newmark J. Nerve agents. In: Dobbs MR. *Clinical Neurotoxicology: syndromes, substances, environments.* Philadelphia, PA, Saunders-Elsevier, 2009; 646–659.

17. Newmark J. The birth of nerve agent warfare: lessons from Syed Abbas Foroutan. *Neurology* 2004; 62: 1590–1596.

18. Rotenberg J, Newmark J. Nerve agents in children: diagnosis and management. *Pediatrics* 2003; 112(3): 648–658.

19. Silbergleit R, Durkalski V, Lowenstein D, Conwit R, Pancioli A, Palesch Y, Barsan W, NETT Investigators. Intramuscular versus intravenous therapy for prehospital status epilepticus. *N Engl J Med* 2012; 366(7): 591–600.

20. Stern JE. The covenant, the sword, and the arm of the Lord. In: Tucker J, ed. *Toxic Terror: Assessing Terrorist Use of Chemical and Biologic Weapons.* Cambridge, MA, MIT Press, 2000; 139–157.

21. Yanagisawa N, Morita H, Nakajima T. Sarin experiences in Japan: acute toxicity and long-term effects. *J Neurol Sci* 2006; 249: 76–85.

22. Morita H, Yanagisawa N, Nakajima T, Shimizu M. Sarin poisoning in Matsumoto, Japan. *Lancet* 1995; 346: 290–294.

23. Murakami H. *Underground.* New York, Random House, 2001; 11 and elsewhere.

24. Ohbu S, Yamashina A, Takasu N, et al. Sarin poisoning on Tokyo subway. *South Med J* 1997; 90: 587–593.

25. Kaplan DE. Aum Shinrikyo. In: Tucker J, ed. *Toxic Terror: Assessing Terrorist Use of Chemical and Biologic Weapons.* Cambridge, MA, MIT Press, 2000; 207–226.

26. Monterey WMD Terrorism Database. http://cns.miis.edu/wmdt (Restricted access November 18, 2008).

27. Cannard K. The acute treatment of nerve agent exposure. *J Neurol Sci* 2006; 249: 86–94.

28. Loh Y, Swanberg MM, Ingram MV, Newmark J. Case report: long-term cognitive sequelae of sarin exposure. *Neurotoxicology* 2010; 31(2): 244–246.

29. Sarin, Mustard Gas Discovered Separately in Iraq, Monday, May 17, 2004. http://www.foxnews.com (Accessed November 18, 2008).

30. Wesley R. Chlorine attack reflects ongoing militant strategy in Iraq. The Jamestown Foundation. *Terrorism Focus* 2007; 4:3.

31. California Governor's Office of Emergency Services. Golden Guardian Exercise November 15, 2005. http://www.oes.ca.gov/Operational/OESHome.nsf (Accessed November 18, 2008).

32. Mattson J. Derailment disaster. *Minot Daily News.* http://www.minotdailynews.com (Accessed November 18, 2008).

33. Wagner SP. Lost in the cloud: ammonia spill leaves Minot in blind panic. *The Forum.* August 18, 2002.

34. Selected Stories 1/18/02–3/21/02. *Minot Daily News.* http://www.minotdailynews.com (Accessed November 18, 2008).

35. National Transportation Safety Board. Derailment of Canadian Pacific Railway Freight Train 292–16 and Subsequent Release of Anhydrous Ammonia Near Minot, North Dakota. January 18, 2002. Railroad Accident Report NTSB/RAR-04/01. 2004

36. Mitchell JK, ed. Long-term recovery from the Bhopal crisis. In: *The Long Road to Recovery: Community Responses to Industrial Disaster.* New York, United Nations University Press, 1996.

37. http://www.fema.gov/pdf/emergency/nrf/nrf-core.pdf (Accessed May 1, 2013).

38. Miyaki K, Nishiwaki Y, Maekawa K, et al. Effects of sarin on the nervous system of subway workers seven years after the Tokyo subway sarin attack. *J Occup Health* 2005; 47(4): 299–304.

39. Yamasue H, Abe O, Kasai K, et al. Human brain structural change related to acute single exposure to sarin. *Ann Neurol* 2007; 61(1): 37–46.

40. Clarke SF, Chilcott RP, Wilson JC, Kamanvire R, Baker DJ, Hallett A. Decontamination of multiple casualties who are chemically contaminated: a challenge for acute hospitals. *Prehosp Disaster Med* 2008; 23(2): 175–181.

41. Domres BD, Rashid A, Grundgeiger J, Gromer S, Kees T, Hecker N, Peter H. European survey on decontamination in mass casualty incidents. *Am J Disaster Med* 2009; 4(3): 147–152.

42. Tuorinsky SR, ed. Medical Aspects of Chemical Warfare. In: *Textbook of Military Medicine* series. Washington, DC, Office of the Surgeon General and Borden Institute, Walter Reed Army Medical Center, 2008.

43. http://ccc.apgea.army.mil (Accessed May 2, 2013).

32

BIOLOGICAL EVENTS

Zygmunt F. Dembek and Theodore J. Cieslak

The opinions and assertions contained herein are the private views of the authors and are not to be construed as official or as necessarily reflecting the views of the U.S. Department of Defense (DOD), Department of Health and Human Services (HHS), or any of their component institutions, including the Uniformed Services University of the Health Sciences and all others.

OVERVIEW

A Brief History of Biological Warfare

Ancient cultures used biological weapons through an empirical understanding of cause and effect of infection. The Hittites drove infected animals and a syphilitic woman into their enemy's camps with the intent of disease initiation. Deliberate poisoning of wells and water supplies with toxic plants occurred in sixth-century Greece. Kautilya's *Arthashastra*, a fourth-century text written in India, describes recipes for transmitting infectious disease to an enemy.

In 1346, Tatar invaders under the command of de Mussis laid siege to the city of Kaffa (now Feodosiya, Ukraine). When an outbreak of bubonic plague afflicted the Tatar invaders, they then catapulted the bodies of their own victims over the city walls in an attempt to intentionally spread plague within the city. The plan appeared to succeed. Genoese and Venetian merchants stranded within the city contracted plague, fled the city, sailed home, and took the disease with them, thus firmly establishing the "Black Death" in continental Europe.[1] Current understanding suggests that catapults fail to explain the extension of plague into Kaffa; bubonic plague is now known to be transmitted by fleas, which rapidly abandon the cooling cadaver, making it unlikely that corpses would remain infectious.

The American experience with biological warfare dates back at least as far as 1763. During the French and Indian Wars, the British Colonial Commander, Sir Jeffrey Amherst, recommended the use of smallpox to "reduce" Native American tribes hostile to the British. A subordinate of Amherst, Captain Simeon Ecuyer, gave blankets and a handkerchief from a smallpox hospital to the Native Americans, and recorded in his journal "I hope it will have the desired effect."[2]

In the nineteenth century, the advent of modern microbiology, germ theory, and Koch's postulates opened the way for a stockpiling of infectious pathogens and more robust efforts at state-sponsored biological weapons programs. Imperial Germany, during World War I, experimented with the causative agents of anthrax (*Bacillus anthracis*) and glanders (*Burkhoderia mallei*), intending them as anti-animal weapons directed at adversaries' livestock food sources and beasts of burden.[3] At a private home in Chevy Chase, Maryland, Dr. Anton Dilger, a German-American physician, established a secret biological warfare laboratory. Considerable amounts of *B. anthracis* and *B. mallei* were grown from seed cultures brought by Dilger to the United States from Germany. Dilger and his associates spread his cultures among horses being shipped to England from the ports of Baltimore, Norfolk, Newport News, and New York City. They also poured anthrax cultures into the animals' food and water.[3] Some have asserted that Germany continued biological warfare research between the world wars, and released the microbiological warfare stimulant *Serratia marcescens* in the London Tube and Paris Metro in order to study its flow in such settings.[4] From 1932–1945, Japan employed many different biological agents (including *B. anthracis*, *Vibrio cholera*, and *Yersinia pestis*) to conduct extensive macabre human biological warfare experiments on civilians and prisoners of war in occupied Manchuria in a covert biological and chemical warfare research and development facility known as Unit 731.[4] Additionally, field trials and attacks on at least eleven Chinese cities with biological agents, including attacks on water supplies and the release of fleas infected with *Y. pestis*, were conducted in an effort to initiate plague outbreaks. Largely in response to this history, and a perceived threat of biological warfare from Axis powers, the United States established its own biological warfare research center at Camp Detrick in Maryland in 1943. In 1953, a defensive medical countermeasures program (which continues today) was added to Camp Detrick's previously offensive-oriented efforts.

The United States examined *Y. pestis* as a potential biological warfare agent in the 1950s and 1960s before the offensive biowarfare program was terminated; other countries are suspected of weaponizing this organism as well. The former Soviet Union had more than ten institutes and thousands of scientists who worked with *Y. pestis*. During World War II, Unit 731, a battalion of the Japanese Army, reportedly released *Y. pestis*-infected fleas from aircraft over Chinese cities, but this method of dissemination proved cumbersome and unpredictable. The United States and Soviet Union developed the more reliable and effective method of aerosolizing the organism.[5] Interest in the terrorist potential of plague was brought to light in 1995 when Larry Wayne Harris was arrested in Ohio for the illicit procurement of a *Y. pestis* culture through the mail.[6]

In 1925, in response to the horrors produced by chemical weapons in the trenches during World War I, the Geneva Gas Protocol was promulgated. It prohibited, among other things, the "practice of bacteriological warfare."[7] Some have noted that this protocol did not include toxin warfare, nor did it prohibit production and storage of biological agents. A lack of the latter provision is understandable, given the growth in bacteriological research during that era following the initial discoveries of Koch and Pasteur. Furthermore, the ability for a state to conduct "bacteriological warfare" was poorly understood at the time. The work of Anton Dilger and others was largely unknown until almost twenty years later. The lack of a prohibition against toxin weapons is more troubling. Although the mechanism of action for toxins was incompletely understood at the time, according to a 1918 research report, bullet shrapnel could be made toxic through an application of ricin. In 1969, however, President Nixon, speaking for the nation, unilaterally renounced the use of biological weapons. Moreover, he ordered that the U.S. offensive program be halted and existing weapons stockpiles be destroyed. This destruction occurred during the period from 1969–1972, and culminated in the signing of the Biological Weapons Convention (BWC) by the Soviet Union, the United Kingdom, and the United States. This treaty has since been ratified by over 140 nations, and prohibits the possession, stockpiling, and use of biological weapons. The United States ratified both the Geneva Gas Protocol and the BWC in 1975.

Developing a Threat List

Biological warfare, according to language used during crafting of the BWC, is the "use, for hostile purposes, of living organisms, whatever their nature, or infective material derived from them, which are intended to cause disease or death in man, animals, or plants."[8] Little about the topics of biowarfare and bioterrorism is as straightforward as this definition might make it appear. In fact, the wording of the BWC has complicated attempts to develop a universally accepted list of biological agents of concern. For example, the Soviet Union accused the U.S. government of violating the terms of the BWC by employing defoliant agents

Table 32.1. Components of the Former U.S. Biological Arsenal

Lethal Agents	Incapacitating Agents	Anti-Crop Weapons
Bacillus anthracis	Venezuelan Equine Encephalitis	Wheat-Stem Rust
Botulinum Toxin	Staphylococcal Enterotoxin B	Rye-Stem Rust
Francisella tularensis	*Brucella suis*	Rice-Blast Spore
	Coxiella burnetii	

Table 32.2. Russian Rating System of Bioagent Distribution According to Probability of Use as a Bioweapon[10]

Smallpox Virus

Yersinia pestis

Bacillus anthracis

Botulinum Toxin

Venezuelan Equine Encephalitis Virus

Francisella tularensis

Coxiella burnetii

Marburg Virus

Influenza Virus

Burkholderia mallei

Rickettsia typhi

such as "Agent Orange" during the Vietnam War. The U.S. government, for its part, considered this to be a non-prohibited use of a chemical agent. Similarly, during the 1970s and 1980s, the United States accused the Soviets of waging biological warfare by employing trichothecene mycotoxins ("Yellow Rain"), a charge the Soviets denied. Moreover, they apparently considered toxins to be chemical, rather than biological, weapons. As science advances, consideration of novel substances such as biomodulators (e.g., kinins, leukotrienes, substance P, δ-sleep inducing peptide) as potential agents of warfare will likely heighten various semantic controversies.

In order to gain insight into prospective biological weapons candidates, a review of agents contained within the U.S. arsenal during the 1943–1969 period of offensive weapons research and development is useful. Ten agents were weaponized in the 1950s and 1960s (Table 32.1). These can be divided into antipersonnel (7) and anti-crop agents (3); the antipersonnel agents can be further subdivided into lethal agents and incapacitants.[9] A second opinion is found in Russian sources.[10] A list, in some order of priority, of agents considered for weaponization by Russian (and presumably, Soviet) scientists is provided in Table 32.2.

Biological Warfare versus Bioterrorism

Although the biological weapon caches of the Cold War superpowers provide an interesting starting point, it is useful to examine the biological threat in other ways. Strategically speaking, biological agents might be used to strike fear into a nation's inhabitants and to diminish the resolve of the citizenry. As such, strategic biological weapons, in this context at least, need only be effective enough to create such fear. Perception of a weapon's abilities might thus be more important than its actual ability to cause disease. Strategic weapons might also be used against domestic targets important to the conduct of a foreign war, such as command and control locations, staging bases, and ports of embarkation. Thus, even biological agents capable of infecting a few key personnel (and not causing widespread death) might be strategically beneficial to an enemy.

Conversely, the ability of an infection to spread from person-to-person might be a useful property in a strategic weapon, permitting its propagation among a population. Such contagion, however, might limit a commander's enthusiasm for employing the same weapon on the battlefield, where friendly forces might contact it inadvertently. This property of contagion likely explains the inclusion of smallpox, plague, and Marburg virus in the Soviet arsenal (the Soviets favored strategic use of biological agents)[11] and, perhaps, their exclusion from the U.S. arsenal (as the United States saw these primarily as operational agents).

A number of biological agents might be adapted for operational use. That is, they possess characteristics (such as atmospheric stability) that could enable their use over large geographical areas. The list of such agents is short, enabling public health authorities to concentrate countermeasure efforts on a finite number of threats. Anthrax, plague, tularemia, and perhaps a few other agents might pose viable operational threats. In one regard, the threat posed by tactical employment of biological agents is more problematic than the operational threat, in that certain viruses and toxins, which lack the stability necessary for effective operational employment, might nonetheless be used effectively against smaller, more concentrated targets (such as individual buildings or smaller areas of terrain). Conversely, some strategists would argue that biological agents are a poor choice for such tactical employment. This contention stems from a unique characteristic not typically shared by conventional, chemical, and nuclear weapons, namely, the incubation periods normally inherent with infectious agents. These incubation periods might vary from hours in the case of staphylococcal enterotoxin B (SEB) to weeks with diseases such as brucellosis or Q-fever, but are more typically several days in duration. Commanders tasked with tactical objectives (such as seizing an important terrain feature) would likely reject the idea of pausing for several days while waiting for biological agents to slowly produce their effects. Even if one could conceive of a tactical use for biological weapons, the list of viable candidates is short, with only a small handful of agents possessing the desirable characteristics.

In addressing the terrorist threat, public perception is of paramount importance, and any attack capable of generating headlines (and publicity for an extremist group) might be considered "viable." Moreover, the delay induced by the incubation periods of biological agents would not dissuade the terrorist from their use. The list of potential agents of terrorism thus becomes quite lengthy. Designing effective countermeasures and defensive strategies against such a large inventory of possible threats accordingly becomes a daunting task. Agents and diseases such as HIV, *E. coli*, "mad cow," rabies, and Ebola, which might otherwise lack characteristics desirable in a biological weapon, possess the "brand-name" recognition sought by certain terrorists. Similarly, terrorists might select "weapons of opportunity," that is, weapons that might be widely available or readily procured by a member of the group. This then creates an extensive selection of potential agents. The intentional contamination of restaurant salad bars in The Dalles, Oregon, with *Salmonellae* in 1984 highlights this problem,[12] as does the 1996 use of *Shigella*-laden pastries in a notable biocrime.[13] Although not considered credible military threats by most planners, these two common gastrointestinal pathogens were, nonetheless, effective in the hands of criminals. Presumably, dozens of similar organisms and many toxins might be employed in an analogous manner. Therefore, many intelligence and law enforcement professionals contend that the magnitude of the terrorist threat surpasses, in some ways, that of the military threat. Moreover, this threat remains nebulous and difficult to monitor. Finally, while response to the military use of such weapons might occupy defense planners, it is the civilian medical and public health community that must shoulder the responsibility of reacting to a terrorist release. Consequently, the remainder of this chapter focuses on this terrorist threat.

CURRENT STATE OF THE ART

The Terrorist Threat

Examples of terrorist uses of conventional weapons abound. Beirut, Oklahoma City, the Khobar Towers, the first World Trade Center attacks, the bombing of American embassies in Nairobi and Dar es Salaam, the Mumbai bombings, the Boston Marathon bombing, and the Paris bombings all highlight the conventional threat. The use of airplanes in the second attack on the World Trade Center and on the Pentagon on September 11, 2001, gives a new meaning to unconventional weaponry without requiring access to nuclear, chemical or biological arms. The release of sarin in the Tokyo subway system by members of the Aum Shinrikyo cult is a reminder that terrorists may have the ability to procure and deploy chemical weapons. By comparison, the intentional mailing of anthrax-laced letters[14] in October 2001 sickened twenty-two and resulted in a relatively modest (by comparison) death toll of five. Why, then, might biological weapons interest terrorist factions? Multiple characteristics make biological weapons potentially attractive to such groups.

First, biological weapons are relatively easy to procure. For example, *Clostridium botulinum* is ubiquitous in soil, and easily cultured by anyone with modest training in microbiology. *Bacillus anthracis* is similarly readily cultivatable from soil in many parts of the United States and the world. Ricin extraction from castor beans, readily available throughout the world, is easily accomplished using recipes widely published on the Internet. Multiple putative biological weapons, such as *Coxiella burnetii*, the encephalitic alphaviruses, the *Brucellae*, *Francisella tularensis*, *Yersinia pestis*, and *Bacillus anthracis* continue to cause endemic disease in many parts of the world. Clinical laboratories in those locales handle cultures of such organisms and constitute a potential source for their acquisition. Culture repositories organized for legitimate scientific purposes might be accessed by those with sinister motives. While the U.S. Centers for Disease Control and Prevention-managed Select Agent Program[15] seeks to limit access to particularly hazardous pathogens and toxins (regulated agents are listed in Table 32.3), hundreds of such repositories exist in dozens of foreign nations; many sell and ship these hazardous agents.[16] Devices able to disseminate biological agents are also widely available. Crop-dusting assemblies can be adapted by terrorists for sinister purposes and can, in some cases, generate aerosolized particles of 2–6 μm in diameter, the ideal size for impinging on the human lower respiratory tract.

Second, biological weapons are potentially inexpensive to produce. In 1969, a United Nations study considered the cost to a belligerent of producing mass (defined as 50%) casualties and found crude biological weapons to be far less costly than chemical, nuclear, or even conventional arms on a "casualties per square kilometer" basis.[17]

Third, unless terrorists announced the release of a biological agent, detection of a biological attack would be challenging. Aerosolized biological agents would likely be odorless, colorless, tasteless, and otherwise invisible (in contrast to chemical agents, which often have characteristic odors). Standoff detection

Table 32.3. HHS and U.S. Department of Agriculture (USDA) Select Agents and Toxins (7 CFR Part 331, 9 CFR Part 121, and 42 CFR Part 73)

HHS Select Agents and Toxins

Abrin

Cercopithecine herpesvirus 1 (Herpes B virus)

Coccidioides posadasii

Conctoxins

Crimean-Congo hemorrhagic fever virus

Diacetoxyscirpenol

Ebola virus

Lassa fever virus

Marburg virus

Monkeypox virus

Reconstructed replication competent forms of the 1918 pandemic influenza virus containing any portion of the coding regions of all eight gene segments (Reconstructed 1918 influenza virus)

Ricin

Rickettsia prowazekii

Rickettsia rickettsii

Saxitoxin

Siiga-like ribosome inactivating proteins

South American hemorrhagic fever viruses

Flexal

Guanarito

Junin

Machupo

Sabia

Tetrodotoxin

Tick-borne encephalitis complex (flavi) viruses

Central European tick-borne encephalitis

Far Eastern tick-borne encephalitis

Kyasanur Forest disease

Omsk hemorrhagic fever

Russian Spring and Summer encephalitis

Variola major virus (smallpox virus) and

Variola minor virus (Alastrim)

Yersinia pestis

Overlap Select Agents and Toxins

Bacillus anthracis

Botulinum neurotoxins

Botulinum neurotoxin producing species of Clostridium

Brucella abortus

Brucella melitensis

Brucella suis

Burkholderia mallei (formerly *Pseudomonas mallei*)

Burkholderia pseudomallei (formerly *Pseudomonas pseudomallei*)

Clostridium perfringens epsilon toxin

Coccidioides immitis

Coxiella burnetii

Eastern equine encephalitis virus

Francisella tularensis

Hendra virus

Nipah virus

Rift Valley fever virus

Shigatoxin

Staphylococcal enterotoxins

1–2 toxin

Venezuelan equine encephalitis virus

USDA Select Agents and Toxins

African horse sickness virus

African swine fever virus

Akabane virus

Avian influenza virus (highly pathogenic)

Bluetongue virus (exotic)

Bovine spongiform encephalopathy agent

Camel pox virus

Classical swine fever virus

Cowdria ruminantium (Heartwater)

Foot-and-mouth disease virus

Goat pox virus

Japanese encephalitis virus

Lumpy skin disease virus

Malignant catarrhal fever virus (Alcelaphine herpesvirus type 1)

Menangle virus

Mycoplasma capricolumi M.F38//M. mycoides Capri (contagious caprine pleuropneumonia)

Mycoplasma mycoides mycoides (contagious bovine pleuropneumonia)

Newcastle disease virus (velogenic)

Peste des petits ruminants virus

Rinderpest virus

Sheep pox virus

Swine vesicular disease virus

Vesicular stomatitis virus (Exotic)

USDA Plant Protection and Quarantine (PPQ) Select Agents and Toxins

Candidatus Liberobacter africanus

Candidatus Liberobacter asiaticus

Peronosclerospora philippinensis

Ralstonia soianacearum race 3, biovar 2

Schlerophthora rayssiae var zeae

Synctiytrium endobioticum

Xanthomonas oryzae pv. oryzicola

Xylella fastidiosa (citrus variegated chlorosis strain)

systems have been developed and efforts to improve their capabilities are ongoing; these have been employed during certain high-profile public events. The current favored technology for standoff biological detection is ultraviolet laser-induced fluorescence LIDAR (light detection and ranging).[18] The initial detection of a bioterrorist attack may not be dependent on the finding of delivery devices such as explosive devices, missiles, or even crop-dusting equipment. Nor would it likely involve environmental detection or meteorological perturbations. Rather, it more likely will involve the presentation (perhaps widely dispersed geographically) of patients with nonspecific symptoms to various practitioners, clinics, and emergency departments. This makes effective management particularly difficult, as treatment of diseases such as anthrax, plague, and botulism is most effective when begun early (when nonspecific symptoms predominate), ideally during the incubation period. By the time hallmark findings (hemorrhagic mediastinitis and related chest findings in the case of anthrax, hemoptysis in plague victims, neuromuscular symptoms of botulism) appear, treatment is of dubious benefit and prognosis often poor. Moreover, with easy access to jet travel, incubation periods ensure that perpetrators can safely depart for any foreign land before detection. Additionally, contagious biological agents (smallpox and pneumonic plague) can continue to propagate among successive generations of victims prior to discovery and diagnosis.

Finally, victims of a biological attack, more so than conventional or chemical casualties, can potentially overwhelm medical response capabilities. Botulism provides an instructive example. A survivable disease in isolated cases with early diagnosis and access to modern medical interventions (such as lengthy courses of mechanical ventilation and other intensive care modalities), the sudden requirement for hundreds or thousands of patients requiring ventilation in a given city would render a large botulism outbreak difficult to manage.

With these considerations in mind, it is clear that the spectrum of biological terrorism warrants a level of planning and preparedness at least as great as that devoted to conventional and chemical terrorism. In fact, it is precisely a lack of preparedness that might amplify the allure of biological weapons in the minds of some terrorists. Capitalizing on this lack of preparedness, a terrorist might simply threaten the release of a biological agent. Such a threat may suffice to influence policy-making and engender a massive commitment of resources. For example, many hundreds of anthrax threats have come to the attention of law-enforcement agencies over the past decade. With the notable exception of the anthrax mailings of October 2001, however, virtually all of these threats have been unfounded.[19] Yet, even the most amateur hoax or innocent but unwarranted concern has resulted in a response expending hundreds of thousands of dollars.

For bioterrorism defense planning and preparedness purposes, it is necessary to be familiar with the specific agents that might be employed by terrorists. The agents developed and studied by the Cold War superpowers (Tables 32.1 and 32.2) provide a starting point for consideration. An examination of a terrorist's potential motives permits further refinement of these lists. A World Health Organization (WHO) study[20] showed that anthrax is somewhat unique in its ability to produce widespread mortality. This study considered a release of 50 kg of agent along a 2-km line upwind of a city of 500,000 inhabitants. In this scenario, 250,000 persons would contract the disease, and 100,000 would die. Thus, for a terrorist group interested in producing widespread lethality, anthrax would be an ideal choice of weapon

(assuming it could be procured, weaponized, and delivered optimally). Smallpox, a disease not considered in the WHO study, could produce similar or even greater magnitude health effects. Smallpox and pneumonic plague (and, to a lesser degree, certain viral hemorrhagic fevers) are noteworthy in that they, in contrast to other agents already mentioned in this chapter, are contagious. Terrorists might thus leverage the results of an attack by weaponizing smallpox or plague, infecting a modest number of persons in a "first wave" and depending on contagion to assist the agent in propagating through a population, thereby overcoming some of the technical challenges of widespread aerosol delivery.

While certain assumptions and generalizations can be made in attempting to define and combat the terrorist threat, the motives and rationale of terrorists are sometimes unpredictable. *Shigella*, giardia, and even roundworms have been employed as "weapons" by terrorists, criminals, or other disgruntled individuals.[21] Envisioning and preparing for all these scenarios in advance would have been impractical. Given this factor and the constraint of limited resources, it is most useful to focus on agents both most likely to be used and also to produce the most devastating consequences. In June 1999, U.S. public health experts met in Atlanta and used this rationale to develop a list[18,22] of "critical biological agents for health preparedness" (Table 32.4). Agents in Category A are those that, if effectively dispersed, would be expected to have a high overall public health impact. Consequently, significant medical intervention would be required and intensive public health preparedness is needed. Such preparedness includes stockpiling of medications and supplies as well as improvements in disease surveillance and response capabilities of local, state, federal, and international health authorities. Category B agents present a somewhat lesser requirement for preparedness, while Category C agents require vigilance in order to guard against their future development as threat agents, but might otherwise be adequately managed within the framework of the existing public health infrastructure. Because they are of most concern, category A agents will be discussed in more detail; a concise guide to the treatment of (and prophylaxis against) diseases caused by these agents is provided in Table 32.5.

Category A Agents

Anthrax

The causative agent of anthrax, *Bacillus anthracis*, is a Gram-positive, sporulating, rod-shaped bacterium. Anthrax is primarily an endemic and epidemic disease of livestock. Ungulates such as sheep, goats, and cattle are exposed through the ingestion of soil-borne spores while grazing. These spores germinate within the animal, multiply rapidly in the bloodstream, and lead to death within days. At the time of death, the animal's blood may contain as many as 10^8 bacterium per cubic centimeter; these bacteria, once exposed to oxygen as the animal decomposes, sporulate, enter the soil, and continue the cycle.

B. anthracis has several characteristics that make it a useful biological weapon: 1) it is easy to obtain – the organism can be found virtually anywhere in the world where livestock are kept but are not routinely immunized against anthrax; 2) it grows readily in easily-prepared media; 3) it can easily be induced to form spores, which are not only highly infective via the aerosol route, but can be stored for an extended time with minimal degradation; 4) spore size and durability facilitate highly efficient aerosol delivery as a biological weapon.

Table 32.4. Critical Agents for Public Health Preparedness

Category A	Category B	Category C
Variola virus	Coxiella burnetii	Emerging threat agents (e.g., Nipah virus, hantaviruses, pandemic influenza viruses)
Bacillus anthracis	Brucellae	
Yersinia pestis	Burkholderia mallei	
Botulinum toxin	Burkholderia pseudomallei	
Francisella tularensis	Alphaviruses	
Filoviruses & Arenaviruses	Rickettsia prowezekii	
	Certain toxins (Ricin, SEB)	
	Chlamydia psittaci	
	Food safety threat agents (Salmonellae, E. coli O157:H7)	
	Water safety threat agents (e.g., Vibrio cholera)	

Category A: Agents with high public health impact requiring intensive public health preparedness and intervention; Category B: Agents with a somewhat lesser need for public health preparedness; Category C agents are emerging infections that may pose a threat in the future.

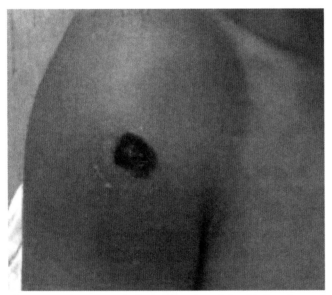

Figure 32.1. Cutaneous Anthrax. Note the painless black eschar and moderate surrounding erythema. Photo courtesy of the Centers for Disease Control and Prevention, Atlanta, Georgia, www.bt.cdc.gov/agent/anthrax/anthrax-images/cutaneous.asp.

Human anthrax takes three primary forms – cutaneous, gastrointestinal, and inhalational. Cutaneous anthrax is the most common naturally occurring form of human disease. Approximately 7 days (range 1–12 days) following exposure to infected hides or meat, a painless or mildly pruritic papule forms at the site of exposure. The lesion rapidly enlarges and ulcerates, often developing vesicles or bullae at the margins, and often accompanied by significant surrounding edema and regional lymphadenopathy. As the ulcer dries, it forms a coal-black scab (hence the name, "anthrax," from the Greek anthracis meaning coal) which resolves over 1–2 weeks (Figure 32.1). Up to

20% of untreated cutaneous anthrax cases progress to systemic disease and result in death. Notably, eleven of the twenty-two suspected or documented cases of anthrax from the 2001 "Amerithrax" mailings were cutaneous in nature.[14] In addition, cutaneous, inhalational, and gastrointestinal anthrax have been reported since 2006 from exposure to imported African animal skins.[23,24]

Oropharyngeal anthrax is a variation of cutaneous anthrax in which ingestion of contaminated meat leads to an oropharyngeal lesion and associated neck edema and adenopathy; the mortality rate in oropharyngeal anthrax can be much higher than that for other forms of cutaneous anthrax, likely due to the increased incidence of systemic spread as well as airway compromise resulting from oropharyngeal edema.[25]

Gastrointestinal anthrax results from consumption of insufficiently cooked meat from infected animals. Between 1 and 6 days following ingestion, fever, nausea, vomiting, and focal abdominal pain ensue. Victims then typically develop massive gastrointestinal bleeding and sepsis, with a fatal outcome occurring in more than 50% of cases.[25]

Historically, inhalational anthrax has been an extraordinarily rare disease found only in wool or hide mill workers after exposure to high concentrations of anthrax spores that are aerosolized by manipulation of contaminated animal products. Disease is the result of inhalation of aerosolized spores, which are then ingested by alveolar macrophages and carried to mediastinal lymph nodes, where they multiply and release toxins. Typically 1–6 days after exposure (but possibly up to several months later) disease onset is heralded by a nonspecific febrile illness, often accompanied by malaise, fatigue, and drenching sweats. Pneumonia is rare, and an auscultatory exam of the lungs is often normal at this phase of the illness, although radiologic studies may demonstrate pleural effusions and the classic widened mediastinum of hemorrhagic mediastinitis. Upper respiratory symptoms such as rhinorrhea or nasal congestion are rare in inhalational anthrax. Cough, if present, is generally non-productive. If untreated, disease that

Table 32.5. Recommended Therapy and Prophylaxis for Diseases caused by 'Category A' Biothreat Agents, 2015 Version

Condition	Adults	Children
Anthrax, Inhalational, Therapy[1] (patients who are clinically stable after 14 days can be switched to a single oral agent [ciprofloxacin or doxycycline] to complete a 60-day course[2])	Ciprofloxacin 400 mg IV q12h OR Levofloxacin 500 mg IV/PO qd OR Doxycycline 100 mg IV q12h AND Clindamycin[3] 900mg IV q8h AND Penicillin G[4] 4 mil U IV q4h AND Consider: Raxibacumab 40 mg/kg IV	Ciprofloxacin 10-15 mg/kg IV q12h OR Levofloxacin 8 mg/kg PO q12h OR Doxycycline 2.2 mg/kg IV q12h AND Clindamycin[3] 10-15 mg/kg IV q8h AND Penicillin G[4] 400-600k U/kg/d IV q4h AND Consider: Raxibacumab ($>$50 kg: 40 mg/kg IV; 15–50 kg: 60 mg/kg IV; $<$15 kg: 80 mg/kg IV)
Anthrax, Inhalational, Post-Exposure Prophylaxis (60-day course[2])	Ciprofloxacin 500 mg PO q12h OR Levofloxacin 500 mg PO qd OR Doxycycline 100 mg PO q12h	Ciprofloxacin 10-15 mg/kg PO q12h OR Levofloxacin 8 mg/kg PO q12h OR Doxycycline 2.2 mg/kg PO q12h
Anthrax, Cutaneous in setting of Terrorism, Therapy[5]	Ciprofloxacin 500 mg PO q12h OR Levofloxacin 500 mg PO qd OR Doxycycline 100 mg PO q12h	Ciprofloxacin 10-15 mg/kg PO q12h OR Levofloxacin 8 mg/kg PO q12h OR Doxycycline 2.2 mg/kg PO q12h
Plague, Therapy	Gentamicin 5 mg/kg IV qd OR Doxycycline 100 mg IV q12h OR Ciprofloxacin 400 mg IV q12h OR Levofloxacin 500 mg IV/PO qd OR Moxifloxacin 400 mg PO/IV qd x10-14 days	Gentamicin 2.5 mg/kg IV q8h OR Doxycycline 2.2 mg/kg IV q12h OR Ciprofloxacin 15 mg/kg IV q12h OR Levofloxacin 8 mg/kg IV/PO q12h
Plague, Prophylaxis	Doxycycline 100 mg PO q12h OR Ciprofloxacin 500 mg PO q12h OR Levofloxacin 500 mg PO qd OR Moxifloxacin 400 mg PO/IV qd x10-14 days	Doxycycline 2.2 mg/kg PO q12h OR Ciprofloxacin 20 mg/kg PO q12h OR Levofloxacin 8 mg/kg PO q12h
Tularemia, Therapy & Prophylaxis	Same as for Plague[6]	Same as for Plague[6]
Smallpox, Therapy	Supportive Care	Supportive Care
Smallpox, Prophylaxis	Vaccination may be effective if given within the first several days after exposure.	Vaccination may be effective if given within the first several days after exposure.
Botulism, Therapy	Supportive Care; Antitoxin may halt the progression of symptoms but is unlikely to reverse them.	Supportive Care; Antitoxin may halt the progression of symptoms but is unlikely to reverse them.
Viral Hemorrhagic Fevers, Therapy	Supportive Care; Ribavirin may be beneficial in select cases.	Supportive Care; Ribavirin may be beneficial in select cases.

[1] In a mass casualty setting, where resources are constrained, oral therapy may need to be substituted for the preferred parenteral option.

[2] If the organism is sensitive, children may be switched to oral amoxicillin (80 mg/kg/d q8h) to complete a 60-day course. Current recommendations, however, are that the first 14 days of therapy or post-exposure prophylaxis include ciprofloxacin, levofloxacin, or doxycycline regardless of age. A three-dose series of Anthrax Vaccine Adsorbed (AVA) may permit shortening of the antibiotic course to 30 days.

[3] Rifampin or clarithromycin also target bacterial protein synthesis may thus be acceptable alternatives to clindamycin. If ciprofloxacin or another quinolone is employed, doxycycline may be used as a second agent, as it also targets protein synthesis.

[4] Ampicillin, imipenem, meropenem, or chloramphenicol penetrate the CSF well and may thus be acceptable alternatives to penicillin.

[5] Ten days of therapy may be adequate for endemic cutaneous disease. Current recommendations, however, recommend a full 60-day course in the setting of terrorism because of the possibility of a concomitant inhalational exposure.

[6] Levofloxacin is licensed by the U.S. Food and Drug Administration for the prophylaxis and treatment of plague in the setting of a bioterror attack, but not tularemia.

[7] On May 8, 2015, the Food and Drug Administration approved moxifloxacin for the prevention and treatment of plague in adults (http://www.fda.gov/NewsEvents/Newsroom/PressAnnouncements/ucm446283.htm (Accessed August 27, 2015)).

has progressed this far will typically lead to severe respiratory distress, shock, and death within 2–5 days. Historically, mortality for inhalational anthrax was greater than 85%, although only five of the eleven victims with inhalational anthrax (45%) succumbed in the Amerithrax mailings of 2001. This improvement in outcome likely reflects the aggressive management of the recent cases with modern intensive care resources, but might also be skewed simply because of the small numbers. Patients with all forms of anthrax disease should be managed using standard infection control precautions. Person-to-person spread of anthrax is extremely rare, even in inhalational cases. Invasive procedures that can generate infectious aerosols should, however, be avoided in patients who may be bacteremic. In addition, it is at least theoretically possible for person-to-person transmission of cutaneous anthrax to occur via nonintact skin; therefore standard precautions should be followed for individuals with open skin or mucosal lesions.

Effective diagnosis of anthrax relies on a strong clinical suspicion to drive appropriate confirmatory laboratory studies. For systemic febrile disease resulting from any form of anthrax, blood cultures may be diagnostic if performed prior to antibiotic administration. For mild cutaneous disease, culture of the lesion (ideally vesicle fluid) may be positive; Gram stain of vesicle fluid may show large, Gram-positive bacilli; and immunohistochemical stains can identify anthrax in culture-negative lesions. In patients with gastrointestinal anthrax, stool cultures are sometimes positive; hemorrhagic peritoneal fluid can also be cultured or immunostained for *B. anthracis*. A widened mediastinum with or without pleural effusions on chest radiograph or computerized tomography suggests inhalational anthrax (Figure 32.2). Gram stain of pleural fluid or cerebrospinal fluid (in the presence of meningitis, seen in up to 50% of inhalational anthrax cases and hemorrhagic in character) is often positive, and specific immunostaining or polymerase chain reaction of these fluids can be diagnostic.[25] Furthermore, newer treatment guidelines recommend that fluid drainage be performed on anthrax patients with ascites or pleural effusions. In the event of pericardial effusions, drainage should only be performed when hemodynamic compromise is present.[26]

The key clinical decision point for the treatment of anthrax is based on the presence or absence of meningitis (Figure 32.3). Meningitis is frequently present in inhalational anthrax cases, is often fatal, and an enhanced therapy of three drugs is recommended: one with a high central nervous system (CNS) penetration (e.g., meropenem), a protein synthesis inhibitor (e.g., linezolid), and a bactericidal agent (e.g., ciprofloxacin). In the absence of meningitis, the CNS penetrating agent can be omitted.[26]

Uncomplicated cutaneous anthrax disease should be treated initially with either ciprofloxacin (500 mg PO bid for adults or 10–15 mg/kg/d divided bid [up to 1,000 mg/d] for children) or doxycycline (100 mg PO bid for adults, 5 mg/kg/d divided bid for children less than 8 years [up to 200 mg/d]). If the strain proves to be penicillin-susceptible, then the treatment may be switched to amoxicillin (500 mg PO tid for adults or 80 mg/kg PO divided tid [up to 1,500 mg/d] for children) (Table 32.5). Antitoxin antibody should also be administered to patients with systemic illness.[26]

While the *B. anthracis* genome encodes for beta-lactamases, the organism may still respond to penicillins (such as amoxicillin) if slowly growing, as in localized cutaneous disease. In the event that the exposure route is unknown or suspected to be

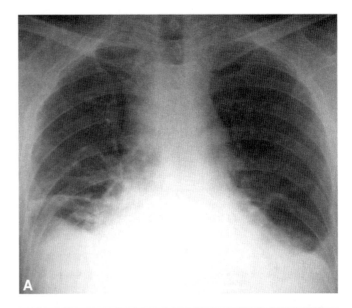

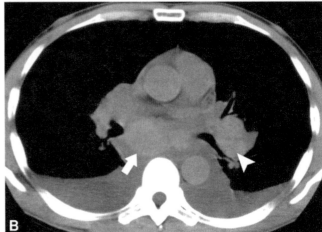

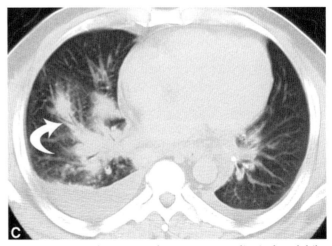

Figure 32.2. (A) Chest X-ray demonstrates mediastinal and hilar widening and bilateral pleural effusions. (B) Chest computed tomography scan demonstrates enlarged, hyperdense subcarinal (arrow) and left hilar (arrowhead) lymph nodes probably secondary to intranodal hemorrhage. (C) Note the peribronchial consolidation, which reflects lymphatic spread of anthrax infection. Images courtesy of JR Garvin, MD, and AA Frazier, MD, Department of Radiologic Pathology, Armed Forces Institute of Pathology, Washington, DC.

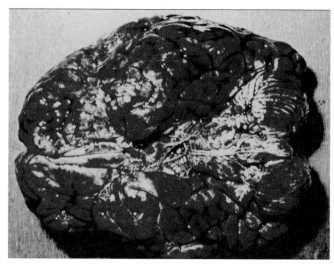

Figure 32.3. Meningitis with subarachnoid hemorrhage in a man from Thailand who died 5 days after eating undercooked carabao (water buffalo). Reproduced from: Binford CH, Connor DH, eds. *Pathology of Tropical and Extraordinary Diseases*, Vol. 1. Washington, DC: Armed Forces Instituted of Pathology, 1976: 121. AFIP Negative 75-12374-3.

intentional, antibiotics should be continued for at least 60 days. If the exposure is known to have been due to contact with infected livestock or their products, then 7–10 days of antibiotics may suffice. For patients with significant edema, non-steroidal anti-inflammatory drugs (NSAIDs) or corticosteroids may be of benefit. Debridement of lesions is not indicated. If systemic illness accompanies cutaneous anthrax, then intravenous (IV) antibiotics should be administered as per the inhalational anthrax recommendations discussed previously.[27,28,29]

While fluoroquinolone and tetracycline antibiotics are generally not recommended for use in children and pregnant women, a U.S. consensus group, as well as the American Academy of Pediatrics,[30,31] recommended ciprofloxacin or doxycycline as first-line therapy in life-threatening anthrax disease or in disease suspected to be of sinister origin (because penicillin-resistant strains can readily be selected for in the laboratory) until strain susceptibilities are known. The U.S. Food and Drug Administration (FDA) approved ciprofloxacin for prophylaxis and treatment of anthrax in children; it is the first choice for antibiotics in pregnant women.[27] If the infecting strain later proves to be penicillin-susceptible, transition to oral penicillin VK or amoxicillin is acceptable for cases of mild cutaneous anthrax.

For all forms of symptomatic anthrax aside from mild cutaneous disease (including inhalational, gastrointestinal, oropharyngeal, and severe cutaneous forms), combination IV antibiotics are strongly advised. Initial empiric therapy should include ciprofloxacin or doxycycline plus one or two additional antibiotics effective against anthrax. *B. anthracis*-susceptible antibiotics include: imipenem, meropenem, daptomycin, quinupristin-dalfopristin, linezolid, vancomycin, rifampin, the macrolides, clindamycin, chloramphenicol, and the aminoglycosides. Oral therapy should replace IV antibiotics when the patient's clinical course dictates, although in most situations, the optimal duration of therapy and antibiotic combination is not known. A monoclonal antibody, raxibacumab, was approved in 2012 as an adjunct to antibiotics in the treatment of inhalational anthrax. Finally, human anthrax immune globulin, collected from recip-

ients of Anthrax Vaccine Adsorbed (AVA),[32,33] is a potential adjunctive therapy that is FDA-licensed.

AVA is a protein vaccine produced from the supernatant of a culture of an attenuated strain of *B. anthracis*. In the United States, it is licensed for the prevention of anthrax, and is provided to certain laboratory workers, selected first responders, and military personnel. It is administered subcutaneously in an initially five-dose series over 18 months (0 and 4 weeks; then 6, 12, and 18 months), followed by annual boosters. While AVA is only licensed for preexposure prophylaxis of anthrax in adults aged 18 to 65 years, it is available under Investigational New Drug (IND) protocol for preexposure use in children, and post-exposure prophylaxis in adults and children. Its safety and efficacy in post-exposure prophylaxis, however, has not been established.[32,33] Patients with a history of hypersensitivity reactions to previous doses should not receive AVA; the vaccine should be deferred in pregnancy, persons with a febrile infectious disease, and those taking immunosuppressant drugs such as corticosteroids. FDA reports that AVA is "safe and effective" in preventing all forms of anthrax disease.[32]

Following an aerosolized attack with *B. anthracis*, exposed persons should receive antibiotic prophylaxis to prevent development of disease. Even previously immunized victims should immediately receive oral ciprofloxacin, levofloxacin, or doxycycline, all of which have been licensed for this application. Should the offending strain later be determined to be penicillin-sensitive, penicillin VK or amoxicillin can be substituted for those who cannot tolerate first-line antibiotics. Antibiotics should be continued for at least 60 days, as spores can remain dormant within a victim's lungs for extended periods only to germinate later, after the victim has completed weeks of prophylaxis. After completing antibiotics, patients should receive close follow-up for development of fever or other signs and symptoms of anthrax infection.[34]

Smallpox

Smallpox is a disease limited to humans and caused by the Orthopox virus *Variola major*. A related strain, *Variola minor*, causes a milder form of disease termed alastrim. Historically, smallpox was a significant cause of human suffering and death worldwide, responsible for as many as 50 million cases per year in the 1950s. WHO declared smallpox to be eradicated in 1980 after a monumental worldwide vaccination campaign. However, significant concern remains that existing laboratory-based Variola virus isolates could be reintroduced as weapons into an increasingly susceptible population. Variola is easily grown in cell culture or chicken eggs, and is readily dried into a stabile form, which can survive prolonged storage and is suitable for aerosolization. Contagious via droplet nuclei, smallpox can spread readily through a susceptible population, with secondary attack rates as high as 50% in nonimmune household contacts.[35]

People typically acquired smallpox via mucous membrane contact with infectious respiratory droplet nuclei from an infected, coughing individual. Less commonly, disease was transmitted via direct contact with lesions or secretions, fomites, or via infectious aerosols. Approximately 12 days (range 7–19 days) after inoculation, an infected person experienced the sudden onset of high fever (38.8–40.0° C), malaise, headache, and shaking chills. The patient would often be bedridden with severe backache, abdominal pain, and vomiting. Within 2–3 days after symptom onset, the patient would experience mild improvement, with decreased fever, and develop an enanthem in the

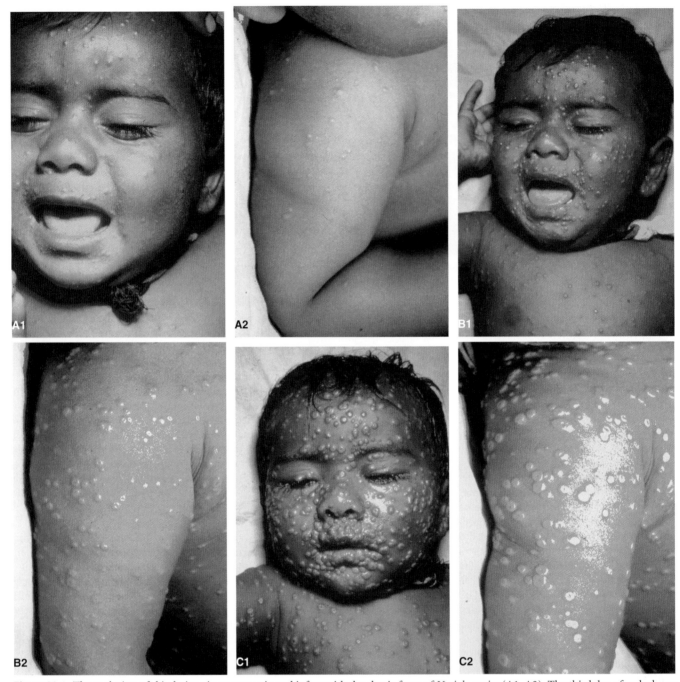

Figure 32.4. The evolution of skin lesions in an unvaccinated infant with the classic form of *Variola major* (A1, A2). The third day of rash shows synchronous eruption of skin lesions; some are becoming vesiculated (B1, B2). On the fifth day of rash, almost all papules are vesicular or pustular (C1, C2). On the seventh day of rash, many lesions demonstrate central umbilication, and all lesions are in the same general stage of development. Reproduced with permission from Fenner FHD, Arita I, Jezek Z, Ladnyi ID. *Smallpox and its eradication.* Geneva, World Health Organization, 1988.

form of small, painful ulcerations of the tongue and oropharynx (Figure 32.4). Oral secretions at this phase of illness are teeming with Variola virus, and the patient is a significant infectious risk. Within a day of enanthem onset, 2–3-mm erythematous macules appear on the face and distal extremities. The macules progress to papules, and then to clear vesicles over the next 3–5 days, and finally to tense, painful, centrally umbilicated pustules shortly thereafter, often accompanied by a second fever spike. As the lesions evolve, they spread centrally, although they typically remain more pronounced and abundant on the face

and distal extremities. Death, if it occurs, typically does so during this second week of infection. Among survivors, pustules further progress to scabs, which separate to leave depressed, hypopigmented, permanent scars that are often quite disfiguring.[36] Scabs contain viable virus; the patient is thus considered contagious and requires strict isolation until scabs are entirely shed.

The severity of smallpox disease in the past was quite variable, with several forms of disease described. Morbidity, and ultimate mortality, were directly related to the number and concentration

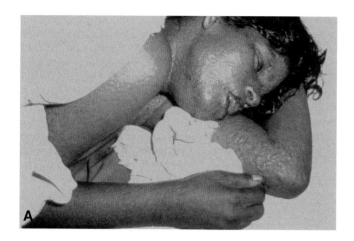

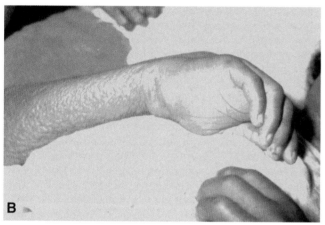

Figure 32.5. Flat-type smallpox in an unvaccinated woman on the sixth day of rash. Extensive flat lesions (A and B) and systemic toxicity with a fatal outcome were typical. Reproduced with permission from Fenner FHD, Arita I, Jezek Z, Ladnyi ID. *Smallpox and its eradication.* Geneva, World Health Organization, 1988.

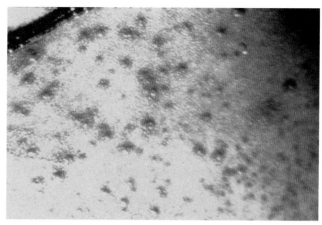

Figure 32.6. Early hemorrhagic-type smallpox with cutaneous signs of hemorrhagic diathesis. Death usually intervened before the complete evolution of pox lesions. Reproduced with permission from Herrlich A, Munz E, Rodenwaldt E. *Die pocken; Erreger, Epidemiologie und Klinisches Bild.* 2nd ed. Stuttgart, Germany: Thieme, 1967.

of skin lesions; confluent lesions portended a particularly bad outcome. Disease was generally more severe in women (especially if pregnant), children, the elderly, certain ethnic groups (e.g., Native Americans and Pacific Islanders), and immunocompromised individuals. Partially immune individuals (i.e., vaccinated) tended to have mild disease, with few lesions and lower mortality – a syndrome closely resembling that seen in Variola minor. Flat-type smallpox (Figure 32.5) probably represented an extreme form of confluent smallpox in which the skin took on a uniform "crepe rubber" appearance instead of forming classic lesions; it was seen most commonly in children. Hemorrhagic smallpox (Figure 32.6) was a rare form of fulminant disease with associated bleeding diatheses seen predominantly during pregnancy and in immunocompromised individuals. Mortality from classic smallpox varied from 10–30% in nonimmune individuals, to roughly 3% in the immunized. Among pregnant women, the mortality rate was as high as 65%, and flat and hemorrhagic forms of disease were fatal in 95% of cases. Long-term complications of smallpox included blindness from corneal scarring (1–4% of cases),[37] growth abnormalities in children secondary to Variola osteomyelitis (2–5% of child cases),[38] and disfiguring or physically debilitating dermal scarring from the pox lesions themselves.

Since routine immunization of U.S. civilians against smallpox ceased in 1972, there is an increase in the immunologically naive population. This coupled with the ease of global travel means that smallpox would likely spread faster than it did in the past. Historically, close person-to-person contact was required for transmission to occur reliably. Spread was greatest after exposure to persons with confluent rash or severe enanthem and to those with bronchiolitis and cough. While person-to-person contact is typically required, spread via aerosol is well-documented in hospital outbreaks.[39] Thus Variola can also be spread by contact with contaminated bedding, especially in the hospital setting, although such factors typically played a small role in overall transmission through a population. In past outbreaks, environmental conditions are thought to have factored prominently in disease propagation. Smallpox spread more quickly in conditions of low humidity, and during winter or rainy seasons, when people would crowd together in their homes. The disease tended to spread slowly through partially immune communities, but could become endemic in densely populated regions, even in a population with up to 80% vaccination rates.[35]

Historically, the diagnosis of smallpox was largely based on characteristic clinical findings, particularly the rash. In some cases, such clinical diagnosis could be problematic. Prodromal smallpox is difficult to differentiate from other febrile syndromes. The early rash of smallpox has been commonly mistaken for varicella, and other viral exanthems (e.g., adenovirus), as well as conditions, such as erythema multiforme, that may cause febrile illness with rash. Flat type and hemorrhagic smallpox may be difficult to differentiate clinically from other fulminant infectious syndromes presenting with shock and disseminated intravascular coagulation.

Monkeypox, another Orthopox virus closely related to smallpox, occurs naturally in equatorial Africa. While monkeypox is not a Category A agent, it can be clinically indistinguishable from smallpox. The differences are a much lower case fatality rate (11% or less in non-immunized) and the presence of cervical and inguinal lymphadenopathy, appearing 1–2 days before the rash in 90% of cases.[40] An outbreak involving eighty-one human cases of monkeypox occurred in 2003 in the United States due to exposure to exotic pets (such as Gambian rats) imported from West Africa. These cases demonstrated only localized lesions and mild disease, with no secondary transmission occurring among humans.[41] Past data from Africa suggests that the smallpox vaccine is at least 85% effective in preventing monkeypox. It is recommended that the vaccine be given within 4 days from the date of exposure in order to prevent onset of the monkeypox. If given between 4 and 14 days after the date of exposure, vaccination may reduce the symptoms of the disease, but may not prevent the disease.[42]

There are no proven specific therapies for smallpox (Table 32.5). Parenteral cidofovir is an antiviral drug (licensed for use in cytomegalovirus retinopathy) that shows in-vitro activity against a broad range of poxviruses, and potential in-vivo benefit in animal studies of poxvirus infections. Additional studies are underway to determine whether parenteral or oral cidofovir might be efficacious in the treatment of human Orthopox virus infections.[43] Patients with ocular smallpox may benefit from treatment with topical antivirals such as trifluridine or idoxuridine. Aggressive supportive care is the cornerstone of successful management of smallpox disease and includes maintenance of hydration and nutrition, pain control, and prevention and treatment of secondary infections.

Infection control within healthcare facilities could represent a significant challenge; smallpox patients should be isolated under contact and airborne precautions. Caregivers should be immunized and wear appropriate personal protective equipment (PPE), regardless of their immunization status. Providers who collect or process specimens should only do so under the direction of public health officials.[44] Patients should be considered infectious until all scabs separate. The U.S. Centers for Disease Control and Prevention (CDC) maintain planning guidance for smallpox and other contagious infectious diseases on their bioterrorism website (http://emergency.cdc.gov/agent/smallpox/prep). Victims of an attack using weaponized smallpox, as well as contacts of known smallpox cases, should be immunized and monitored for at least 17 days following the last known exposure, regardless of their vaccination status. If fever manifests, they should be immediately isolated using contact and airborne precautions. Isolation should continue until smallpox is either ruled out or confirmed, and, if confirmed, until all scabs separate.

In 2007, the FDA licensed ACAM2000™ for smallpox vaccination, replacing the previously licensed vaccine (Dryvax®). In addition, the U.S. government purchased and stockpiled IMVAMUNE® smallpox vaccine for use in a public health emergency involving smallpox. ACAM2000, unlike previous smallpox vaccines, is grown in cell culture. It is administered via intradermal inoculation using a bifurcated needle – a process known as scarification. Primary vaccinees receiving ACAM2000 are given three punctures with the needle, while repeat vaccinees receive fifteen. The typical reaction to the vaccine includes appearance of a pruritic vesicle at the inoculation site 5–7 days following administration. Local erythema, pain, and induration as well as fatigue, axillary lymphadenopathy, and mild systemic symptoms to include fever, malaise, headache, and myalgias are common. Over the ensuing several days, the vesicle progresses to form a pustule, then a 3–10-mm scab which sloughs within 1–2 weeks, leaving a permanent scar. The lesion contains live vaccinia virus and spread of infection via contact is possible until the scab has separated.

Historically, with the previously employed Dryvax vaccine, serious adverse reactions occurred in approximately 1 per 1,000 patients immunized, with 1–5 of 10,000 immunizations leading to life-threatening complications, and 1 in a million leading to death. Serious reactions were approximately ten times more common in those being immunized for the first time than in those undergoing re-immunization. Adverse events have occurred with ACAM2000 vaccine, and are expected to occur at similar rates as Dryvax, since the same viral strain is used in both vaccines.[45] Inadvertent autoinoculation of the virus to distant skin sites, as well as transfer of virus to contacts, has occurred historically in about 6 per 10,000 vaccines; ocular vaccinia is the most common form of inadvertent inoculation and can result in permanent corneal scarring. Generalized vaccinia results from systemic spread of the virus to produce lesions removed from the primary vaccination site; it occurs in 3 of 10,000 vaccinees. Post-vaccinial encephalitis is seen in approximately 1 per 100,000 primary vaccinees and has a 25% mortality rate, with another 25% developing permanent neurologic sequelae. Fetal vaccinia is a rare (<50 reported cases) but often fatal complication of maternal vaccination, most commonly reported in the third trimester of pregnancy. During a smallpox vaccination campaign in 2003, myopericarditis was reported in approximately 1 in 10,000 primary vaccinees in the United States, a rarely reported adverse event in previous programs.[46–48] Eczema vaccinatum (generalized cutaneous spread of vaccinia in patients with eczema), a potentially lethal complication, can occur after vaccination in patients with a history of eczema. For this reason, CDC states that eczema is a contraindication to vaccination. Progressive vaccinia is the systemic spread of vaccinia virus in immunocompromised individuals, seen in 1 per million primary vaccinees and almost uniformly fatal.[46–48]

CDC's Advisory Committee on Immunization Practices recommends that laboratory workers who directly handle live, unattenuated Orthopox virus cultures or infected animals, as well as select healthcare workers who are members of smallpox response teams, receive ACAM2000. Vaccination with a verified clinical "take" (vesicle with scar formation) within the past 3 years is considered to render a person immune to natural variola.

Preexposure vaccination is contraindicated in persons with the following conditions: immunosuppression (including those taking immunosuppressive drugs such as corticosteroids or alkylating agents), HIV infection, clinical evidence or history of eczema or other chronic exfoliative skin disorders, pregnancy or breastfeeding, and age less than 1 year. Additionally, the presence of household, sexual, or other close physical contacts with these conditions are contraindications to preexposure vaccination. There are no absolute contraindications to vaccination after bona fide exposure to variola. Vaccination after exposure to weaponized smallpox or to a person with smallpox may prevent or ameliorate disease if given promptly. Vaccination is likely to be most effective if given within 24 hours, but may still be somewhat effective from 4–7 days after exposure.[49]

A formulation of intravenous Vaccinia Immune Globulin (VIG) is licensed by FDA for treatment of certain complications of smallpox (vaccinia) vaccination, including generalized vaccinia, eczema vaccinatum, and progressive vaccinia. Public health professionals must have ready access to VIG when initiating vaccination programs. VIG is available as an IND through both DOD and CDC for intramuscular (IM) injection. An intravenous formulation of VIG (IV-VIG) is being produced to support the treatment of adverse events that may result from smallpox vaccination, and is also available under IND protocols from both CDC and DOD. The dose is 100 mg/kg for the intravenous formulation termed VIG-IV (first line, if available). If VIG-IV is unavailable, cidofovir can be used for treatment of vaccine adverse events (second line). The VIG-IM formulation is dosed at 0.6 ml/kg (third line), and due to its large volume (42 ml in a 70 kg person), should be given in multiple sites over 24–36 hours. Limited data suggest that VIG may also be of value in post-exposure prophylaxis against smallpox when given within the first week after exposure, and concurrently with vaccination. Concomitant administration of VIG may be particularly useful for pregnant and eczematous persons in such circumstances.[50,51] Early vaccination alone is recommended for those without contraindications to the vaccine. If more than 1 week has elapsed after exposure, administration of both products (vaccine and VIG), if available, is a reasonable approach.[52]

Plague

Yersinia pestis, the causative agent of plague, is a rod-shaped, non-motile, non-sporulating, Gram-negative bacterium of the family *Enterobacteriaceae*. Plague is principally a zoonotic disease of rodents. Fleas that live on the rodents can transmit the bacteria to humans via biting. These exposed persons may then develop the bubonic form of plague within the lymphatic distribution after the flea bite. The bubonic form may progress to the septicemic and/or secondary pneumonic forms, discussed in detail later. Primary pneumonic plague would likely be the predominant form encountered following the purposeful aerosol dissemination of a weaponized form of *Y. pestis*. All human populations are thought to be susceptible to plague, and recovery from the disease does not confer lasting immunity. *Y. pestis* can remain viable in water, moist soil, and grain for several weeks. It can also remain infectious for some time in dry sputum, flea feces, and cadavers, but is killed within several hours of exposure to sunlight.

The contagious nature of pneumonic plague makes it particularly dangerous as a biological weapon. Plague may present three distinct clinical syndromes: bubonic (~85% of naturally occurring cases), septicemic (~13%), and pneumonic (~1–2%). The bubonic form begins after an incubation period of 2–10 days, with acute and fulminant onset of nonspecific symptoms, including high fever, malaise, headache, myalgias, and sometimes nausea and vomiting. Up to 50% of patients have abdominal pain. Simultaneous with or shortly after the onset of these nonspecific symptoms, the bubo develops – a swollen, very painful, infected lymph node (Figure 32.7). Buboes are normally seen in the femoral or inguinal lymph nodes, as the legs are the most common flea-bitten part of the adult human body. The liver and spleen of bubonic plague victims are often tender and palpable. One-quarter of patients will have a pustule, vesicle, eschar, or papule (containing leukocytes and bacteria) in the lymphatic drainage of the bubo, presumably representing the site of the inoculating flea bite. Bacteremia is common, and greater than 80% of blood cultures are positive for the organism in patients with bubonic plague. However, only about a quarter of bubonic plague patients progress to clinical septicemia.[53]

Among those who progress to secondary septicemia, as well as those presenting initially with septicemia without lymphadenopathy (primary septicemia), symptoms are similar to those seen in other Gram-negative septicemias (i.e., high fever, chills, malaise, hypotension, nausea, vomiting, and diarrhea). Plague septicemia, however, is distinctive in that it is also characterized by thromboses in the acral vessels, with necrosis, gangrene, and disseminated intravascular coagulation (DIC). Black necrotic appendages and more proximal purpuric lesions caused by endotoxemia are often present (Figure 32.8). Organisms in the bloodstream can gain access to the central nervous system,

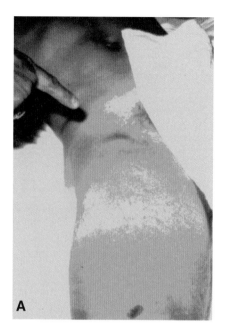

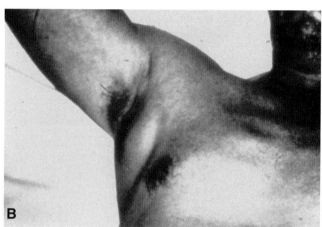

Figure 32.7. A femoral bubo (A) is the most common site of an erythematous, tender, swollen lymph node in patients with plague. The next most common lymph node regions involved are the inguinal, axillary (B), and cervical areas. Bubo location is a function of the region of the body in which an infected flea inoculates the plague bacilli. Photos courtesy of Kenneth L Gage, PhD, Centers for Disease Control and Prevention Laboratory, Fort Collins, Colorado.

lungs, and elsewhere; plague meningitis occurs in about 6% of septicemic and pneumonic cases.

Pneumonic plague is an infection of the lungs due to either inhalation of organisms (primary pneumonic plague), or spread to the lungs from septicemia (secondary pneumonic plague, seen in about 12% of U.S. bubonic cases over the past 50 years).[54] After an incubation period varying from 1–6 days for primary pneumonic plague (usually 2–4 days, and presumably dose-dependent), onset is acute and often fulminant. The first signs of illness include high fever, chills, headache, malaise, and myalgias, followed within 24 hours by cough with bloody sputum. Although bloody sputum is characteristic, it can sometimes be watery or, less commonly, purulent. Gastrointestinal symptoms, including nausea, vomiting, diarrhea, and abdominal pain, may be present. Rarely, a cervical bubo might result from an inhalational exposure. Radiographic findings are variable, but most

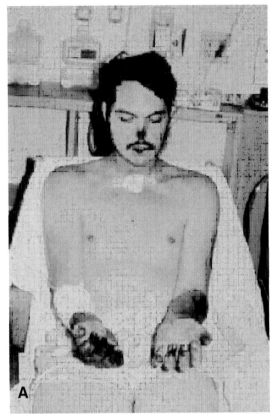

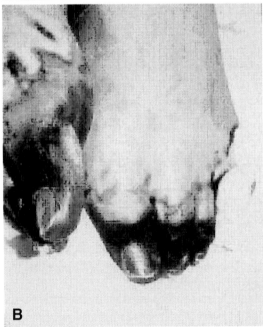

Figure 32.8. (A) This patient developed bubonic plague that progressed to the septicemic and pneumonic forms after the causative organism, *Y. pestis*, disseminated from his buboes into his bloodstream. (B) Note the necrosis of tissue involving the tip of the nose, the fingers, and the toes. This is due to thrombosis of distal arterioles and is a known complication of septicemic plague. Photos courtesy of Kenneth L Gage, PhD, Centers for Disease Control and Prevention Laboratory, Fort Collins, Colorado.

commonly include bilateral pulmonary infiltrates, which may be patchy or consolidated. Plague pneumonia progresses rapidly, resulting in dyspnea, stridor, and cyanosis. The disease terminates with respiratory failure and circulatory collapse. In humans, the mortality of untreated bubonic plague is approximately 60% (reduced to <5% with prompt effective therapy), whereas in untreated pneumonic plague the mortality rate is nearly 100%; survival is unlikely if treatment is delayed beyond 18–24 hours of the symptom onset.[53,55]

Patients with plague exhibit leukocytosis, with a predominance of polymorphonuclear cells. Increased fibrin split products in the blood indicate low-grade DIC. The serum blood urea nitrogen, creatinine, alanine aminotransferase, aspartate aminotransferase, and bilirubin may also be elevated, consistent with multi-organ failure[53,55] Nonetheless, a prompt diagnosis must often be based primarily on clinical suspicion. The presentation of large numbers of previously healthy patients with sudden, severe, rapidly progressive pneumonia with hemoptysis strongly suggests plague. A presumptive diagnosis can be made microscopically by identification of the coccobacillus with bipolar "safety-pin" morphology in Gram, Wright, Giemsa, or Wayson's stained smears from lymph node needle aspirate, sputum, blood, or cerebrospinal fluid samples. When available, immunofluorescent staining is very useful. Definitive diagnosis relies on culturing the organism from blood, sputum, cerebrospinal fluid, or bubo aspirates. Most clinical assays can be performed in Biosafety Level 2 (BSL-2) labs, whereas procedures producing aerosols or yielding significant quantities of organisms require BSL-3 containment.[55]

Standard precautions are adequate when caring for bubonic plague patients. Suspected pneumonic plague cases (those who have potentially inhaled *Y. pestis* organisms) require strict isolation with droplet precautions for at least 48 hours following the initiation of antibiotic therapy, or until sputum cultures are negative in confirmed cases. If replication-competent vectors (fleas) and reservoirs (rodents) are present in the environment, measures must be taken to prevent disease from becoming enzootic. These measures might include, but are not limited to, the use of flea insecticides, rodent control measures (after or during flea control), and flea barriers for patient care areas.

Streptomycin, gentamicin, doxycycline, and chloramphenicol are highly effective in the treatment of plague, if therapy is initiated early; although streptomycin is not generally available in the United States (Table 32.5). Results obtained from animal studies indicate that quinolone antibiotics, such as ciprofloxacin, levofloxacin, and moxifloxacin, would also be effective. Chloramphenicol is recommended for the treatment of plague meningitis.[52] Usual supportive therapy includes IV administration of crystalloids and hemodynamic monitoring. Although low-grade DIC may occur, clinically significant hemorrhage is uncommon, as is the need to treat with heparin. Endotoxic shock is common, but pressor agents are rarely needed. Finally, buboes rarely require any form of local care, but instead recede with systemic antibiotic therapy. In fact, incision and drainage poses a risk of disease transmission to others in contact with the patient; aspiration is recommended for diagnostic purposes and may provide symptomatic relief.

At the time of this writing, no vaccine is available for plague prophylaxis. A licensed, killed whole cell vaccine was previously available in the United States; it offered protection against bubonic plague, but would not likely have been effective against aerosolized *Y. pestis*. An F1-V antigen (fusion protein) vaccine is in development at the U.S. Army Medical Research Institute of Infectious Diseases (USAMRIID). It protects mice against an inhalational challenge, and is undergoing testing in primates.

Persons having face-to-face contact (within 2 meters) with pneumonic plague victims, or persons possibly exposed to a plague aerosol during a biological attack, should receive antibiotic prophylaxis for at least 7 days following the cessation of exposure. Doxycycline (100 mg orally twice daily), ciprofloxacin (500 mg orally twice daily) and levofloxacin (500 mg orally once daily) have been shown effective in preventing disease in mice exposed to aerosolized plague bacilli and, in fact, all are licensed for post-exposure prophylaxis in humans. Tetracycline (500 mg orally four times daily) and chloramphenicol (25 mg/kg orally four times daily) are acceptable alternatives. Contacts of bubonic plague patients should be observed for symptoms for at least 1 week. Should such symptoms occur, antibiotic therapy should be instituted pending the results of diagnostic studies.

Botulism

Botulism is a toxin-mediated disease (rather than a true infection), which occurs following exposure to one of seven related botulinum neurotoxins (A–G) produced by certain strains of *Clostridium botulinum* and closely related bacteria. These organisms are strictly anaerobic spore-forming Gram-positive bacilli ubiquitously found in soil. The neurotoxins they produce are the most toxic substances known, with a lethal dose (LD_{50}) for type A toxin of approximately 0.001 µg/kg. On a weight basis, this is approximately 15,000 times more lethal than VX, the most potent chemical warfare agent. The botulinum neurotoxins function at the presynaptic nerve terminal, preventing the release of acetylcholine, interrupting neuronal transmission at cholinergic autonomic (muscarinic) and motor (nicotinic) receptors, thereby leading to a generalized flaccid paralysis and autonomic dysfunction. Binding of toxin within the presynaptic neuron is permanent; recovery is thus predicated on development of new axons, which may require several months.

Only types A, B, and E toxin are significant causes of naturally occurring human botulism. Exposure to type C toxin appears to be a prevalent cause of botulism among poultry and other avian species, while types C and D are associated with disease in cattle. Neither type C nor D appears to affect humans in nature, although all serotypes have the potential to cause human disease. In 1981, a single small outbreak of botulism due to type G toxin was reported in Argentina.[56] More recently, several cases of neonatal botulism due to type F toxin associated with *C. baratii* have been described,[57] and a few cases of infant botulism (type E) have been associated with *C. butyricum*.[58]

Sinister use of botulinum toxin might involve its aerosolization or the intentional contamination of food and water supplies. Iraq weaponized botulinum toxin for aerosol delivery and declared such weapons under the auspices of the BWC in the aftermath of the 1990–1991 Gulf War. The Japanese doomsday cult Aum Shinrikyo made several unsuccessful attempts to use botulinum toxin as a weapon prior to their sarin attacks on the Tokyo subway system. Naturally occurring botulism, however, is generally acquired in one of three ways:

1. Food-borne botulism occurs as a result of the consumption of improperly canned food. As *C. botulinum* is ubiquitous in soil, contamination of food with small amounts of soil provides the nidus of bacteria. Failure to properly sterilize food during canning allows for bacterial survival. The canning process then provides for the strict anaerobic environment necessary for bacterial proliferation and toxin production. Subsequent heating or cooking (such as might occur after opening the previously canned goods) may kill bacteria but does not destroy the toxin. Consuming contaminated canned goods allows for the gastrointestinal absorption and hematogenous circulation of toxin, which ultimately reaches its target at the peripheral cholinergic synapse. While types A and B toxin are traditionally associated with foodborne outbreaks, type E toxin is particularly associated with botulism resulting from improperly canned fish products.

2. Wound botulism occurs when soil contaminates a wound and is contained within an anaerobic pocket beneath the skin. *C. botulinum* proliferates in this environment and produces toxin. A large number of wound botulism cases have been associated with the injection of "black-tar" heroin.[59]

3. Infant botulism occurs when newborns ingest dirt or substances (typically raw honey) heavily contaminated with *C. botulinum* spores.[60] Under normal circumstances, the acidity of the stomach would destroy these spores, but the relatively weak acid levels of the neonatal stomach are thought to permit some spores to survive and transit the intestinal tract, where the relative lack of competing bowel flora allows them to colonize and germinate in the large intestine and begin to produce toxin, which is then absorbed.

Regardless of the original route of acquisition of botulinum toxin (via any of the three aforementioned routes or via inhalation following a deliberate aerosol attack), the final common pathway is the same. Following exposure to botulinum toxin, a latent period ranging from 24 hours to several days occurs before clinical manifestations develop. Signs and symptoms initially involve cranial nerve dysfunction, manifested as bulbar palsies, ptosis, photophobia, and blurred vision caused by a difficulty in accommodation. The autonomic effects of botulism may include dry mouth, ileus, constipation, and urinary retention. Nausea and vomiting may occur as nonspecific sequelae of an ileus. Hence the combination of neurological and gastrointestinal symptoms should lead clinicians to suspect botulism. Symptoms progress to include dysarthria, dysphonia, and dysphagia. Finally, a descending symmetric flaccid paralysis develops and, in the absence of ventilatory support, death results from respiratory muscle failure.

The diagnosis of botulism is principally clinical. The extreme potency of the toxin is such that the LD_{50} is below the threshold of human immune response. Detectable antibody production is thus absent in cases of human botulism, and clinical botulism does not confer immunity to subsequent intoxications. It is possible to detect toxin in clinical or environmental samples using enzyme-linked immunosorbent assays, but the mouse neutralization bioassay remains the gold standard for botulinum neurotoxin detection. In cases of foodborne botulism, therefore, it is critical to obtain implicated food for testing in such assays.

Clinically, a solitary case of botulism must be differentiated from other uncommon neurological disorders such as myasthenia gravis, tick paralysis, Guillain-Barre and Eaton-Lambert syndromes, and others. The presence of multiple casualties with similar symptoms as those described, clustered in time and space, strongly suggests a botulism outbreak. In the setting of terrorism, botulism might superficially be confused with nerve agent intoxication, owing to the preponderance of neuromuscular symptomatology in both conditions. The two are easy to differentiate, however; organophosphate nerve agents inhibit acetylcholinesterase, leading to excessive cholinergic activity at neuronal synapses, in contrast to the lack of cholinergic activity seen in botulism. The "paralysis" of nerve agents, then, is spastic, rather than flaccid, and autonomic hyperarousal is seen.

Supportive care, including meticulous attention to ventilatory support (but typically not oxygenation), is the mainstay of botulism management. Patients may require such support for several months, making the management of a large-scale botulism outbreak especially problematic in terms of medical and health resources. Planners should anticipate the need for mass ventilation, but not necessarily large supplies of oxygen as might be needed for management of other public health emergencies such as influenza pandemics. Recognition of the utility of tracheostomy and improvements in mechanical ventilation have reduced the mortality rate for isolated cases in the United States from greater than 60% prior to 1950 to less than 5% in modern times. Attention to hydration status, as well as bowel and bladder care and cognizance of the need to prevent decubitus ulcers and deep vein thromboses, also play a large role in patient outcome. If antibiotics are prescribed in the treatment of wound botulism, no aminoglycosides or clindamycin should be administered because of their weak pharmacological effects as neuromuscular blocking agents. This could acutely worsen paralysis and precipitate respiratory arrest.

A licensed heptavalent antitoxin (types A–G) is available through CDC. Administration of this antitoxin is unlikely to reverse disease in symptomatic patients, but may prevent further progression. Additionally, an anti-type A/B product, Botulism Immune Globulin Intravenous (Human), BabyBIG®, is available through government sources, such as the California Department of Health Services in the United States, for the treatment of infant botulism (Table 32.5).[61]

Although no licensed vaccine is available to protect against botulism, considerable experience exists with an investigational pentavalent (types A–E) vaccine, available through USAMRIID. A theoretical concern, given the expansion of indications for therapeutic use of botulinum toxins, surrounds the possibility that vaccine recipients may be immune to the beneficial effects of such treatment. Of note, therapeutic botulinum toxin is produced from type A (Botox®) or type B (Myobloc®) toxin.

Viral Hemorrhagic Fevers

The term "viral hemorrhagic fever" (VHF) is a clinically descriptive one, referring to a group of widely heterologous diseases caused by lipid-enveloped, single-stranded RNA viruses of four taxonomic families: the arenaviruses, bunyaviruses, filoviruses, and flaviviruses. Although "brand-name recognition" (i.e., the notoriety of diseases such as Ebola virus disease and the consequent ability of these diseases to capture public attention and create concern) is somewhat responsible for their inclusion among the Category A agents, actual weaponization of these agents would likely be challenging, owing to difficulties in mass production, and rapid inactivation of the various causative viruses by environmental heat, desiccation, and ultraviolet light.[62] Nonetheless, several have been examined as weapons candidates.

VHFs would be expected to present as acute febrile illnesses with a host of nonspecific features such as malaise, fatigue, nausea, vomiting, diarrhea, abdominal pain, and headache. Hypotension and shock can rapidly ensue and death occurs frequently among patients with certain VHFs. As the name implies, vascular involvement constitutes the defining characteristic of this broad group of infectious diseases, and can manifest as hypotension, flushing, edema, petechiae, bruising, and bleeding. Such findings can vary from subtle to overt in their presentation.

The pathogenesis of the VHFs is complex and variable (Figure 32.9). While some VHF viruses cause vascular damage and DIC through direct endothelial infection, others result in immune complex deposition, thereby activating complement and inflammatory cascades. Vascular endothelial damage, however, is a "final common pathway," and results in vascular leak, with secondary hypotension, edema, and hemorrhage, often resulting in shock and end-organ failure. While the various VHFs share common manifestations, many clinical findings vary among the different diseases, and among patients with the same disease. Lassa fever, caused by an Old World arenavirus, typically presents with edema, without hemorrhage, while diseases due to the New World arenaviruses (the agents of Argentinean, Bolivian, and Venezuelan hemorrhagic fevers) are notable for prominent petechiae, purpura, ecchymoses and mucosal hemorrhage.

The hantaviruses are members of the bunyavirus family. Hemorrhagic fever with renal syndrome (HFRS), usually caused by Old World (and occasionally New World) hantaviruses, begins with a nonspecific prodrome, followed by the development of facial edema. A morbilliform eruption, flushing of the upper body, and dermatographism may appear. Hemorrhagic manifestations range from subtle petechiae to massive hemorrhage. Congo-Crimean hemorrhagic fever (CCHF), caused by another bunyavirus, is often characterized by severe ecchymoses and hemorrhage, although some cases may present with only nonspecific, minor hemorrhagic manifestations (Figure 32.10).

The filoviral fevers, Ebola and Marburg, are characterized by an acute severe prodrome, followed by a papular exanthem which rapidly progresses into large, coalescent papules, purpura, and ecchymoses. Patients often develop gross hemorrhage and shock. Mortality rates range from 23% in some Marburg disease outbreaks to as high as 90% for certain Ebola outbreaks. Most of these deaths occur during the second week of illness.

Flavivirus infections also produce manifestations which are quite variable. Dengue fever, also known as "breakbone" fever due to its severe muscle and joint pains, typically presents as a nonspecific febrile illness, sometimes accompanied by a diffuse morbilliform rash. While infection due to one of the four dengue virus serotypes confers lifelong immunity to that particular serotype, reinfection with another (heterologous) strain may result in immune amplification. This leads to a more severe clinical outcome, termed dengue hemorrhagic fever or dengue shock syndrome. Severe ecchymoses and hemorrhage can occur in cases of dengue hemorrhagic fever. Two other flaviviral hemorrhagic fevers, Omsk hemorrhagic fever and Kyasanur Forest disease, also feature a wide range of hemorrhagic manifestations.

Clinical diagnosis is essential in the case of the viral hemorrhagic fevers. Since the endemic range of the various causative viruses is frequently unique and limited, naturally occurring cases are often suspected on geographic and epidemiologic grounds; a detailed travel history should be sought when VHF is considered. Clinical laboratory findings of proteinuria, thrombocytopenia, leucopenia, elevated serum transaminase levels, and abnormal coagulation studies may be sought, but are nonspecific. Specific etiologic diagnosis by serologic testing or viral isolation requires sending clinical specimens to a limited number of laboratories with high-level biosafety containment capabilities. In fact, many of the VHF viruses (the filoviruses and arenaviruses,

A

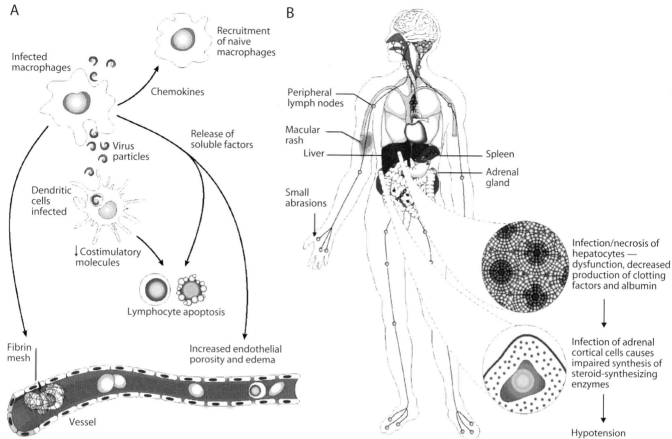

B

Figure 32.9. Model of VHF Pathogenesis. (A) Virus spreads from the initial infection site to regional lymph nodes, liver, and spleen. At these sites, the virus infects tissue macrophages (including Kupffer cells) and dendritic cells. Soluble factors released from virus-infected monocytes and macrophages act locally and systemically. Release of chemokines from these virus-infected cells recruits additional macrophages to sites of infection, making more target cells available for viral exploitation and further amplifying the dysregulated host response. Although none of these viruses infect lymphocytes, the rapid loss of these cells by apoptosis is a prominent feature of disease. The direct interaction of lymphocytes with viral proteins cannot be discounted as having a role in their destruction, but the marked loss of lymphocytes is likely to result from a combination of factors, including viral infection of dendritic cells and release of soluble factors from virus-infected monocytes and macrophages. For example, viral infection of dendritic cells impairs their function by interfering with the upregulation of costimulatory molecules, which are important in providing rescue signals to T lymphocytes. Additionally, release of soluble factors from infected monocytes and macrophages results in deletion of lymphocytes, both directly by release of mediators such as nitric oxide, and indirectly by contributing to upregulation of proapoptotic proteins such as Fas and tumor necrosis factor–related apoptosis-inducing ligand. The coagulation abnormalities vary in nature and magnitude among the VHFs. For example, Ebola virus induces the overexpression of tissue factor that results in activation of the clotting pathway and the formation of fibrin in the vasculature. As another example, coagulation disorders are less marked in Lassa fever, and impairment of endothelial function contributes to edema, which seems to be a more prominent finding in Lassa fever than in other VHFs. (B) The hemodynamic and coagulation disorders common among all of the VHFs are exacerbated by infection of hepatocytes and adrenal cortical cells. Infection of hepatocytes impairs synthesis of important clotting factors. At the same time, reduced synthesis of albumin by hepatocytes results in a reduced plasma osmotic pressure and contributes to edema. Impaired secretion of steroid-synthesizing enzymes by VHF-infected adrenal cortical cells leads to hypotension and sodium loss with hypovolemia. Macular rashes are often seen in VHFs. Reproduced with permission from: Geisbert TW, Jahrling PB. Exotic emerging viral diseases: progress and challenges. *Nat Med.* 2004; 10(12 suppl): S110–121.

as well as CCHF, Omsk, and Kyasanur Forest disease viruses) are assigned to Biosafety Level 4. Clinical specimens potentially containing these viruses should thus be handled only at facilities that possess BSL-4 laboratories, including CDC or USAMRIID.

Supportive care is the mainstay of therapy in most cases of VHF, and many severely affected individuals require intensive resuscitation (Table 32.5). Vigorous fluid, as well as vasoactive agent and inotropic administration may be necessary; the provision of such modalities is especially problematic in developing nations where many of these diseases are endemic. Sedative and anxiolytic therapy, analgesia, anticonvulsant therapy, antibacterial therapy (for secondary infections), mechanical ventilation,

and renal dialysis are often required. As coagulopathy is an integral component of the pathogenesis of many VHF cases, particular attention should be paid to clotting studies, and blood products (red blood cells, platelets, clotting factors) should be provided as clinically indicated. As with any case of significant coagulopathy, intramuscular injections and anticoagulating drugs (such as aspirin) should be avoided.

Intravenous ribavirin shows promise in the treatment of many of the viral hemorrhagic fevers, including CCHF, Lassa fever, HFRS, and Rift Valley fever.[63] Ribavirin is available for therapy of CCHF, Lassa fever, and HFRS under an IND protocol. A clinical trial concluded that parenteral ribavirin reduces

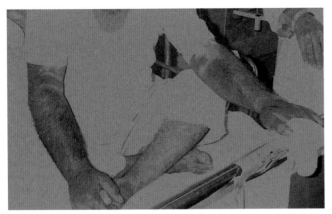

Figure 32.10. Ecchymosis associated with late-stage CCHF infection 1 week following development of clinical signs and symptoms. Ecchymosis indicates significant impairment of the patient's coagulation system and loss of vascular integrity. Photo courtesy of Dr. Sadegh Chinikar, Pasteur Institute of Iran, Tehran, Iran.

mortality in HFRS.[64,65] In addition, several trials have suggested that ribavirin reduces both morbidity and mortality of Lassa fever.[66,67] In HFRS field trials, treatment was effective if begun within the first 4 days of fever, and continued for a 10-day course. In the United States, both CDC and USAMRIID have IND protocols for the treatment of VHFs with IV and oral ribavirin. Since supplies of the preferred IV formulation are limited, oral ribavirin may be required in a mass casualty event. Ribavirin has poor in vitro and in vivo activity against the filoviruses and the flaviviruses. As of the end of 2015, the 17-D yellow fever vaccine is the only FDA-approved immunization available against a hemorrhagic fever virus.[68] Vaccine candidates effective against HFRS and Rift Valley, Argentine hemorrhagic, Lassa, Marburg, and Ebola fevers are in various stages of study or development.

Patients with certain VHFs present infection control and public health challenges because they are highly contagious and are commonly transmitted to healthcare workers. The arenaviruses, CCHF, and the filoviruses are communicable, primarily by contact with blood and body fluids. Specific infection control guidelines for hospitalized patients with these diseases include contact precautions, augmented in some circumstances with airborne precautions, with special attention to disposal of body waste. Patients with HFRS and those with flavivirus infections can be managed using standard precautions unless aerosolized procedures are being performed.

Tularemia

Tularemia, a plague-like zoonotic illness that occasionally affects humans, is caused by the Gram-negative facultative intracellular coccobacillus, *Francisella tularensis*. First discovered in ground squirrels in Tulare County, California, in 1911, two biovars of *F. tularensis* are now known. *F. tularensis tularensis*, the causative agent of Biovar A tularemia, is found primarily in temperate areas of North America, where it is typically transmitted by ticks among lagomorph reservoirs (hence the name "rabbit fever"), although many other wild animals may serve as reservoirs and many insects are vectors. Humans are coincidental "dead end" hosts who cannot transmit disease. Natural infection in humans occurs through inoculation by an infected arthropod, contact with contaminated animal tissue, inhalation of aerosolized bacterium, or ingestion of contaminated water or meat. Approximately half of all naturally occurring U.S. cases originate in Missouri, Arkansas, or Oklahoma.[69]

The number of reported cases of tularemia in the United States has decreased from several thousand per year prior to 1950, to about 125 cases per year during 2000–2008. A diminishing fondness for rabbit hunting may be responsible, in part, for this finding. Occupational exposure and environmental factors are major risk factors in disease acquisition, and tularemia generally affects more men than women, likely owing to its association with hunting. Naturally occurring tularemia occurs in two seasonal peaks: during the summer (when ticks are active) and the winter (during hunting season).

F. tularensis tularensis is an organism of extraordinarily high virulence, and as few as ten cells constitute the rabbit LD_{50} and human infectious dose (ID_{50}). *F. tularensis palearctica*, the causative agent of type B tularemia, on the other hand, is a low-virulence organism found in Europe and the former Soviet Union. The rabbit LD_{50} of this organism is on the order of 10 *million* cells. While these differences have epidemiologic and vaccine development implications, immunity against one biotype appears to be cross-protective.

Widespread waterborne outbreaks of tularemia in the former Soviet Union prior to and during WWII led to a more thorough study of the bacterium and its potential as a biological weapon. Its high infectivity, ability to produce severe or fatal human illness, relative heartiness and ease of dissemination, and nonspecific clinical presentation apparently argued convincingly for such a role. In fact, the United States developed tularemia aerosols during human exposure experiments and, by the 1950s, had stockpiled tularemia as one of the first entries in its biologic arsenal. Some, including Ken Alibek, a former Soviet biological weapons scientist, have alleged that tularemia was intentionally deployed by the Soviets at the Battle for Stalingrad in 1942–1943.[70,71] Unusual epidemiology and an overwhelming preponderance of pneumonic disease, which occurred during a large outbreak between the Don and Volga Rivers during that period,[70] lend credence to these allegations, although others dispute a sinister explanation for the outbreak.[71] Finally, Alibek also detailed the Soviet Union's attempts to engineer drug resistance into *F. tularensis* weapons during the 1990s.[72]

Tularemia presents in at least six different clinical forms, all heralded by the onset of a nonspecific influenza-like syndrome. The terms ulceroglandular, glandular, oculoglandular, pharyngeal, typhoidal, and pneumonic, describe these clinical presentations. In many ways, however, glandular and oculoglandular disease can be thought of as variants of the ulceroglandular form, and the six clinical syndromes can be more simply described as two broader clinical pictures, analogous in many ways to plague. Ulceroglandular tularemia is similar in many regards to the bubonic form of plague (or, in some respects, to the cutaneous form of anthrax). Pneumonic tularemia, on the other hand, is likely to be the predominant presentation following an intentional aerosolized release, and can be thought of as somewhat analogous to the pneumonic form of plague (or the inhalational form of anthrax).

Ulceroglandular tularemia results from arthropod bites or from exposure of skin and mucous membranes to the hides and meat of infected animals. Onset of fever and systemic symptoms (which may include chills, headache, cough, myalgias, chest pain, vomiting, arthralgia, sore throat, and abdominal pain) occur following a 3–6 day incubation period.[72] Within 48–72 hours an erythematous maculopapular lesion develops at the site of inoculation and soon ulcerates. This characteristic chancre-like ulcer is typically 0.4–3.0 cm in diameter with raised edges. Bacteria present at the ulcer site subsequently gain access to lymphatic vessels and travel to regional lymph nodes, producing the lymphadenitis, which, in combination with the ulcer, constitutes the hallmark dyad of ulceroglandular tularemia. The lymphadenopathy of ulceroglandular tularemia is often pronounced and persistent. Involved lymph nodes can grow as large as 10 cm in diameter, and frequently become fluctuant, draining spontaneously despite appropriate antibiotic therapy. From the lymph node, bacteria may secondarily gain access to the systemic circulation and ultimately seed the liver, spleen, and other distant organs.

Pneumonic tularemia results from inhalation of aerosolized bacteria, but may also occur secondarily following seeding of the lungs in complicated cases of ulceroglandular and typhoidal tularemia. Aerosolization of bacteria can occur intentionally, through the actions of belligerents or terrorists, but may occur naturally in circumstances where infected blood and other animal products are mishandled. Some reports attribute cases of inhalational (pneumonic) tularemia to aerosolization of rabbits by lawnmowers.[73,74] Symptoms of pneumonic tularemia include cough (which may be productive), dyspnea, and pleuritic chest pain. Pleural effusions, cavitary lesions, bronchopleural fistulae, and pulmonary calcifications occur less commonly.

Most diagnoses of tularemia are made serologically using bacterial agglutination or enzyme-linked immunosorbent assay. *F. tularensis* may be cultured from the blood of infected individuals, but such culturing should only be attempted by experienced technicians in laboratories equipped with BSL-3 safety systems. The extreme infectivity of *F. tularensis* in laboratory settings is evident given that it was the most common cause of laboratory-acquired infection at Fort Detrick in the United States prior to the immunization of laboratory workers.[75] Identification of *F. tularensis* is also possible by microscopic examination of secretions or biopsy specimens using direct fluorescent antibody or immunohistochemical staining techniques. Detectable levels of agglutinating antibodies against *F. tularensis* typically appear in blood within approximately 7 days of infection, although higher levels and improved diagnostic sensitivity (i.e., serology titer >1:160) may be obtained by sampling at 2 weeks following suspected infection. Moreover, the serologic response may be blunted by the administration of antibiotics, making diagnosis more problematic. Due to cross-reactivity of *F. tularensis* with *Brucellae*, *Proteus* OX19, and *Yersinia* organisms, acute infection should ideally be diagnosed only in the presence of a fourfold or greater increase in titer following an acute infection.[69]

As with plague, streptomycin (1 g IM twice daily) has traditionally been considered the drug of choice in the treatment of all forms of tularemia. A literature review reports a 97% cure rate with no relapses with streptomycin use.[76] Patients treated with streptomycin usually demonstrate a clinical response within 48 hours. Gentamicin (5 mg/kg daily IM or IV) was an acceptable alternate in this same review, and, given the difficulty in procuring streptomycin in some countries, has become a widely used therapy for this condition. Duration of therapy using either antibiotic is a minimum of 10 days. Ciprofloxacin (400 mg IV twice daily) given for 10 days is a potential alternate to aminoglycoside therapy. Bacteriostatic drugs such as chloramphenicol (15 mg/kg IV four times daily) and doxycycline (100 mg IV twice daily) are effective, but should be administered for at least 14–21 days to prevent relapse. Post-exposure prophylaxis may be accomplished using oral doxycycline (100 mg twice daily) or ciprofloxacin (500 mg twice daily) for 14 days (Table 32.5).

The prevention of tularemia among hunters and other persons handling animals, animal hides, or carcasses is best achieved by the wearing of gloves, attention to hand hygiene, and avoidance of mucosal exposure. Laboratory technicians working with cultures or potentially infectious clinical material should use BSL-3 precautions, including facemasks, rubber gloves and biologic containment hoods. In the event of a laboratory spill or surface contamination, decontamination can be accomplished with ordinary bleach solution. Although over half a century of experience exists with investigational tularemia vaccines and a live vaccine strain has been administered by scarification to more than 5,000 persons with no significant adverse reactions, none are licensed in the United States at the time of this writing.[77]

RECOMMENDATIONS FOR FURTHER RESEARCH

While preparedness programs increase after actual events, such as the 2011 Amerithrax events, and many knowledge gaps described in the previous edition of this book as potentially problematic have been closed, continuing focused research on biological event management remains important.

As an example, the public health preparedness system in the United States has made many advances. The Strategic National Stockpile (SNS) has been further developed and is maintained by CDC. It contains stockpiles of large quantities of pharmaceutical and medical supplies that can be deployed throughout the United States in response to a bioterrorism attack or disaster. Diseases reported to public health authorities through laboratory surveillance, case reporting, and syndromic surveillance systems are integrated and monitored 24/7 nationally by CDC. The global SARS outbreak (2002–2003), H1N1 pandemic (2009), Ebola virus disease (2014–2015), as well as individual cases of diseases caused by other Category A agents (e.g., anthrax, plague, and tularemia), have all stressed the public system, leading to improvements in disease detection capabilities and public health emergency response systems.

Highly specialized laboratory facilities to conduct biodefense medical countermeasure research exist, many of which were not operational prior to the anthrax letter attacks in the fall of 2001. At the time of this writing, there are six operational BSL-4 (the highest level of biocontainment) laboratories in the United States: at CDC in Atlanta, Georgia; USAMRIID in Frederick, Maryland; the Southwest Foundation for Biomedical Research in San Antonio, Texas; the Center for Biodefense and Emerging Infectious Disease at the University of Texas Medical Branch at Galveston; the Center for Biotechnology and Drug Design at Georgia State University in Atlanta; and Rocky Mountain Laboratories Integrated Research Facility at the National Institute of Allergy and Infectious Diseases in Hamilton, Montana. Additional BSL-4 labs under construction include: Integrated Research Facility at the National Institute of Allergy and Infectious Disease in Fort Detrick; the Galveston National Laboratory of the University of Texas Medical Branch; the Battelle National Biodefense Institute (National Biodefense Analysis and Countermeasures Center) of the Department of Homeland Security in Fort Detrick; the National Bio- and Agro-Defense Facility of the Department of Homeland Security in Manhattan, Kansas;

the National Biocontainment Laboratory at Boston University in Massachusetts; and the Virginia Division of Consolidated Laboratory Services of the Department of General Services of the Commonwealth of Virginia in Richmond.

Despite these advances, vulnerabilities persist that would enable a bioterrorist to carry out a nefarious mission. During the twenty-first century, the threat from biological weapons and bioterrorism has become more complex because of increased biological agent variety, further development of laboratory-based scientific expertise, and the potential of in vitro genetic modification of these agents. Due to its bacteriological characteristics, etiology, and epidemiology, *B. anthracis* will likely always remain a pathogen of choice for many potential perpetrators. Potential terrorists may be motivated to focus on new types of viral and bacterial agents, with the increasing availability of relevant technology, materials, information, and expertise, along with publicity about potential vulnerabilities. Novel genetic engineering and other advances in biotechnology provide powerful capabilities to modify virtually any biological agent, so as to attempt to create enhanced agent virulence, increased environmental stability, resistance to medical countermeasures, and the defeat of physical barriers and biological detectors. In addition, readily obtained pathogens such as *Salmonella* and *Shigella* sp. could be used to cause illness in targeted populations, as has already occurred in deliberate foodborne contamination events.

Various government-funded initiatives with respect to biological agent detection, patient identification and treatment, and public health emergency response and mitigation have provided a higher level of preparedness than previously existed. However, as Thomas Jefferson said: "eternal vigilance is the price we pay for liberty."[78] Those measures to maintain and increase biological terrorism and public health preparedness will continue to be of primary importance to prevent, deter, and, if necessary, rapidly respond to a bioterrorism event or biological disaster.

Conclusion

Biological warfare has been a threat to humanity since antiquity and crude attempts at bioterrorism have been a concern for over a century. A renewed appreciation of the sinister potential of biological weapons resulted from the glasnost which followed the end of the Cold War and the migration of ex-Soviet scientists to the west. Similarly, an escalation of terrorist capabilities in the area of chemical and biological weapons was brought to public attention with Aum Shinrikyo's use of sarin in the Tokyo subway system, their attempts to use anthrax and botulinum toxin, the subsequent use of anthrax-contaminated letters in October 2001, and many other events. Needed preparedness efforts include analysis of the wide spectrum of surveillance initiatives; assessing efficacy of security and biosafety measures; further development of countermeasures; research and development; and improved intelligence gathering, public health preparedness, and education. Given the character of advances in scientific capabilities, the interconnectedness of world societies, and the nature of world events, all of these preparedness efforts need to continue for the foreseeable future.

REFERENCES

1. Derbes VJ. De Mussis and the great plague of 1348. A forgotten episode of bacteriological warfare. *JAMA* April 4, 1966; 196(1): 59–62.

2. Parkman F. *The Conspiracy of Pontiac and the Indian War after the Conquest of Canada*. vol. 2. Boston MA, Little, Brown, and Co, 1901.

3. Koenig R. *The Fourth Horseman: One man's secret campaign to fight the Great War in America*. New York: Public Affairs, 2006.

4. Hugh-Jones M. Wickham Steed and German biological warfare research. *Intell Natl Secur* 1992; 7: 379–402.

5. Harris S. Japanese biological warfare research on humans: a case study of microbiology and ethics. *Ann N Y Acad Sci* December 31, 1992; 666: 21–52.

6. Christopher GW, Cieslak TJ, Pavlin JA, Eitzen EM, Jr. Biological warfare. A historical perspective. *JAMA* August 6, 1997; 278(5): 412–417.

7. Carus W. *Bioterrorism and biocrimes: the illicit use of biological agents in the 20th century*. Washington, DC, National Defense University, 1999.

8. Protocol for the Prohibition of the Use in War of Asphyxiating, Poisonous or Other Gases, and of Bacteriological Methods of Warfare. Signed at Geneva June 17, 1925. http://www.un.org/disarmament/WMD/Bio/pdf/Status_Protocol.pdf (Accessed August 27, 2015).

9. Sims N. *The diplomacy of biological disarmament*. vol. 18. New York, St Martin's Press, 1988.

10. Army UDot. *US Army activity in the US biological warfare programs*. Washington, DC, U.S. Dept of the Army, February 24, 1977; 2.

11. Vorobjev A, Cherkassky B, Stepanov A, Kyuregyan Y, Fjedorov M. Key problems of controlling especially dangerous infections. Paper presented at: Proceedings of an International Symposium: Severe infection diseases: epidemiology, express-diagnostics and prevention. Kirov, Russia, 1997.

12. Alibek K, Handelman S. *Biohazard : the chilling true story of the largest covert biological weapons program in the world, told from the inside by the man who ran it*. 1st ed. New York, Random House, 1999.

13. Torok TJ, Tauxe RV, Wise RP, et al. A large community outbreak of salmonellosis caused by intentional contamination of restaurant salad bars. *JAMA* August 6, 1997; 278(5): 389–395.

14. Kolavic SA, Kimura A, Simons SL, Slutsker L, Barth S, Haley CE. An outbreak of Shigella dysenteriae type 2 among laboratory workers due to intentional food contamination. *JAMA* August 6, 1997; 278(5): 396–398.

15. Jernigan DB, Raghunathan PL, Bell BP, et al. Investigation of bioterrorism-related anthrax, United States, 2001: epidemiologic findings. *Emerg Infect Dis* October 2002; 8(10): 1019–1028.

16. *7 CFR Part 331, 9 CFR Part 121, 42 CFR Part 73*.

17. Atlas R. Biological weapons pose challenge for microbiology community. *ASM News* 1998; 64: 383–389.

18. *NATO Handbook on the Medical Aspects of NBC Defensive Operations (AmedP-6)* Departments of the Army, Navy, and Air Force, February 1996. http://fas.org/irp/doddir/army/fm8-9.pdf

19. Joshi D, Kumar D, Maini AK, Sharma RC. Detection of biological warfare agents using ultra violet-laser induced fluorescence LIDAR. *Spectrochim Acta A Mol Biomol Spectrosc* August 2013; 112: 446–456.

20. *Bioterrorism alleging use of anthrax and interim guidelines for management – United States, 1998*. MMWR, February 5, 1999; 48(4): 69–92.

21. *Health aspects of chemical and biological weapons*. Geneva, World Health Organization, 1970.

22. Rotz LD, Khan AS, Lillibridge SR, Ostroff SM, Hughes JM. Public health assessment of potential biological terrorism agents. *Emerg Infect Dis* February 2002; 8(2): 225–230.

23. CDC. Inhalation anthrax associated with dried animal hides – Pennsylvania and New York City, 2006. *MMWR* 2006; 55(10): 280–282.

24. CDC. Cutaneous anthrax associated with drum making using goat hides from West Africa – Connecticut, 2007. *MMWR* 2008; 57(23): 628–631.

25. Jernigan JA, Stephens DS, Ashford DA, et al. Bioterrorism-related inhalational anthrax: the first 10 cases reported in the United States. *Emerg Infect Dis* November–December 2001; 7(6): 933–944.

26. Sprenkle MD, Griffith J, Marinelli, W, Boyer AE, Quinn CP, Pesik NT, et al. Lethal factor and anti-protective antigen IgG levels associated with inhalation anthrax, Minnesota, USA. *Emerg Infect Dis* February 2014. http://dx.doi.org/10.3201/eid2002 .130245 (Accessed March 13, 2014).

27. Updated recommendations for antimicrobial prophylaxis among asymptomatic pregnant women after exposure to Bacillus anthracis. *MMWR Morb Mortal Wkly Rep* 2001; 50(43): 960.

28. CDC. Use of vaccine in the United States: Recommendations of the Advisory Committee on Immunization Practices (ACIP), 2009. *MMWR* 2010; 59(RR-6): 1–30.

29. CDC. Use of vaccine in the United States: Recommendations of the Advisory Committee on Immunization Practices (ACIP), 2009. *MMWR* 2010; 59(RR-6): 1–30.

30. Stern EJ, Uhde KB, Shadomy SV, Messonnier N. Conference report on public health and clinical guidelines for anthrax [conference summary]. *Emerg Infect Dis* April 2008. http://wwwnc .cdc.gov/eid/article/14/4/07–0969.htm (Accessed September 9, 2013).

31. Inglesby TV, O'Toole T, Henderson DA, et al. Anthrax as a biological weapon, 2002: updated recommendations for management. *JAMA* May 1, 2002; 287(17): 2236–2252.

32. Department of Health and Human Services. Biological Products; Bacterial Vaccines and Toxoids; Implementation of Efficacy Review; Anthrax Vaccine Adsorbed; Final Order. *Federal Register* 2005; 70(242): 75180–75198.

33. Biothrax™ (Anthrax Vaccine Absorbed). Prescribing information. Emergent Biosolutions, Rockville, MD. Revised May 2012. http://www.biothrax.com/prescribinginformation_ biothrax_us.pdf (Accessed August 27, 2015).

34. Use of anthrax vaccine in response to terrorism: supplemental recommendations of the Advisory Committee on Immunization Practices. *MMWR Morb Mortal Wkly Rep* 2002; 51(45): 1024–1026.

35. Fenner FHD, Arita I, Jezek Z, Ladnyi ID. *Smallpox and its eradication*. Geneva, World Health Organization, 1988.

36. Henderson DA, Inglesby TV, Bartlett JG, et al. Smallpox as a biological weapon: medical and public health management. Working Group on Civilian Biodefense. *JAMA* June 9, 1999; 281(22): 2127–2137.

37. Smith JA, Casey CG, Tierney BC. The ocular complications of smallpox and smallpox immunization. *Arch Ophthalmol* September 2004; 122(9): 1407; author reply 1407–1408.

38. Eeckels R, Vincent J, Seynhaeve V. Bone Lesions Due to Smallpox. *Arch Dis Child* December 1964; 39: 591–597.

39. Wehrle PF, Posch J, Richter KH, Henderson DA. An airborne outbreak of smallpox in a German hospital and its significance with respect to other recent outbreaks in Europe. *Bull World Health Organ* 1970; 43(5): 669–679.

40. Jezek Z, Szczeniowski M, Paluku KM, Mutombo M. Human monkeypox: clinical features of 282 patients. *J Infect Dis* August 1987; 156(2): 293–298.

41. Update: multistate outbreak of monkeypox – Illinois, Indiana, Kansas, Missouri, Ohio, and Wisconsin, 2003. *MMWR Morb Mortal Wkly Rep* July 11, 2003; 52(27): 642–646.

42. http://www.cdc.gov/ncidod/monkeypox/vaccineqa.htm (Accessed August 27, 2015).

43. Buller RM, Owens G, Schriewer J, Melman L, Beadle JR, Hostetler KY. Efficacy of oral active ether lipid analogs of cidofovir in a lethal mousepox model. *Virology* January 20, 2004; 318(2): 474–481.

44. *Acute, Generalized Vesicular or Pustular Rash Illness Testing Protocol in the United States*. Centers for Disease Control and Prevention, Atlanta, GA, 2006. http://www.bt.cdc.gov/agent/smallpox/ diagnosis/rashtestingprotocol-chart2.asp (Accessed August 27, 2015).

45. Beachkofsky TM, Carrizales SC, Bidinger JJ, Hrncir DD, Whitemore DE, Hivnor CM. Adverse events following smallpox vaccination with ACAM2000 in a military population. *Arch Dermatol* 2010; 146(6): 656–661.

46. *Smallpox Vaccine. Dried, Calf Lymph Type. Dryvax. Dried Smallpox Vaccine. Package Insert*. Philadelphia, Wyeth Pharmaceuticals, Inc., June 2007.

47. Casey CG, Iskander JK, Roper MH, et al. Adverse events associated with smallpox vaccination in the United States, January-October 2003. *JAMA* December 7, 2005; 294(21): 2734–2743.

48. Smallpox vaccination and adverse reactions: guidance for clinicians. *Ann Pharmacother* March 2003; 37(3): 467–468.

49. Grabenstein JD, Winkenwerder W, Jr. US military smallpox vaccination program experience. *JAMA* June 25, 2003; 289(24): 3278–3282.

50. Centers for Disease Control and Prevention. Supplemental recommendations on adverse events following smallpox vaccine in the pre-event vaccination program: recommendations of the Advisory Committee on Immunization Practices. *JAMA* April 23–30, 2003; 289(16): 2064.

51. Parrino J, Graham BS. Smallpox vaccines: Past, present, and future. *J Allergy Clin Immunol* December 2006; 118(6): 1320–1326.

52. Wittek R. Vaccinia immune globulin: current policies, preparedness, and product safety and efficacy. *Int J Infect Dis* May 2006; 10(3): 193–201.

53. Inglesby TV, Dennis DT, Henderson DA, et al. Plague as a biological weapon: medical and public health management. Working Group on Civilian Biodefense. *JAMA* May 3, 2000; 283(17): 2281–2290.

54. Dembek ZF, et al., eds. *Medical Management of Biological Casualties Handbook. The USAMRIID "Blue Book."* 7th ed. Fort Detrick, MD, USAMRIID, September 2011.

55. Perry RD, Fetherston JD. Yersinia pestis–etiologic agent of plague. *Clin Microbiol Rev* January 1997; 10(1): 35–66.

56. Sonnabend O, Sonnabend W, Heinzle R, Sigrist T, Dirnhofer R, Krech U. Isolation of Clostridium botulinum type G and identification of type G botulinal toxin in humans: report of five sudden unexpected deaths. *J Infect Dis* January 1981; 143(1): 22–27.

57. Barash JR, Tang TW, Arnon SS. First case of infant botulism caused by Clostridium baratii type F in California. *J Clin Microbiol* August 2005; 43(8): 4280–4282.

58. Aureli P, Fenicia L, Pasolini B, Gianfranceschi M, McCroskey LM, Hatheway CL. Two cases of type E infant botulism caused by neurotoxigenic Clostridium butyricum in Italy. *J Infect Dis* August 1986; 154(2): 207–211.

59. Passaro DJ, Werner SB, McGee J, Mac Kenzie WR, Vugia DJ. Wound botulism associated with black tar heroin among

injecting drug users. *JAMA* March 18, 1998; 279(11): 859–863.

60. Spika JS, Shaffer N, Hargrett-Bean N, Collin S, MacDonald KL, Blake PA. Risk factors for infant botulism in the United States. *Am J Dis Child* July 1989; 143(7): 828–832.

61. Arnon SS, Schechter R, Maslanka SE, Jewell NP, Hatheway CL. Human botulism immune globulin for the treatment of infant botulism. *N Engl J Med* February 2, 2006; 354(5): 462–471.

62. Borio L, Inglesby T, Peters CJ, et al. Hemorrhagic fever viruses as biological weapons: medical and public health management. *JAMA* 2002; 287: 2391–2405.

63. Snell NJ. Ribavirin–current status of a broad spectrum antiviral agent. *Expert Opin Pharmacother* 2001; 2: 1317–1324.

64. H. Rusnak, JM, Byrne WR, Chung KN, et al. Experience with ribavirin in the treatment of hemorrhagic fever with renal syndrome in Korea. *Antiviral Res* January 2009; 81(1): 68–76.

65. Mertz GJ, Miedzinski L, Goade D, et al. Placebo-controlled, double-blind trial of intravenous ribavirin for the treatment of hantavirus cardiopulmonary syndrome in North America. *Clin Infect Dis* 2004; 39: 1307–1313.

66. Gowen BB, Bray M. Progress in the experimental therapy of severe arenaviral infections. *Future Microbiol* December 2011; 6(12): 1429–1441.

67. McCormick JB, King I, Webb P, et al. Lassa fever: Effective therapy with Ribavirin. *N Engl J Med* 1986; 314: 20–26.

68. Cetron MS, Marfin AA, Julian KG, et al. Yellow fever vaccine. Recommendations of the Advisory Committee on Immunization Practices (ACIP). *MMWR* 2002; 51(RR-17): 1–11.

69. Dennis DT, Inglesby TV, Henderson DA, et al. Tularemia as a biological weapon, medical and public health management. *JAMA* 2001; 285: 2763–2773.

70. Rogozin II. Tularemia prevention during the Second World War. *Zh Mikrobiol Epidemiol Immunobiol* 1970; 47: 23–26.

71. Croddy E, Krcalova S. Tularemia, biological warfare, and the battle for Stalingrad (1942–1943). *Mil Med* 2001; 166: 837–838.

72. Alibek K. *Biohazard.* New York, Random House, 1999; 29–38.

73. Feldman KA, Enscore RE, Lathrop SL, et al. An outbreak of primary pneumonic tularemia on Martha's Vineyard. *New Engl J Med* 2001; 345: 1601–1606.

74. Feldman KA, Stiles-Enos D, Julian K, et al. Tularemia on Martha's Vineyard: Seroprevalence and occupational risk. *Emerg Infect Dis* 2003; 9: 350–354.

75. Rusnak JM, Kortepeter MG, Hawley RJ, et al. Risk of occupationally acquired illnesses from biological threat agents in unvaccinated laboratory workers. *Biosecur Bioterror* 2004; 2: 281–293.

76. Enderlin G, Morales L, Jacobs RF, Cross JT. Streptomycin and alternative agents for the treatment of tularemia: review of the literature. *Clin Infect Dis* 1994; 19: 42–47.

77. Marohn ME, Barry EM. Live attenuated tularemia vaccines: Recent developments and future goals. *Vaccine* 2013; 31: 3485–3491.

78. 4th July, 1817, 42d year. [Bennington]. *Vermont Gazette.* July 8, 1817; 2: "let your motto be 'eternal vigilance is the price we pay for liberty.'"

33

RADIATION ACCIDENTS AND THE MEDICAL MANAGEMENT OF ACUTE RADIATION INJURY

Richard J. Hatchett, David M. Weinstock, and Ronald E. Goans

OVERVIEW

Large-scale Radiation Events: An Evolving Risk

Mass exposure to radiation does not occur frequently. When it does, such events present significant logistical, operational, and medical challenges that may be compounded by a lack of familiarity among most first responders and healthcare personnel with the manifestations and management of radiation injury. It appears that the risk of deliberate mass exposures to radiation has increased in recent years due to the proliferation of nuclear states, the occurrence of at least one well-documented case of nuclear technology smuggling, the widespread availability of radioactive materials, and continuing concerns about the risk of nuclear or radiological terrorism. Additionally, there is an ever-present risk of accidental mass exposures, such as occurred after the Chernobyl accident and the Cesium 137 (^{137}Cs) dispersion event in Goiânia, Brazil.[1,2] The recent efforts of the United States and other nations to improve their capabilities to prevent or interdict nuclear smuggling, to enlarge the armamentarium of radiation countermeasures, and to disseminate information about the management of radiation casualties suggest the seriousness with which the threat of deliberate attack is regarded.[3] Numerous authors have summarized the publicly available information related to this threat, and the interested reader is referred to these sources for more detailed accounts.[4,5,6,7]

Scenarios of Concern

Mass exposures to radiation may be accidental or deliberate in origin. Heretofore, all such incidents have been the result of accidents, with the notable exceptions of the atomic bombings in Hiroshima and Nagasaki and the exposure of more than a hundred people to [210]Po in the wake of the Alexander Litvinenko poisoning.[7] The causes of accidental exposure have varied dramatically, ranging from criticality events or "excursions" (in which transient fission occurs) to the dispersion of radioactive materials (whether on a small or large scale) to the misadministration of radiation therapy. Selected incidents that represent the types of accidental exposures encountered, in terms of both causation and the radiation injury produced, will be discussed in detail later in this chapter. Presented here are the general features of such accidents. Many of the deliberate exposures that could occur as a consequence of terrorist acts are comparable in scope and effect to some of the accidents. Therefore, it is useful to summarize the nature of such threats. The threat of nuclear terrorism, however, is unique. The detonation of a moderate-sized (10–15 kiloton) device in a densely populated urban area would be similar to the bombings of Hiroshima and Nagasaki and likely result in tens of thousands of fatalities.

Criticality Accidents

Criticality accidents have occurred during the assembly or disassembly of nuclear weapons, the processing of solutions containing fissionable materials, and as a result of accidents within nuclear reactors.[8–12] Criticality accidents are typically associated with significant mixed field exposures (i.e., neutron and gamma radiation) but are not associated with blast or thermal injury. Such events do not directly result in contamination of the environment or geographically extensive exposures, and pose a threat mainly to workers in the immediate vicinity of the causative nuclear materials. Victims of some criticality accidents received exceptionally high doses (> 40 Gy), and these exposures were associated with highly accelerated mortality, with death occurring 1–7 days post-exposure.[9] The terms (Gy) and rad measure the radiation energy absorbed with 1 Gy equivalent to 100 rads. Since 1945, approximately sixty such accidents have occurred, not all of which have resulted in significant human exposures.[9] Mettler and colleagues cited eighteen known deaths from the acute radiation syndrome (ARS) caused by such accidents over this period.[12] Several of these accidents will be summarized at the end of this chapter.

Nuclear Power Plant Accidents

The explosion and subsequent fire in a graphite-moderated reactor at the Chernobyl nuclear power station on April 26, 1986, remains the most significant radiation accident in history, in terms of amount of radioactivity released, area affected, and number of people exposed. Approximately 50 megacuries of radioactivity (representing < 4% of the reactor's total radionuclide inventory) were released into the environment before the fire in the reactor was extinguished on May 6, 1986, resulting in serious contamination of local regions and trace contamination throughout Eastern and Western Europe. The primary contributors to the released radioactivity were radiocesiums and radioiodines. Within ten days of the accident, elevated levels of radioactivity were detected as far away as Israel, Kuwait, China, Japan, and the United States.[13] A summary of the salient features of the accident follow; the acute and long-term health effects of the accident have received comprehensive assessment elsewhere.[1]

The accident and subsequent release of radioactivity at Chernobyl were directly related to the design of the reactor, which had a water-cooled graphite core. In such reactors, graphite is used to moderate the chain reaction initiated by the decay of uranium 235 (^{235}U), slowing the emitted neutrons and increasing their propensity to strike other ^{235}U nuclei. Graphite is a very efficient moderator and offers two advantages over water, which can also be used as a moderator. First, it is so efficient that it can sustain fission in naturally occurring, unprocessed uranium. Water-moderated reactors require enrichment of ^{235}U from its natural 0.7% up to at least 3%. Second, graphite-moderated reactors produce more weapons-grade plutonium than water-moderated reactors, and the plutonium is easier to recover. Water has one major advantage over graphite: reactors using water as a moderator have a built-in fail-safe mechanism. Graphite-moderated reactors use water as a critical coolant to slow down and control the chain reaction. As such, a failure in the water cooling system can lead to an escalation of fission (as occurred at Chernobyl). The water in a water-moderated reactor directly facilitates the fission itself. Any change in conditions within the reactor resulting in increased fission and heat causes the water to boil, reducing its availability to serve as a neutron moderator, slowing down the chain reaction and reducing the temperature. Water-moderated reactors thus have a natural negative-feedback mechanism built into their design that functions independently of any human operator.[8] Reactor types and their governing regulations vary by country. For example, regulations in the United States require that all nuclear reactors use water as a moderator. Other regulations mandate broader shutdown margins, more robust containment structures, and more stringent procedural controls than were operative at Chernobyl.[13] These layered safety mechanisms are the basis of the common assertion that a Chernobyl-like accident could not occur in the United States.

There have been three other significant nuclear power plant accidents resulting in the release of radioactivity into the environment. The first, a fire in the graphite-moderated, air-cooled Windscale facility in Cumbria, England, in October 1957, resulted in the release of approximately 20,000 Ci of radioactive material into the surrounding countryside. The isotopes released were primarily iodine 131 (^{131}I), ^{137}Cs, and polonium 210 (^{210}Po). No acute injuries were attributed to the accident.[16] The second event involved a partial meltdown of the water-moderated Three Mile Island 2 reactor in March 1979 in the United States. This was attributed to a sequence of equipment malfunctions, design-related problems, and human errors. Although approximately half of the core melted in the accident, it did not result in a breach of the containment system. The amount of radiation released had trivial public health consequences, with the average dose to population in the area being about 1 millirem and the maximum doses estimated at less than 100 millirem. A CT scan, by comparison, can result in an effective dose of up to 1 rem or 10 mSv.[17] The terms rem and Sievert quantify the biological effect of radiation energy. One rem of injury is standardized to the effect from 1 rad of gamma exposure. One Sievert (Sv) equals 100 rem.

The third and most recent major accident occurred at the Fukushima Daiichi Nuclear Power Plant in Japan in the wake of the Tōhoku Earthquake and Tsunami on March 11, 2011. The disaster resulted in the sequential failure and partial meltdown of the three nuclear reactor units in operation at the time, leading to the atmospheric release of approximately 1,020 PBq ($\sim 2.75 \times 10^7$ Ci) of radioactive material, primarily as inert Noble gases ^{131}I, ^{137}Cs, and ^{134}Cs.[18] Japanese authorities implemented mandatory evacuations, established an exclusion zone in Fukushima prefecture, and placed restrictions on agricultural products, meat, and fish from certain areas in Fukushima and surrounding prefectures. No deaths or cases of ARS occurred as a result of the accident, which was the second largest on record. In 2013, a WHO Health Risk Assessment concluded that the radiation doses in Fukushima prefecture were well below the threshold for the deterministic effects of radiation exposure (i.e., acute injury) and were also too low to affect fetal development and the outcome of pregnancy. In the two most affected locations within Fukushima prefecture, the preliminary effective doses for the first year following the accident ranged from 12–25 mSv, which may be high enough to increase lifetime risks for leukemia and solid tumors (including thyroid cancer) over baseline rates, especially in younger individuals.[18,19]

In the United States, potential for the accidental release of spent nuclear fuel from temporary storage facilities has led to plans for the establishment of a centralized geological repository. Currently, more than 45,400 metric tons (50,000 short tons) of high-level nuclear waste and spent fuel are stored in pools or dry casks at seventy-two sites in thirty-three states.[20] Three-quarters of these locations are within 80 km (50 miles) of major population centers and more than 160 million people live within 120 km (75 miles) of a nuclear waste storage facility.[20]

Radionuclide Exposures

As described previously, nuclear power plant accidents leading to the release of radioactive materials could cause widespread environmental contamination with a variety of radionuclides. There are also numerous non-nuclear scenarios that could lead to the dispersion of radionuclides and the external or internal contamination and exposure of affected populations. External contamination is defined as deposition of radioactive material on body surfaces. Internal contamination occurs when radionuclides are inhaled, ingested, or injected. A form of this contamination type is called incorporation and results when radionuclides are used by cells to synthesize organic molecules. The incorporation of ^{131}I into thyroid hormone is an example. Three non-nuclear scenarios resulting in human exposures occurred in Lilo, Georgia; Goiânia, Brazil; and along the Techa River in Russia.

The accident in Lilo, Georgia, involved orphaned (abandoned) radiation sources that had been left behind at a civil defense training site by the Soviet Army when Georgia gained its independence in 1991. Between July 1996 and October 1997, eleven young military recruits presented for evaluation with nausea, headache, weakness, and skin lesions that evolved to ulceration and necrosis requiring prolonged medical care. Because they received medical care in a variety of facilities, recognition of the links between the cases and the location of the lost radiation sources was significantly delayed. Ultimately, investigators discovered multiple ^{137}Cs, cobalt 60 (^{60}Co), and radium 226 (^{226}Ra) sources during radiation surveys of the training facility. Apparently, the Georgian recruits found some of these sources and at least one was placed into the pocket of a soldier's winter jacket. It was evidently shared among several recruits who subsequently developed symptoms of radiation sickness.[22]

More widespread dispersion of radioactive material occurred as a result of an accident involving another orphan source in Goiânia, Brazil, in 1987. On September 13 of that year, two peddlers removed a medical teletherapy source containing 50.9 terabecquerels (TBq) (1,375 Ci) of ^{137}Cs from an abandoned radiotherapy clinic. They removed the rotating assembly of the device's shielding head and subsequently ruptured the source canister itself before selling the assembly containing the damaged source to the owner of a junkyard. This individual, noticing the blue glow emanating from the device, brought it home, where the cesium chloride salt it contained became widely dispersed. Sixteen days passed before health authorities recognized that a radiation exposure had occurred, during which time a significant number of homes, public places, and vehicles became contaminated. Disclosure of the accident produced a significant amount of public anxiety and ultimately almost 113,000 people out of a local population of approximately 1 million presented for screening. Eventually, 249 victims showed evidence of contamination and 49 required medical treatment. Four persons died as a result of the accident.[23]

During the period 1949–1956, exposures along the Techa River in the former Soviet Union occurred as a result of the continuous discharge of radiochemical waste [primarily strontium 90 (^{90}Sr) and ^{137}Cs] into the river from the Mayak weapons processing facility. The most significant exposures (up to 2 Gy/year for some individuals) occurred prior to 1952. Nearly 30,000 people were exposed, with an average effective equivalent dose of 320 mSv in the Chelyabinsk region and approximately 70 mSv in the Kurgan region. Inhabitants of villages along the upper Techa River were relocated over several years beginning in 1951. The affected populations have been followed medically since that time, now forming (with the atomic bomb survivors in Hiroshima and Nagasaki) one of the most important cohorts for the study of radiation carcinogenesis.[24]

These incidents varied tremendously in the duration and magnitude of the exposures that occurred. They provide valuable data regarding the possible scenarios that could result from the accidental or deliberate release of radionuclides into the environment in the future.

Radiotherapy and Industrial Radiography Accidents

Accidents may result from the failure of procedural safeguards against excess exposure during legitimate uses of radiation sources. Dozens of radiotherapy accidents, some involving hundreds of patients, have occurred in the last several decades, with several resulting in iatrogenic deaths. One incident, for example, caused by an error in maintenance of a linear accelerator in a radiotherapy clinic in Zaragoza, Spain, resulted in significant overexposure of twenty-seven patients with fifteen deaths. Another notable accident attributed to the miscalibration of a ^{60}Co teletherapy device in Costa Rica, resulted in the overexposure of at least 114 patients and 17 deaths.[26] Accidents at commercial irradiator facilities have occurred sporadically, typically involving one or at most a few individuals, and have occasionally resulted in fatalities.[27]

Terrorist Threat Scenarios

Authorities have frequently expressed concern that motivated terrorists could employ radioactive materials in attacks on civilian populations. Radiation sources are comparatively accessible and implementing many of the potential scenarios would not require a great deal of technical sophistication on the part of the perpetrators.

RADIOLOGICAL TERRORISM

A frequently discussed scenario is the detonation or deployment of a so-called radiological dispersion device. Such a device can disperse radioactive material overtly, as would be the case with the detonation of a "dirty bomb" (an improvised explosive device containing radioactive material). It could also be achieved covertly, as would be the case if radioactive materials were dispersed surreptitiously, perhaps through ventilation systems or through food and water supplies. Some experts have argued that the public health threat from dirty bombs relates mainly to the conventional explosives they contain, and that the effect from any radioactive materials dispersed by a dirty bomb would be minimal. Such experts have classified these devices as "weapons of mass disruption" rather than "weapons of mass destruction." Other authorities have disagreed, believing that such weapons, if properly constructed and delivered, would pose a significant radiation risk to affected civilian populations.[28,32]

The clandestine placement of a radiation source in environments where prolonged human exposure is likely (such as on airplanes, subways, or in movie theaters) could result in the irradiation of significant numbers before the hidden source (a "radiological exposure device") is discovered. In an unusual demonstration, Chechen rebels placed a ^{137}Cs radiation source in a Moscow park in 1995, then notified authorities. No one was harmed in this incident, which nevertheless remains one of the most well-known acts of radiological terrorism.[29]

NUCLEAR TERRORISM

The most ominous scenario involves the detonation of a nuclear weapon. Although it is unlikely that a terrorist group would ever have the wherewithal to establish a uranium enrichment program (such programs being phenomenally expensive and requiring a great deal of specialized equipment and technical expertise), it is not impossible that terrorists could acquire fissionable materials in sufficient quantities to fashion a crude nuclear device (a so-called improvised nuclear device). It is also theoretically possible that terrorists could obtain a device from a sympathetic, corrupt, or incompetent regime that possessed such weapons. The possibility that such illicit transfers might occur in the period immediately following the collapse of the Soviet Union inspired the U.S. Nunn-Lugar Cooperative Threat Reduction Program, which has helped secure and deactivate thousands of nuclear warheads since its inception in 1991.[30] More recently, the activities and Islamist sympathies of A. Q. Kahn, the "father" of Pakistan's nuclear weapons program, raised concerns about the possibility of al-Qaeda's obtaining a device.[31] In terms of casualties and economic costs, detonation of a nuclear weapon in an urban environment would dwarf the events of September 11, 2001. Although the likelihood of such an event is undoubtedly remote, the potential consequences have led many elected officials to regard nuclear terrorism as the single greatest threat to U.S. national security.[33]

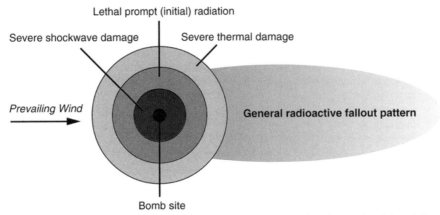

Figure 33.1. Flat-plain damage patterns from a ground-level nuclear detonation (viewed from above). The "cigar-shaped" fallout pattern is a simplification, as the fallout pattern will be determined by the direction and speed of upper-level winds at the time of the detonation.

Nuclear Detonation Effects

This section summarizes the prompt and delayed effects of fission explosions in the range of energy yields (10–15 kilotons) expected from an improvised nuclear device. Almost uniformly, nuclear security experts believe that the need for specialized and strictly controlled nuclear materials and highly sophisticated, industrial-level engineering capabilities preclude terrorists from obtaining, constructing, or using high-yield (megaton-range) thermonuclear devices. Consequently, the effects of these devices are not discussed here.

General Considerations

The yield of a nuclear detonation is described in terms of the conventional high explosive mass required to produce comparable effects. The typical explosive used as a reference is trinitrotoluene (TNT). The detonation of a 1 kiloton (kT) device generates 10^{12} calories and is equivalent to 1,000 metric tons of TNT. It releases neutrons and gamma radiation from the fissioning nuclei and heats the other weapon components to tens of millions of degrees.[34] This intense heat causes any matter in the immediate vicinity of the detonation to emit radiation, mainly in the form of X-rays, which heat the surrounding air. These X-rays produce an expanding sphere of heated gas, which in turn heats and vaporizes materials, releasing additional radiation for a considerable distance from the detonation point. The shock wave produced by the detonation topples or severely damages buildings, shatters windows, turns loose objects into projectiles, and causes profound trauma to persons in its path. Simultaneously, radioactive fission products and neutron-activated debris are propelled upward into the atmosphere by the explosion. This material ultimately deposits downwind of the detonation as radioactive fallout.

A nuclear detonation will produce two kinds of casualties: 1) victims with "prompt" injuries, reflecting the immediate blast, thermal, and radiation effects of the detonation; and 2) victims with radiation injuries occurring as a result of exposure to fallout. Although the regions associated with the prompt and fallout effects partially overlap, in general they demonstrate significant spatial separation (Figure 33.1).

Exposures to fallout after a nuclear detonation will vary according to distance, meteorological conditions, and available shelter. If the graphic depicted in Figure 33.1 represented a

Table 33.1. Estimated Dose Rates at Different Time Intervals at a Point 2.5 km Downwind from 10 kT Nuclear Detonation

Time Post-Detonation	Outdoor Exposure Rate from Fallout
1 min	300 Gy/min
15 min	0.25 Gy/min
120 min	0.03 Gy/min
480 min	0.001 Gy/min

10 kT ground detonation, fallout would arrive at a location 2.5 km downwind after approximately 1 minute. Estimated dose rates that might be measured 2.5 km downwind at different time intervals after the detonation are provided in Table 33.1.[34,35]

As Table 33.1 demonstrates, dose rates decline rapidly over time as fission products with a short half-life decay, so the importance of obtaining shelter cannot be overstated. Underground shelters can substantially reduce doses from fallout. However, if basement shelters are not available, sheltering away from the ground in the upper floors of buildings (assuming windows are intact and ventilation systems are off) can also provide enhanced protection when compared with ground-level shelters. The quality of a shelter's building materials influences the degree of protection it affords, with stone office buildings providing more shelter than a wood frame house.

Prompt Effects

Prompt effects are those occurring as a direct result (and within the first minutes) of the detonation. They encompass radiation, blast, and thermal effects, which are described briefly in the next sections.

Radiation Effects

Prompt radiation includes: 1) neutrons and gamma rays emitted as a direct result of fission; 2) alpha and beta particles and gamma radiation emitted by unstable fission products; and 3) radiation emitted by neutron-activated debris swept up into the fallout cloud from the immediate vicinity of the detonation.

Prompt radiation doses decline according to the inverse square law (doubling the distance from the detonation site reduces the dose by a factor of 4), but are sufficient to produce signs and symptoms of ARS at distances up to approximately 1.5 km from a 10-kT detonation. Within this radius, terrain and building structures may provide shielding from the thermal radiation but will not greatly attenuate the neutron and gamma radiation.

Blast Effects

The blast wave accounts for approximately 50% of the energy released by a nuclear detonation. Consequently, blast effects make the greatest single contribution to the immediate damage caused by the detonation. The blast wave moves outward from the point of detonation at supersonic velocity, generating winds of up to several hundred kilometers per hour. Injury and lethality due to blast effects are very difficult to predict because of the varied and complex mechanisms whereby the shock wave can interact with structures and people. Modeling suggests that many or most casualties receiving a prompt radiation dose exceeding a few hundred centigray (cGy) will probably die from blast effects.

Thermal Effects

Thermal radiation (heat) accounts for approximately 35% of the energy released by air bursts such as those at Hiroshima and Nagasaki (this percentage will be reduced if the detonation occurs at ground level). Thermal radiation will produce primary and secondary burn injuries: primary burns are caused by direct exposure to the thermal pulse; and secondary burns result from the incendiary effects of the radiation on flammable items. In certain environments, fire storms may ensue as individual fires coalesce. Modeling suggests that burns will be severe at distances of up to 1 km for a 1-kT burst and up to 3–4 km for a 10-kT detonation. Within these zones, burn lethality will be enhanced in victims experiencing blast and radiation effects.

Fallout

Ground bursts aerosolize more radioactive debris with a wider range of particle sizes than air bursts. The particles of larger size tend to fall sooner. Ground bursts thus produce more concentrated fallout in larger amounts than air bursts. Such fallout poses an extreme radiological hazard to downwind populations. The deposition of fallout will be heavily influenced by weather patterns and may not be uniform. Some areas ("hotspots") receive greater amounts than others as a result of local meteorological conditions.

FALLOUT COMPOSITION

Fission of nuclear weapons materials may generate more than 300 isotopes of thirty-six different elements, with each isotope having a unique specific activity and half-life. Precise fission yields are dependent on the involved isotope and the energy of the neutrons causing fission.[34,36] In addition to these fission products, the fallout cloud produced by a ground burst will carry a substantial amount of neutron-activated debris. Table 33.2 provides estimates of fission yields for some of the more prevalent elements produced from ^{235}U by slow neutrons (the combined yield exceeds 100% because each fission results in two products).[36] Elements listed by name only are represented by multiple isotopes. Due to the differential radioactive decay as the fallout cloud travels downwind, the isotopic composition of deposited fallout will change from location to location and over time.

Table 33.2. Yield of Fission Products

Element	Percentage Yield
Rubidium	7
^{90}Sr	5.8
Yttrium	24
Zirconium	12.5
Molybdenum	11.3
Iodine	21.7
^{135}Xe	6.5
^{137}Cs	6.2
Barium	12.6
Cerium	9.3

Most of the isotopes occurring in fission products emit beta particles, with a high percentage of these also emitting gamma radiation. Beta particles emitted by fallout can produce cutaneous burns when this radioactive material remains in contact with skin for extended periods. Beta burns were the most prominent clinical manifestation in Marshall Islanders after exposure to fallout in the early 1950s, for example. Because beta particles are not penetrating, however, beta exposure will not contribute significantly to bone marrow doses and thus will not produce many of the systemic features of radiation exposure. Gamma rays, which are penetrating, make the greatest contribution by far to bone marrow irradiation from fallout. Few if any of the fission products are alpha emitters. However, alpha emitters will be represented in fallout in the form of unfissioned ^{235}U or plutonium 239 (^{239}Pu). That being said, the radioactivity of the fission products is far greater in aggregate than the activity of the dispersed fissile material and constitutes a much greater threat to downwind populations. Neutron radiation is not a component of fallout.

Among the isotopes in fallout of greatest concern are ^{90}Sr, ^{137}Cs, and the iodine isotopes. ^{90}Sr has a long half-life, is concentrated in bones and teeth, and emits a high-energy beta particle. ^{137}Cs also has a long half-life, emits gamma rays, and behaves biologically like potassium (and thus can be passed up the food chain). The iodine isotopes, which have moderate half-lives (8 days for ^{131}I), are avidly taken up by the thyroid gland and produce a significant cancer risk in younger individuals.

Dynamic Dose Rates Due to Fission Product Decay

Doses and dose rates due to fallout reflect patterns of deposition and thus are heavily influenced by meteorological conditions and other factors. The behavior, and to some extent the composition, of fallout produced by a ground burst in an urban environment affected by microclimate features is difficult to model precisely. Table 33.3 gives approximate predicted radiation doses received by fully exposed individuals directly under the fallout plume at various distances from the point of detonation for the first hour following a 1- or 10-kT surface blast.[34,35] It is clear from the calculated doses that the initial dose rates produced by fallout are extremely high. The low doses at large distances will increase as the major part of the fallout plume passes overhead. Therefore, early evacuation and/or sheltering are

Table 33.3. Fallout Doses in First Hour

Range (km)	1 kT detonation (Sv)	10 kT detonation (Sv)
1	4,100	32,000
2	58	930
4	14	79
8	3.3	13
10	1.9	7.3
20	.12	.64
40	minimal	minimal

Table 33.4. Fallout Decay

Time after detonation (hours)	Percentage of dose rate at 1 hour
1	100
2	43
4	19
6	11
8	8
10	6
12	5

among the most important and effective strategies for reducing exposure.

Fortunately, most of the radioactive isotopes in fallout decay rapidly. Table 33.4 shows the rate of fallout decay, expressed as a percentage of the dose rate at 1 hour, during the first 12 hours following detonation.[35]

Because of the high early dose rates, the cumulative doses observed in exposed populations can still be quite large. Figure 33.2 shows estimated cumulative doses at different distances for fully and continually exposed populations for the first 24 hours following a detonation.[34,35] Such dose estimates are

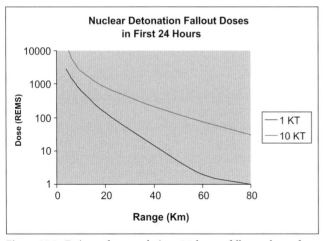

Figure 33.2. Estimated cumulative 24-hour fallout dose from HOTSPOT model.

Table 33.5. Shelter Dose Reduction Factors

Type of Shelter	Dose Reduction Factor
1 meter underground	0.0002
Frame house	0.3–0.6
Basement	0.05–0.1
Upper stories of apartment	0.01
Shelter with 0.6 meter earth cover	0.005–0.02

considered merely illustrative, as individuals almost certainly will move in and out of shelters and through areas with different degrees of fallout deposition during this time period.

Benefits of Shielding

The most effective way to reduce fallout exposure is evacuation. For a variety of reasons, this may be difficult to accomplish within the appropriate timeframe, especially in areas close to the detonation where fallout could reach the ground within minutes and the doses of radiation would be highest. Sheltering-in-place may be more feasible and can provide substantial protection against exposure. Table 33.5 shows the estimated dose reduction factors for different types of shelter.[34,35]

CURRENT STATE OF THE ART

Basics of Radiation Biology

Ionizing radiation exists in two forms: electromagnetic (gamma rays and X-rays) and particulate (alpha particles, beta particles, and neutrons). Both electromagnetic and particulate forms of ionizing radiation can contribute to the radiation injury sustained after accidental or deliberate exposures. Depending on the nature of the precipitating event, the radiation exposure for a given individual may be classified as localized or whole-body. In addition, when fallout or other radioactive substances are involved, internal or external deposition of these materials can result (causing radioactive contamination inside the human body or on its surface).

ARS encompasses a set of complex pathophysiological processes precipitated by exposure to high doses of radiation.[39] The latency, severity, and duration of the various manifestations of ARS are a function of the organ system affected, the radiation dose and dose rate, and the "quality" (particulate or electromagnetic) of the precipitating exposure. Much of the immediate damage at the cellular level caused by radiation is nonspecific, mediated through the generation of free radicals and peroxides. Nonspecific lipid peroxidation, DNA damage, and protein oxidation lead to alterations of gene transcription and messenger RNA translation as part of the cellular stress response. This promotes inflammation and other changes in the tissue microenvironment that contribute to cell death. In patients receiving sufficiently high doses of radiation, the resulting cellular, tissue, and organ damage can trigger a cascade of events leading to multi-organ failure and death. It is clear from both animal experiments and accidental high-dose exposures in humans that the kinetics of lymphocyte, neutrophil, and platelet depletion – and the time course of ARS symptoms in general – are accelerated at higher doses.

Knowledge of ionizing radiation's acute effects on human subjects has been derived from:

1. Animal studies;
2. Studies of Japanese populations exposed to radiation from atomic weapons;
3. Studies of normal tissue injury in patients receiving radiation therapy, typically for cancer; and
4. Accidents involving radiation workers, radiotherapy patients, and (rarely) civilian populations.

The relative value of the first data source is limited by inherent uncertainties regarding interspecies extrapolations. Studies of Japanese atomic bomb survivors have helped quantify the risk of subsequent malignancies and other delayed effects of radiation exposure. However, this population has provided less insight into ARS because little detailed clinical or laboratory data were collected immediately after the attacks. Radiation oncologists have gained extensive experience managing side effects in radiotherapy patients, but such patients are typically treated with fractionated and highly focal therapy, minimizing systemic impacts. In addition, these patients often receive cytotoxic chemotherapy in addition to radiation, so their clinical presentations may be complicated by effects from their primary disease or other concurrent therapy. Thus, it has been difficult to use this clinical experience to develop protocols for the management of ARS.

The most reliable information about ARS is derived from victims of radiation accidents. Not surprisingly, accidental exposures have been highly variable, ranging from alpha emitter inhalation in plutonium production and processing facilities to mixed gamma/neutron field exposures produced by criticality accidents. The largest and most contemporary cohort of patients with ARS consists of Chernobyl emergency workers who received exposures in the deterministic range (doses high enough to produce acute injury). These workers were subjected to the combined effect of radiation from several sources: 1) short-term external gamma/beta radiation from the gas emission cloud in the immediate area surrounding the reactor at the time of the explosion; 2) external gamma/beta radiation of decreasing intensity, from fragments of the damaged reactor core scattered over the site; 3) inhalation of gases and aerosol dust particles containing a mixture of radionuclides reflecting the isotope inventory of the reactor core at the time of the accident; and 4) deposition of these particles on the skin and mucous membranes.[37] Few of these accidents have been good surrogates for the types of exposures that would occur following detonation of a nuclear device or the deposition of fallout. A notable exception was the accidental exposure of Marshall Island inhabitants to fallout from the detonation of a nuclear device in 1954. Estimates of exposure prior to evacuation were less than 2 Gy in the most severely irradiated, with beta burns and mild depression of blood counts being the predominant acute effects.[38]

An estimate of the gamma radiation dose that is lethal to 50% of the population within 60 days of exposure is known as the $LD_{50/60}$. It ranges from approximately 350 cGy for unsupported adults to 600–700 cGy in persons receiving extensive supportive care, including antimicrobials and blood product transfusions.[39] In medically austere environments, or in the presence of combined injuries, the $LD_{50/60}$ will likely decrease substantially. For example, it has been estimated that the $LD_{50/60}$ for victims of the atomic bombings was approximately 220 cGy.[39,40]

Determinants of Biological Effects

DOSE RATE

The frequency and dosage fractionation (amount administered during any one exposure) with which radiation is delivered is an important determinant of the overall biological effects. This fact is exploited by radiation oncologists who seek to maximize tumor destruction while minimizing normal tissue injury by administering the prescribed radiation to target tissues in a series of small doses delivered daily over several weeks. In terms of lethality, studies in small animals have demonstrated that for continuous exposures, the gamma/x-ray $LD_{50/30}$ declines as dose rates increase.[43] For example, Neal found that the $LD_{50/30}$ in mice declined from 1,100 cGy to 790 cGy as the dose rate increased from 2.5 cGy/min to 706 cGy/min.[42] These findings are generally consistent with observations in humans, although it has not been possible to test this hypothesis systematically.

RADIATION QUALITY

The quality of radiation received (alpha, beta, gamma, or neutrons) is an important determinant of the biological effects observed for a given dose. Neutron radiation, for example, is more penetrating than alpha or beta radiation but less penetrating than gamma radiation. Because neutrons are comparatively heavy particles with a moderate degree of penetration, neutron radiation has a high relative biological effectiveness (RBE). In other words, they cause a greater degree of injury than other types of radiation with the same energy. The RBE in canines for an exposure with a mixed radiation field having a neutron-gamma ratio of 5.4:1 is about 1.7 (i.e., the ratio of the $LD_{50/30}$ with gamma radiation alone to the $LD_{50/30}$ of the mixed field is 1.7:1).[44,45] Consistent with the higher RBE observed for neutrons, increasing the neutron-gamma ratio at a fixed exposure (increasing the neutron component of the radiation while holding the energy level constant) has been shown to accelerate and prolong the suppression of white blood cell (WBC) counts.[43] The effect of increasing fractions of fission neutrons on survival in rodents with and without combined injuries is illustrated in Figure 33.3.

Alpha particles, which consist of two protons and two neutrons (and thus are identical to the nucleus of a helium atom),

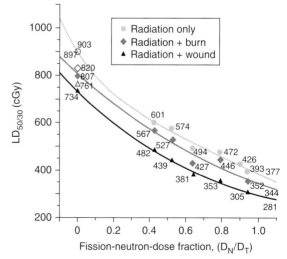

Figure 33.3. Effect of fission-neutron dose fraction on LD_{50} in mice. Data provided by the Armed Forces Radiobiology Research Institute.

are charged and relatively heavy. They interact intensely with atoms in materials they encounter, dissipating their energy over a very short range. As such, they are not highly penetrating and adequate shielding against alpha particles can be provided by a single sheet of paper. External exposures do not represent a significant hazard. However, their RBE is substantially greater than that of gamma rays because they are highly ionizing and they can significantly damage cells and tissues if taken internally.

Beta particles are electrons emitted from the nucleus of a radionuclide by the decay of a neutron into a proton, an electron, and an antineutrino. The energy of the ejected beta particle can vary. Some energetic beta particles may penetrate tens of millimeters into the skin and thus pose both an external and an internal hazard. "Beta burns" are characteristic of exposure to fallout, which contains a high number of beta-emitting radionuclides.[34,40,46]

Differences in radiation quality may have implications for the development of radiation countermeasures. Neutrons, for example, are more likely to cause damage by direct effects on cellular macromolecules than gamma radiation (which mediates its effects indirectly through the generation of free radicals). Consequently, fission-spectrum neutrons appear to be significantly more mutagenic and thus potentially more carcinogenic than gamma radiation. In hybrid B6CF$_1$ mice, a 97% neutron exposure of 150 cGy is approximately equivalent in mutagenic potential to 750 cGy of ^{60}Co gamma rays. For this strain of mice, amifostine administered prior to neutron exposure had a dose reduction factor (DRF) of 1.4 for mutagenic endpoints, whereas for gamma exposures, the DRF was 2.4.[47] Therefore the radiation-induced biological impact was reduced for a given neutron dose by 1.4 and for a given gamma dose by 2.4.

PHYSIOLOGICAL VARIABLES

Cells are most sensitive to ionizing radiation during mitosis. One of the chief determinants of individual tissue sensitivity (and thus of organs) is the rapidity of cell division occurring at the time of irradiation. Consequently, tissues with high rates of cellular turnover, such as bone marrow and the gastrointestinal epithelium, are exquisitely sensitive to radiation while tissues with low rates of turnover (e.g., muscle, kidney) are intrinsically radioresistant.

In individuals, specific genetic defects that cause impaired DNA damage recognition and repair, such as mutations in the ATM (ataxia-telangiectasia mutated) or NBS1 (Nijmegen breakage syndrome) gene loci, are associated with profound hypersensitivity to ionizing radiation and a predisposition to malignancy.[48,49] These and other genetic lesions associated with radiosensitivity are extremely rare. Most of the variability observed in radiosensitivity between individuals is not currently understood and does not appear to result directly from known single nucleotide polymorphisms or other genetic defects.

Studies (primarily in rodents) on the contribution of physiological variables to radiosensitivity demonstrate that significant differences are observed between animal strains in this regard, confirming that complex genetic factors are important determinants of radiation injury. Age and sex also appear to account for observed differences in the lethality of radiation exposures, with animals at the extremes of age and females exhibiting lower LD$_{50/30}$ values.[24,26,51,52] Whether such variables influence outcomes after acute exposures for large animals or humans has not been determined.

Biodosimetry and Radiological Triage

Cytogenetic Biodosimetry

The major determinants of clinical outcome following an acute radiation exposure are the dose received by the affected individual and the section of the body that is irradiated. Estimating this dose (in a process termed "biodosimetry") thus becomes a critical part of clinical management of such individuals.[53]

Prior to 1960, determination of dose relied on reconstruction of the accident. This included health physics studies, time and motion simulation, and analysis of any physical dosimeters that might have been present. Medical management was reactive, heavily weighted toward clinical response to the evolution of various ARS characteristics or of acute local cutaneous injury.

Over the next 50 years, many biodosimetry techniques that have been evaluated. However, the gold standard for radiation dose estimation remains the measurement of cytogenetic changes evaluated by the lymphocyte metaphase-spread dicentric assay (Figure 33.4). This test utilizes dividing lymphocytes arrested in metaphase. The number of chromosomes with 2 centromeres (dicentrics) is counted and this yields an accurate estimate of the radiation dose. The dicentric chromosome assay has been extensively developed and harmonized to international standards. However, the assay remains both time-consuming and labor intensive. Therefore, less precise techniques have been developed that enable the treating physician to estimate the relative magnitude of a patient's exposure relatively quickly and with some degree of confidence. The early initiation of therapy based on such techniques may offer critical benefits, as studies indicate that the likelihood of survival can be significantly increased with appropriate aggressive medical intervention and care.[54,55]

For acute triage after a radiation event, some authorities have recommended that medical personnel rely heavily on

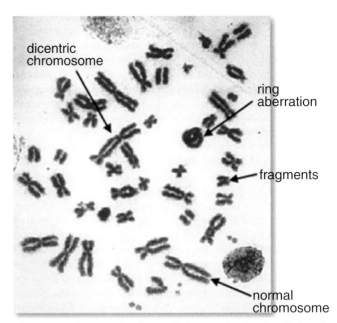

Figure 33.4. Cytogenetic abnormalities noted after irradiation in peripheral blood lymphocytes of a patient exposed to high-dose radiation. Dicentric chromosomes and ring abnormalities are relatively radiation-specific and are characteristic of changes observed. Used with permission from REAC/TS.

Table 33.6. Proposed Biodosimetry Technique as a Function of Expected Dose BM = bone marrow; GI = gastrointestinal; PCC = premature chromosome condensation. Used with permission from NATO/RTO and Prasana

Dose Range (Gy)	Proposed Validated Dosimetry Method	Prodromal Effects	Manifest Symptoms	Survival Expectancy
0.1–1	Dicentrics/PCC	none to mild (1–48 h)	none to slight decrease in blood count	almost certain
1.0–3.5	Lymphocyte depletion kinetics/dicentrics/PCC	mild to moderate (1–48 h)	mild to severe bone marrow damage	0–10% death
3.5–7.5	Lymphocyte depletion kinetics/PCC	severe (1–48 h)	pancytopenia, mild to moderate GI damage	10–100% death within 2–6 weeks
7.5–10.0	Lymphocyte depletion kinetics/PCC	severe (<1 h–48 h)	combined BM and GI damage	90–100% death within 1–3 weeks
>10.0	PCC	severe (minutes to <48 h)	GI, neurological, cardiovascular damage	100% death (within 2–12 days)

clinical signs, lymphocyte kinetics, the time to emesis, and cytogenetic biodosimetry.[55–58] The Biological Dosimetry Team at the U.S. Armed Forces Radiobiology Research Institute (AFRRI) has developed a multi-parameter triage scheme that provides an immediate statistical evaluation of dose.[59] These techniques have been incorporated into a diagnostic computer algorithm called the Biodosimetry Assessment Tool (BAT). It and related decision support tools are available online at http://www.afrri.usuhs.mil/ outreach/biodostools.htm. The algorithms developed for these tools are also the basis for the online dose estimators maintained on the U.S. National Library of Medicine's Radiation Emergency Medical Management (REMM) website (http://www.remm.nlm .gov/ars_wbd.htm).

Harmonized international protocols have been established for the conventional lymphocyte metaphase-spread dicentric assay, which has been used over several decades to guide the management of victims with severe radiation overexposure. Another cytogenetic test, the premature chromosome condensation (PCC) assay, may offer certain advantages over conventional metaphase-spread chromosome-aberration biodosimetry techniques.[60–70] The latter techniques are robust, but as mentioned previously, they are laborious and time-consuming.

For potential high-dose irradiation above the median lethal dose, it is expected that radiation-induced cell death and delay in cell cycle progression into mitosis will interfere with dose estimation. To overcome this limitation, quantitative analysis of radiation-induced damage may be performed using resting peripheral lymphocytes in lieu of metaphase spreads. Use of interphase cytological assays, such as the PCC assay, can eliminate the inherent problems associated with the use of metaphase-spread cytogenetic assays. The PCC assay requires only a small amount of blood (0.5 ml) and chromosomal damage may be visualized within a few hours after obtaining the blood sample. A modification of the PCC assay, the interphase-based rapid interphase chromosome aberration (RICA) assay, is a simple alternate to the metaphase-spread based dicentric analysis. In the RICA assay, damage involving specific chromosomes is examined in chemically induced PCC spreads after fluorescence in situ hybridization (FISH) with specific whole-chromosome DNA hybridization probes. The use of FISH greatly expands the dose range over which the PCC technique can be used and facilitates the recognition of chromosome exchange aberrations.[62] In

summary, PCC techniques are reliable at a wide range of doses. The assay may be used to characterize low dose exposures as well as life-threatening acute high doses of both electromagnetic (gamma rays) and particle (neutrons, alpha) radiation.[60,70] In addition, PCC assays can discriminate between total and partial-body exposures.

Radiation experts have suggested that the dicentric assay could be adapted for the triage of mass casualties.[64,65,66,69] Lloyd and colleagues described an *ex vivo* simulation of an accident with mass casualties receiving whole- or partial-body irradiation in the 0–8 Gy range. Faced with a hypothetically urgent need for rapid results, clinical triage was accomplished by scoring as few as 20 metaphase spreads per subject, compared with the typical 500 to 1,000 spreads scored in routine analyses. In such a situation, twenty cells could be scored per person initially, and a preliminary dose communicated to the treating physicians. If the patient's clinical symptoms suggested a dose significantly higher than the preliminary estimate, the assessment could be improved by scoring up to fifty cells. Using the dicentric assay in this triage mode, a throughput of 500 or more samples per week per laboratory may be feasible.[67] WHO has performed surveys of the capabilities and needs of member nations with respect to cytogenetic biodosimetry. A European network for biological dosimetry has been created to strengthen regional emergency preparedness and response capabilities for a large-scale nuclear accident or radiological emergency.[66,69,70] Similar proposals have been made to create a comparable network in North America, but no such organization exists to date. Table 33.6 lists current AFRRI recommendations on the type of definitive biodosimetry to use when a preliminary estimate of a given dose has been obtained.[60,70]

Several new approaches to biodosimetry are under investigation that utilize either changes in the transcriptome or proteome of peripheral blood in response to radiation. These may offer greater throughput, assuming the availability of equipment for processing large numbers of samples in parallel. For example, Meadows et al.[86] developed gene expression signatures for radiation exposure in mice and demonstrated that genotype differences did not affect the accuracy of the signatures to predict radiation exposure. The signatures could completely distinguish the response to sepsis from radiation response. In addition, human peripheral blood signatures of radiation

Table 33.7. Selected Use of Acute Phase Cytogenetic Assays in Radiation Accidents

Accident Location	Year of Accident	Number of People Exposed	Dicentrics (Chromosomal Abnormalities)	PCC
Cuidad Juarez, Mexico[71]	1984	7?	7?	N/A
Chernobyl, Russia[72]	1986	116,000	158	N/A
Goiânia, Brazil[73]	1987	250	129	N/A
Lilo, Georgia[74]	1986–1987	multiple	4	N/A
Kiisa, Estonia[75]	1994	4	4	N/A
Istanbul, Turkey (multiple cases)[64]	1995	21	21	?18
Tokaimura, Japan[77–79]	1999	3	1	3
		unknown	43	
Meet Halfa, Egypt[80]	2000	7	5	N/A
Bangkok, Thailand[81]	2000	28?	28	28
Ghent, Belgium[82]	2005	1	1	1
Referral Laboratory – incident summary[73]	2003–2005	23	18	uncertain
Referral Laboratory – incident summary[83,84]	1968–2003	996	996	uncertain
Cytogenetic Reference Standards[68,69,83,84,85]	2002–2014	uncertain		
Acute Phase Dosimetry[53,69,83,86]	2002–2014	uncertain		

exposure and chemotherapy treatment differed and could identify patients exposed to radiation with 90% accuracy.

Historical Experience with Early Phase Acute Biodosimetry

Table 33.7 (adapted from Reference 49) lists selected radiation accidents where the dicentric and PCC biodosimetry techniques have played an important role in the clinical management of radiological casualties. More detailed summaries of some notable applications of the techniques are provided in the next section.[71–79]

Cytogenetic study results from the 1986 Chernobyl accident have been summarized.[72] Investigators used chromosomal aberration dosimetry in the acute phase of the Chernobyl accident as a method of dose assessment. A good clinical correlation was observed between doses calculated based on chromosomal aberrations (dicentrics) and severity of ARS.

Soon after the Chernobyl accident, a radiation accident involving a ^{137}Cs therapy source occurred in Goiânia, Brazil, in September 1987. More than fifty individuals received moderate to high doses (0.2–7 Gy) of gamma radiation. A cytogenetic technique (i.e., frequencies of dicentrics and rings in peripheral lymphocytes) was employed in the acute phase to estimate absorbed dose.[73] Ramalho and Nascimento have described a follow-up study in which they found a two-log decline in the dicentric lymphocyte frequency. They reported an average disappearance half-time of lymphocytes containing dicentric and centric rings of approximately 130 days, which is significantly shorter than the value of 3 years usually cited in the literature.[73]

The radiation accident at Tokai-mura in 1999 is a famous and well-studied uranium criticality accident. It is an important event because it was witnessed, allowing careful reconstruction of the event, and because multi-parameter triage techniques were employed in the acute phase medical management of the victims. Despite the very high radiation doses received by two of the victims (approximately 8 and 20 Gy, respectively), the frequency of chromosome aberrations in circulating lymphocytes was found to be a reliable indicator of the absorbed radiation dose. Chromosome-painting techniques were found to be accurate in the evaluation of both dicentrics and translocations.[77–79]

Table 33.8 presents a comparison between various acute phase techniques for this criticality event. All table entries represent data contemporaneous with acute patient care and not from a retrospective analysis. Lymphocyte kinetics and the time to emesis were evaluated in real-time, and the results of chromosome biodosimetry were available quickly enough to impact clinical decisions when taken in the context of the patients' evolving ARS. These different techniques provided useful and generally consistent dose estimates that allowed meaningful inferences about each patient's prognosis. The proceedings from a Tokai-mura-related symposium is available that includes a retrospective

Table 33.8. Acute Phase Estimates of Dose (Gy) after the Tokai-mura Event (1999)

Method	Patient O	Patient S	Patient Y
Na-24 blood (n only)	9.1	5.0	1.2
Rings + dicentrics	21	6.6	2.8
PCC (γ equivalent)	>20	7.8	2.6
Na-24 WBC			1.6
Lymphocyte kinetics	>10	6–10	1–4.5
Survival	Death 82 days post-exposure	Death 210 days post-exposure	Survival

Table 33.9. Selected Use of Acute Phase Electron Paramagnetic Resonance (EPR) in Radiation Accidents. A Radioactive Exposure Device (RED) is a bare radioactive source emitting external radiation

Place of Accident	Date	Type of Accident	Materials
United States[88–92]	1991	Accelerator; various radiation accidents	EPR (bone; digits)
San Salvador[88]	1991	^{60}Co irradiator	EPR (bone; femur)
Tammiku, Estonia[91]	1994	RED	Thermoluminescence or TL (quartz pots) EPR (sugar samples)
Georgia[82]	2001	RED	EPR (bone; vertebra, ribs)
Review of General and Combined Acute Phase Accident Dosimetry[53,78–81]	2005	Overview of Acute Phase Dosimetry	

improved analysis of the source term, power spectra, and medical treatment in this accident.[87]

Electron Paramagnetic Resonance Physical Dosimetry

Electron paramagnetic resonance (EPR) or electron spin resonance spectroscopy is a technique for studying chemical species that have one or more unpaired electrons. Paramagnetic centers (molecules or atoms with unpaired electrons) are produced by the action of radiation on materials. The paramagnetic centers created by ionizing radiation are proportional to the absorbed dose and EPR can be used as a non-destructive probe of the structure and concentration of these paramagnetic centers. In the EPR measurement, irradiated materials are placed in a magnetic field of the appropriate frequency (typically in the GHz range). Electron spin transitions are induced by exposure to this field and then quantitated.

Electron paramagnetic resonance differs from nuclear magnetic resonance in that EPR measures excited electron spins rather than the spins of atomic nuclei. Most stable molecules have all their electrons paired and thus are not detected by EPR techniques, which are sensitive only to paramagnetic species. From the perspective of biological dosimetry, this limitation is actually an advantage in that ordinary chemical solvents and matrices do not give rise to EPR spectra. Thus, the EPR technique is one of great specificity. Bone and teeth have been found to provide the EPR signals of greatest stability, and so serve as natural physical dosimeters.

EPR dosimetry has been used primarily in the retrospective analysis of radiation accidents and is quite valuable in this regard. It is particularly helpful in events where an amputation has occurred and bone fragments are available from a site of severe local irradiation. These samples are often obtained after surgical amputation days to weeks post-accident. Table 33.9 presents selected cases where EPR has been useful in radiation accidents.

EPR has received increased consideration as a health physics and medical tool for the acute phase analysis of radiation incidents. In the United States, various reports are available describing accelerator accidents and cases of severe, acute, local injury in which EPR dosimetry has been performed.[88–93] A 1991 San Salvador accident involving a ^{60}Co source was characterized by significant heterogeneity of exposure, with the highest doses being delivered to the feet and lower legs of the victims. Desrosiers presented a detailed EPR analysis of a femur available from that accident.[92] Evaluation of the multi-casualty radiation accident

in Lilo, Georgia, employed EPR techniques to analyze vertebra and rib samples removed from a victim for medical reasons to reconstruct the dose received by this individual.[93]

In the 1994 radiation accident in Tammiku, Estonia, three brothers stole a large ^{137}Cs source from a poorly guarded radioactive waste depository and took it to their home. Various members of the family were exposed to this source in a chronic and non-uniform manner. In particular, the most severely injured patient received 1,830 Gy to the femur and thigh, and an approximately 4 Gy acute whole-body dose. He soon died of multi-organ failure. Other members of the family received a 0–4 Gy whole-body dose over 28 days and up to a 20–30 Gy acute local dose to the hands. This case is interesting because various acute phase modalities were employed in dose reconstruction: 1) chromosome aberration dicentric analysis; 2) Glycophorin A somatic mutation assays; 3) thermoluminescence dosimetry; 4) optically stimulated luminescence; 5) EPR; 6) chemiluminescence; and 7) Monte Carlo modeling of spatial effects. The use of EPR in this event was a valuable adjunct to clinical analysis of the ARS and of acute local injury.[94,95]

Acute Radiation Syndrome

General Considerations

ARS or "radiation sickness," occurs when individuals are exposed over a short time period to high energy penetrating radiation with doses of ≥ 1 Gy to the whole body.[99–101] Significant partial body exposures can also result in the development of ARS. ARS affects multiple organ systems. Symptoms associated with dysfunction of different organ systems will predominate at varying doses. The most frequently recognized components of ARS are the hematopoietic, gastrointestinal, and neurovascular syndromes, which result from cellular dysfunction or cell death within each of these tissue compartments. Cutaneous injury from trauma, radiation and/or thermal burns is also frequently encountered in radiation accidents. The so-called cutaneous radiation syndrome, where cutaneous injury is solely attributable to radiation exposure, represents a clinical entity distinct and separate from systemic ARS. In other cases, radiation exposure in conjunction with trauma or thermal injury will directly impact multiple organs, resulting in a "radiation combined injury." This extremely complicated physiological state is associated with high mortality and the multi-organ failure syndrome. The complexities presented by individual patients notwithstanding, categorizing the syndromes is still useful, both

Table 33.10. Phases of Radiation Injury (Adapted from Reference 86)

Dose (Gy)	Prodromal Phase	Manifest Phase	Prognosis without Supportive Care
0.5–1.0	Mild	Modest decline in blood counts	Survival
1.0–2.0	Mild to Moderate	Some bone marrow damage	Survival > 90%
2.0–3.5	Moderate	Moderate to severe bone marrow damage	Probable survival
3.5–5.5	Severe	Severe bone marrow damage; modest GI damage	Death within 3.5–6 weeks (50% of victims)
5.5–7.5	Severe	Pancytopenia and moderate GI damage	Death probable within 2–3 weeks
7.5–10.0	Severe	Severe GI and bone marrow damage	Death probable within 2 weeks
>10.0	Severe	Severe GI damage, radiation-induced lung injury, altered mental status; at higher doses (>20.0 Gy), cardiovascular collapse, fever, shock	Death within 2 weeks

for discussion purposes and because such categorizations enable the clinical team to identify the most life-threatening injuries and make better triage and management decisions. A recent review is available of ARS and irradiated victim triage in a military environment.[100,101]

In the absence of cutaneous or non-radiation related injuries, ARS follows a relatively predictable (or deterministic) course for each of its constituent syndromes. The hematopoietic syndrome is associated with the lowest threshold dose and the neurovascular syndrome is seen at the highest dose (Table 33.10). In general, the severity of ARS is directly proportional to dose, while the timing of symptom onset is inversely proportional. For example, ARS has a hematological threshold dose of about 0.7 Gy with severe reductions in blood counts occurring above 3 Gy.[9] As previously noted, the $LD_{50/60}$ for persons receiving no supportive care is about 3.5 Gy. This is primarily due to infection in the setting of neutropenia or hemorrhage in the setting of thrombocytopenia. The $LD_{50/60}$ increases to 6–7 Gy with optimal supportive care (e.g., antibiotics, hematopoietic growth factors, and transfusions). Human mortality resulting from hematological insult has a peak incidence at about 30 days but continues through day 60. Since humans recover from hematological damage more slowly than other mammals, an $LD_{50/60}$ (lethal to 50% of the population within 60 days of exposure) is used, in contrast to the $LD_{50/30}$ for animals.[39] A marked reduction in both the $LD_{50/60}$ and the time from radiation exposure to death would likely occur following a nuclear detonation. This is due to the complex patterns of ARS, radiation combined injury, and cutaneous radiation syndrome that would occur.

Clinical Progression
PRODROMAL PHASE

In terms of its temporal progression, ARS is divided into four sequential phases: prodromal, latent, manifest (illness), and recovery or death. These stages are described in detail. As listed in Table 33.11, a variety of symptoms and signs that characterize the prodromal phase may result within minutes to hours after radiation exposure, depending on the dose received. These symptoms and signs can be divided into two main groups: gastrointestinal and neuromuscular. The gastrointestinal symptoms include vomiting, diarrhea, intestinal cramps, dehydration, and anorexia, while the neuromuscular symptoms include fever, sweating, headache, hypotension, apathy, and easy fatigability.[100] The prodromal symptoms indicative of doses fatal to 50% of the population are nausea, vomiting, anorexia, and easy fatigability.

The presence of initial fever, headache, immediate vomiting and diarrhea, hypotension, and/or disorientation after exposure portends a fatal outcome. As a guideline, persons who vomit within 2 hours of irradiation are at risk for at least moderate ARS. However, one should be cautious as it is difficult to distinguish radiation-induced vomiting from emesis due to psychological factors resulting from environmental stressors.

LATENT PHASE

The latent stages of ARS (Table 33.12) are characterized by a relatively asymptomatic period. With a 2–3 Gy exposure, the prodromal symptoms abate after a few days and the latent period ensues for 2–3 weeks with continued declines in lymphocytes, neutrophils, and platelets. When the dose is high enough to induce the gastrointestinal and neurovascular forms of ARS, the latent phase is shortened or frequently eliminated, respectively.

MANIFEST (ILLNESS) PHASE

During this stage (Table 33.13) the tissue compartments that are damaged become dysfunctional, thereby dictating the form of ARS. At very high doses (e.g., 100 Gy) all organ systems are severely compromised and death quickly ensues from neurovascular dysfunction.

RECOVERY OR DEATH

Recovery or death follows the manifest (illness) phase. At higher doses, the time to recovery can be prolonged, with substantial residual deficits due to late fibrosis and other complications. Patients receiving high doses may experience other delayed effects of acute radiation exposure, such as radiation pneumonitis, radiation nephropathy, cataracts, and cognitive decline.[39,99,100]

Acute Hematopoietic Syndrome

The hematopoietic syndrome is usually encountered with doses that exceed 2 Gy, although the dose thresholds may be lower under compromising conditions, such as significant cutaneous damage.[105,108] This syndrome follows the four well-characterized sequential phases described previously. The prodromal symptoms are nonspecific and include nausea, vomiting, and anorexia. Rapid declines in lymphocytes herald the onset of full-blown hematopoietic syndrome. A latent period follows over 1–2 weeks with continued declines in the peripheral blood cell counts, possibly resulting in infection and hemorrhage during the manifest phase.

Table 33.11. Prodromal Phase: Severity/Dose and Medical Response

Signs/Symptoms after Exposure	Mild (1–2 Gy)	Moderate (2–4 Gy)	Severe (4–6 Gy)	Very severe (6–8 Gy)	Lethal* (>8 Gy)
Vomiting					
Onset	≥2 h	1–2 h	<1 h	<30 min	<10 min
Incidence (%)	10–50	70–90	100	100	100
Diarrhea	None	None	Mild	Heavy	Heavy
Onset	–	–	3–8 h	1–3 h	<1 h
Incidence (%)	–	–	<10	>10	~100
Headache	Slight	Mild	Moderate	Severe	Severe
Onset	–	–	4–24 h	3–4 h	1–2 h
Incidence (%)	–	–	50	80	80–90
Temperature	Normal	Increased	Fever	High fever	High fever
Onset	–	1–3 h	1–2 h	<1 h	<1 h
Incidence (%)	–	10–80	80–100	100	100
Consciousness	Normal	Normal	Normal	Possibly altered	Unconscious
Onset	–	–	–		Sec to min
Incidence (%)	–	–	–		100 (>50 Gy)
Medical Response	Outpatient	Observation or treatment at a specialized hospital if needed	Treatment at a specialized hospital	Treatment at a specialized hospital	If dose <10–12 Gy consider treatment ≥12 Gy palliative

* Individuals may survive with exposures as high as 12 Gy with appropriate medical management for greater than 6 months. Modified from the International Atomic Energy Agency, Diagnosis and Treatment of Radiation Injuries, Safety Report Series No. 2, Vienna; 1998.

Hematopoietic cells are among the most radiosensitive cells in the body. Mitotically active precursor cells are substantially reduced after a 2–3 Gy dose, resulting in a decreased supply of red blood cells, white blood cells, and platelets. At these doses, the supply of mature cells from the diminished precursor pools may be insufficient to maintain an adequate number for proper physiologic function, thereby resulting in the cytopenias characteristic of the hematopoietic syndrome. Certain subpopulations of the precursor cells are more radioresistant, presumably because the cells are in the non-cycling (G0) or radioresistant stage (late S) of the cell cycle.[109] This population may play a vital role in hematological reconstitution with exposures as high as 7–8 Gy. Fortunately, most individuals involved in radiation accidents receive inhomogeneous exposures due to: 1) the radiation mixture (e.g., photons, beta or alpha particles); 2) the energy of the radiation (i.e., penetrating or not); 3) the individual's distance from the source; 4) the physical environment; and/or 5) the degree of internal or external contamination that occurs. As a consequence, persons receiving potentially lethal doses of radiation may still survive due to sparing of small areas

Table 33.12. Latent Phase

Signs/Symptoms after Exposure	Mild (1–2 Gy)	Moderate (2–4 Gy)	Severe (4–6 Gy)	Very severe (6–8 Gy)	Lethal* (>8 Gy)
Latency period (d)	21–35	18–28	8–18	≤7	None
Lymphocytes					
(10⁹ cells/L), days 3–6	0.8–1.5	0.5–0.8	0.3–0.5	0.1–0.3	0.0–0.1
Granulocytes	>2.0	1.5–2.0	1.0–1.5	≤0.5	≤0.1
Diarrhea	None	None	Uncommon	Days 6–9	Days 4–5
Epilation (d)	None	Moderate, ≥15	Moderate, 11–21	Complete, <10	Complete, <10
Medical response	Outpatient	Hospitalization recommended	Hospitalization required	Hospitalization required	Hospitalization required, palliative treatment if ≥12 Gy

* Individuals may survive with exposures as high as 12 Gy with appropriate medical management for greater than 6 months. Modified from the International Atomic Energy Agency, Diagnosis and Treatment of Radiation Injuries, Safety Report Series No. 2, Vienna, 1998.

Table 33.13. Manifest (Illness) Phase

Signs/Symptoms after Exposure	Mild (1–2 Gy)	Moderate (2–4 Gy)	Severe (4–6 Gy)	Very severe (6–8 Gy)	Lethal* (>8 Gy)
Onset (d)	21–35	18–28	8–18	≤7	0
Lethality (%)	0	0–50	20–70	50–100	~100
Onset (weeks)	–	6–8	4–8	1–2	≥1 day to 2 weeks
Clinical Manifestations					
Fatigue	Yes	Yes	Yes	Yes	Yes
Epilation	–	Yes	Yes	Yes	Yes
Infection	–	Yes	Yes	Yes	Yes
Bleeding	–	Yes	Yes	Yes	Yes
Shock	–	–	–	–	Yes
Coma	–	–	–	–	Yes
Lymphocytes (10^9 cells/L)	0.8–1.5	0.5–0.8	0.3–0.5	0.1–0.3	0.0–0.1
Platelets (10^9 cells/L)	60–100	30–60	25–35	15–25	<20
Medical Response	Outpatient	Hospitalization recommended	Hospitalization required	Hospitalization required	Hospitalization required, palliative treatment if ≥12 Gy

* Individuals may survive with exposures as high as 12 Gy with appropriate medical management for greater than 6 months. Modified from the International Atomic Energy Agency, Diagnosis and Treatment of Radiation Injuries, Safety Report Series No. 2, Vienna, 1998.

of bone marrow, especially if located in the central axial skeleton, that can serve as a reservoir for the rapid reestablishment of hematopoiesis.[110]

The rates of decline for the various circulating cells depend on the sensitivity of the cell type (i.e., stem, precursor, and fully differentiated cells) and their turnover time. Lymphocytes decline the most rapidly, while platelets and other leukocytes are depressed less quickly. Having the longest circulating half-life and being resistant to apoptosis, erythrocytes demonstrate the slowest decline. Thus, the acute hematopoietic syndrome predisposes an individual to infection, hemorrhage, and anemia that follow the decline in leukocytes, platelets, and erythrocytes from as early as 5–10 days to several weeks after a high-dose exposure.[111] Due to the long circulating half-life of erythrocytes, the body's compensation mechanisms, and the general availability of transfusions, anemia is seldom life threatening unless other trauma or bleeding results secondary to thrombocytopenia.

Lymphocytes demonstrate a somewhat unusual response to radiation. Terminally differentiated cells (e.g., rhabdomyocytes) are usually more radioresistant than intermitotic cells (e.g., intestinal crypt cells, erythroblasts). However, lymphocytes, which are long-lived and highly differentiated, are nonetheless significantly radiosensitive and undergo rapid apoptosis when exposed to comparatively low doses of radiation. Therefore, lymphopenia occurs more rapidly than the other cytopenias, and assuming no other insult, a predictable dose-dependent decline is expected after radiation. For example, a potentially lethal radiation dose is characterized by a 50% drop in lymphocyte count within the first 24 hours followed by a more severe decline over the next day.[108,110,112]

Neutrophils are part of the innate immune system and are the first responders to infection. Thus, they are the most critical blood cell type in combating an acute threat from microorganisms. Circulating neutrophils have a half-life of about 7 hours before entering the tissue pools where they survive for an additional 1–2 days. In cases of infection, these cells are recruited from the circulation into the tissue and consumed, resulting in a marked reduction in their half-life. Maturation of neutrophil precursors to mature neutrophils in the bone marrow normally takes about 2 weeks. Following irradiation, declines in circulating neutrophils result from depletion of the marrow reserves of mature cells and death of rapidly dividing, early progenitor cells. Thus, the loss of progenitor cells and the unusual kinetics of neutrophil production and release account for the delayed onset of the hematopoietic syndrome.[39,108] To complicate matters, a transient increase in the granulocyte count may occur due to remobilization from the venous, splenic, and bone marrow pools with exposures of less than 5 Gy. A second abortive rise or stabilization in the granulocytes counts may occur in days 5–10 post-exposure, reflecting the production and release of granulocytes from residual hematopoietic tissue. This abortive rise in the peripheral granulocyte counts may suggest a survivable exposure.

The loss of progenitor cells with radiation exposure also results in a decrease in platelets, which have a mean survival time of 8–11 days. The resultant thrombocytopenia contributes to hemorrhage that occurs with the hematopoietic syndrome. Most authorities recommend platelet transfusion: 1) to reduce the risk of spontaneous hemorrhage when platelet counts fall below 10×10^9 cells/L in asymptomatic patients; and 2) for counts in the $10–50 \times 10^9$ cells/L range if there is clinical bleeding or if invasive procedures are anticipated. The final component of the hematopoietic syndrome, anemia, is characterized by a hemoglobin mass of less than 10 g/dl. The long mean lifespan of red cells (which approaches 120 days) makes anemia less of an immediate problem in the hematopoietic syndrome than the other cytopenias.

Acute Gastrointestinal Syndrome

The gastrointestinal (GI) syndrome also has four sequential stages but occurs at higher radiation doses than the hematopoietic syndrome (typically becoming manifest at total body irradiation doses of ≥ 6 Gy). The full syndrome will usually occur with a dose greater than approximately 10 Gy although some symptoms may occur as low as 6 Gy. The GI mucosa is a self-renewing tissue; the morbidity and mortality observed in the GI syndrome reflect the destruction of this mucosal lining in the setting of concurrent myelosuppression. The prodromal stage is characterized by prompt nausea, vomiting, and diarrhea, which are typically more severe than the symptoms observed with the hematopoietic syndrome due to the higher initiating radiation doses. In some cases, this may be followed by a latent period lasting several days, although the duration of latency declines as the exposure dose increases. The manifest stage then follows with severe diarrhea, nausea, vomiting, and fevers. Other systemic effects may include dehydration, ileus, malabsorption, electrolyte derangements, gastrointestinal bleeding, renal impairment, and eventual cardiovascular collapse. As with the hematopoietic system, the dividing precursor cells are more radiosensitive than the differentiated cells. The radiosensitive epithelial stem cells are confined to the crypts and provide a continuous supply of new cells. These new cells differentiate as they move up the villi or luminal surface to become functionally mature cells, which are then extruded. Hence, sufficient radiation sterilizes the dividing crypt cells, eventually disrupting the mucosal barrier resulting in septicemia and usually death. Kolesnick, Fuks, and colleagues have argued that endothelial damage is the primary lesion regulating crypt cell survival and intestinal injury, but this hypothesis remains controversial.[113]

Acute Neurovascular Syndrome

Neurovascular syndrome may be observed at acute doses of greater than 10–20 Gy and is thought to reflect cerebral edema and cardiovascular collapse, although hypotension may also be seen at lower doses. The full syndrome will usually occur with a dose greater than approximately 50 Gy although some symptoms may occur as low as 10 Gy. Death occurs within 3 days and is due to collapse of the circulatory system as well as increased intracranial pressure from edema due to vasculitis and meningitis. As with the hematopoietic and gastrointestinal syndromes, the prodromal phase is characterized by nausea, vomiting, and diarrhea, but this typically occurs within minutes of exposure in persons suffering acute neurovascular syndrome. Disorientation, confusion, and prostration are characteristic of the prodromal phase. Loss of balance and seizures may also occur. Papilledema, ataxia, and reduced or absent deep tendon and corneal reflexes may be noted during the physical examination. This phase is followed, possibly without a latent period, by a severe manifest phase of fever, respiratory distress, disorientation, ataxia, persistent diarrhea, seizures, cardiovascular collapse, and coma. The course is inexorable and death invariably follows within a few days. The clinical course of rapid deterioration mimics that of acute sepsis and septic shock, both of which must also be considered in the differential diagnosis.

Acute Cutaneous Radiation Injury (≤ 90 days)

The skin is composed of the epidermis and dermis. The epidermis provides a durable waterproof protective barrier of stratified squamous epithelium between the body and external environment. The stratum germinativum (or basal layer),

containing the basal stem cells, is the innermost layer of the epidermis. Cells produced in the basal layer differentiate and migrate toward the surface, where they maintain some proliferating potential in the stratum spinosum (squamous layer). The cells then pass through additional layers where they finally make their way to the stratum corneum, where they eventually slough off. The turnover time ranges from 4–7 weeks. The dermis, connected to the epidermis by a basement membrane, contains a dense network of connective tissue, hair follicles, capillaries, lymphatics, sweat glands, nerve endings, sebaceous glands, and apocrine glands. The highly radiosensitive epithelial stem cells, follicular, sebaceous, and sweat germinal cells provide a continuous supply of new cells to their respective structures. These new cells differentiate as they become functionally mature cells and are eventually lost. With irradiation, a large proportion of these cells may die. Unless replenished, the loss of these cells will result in disruption of skin integrity, epilation, dry skin, and if the dose is high enough, failure of thermal regulation. The late effects of radiation are mainly attributable to endothelial cell death within the papillary vasculature and are discussed in detail elsewhere.[116–118]

Significant cutaneous radiation injury independently predicts lethality, thus increasing the risk of death when combined with other trauma.[119,120] Cutaneous radiation injury will usually be combined with other aspects of ARS but it may occur in isolation if the exposure is restricted to low-energy X-rays or beta radiation. Mechanical, chemical, and thermal injuries may accelerate and exacerbate the cutaneous radiation injury. In cases where multiple mechanisms have contributed to the skin damage, a more appropriate term for the clinical syndrome encountered might be "combined skin injury." Moreover, the damage to the skin is almost invariably inhomogeneous due to factors such as the position of the individual in relationship to the radiation source and/or the presence of physical barriers providing partial body protection.

The effects of radiation on the skin are dose, depth, and volume dependent. Most individuals receiving a radiation dose to the skin of 5 Gy or higher will experience a transient skin reaction of erythema, edema, itching, and/or tingling within 24 hours of exposure. This prodromal period is followed by a latent period of 2–3 weeks. Next, an orderly progression occurs of erythema, hyperpigmentation, and finally dry followed by wet desquamation if the focal dose to skin is approximately 15–24 Gy. In the case of extremely high doses (≥ 50 Gy), the period of latency may not occur and the injury may progress from erythema to necrosis within days (Table 33.14).[117] Figure 33.5 demonstrates the progressive stages of cutaneous injury in a patient receiving a focal high-dose exposure to the right hand. Clinicians should remember to include radiation injury as part of the differential diagnosis of desquamation or ulceration of unclear etiology, particularly when the patient lacks a history of a burn injury.

Radiation Combined Injury

In many potential scenarios, burns and/or wounds in combination with radiation are highly likely. It is estimated that 60–70% of persons exposed to significant radiation doses from the atomic bombings of Hiroshima and Nagasaki also sustained traumatic injury. Similarly, in the Chernobyl accident, approximately 10% of the 237 acutely exposed first responders received both significant radiation doses and burns.[119] The combination of radiation exposure with other injuries results in high lethality,

Table 33.14. Skin Injury and Time of Onset

Stage/symptoms*	Dose range (Gy)	Time of Onset (d)*
Erythema	3–10	14–21
Epilation	>3	14–18
Dry desquamation	8–12	25–30
Moist desquamation	15–20	20–28
Blister formation	15–25	15–25
Ulceration (without skin)	>20	14–21
Necrosis	>25	>21

* The time to progression of each stage (erythema, epilation, dry desquamation, etc.) is shortened with increasing dose (not shown). Modified from the International Atomic Energy Agency, Diagnosis and Treatment of Radiation Injuries, Safety Report Series No. 2, Vienna, 1998.

Table 33.15. Data Summarized from the Literature by the Armed Forces Radiobiology Research Institute (AFRRI)

Model	Injury	Mortality
Dog	20% burn	12%
	100 cGy total body irradiation	0%
	combined burn + total body irradiation	73%
Pig	10–15% burn	0%
	400 cGy total body irradiation	20%
	combined burn + total body irradiation	90%
Rat	31–35% burn	50%
	250 cGy total body irradiation	0%
	combined burn + total body irradiation	95%
Guinea pig	1.5% burn	9%
	250 cGy total body irradiation	11%
	combined burn + total body irradiation	38%

whether the etiology is blast, burn, trauma, or infectious. The LD$_{50/30}$ and the time from exposure to death for irradiated animals at a given dose both decrease significantly in the setting of combined injury.[120] This effect has been observed for the combination of radiation injury with burns, wounds, and experimentally induced infections across multiple species. Data derived from studies involving the combination of sublethal radiation exposure and thermal injury are summarized in Table 33.15 and are representative of findings with other permutations of radiation combined injury.

Delayed Effects of Acute Radiation Exposure

In persons surviving the initial phases of ARS, or receiving substantial partial-body exposures, tissue and organs other than those mentioned previously can manifest late radiation effects, referred to collectively as the delayed effects of acute radiation exposure (DEARE). For example, persons exposed to high doses of radiation (typically in excess of 6–8 Gy) often

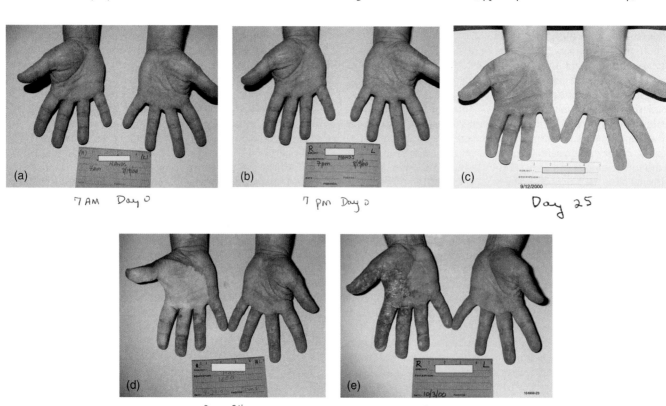

Figure 33.5. Progression of skin lesions in a patient receiving a focal high-dose exposure to the right hand. (a) Minutes after exposure, (b) approximately 12 hours post-exposure, (c) day 25 post-exposure, (d) day 34 post-exposure, and (e) day 46 post-exposure. Images provided by REAC/TS.

develop impairment of lung or kidney function, starting approximately 3 months after the exposure event. Acute, subacute, and chronic radiation syndromes may present as a clinical continuum or there can be a prolonged latency between exposure and the manifestation of radiation-induced organ dysfunction. Although the hematopoietic and gastrointestinal syndromes are largely attributable to the direct cytotoxic effects of radiation on rapidly dividing tissues, DEARE are thought to reflect chronic inflammation induced by vascular damage or other injury to the connective tissue. The interested reader may refer to several reviews on this topic for additional information.[121–124]

Radiation-Induced Malignancy

Individuals exposed to doses of radiation that do not produce immediate acute effects are still likely to be concerned about their risk of developing radiation-induced cancer. In general, the risk of secondary cancer increases with increasing dose, although outcomes for specific individuals cannot be predicted with any certainty. This is in contrast to organ injury, where the severity of dysfunction increases with increasing dose once the threshold dose for injury is surpassed. Among atomic bomb survivors, the observed excess relative risk was greatest for the development of hematologic malignancies (primarily acute myeloid leukemia), with incidence peaking approximately 10 years after exposure.[124,125] Long-term follow-up of participants in the lifespan study cohort of Hiroshima and Nagasaki atomic bomb survivors has shown that excess risk for solid cancers exhibits significant variation with gender, attained age, and age at the time of exposure. According to the latest summary report, it was estimated that solid cancer rates increase by about 35%/Gy for men and 58%/Gy for women, at age 70 after exposure at age 30. In addition, statistically significant radiation-associated increases in risk are seen for cancers of the oral cavity, esophagus, stomach, colon, liver, lung, skin (non-melanoma), breast, ovary, bladder, nervous system, and thyroid.[125]

In the future, it may be possible to estimate an individual's risk of radiation-induced cancer more precisely by assessing the radiation exposure in light of other pertinent factors, such as the volume of tissue irradiated, the individual's history of exposure to other carcinogens (e.g., smoking), and the victim's age and family history. At present, however, there is no way to reduce an individual's risk of radiation-induced cancer after the radiation exposure has occurred.

Treatment of Acute Radiation Syndrome

Medical Management of Acute External Radiation Syndrome

Treatment for ARS in the absence of combined injury is usually required only in those who have received radiation doses ≥ 2 Gy.[99] Patients who present with combined injuries due to mechanical, thermal, and/or chemical causes should be triaged as described elsewhere in the chapter and managed using relevant burn or trauma protocols. Since radiation is not immediately life-threatening, the non-radiation-related injuries should be addressed first. The management of acute radiation injury depends on multiple factors including the location of exposure (external or internal), the extent of exposure (partial or whole body), the dose and type of radiation, concurrent injuries or illnesses, age and weight of the patient, pregnancy status, and the particular radionuclides involved in the case of internal contamination.

Infection is a major cause of death in patients with ARS. Therefore, supportive care including wound care, antimicrobial treatment and prophylaxis for infection, and mitigation of neutropenia with myeloid cytokines and possibly stem cell transplantation all play vital roles in proper management.[130–137] Several cases of high-dose exposure illustrate that restoration of bone marrow function may be possible even after exposures as high as 10–12 Gy with aggressive supportive care. Hematopoietic recovery has not translated into long-term survival, however, due to progressive gastrointestinal and pulmonary dysfunction.[11] As a result, it is appropriate to withhold aggressive treatment for victims who have received a supralethal dose of radiation, especially in a setting of mass casualties, where resource allocation constraints may be significant.[99,101,131–137] Exactly what constitutes a supralethal dose remains contentious, but whole body doses over 12 Gy have universally been fatal.

Radiation injury management can be divided into three categories: acute (≤ 72 hours), intermediate (3–30 days), and late (> 30 days). A discussion follows highlighting the management of radiation injury during the acute and intermediate periods.

ACUTE MANAGEMENT

Both external and internal decontamination should be performed along with medical and surgical stabilization as soon as possible (methods of internal decontamination are discussed later). External decontamination is achieved for most victims by removal of clothing and showering with soap and water. Achieving a reading of no more than two times background levels of radiation on a survey instrument indicates effective decontamination. The presence of persistent radioactive material should not delay critical medical interventions. Additional information on decontamination can be found in Chapter 16.

Prodromal symptoms such as nausea, vomiting, diarrhea, and headache may be controlled with conventional agents such as 5-hydroxytryptamine (5-HT3) receptor antagonists (ondansetron) and fluids, loperamide, and acetaminophen (paracetamol), respectively. All blood products should be leuko-reduced and irradiated to minimize transfusion-associated graft-versus-host disease (GVHD). Not only can GVHD cause significant morbidity and mortality, it can also pose a clinical dilemma as some of the signs and symptoms are similar to those of severe ARS (e.g., diarrhea, fever, hyperbilirubinemia, and pancytopenia).

Table 33.16 outlines general recommendations for pharmacologic management of hematologic ARS. Similar guidelines have been published elsewhere and reflect differences in appropriate care based on the size of the incident.[126–130,132] Patients susceptible to severe life-threatening infections should receive prompt antibiotic treatment on an empirical basis if they show clinical evidence of infection. In casualties who have become neutropenic (peripheral blood absolute neutrophil count less than 0.5×10^9 cells/L) but do not have evidence of active infection, it is appropriate to administer acyclovir for prophylaxis against herpes simplex virus. Based on guidelines for patients with cancer receiving chemotherapy from the National Comprehensive Cancer Network (www.nccn.org) and Infectious Disease Society of America, patients who are expected to have neutropenia lasting longer than 3–5 days may also benefit from prophylaxis against bacteria and *Candida*.[132] This can be accomplished with the combination of a fluoroquinolone such as levofloxacin and a triazole such as fluconazole. These agents can all be discontinued upon the resolution of neutropenia.

Table 33.16. Treatment Guidelines for Radiation Exposure Based on Estimates of Whole-Body Dose

Dose (Gy)

	Cytokine Treatment	^Antibacterial/Viral/Fungal Treatment#	Consider Allogeneic Stem Cell Transplant
>100 Casualties			
Healthy person, no injuries	3–7*	2–7#	7–10
Combined injuries	2–6*	2–6#	–
≤100 casualties			
Healthy person, no injuries	3–10*	2–10#	>7
Combined injuries	2–6	2–6#	–

^ Prophylactic antibiotic, antiviral, and antifungal therapy: fluoroquinolone, acyclovir, and fluconazole,

* In the elderly (> 60) and non-adolescent children, consider initiating therapy at a lower dose, i.e., 2 Gy. Also, G-CSF should be started in those who develop neutropenia (< 0.5 x 10^9 cell/L) and are not already receiving it.

Therapy should be continued until no longer neutropenic. Follow the Infectious Diseases Society of America Guidelines if the patient develops neutropenic fever while on prophylactic therapy.

In those who are expected to develop neutropenia, hematopoietic colony stimulating factor (CSF) treatment should be initiated as quickly as possible assuming that the radiation- and non-radiation-related injuries are potentially survivable.[87] Data from non-human primates suggests that the greatest survival benefit from CSFs requires instituting treatment within 24 hours after exposure.[135] The only cytokines approved by the U.S. Food and Drug Administration (FDA) for management of treatment-associated neutropenia are the recombinant forms of granulocyte CSF (G-CSF, filgrastim and Tbo-G-CSF), the pegylated form of G-CSF (pegfilgrastim), and granulocyte macrophage colony stimulating factor (GM-CSF, sargramostim). These hematopoietic factors enhance neutrophil recovery following chemotherapy, resulting in a reduction in the frequency of both neutropenic fever and hospitalization.[133–135] These agents have also been utilized to treat radiation accident victims, and may have shortened their duration of neutropenia. Several other cytokines such as interleukin-11, thrombopoietin, Fms-related tyrosine kinase 3 (FLT-3) ligand, and keratinocyte growth factor (KGF) have shown preclinical efficacy but cannot be recommended for broad use.

Besides addressing the victim's physical symptoms and injuries, physicians should be sensitive to the potentially profound psychological impact of radiation injury. Patients and their families are likely to have concerns and anxieties that should be addressed, particularly in the case of high-dose exposures where the prognosis may be poor.

General skin management guidelines have emerged to minimize desquamation and/or infection.[134–136] Areas of acute erythema and dry desquamation (Radiation Therapy Oncology Group [RTOG] Grade I) should be washed with lukewarm water or with mild soap, avoiding temperature extremes and mechanical irritation. Moisturizing cream – such as one containing unscented, lanolin-free, hydrophilic ingredients – may be helpful in early or minor reactions, but should be discontinued if wet desquamation occurs. Moist desquamation (RTOG Grade II–III) is managed by keeping the wounds clean and using antiseptic dressings to minimize infection, desiccation, and further trauma to the wound. Skin necrosis and ulceration (RTOG Grade IV) may require skin grafts with non-irradiated skin. Alternatively,

smaller defects may be treated with hyperbaric oxygenation to stimulate reepithelialization.

Selected patients without significant combined injuries who receive doses that fully ablate the marrow but may otherwise be survivable (i.e., > 7 Gy but < 10–12 Gy) may benefit from stem cell transplantation. For those receiving total body doses of greater than 10–12 Gy, stem cell transplantation is probably of no benefit since death would result from non-bone marrow related multi-organ dysfunction. The accurate determination of whether a patient would likely improve with stem cell transplantation is difficult because the benefits of transplantation appear to occur within a narrow radiation dose window. Problems with patient selection are further compounded by the likely heterogeneous radiation exposure to the various body parts. Liberal use in uncertain situations may result in unnecessary mortality since allogeneic stem cell transplantation may result in death from GVHD. The Radiation Injury Treatment Network (www.ritn.net) has established guidelines for human leukocyte antigen (HLA)-typing, donor recruitment and stem cell transplantation for radiation victims. Patients should undergo bone marrow aspiration 14–21 days after exposure and after a trial of myeloid cytokines to demonstrate aplasia prior to transplantation. In the rare cases of patients with an identical twin or who have previously stored autologous hematopoietic stem cells, syngeneic or autologous stem cell transplantation may be beneficial and should be considered.

After recovery of neutrophils, casualties who have received doses greater than 3 Gy may experience prolonged lymphopenia that places them at risk for opportunistic infections including cytomegalovirus (CMV) and Pneumocystis. Thus, patients with exposures greater than 3 Gy and/or peripheral blood CD4 counts less than 0.2 × 10^9 cells/L may benefit from prophylaxis against Pneumocystis beginning 30 days after exposure. Preemptive monitoring of CMV in the peripheral blood is also indicated with rapid institution of gancyclovir or valgancyclovir treatment if CMV is detected.

Medical Countermeasures and Treatments

In recent years, medical countermeasures against radiation have typically been classified according to the following schema:

- Radioprotectants – given before exposure (or in the midst of ongoing exposure) as prophylaxis against radiation injury
- Radiation mitigators – given after exposure and prior to the onset of symptoms to reduce the biological consequences of radiation exposure
- Therapeutics – given after the radiation effect is manifest
- Decorporation – given to reduce the total body burden of an isotope following its internalization
- Blocking agents – given to reduce organ uptake of an isotope following its internalization

Elucidation of the complex nature and evolution of radiation injury has dissipated hopes for a medical panacea. Antioxidants and radioprotectants such as amifostine must be present at the cellular level at the time of irradiation to offer tangible benefits in reducing acute injury. Therapeutics targeting specific signaling pathways will likely demonstrate time-sensitive windows of opportunity during which administration may provide clinical benefit and outside of which efficacy may erode fairly sharply. Modulation of cytokine activity through the use of anti-inflammatory agents or monoclonal antibodies may offer organ-specific or more general benefits but whether these compounds will improve overall outcomes remains unknown. Developing and confirming the efficacy of such combinations will be one of the more challenging tasks investigators face in coming years. To complicate matters further, the manifestations of ARS reflect a molecular and physiological cascade of events unfolding over time. This may afford opportunities for intervention at multiple time points, and how medical countermeasures are sequenced may prove to be an important determinant of a regimen's overall efficacy.

Table 33.17 lists the various organ-specific syndromes associated with acute radiation exposure and the currently available countermeasures for prophylaxis, mitigation, and treatment of these entities. None of the likely drugs used in the management of patients with ARS or DEARE are FDA-approved for radiation injury. Currently, only potassium iodide (KI), Prussian Blue, Ca-DTPA and Zn-DTPA (see Treatment for Internal Radionuclide Contamination section to follow) are specifically FDA-approved in the United States as countermeasures for radiation injury from internal radionuclide contamination.

Internally Deposited Radionuclides

Internal contamination of individuals can occur any time radioactive materials are free to spread in an environment, with the most common routes of intake being inhalation and absorption through wounds. Despite engineering and health physics controls, activities during the various stages of the nuclear fuel cycle and other industrial processes occasionally result in the accidental release of radioactive material. Such activities include mining and processing of nuclear fuel, fabrication of fuel elements, reactor operations and repair, decommissioning, fuel reprocessing, and waste management. Unless heralded by fires and explosions, gaseous and particulate releases might not be evident until detected by air monitors. The ingestion pathway is uncommon in industrial settings, but may become critical for the general public after an accidental release of airborne or liquid radioactive material into the environment. Various documents give an overview of current thoughts on techniques pertinent to the mitigation of internal contamination.[138–141]

Following an accidental intake of radioactive material, the radiation dose, toxicity, and treatment methods are dependent on various factors. These include the identity of the radionuclide and its physical and chemical characteristics (physical and biological half-life, particle size, chemical composition, solubility, tissue tropism, etc.). For radionuclides internalized through the inhalation pathway, particle characteristics (size, chemical composition, and chemical solubility in body fluids) are important determinants of the radiation dose received. The size of aerosol particles determines the region of the respiratory tract where deposition occurs, but the ultimate fate of inhaled particles is also critically dependent on their physicochemical properties. Highly insoluble particles, for example, may remain in the lung for long periods of time, during which a small fraction will be transported to the tracheobronchial lymph nodes by pulmonary macrophages. Insoluble particles may also be swallowed and therefore are often excreted primarily in the feces.

General medical and health physics assessment after an inhalation event should include initial attempts to determine the maximum credible amount internalized. Nasal swabs taken within a few minutes post-accident, if positive, can aid in nuclide identification and in estimating the amount of material inhaled. If there is evidence for significant intake, preparations should be considered for urine and fecal bioassay and whole-body or lung counting. There is a high false-negative rate when using nasal swabs due either to the elapsed time post-event, sampling technique, or clearance from the nasal region. However, positive nasal smears bilaterally and/or a history of external contamination above the waist and contamination around the nose, can be clues to possible intake. Mansfield has offered a rough rule of thumb that the combined activity of both nasal swabs totals approximately 5% of deeper lung deposition, using the International Commission on Radiological Protection (ICRP) 30 lung model as a reference.[142] Experience has shown that this technique generally overestimates deep lung deposition (sometimes substantially) but is useful for initial estimates and decisions about the initiation of therapy, pending the results of bioassays. Current practice at the Radiation Emergency Assistance Center/Training Site (REAC/TS) is to assume that the combined activity of nasal swabs represents approximately 10% of deeply deposited activity.

Whole body or wound counting may be useful to identify those nuclides that emit penetrating X-rays or gamma rays. It may also be utilized for nuclides emitting energetic beta particles that can be detected by their bremsstrahlung. The initial problem for the health physicist and for the treating physician is to estimate the maximum credible amount internalized. This estimate directs further medical care.

In all cases involving internal contamination, it is the chemistry of the stable element in the human body that determines radionuclide biokinetics. The biological half-life (T_B) of the stable element (which is equivalent to that of the radioisotope) and the physical half-life (T_P) of the radioisotope act in concert to produce the effective half-life (T_{eff}) of an isotope, which is given by:

$$1/T_{eff} = 1/T_p + 1/T_B$$

Thus, the effective half-life is less than either the physical or biological half-lives. As an illustrative example, radioactive iodine is chemically identical to non-radioactive iodine, and the biological clearance of the radioactive and normal isotopes is indistinguishable. The toxicity of ^{131}I, however, derives from its radioactivity. The biological effects and toxicities of ^{131}I are therefore a function

Table 33.17. Currently Available Medical Countermeasures for ARS and DEARE

Syndrome		Timing	Treatment	Comment
Hematopoietic	Neutropenia	Prophylaxis	None	
		Mitigation	Colony stimulating factors (G-CSF, GM-CSF, pegylated G-CSF) to decrease duration and intensity of neutropenia	Treatment for radiation exposure > 2Gy should begin within 1–2 days[87] CSF use has been associated with rare fatal splenic rupture[96]
			Antibiotics at time of neutropenia	Consider antibacterial, antifungal, and HSV-directed prophylaxis when prolonged neutropenia is anticipated[97,115]
		Therapeutic	Colony stimulating factors as above	
			Supportive care: antibiotics for febrile neutropenia	
			Allogeneic stem cell transplantation	Limited utility due to severe morbidity and mortality associated with concurrent non-hematopoietic injuries sustained at marrow-lethal doses of radiation[87]
	Thrombocytopenia	Prophylaxis	None	
		Mitigation	Cytokines (oprelvekin [recombinant human IL-11]), eltrombopag, romiplostim	Limited if any human experience with irradiated patients. Oprelvekin is indicated for prevention/mitigation of thrombocytopenia following myelosuprressive chemotherapy in adult patients with nonmyeloid malignancies. Eltrombopag and romiplostim are thrombopoietin receptor agonists that are indicated for the treatment of chronic immune thrombocytopenia
		Therapeutic	Supportive care: platelet transfusion	
	Anemia	Prophylaxis	None	
		Mitigation	Cytokines (erythropoietin)	
		Therapeutic	Cytokines (erythropoietin)	
			Supportive care: red blood cell transfusion	
			Allogeneic stem cell transplantation	
	Lympho-penia	Prophylaxis	None	
		Mitigation	None	
		Therapeutic	Allogeneic stem cell transplantation	
Gastrointestinal	Nausea/vomiting	Prophylaxis	Oral and IV antiemetics: 5HT3 receptor antagonists ± dexamethasone	
		Therapeutic	5-HT3 receptor antagonists	Preferred[98]
			Dopamine antagonists	
			Benzodiazepines	
			Corticosteroids	
	Mucosal injury	Prophylaxis	Keratinocyte growth factor (KGF)	KGF decreases the incidence and duration of severe oral mucositis in patients with hematologic malignancies receiving myelotoxic therapy requiring hematopoietic stem cell support. The safety and efficacy of KGF have not been established in patients with non-hematologic malignancies or radiation casualties.

Table 33.17. (*continued*)

Syndrome		Timing	Treatment	Comment
		Mitigation	Cytokines (G-CSF, GM-CSF, peg-G-CSF)	Mixed results in small human trials with fractionated radiotherapy[99,100]
		Therapeutic	Gastrointestinal decontamination: fluoroquinolones, vancomycin, polymyxin B sulfate, antifungals	Very limited human data; animal data demonstrates reduction in bacteremia[101]
			L-Glutamine	Very limited human data[102]
			Supportive care: total parenteral nutrition, elemental diets, fluids, electrolyte repletion	
	Diarrhea	Prophylaxis	None	
		Mitigation	None	
		Therapeutic	Antidiarrheals: loperamide, diphenoxylate/atropine, tincture of opium	
	Hemorrhage	Prophylaxis	Antacids: proton pump inhibitors, H2 receptor antagonists, sucralfate, other antacids	Reduces risk of upper gastrointestinal bleeding in critically ill patients; limited data in patients with ARS[103]
		Mitigation	None	
		Treatment	Supportive care: transfusions	
Cardiovascular CNS		Prophylaxis	None	
		Mitigation	None	
		Therapeutic	Palliative care	
Chronic organ injury		Prophylaxis	None	
		Mitigation	Pentoxifylline for early and late pulmonary toxicity	Single randomized clinical trial in patients with lung or breast cancer[104]
		Therapeutic	Pentoxifylline + α-tocopherol for radiation-induced superficial fibrosis (RIF)	Randomized clinical trial in patients with RIF after radiotherapy[105]
			Suppression of renin-angiotensin system for radiation nephropathy: Angiotensin converting enzyme (ACE) inhibitors, angiotensin II, type I receptor antagonists	Anecdotal human evidence of efficacy[106]
Combined injury – blast, thermal effects		Prophylaxis	None	Experimental models suggest that mortality from combined injuries will be significantly higher than mortality from pure radiation injury for any given dose of radiation[105]
		Mitigation	None	
		Therapeutic	Surgical interventions should be performed within 48 hours or delayed 5–6 weeks	

of both its half-life (8 days) and its concentration in the serum and thyroid. These effects and toxicities decline as a function of both the radioisotope's clearance and its radioactive decay.

Treatment for Internal Radionuclide Contamination

Hospital emergency personnel should triage victims of a radiation incident using traditional medical and trauma criteria. In general, personal protective equipment (PPE) appropriate for managing blood-borne/airborne pathogens (e.g., N95 respirators, gloves, and suitable surgical gowns) are all that is necessary for treating patients with external contamination, internal contamination, or radiation-related injury from external sources. In some cases, however, Level C or even Level B PPE is recommended (see Chapter 15). In the history of radiation accidents, no healthcare provider has received an external dose of more than 0.005 Sv while delivering normal patient care. Healthcare workers may perceive a large risk in treating patients with radiation injury but this is not substantiated by actual experience. It is, however, necessary to practice appropriate contamination controls to minimize dose to providers.

Table 33.18. Decorporation Therapy Recommendations for Radionuclides of Concern

Radionuclide	Treatment	Preferred Rx
Actinium (Ac)	DTPA	DTPA
Americium (Am)	DTPA*	DTPA*
Arsenic (As)	BAL; Penicillamine; DMSA?	BAL
Barium (Ba)	Strontium therapy[†]	Strontium therapy[†]
Berkelium (Bk)	DTPA	DTPA
Bismuth (Bi)	BAL?	BAL?
Cadmium (Cd)	DTPA; EDTA; DMSA	DMSA
Californium (Cf)	DTPA	DTPA
Calcium (Ca)	Strontium therapy[†]	Strontium therapy[†]
Carbon	No treatment available	N/A
Cerium (Ce)	DTPA	DTPA
Cesium (Cs)	Prussian Blue*	Prussian Blue*
Chromium (Cr)	DTPA; DMSA	DMSA
Cobalt (Co)	Penicillamine; DTPA; EDTA; DMSA; N-Acetylcysteine; Penicillamine; BAL	DTPA and EDTA
Copper (Cu)	Penicillamine*; Trientine*	Penicillamine*
Curium (Cm)	DTPA*	DTPA*
Einsteinium (Es)	DTPA	DTPA
Europium	DTPA	DTPA
Fission products (mixed)	See text in next section	N/A
Fluorine	Aluminum Hydroxide	Aluminum Hydroxide
Gallium	Penicillamine	Penicillamine
Gold (Au)	Penicillamine; BAL	BAL
Indium (In)	DTPA	DTPA
Iodine (I)	KI*; Propylthiouracil; Methamizole; Potassium perchlorate	KI*
Iridium	DTPA; Penicillamine	Penicillamine?
Iron	Deferoxamine*; Deferiprone*; Deferasirox*	Deferoxamine
Lanthanum (La)	DTPA	DTPA
Lead (Pb)	DMSA; BAL with EDTA	DMSA
Manganese (Mn)	DTPA; EDTA	EDTA
Magnesium (Mg)	EDTA	EDTA

Table 33.18. (*continued*)

Radionuclide	Treatment	Preferred Rx
Mercury (Hg)	BAL; Penicillamine; DMSA?	BAL
Molybdenum (Mo)	?	?
Neptunium (Np)	Deferoxamine	Deferoxamine
Nickel (Ni)	DTPA; Imuthiol	Imuthiol
Niobium (Nb)	DTPA	DTPA
Palladium (Pd)	Penicillamine; DTPA	Penicillamine
Phosphorus (P)	Phosphorus therapy[†]	Phosphorus therapy[†]
Plutonium (Pu)	DTPA*	DTPA*
Polonium (Po)	BAL; DMSA?; Penicillamine?	BAL
Potassium (K)	Diuretics	Diuretics
Promethium (Pm)	DTPA	DTPA
Radium (Ra)	Strontium therapy[†]	Strontium therapy[†]
Rubidium (Rb)	Prussian Blue	Prussian blue
Ruthenium (Ru)	DTPA	DTPA
Scandium (Sc)	DTPA, EDTA	DTPA
Silver (Ag)	No treatment available	N/A
Sodium (Na)	Diuretic	Diuretic
Strontium (Sr)	Strontium therapy[†]	Strontium therapy[†]
Sulfur (S)	No treatment available	N/A
Technetium	Potassium perchlorate	Potassium Perchlorate
Thorium (Th)	DTPA	DTPA
Tritium (H-3)	Force fluids	Water diuresis
Uranium (U)	Bicarbonate	Bicarbonate
Yttrium (Y)	DTPA; EDTA	DTPA
Zirconium (Zr)	DTPA	DTPA

* Approved by the U.S. FDA
[†] For strontium and phosphorus therapy, see Table 33.19.
BAL = British anti-Lewisite (dimercaprol; 2,3-dimercaptopropanol)
DMSA= Dimercaptosuccinic acid (succimer)
DTPA = Diethylenetriaminepentaacetate
EDTA= Ethylenediaminetetraacetic acid

After immediately life-threatening injuries are stabilized, radionuclide-specific therapy may be considered. The major goal of radionuclide-specific therapy after internal contamination is decorporation (removal from the body) of the internally deposited radionuclide. Early and effective decorporation can substantially reduce the overall committed dose of radiation the internally contaminated individual receives as a result of the radionuclide exposure. In general, treatment strategies for internal contamination fall into one of several major categories.[138,140]

- Reducing and/or inhibiting absorption of the isotope in the GI tract. Example: inducing emesis, performing gastric lavage, or administering cathartics.
- Blocking uptake to the organ of interest. Example: administering potassium iodide to block uptake of radioactive iodine by the thyroid.
- Diluting the ingested radionuclide. Example: administering fluids for internal contamination with tritium.
- Altering the chemistry of the substance. Example: administering sodium bicarbonate to convert uranyl ions to uranium bicarbonate (a less nephrotoxic form of uranium) in the renal tubules.
- Displacing the isotope from receptors. Example: administering calcium to compete with radiothorium.
- Utilizing traditional chelation techniques. Example: administering Diethylenetriaminepentaacetate (DTPA) to enhance excretion of internalized plutonium or americium.

Early identification of the radionuclide is crucial in the medical management of the acute phase. From medical experience with industrial radiation accidents, decorporation therapy is generally recommended for intakes of 5–10 times the recommended annual limit of intake (ALI) and strongly recommended for intakes exceeding 10 ALI. The ALI is defined as the inhalation intake necessary to give a committed effective dose equivalent 0.05 Sv (5 rem). It would be unusual to treat a non-pregnant adult with an intake below 1 ALI. If, however, the patient requests treatment and there are sufficient resources available, physicians may justify therapy for intakes below 1 ALI according to the radiation safety principle that exposures should be "as low as reasonably achievable." In an extreme event involving thousands of contaminated individuals, the radiation dose received by the population can be reduced by a factor of 2–10 or more simply by sheltering-in-place, depending on the quality of the shelter. In comparison, medical decorporation therapy can only affect the dose by a factor of 2–3.[143]

Since internal contamination by radionuclides is often considered as a type of poisoning by physicians, poison control centers are occasionally contacted initially for information on reducing the body burden of the specific radioactive element. It is therefore important that toxicologists and all physicians in poison control centers have access to the most current treatment modalities. Table 33.18 lists decorporating, chelating, and blocking agents available for treating or blocking internal radionuclide deposition. Table 33.19 provides dosing recommendations for these drugs. The information in Tables 33.18 and 33.19 is currently consistent with recommendations from the National Council on Radiation Protection (NCRP Report No. 161). In the United States, however, there are relatively few drugs actually approved by the FDA for these indications. The drugs that are approved in the United States are noted with an asterisk in Table 33.18. Uses of these drugs for other indications and other radionuclides must be considered "off-label." Other countries, such as those within the European Union, have additional approved drugs.

Treating physicians should remember that most chelating and decorporating agents are radionuclide-specific and that the value of decorporation therapy may be dependent on the context of the patient's exposure. One example is the FDA guidelines for use of potassium iodide.[144] Another example is using radionuclide chelators/blockers in an effective and targeted manner following a nuclear detonation. This would present significant chal-

lenges, and may not be feasible or desirable. Internal exposures will vary considerably and it is likely that only a comparatively small number of people might incur doses that actually warrant treatment. It is also likely that this population will have received higher external doses from fallout and that this external exposure will be the predominant cause of morbidity and mortality for these victims. Internal contamination from radionuclides in fallout will, therefore, be a secondary health concern compared to the thermal, blast, and prompt radiation injuries associated with the detonation. An additional consideration is that the composition of fallout will be complex, reflecting a disparate mix of radionuclides. This mixture will likely include compounds for which no or only minimally effective decorporating or blocking agents exist.

The Psychological and Behavioral Consequences of Radiation Events

Incidents resulting in the release of radiation, particularly if the event represents a deliberate attack, will produce uncertainty, anxiety, and fear in many otherwise psychologically normal and healthy individuals. These feelings may manifest directly or be expressed indirectly as anger, disbelief, sadness, irritability, arousal, sleep disturbance, dissociation, or increased use of alcohol and drugs. In general, such feelings and the behavioral symptoms associated with them represent normal responses to profoundly abnormal events.[145] For most persons, acute post-traumatic psychiatric and behavioral symptoms will subside with time. Individuals exposed to risks that actually threaten their lives or who sustain injuries are at the highest risk of psychiatric morbidity. Such individuals may develop symptoms meeting the criteria for psychiatric diagnoses such as acute stress disorder or post-traumatic stress disorder (PTSD).[146] For many persons, knowledge that one has been exposed to a toxin such as radiation can be a potent traumatic stressor.[145–148] Terrorist attacks are likely to produce substantial levels of persistent psychiatric illness and morbidity in the persons targeted. Among 267 Pentagon staff surveyed 2 years after the attacks of September 11, 2001, 14% had probable PTSD and 7% had probable depression. Direct exposure to the September 11 terrorist attack on the Pentagon, injury during the attack, and exposure to dead bodies were associated with higher frequencies of persistent psychiatric illness and psychological distress.[147]

In the aftermath of an event, the public will seek advice from healthcare providers and the scientific community to determine the extent of internal and external contamination. Those who have been exposed or anticipate possible exposure are likely to experience feelings of vulnerability, anxiety, and lack of control. Internal contamination with radionuclides may be particularly anxiety-provoking since the patient has little control over isotope decorporation therapy and must rely on evaluation from the medical community. In addition, if there is a lack of consensus among experts, this can increase the fear and anger of exposed individuals.

The stress of radiation exposure may also cause some victims to seek medical treatment, even when none is indicated or risk is minimal. For example, there have been many cases at industrial sites where workers have been exposed to accidental inhalation of actinides in minimal quantities. Some of these workers have requested treatment with DTPA and other medications for years after the event, even when assured that chelation therapy would provide little medical efficacy. Psychological distress after

Table 33.19. Dose Schedules by Drug or Treatment Modality

Drug or Treatment Modality	Dosage
BAL	**IM:** 300 mg/vial for deep IM use, 2.5 mg/kg (or less) every 4 hours (q4h) x 2 days, then bid for 1 day, then every day (QD) for days 5–10
DTPA (Ca or Zn)	**IV:** 1 g in 250 ml normal saline (NS) or 5% glucose, given in 1–2 h, or IV push over 3–4 min
	IM: 1 g can be given with procaine to reduce pain(not FDA approved)
	Inhalation: 1g in 1:1 dilution with water or NS over 15–20 min (not FDA approved)
	Pediatrics (< 12 years old): 14 mg/kg IV, IM or by inhalation as described for adults but, not to exceed 1.0 g
D-Penicillamine	**Orally (PO):** 250 mg, QD between meals & at bedtime. May increase to 4 or 5 g QD in divided doses.
Deferoxamine	**IM or IV (IM is preferred):** 1 g IM or IV (2 ampules) slowly (15 mg/kg/h); Repeat as indicated as 500 mg IM or IV q 4 h x 2 doses; then 500 mg IV every 12 hours (q12h) for 3 days.
DMSA	**PO (for lead poisoning in pediatric patients):** Start dosage at 10 mg/kg or 350 mg/m^2 orally every 8 hours (q8h) x 5 days. Reduce frequency of administration to 10 mg/kg or 350 mg/m^2 q 12 h (two-thirds of initial daily dosage) for an additional 2 weeks of therapy (course of treatment = 19 days).
EDTA (Ca)	**IV:** Ca-EDTA 1,000 mg/m^2/d added to 500 ml D$_5$NS infused over 8–12 h.
Imuthiol	**IV:** For mild to moderate poisoning, the recommended dose is 2 g QD in divided doses. Titrate upward in dose if indicated.
PHOSPHORUS THERAPY	**PO:** 250 mg phosphorus per tablet.
Potassium phosphate, dibasic	
	Adult: 1–2 tabs p.o. taken four times per day (qid), with full glass of water each time, with meals and at bedtime.
	Children over 4 y: 1 tab qid.
Potassium Iodide (KI)	**All PO**
	Adults > 40 years of age: with thyroid exposure >500 cGy: 130 mg/d
	Adults 18–40 years of age: with thyroid exposure > 50 cGy: 130 mg/d
	Pregnant or lactating women: 130 mg/d
	Children and adolescents 3–18: with thyroid exposure > 5 cGy:65 mg/d
	Infants 1 month to 3 years: 32.5 mg/d
	Neonates from birth to 1 month: 16 mg/d
Propylthiouracil (PTU)	**PO:** 50 mg tabs, 2 tabs three times per day (TID) × 8 days
Prussian Blue	**PO:** Begin with 1 g TID PO with 100–200 ml water; may titrate up to 4 g QID for thallium or high ^{137}Cs intake. FDA drug label 3 g PO TID.
	Pediatrics, 2–12 years old: 1 g PO TID
Sodium Bicarbonate	**IV:** 2 ampules sodium bicarbonate (44.3 meq each, 7.5%) in 1,000 ml NS, 125 ml/L, or 1 ampule of sodium bicarbonate (44.3 meq, 7.5%) in 500 ml NS, 500 ml/h
	PO: 2 tablets q 4 h until urine pH = 7–8, or 4 g (8 tablets) 3 TID
STRONTIUM THERAPY	**PO:** 60–100 ml. once
Aluminum hydroxide	**PO:** 100 ml immediately after exposure once
Aluminum phosphate gel	**PO:** 1–2 g QID for 6 d
Ammonium chloride	**PO:** Generous doses; at least 1.5– 2 g daily
Calcium	**IV:** 5 ampules (500 mg calcium each) in 500 ml of 5% dextrose in water (D5W) over 4 h; continue × 6 d
Calcium gluconate	**PO:** 10 g powder in a 30 cc vial, add water and drink
Sodium Alginate	
Water diuresis	**PO:** >3–4 L per day

a radiological incident may also manifest as nonspecific somatic complaints (a presentation sometimes referred to as "MIPS," multiple idiopathic physical symptoms).[145]

Acute stress disorder and PTSD are the conditions most commonly associated with the public's response to a radiation event. Additional illnesses that may occur include major depression, increased substance use, family conflict, and generalized anxiety disorder. In the acute aftermath of a radiation event, many unexposed patients will fear that they have been exposed and will misattribute signs and symptoms of autonomic arousal to radiation contamination (after the ^{137}Cs contamination in Goiânia, Brazil, only 8.3% of the first 60,000 people screened presented with signs and symptoms of autonomic arousal consistent with acute radiation sickness).[149,150] In the longer term, patients may present to primary care providers with multiple somatic complaints for which no etiology can be determined. Such effects can be very widespread. In 2006, for example, the United Nations Chernobyl Forum stated that the "mental health impact of Chernobyl is the largest public health problem caused by the accident to date." It concluded that the accident had a serious impact on the mental health and well-being of the general populations in the countries most affected by the event (Belarus, Ukraine, and Russia).[1]

A well-organized and effective medical response will instill hope and confidence in the impacted population, reduce fear and anxiety, and support the continuity of basic community functions. Mental health professionals including psychologists and psychiatrists should be an integral part of the teams that perform initial screening and triage. When feasible, the establishment of an Emergency Services Extended Care Center may provide a functional mechanism for monitoring patients who remain fearful and are not reassured by negative findings on clinical laboratory studies.[134] Reinforcing individuals' self-sufficiency and providing actionable information useful for protecting oneself and one's family can decrease distress. Distributing appropriate medical countermeasures can also provide substantial reassurance, with concomitant psychological benefits.

Case Studies in Radiation Medicine

Goiânia (Large [137]Cs Source in the Public Domain)

On the afternoon of September 29, 1987, a physicist in the town of Goiânia, Brazil notified the country's National Nuclear Energy Commission about the possible occurrence of a serious radiation accident. Three men had removed a 50.9 TBq (1,375 Ci) ^{137}Cs radiation therapy device from an abandoned radiotherapy clinic on or about September 13, 1987, and sold it to a junkyard as scrap.[149] It is believed that the source capsule was ruptured on September 18. The relatively soluble cesium chloride mass was divided into smaller pieces and distributed among various friends and neighbors. The accident became known 16 days later. A physicist contacted by medical authorities was able to identify the nature of the source and subsequent widespread contamination. The physicist's involvement was prompted when the wife of the junkyard owner brought a piece of the source to the attention of her physician, saying that it was responsible for illness in many of her friends.

In total, approximately 110,000 residents of Goiânia were monitored in Olympic Stadium, and 249 were found to be contaminated either internally, externally, or both. Four main foci of contamination were noted: three junkyards and the residence where the source was ruptured. Handling of the radioactive cesium generally caused internal contamination by ingestion.

Four individuals died in the accident, three from external exposure and one, a 6-year-old child, from ingestion of powdered cesium. In addition, the town was extensively contaminated. During decontamination efforts, a total of 12,500 drums and 1,470 boxes were filled with contaminated debris. More recent developments from this accident have been described in a subsequent International Atomic Energy Agency publication.[150]

The Radiation Accident in Estonia (Large [137]Cs Source in a Private Home)

On October 21, 1994, an Estonian citizen (RiH), along with his two brothers, visited a radioactive waste facility to scavenge for scrap metal, overriding the electrical alarm system and cutting various padlocks. RiH climbed into one of the vaults to obtain salvageable metal and passed a large ^{137}Cs source to his brothers. At this time, none of the brothers realized that this metallic object was highly radioactive. During the theft, RiH injured his leg slightly when an aluminum drum fell against it. Shortly after entry into the repository, RiH began to feel ill and went home. Other occupants of the house were the man's stepson (RT), the boy's mother, and the boy's great-grandmother. The cesium source was initially placed in the pocket of RiH's coat, which was hanging in the hall. Eventually, it was placed in a kitchen drawer along with various tools. Details of the radiation injury to members of the household and the resulting radiation-induced pathology are described in an International Atomic Energy Agency publication.[151]

Soon thereafter, RiH was hospitalized with severe injury to his leg. During the initial medical history, RiH claimed that he received the injury while working in the nearby forest. As a consequence, he was treated for crush injury. On November 2, 1994, RiH died without medical authorities having any suspicion of radiation exposure as the etiology of his terminal illness. Meanwhile, by November 9, 1994, the stepson RT had developed signs and symptoms that indicated he had come in contact with the source multiple times.

Shortly thereafter, the 4-month old pet dog died. The dog had slept much of the time in the kitchen near the cesium source. RT was also eventually admitted to the hospital with severe hand burns, which physicians correctly diagnosed as radiation-induced cutaneous injury. As a result of this diagnosis, the police were notified, and in turn, notified the Estonia Rescue Board, which immediately dispatched staff. A Russian medical delegation also arrived soon thereafter to provide medical and health physics consultation.

After an extensive radiation dose reconstruction, the investigators estimated that RiH received a dose of approximately 1,830 Gy to his thigh and approximately 4 Gy to the rest of his body. Clinically, RiH experienced many of the acute hematopoietic syndrome effects along with severe, extensive local injury to his thigh (the dose rate of the stolen source was estimated to be 2,000–3,000 Gy/hour). He died from neutropenic sepsis and acute renal failure 12 days following his exposure. An autopsy showed acute radiation necrosis of the right thigh and hip, along with hemorrhage and thinning of the intestinal wall. The cause of death was ARS with both hematopoietic and gastrointestinal components, along with severe local radiation necrosis.

The investigators estimated that the stepson, RT, received 20–30 Gy to his left hand, 8–10 Gy to his right hand, and approximately 2.5 Gy to his whole body during various episodes of bicycle maintenance. Other family members received hand doses in the range of 8–20 Gy and whole-body doses in the range of

1–2.5 Gy. The dose estimations were based on each individual's recollection of the time spent occupying various locations within the house. In addition, spatial computer analysis, chromosome aberration analysis, and other specialized assays were employed.

Criticality Accidents in the United States

LOS ALAMOS PLUTONIUM SPHERE CASES

Two criticality events occurred with the same 6.2-kg delta-phase plutonium sphere at Los Alamos National Laboratory (LANL).[9,152–154] The first incident occurred on August 21, 1945, when a worker was preparing a critical assembly by stacking tungsten carbide bricks around the plutonium core as a reflector. He moved the final block over the assembly but, noting that this block would make the assembly supercritical, he withdrew it. The brick fell onto the center of the assembly, resulting in a super-prompt critical state of approximately 6×10^{15} fissions.[9] The worker sustained an average whole-body dose of approximately 5.1 Gy and a dose to the right hand of approximately 100–400 Gy. The patient died of sepsis 28 days after the accident. Lymphocyte depletion kinetics from the 1945 LANL-1 criticality accident are shown in Figure 33.6.

The second criticality accident occurred in 1946 during an approach to criticality demonstration at which several observers were present. The operator used a screwdriver as a lever to lower a hemispherical beryllium shell reflector into place. While holding the top shell with his left thumb using an opening at the spherical pole, the screwdriver slipped and caused a critical configuration. The fission yield in this accident was estimated at 3×10^{15} fissions. The operator received an estimated acute whole-body dose of approximately 21 Gy, with a dose to the left hand 150 Gy and somewhat less to the right hand. Seven observers were exposed in the range 0.27–3.6 Gy. The operator died 9 days later.

LOS ALAMOS LIQUID CRITICALITY EVENT

On December 30, 1958, during purification and concentration of plutonium, unexpected plutonium-rich solids were washed from two vessels into a single large vessel that contained layered, dilute, aqueous and organic solutions. The tank contained approximately 295 liters of a caustic stabilized organic

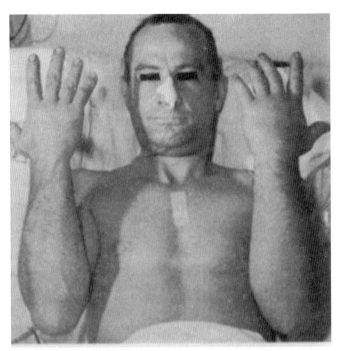

Figure 33.7. Wood River Valley patient 24 hours post-accident. Note edema in the left arm. Figure reprinted by permission of the *New England Journal of Medicine*.

emulsion. The added nitric acid wash is believed to have separated the liquid phases. Accident analysis shows that the aqueous layer initially was slightly below delayed critical activity (approximately 203 mm wide, critical thickness being 210 mm). When the stirrer was started, the central portion of the liquid system was thickened, changing system reactivity to super-prompt critical. The excursion yield was approximately 1.5×10^{17} fissions. Bubble generation was the negative feedback mechanism for terminating the first neutron spike. The system was driven permanently subcritical by mixing of the two layers. This accident resulted in the death of the operator 36 hours post-event. The dose to the upper extremity was estimated at 120 Gy ± 50%. Two other persons received acute doses of 1.34 Gy and 0.53 Gy.

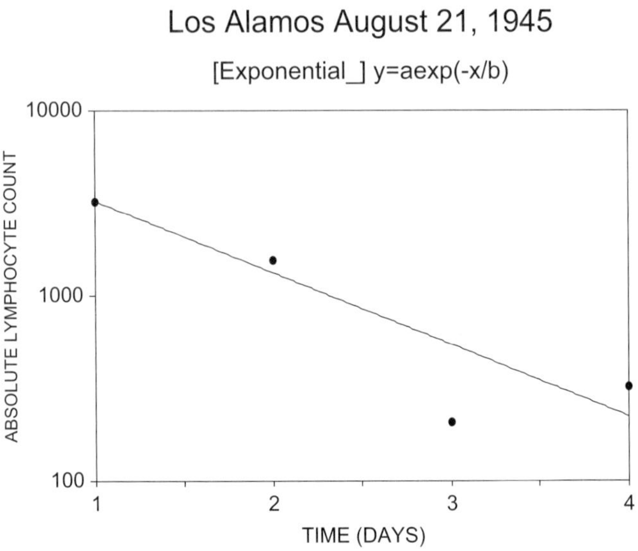

WOOD RIVER JUNCTION CRITICALITY EVENT

This liquid process accident occurred on July 24, 1964, at the United Nuclear Fuels Recovery Plant in Wood River Junction, Rhode Island.[155,156] A chemical processing plant was designed to recover highly enriched uranium from scrap material left over from the production of fuel rods. Uranyl nitrate solution U(93) was poured into a carbonate reagent vessel. The critical excursion occurred when nearly all of the uranium had been transferred, resulting in approximately 1.1×10^{17} fissions. It is probable that the system oscillated, resulting in a series of excursions with total energy release equivalent to 1.3×10^{17} fissions. The acute dose to the operator was estimated to be 100 Gy. Two supervisory personnel received approximately 1 Gy and 0.6 Gy. The operator died 49 hours after the accident (Figure 33.7).

Clinical Course of the Criticality Cases

Case 1 – Los Alamos plutonium sphere (hematopoietic syndrome; cutaneous radiation injury syndrome; whole-body dose approximately 5.1 Gy, dose to right hand 100–400 Gy)

Los Alamos August 21, 1945

[Exponential_] y=aexp(-x/b)

Figure 33.6. Lymphocyte depletion kinetics in the 1945 LANL-1 criticality accident. Reprinted from Reference 152.

The patient was a 26-year-old male whose past medical history was significant only for Wolff-Parkinson-White Syndrome diagnosed 3 years prior to the incident. On admission to the hospital, his vital signs were within normal limits and his only initial complaint was numbness and tingling of both hands. The initial physical exam was also within normal limits.

Within 30 minutes post-accident, the patient's right hand had become diffusely swollen. Emesis began approximately 1.5 hours post-event, and nausea continued intermittently for the next 24 hours. The patient experienced subjective improvement but had a low grade fever, gastric distress, and fatigue during days 3–6. By day 5, the patient experienced a distinct rise in temperature with tachycardia, and began to appear increasingly toxic. On day 10, he developed severe stomatitis, a paralytic ileus, and diarrhea. Clinical signs of pericarditis were noted on day 17, and the patient's mental status deteriorated. The clinical course was notable for progressive pancytopenia. Figure 33.6 demonstrates an exponential decrease of lymphocytes during the first 4 days post-accident.

Within 36 hours of the accident, blisters were noted on the volar aspect of the right third finger, and within another day extensive blistering was noted on both palmar and volar surfaces of the hand. A decision was made on day 3 to surgically drain the blisters but by the third week, the right hand had progressed to a dry gangrene. Desquamation of the epidermis involved almost all of the skin covering the dorsal forearm and hand. In addition, epilation was almost complete at the time of death.

On day 24, the patient's temperature had risen to $41.1°$C. He had lost a great deal of weight, developed thoracoabdominal erythema, and showed signs of sepsis. The patient became comatose and died on the same day. During the patient's clinical admission, treatment consisted of fluid support, penicillin antibiotic therapy, thiamine, and two blood transfusions.

On autopsy, severe skin necrosis was observed as well overt dry gangrene. The cardiopulmonary system was significant for pericarditis, cardiac hypertrophy, pulmonary edema, and alveolar hemorrhage. The spleen was noted to have no germinal centers and the mucosa of the large bowel and buccal surfaces was ulcerated. The bone marrow was noted to be hypoplastic and lymph nodes also showed significant lymphocyte depletion. The testes demonstrated significant atrophy with aspermia. A solitary ulcer was noted in the large colon as well as a right renal infarct.[154]

Case 2 – Los Alamos plutonium sphere (gastrointestinal syndrome; cutaneous radiation syndrome; acute dose approximately 21 Gy, dose to the left hand 150 Gy)

The patient was a 32 year-old male, admitted to the hospital within 1 hour of the accident. His medical history was generally unremarkable. His occupational history was significant only for several prior, generally chronic occupational exposures, none exceeding 0.005 Gy in a week. The patient complained of nausea in the hour prior to admission and vomited once in the first hour after the accident.

The general condition of the patient was quite good in the first 5 days post-accident. On the fifth day there was a precipitous drop in his leukocyte count, and his condition quickly deteriorated. The patient rapidly lost weight, developed mental confusion on the seventh day, ultimately became comatose, and died on the ninth day.

Medical therapy during the 9-day course was largely supportive. Penicillin (50,000 U) was given intramuscularly every 3 hours beginning on day 5 because of granulocytopenia. Blood transfusions were also given daily after the fifth day. On day 6, fever and tachycardia developed, and on day 7, the patient developed a severe paralytic ileus. The patient died on day 9 in cardiovascular shock. At the time of death, both hands showed extensive radiation damage.

On autopsy, examination of the skin on the abdomen revealed early vesicle formation and marked epidermal damage. The cardiopulmonary system was remarkable for cardiac hemorrhage and myocardial edema, and the terminal bronchi showed features of aspiration pneumonia. The spleen exhibited no germinal centers and most of the GI tract mucosa showed sloughing, most pronounced in the jejunum and ileum. Widespread degenerative changes were noted in the adrenal cortex as well as hyaline degeneration in the renal tubular epithelium. Examination of the red bone marrow (myeloid tissue) showed it to be of liquid consistency.[154]

Case 3 – Los Alamos Liquid Criticality Event (Central nervous system syndrome; dose to the upper extremity 120 Gy ± 50%)

The patient was a 50-year-old male with no significant past medical history. The clinical course can be divided into four separate phases:

- Phase 1 (20–30 minutes post-event): immediate physical collapse and mental incapacitation, progressing eventually into semi-consciousness
- Phase 2 (90 minutes): signs and symptoms of cardiovascular shock accompanied by severe abdominal pain
- Phase 3 (28 hours): subjective minimal clinical improvement
- Phase 4 (2 days): rapidly developing irritability and mania, progressing to coma and death.

The clinical course was remarkable for continuing, profound hypotension, tachycardia, and intense dermal and conjunctival hyperemia. The patient died 35 hours after exposure.

On autopsy, examination of the bone marrow was most significant for absence of mitotic activity. The lungs showed pyknotic, degenerating cells in the pleura, degenerating lymphocytes and neutrophils in the subpleural connective tissue, and many areas of focal atelectasis interspersed with foci of emphysema. All lymph nodes were markedly atrophic and lymphoid follicles in the spleen were greatly depleted.

Examination of the heart showed acute myocarditis, myocardial edema, cardiac hypertrophy, and a fibrinous pericarditis. Examination of the brain demonstrated cerebral edema, diffuse vasculitis, and cerebral hemorrhage. The GI system showed necrosis of the anterior gastric wall parietal cells, acute upper jejunal distention, mitotic suppression throughout the entire gastrointestinal tract, and acute jejunal and ileal enteritis.[154]

Case 4 –Wood River Junction (Central nervous system syndrome; approximately 100 Gy)

The patient was a 38-year-old male with no significant medical history. Following the initial criticality excursion, the patient appeared stunned, ran from the building, and immediately vomited. He also experienced instantaneous diarrhea and complained of severe abdominal cramping, headache, and thirst associated with profuse perspiration. His initial vital signs showed borderline blood pressure elevation and tachycardia. Approximately 4 hours after the accident, the patient experienced transient difficulty in speaking, hypotension, and tachycardia. A portable chest X-ray 16 hours after admission revealed hilar congestion. Physical examination showed an edematous left hand and forearm and also demonstrated left-sided conjunctivitis and periorbital edema (Figure 33.7). On day 2, the patient became very disoriented, hypotensive, and anuric. The patient died 49 hours after the accident in cardiovascular shock.

At autopsy, interstitial edema of the left hand, arm, and abdominal wall was noted. Examination of the heart, lungs, and abdominal cavity revealed acute pulmonary edema, bilateral pleural effusions, a pericardial effusion, abdominal ascites, acute pericarditis; interstitial myocarditis, and inflammation of the ascending aorta. Examination of the gastrointestinal tract showed severe subserosal edema of the stomach, transverse colon, and descending colon. Inspection of the hematopoietic system demonstrated an aplastic bone marrow with the lymph nodes, spleen, and thymus depleted of lymphocytes. The brain showed minimal effects, with rare foci of microglial change. The testes showed interstitial edema and overt necrosis of the spermatogonia.[155,156]

RECOMMENDATIONS FOR FUTURE RESEARCH

New treatments for radiation injury are emerging that may accelerate healing of acute radiation injuries and/or minimize the delayed effects of acute radiation exposure. Examples include mitigation of fibrosis, radiation nephropathy, and other complications. Current research is exploring the possibility of translating therapies that have been efficacious in the treatment of chemotherapy-induced myelosuppression, GVHD, thermal burns, ischemic injury (e.g., diabetes), and other disorders for use in the management of radiation-induced injury.

Many of the therapies currently under consideration as potential radiation countermeasures were developed as supportive care for oncology patients. Multiple chemotherapeutic agents share with radiation the property of killing rapidly dividing cells and thus producing toxicity profiles. Some of these profiles, including pronounced bone marrow and GI toxicity, mimic the effects of radiation. Drugs and therapeutics that have demonstrated efficacy in preventing, mitigating, or treating such toxic effects are obvious candidates for development as radiation countermeasures. The efficacy of CSFs such as filgrastim, pegfilgrastim, and sargramostim in shortening the duration of neutropenia after chemotherapy is well established and these products are widely used clinically for this purpose. In May 2013, a Joint Meeting of the FDA Medical Imaging Drugs and Oncologic Drugs Advisory Committees evaluated the available data supporting the use of such products as a treatment for radiation-induced neutropenia. These committees concluded that filgrastim was reasonably likely to produce clinical benefits in humans exposed to myelosuppressive doses of radiation. In addition, the probable safety and efficacy of filgrastim in this setting could be generalized to other approved CSFs.[180] As of July 2014, however, FDA has not approved any CSFs for the treatment of radiation-induced neutropenia on the basis of these recommendations. Second-generation thrombopoietin receptor agonists have been approved for the treatment of chronic immune thrombocytopenia refractory to other therapy. These agents show promise for the mitigation of chemotherapy-induced thrombocytopenia, and may be helpful in the treatment of the acute hematopoietic syndrome. Oral beclomethasone dipropionate was initially investigated as a treatment for acute gastrointestinal GVHD and has shown promise as a treatment for the GI syndrome.[181] Such agents are now being studied in animal models of acute radiation exposure. It is possible that the benefits observed from the use of these drugs to reduce the toxicity of chemotherapy or other cancer treatments will translate to the management of radiation victims. It should be underscored that none of these agents are presently licensed in the United States for the treatment of radiation injury and the off-label use of such products cannot be recommended.

Other forms of injury not directly targeting rapidly dividing cell populations also appear to share common mechanistic pathways with radiation injury. Trauma, for example, appears to up-regulate many of the same pro-inflammatory cytokines and matrix metalloproteinases as acute radiation exposure (e.g., transforming growth factor–β and tumor necrosis factor–α). Other cytokines (e.g., platelet-derived growth factor and fibroblast growth factor), however, might be at insufficient levels for maximal healing.[160–162] Treatments that affect cytokine levels have demonstrated significant efficacy at mitigating the acute effects of many kinds of injury in clinical studies and preclinical models. It is reasonable to hypothesize that they might demonstrate efficacy in the treatment of radiation-induced injury and/or radiation combined injury. The role that individual cytokines play in the healing process is complex, however. Applications or generalized class inhibition of some cytokines may have either beneficial or deleterious properties depending on the stage of the healing process.[164–166] Commercially available tissue-engineered products have also demonstrated efficacy in wound repair by providing a protective barrier and possibly an environment rich in cytokines for the treated wound.

The administration of multiple cytokines simultaneously also appears to offer great promise. Combination therapy with cytokines clearly shortens the duration of hematopoietic pancytopenia in preclinical models. Herodin et al. demonstrated that in animal models the combination of stem cell factor + FLT-3-ligand + thrombopoietin + interleukin 3 (regimen name: SFT3) reduced the period of thrombocytopenia and blood transfusions required after 7 Gy of total-body irradiation. Furthermore, the addition of pegfilgrastim to the combination shortened the period of neutropenia compared with the control and SFT3 groups. Bone marrow activity recovered faster in the SFT3 groups compared with the control. Of note, no long-term mutagenic toxicity appears associated with SFT3.[167] Herodin et al. also demonstrated that post-radiation administration of KGF and SFT3 resulted in 75% survival at 30 days compared to the controls of less than 10% (p < 0.01). Thus, treatments that address multi-organ failure appear promising.[159]

The role of allogeneic stem cell transplantation in the treatment of ARS remains limited, but new approaches to cell therapy show promise and are under active investigation. A number of preclinical studies have demonstrated that systemically administered mesenchymal stem cells (MSCs) can speed the recovery of autologous hematopoietic function and salvage lethally irradiated mice. Case reports suggest that the topical application of MSCs to severe radiation burns may improve wound healing and cosmetic outcomes.[182,183] Committed myeloid progenitor cells have also shown promise as a radiation countermeasure. Life-saving benefits are observed even in the setting of extremely high doses of radiation (up to 15 Gy) or when administered up to a week after exposure.[184] A common theme seen in treatment with cell therapy is that it appears to provide benefits across multiple organ systems. For example, conventional bone marrow transplantation has been shown to speed recovery of the mucosal immune system and enhance intestinal mucosal barrier function compared to untreated animals, in addition to facilitating recovery of hematopoietic function.[185] At present, the mechanisms by which these benefits are conferred are incompletely understood.

Therapies that treat or mitigate both the acute and late effects of radiation exposure are being investigated. For example, angiotensin-converting enzyme inhibitors and angiotensin II receptor antagonists have been shown to decrease chemical, mechanical, and radiation acute and/or late effects in a variety of organs.[168–172] Suppressing or regulating the acute or chronic inflammatory response also appears to expedite the healing process. Neutrophil-depleted mice, for example, have demonstrated more rapid wound closure, presumably as a result of the suppression of neutrophil-mediated inflammation (although the mice are more susceptible to infection).[173] Emerging evidence suggests that treatments suppressing the ongoing inflammatory response may accelerate repair while minimizing late sequelae such as fibrosis and scarring.[174]

Another area of concern and controversy is the exposure of large numbers of people to low doses of ionizing radiation from an atomic bomb explosion or from diagnostic medical procedures. This can result in stochastic late effects, specifically cancer. One area of current interest is the population effect from the widespread use of CT scans. In a prominent 2007 article, Brenner and Hall suggest that 1.5–2% of all cancers in the United States may be attributable to radiation from CT studies.[175] The study is mainly based on the linear no-threshold model for cancer induction and extrapolates medical data from atomic bomb survivors. The linear no-threshold (LNT) model, however, has been the subject of continuing controversy because no increased evidence of cancer has been observed at doses of less than 10 cGy in adults and infants.

Some authorities have rejected the LNT model as the basis for radiation exposure risk assessment at very low doses. For example, the French Academy of Medicine "denounces utilization of the linear no-threshold (LNT) relation to estimate the effect of low doses to a few mSv."[176] A second issue involves utilizing the medical data on atomic bomb survivors for estimating the effects of diagnostic radiation. Although absolute energy exposure may be similar, the qualities of the ionizing radiation that produce such exposures are different. Diagnostic medical devices use X-rays and typically result in highly non-uniform exposures, whereas the prompt radiation associated with fission and delayed radiation from fallout results in more nearly uniform exposures to both electromagnetic (gamma rays and X-rays) and particulate (alpha particles, beta particles, and neutrons) forms of radiation. It remains to be demonstrated that the carcinogenic potential of these different kinds of exposure are identical. Uncertainty also remains as to the risk imposed by in utero exposures below 10 cGy because of the contradictory epidemiological data.[177] Regardless, the development of highly safe therapies for use in large exposed populations to minimize stochastic effects is warranted, especially at doses at which there is clear evidence for increased cancer induction above the 10–20 cGy threshold.

The 2006 poisoning of Russian dissident Alexander Litvinenko in London with ^{210}Po underscored the lethality associated with the internalization of radioactive elements and,

therefore, the importance of developing new and improved methods of decorporating radionuclides. In recent years, the Radiation Countermeasures Program at the U.S. National Institutes of Allergy and Infectious Diseases has funded research to support the development of orally available DTPA, nano-engineered sorbents, chitosan-based materials, and other novel chelating agents. Several of these projects have demonstrated improved decorporation and toxicity profiles in preclinical models and work is continuing at the time of this writing.

Finally, for countermeasures such as those described herein to be useful, emergency management officials must have reliable mechanisms for delivering them to exposed individuals in a timely fashion. Delivery of products from centralized stockpiles may be sufficient for countermeasures that can be administered 24–48 hours after exposure but will likely be inadequate for highly time-sensitive countermeasures such as potassium iodide. The U.S. National Academy of Sciences reported on strategies for stockpiling and distributing potassium iodide, and other authors have proposed alternate solutions for forward deployment that could facilitate the rapid distribution of other time-sensitive countermeasures.[178,179]

Conclusions

As noted in the Overview, mass exposure to radiation does not occur frequently. When such events do occur, however, they present tremendous challenges to affected communities. With the concerns in recent years regarding nuclear or radiological terrorism, it would also appear that the risk of deliberate mass exposures to radiation has increased. Nations, regions, and communities must maintain their primary focus on preventing the occurrence of radiological and nuclear accidents but should also engage in prudent consequence management planning as well. Planning must include provision for the medical and public health response to radiation emergencies, including: 1) the management of large numbers of potentially contaminated patients; 2) the performance of accurate biodosimetry and dose assessment; 3) the rapid delivery and distribution of pertinent medical countermeasures; 4) the clinical care of radiological casualties; and 5) the extension of emergency psychological and social services to traumatized communities. State of the art symposia on radiation medicine are presented approximately every 10 years by REAC/TS, the U.S. Department of Energy's asset for emergency response to radiation events.[186,187]

In future years, the application of novel scientific tools and techniques to the challenges of radiobiology and normal tissue injury will likely result in significant advances in the ability to diagnose, mitigate, and treat both the immediate and delayed effects of acute radiation exposure. The application of genomic, proteomic, and metabolomic probes to irradiated tissue may result in new ways to perform rapid dose assessments and the development of a truly predictive biodosimetry. In the realm of therapeutics, a better understanding of the systems biology of radiation injury will likely lead to the rational design of targeted radiation countermeasures, an enhanced understanding of the role of growth factors, and the use of pleiotropic cytokines in mitigating radiation injury. Improved methods for promoting immune reconstitution and tissue repair after high-dose irradiation are on the horizon, perhaps involving novel approaches to cell therapy and regenerative medicine. After a period of comparative neglect, the future for the fields of radiobiology and normal tissue injury appears to be bright.

REFERENCES

1. Bennett B, Repacholi M, Carr Z, eds.*Health Effects of the Chernobyl Accident and Special Health Care Programmes: Report of the UN Chernobyl Forum Health Expert Group.* Geneva, World Health Organization, 2006. http://www.who.int/ionizing_radiation/chernobyl/WHO%20Report%20on%20Chernobyl%20Health%20Effects%20July%2006.pdf (Accessed June 22, 2013).

2. Oliveira AR, Hunt JG, Valverde NJ, Brandao-Mello CE, Farina R. Medical and related aspects of the Goiania accident: an overview. *Health Physics* 1991; 60: 17–24.

3. The efforts cited include but are not limited to the establishment of the Domestic Nuclear Detection Office, the development of medical countermeasures against radiation by the National Institute of Allergy and Infectious Diseases and the Biomedical Advanced Research and Development Authority, and the Radiation Event Medical Management website available online at www.remm.nlm.gov. The latter programs are discussed later in this chapter.

4. Tenet G. *At the Center of the Storm: My Years at the CIA.* New York, Harper Collins Publishers, 2006; see particularly chapters 14 and 15.

5. Allison G. *Nuclear Terrorism: The Ultimate Preventable Catastrophe.* New York, Henry Holt and Company, 2004.

6. Williams PL. *Osama's Revenge: The Next 9/11.* Amherst, NY, Prometheus Books, 2004.

7. Ferguson CD, Potter WC. *The Four Faces of Nuclear Terrorism.* Monterey, CA, Monterey Institute for International Studies, 2004.

8. Bailey MR, Birchall A, Etherington G, et al. *Individual monitoring conducted by the Health Protection Agency in the London Polonium-210 Incident. HPA-RPD-067.* Oxford, Health Protection Agency Centre for Radiation, Chemical and Environmental Hazards Radiation Protection Division, 2010. http://www.hpa.nhs.uk/webc/HPAwebFile/HPAweb_C/1274089667322 (Accessed June 22, 2013).

9. McLaughlin TP, Monahan SP, Pruvost NL, Frolov VV, Ryazanov BG, Sviridov VI. *A Review of Criticality Accidents, 2000 Revision.* Los Alamos National Laboratory, Los Alamos, NM, 2000. http://www.orau.org/ptp/library/accidents/la-13638.pdf (Accessed June 22, 2013).

10. Andrews GA. Criticality accidents in Vinca, Yugoslavia, and Oak Ridge, Tennessee. Comparison of radiation injuries and results of therapy. *JAMA* 1962; 179: 191–197.

11. Tanaka SI. Summary of the JCO criticality accident in Tokaimura and a dose assessment. *J Radiat Res (Tokyo)* 2001; 42 Suppl: S1–S9.

12. Mettler FA, Voelz GL, Nenot J-C, Gusev IA. Criticality accidents. In: Gusev IA, Guskova AK, Mettler FA, eds., *Medical Management of Radiation Accidents.* Boca Raton, FL, CRC Press, 2001.

13. Guskova AK, Gusev IA. Medical aspects of the accident at Chernobyl. In: Gusev IA, Guskova AK, Mettler FA, eds., *Medical Management of Radiation Accidents.* Boca Raton, FL, CRC Press, 2001.

14. Cohen BL. *The Nuclear Energy Option: An Alternative for the 90s.* New York, Plenum Puiblishing, 1990. http://www.phyast.pitt.edu/~blc/book/BOOK.html (Accessed June 22, 2013).

15. U.S. Nuclear Regulatory Commission. Backgrounder on Chernobyl Nuclear Power Plant Accident. http://www.nrc.gov/reading-rm/doc-collections/fact-sheets/chernobyl-bg.html (Accessed June 22, 2013).

16. Crick MJ, Linsley GS. An assessment of the radiological impact of the Windscale reactor fire, October 1957. *Int J Radiat Biol Rela Stud Phys Chem Med* 1984; 46: 479–506.

17. U.S. Nuclear Regulatory Commission. Backgrounder on the Three Mile Island Accident. http://www.nrc.gov/reading-rm/doc-collections/fact-sheets/3mile-isle.html (Accessed June 22, 2013).

18. Tokyo Electric Power Company. Estimation of Radioactive Material Released to the Atmosphere during the Fukushima Daiichi NPS Accident. May 2012. http://www.tepco.co.jp/en/press/corp-com/release/betu12_e/images/120524e0205.pdf (Accessed June 22, 2013).

19. World Health Organization. Health risk assessment from the nuclear accident after the 2011 Great East Japan Earthquake and Tsunami, based on a preliminary dose estimation. 2013. http://apps.who.int/iris/bitstream/10665/78218/1/9789241505130_eng.pdf (Accessed June 22, 2013).

20. United States General Accounting Office. Spent nuclear fuel: options exist to further enhance security. GAO Report No. 03–426. 2003. www.gao.gov/new.items/d03426.pdf (Accessed September 5, 2015).

21. Pilkey OH, Pilkey-Jarvis L. *Useless Arithmetic: Why Environmental Scientists Can't Predict the Future.* New York, Columbia University Press, 2007; 20. Langewiesche W. *The Atomic Bazaar: The Rise of the Nuclear Poor.* New York, Farrar, Straus and Giroux, 2007.

22. Peter RU, Arsin H, Cosset J-M, Clough K, Gourmelon P, Nenot J-C. Accident involving abandoned radioactive sources in Georgia, 1997. In: Gusev IA, Guskova AK, Mettler FA, eds. *Medical Management of Radiation Accidents.* Boca Raton, FL, CRC Press, 2001.

23. De Oliveira CN, Melo DR, Liptzstein JL. Internal contamination in the Goiânia accident, Brazil, 1987. In: *Medical Management of Radiation Accidents.*

24. Guskova AK. Epidemiological evaluation of populations accidentally exposed near the Techa River, Russia. In: *Medical Management of Radiation Accidents.*

25. Guskova AK, et al. Acute radiation effects in victims of the Chernobyl accident. UNSCEAR 1988 Report, Appendix to Annex G. http://www.unscear.org/docs/reports/1988annexgappx.pdf (Accessed July 6, 2013).

26. Mettler FA, Ortiz-Lopez P. Accidents in radiation therapy. In: *Medical Management of Radiation Accidents.*

27. Mettler FA. Accidents at industrial irradiation facilities. In: *Medical Management of Radiation Accidents.*

28. Zimmerman PD, Loeb C. Dirty bombs: the threat revisited. *Defense Horizons* 2004; 38: 1–11.

29. Bale JM. The Chechen resistance and radiological terrorism. Nuclear Threat Initiative Issue Brief. http://www.nti.org/e_research/e3_47a.html (Accessed September 5, 2015).

30. The Nunn-Lugar Cooperative Threat Reduction (CTR) Program. http://www.nti.org/db/nisprofs/russia/forasst/nunn_lug/overview.htm (Accessed September 5, 2015).

31. Langewiesche W. *The Atomic Bazaar: The Rise of the Nuclear Poor.*

32. Bush, Kerry: nukes most serious threat. *CNN Newswire.* October 9, 2004. http://www.cnn.com/2004/ALLPOLITICS/09/30/debate.main/index.html (Accessed September 5, 2015).

33. Jackson D. Obama: nuclear terrorism is 'the single biggest threat' to U.S. *USA Today.* http://content.usatoday.com/communities/theoval/post/2010/04/obama-kicks-off-nuclear-summit-with-five-leader-meetings/1 (Accessed June 23, 2013).

34. Glasstone S, Dolan P. *The Effects of Nuclear Weapons. Department of the Army Pamphlet No. 50–3.* Washington, DC, Department of the Army, 1997.

35. HOTSPOT Version 2.06 Nuclear Explosion Program. Lawrence Livermore National Laboratory. http://www.llnl.gov/

nhi/hotspot (Accessed September 5, 2015). Documentation is within the "Help" function of the computer program.

36. Martin JE. *Physics for Radiation Protection.* New York, John Wiley & Sons, 2000.

37. Guskova AK, et al. Acute radiation effects in victims of the Chernobyl accident. UNSCEAR 1988 Report, Appendix to Annex G. http://www.unscear.org/docs/reports/1988annexgappx.pdf (Accessed September 5, 2015).

38. A notable exception was the accidental exposure of inhabitants of the Marshall Islands to fallout from the detonation of a nuclear device in 1954. Exposures prior to evacuation were estimated to be < 2 Gy in the most severely exposed, with beta burns and mild depression of blood counts being the predominant acute effects. See Cronkite EP, et al. Medical effects of exposure of human beings to fallout radiation from a thermonuclear explosion. *Stem Cells* 1995; 13(Suppl. 1): 49–57.

39. Hall EJ. Acute effects of total-body irradiation. In: Hall EJ, ed. *Radiobiology for the Radiologist.* Philadelphia, PA, Lippincott Williams & Wilkins, 2000;124–135. Of note, however, only one (5%) of the twenty-one Chernobyl emergency workers receiving doses in excess of 650 cGy survived, despite aggressive supportive care (thirteen received allogeneic bone marrow transplants). Fifteen (68%) of the twenty-two emergency responders receiving doses between 420 and 640 cGy survived. See United Nations Scientific Committee on the Effects of Atomic Radiation. Sources and Effects of Ionizing Radiation. Annex J: Exposures and effects of the Chernobyl Accident. New York, United Nations, 2000. http://www.unscear.org/docs/reports/annexj.pdf (Accessed September 5, 2015).

40. Rotblat J. Acute radiation mortality in a nuclear war. In: Soloman F, Marston RQ, eds. *The Medical Implications of Nuclear War.* Washington, DC, Institute of Medicine, National Academy of Sciences, 1986: 233–250. This calculated dose reflected a neutron-dose fraction of < 0.06.

41. Kallman RF. The effect of dose rate on mode of acute radiation death of C57BL and BALB/c mice. *Radiat Res* 1962; 16: 796–810.

42. Neal FE. Variation of acute mortality with dose-rate in mice exposed to single large doses of whole-body x-irradiation. *Int J Radiat Biol* 1960; 2: 295–300.

43. Broyles AA. The effect of dose rate on radiation injury. *Health Physics* 1989; 56: 933–937.

44. MacVittie TJ, et al. The relative biological effectiveness of mixed fission-neutron-gamma radiation on the hematopoietic syndrome in the canine: effect of therapy on survival. *Radiat Res* 1991; 128(1 Suppl.): S29–S36.

45. Wang J, et al. The response of dogs to mixed neutron-gamma radiation with different neutron/gamma ratios. *Radiat Res* 1991; 128(1 Suppl.): S42–S46. In this study, the WBC nadir after a 90% neutron exposure of 265 cGy occurred at 5 days while the WBC nadir at the same dose with 15% neutrons occurred at 15–17 days.

46. Cronkite EP, et al. Medical effects of exposure of human beings to fallout radiation from a thermonuclear explosion. *Stem Cells* 1995; 13(1 Suppl.): 49–57.

47. Kataoka Y, et al. Antimutagenic effects of radioprotector WR-2721 against fission-spectrum neutrons and 60Co gamma rays in mice. *Int J Radiat Biol* 1992; 61: 387–392.

48. Su Y, Swift M. Mortality rates among carriers of ataxia-telangiectasia mutant alleles. *Ann Intern Med* 2000; 133: 770–778.

49. Carlomagno F, Chang-Claude J, Dunning AM, Ponder BA. Determination of the frequency of the common 657Del5 Nijmegen breakage syndrome mutation in the German population: no association with risk of breast cancer. *Genes Chromosomes Cancer* 1999; 25: 393–395.

50. Thomson JF, Tourtellotte WW, Carttar MS, Cox RS, Wilson JE. Studies on the effects of continuous exposure of animals to gamma radiation from cobalt 60 sources. *Am J Roentgenol Radium Ther Nucl Med* 1953; 69: 830–838.

51. Garner RJ, et al. Effect of age on the acute lethal response of the beagle to cobalt-60 gamma radiation. *Radiat Res* 1974; 58: 190–195.

52. Casarett AP. Modification of Radiation Injury. In: *Radiation Biology.* Englewood Cliffs, NJ, Prentice-Hall, Inc., 1968; 236–265.

53. Alexander GA, Swartz HM, Amundson SA, et al. BiodosEPR-2006 Meeting: Acute dosimetry consensus committee recommendations on biodosimetry applications in events involving uses of radiation by terrorists and radiation accidents. *Radiat Measurements* 2007; 42: 972–996.

54. Anno GH, Young RW, Bloom RM, Mercier JR. Dose response relationships for acute radiation lethality. *Health Phys* 2003; 84: 565–575.

55. Goans RE. Clinical care of the radiation patient. In: Ricks RC, Berger ME, O'Hara FM, eds. *The Medical Basis for Radiation-Accident Preparedness: The Clinical Care of Victims.* Nashville, TN, Parthenon Publishing, 2002.

56. Goans RE, Waselenko JK. Medical management of radiation casualties. *Health Phys* 2005; 89: 505–512.

57. Coleman CN, Weinstock DM, Casagrande R, et al. Triage and treatment tools for use in a scarce resources-crisis standards of care setting after a nuclear detonation. *Disaster Med Public Health Prep* March 2011; 5 Suppl. 1): S111–S121.

58. Dainiak N, Gent RN, Carr Z, et al. First global consensus for evidence-based management of the hematopoietic syndrome resulting from exposure to ionizing radiation. *Disaster Med Public Health Prep* October 2011; 5(3): 202–212.

59. Sandgren DJ, Salter CA, Levine IH, Ross JA, Lillis-Hearne PK, Blakely WF. Biodosimetry Assessment Tool (BAT) software-dose prediction algorithms. *Health Phys* 2010; 99(Suppl. 5): S171–S183.

60. Blakely WF, Salter CA, Prasanna PG. Early-response biological dosimetry - recommended countermeasure enhancements for mass-casualty radiological accidents and terrorism. *Health Phys* 2005; 89: 494–504.

61. Pantelias GE, Maillie HD. The use of peripheral blood mononuclear cell prematurely condensed chromosomes for biological dosimetry. *Radiat Res* 1984; 99: 140–150.

62. Evans JW, Chang JA, Giaccia AJ, Pinkel D, Brown JM. The use of fluorescence in situ hybridization combined with premature chromosome condensation for the identification of chromosome damage. *Br J Cancer* 1991; 63: 517–521.

63. Prasanna PGS, Kolanko CJ, Gerstenberg HM, Blakely WF. Premature condensation assay for biodosimetry: studies with fission neutrons. *Health Phys* 1997; 72: 594–600.

64. Lloyd DC, Edwards AA, Moquet JE, Guerrero-Carbajal YC. The role of cytogenetics in triage of radiation casualties. *Applied Radiation and Isotopes* 2000; 52: 1107–1112.

65. Voisin P, Benderitter M, Claraz M, et al. The cytogenetic dosimetry of recent accidental overexposure. *Cell Mol Biol (Noisy-le-grand)* 2001; 47: 557–564.

66. Blakely WF, Carr Z, Chu MC, et al. WHO 1st consultation on the development of a global biodosimetry laboratories network for radiation emergencies (BioDoseNet). *Radiat Res* 2009; 171: 127–139.

67. Prassanna PGS, Subramanian U, Greenhill RG, Jacocks JM, Jackson WE, Blakely WF. Proceedings of the 36th Health Physics Society Topical Meeting: Radiation Safety Aspects of Homeland Security. San Antonio, TX, 2003; 218–222.

68. Maznyk NA, Wilkins RC, Carr Z, Lloyd DC. The capacity, capabilities and needs of the WHO Biodosenet member laboratories. *Radiat Prot Dosimetry* 2012; 151: 611–620.

69. Kulka U, Ainsbury L, Atkinson M, et al. Realising the European Network of Biodosimetry (RENEB). *Radiat Prot Dosimetry* 2012; 151: 621–625.

70. Prasanna PGS, Muderhwa JM, Miller AC, Grace MB, Salter CA, Blakely WF. Diagnostic biodosimetry for radiation disasters: current research and service activities at AFRRI. In: *NATO Medical Surveillance and Response: Research and Technology Opportunities and Options.* Neuilly-Sur-Seine, North Atlantic Treaty Organization, 2004.

71. Littlefield LG, Joiner EE, Sayer AM. Cytogenetic analysis of the Juarez radiation accident. In: Mettler FA, Kelsey CA, Ricks RC, eds. *Medical Management of Radiation Accidents.* Boca Raton, FL, CRC Press, 1989.

72. Sevan' kaev AV. Results of cytogenetic studies of the consequence of the Chernobyl accident. *Radiation Biology Radioecology* 2000; 40: 589–595.

73. Ramalho AT, Nascimento AC. The fate of chromosomal aberrations in 137Cs-exposed individuals in the Goiania radiation accident. *Health Phys* 1991; 60: 67–70.

74. Roy L, Gregoire E, Durand V, et al. 2006. Study of the tools available in biological dosimetry to estimate the dose in cases of accidental complex exposure to ionizing radiation: the Lilo accident. *Int J Radiat Biol* 2006; 82: 39–48.

75. Lindholm C, Romm H, Stephan G, Schmid E, Moquet J, Edwards A. Intercomparison of translocation and dicentric frequencies between laboratories in a follow-up of the radiological accident in Estonia. *Int J Radiat Biol* 2002; 78: 883–890.

76. Koksal G, Pala FS, Dalci DO. In vitro dose response curve for chromosome aberrations induced in human lymphocytes by 60Co irradiation. *Mutat Res* 1995; 329: 57–61.

77. Hayata I, Kanda R, Minamihisamatsu M, Furukawa M, Sasaki MS. Cytogenetic dose estimation for 3 severely exposed patients in the JCO criticality accident in Tokai-mura. *Journal of Radiation Research* 2001; 42: S149–S155.

78. Sasaki MS, Hayata I, Kamada N, Kodama Y, Kodama S. Chromosome aberration analysis in persons exposed to low-level radiation from the JCO criticality accident in Tokai-mura. *Journal of Radiation Research* 2001; 42: S107–S116.

79. Kanda R, Minamihisamatsu M, Hayata I. Dynamic analysis of chromosome aberrations in three victims of the Tokai-mura criticality accident. *Int J Radiat Biol* 2002; 78: 857–862.

80. El-Naggar AM, Mohammad MHM, Gomaa MA. The radiological accident at Meet Halfa, Qaluobiya, Egypt. In: *The Medical Basis for Radiation-Accident Preparedness: The Clinical Care of Victims.*

81. Jinaratana, V. The radiological accident in Thailand. In: *The Medical Basis for Radiation-Accident Preparedness: The Clinical Care of Victims.*

82. Thierens H, De Ruyck K, Vral A, de Gelder V, Whitehouse CA, Tawn EG, Boesman I. Cytogenetic biodosimetry of an accidental exposure of a radiological worker using multiple assays. *Radiat Prot Dosimetry* 2005; 113: 408–414.

83. Lloyd DC, Edwards AA, Moquet JA, Hone PA, Szluinska M. Doses in radiation accidents investigated by chromosome aberration analysis. XXIV. In: *Center for Radiation, Chemical and Environmental Hazards, Review of Cases Investigated, 2003–2005.* 2006; London, Health Protection Agency, 2006.

84. Voisin P, Barquinero R, Blakely B, et al. Towards a standardization of biological dosimetry by cytogenetics. *Cell Mol Biol (Noisy-le-grand)* 2002; 48: 501–504.

85. Blakely WF, Brooks AL, Lofts RS, van der Schans GP, Voisin P. Overview of low-level exposure assessment. *Mil Med* 2002; 167(2 Suppl.): 20–24.

86. Meadows SK, Dressman HK, Muramoto GG, et al. Gene expression signatures of radiation response are specific, durable and accurate in mice and humans. *PLoS One* April 2, 2008; 3(4): e1912.

87. Tsujii N, Akashi M, eds. *Proceedings of an International Symposium on the Criticality Accident in Tokai-mura: Medical Aspects of Radiation Emergency.* Chiba, National Institute of Radiological Sciences, 2001.

88. Schauer DA, Coursey DM, Dick CE, McLaughlin WL, Puhl JM, Desrosiers MF, Jacobson AD. A radiation accident at an industrial accelerator facility. *Health Phys* 1993; 65: 131–140.

89. Schauer DA, Desrosiers MF, Le FG, Seltzer FM, Links JM. EPR dosimetry of cortical bone of tooth enamel irradiated with X and gamma rays: study of energy dependence. *Radiat Res* 1994; 138: 1–8.

90. Schauer DA, Desrosiers MF, Kuppusamy P, Zwier JL. Radiation dosimetry of an accidental overexposure using EPR spectrometry and imaging of human bone. *Appl Radiat Isot* 1996; 47: 1345–1350.

91. Romanyukha AA, Schaur AA, Thomas JA, Regulla DF. Parameters affecting EPR dose reconstruction in teeth. *Appl Radiat Isot* 2005; 62: 147–154.

92. Desrosiers ME. In vivo assessment of radiation exposure. *Health Phys* 1991; 61: 859–861.

93. Clairand I, Trompier F, Bottollier-Depois JF, Gourmelon P. Ex vivo ESR measurements associated with Monte Carlo calculations for accident dosimetry: application to the 2001 Georgian accident. *Radiat Prot Dosimetry* 2006; 119: 500–505.

94. Lindholm C, Salomaa S, Tekkel M, Paile W, Koivistoinen A, Ilus T, Veidebaum T. Biodosimetry after accidental radiation exposure by conventional chromosome analysis and FISH. *Int J Radiat Biol* 1996; 70: 647–656.

95. Hutt G, Brodski L, Polyakov V. Gamma ray assessment after the 1994 radiation accident in Kiisa (Estonia): preliminary results. *Applied Radiat Isot* 1996; 45: 1329–1334.

96. Swartz HM, Iwasaki A, Tazeusz W, et al. Measurements of clinically significant doses using non-invasive EPR spectroscopy of teeth in situ. *Applied Radiat Isot* 2005; 62: 293–299.

97. Trompier F, Tikunov DD, Ivannikov A, Clairand, I. ESR investigation of joint use of dentin and tooth enamel to estimate photon and neutron dose components of a mixed field. *Radiat Prot Dosimetry* 2006; 120: 191–196.

98. Kleinerman RA, Romanyukha AA, Schauer DA, Tucker JD. Retrospective assessment of radiation exposure using biological dosimetry: chromosome painting, electron paramagnetic resonance, and the glycophorin A mutation assay. *Radiation Research* 2006; 166: 287–302.

99. Waselenko JK, MacVittie TJ, Blakely WF, et al. Medical management of the ARS: recommendations of the Strategic National Stockpile Radiation Working Group. *Ann Intern Med* 2004; 140: 1037–1051.

100. Goans RE, Flynn DF. ARS in Humans. In: *Textbook of Military Medicine.* Office of the Surgeon General, Department of the Army, Borden Institute, 2012; 17–38.

101. Flynn DF, Goans RE. Triage and Treatment of Radiation and Combined-injury Casualties. In: *Textbook of Military Medicine;* 39–72.

102. Hogan DE, Kellison T. Nuclear terrorism. *Am J Med Sci* 2002; 323: 341–349.

103. Barnett DJ, Parker CL, Blodgett DW, Wierezba RK, Links JM. Understanding radiologic and nuclear terrorism as public health

threats: preparedness and response perspectives. *J Nucl Med* 2006; 47: 1653–1661.

104. U.S. Centers for Disease Control and Prevention. ARS: Fact Sheet for Physicians. http://www.bt.cdc.gov/radiation/arsphysicianfactsheet.asp (Accessed July 6, 2013).

105. Hall EJ. Acute effects of total-body irradiation. In: Hall EJ, ed. *Radiobiology for the Radiologist*. Philadelphia, PA, Lippincott Williams & Wilkins, 2000.

106. Leikin JB, McFee RB, Walter FG, Edsall K. A primer for nuclear terrorism. *Dis Mon* 2003; 49: 485–516.

107. Berger ME, Christensen DM, Lowry PC, Jones OW, Wiley AL. Medical management of radiation injuries: current approaches. *Occup Med (Lond)* 2006; 56: 162–172.

108. Dainiak N, Waselenko JK, Armitage JO, MacVittie TJ, Farese AM. The hematologist and radiation casualties. *Hematology Am Soc Hematol Educ Program* 2003: 473–496.

109. van Bekkum DW. Radiation sensitivity of the hemopoietic stem cell. *Radiat Res* 1991; 128(1 Suppl.): S4–S8.

110. Koenig KL, Goans RE, Hatchett RJ, Mettler FA, Schumacher TA, Noji EK, Jarrett DG. Medical treatment of radiological casualties: current concepts. *Ann Emerg Med* 2005; 45: 643–652.

111. Walker RJ, Willemze R. Neutrophil kinetics and the regulation of granulopoiesis. *Rev Infect Dis* 1980; 2: 282–292.

112. Chao NJ. Accidental or intentional exposure to ionizing radiation: biodosimetry and treatment options. *Exp Hematol* 2007; 35(4 Suppl. 1): 24–27.

113. Paris F, Fuks Z, Kang A, et al. Endothelial apoptosis as the primary lesion initiating intestinal radiation damage in mice. *Science* 2001; 293: 293–297.

114. Maj JG, Paris F, Haimovitz-Friedman A, Venkatraman E, Kolesnick R, Fuks Z. Microvascular function regulates intestinal crypt response to radiation. *Cancer Res* 2003; 22: 5897–5906.

115. Schuller BW, Rogers AB, Cormier KS, et al. No significant endothelial apoptosis in the radiation –induced gastrointestinal syndrome. *Int J Radiat Oncol Biol Phys* 2007; 68: 205–210.

116. Seegenschmiedt H. Management of skin and related reactions to radiotherapy. *Front Radiat Ther Oncol* 2006; 39: 102–119.

117. Hymes SR, Strom EA, Fife C. Radiation dermatitis: clinical presentation, pathophysiology, and treatment 2006. *J Am Acad Dermatol* 2006; 54: 28–46.

118. Barabanova AV. ARS with cutaneous syndrome. In: *The Medical Basis for Radiation-Accident Preparedness: The Clinical Care of Victims.*

119. Pellmar TC, Ledney GD. Combined injury: radiation in combination with trauma, infectious disease, or chemical exposures. Presented at the Human Factors and Medicine Panel Research Task Group 099 (NATO RTG-099 2005), Radiation and Bioeffects and Countermeasures Meeting, Bethesda, Maryland, June 21–23, 2005. Published in Armed Forces Radiobiology Research Institute (AFRRI)-CD-05–2, 2005; 19-1-19-9. Summary at http://www.usuhs.edu/afrri/www/rtg-099/4_combined/sg4_PellmarChap12.pdf (Accessed July 7, 2013).

120. Pellmar TC, Ledney GD. Combined injury: radiation in combination with trauma, infectious disease, or chemical exposures. NATO RTG. 2005;099:1–9.

121. Brush J, Lipnick SL, Phillips T, Sitko J, McDonald JT, McBride WH. Molecular mechanisms of late normal tissue injury. *Semin Radiat Oncol* 2007; 17: 121–130.

122. Moulder JE, Cohen EP. Future strategies for mitigation and treatment of chronic radiation-induced normal tissue injury. *Semin Radiat Oncol* 2007; 17: 141–148.

123. Robbins ME, Diz DI. Pathogenic role of the renin-angiotensin system in modulating radiation-induced late effects. *Int J Radiat Oncol Biol Phys* 2006; 64: 6–12.

124. Richardson D, Sugiyama H, Nishi N, et al. Ionizing radiation and leukemia mortality among Japanese Atomic Bomb Survivors, 1950–2000. *Radiat Res* 2009; 172: 368–382.

125. Preston DL, Ron E, Toruoka S, Funamoto S, Nishi N, Soda M, Mabuchi K, Kodama K. Solid cancer incidence in atomic bomb survivors: 1958–1998. *Radiat Res* 2007; 168: 1–64.

126. Weisdorf D, Chao N, Waselenko JK, Dainiak N, Armitage JO, McNiece I, Confer D. Acute radiation injury: contingency planning for triage, supportive care, and transplantation. *Biol Blood Marrow Transplant* 2006; 12: 672–682.

127. Flynn DF, Goans RE. Nuclear terrorism: triage and medical management of radiation and combined-injury casualties. *Surg Clin North Am* 2006; 86: 601–636.

128. Casagrande R, Wills N, Kramer E, et al. Using the model of resource and time-based triage (MORTT) to guide scarce resource allocation in the aftermath of a nuclear detonation. *Disaster Med Public Health Prep* 2011; 5(Suppl. 1): S98–S110.

129. Caro JJ, DeRenzo EG, Coleman CN, Weinstock DM, Knebel AR. Resource allocation after a nuclear detonation incident: unaltered standards of ethical decision making. *Disaster Med Public Health Prep* 2011; 5(Suppl. 1): S46–S53.

130. DiCarlo AL, Maher C, Hick JL, et al. Radiation injury after a nuclear detonation: medical consequences and the need for scarce resources allocation. *Disaster Med Public Health Prep* 2011; 5(Suppl. 1): S32–S44.

131. Dainiak N, Gent RN, Carr Z, et al. Literature review and global consensus on management of acute radiation syndrome affecting nonhematopoietic organ systems. *Disaster Med Public Health Prep* October 2011; 5(3): 183–201.

132. http://www.idsociety.org/uploadedFiles/IDSA/Guidelines-Patient‐Care/PDF‐Library/FN.pdf (Accessed September 5, 2015).

133. Barbour SY, Crawford J. Hematopoietic growth factors. In: Pazdur R, Coia LR, Hoskins WJ, Wagman L, eds. *Cancer Management: A Multidisciplinary Approach*. New York, CMP Healthcare Media, 2006.

134. Bolderston A, Lloyd NS, Wong RK, Holden L, Robb-Blenderman L. Supportive Care Guidelines Group of Cancer Care Ontario Program in Evidence-Based Care. The prevention and management of acute skin reactions related to radiation therapy: a systematic review and practice guideline. *Support Care Cancer* 2006; 14: 802–817.

135. Farese AM, Cohen MV, Katz BP, Smith CP, Gibbs A, Cohen DM, MacVittie TJ. Filgrastim improves survival in lethally irradiated nonhuman primates. *Radiat Res* 2013; 179: 89–100.

136. Radiation Injury Treatment Network. ARS Treatment Guidelines. Powerpoint presentation. http://www.ritn.net/Treatment (Accessed July 7, 2013).

137. Herodin F, Drouet M. Cytokine-based treatment of accidentally irradiated victims and new approaches. *Exp Hematol* 2005; 33: 1071–1080.

138. Goans, RE. Update on the Treatment of Internal Contamination. In: *The Medical Basis for Radiation-Accident Preparedness: The Clinical Care of Victims.*

139. Bhattacharyya MH, Breitenstein BD, Metivier H, Muggenburg BA, Stradling GN, Volf V. Guidebook for the Treatment of Accidental Internal Radionuclide Contamination of Workers. eds. GB Gerber, and RG Thomas. A Joint Publication for the Commission of the Commission of the European Communities and the US DOE Office of Health and Environmental Research. *Radiat Prot Dosim* 1992; 41(1): 1–49.

140. National Council on Radiation Protection & Measurements. Report Number 161. I – Management of Persons Contaminated with Radionuclides: Handbook. 2008.

141. National Council on Radiation Protection & Measurements. Report Number 161. II – Management of Persons Contaminated with Radionuclides: Scientific and Technical Basis. 2008.

142. Mansfield WG. *Nuclear Emergency and Radiological Decision Handbook*. Livermore, CA, Lawrence Livermore National Laboratory, 1997.

143. Mettler F. Personal communication. 2007.

144. Potassium iodide as a thyroid blocking agent in radiation emergencies. FDA Center for Drug Evaluation and Research Procedural, Rockville, MD, December 2001. http://www.fda.gov/downloads/Drugs/.../Guidances/ucm080542.pdf (Accessed July 7, 2013).

145. Norwood AE, Ursano RJ, Fullerton CS. Disaster psychiatry: principles and practice. *Psychiatr Q* 2000; 71: 207–226.

146. Boudreaux E, Kilpatrick DG, Resnick HS, Best CL, Saunders BE. Criminal victimization, posttraumatic stress disorder, and comorbid psychopathology among a community sample of women. *J Trauma Stress* 1998; 11: 665–678.

147. Grieger TA, Waldrep DA, Lovasz MM, Ursano RJ. Follow-up of Pentagon employees two years after the terrorist attack of September 11, 2001. *Psychiatr Serv* 2005; 56: 1374–1378.

148. Koenig KL, Hatchett R, Crail S, et al. *Report of the Department of Homeland Security Working Group on Radiological Dispersal Device (RDD) Preparedness Medical Preparedness and Response Sub-Group*. Washington, DC, Department of Homeland Security, 2003. http://www.acr.org/~/media/ACR/Documents/PDF/Membership/Legal%20Business/Disaster%20Preparedness/Counter%20Measures.pdf (Accessed July 7, 2013).

149. International Atomic Energy Agency. *The Radiation Accident in Goiania*. STI/PUB/815. Vienna, IAEA, 1988.

150. International Atomic Energy Agency. *Dosimetric and Medical Aspects of the Radiological Accident in Goiana in 1987*. IAEA-TECDOC-1009. Vienna, IAEA, 1998.

151. International Atomic Energy Agency. *The Radiation Accident in Tammiku*. STI/PUB/1053. Vienna, IAEA, 1998.

152. Goans RE, Wald N. Radiation accidents with multi-organ failure in the United States. *BJR Suppl* 2005; 27: 41–46.

153. McLaughlin TP, Monahas SP, Pruvost NL, Frolov VV, Ryazanov BG, Sviridov VI. *A Review of Criticality Accidents: 2000 Revision*. LA-13638. Los Alamos, NM, Los Alamos National Laboratory, 2000. http://www.orau.org/ptp/Library/accidents/la-13638.pdf (Accessed July 7, 2013).

154. Hempelmann LH, Lisko L, Hoffman JG. The ARS: a study of nine cases and a review of the problem. *Ann Intern Med* 1952; 36: 279–510.

155. Shipman TL, Lushbaugh LL, Peterson DF, Langham WH, Harris PS, Lawrence JNP. Acute radiation death resulting from an accidental nuclear critical excursion. *J Occup Med Special Supplement* 1961: 145–192.

156. Karas JS, Stanbury JB. Fatal radiation syndrome from an accidental nuclear excursion. *N Engl J Med* 1965; 272: 755–761.

157. Farrell CL, Bready JV, Rex KL, et al. Keratinocyte growth factor protects mice from chemotherapy and radiation-induced gastrointestinal injury and mortality. *Cancer Res* 1998; 58: 933–939.

158. Dörr W, Noack R, Spekl K, Farrell CL. Modification of oral mucositis by keratinocyte growth factor: single radiation exposure. *Int J Radiat Biol* 2001; 77: 341–347.

159. Hérodin F, Grenier N, Drouet M. Revisiting therapeutic strategies in radiation casualties. *Exp Hematol* 2007; 35(4 Suppl. 1): 28–33.

160. Miller MC, Nanchahal J. Advances in the modulation of cutaneous wound healing and scarring. *Bio Drugs* 2005; 19: 363–381.

161. Jurjus A, Atiyeh BS, Abdallah IM, et al. Pharmacological modulation of wound healing in experimental burns. *Burns* 2007; 33: 892–907.

162. Denham JW, Hauer-Jensen M. The radiotherapeutic injury – a complex 'wound.' *Radiother Oncol* 2002; 63: 129–145.

163. Mustoe TA, Purdy J, Gramates P, Deuel TF, Thomason A, Pierce GF. Reversal of impaired wound healing in irradiated rats by platelet-derived growth factor-BB. *Am J Surg* 1989; 158: 345–350.

164. Amendt C, Mann A, Schirmacher P, Blessing M. Resistance of keratinocytes to TGFβ-mediated growth restriction and apoptosis induction accelerates re-epithelialization in skin wounds. *J Cell Sci* 2002; 115: 2189–2198.

165. Anand P, Terenghi G, Warner G, Kopelman P, Williams-Chestnut RE, Sinicropi DV. The role of endogenous nerve growth factor in human diabetic neuropathy. *Nat Med* 1996; 2: 703–707.

166. Kanaan SA, Saad´eNE, Karam M, Khansa H, Jabbur SJ, Jurjus AR. Hyperalgesia and upregulation of cytokines and nerve growth factor by cutaneous leishmaniasis in mice. *Pain* 2000; 85: 477–482.

167. Hérodin F, Roy L, Grenier N, et al. Antiapoptotic cytokines in combination with pegfilgrastim soon after irradiation mitigates myelosuppression in nonhuman primates exposed to high irradiation dose. *Exp Hematol* 2007; 35: 1172–1181.

168. Candan F, Alaqözlü H. Captopril inhibits the pulmonary toxicity of paraquat in rats. *Hum Exp Toxicol*. 2001;20:637–641.

169. He X, Han B, Mura M, et al. Angiotensin-converting enzyme inhibitor captopril prevents oleic acid-induced severe acute lung injury in rats. *Shock* 2007; 28: 106–111.

170. Jiang JS, Wang LF, Chou HC, Chen CM. Angiotensin-converting enzyme inhibitor captopril attenuates ventilator-induced lung injury in rats. *J Appl Physiol* 2007; 102: 2098–2103.

171. Moulder JE, Fish BL, Cohen EP. Treatment of radiation nephropathy with ACE inhibitors and AII type-1 and type-2 receptor antagonists. *Curr Pharm Des* 2007; 13: 1317–1325.

172. Robbins ME, Diz DI. Pathogenic role of the renin-angiotensin system in modulating radiation-induced late effects. *Int J Radiat Oncol Biol Phys* 2006; 64: 6–12.

173. Dovi JV, He LK, DiPietro LA. Accelerated wound closure in neutrophil-depleted mice. *J Leukoc Biol* 2003; 73: 448–455.

174. Martin P, Leibovich SJ. Inflammatory cells during wound repair: the good, the bad and the ugly. *Trends Cell Biol* 2005; 15: 599–607.

175. Brenner DJ, Hall EJ. Computed tomography–an increasing source of radiation exposure. *N Engl J Med* 2007; 357: 2277–2284.

176. French Academy of Medicine. Medical Irradiation, Radioactivity Releases, and Disinformation: An Opinion by the Academy of Medicine, December 4, 2001. http://www.radscihealth.org/rsh/docs/academy_of_medicine_of_france.htm (Accessed September 5, 2015).

177. International Agency for Research on Cancer. *Ionizing Radiation, part I: x- and gamma (γ) radiation and neutrons. IARC Monographs on the evaluation of carcinogenic risks to humans*. vol. 75. Lyon, International Agency for Research on Cancer, 2000.

178. National Research Council, Board on Radiation Effects Research. *Distribution and Administration of Potassium Iodide in the Event of a Nuclear Accident*. Washington, DC, National Academies Press, 2004.

179. Koenig KL, Bey T, Bradley D, Kahn CA, Schultz C. The RAD-PACK: a new concept for stockpiling medical countermeasures

for a radiation disaster at the local level. *West J Emerg Med* 2008; 9(1). http://repositories.cdlib.org/uciem/westjem/vol9/iss1/art49 (Accessed September 5, 2015).

180. Summary Minutes of the Joint Meeting of the Medical Imaging Drugs Advisory Committee and the Oncologic Drugs Advisory Committee. May 3, 2013. http://www.fda.gov/downloads/advisorycommittees/committeesmeetingmaterials/drugs/medicalimagingdrugsadvisorycommittee/ucm363898.pdf (Accessed July 3, 2014).

181. Castilla C, Perez-Simon JA, Sanchez-Guijo FM, et al. Oral beclomethasone dipropionate for the treatment of gastrointestinal acute graft-versus-host disease (GVHD). *Biol Blood Marrow Transplant* 2006; 12: 936–941.

182. Lange C, Brunswig-Spickenheier B, Cappallo-Obermann H, et al. Radiation rescue: mesenchymal stromal cells protect from lethal irradiation. *PLoS One* 2011; 6(1): e14486.

183. Bey E, Prat M, Duhamel P, et al. Emerging therapy for improving wound repair of severe radiation burns using local bone marrow-derived stem cell administration. *Wound Repair Regen* 2010; 18: 50–58.

184. Singh VK, Christensen J, Fatanmi OO, et al. Myeloid progenitors: a radiation countermeasure that is effective when initiated days after irradiation. *Radiat Res* 2012; 177: 781–791.

185. Garg S, Wang W, Biju PG, et al. Bone marrow transplantation helps restore the intestinal mucosal barrier after total body irradiation in mice. *Radiat Res* 2014; 181: 229–239.

186. Goans RE. Cytogenetic Biodosimetry and Clinical Hematology in the Management of Radiation Injury. Wiley A, Christensen D, eds. Fifth REACTS' Symposium on the Medical Management of Radiation Injury. Miami, FL, 2011. Oak Ridge Associated Universities. ORAU 12–1771, 2013.

187. Goans RE, Iddins CJ, Christensen DM. Ultrasound & Thermography for Diagnosis of Extent & Magnitude of Acute Local Radiation Injury (LRI). Fifth REACTS' Symposium on the Medical Management of Radiation Injury. Miami, FL, 2011. Oak Ridge Associated Universities. ORAU 12–1771, 2013.

34

Hazardous Material, Toxic, and Industrial Events

Hoon Chin Lim and Hock Heng Tan

OVERVIEW

Hazardous material (hazmat) incidents are increasingly prevalent due to the continuing rapid growth and globalization of the chemical industry and use of chemicals worldwide. In a recent document by World Health Organization (WHO), more than 15 million chemical substances are commercially available with approximately 60,000 to 70,000 chemical substances in regular use.[1–3] This number is increasing yearly, with an exponential growth of new chemicals. Globally, chemical production and use has increased nearly tenfold over the last 30 years, and this is particularly true in developing countries.[4]

The presence of such large quantities of toxic chemicals and hazardous substances among populations poses a significant threat to global health and the environment. In a systematic review of the literature for global burden of disease estimates from chemicals, 4.9 million deaths and 86 million disability-adjusted life years (DALYs) were attributable to environmental exposure and management of selected chemicals in 2004.[5] The study concluded that the known burden due to chemicals is considerable. Effective public health interventions can successfully manage chemicals and limit their public health impacts, and should be implemented at national and international levels.

In Organization for Economic Cooperation and Development's (OECD) Environmental Outlook to 2050, one of the "red light" key environmental challenges is the high burden of disease from exposure to hazardous chemicals, particularly in non-OECD countries.[6] The report warns that although many OECD governments have changed or are in the process of changing, enforcement of legislation to expand regulatory coverage of chemicals is still incomplete.

This chapter will focus on industrial hazmat events. Hazards of a biological nature or those with radioactive properties are discussed in Chapters 32 and 33. Harm can also result from deliberate release of hazardous materials in an act of terrorism. Chemical emergencies related to the use of substances such as nerve agents are described further in Chapter 31. Practical advice is provided based on best available evidence and any guidance is intended to undergo local interpretation.

Epidemiology of Acute Hazardous Material Events

Acute releases of hazardous materials are common and occur on a daily basis. Although the frequency of chemical incidents increased during the twentieth century, the consequences of these industrial disasters have decreased. This reduction in severity is due to improvements in the management of chemical emergencies in many developed nations.[1]

A total of 2,981 acute toxic substance incidents were reported in seven U.S. states in a 2010 annual report by the National Toxic Substance Incidents Program (NTSIP).[7] For 2009, the Chemical Surveillance Report by the Health Protection Agency (HPA) in the United Kingdom noted 967 chemical incidents. An unusually high number of fatalities occurred (twenty-two) resulting from nineteen separate acute chemical incidents reported in this period. Sixteen percent of acute chemical incidents resulted in evacuation of the nearby population.[8] In a study analyzing hazardous chemical accidents in China from 2000 to 2006, there were many accidents and fatalities recorded. The number of accidents with injuries fluctuated between 200–600/year while the number of fatalities fluctuated between 220–1,100/year.[9]

The numbers from various databases will differ depending on surveillance methodology and the reliability of sources that report such events. With regard to chemical emergencies, WHO recognizes that wide-scale major industrial accidents or attacks using chemical weapons give an incomplete picture of the disease burden from chemical incidents. Generally, it is uncommon for acute hazmat events to cause mass casualty scenarios.

The majority of exposure-related deaths and illnesses are attributable to the many medium-sized and small-scale chemical incidents that occur every year around the world. This is supported by the findings from a Chinese study that noted that nearly 80% of dangerous chemical accidents occurred in small and medium-sized enterprises.[9] It is possible that in some countries, these are the same incidents that go unreported due to poor or nonexistent injury surveillance systems. This may lead to an underestimation of disease burden.

An industrial chemical disaster is defined as the release or spill of a toxic chemical that results in an abrupt and serious functional disruption of a society. It causes widespread human, material, or environmental losses that exceed the ability of the affected society to cope using only its own resources.[10] One example, possibly the worst incident in history, is the 1984 Bhopal disaster in which more than 2,500 people were killed and an additional 200,000–300,000 individuals were affected.[11] In contrast, most acute events (92%) that were previously reported by the now defunct U.S. Hazardous Substances Emergency Events Surveillance (HSEES) system in 2004, do not result in patient injury. The majority of events that do produce casualties (75%) result in only one or two injured victims.[12]

Nevertheless, these incidents call for special planning and preparedness due to the challenges of managing a chemically injured victim and the potential for hazmat incidents to harm emergency healthcare providers. Employees are most often injured, followed by the general public. Within the group of first responders, police, career firefighters, and volunteer firefighters were frequently victims of both fixed facility and transportation-related events.

Many factors can contribute to a chemical incident. They include poor maintenance of manufacturing and storage equipment, lack of regulation and poor enforcement of existing safety standards, motor vehicle collisions, and human error. Additional challenges result from meteorological and geological events such as heavy rain, earthquakes, hurricanes, floods, and terrorism.[13] As a consequence of these factors, incidents could be associated with fires, explosions, spills and leaks, and structural collapse. Industrial accidents can also be described by the initiating event, which can be one or more of the following: human error, environmental conditions, and container or equipment failure.[14]

The majority of hazmat events occur in fixed facilities with most incidents involving the release of only one substance.[15] By comparison, transportation-related events are less common. In the United States, hazardous materials transportation (all modes, including pipelines) accounts for an average of twenty-eight deaths each year.[16] Of the 7,169 transportation-related events from 1998 to 2001 reported by HSEES, 85% occurred during ground transport; 9% during rail transport, and 6% during a combination of air, pipeline, water, or other types of transport.[15]

Most acute hazmat events affect public health within the nation of their occurrence. Occasionally, these chemical incidents become events of international public health concern. In August 2002, WHO initiated a pilot project sponsored by the International Programme on Chemical Safety (IPCS) to determine whether a system comparable to that for communicable disease surveillance and response could be developed for chemical incidents and related illnesses. Using several informal (Internet-based resources) and formal (various networks of organizations) sources, incidents were assessed against criteria for international public health emergencies using the then proposed revised International Health Regulations (IHR). During the 17 months of the project, from August 1, 2002 to December 31, 2003, thirty-five chemical incidents from twenty-six countries met one or more of the IHR criteria. The WHO European Region accounted for 43% (15/35) of reports.[17]

Bhopal Methyl Isocyanate Event: Example of a Fixed Facility Industrial Disaster

On December 2–3, 1984, approximately 37 metric tons (41 short tons) of highly toxic gaseous methyl isocyanate was released into the air from a Union Carbide plant in the city of Bhopal, located in the Indian state of Madhya Pradhesh. Additionally, other sub-

Table 34.1. Factors Contributing to the 1984 Bhopal Disaster

◾ Multinational industrial producer of chemicals operates in a developing nation and does not adhere to accepted international safety standards
◾ Financial pressures supersede industrial safety regulations (violation of industrial zoning in the inner city, violation of limits for maximal production)
◾ No enforcement of international safety operational standards
◾ Lack of risk reduction in plant location
◾ Poor public health infrastructure in the vicinity of a major industrial operation
◾ Poor public utility infrastructure such as drinking water, sewer, electricity, and telephone
◾ Absence of an emergency response system for industrial accidents
◾ Lack of infrastructure and technical expertise to manage an industrial incident

Adapted after Broughton[1]

stances such as carbon dioxide, carbon monoxide, hydrogen cyanide, oxides of nitrogen, and phosgene were probably released within the gas cloud.[18] At the time of the disaster, inadequate industrial safety programs were in place at the Bhopal Union Carbide plant (Table 34.1).[18–23] The infrastructure around the plant was deficient and included ineffective roadways and streets, water supply, and medical treatment facilities. Poor to nonexistent urban planning was prevalent for people living extremely close to the industrial plant. Additionally, people in Bhopal were destitute and had little education or training on how to respond as a community to a chemical disaster. The health infrastructure was weak in Bhopal in 1984. No mass casualty emergency response system existed in the city and the community lacked warning devices, shelter-in-place training, public education on the dangers associated with the plant, and joint planning activities by public agencies and the Union Carbide plant.[19]

No consensus exists regarding how many people died, how many were actually exposed, or the numbers who suffered long-term disabilities.[22] The literature describes different numbers of immediate and delayed fatalities as well as exposed individuals. Gupta and Broughton estimate that there were approximately 3,800–4,000 immediate deaths and more than 200,000 injuries.[21] In a report published in 2004, Sharma points out that Amnesty International estimated that between 7,000 and 10,000 people lost their lives within the first 3 days of the Bhopal chemical release. Additionally, Amnesty International estimated that another 15,000–20,000 people succumbed to their exposures between 1985 and 2003.[22] Eckerman suggests that approximately 500,000 people were exposed.[18] This makes the Bhopal incident the largest industrial disaster in history to date in terms of deaths and disabilities related to pulmonary, ophthalmological, neurological, reproductive, gastrointestinal, and psychiatric effects.[22]

Numerous articles were published in the aftermath, analyzing the event.[18–23] Broughton points out that many safety measures and precautions that were normally in place in a highly industrialized country were absent in the Bhopal scenario. The Bhopal industrial disaster stands as a classic example of the consequences when pressure to expand industrialization in a developing nation leads to negligent enforcement of concurrent safety regulations.

The Bhopal disaster changed the chemical process industry permanently. Gupta emphasizes that improvements in the chemical process industry resulting from this event have saved lives and money by reducing accident damages.[21] These improvements include:

- New legislation resulting in better enforcement and harsher sentencing;
- Enhancement in process safety;
- Development of safer industrial plants;
- Monitoring by the media, nongovernmental organizations, and the public; and
- Chemical process industry management's willingness to invest in safety equipment, education, and training.

The Bhopal incident had a major effect on legislation and public political consciousness about chemical safety in the United States. It resulted in the formation of the American Institute of Chemical Engineers (AICHE), Center for Chemical Process Safety, and the Safety and Chemical Engineering (SACHE) program. These organizations orchestrated a change in the practice and education of chemical engineers.[23]

Graniteville Chlorine Event: Example of a Transportation Incident

Transportation hazmat incidents pose challenges that are different from fixed facility events like the one at Bhopal. Hazardous material can be transported through densely populated regions as well as over rugged terrain in rural areas with limited access for emergency responders. On January 6, 2005, at 2:39 AM, a train derailed in the small rural U.S. town of Graniteville, South Carolina, releasing 55 metric tons (60 short tons) of liquefied chlorine. It resulted in 9 deaths, 75 hospital admissions, and the evacuation of 5,400 residents.[24,25] The problems identified after review of the crash included inadequate information, communication, and training for residents and the rail transport crew in managing a hazmat response. The limited capacity of rural areas to direct evacuations and large-scale emergencies was also a challenge. Since the need for evacuation would arise spontaneously, deciding whether to shelter-in-place or leave would depend on the scenario, chemical properties of the toxic agent, ambient environmental conditions, topography of the crash site, and the means to successfully evacuate local residents. For example, chlorine is denser than air and, therefore, concentrates in low-lying areas. In a cold environment, it could flow like a liquid through a valley, covering long distances.[25] Multiple interventions should be explored to enhance management of transit-associated hazardous substance releases.[26] Proposed solutions by Henry et al. include:

- Select transportation route through less populated areas;
- Develop emergency response plans that involve the community;
- Have public warning systems;
- Ensure maintenance of vehicles;
- Ensure transport personnel are properly trained and have protective equipment; and
- Ensure that responders are equipped to address hazardous material incidents.[26]

Hazardous Wastes and the Environment

Hazardous wastes are dangerous substances intended for disposal. Their covert or deliberate release into the environment may not cause "disasters" that are immediately evident. However, being insidious and cumulative in effect, the damage they cause to the environment and subsequently public health is potentially great.

Since the adoption of Agenda 21 at the United Nations (UN) Conference on Environment and Development in 1992, the attention of policymakers has been drawn to the links between health and the environment.[27] Recently, attendees at the UN Conference on Sustainable Development in 2012 reaffirmed their commitment to Agenda 21 in their outcome document called "The Future We Want."[28] It states that the sound management of chemicals is crucial for the protection of human health and the environment, and calls for a comprehensive management strategy for chemicals and waste at all levels. There should be effective implementation and strengthening of the Strategic Approach to International Chemicals Management (SAICM).[29] This endeavor should be part of a robust, coherent, effective, and efficient system for the safe management of chemicals throughout their life cycle, including the response to emerging challenges.

The case of hazardous waste disposal into Minamata Bay, Japan, illustrates the consequences of chemical waste mismanagement and represents one of the worst chemical disasters in modern history. It was characterized by the chronic release of hazardous materials into the environment, poisoning a large number of victims. Between 1932 and 1968, Chisso Corporation, a company located in Kumamoto, Japan, deposited large amounts of mercury compounds into Minamata Bay. It was not until the mid-1950s that people began to notice a "strange disease." Thousands of people whose normal diet included fish from the bay unexpectedly developed a neurological syndrome characterized by ataxia, numbness, muscle weakness, and visual disturbances. The illness became known as "Minamata disease." The illness was ultimately diagnosed as methyl mercury poisoning. The public health impact was devastating. The resultant manifestations of congenital exposure to methyl mercury resulted in children with intellectual disability, primitive reflexes, hyperkinesis, deafness, blindness, cerebral palsy, cerebellar ataxia, seizures, strabismus, dysarthria, and limb deformities.[30] At the end of March 2001, more than 2,200 persons have been recognized as having Minamata disease.[31]

The Basel Convention controlling the trans-boundary movement of hazardous wastes and their disposal became effective in 1992, and to date has 170 member countries. It aims to protect human health and the environment from the adverse effects produced by the generation, management, trans-boundary movements, and disposal of hazardous and other wastes.[32] Hazardous waste cannot be indiscriminately transported from industrialized countries with strict waste control measures to developing countries for disposal without prior agreement. In addition, the waste must be managed in an environmentally sound manner.

Chemical Incidents and Environmental Justice

A study in the United States investigated the relationship between incidents at chemical facilities and characteristics of the surrounding communities. It revealed that larger facilities with higher risk for hazmat incidents are located in counties with larger African-American populations and higher levels of income disparity.[33] The relationship between chemical facility risk and the demographics of the surrounding community is complex.

Higher-risk facilities are more frequently found in counties with sizeable poor and/or minority populations who disproportionately bear the collateral environmental, property, and health risks.[33] In the light of such findings, environmental justice seeks to redress the inequitable distribution of this burden. The U.S. Environmental Protection Agency (EPA) defines environmental justice as the fair treatment and meaningful involvement of all people regardless of race, color, national origin, culture, education, or income with respect to the development, implementation, and enforcement of environmental laws, regulations, and policies.[34] Legislation such as the Emergency Planning and Community Right-to-Know Act (EPCRA) mandates the community be informed regarding the risks of chemical incidents that could arise from nearby facilities.[35]

CURRENT STATE OF THE ART

Hazardous Materials Identification and Classification

Hazardous materials are substances that pose a potential risk to life, health, the environment, or property when not properly contained because of their chemical, physical, or biological properties.[36] Different government agencies may define hazmat differently for operational reasons; some use it loosely to describe specialized first responder teams equipped to handle on-site control and containment of hazardous chemicals.

Apart from its inherent toxicity, the sheer quantity or concentration of the hazardous material in an acute release will also determine its ability to cause harm. These substances can be in solid, liquid, or gaseous form. Knowledge of a hazardous substance's physical properties (such as vapor pressure) during an acute event is useful because it will help to determine the route of victim exposure, the likelihood of secondary contamination, and the most effective method of protection and decontamination.

Chemicals may be known by their common, generic, chemical, or brand names. The Chemical Abstracts Service (CAS) of the American Chemical Society numbers chemicals to overcome the confusion regarding multiple names for a single chemical. The CAS assigns a unique CAS registry number (CAS#) to atoms, molecules, and mixtures. Currently, there are more than 71 million unique organic and inorganic substances in the database, making it the most comprehensive collection in the world. These numbers provide a unique identification for chemicals and a means for cross-checking chemical names. Identifying a chemical by name and CAS# is critical because one must be as specific as possible about the hazardous material in question. Trade or brand names can be misleading.[37,38] Another method for identifying hazardous substances is the globally recognized four-digit United Nations Substance Identification Number (UN SIN or UN Number), which is used for the transportation of dangerous goods. The North American (NA) Number is identical to the UN Number except that some material without a UN Number may be assigned an NA Number.

Many countries have their own standard for classification and communication regarding hazardous materials. These different systems are frequently inconsistent in their use of terminology and safety standards, leading to confusion and increasing the risk of accidents and injuries. The need to comply with multiple regulations reflected in these systems also increases the economic cost of international trade. One positive step comes from the continuing development of a Globally Harmonized System for the Classification and Labeling of Chemicals (GHS).[39] An inter-nationally synchronized approach to classification and labeling exemplified by GHS would provide the foundation for national programs to ensure safe use, transport, and disposal of hazardous substances. It would also provide a basis for harmonizing rules and regulations on chemicals at national and international levels, an important step to facilitate trade and improve hazard risk management. Although country participation in this program is voluntary, at least sixty-seven countries are supportive and are in various stages of implementation. These governments have either incorporated GHS into their existing regulations or established workgroups to reconcile existing legislation with GHS. The first version was published in 2003 and now the fourth revised edition of GHS was released in 2011.[40]

The objectives of GHS are: 1) harmonized criteria for classifying substances and mixtures according to their hazard class; and 2) harmonized hazard communication elements, including requirements for labeling and safety data sheets. Classification under GHS lists sixteen physical hazard classes, ten health hazard classes, and two environmental hazard classes. Each hazard class has a unique pictogram (Figure 34.1). Within each class, the hazard is further categorized according to severity, with the smaller number being more severe. The classes and categories are then applied to single substances and mixtures based on the prescribed definitions.

Various systems have been devised for the actual labeling of hazardous materials. Labels or placards contain information alerting people to the presence of dangerous materials using a pictogram or symbol. The placard may have words such as "flammable liquid" or "toxic gas," a product identifier, hazard classification number, or an emergency assistance number to call (Figure 34.2). Some identification systems are permanent and cannot be modified once attached to a container. Others can be changed with fitted slots or interchangeable placards. GHS prescribes a standard format and content for labeling of chemicals with product identifier, hazard pictograms, signal words, hazard statements, precautionary statements, and supplier information.

In some countries, material safety data sheets (MSDS) containing basic substance information are legally required to accompany each product supplied to an end user. MSDS are not necessarily intended for emergency responders, but they can be used by professional staff to advise such individuals. MSDS have existed for many years in a wide variety of formats, with a broad range of data quality and quantity. Under GHS, MSDS are now termed safety data sheets (SDS) and have sixteen subcategories that include product identification, company information, ingredient information, and hazard identification. A complementary hazard communication information source is found in the International Chemical Safety Cards (ICSC) produced by IPCS and the European community, and these are translated into various languages.[41,42]

The transport of dangerous goods has a different system of hazard classification under the UN. The first version was issued in 1956 and now the UN has published the seventeenth edition of its Recommendations on the Transport of Dangerous Goods – Model Regulations in 2011.[43] Its focus is on the risk associated with transport of the hazard whereas the GHS focus is on the inherent toxicity of the chemicals. The UN groups hazards into nine classes and hazard severity is classified into packing groups. It provides a system of classification in listing, packing, marking, labeling, placarding, and documentation. This is modified by various international aviation, maritime, and rail organizations for

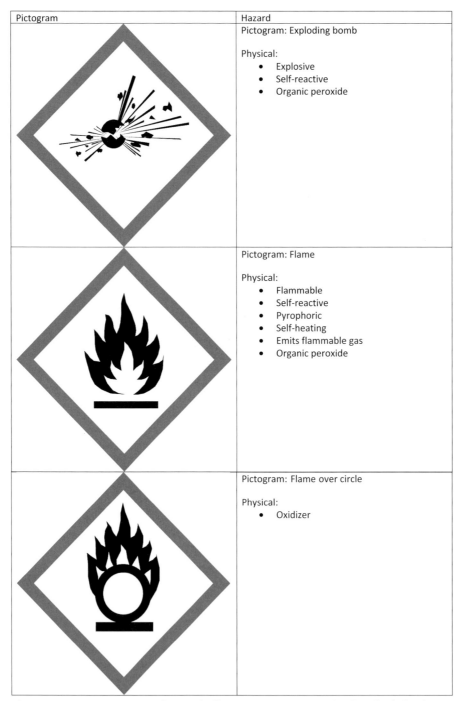

Pictogram	Hazard
	Pictogram: Exploding bomb Physical: • Explosive • Self-reactive • Organic peroxide
	Pictogram: Flame Physical: • Flammable • Self-reactive • Pyrophoric • Self-heating • Emits flammable gas • Organic peroxide
	Pictogram: Flame over circle Physical: • Oxidizer

Figure 34.1. GHS Pictogram and Hazard Allocation. Pictogram can be downloaded at http://www.unece.org/trans/danger/publi/ghs/pictograms.html.

adoption into their regulations. There are various forms of hazard communication systems used by transportation industries and fixed facilities in different countries and these are illustrated in the next section. However, these governments are in various stages of implementing and adopting GHS.

Within the European community, regulations require that written emergency instructions be carried in the vehicle cab. The European Chemical Industry Council has produced a series of instructions called TREMCARDS (transport emergency cards). These cards are written using internationally approved standard sentences with appropriate translations. They provide

information on immediate actions required as well as first aid advice.[42,44]

First responders may also encounter other numerical codes such as the Emergency Action Codes and the Hazard Identification Number (also known as the Kemmler Code). Emergency Action Codes (commonly called Hazchem Codes) are designed to assist emergency services providers during the initial contact with a hazmat incident by instructing responders which actions they should perform. They are designed for responding to bulk product incidents. In contrast, the Hazard Identification Number, which is usually found in the United

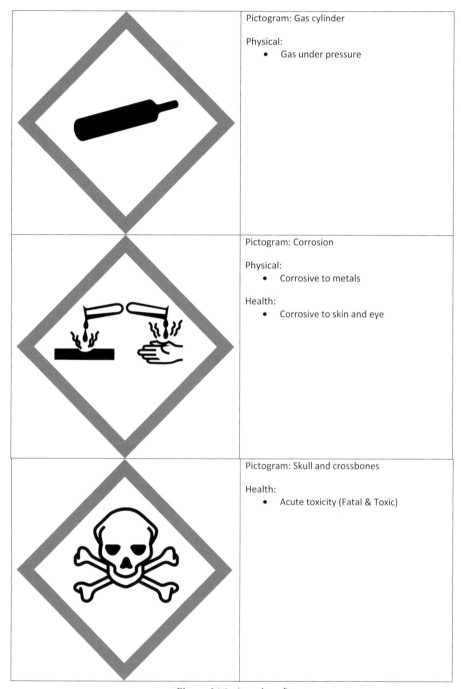

	Pictogram: Gas cylinder **Physical:** • Gas under pressure
	Pictogram: Corrosion **Physical:** • Corrosive to metals **Health:** • Corrosive to skin and eye
	Pictogram: Skull and crossbones **Health:** • Acute toxicity (Fatal & Toxic)

Figure 34.1. (*continued*)

Kingdom on vehicles traveling internationally, gives advice on the nature of the hazard presented by the substance in question, as opposed to the actions required when dealing with the material.[45]

In the United States, the Department of Transportation (DOT) Pipeline and Hazardous Materials Safety Administration uses the Hazard Classification System in its guidebook.[46] This system assigns a chemical to a hazard class based on its most dangerous physical characteristic, such as corrosiveness, flammability, or radioactivity. It is primarily a guide to aid first responders in: 1) quickly identifying the specific or generic classification of the material(s) involved in the incident; and 2) protecting themselves and the general public during the initial response phase of the incident.

In contrast, fixed facilities in the United States use a labeling system that is different from the vehicular placarding system. The National Fire Protection Association (NFPA) 704 system is used at most fixed facilities.[47] This system uses a diamond-shaped sign (commonly referred to as the "fire diamond") that is divided into color-coded quadrants: blue, red, yellow, and the 6 o'clock position which is assigned no special color. The blue color indicates the degree of health hazard, red is used for flammability, yellow for instability, and the last quadrant is reserved for special hazards. These markings assist first

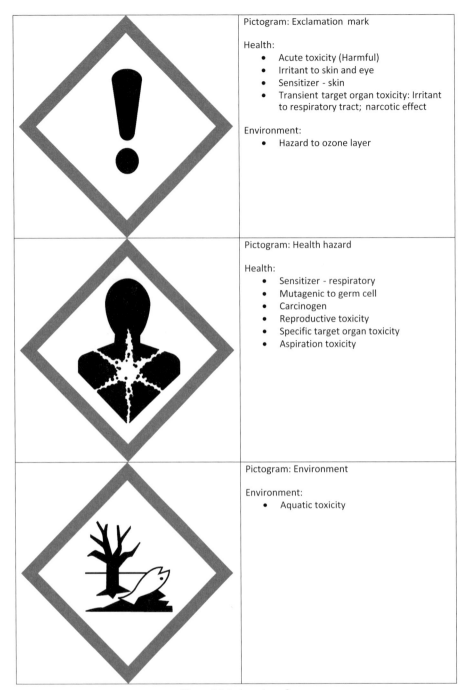

Figure 34.1. (*continued*)

responders to quickly and easily identify the risks posed by the hazmat, helping to determine what specialty equipment should be used, procedures followed, or precautions taken during the first moments at the site of the release. They do not identify the substance.

First responders need to rapidly and precisely identify the chemical or the components of a hazmat mixture. They must be familiar with the local labeling systems and know where to seek further information regarding the chemical. One cannot always rely on the presence of a hazmat placard. Many hazmats may not be placarded because their quantity did not exceed a certain weight limit (such as 450 kg). Placards may also be damaged by fire or explosions during the event. Other sources of information that may aid identification include site of the hazmat incident and the type of business, laboratory, or vehicle involved. SDS, order invoices, shipping documents, inventory sheets, and verbal information from front-line employees and management are potential sources of information.[38] The Internet provides up-to-date resources related to chemical identification and database information (Table 34.2).

Public Health Response Cycle in an Industrial Hazardous Material Incident

Comprehensive emergency management of industrial hazmat incidents involves addressing all the elements of the public health

Table 34.2. Online Resources Related to Chemical Identification and Database Information

Name	Description and Internet Address
Chemical Abstracts Service (CAS)	A division of the American Chemical Society, this group provides the most comprehensive database of disclosed research in chemistry and related sciences, including the world's largest collection of substance information, the CAS REGISTRYSM. http://www.cas.org
Databases for emergency chemical responses:	
CAMEO (Computer-aided Management of Emergency Operations) Chemicals	CAMEO Chemicals is developed jointly by three U.S. federal agencies: National Oceanic and Atmospheric Administration (NOAA), EPA, and Coast Guard. CAMEO Chemicals is an online version of part of the CAMEO A suite of software programs developed by NOAA and EPA. CAMEO supports a number of information management functions, such as retrieval of chemical-specific information to support emergency response activities, threat zone calculation and plotting for risk assessment, organization and management of EPCRA information, and storage and computer display of area maps. http://cameochemicals.noaa.gov
CHEMTREC®	Accessible library of over 5 million MSDS, has 24-hour toxicology specialists, language translation services, and chemical industry experts. http://www.chemtrec.com/Chemtrec
MSDSOnline®	MSDS online develops on-demand products and services to help environmental health and safety professionals around the globe to access, manage and deploy MSDS and safety information. The database contains millions of original MSDS documents in an indexed electronic format. More than 10,000 new or updated MSDS documents are added to their database each week. http://www.msdsonline.com
National Fire Protection Association (NFPA) 704, Standard System for the Identification of the Hazards of Materials for Emergency Response, 2012 Edition	This standard addresses the health, flammability, instability, and related hazards that are presented by short-term, acute exposure to a material under conditions of fire, spill, or similar emergencies. http://www.nfpa.org/aboutthecodes/aboutthecodes.asp?docnum=704
U.S. Department of Transportation (DOT) Pipeline and Hazardous Materials Safety Administration (PHMSA), Emergency Response Guidebook (ERG 2012)	Developed jointly by U.S. DOT, Transport Canada, and the Secretariat of Communications and Transportation of Mexico (SCT) for use by firefighters, police, and other emergency services personnel who may be the first to arrive at the scene of a transportation incident involving a hazmat. http://phmsa.dot.gov/hazmat/library
WISER (Wireless Information System for Emergency Responders)	WISER is a system designed to assist first responders in hazardous material incidents. WISER provides a wide range of information on hazardous substances, including substance identification support, physical characteristics, human health information, and containment and suppression advice. http://wiser.nlm.nih.gov
Databases for clinical toxicology, risk assessment and emergency preparedness:	
Agency for Toxic Substances and Disease Registry (ATSDR)	ATSDR provides comprehensive review of health effects of chemicals. It includes Managing Hazardous Material Incidents (MHMI) series, Medical Management Guidelines (MMGs) for acute chemical exposures and ToxFAQs™, toxicological profiles and interaction profiles. http://www.atsdr.cdc.gov/substances/indexAZ.asp
IPCS InCHEM	InChem is a chemical safety information database produced through cooperation between IPCS and the Canadian Centre for Occupational Health and Safety (CCOHS). It provides rapid access to internationally peer-reviewed information on chemicals commonly used throughout the world. Its databases include references to many others. http://www.inchem.org
Occupational Safety and Health Administration (OSHA) Chemical Sampling Information (CSI)	The CSI pages present, in concise form, data on a large number of chemical substances that may be encountered in industrial hygiene investigations. It is intended as a basic reference for OSHA personnel. http://www.osha.gov/dts/chemicalsampling/toc/toc_chemsamp.html
Toxicology Data Network (TOXNET)	TOXNET is a group of more than ten databases covering chemicals and drugs, diseases and the environment, environmental health, occupational safety and health, poisoning, risk assessment and regulations, and toxicology. It is managed by the Toxicology and Environmental Health Information Program (TEHIP) in the Division of Specialized Information Services (SIS) of the National Library of Medicine (NLM). http://toxnet.nlm.nih.gov

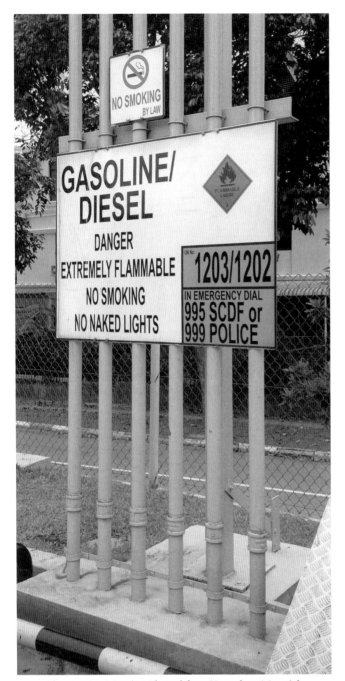

Figure 34.2. Warning Placard for a Hazardous Material.

- Ministries of health, labor, industry, and transportation;
- Regional and local health authorities and inspectors;
- Hospitals and other treatment facilities;
- Providers of toxicological/health information, such as poison information centers and chemical emergency centers;
- Facilities handling, storing, or producing hazardous materials;
- Occupational health centers; and
- Suppliers of pharmaceuticals and medical equipment.

On a national level, the main tasks of the organization are to develop:[1]

- A national chemical emergency coordinating structure, including appropriately trained staff with the right knowledge and skills for dealing with each stage of the disaster cycle;
- A Chemical Incident Response Plan (including public health involvement);
- The necessary policies, legislation, and enforcement strategies for all stages of the disaster cycle;
- Databases on chemicals, sites, transport routes, and expertise;
- Mechanisms for interagency communication and public communication;
- Emergency response guidelines, including environmental protection guidelines;
- Incident exercises, training, and audits;
- Preventive measures;
- National Chemical Incident Surveillance; and
- A structure for independent investigation of chemical incidents.

Risk Management, Prevention, and Mitigation

Risk management is part of disaster prevention and mitigation. The main vulnerability factors are political-institutional, economic, and sociocultural.[49] They include issues such as fragile infrastructure, absent or poorly developed safety policies, low levels of political and social organization, absence of early warning systems, and an increase in population density, especially around chemical facilities. Table 34.3 contains items to be considered when undertaking a risk assessment in a catchment area.[50]

For any community, complete prevention of hazmat incidents is unrealistic. There will always be residual risk of events in the presence of hazards. The approach should be that of managing and reducing risks causing disaster. Risks can be assessed by investigating the cause–effect matrix between hazards and vulnerability (hazard vulnerability assessment [HVA]). A four-step risk assessment process that involves hazard identification, dose-response assessment, exposure assessment, and risk characterization may also be used.[1]

When considering the type of chemical, toxic industrial substances demand extra care and attention. They are defined as industrial chemicals with an LD_{50} (lethal concentration of a substance in 50% of the population exposed over a specific time) of less than 100,000 mg/m^3/min in any mammalian species. In addition, they are produced in quantities exceeding 30 metric tons per year at one production facility.[51] These chemicals have the potential for causing a large number of casualties and should be highly regulated by risk management plans. They have a greater potential for harm if deliberately released.

disaster management cycle – prevention, mitigation, preparedness, response, and recovery. A chemical incident management structure is needed to manage and coordinate the widely differing activities undertaken by the many actors involved at the different stages of the disaster cycle. An organizational structure that includes public health professionals is recommended at the various administrative levels (e.g., national, provincial, and/or local levels).[1]

The aim is to improve prevention of hazmat incidents that might affect the general population and, should an event occur, to minimize adverse effects on human health. Organizations and officials having roles in this management structure include, but may not be limited to, those working in the following areas:[48]

Table 34.3. Items to Be Considered When Undertaking a Risk Assessment in a Catchment Area[50]

- What are the use and storage arrangements for chemicals for all industrial sites?
- What are the on-site capabilities of local industrial sites?
- What are the transport arrangements for hazardous substances?
- What are the historical patterns of local chemical incidents?
- What is the population density, taking into consideration the size and position of the major population centers?
- Are all sites accessible within 20 minutes?
- What and where are the local bodies of water?
- What is the potential for deliberate release of industrial chemicals or chemical warfare agents?
- What is the overall risk?

Other areas of risk assessment include:[49]

- Records of past disasters
- Specific geological, climatic, and other hazards in the local/regional area
- Drafting and updating hazard maps and vulnerability profiles with maximal participation
- Surveys of vulnerable populations
- Surveys of buildings, production activities, roads, vehicles, persons per households

Integrated response plans involving both specialized plant hazmat teams and local community first responders can be devised by following each stage of the chemical life cycle: 1) research and development; 2) site of manufacture; 3) storage at site of manufacture; 4) transportation; 5) storage at site of use; 6) site of use; and 7) disposal of waste products.[52] Reducing human error and equipment failure in each stage will yield the highest return. Community awareness and inclusion of emergency responders in planning has increased through implementation of Responsible Care, a global initiative by the chemical industry to embrace chemical safety.[53] Implementation of the Global Product Strategy has served to increase public and stakeholder awareness and confidence that chemicals in commerce are appropriately managed throughout their lifecycle.[54]

In the United States, the Risk Management Program (RMP) is coordinated by EPA. It requires companies to perform hazard analyses and determinations of "vulnerability zones" and put in place preventive and emergency response plans. The program involves about 14,000 facilities using regulated chemicals that exceed a predetermined threshold quantity established by EPA's RMP.[55] In Europe, the European Commission Seveso Directives I, II, and III oblige member states to ensure that operators have a policy in place to prevent major accidents. The regulations provide a tiered approach to the level of controls: the larger the quantities of dangerous substances present within an establishment, the stricter the rules. "Upper-tier" establishments produce larger quantities than "lower-tier" establishments and are, therefore, subject to tighter controls.[56]

It is much more efficient to implement effective risk-management strategies and avoid the costs of chemical industrial events than to respond to actual incidents. However, one might face reluctance when approaching the topic, due to issues such as cost, poor awareness, resistance to reforms, and minimizing the likelihood of events.[49]

Plans for mitigation should incorporate an all-hazards approach, be location-specific, and be flexible to circumstances surrounding an event. Mitigation planning commonly includes the following areas, which can be considered in the context of hazmat incidents:[49,57]

- Business continuity plans;
- Building design, for example drainage systems for decontamination runoff;
- National and local regulation on land use, locating buildings outside hazard zones;
- Essential building utilities;
- Protection of building contents;
- Mechanisms and instruments for spreading risk and/or risk transfer (insurance and safety reserves);
- Education, such as training the population and local and national institutions on the causes, impacts, and means of disaster prevention;
- Surveillance; and
- Warning and evacuation.

Mitigation measures need not duplicate resources. For example, public warning systems for disaster evacuation are all-hazards and are not only used in chemical releases. Special considerations concerning population protection measures arise from chemicals released as vapor or gas. Shelter-in-place contingencies may be useful when there is insufficient time for evacuation following release or when remaining indoors is safer due to the presence of an outdoor chemical plume. To be effective, public awareness, education, and communication are crucial. The process of sustainable hazards mitigation requires: 1) nonjudgmental debate; 2) full public participation; 3) a willingness to experiment, learn, refine, and alter approaches; and 4) a consensus among stakeholders to stand behind their shared commitment to the goal.[58]

To assist in risk-management planning, emergency exposure limits have been produced by various organizations: 1) the American Industrial Hygiene Association has developed the Emergency Response Planning Guideline; 2) EPA created the Acute Exposure Guideline Level; and 3) the Department of Energy published the Temporary Emergency Exposure Limits. These exposure limits have been used to derive Protective Action Criteria.[59] Such criteria represent the concentration of airborne chemicals at which protective actions are required. These exposure limits can help planners institute preventive measures and estimate the consequences of an uncontrolled chemical release. In the event that an incident occurs, they can be used to evaluate the severity of the release and identify potential outcomes. These emergency limits have additional advantages over industrial limits as they can be applied to the general population.

Predictive modeling of a toxic plume cloud can help estimate the rate and spread of an uncontrolled chemical release during an incident. The Area Location of Hazardous Material computer system (among many others) has been developed to generate models that assist in planning and response.[60] These models identify areas of exposure and the need to evacuate populations at risk, and can be used for training and actual incident management.

Prevention and mitigation efforts should also focus on the transport of dangerous goods. For example, GPS satellite-based technology that tracks ground transportation vehicles carrying hazardous substances provides their exact locations in the event of an acute release. The system can mitigate damage by reducing response time of emergency services to the scene. It also provides surveillance and early warning of any deviation from predetermined routes, be it accidental or deliberate, as in a hijacking by terrorists. With improved situational awareness by drivers, route planning can be optimized and include consideration of hazards such as the weather. In this way, it also assists with disaster prevention. In the event that the vehicle veers off its allocated route or the drivers become intoxicated, the fuel supply for the vehicle can also be shut off.

Preparedness

A systems approach to seamlessly integrate capability is needed for all-hazards incident planning. The same approach should be undertaken with special considerations to the intricacies of a hazmat incident. The 3-S System (staff, stuff, and structure – see Chapter 3) is a reminder of what plans should include to develop optimized and sustainable capability.[61]

Planning and Systems

To deal with residual risks, healthcare authorities, local communities, and hospitals need to plan for acute chemical incidents. At any time, hospitals must be ready to safely and rapidly decontaminate, evaluate, and treat a few chemically injured victims. This is the premise for development of further response capabilities for mass casualty incidents involving chemical or radiological weapons of mass destruction. In a study comparing 1996 and 2000 measures of preparedness among hospitals in a major U.S. metropolitan area, the hospitals were poorly prepared to manage chemical emergency incidents, including terrorism. This lack of hospital preparedness did not change significantly between 1996 and 2000, despite increased funds allocated to bioterrorism preparedness at the local level.[62]

In some countries, such as the United States, extensive legislation, regulation, and standards exist mandating and assisting hospitals to plan for chemical incidents. Examples include:

1. Occupational safety regulations from the Occupational Safety and Health Administration (OSHA) protect healthcare providers during a hazmat response as a worker safety issue.[63]
2. The Emergency Medical Treatment and Active Labor Act requires hospitals to provide a medical screening examination and stabilization (consistent with their capabilities) to anyone presenting to their location for treatment regardless of citizenship, legal status, or ability to pay.[64] It does not make exceptions for contaminated patients.
3. EPCRA is a section of the Superfund Amendments and Reauthorization Act (SARA) Title III.[65] It states that facilities manufacturing or storing hazardous chemicals must report inventories and every hazmat release to public officials and emergency health agencies. The act also requires the establishment of state emergency response commissions and local emergency planning committees.
4. Healthcare accreditation organizations such as the Joint Commission have requirements relating to hazmats.[66]

Planning for toxic incidents involves modification within the framework of existing emergency response plans and incident command systems, rather than creating entirely new protocols. Plans should be established before a hazmat incident occurs. Separate prehospital and hospital plans are needed for first responders and first receivers, respectively, to manage victims. Both plans must be integrated and harmonized.

In addition to areas addressed in general emergency management programs, specific areas to consider when planning for a hospital's hazmat response include:

- Hazards and vulnerabilities identified in an HVA;
- Estimated time before arrival based on location of hazard;
- Casualty care areas;
- Decontamination procedures and protocols;
- Secondary contamination and containment of contaminated equipment and runoff water;
- Safety: personal protection equipment (PPE);
- Communications at decontamination area;
- Heating, ventilating, air conditioning, and in-place protection;
- Medical management – antidotes;
- Interfacility transfers – patients with special needs, burn patients; and
- Knowledge resources for hazardous materials.

Local authorities that develop such plans should consider the following:[67]

- Identify local facilities using hazardous substances.
- Designate community and industrial coordinators.
- Establish mechanisms for emergency notification.
- Establish procedures for determining the occurrence of a release and an estimation of the affected population (location and numbers).
- Identify community emergency equipment facilities.
- Establish evacuation plans.
- Establish and schedule training programs for emergency personnel.

Staff

The hospital's incident command center is responsible for optimal use of staffing resources. It should coordinate medical and auxiliary personnel, direct activities at the various treatment sites, organize equipment and supplies, and maintain contact with outside authorities.[68] Standard operating procedures indicating roles and responsibilities of personnel must be established before an event occurs.

Education and training are important aspects of planning because of specialized procedures and equipment used by prehospital providers and hospital personnel. First responders and first receivers must acquire necessary knowledge, skills, and abilities to respond safely to incidents involving hazardous materials. Because of different work environments and PPE requirements, education and training should be tailored to address their specific needs. It should be structured and standardized, locally relevant to hazards and equipment used, continually revised and updated, and delivered multiple times and across all work shifts to enhance retention.

In a study of paramedic students, retention of proper donning and doffing techniques for PPE was poor at 6 months after initial training. Critical errors were common even in individuals with previous hazmat, firefighter, and emergency medical services training.[69] It appears unrealistic to retrain hospital decontamination teams composed of staff nurses and allied health personnel every 6 months; however, annual refresher courses are achievable.

Table 34.4. Five-Level Scale for Hospital Preparedness According to Existing Threat[68]

Level of Preparation*	Action Required
I – No Threat	1. Prepare a hospital deployment plan for a chemical incident (e.g., due to a motor vehicle collision)
II – Minimal Threat	1. Instruction of the hospital plan and principles of chemical agent diagnosis and treatment once a year 2. Assign specific tasks in the deployment plan to hospital personnel 3. Partial practice drill once in 3 years 4. Consider the need for medical equipment, supplies, and communication systems, and examine their maintenance once a year
III – Existing Threat	1. Full practice drill once in 3–5 years, instruction every year 2. Prepare appropriate medical equipment, supplies, and communication systems, and examine their maintenance every half year
IV – Increased Threat	1. Organize appropriate shifts of hospital personnel to increase their availability and an emergency calling system for the staff and auxiliary personnel according to their assigned tasks 2. Full practice drill once in 1–2 years, instruction and smaller scale review drills on receiving the new threat level and as often as possible 3. Examine maintenance of equipment, protective gear, and communication systems every few months. Increase their availability by storage at or near the sites 4. Prepare arrangements for shifting of patients inside the hospital
V – Maximal Threat	1. Be prepared to receive and treat chemical casualties within minutes or hours 2. Organize equipment, protective gear, and communication systems at all sites 3. Arrange patient transfer and discharge when possible 4. Maintain continuous contact with authorities outside the hospital

* Each level should also include the required actions of the previous levels

The training courses may consist of practical approaches to the management of hazmat casualties, common toxicological agents, triaging contaminated victims, computer searches for information on toxic materials, wearing PPE, and assembling a portable decontamination shower.[70] Hospitals can video record and review drills to critique and refresh the knowledge of their participating staff.

Frequently planned drills are essential for effective implementation of disaster plans. Joint training and education are important ingredients in producing a multidisciplinary team functioning optimally under stressful circumstances. Training must include: 1) communication exercises; 2) small-scale (hospital and emergency service) response exercises; and 3) full-scale simulations involving industry, health professionals, emergency services, and others with responsibilities in the area, such as civil defense services and military authorities.[71] A cost-effective five-level scale for hospital preparedness in accordance with the existing threat has been suggested (Table 34.4).[68]

Stuff and Structure

Hazmat medical response involves mobilization and utilization of equipment and treatment areas that are rarely encountered in the course of routine hospital work. "Structure" can mean physical infrastructure such as a fixed facility for decontamination, assembly, triage and evaluation, and patient care, all of which must be determined pre-event. Decontamination can be conducted in fixed, semi-fixed, or mobile facilities like tents, inflatable structures, and mass decontamination vehicles.

Some of the challenges facing hospitals on the safe treatment of hazmat exposures may be mitigated by engineering controls. Examples include:[62,72]

- Controlled access points to prevent contaminated patients from entering the facility prior to decontamination;
- Designing decontamination shower facilities that can accommodate placement of warm water lines;
- Situating shower nozzles on the building exterior;
- Collection system to control for contaminated water runoff;
- Access fittings for medical gases on the building exterior that will facilitate use by emergency responders when utilizing supplied-air respirators; and
- Design of hospital ventilation systems that takes into account the potential need to isolate the internal hospital environment.

Procurement and acquisition of PPE and decontamination items need to complement the hospital's role and HVA outcomes. Further elaboration on both topics can be found in Chapters 15 and 16. "Stuff" also includes knowledge resources that are needed for medical management of victims. A vast amount of informative resources are web-based, thus underscoring the need for maintenance of Internet access during a crisis. Other resources include poison information centers, ad hoc toxicological advisory teams, in-hospital toxicologists, or textbooks.[73]

Medical field teams deployed from hospitals to the scene of a hazmat mass casualty incident usually conduct their work in the "cold" zone. Nevertheless, they will need to carry PPE that is commensurate with the hazard's risk, in case the zone turns suddenly "warm" without the opportunity for timely evacuation. In addition to general items, an inventory of antidotes and burn care supplies should be considered.

Antidote stockpiling is a critical component of comprehensive medical preparedness in chemical emergencies.[74] A national program for distribution of antidotes from a central stockpile plays a fundamental role; however, demographic, geographical, and economic factors often obstruct the rapid disbursement of

Table 34.5. Available Life-saving Antidotes for Hazmat and Chemical Weapons[74]

Antidote	Chemical
Calcium	Hydrofluoric acid or fluoride
Hydroxocobalamin	Cyanides
Atropine	Organophosphates, carbamates, nerve agents
Amyl nitrite	Cyanides, nitriles, sulfides
Methylene blue	Methemoglobin-forming compounds
Oxygen	Simple asphyxiants, systemic asphyxiants, methemoglobin-forming compounds, carbon monoxide, cyanides, azides and hydrazoic acid, hydrogen sulfide and sulfides
Oximes	Organophosphates, nerve agents
Pyridoxine	Hydrazones

antidotes. Any system of antidote distribution must provide poisoned patients with empirical antidotes based on toxidromic assessment or specific antidotes based on substance identification in appropriate quantities and within the time required for treatment. Local stockpiles of antidotes are limited by factors such as infrequent use, cost, and short shelf life. A push system can be adopted to supplement local stockpiles with antidotes to common poisonings, which can be based on the local HVA. This is important in the initial phase when the substance is unidentified. Larger quantities of specific items or antidotes can follow as the situation becomes clearer. Time-sensitive antidotes such as diazepam, cyanide antidote kits, atropine, and pralidoxime are the most important drugs to stockpile locally for the potential treatment of mass casualties from a chemical emergency (Table 34.5).[74–76] In addition to antidote stockpiling, emergency drugs and essential standard drugs should also be stockpiled because these can be rapidly depleted in a mass casualty situation.[73]

Response

When responding to an acute hazmat incident, the protocols and procedures planned during the preparation phase are followed and executed. The command structure and responsibilities should follow the same approach as that for a major incident.[50] Early recognition that a hazmat situation exists, effective risk communication, wearing appropriate PPE, administration of basic or advanced resuscitation measures, rapid decontamination, and timely evacuation and transport to hospitals that can provide appropriate treatment are crucial factors for improving outcomes. The response phase is usually staged in two locations: the prehospital environment and the hospital site.

Prehospital Response

To recognize a hazmat event, emergency medical services and fire department personnel responding to a motor vehicle collision or structure fire must have a high index of suspicion. They may not receive information on hazardous materials involvement prior to arriving on scene. The ability to recognize that an event has occurred is the key to responder safety.

First responders may immediately suspect a hazmat incident when confronted with a truck rollover and leakage of unknown substances. In the absence of such obvious clues, general indicators of possible hazmat event include:[70]

- Unusual occurrence of dead or dying animals (such as dead birds);
- Unexplained casualties (multiple victims with the similar signs and symptoms such as skin, respiratory, vision, and nervous system involvement);
- Increase in the frequency of those with the aforementioned signs and symptoms in the direction of prevailing winds;
- Unusual liquid or vapor clouds (droplets, unexplained odor or taste); and
- Mass casualties without any conventional injuries.

Binoculars are helpful for ascertaining visible information from a safe distance.

After recognizing the presence of a hazmat, one needs to assess the event. One approach is by performing a three-point incident site assessment of environment, containers, and materials involved (chemical and physical properties).[77] This method builds a framework that enables the responder to see the overall picture and have a manageable span of control over the data, using it to develop and implement an incident action plan. Weather patterns in the immediate area, particularly the local wind direction and speed, are important considerations as these incidents are approached from uphill and upwind. Other weather factors, such as heat and humidity, can greatly affect the behavior of a hazmat. For example, anhydrous ammonia typically moves upward, but a cloud can interact with moisture in the atmosphere and hover along the ground on a humid day.[77]

Once a hazmat incident has been declared, all non-contaminated, non-protected personnel should be evacuated from the scene. The area is then cordoned off, with limited access. When full decontamination is needed, it occurs along a corridor in the "warm zone." This is the area between the site of contamination (the hot zone) and the safe area (the cold zone).[78] The cold zone is uphill and upwind from the hot zone (Figure 34.3).[79] An alternate to evacuation is a shelter-in-place strategy. This involves remaining indoors and securing refuge in a room with no or few windows while waiting for the toxic plume to disperse. This is applicable for selected type of chemicals and in appropriate settings.[80]

Information from the scene should be widely communicated as soon as possible to receiving hospitals to optimize their preparation. If available, the following data should be transmitted: number and type of casualties; chemical substance involved; estimated time of arrival for first casualties (realizing that some patients may bypass the prehospital system and self-present); time and location of the incident; method of contamination (vapor or liquid); and potential hazards to healthcare providers.[79] The development of state of the art computer-based communication and information networks designed especially for mass casualty incident management has provided the means for a more coordinated and effective response by facilitating information flow. Through these systems, first responders can activate web-based cameras to provide live streaming videos of selected incident areas (such as casualty clearing stations) to improve situational awareness at the hospitals.

Identification of the hazardous substance is useful and potential sources of information have been discussed earlier in this

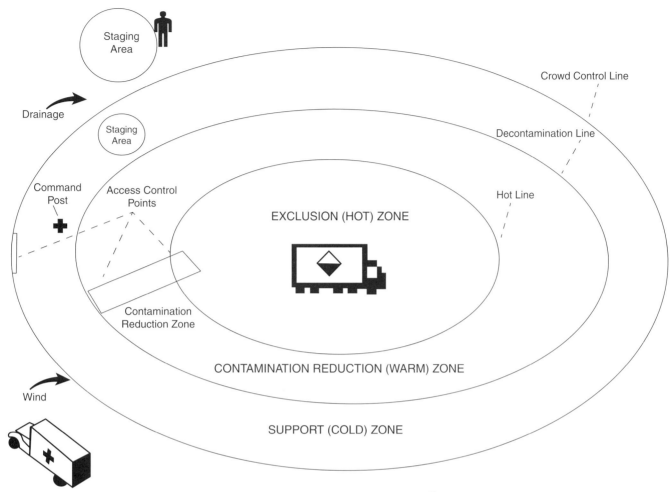

Figure 34.3. Incident site control zones.[79]

chapter. Equipment exists, including chemical detection paper and the Improved Chemical Agent Monitor that allows trained personnel to detect chemicals. A rapid detection device is used first, then followed by confirmation with sophisticated methods in specialized laboratories. Staff must adhere to proper sampling techniques and a list of laboratories should be readily available.[73]

Depending on the scale of the chemical incident and local emergency planning, physicians and nurses from hospitals or organized response teams may be mobilized to provide forward medical care to victims on scene. They usually perform their duties in the cold zone, where it is not contaminated and safe. Hazmat victims may, however, have acute life-threatening respiratory and cardiovascular problems that require aggressive and early definitive care. The problem is amplified should the substance have high persistence in the surroundings. To withhold care until decontamination is completed may lead to unacceptable delays in treatment. Medical personnel in appropriate PPE may provide early, enhanced basic or advanced life support inside the warm zone where decontamination is conducted. Due to an emergent need for care, some medical providers can also function in the contaminated hot zone, where trapped survivors may be located.[81,82] Medical response personnel who enter the contaminated zone should be adequately trained and equipped with appropriate PPE. Safety is the first and foremost consideration. Special knowledge on medical and operational aspects of managing victims in a hostile, contaminated environment is required

for the best results.[83,84] In a situation where decontamination can be conducted quickly, limiting medical attention to opening the airway with spinal precautions, controlling hemorrhage, and terminating seizures can expedite a victim's transport to definitive care.

Triage

When decontamination facilities are saturated, two factors should help to decide patient priority – the principles of field medical triage and the severity of contamination.[78] Casualties who require immediate treatment with antidotes should receive early intervention and be reevaluated at intervals. Triage at this point will also help to identify which patients need immediate, lifesaving care before and during decontamination.

Whichever triage system is used in a hazmat incident, it should be familiar to those responsible for the activity. Physiological methods such as the modified triage sieve have been described for use in the warm zone, although there is some question as to its efficacy.[50,85,86] Other triage methods have factored in aspects such as organ system involvement, area of skin injury, and response to antidotes.[79] Although such criteria may improve triage precision, application of these algorithms may be restricted by their complexity in a situation in which time is limited. One chemical triage algorithm proposed by Cone et al. considers the latency period of some hazardous chemicals like phosgene and uses "breathing" as a simple subjective assessment of patient's overall respiratory status.[87] This system will need further refinement and testing.

Decontamination and PPE

Decontamination of chemically contaminated casualties should be viewed as part of the initial treatment, not as an additional process, and should occur as soon as possible.[50] It also prevents secondary contamination of personnel and equipment. Removal of outer layers of clothing may reduce contamination by up to 85%.[78]

If the exposure is from a vapor or gas, then nearly all of the contaminants will be eliminated when the victim is evacuated and the clothing is removed. They are not likely to pose a secondary contamination risk to hospital personnel.[88-90] Gas or vapor releases can expose victims to toxic concentrations, but tend to dissipate quickly. However, victims whose hair, skin, or clothing is grossly contaminated with solid or liquid material, including condensed vapor or aerosol, can endanger emergency personnel by direct contact or by off-gassing of the toxic substance.[91] Nonetheless, it is unlikely that a living victim could create an "immediately dangerous to life or health" environment at a receiving hospital if contaminated clothing is quickly removed and isolated, and the victim is treated and decontaminated in an area with adequate ventilation.[92] Failure to perform these actions, however, can generate an immediately dangerous to life or health situation during treatment of a viable victim within the hospital, resulting in significant medical consequences for healthcare providers.[93]

Skin decontamination is not needed in a mass casualty situation with limited resources, and removal of clothing may be sufficient if it has been confirmed that the exposure is due only to vapor or gas and no gross contamination of the hair or skin by condensation exists.[36,92,94] Special consideration should be made for highly soluble irritant gases such as ammonia. This substance can dissolve in the moisture of mucous membranes to form ammonium hydroxide, a strong base. It produces a local toxic effect of irritation and burning on mucous membranes. If victims feel skin burning, decontamination should be conducted. All clothing should ideally be removed on scene and double bagged.

Decontamination should be conducted with consideration for privacy. Equipment for medical care including bag-mask-valve devices, oxygen tanks, airway devices, and wound care items must be prepared and mobilized to the warm zone. Further detailed discussion on PPE and decontamination can be found in Chapters 15 and 16, respectively.

Transportation and Evacuation

Prioritizing the transportation of victims from the casualty clearing station to hospitals requires further triage. Transport vehicles should be well ventilated with the windows open if necessary. The importance of improving ventilation in the confined space of a transport vehicle was underscored by the Tokyo sarin attack in 1995, when it was observed that 9.9% of 1,364 emergency medical technicians showed acute symptoms and received medical treatment at hospitals. Most of them experienced the onset of symptoms during transportation, and it is suspected that they were exposed to the vaporized sarin from the victims' clothes in ambulances. The ventilation in ambulances and minivans was poor because the windows were shut.[94] Additionally, patients were not undressed and decontaminated before transport to healthcare facilities.

Hospital-Based Response

Decontamination Again?

It is not easy for first receivers at healthcare facilities to accurately determine whether prehospital decontamination of casualties has been adequately conducted. Casualties can be symptomatic but "clean," and checking individually with chemical detection devices will require too much time. Some hospitals may subject these casualties to a second decontamination procedure. This method is debatable as it delays treatment. Local health authorities, experts, and first responders and receivers should discuss the options and arrive at a consensus.

Wounds should be irrigated and covered with waterproof dressing during decontamination. Following that, attention should be paid to decontamination of the eyes, nose, ears, and oral cavity as necessary. The eyes can be irrigated with the help of a Morgan lens or an improvised device using a nasal cannula placed across the nasal bridge and attached to a 1-liter bag of normal saline.

Medical Treatment

Initial medical attention should be focused on providing basic resuscitation measures by addressing the ABCDEs in a primary trauma survey: airway (with cervical spine control); breathing; circulation; disability (nervous system); and exposure (decontamination, examination for injuries). The possibility of concomitant physical trauma, burns, and smoke inhalation injuries should be considered because many of these incidents involve fires and explosions. Supportive care is more important than specific antidotes. In a seizing victim, opening the airway, providing oxygenation, and aborting the seizure with a benzodiazepine will confer more benefit than any antidote.

Obtaining a concise history can be guided by using the AMPLE mnemonic, which stands for Allergies, Medications, Past medical history, Last meal, and Events leading up to the incident. Any past respiratory condition is significant because inhalation is the most common route of exposure to agents at hazmat incidents. Victims with cardiac conditions may be at greater risk in asphyxiant (carbon monoxide and cyanide) poisoning due to ischemia. With regard to events leading up to the incident, helpful information includes: route of exposure; location of the incident; whether the incident occurred in a confined space; elapsed time since exposure; duration of exposure (entrapment); the presence of fire, explosion, or blast; and whether loss of consciousness occurred.

After the primary survey and resuscitation, hazmat patient assessment involves a secondary survey that focuses on:

- Identifying complications of poisoning;
- Recognizing existing medical problems with potential for exacerbation;
- Assessing for accompanying trauma or burns; and
- Recognizing hazmat toxic syndromes (toxidromes).

Toxidromes are collective sets of signs and symptoms that indicate poisoning with a specific class of agents. They help to simplify the approach to treatment and have both practical and medical relevance. Table 34.6 summarizes the features and treatment of five toxidromes: irritant gases, asphyxiants, cholinergics, corrosives, and hydrocarbons and halogenated hydrocarbons.[95]

The use of PPE in the warm and hot zones limits dexterity, so antidotes are given via auto-injectors that deliver fixed

Table 34.6. Features of Five Toxidromes (Table constructed with information from Advanced Hazmat Life Support/AHLS)[95]

	Irritant gas	Asphyxiant	Cholinergic	Corrosive	Hydrocarbon and Halogenated Hydrocarbon
Common agents. Some may present with characteristics of more than one toxidrome	High water solubility: ammonia, sulphur dioxide, hydrogen chloride Moderate solubility: chlorine Low solubility: phosgene, nitrogen dioxide	Simple: carbon dioxide, methane, propane Systemic: carbon monoxide, cyanides, hydrogen sulphide, isobutyl nitrite, aniline	Organophosphates, carbamates pesticides	Acids (sulphuric, hydrochloric, hydrofluoric), bases (sodium hydroxide), oxidizers (hydrogen peroxide), white phosphorus	Methane, ethane, propane, butane, benzene, phenol, chloroform, chlorofluorocarbons (CFCs), and hydrochlorofluorocarbons (HCFCs)
Industry	Chemical synthesis, bleaching, disinfectant, and dye production	Byproduct of incomplete/complete combustion, chemical synthesis, liquefied petroleum gas (LPG), dye production, fumigant, sewer gas	Pest control at home and agricultural, organophosphate nerve agents	Chemical synthesis, food production, petroleum refining, disinfectant, propellant, fireworks	Natural gas, chemical synthesis, LPG, dye production, preservatives, refrigerants
Routes of exposure	Inhalation, skin, and mucous membranes	Inhalation, skin, and mucous membranes, ingestion	Inhalation, skin, and mucous membranes, ingestion	Inhalation, skin, and mucous membranes, ingestion	Inhalation, skin, and mucous membranes, ingestion
Classification.	Water solubility: High – upper airway affected (lower airway maybe affected with prolonged exposure) Moderate – overlap of upper and lower airway Low – lower airway affected	Simple: displace oxygen from surrounding atmosphere Systemic: affects oxygen transport via hemoglobin, or interferes with aerobic metabolism	Organophosphates, carbamates	Acid, base, and oxidizer	Aliphatic, aromatic, halogenated flammability
Characteristic presentation (signs and symptoms)	Upper airway: coughing and stridor, pharyngitis, laryngeal edema, laryngospasm, dysphonia, rhinorrhea Lower airway: Bronchospasm, delayed noncardiogenic pulmonary edema Others: Lacrimation, conjunctival injection	Simple asphyxiant: Headache, fatigue, anxiety, giddiness, nausea, dyspnea, palpitations, altered mental status, coma, seizure, cardiac ischemia In addition, systemic asphyxiant: cyanosis and unreliable pulse oximetry readings can be due to methemoglobinemia Delayed neuropathy and cognitive effects.	SLUDGE mnemonic (muscarinic): salivation, lacrimation, urination, defecation, gastrointestinal cramping, emesis MTWHF mnemonic (nicotinic): mydriasis, tachycardia, weakness, hypertension, fasciculation CNS (nicotinic and muscarinic): confusion, convulsion and coma	Coughing, dyspnea, dysphonia, stridor, laryngeal edema, nausea and vomiting, bronchospasm, noncardiogenic pulmonary edema, cyanosis, skin burns Others: lacrimation, conjunctival injection, blindness White phosphorus: liver and kidney damage, hypocalcemia Hydrofluoric acid: hypocalcemia	Presents like simple asphyxiant. sensitization of the heart to endogenous catecholamines, arrhythmias Central nervous system depression, narcosis, coma Skin irritation, defatting dermatitis and chemical burns Halogenated hydrocarbon: liver and kidney damage
Main systems affected	Airway and breathing	Cardiovascular and nervous system	Nervous system	Airway, cardiovascular,	Cardiovascular and nervous system
Treatment summary	Consider latency of chemical affecting lower airway Supportive management includes: oxygenation, bronchodilators, corticosteroids	Provide oxygen support Cyanide: antidotes include amyl nitrite (inhaled), sodium nitrite, sodium thiosulfate, hydroxocobalamin Hydrogen sulphide: sodium nitrite Consider hyperbaric oxygen treatment for carbon monoxide, methylene blue for methemoglobinemia	Supportive management Give antidotes early: Atropine, oximes (e.g., pralidoxime), benzodiazepine (for seizure)	Rapid decontamination, water irrigation of eyes and skin, burns management Hydrofluoric acid: local or parenteral calcium replacement	Supportive management includes: oxygenation, control seizures, wound care Avoid sympathomimetics due to cardiac irritability

incremental doses of drugs such as atropine. At the first aid post or hospital setting, a dose–response regime via intravenous route should be adopted. In patients with shock and peripheral vasoconstriction, absorption of drugs via intramuscular injection may be unpredictable and erratic.

Victims with seizures should be examined for intracranial pathology, including traumatic hemorrhage. Attributing such phenomenon simply to central nervous system injury from toxins is not suggested. The common approach to differential diagnosis for clinical symptoms and signs still applies.

The toxic effect of chemicals may be seen acutely or only become apparent after a period of latency. One such example is phosgene. This agent is a gas at room temperature, is poorly soluble in water, and has an odor threshold that is five times higher than the OSHA permissive exposure level.[63] It causes little or no upper respiratory tract symptoms and its odor provides insufficient warning of hazardous concentration, thus prolonging exposure of victims to the chemical. This allows the chemical to enter the lower airways due to a lack of avoidance behavior by victims. It may initially cause no signs or symptoms, or symptoms may be due only to mild irritation of the airways. These symptoms (dryness and burning of the throat and cough) may cease when the patient is removed from exposure. After an asymptomatic interval of 30 minutes to 8 hours, however, respiratory damage becomes evident.[96] This affects the period of observation that may be needed for victims of such exposures. There is an inverse relationship between the dose of most agents and their latent periods. This means a higher dose results in a shorter latency period.

While difficult to measure precisely, in mass casualty incidents, it is thought that there is often a 5:1 or larger ratio of persons who are symptomatic because they think they have been exposed compared to those who have actually been exposed. Those who are psychological casualties assert an extra burden on a healthcare system that must attend to the physically and physiologically injured victims first. It is difficult to identify psychological casualties initially and decontamination will be needed before further clinical assessment can be made. Trained counselors are an important part of the management team and provide needed psychological support.

Recovery

The recovery phase involves decontamination of the facility and certification that it is safe to resume normal operations. Patients, visitors, hospital staff, and the media should be kept informed during this process. Documentation created during the incident is collected for the purposes of archiving, creation of after-action reports, development of corrective action plans, and research purposes to share with the international community. In some countries, such documents are crucial for financial reimbursement purposes.

Public health authorities need to undertake four important roles in the recovery phase:[1]

1. Organization of healthcare to treat victims and support them in regaining control of their lives, including a central access to information and assistance;
2. Risk and health outcome assessment, including exposure, environmental, and human health assessments;
3. Implementing remediation and restoration actions; and
4. Evaluation, including root cause analysis, response, and new knowledge gained.

At the hospitals, equipment and contaminated areas must be decontaminated. PPE such as chemical suits, gloves, and boots may require disposal. It is often difficult to ensure safe reuse due to limitations in the ability to assess the degree that chemicals have penetrated the equipment. Safe disposal of contaminated runoff water and other hazardous waste is necessary, usually with assistance from local fire, health, and environmental authorities. Disposition of the victims' contaminated personal belongings must also be addressed. In some cases, all such items must be retained as evidence for law enforcement investigations of a crime scene.

A separate morgue must be established to prevent cross-contamination between the victims' dead bodies and those who died of other causes. The burial process will require special arrangements with environmental and public health considerations.

Large-scale events engender different types of stressors. These include threats to one's life, confrontation with the injured and dead, bereavement (family member and friends lost), significant loss of property (such as homes), and social and community disruption that have lasting effects. The impact of disasters is usually much broader than the acute health problems that occur.[1] Behavioral health (acute and long-term) services must be provided for staff and victims.

RECOMMENDATIONS FOR FURTHER RESEARCH

Research in Hazardous Material, Toxic, and Industrial Events

The conduct of disaster research is often difficult. It is not possible to "create disasters" for scientific study purposes. Investigators must usually wait for actual events to occur, and when it does, a stressed and altered environment affects the ability collect accurate data. To give a clearer picture, global and national cooperative research involving multiple stakeholders is needed to define problem areas and find solutions.

In the United States, the Hazardous Materials Cooperative Research Program managed by the Cooperative Research Programs of the Transportation Research Board focuses on transportation incidents and has conducted perceived gap analysis and explored research needs.[97] Another program, the National Toxic Substance Incidents Program (NTSIP) sponsored by the Agency for Toxic Substances and Disease Registry receives data from ten state partners, collecting information about spills from the health departments.[98] These national programs are crucial to defining problems and providing feasible, scientific solutions. Future areas of research are expansive, with varied goals and objectives attempting to optimize health and environment outcomes (Table 34.7).

Fundamentally, research in disaster medicine should have a strong public health and epidemiological approach and should be outcomes oriented. At the same time, disaster research should be fiscally responsible and strive to pursue the best scientific evidence. Newer technologies such as computer-based programs and teaching methods such as simulations have greatly expanded the possibilities for facilitating problem-based research and finding solutions in disaster management.

One of the biggest challenges in disaster medicine is accurate data collection before, during, and after an actual event. One of the obstacles to collecting accurate data is the lack of dedicated research staff. When managing disasters, most personnel are

Table 34.7. Future Disaster Research Goals and Objectives for Industrial and Hazmat Incidents

- Epidemiological research and improved data collection before, during, and after incidents
- Strengthening of the research agenda for technology, meteorology, engineering, and the environment. Alignment and synthesis of these activities with the medical and public health research agenda
- Development of best practices for public warning
- Urban and city planning research focusing on the locations of industrial and hazmat facilities and transportation corridors
- Support for infrastructure research and high-technology modeling for preparedness, mitigation, response, and recovery from industrial and hazmat disasters
- Strengthening of the toxicology and occupational medicine research agenda: antidotes, decontamination techniques, analytical methods for rapid detection of toxic chemicals, and mass casualty chemical triage
- Continuous HVA to improve surge capacity based on the latest data for the facility, staff, and current equipment
- Funding for dedicated research staff with existing protocols deployed to incidents as a part of disaster management teams
- Technology research for prevention and monitoring of industrial accidents. Examples: video cameras, surveillance satellites and aerial reconnaissance, and fixed and mobile monitoring units similar to "black boxes" in airplanes. Enhanced medical and technological monitoring of staff and environment
- After events, implementation of improved, harmonized, and synchronized data collection on long-term effects of industrial incidents on health and environment
- Economic research examining the risk/benefit ratio for operation of industrial and hazmat facilities and transports
- Sociological research to study behavioral and psychological patterns during hazmat incidents
- Educational goals and objectives for a research agenda
- Investigate strategies to optimize collaboration among different specialties such as chemists, meteorologists, physicians, and managers

usually engaged in disaster response activities and not available for independent academic research. Additionally, disaster research for complex events such as industrial incidents must be multidisciplinary and use an all-hazards approach. One possibility to increase data collection during and after industrial accidents is the use of newer monitoring technology such as closed-circuit video cameras, aerial and satellite observation, and "black boxes" similar to those used on aircraft mounted on fixed structures that collect data and monitor all events. A high-quality HVA and subsequently designed disaster management plan can only be based on accurate and sufficient data from previous experiences and events. Safety and security protocols for industrial facilities and hazmats should be based on the best scientific evidence and less on financial interests.

Decision makers and disaster managers who are responsible for development and implementation of protocols face a special challenge. They are caught in a conflict between the scientific data depicting the correct approaches and the financial realities of what they can afford. Many of the existing disaster protocols and much of the equipment have not been scientifically tested under the actual conditions for which they were designed. Often theoretical models, policies, and equipment are simply transferred from one disaster scenario to another. In general, there should be more funding from unbiased sources to sup-

port independent and sound scientific research. There should be more collaboration among academic institutions with respect to the collection of research data in a central repository to prevent duplication. A well-developed research agenda will provide the evidence-based science to guide community risk management and enforcement of high safety standards in the chemical industry.

Strengthen Both Regional and Global Public Health Responses

Public health responses must be integrated globally as well as locally. Chemicals released into the environment can spread beyond the local vicinity and, in some cases, cross national borders. Therefore, it is also necessary to coordinate international preparedness and response. Some international agreements already exist, such as the UN Economic Commission for Europe's Convention on the Trans-boundary Effects of Industrial Accidents.[99] Its continuing work helps improve exchanges of information, implementation, and surveillance of programs for monitoring, planning, and research and development addressing chemical production. It fosters mutual assistance on research and training methodologies. The goal is to develop and provide models based on experience from industrial accidents and scenarios that illustrate preventive, preparedness, and response measures. Additional research in international agreements will further strengthen the safety of chemical production, distribution, and disposal.

REFERENCES

1. World Health Organization. WHO Manual: The Public Health Management of Chemical Incidents. 2009.
2. Chemical Abstracts Service. Chemical abstracts service. http://www.cas.org (Accessed June 19, 2013).
3. Public Health and Chemical Incidents – Guidance for national and regional policy makers in the public/environmental health roles. International Programme on Chemical Safety (IPCS), 1999.
4. OECD. Environmental outlook for the chemical industry. http://www.oecd.org/dataoecd/7/45/2375538.pdf (Accessed March 21, 2013).
5. Prüss-Ustün A, Vickers C, Haefliger P, Bertollini R. Knowns and unknowns on burden of disease due to chemicals: a systematic review. *Environmental Health* 2011; 10(9). http://www.biomedcentral.com/content/pdf/1476–069X-10–9.pdf (Accessed June 19, 2013).
6. OECD. OECD Environmental Outlook to 2050: The Consequences of Inaction. June 2012.
7. Agency for Toxic Substances and Disease Registry (ATSDR). National Toxic Substance Incidents Program (NTSIP) Annual Report 2010. 2010. http://www.atsdr.cdc.gov/ntsip/docs/ATSDR_Annual%20Report_031413_FINAL.pdf (Accessed June 19, 2013).
8. Health Protection Agency, Centre for Radiation, Chemical & Environmental Hazards. Chemical Surveillance Report. January 1–December 31, 2009. http://www.hpa.org.uk/Publications/ChemicalsPoisons/ChemicalsSurveillanceReports (Accessed March 21, 2013).
9. Duan W, Chen G, Ye Q, Chen Q. The situation of hazardous chemical accidents in China between 2000 and 2006. *Journal of Hazardous Materials* 2011; 186: 1489–1494.

10. Keim ME. Industrial chemical disasters. In: Ciottone GR, Anderson PD, Auf der Heide E, et al., eds. *Disaster Medicine.* 3rd ed. Philadelphia, PA, Mosby Elsevier, 2006; 556–562.

11. Mehta PS, Mehta AS, Mehta SJ, Makhijani AB. Bhopal tragedy's health effects. *JAMA.* 1990; 264: 2781–2787.

12. ATSDR. Hazardous Substances Emergency Events Surveillance (HSEES) system – Annual report 2004. http://www.atsdr.cdc.gov/HS/HSEES/annual2004.html (Accessed March 21, 2013).

13. WHO. Chemical Incidents – Technical Hazard Sheet – Technological Disaster Profiles. http://www.who.int/hac/techguidance/ems/chemical_insidents/en/index.html (Accessed March 21, 2013).

14. Noll GG, Hildebrand MS, Yvorra JG. *Hazardous materials: managing the incident.* Fire Protection Publications, Oklahoma State University, 1995.

15. ATSDR. Hazardous Substances Emergency Events Surveillance (HSEES) system – Cumulative Report 1998–2001. http://www.atsdr.cdc.gov/HS/HSEES/Cum1998_2001.html (Accessed March 21, 2013).

16. U.S. Department of Transportation. Pipeline and Hazardous Materials Safety Administration, Strategic Plan (2012–2016). http://www.phmsa.dot.gov (Accessed March 21, 2013).

17. Olowokure B, Pooransingh S, Tempowski J, et al. Global surveillance for chemical incidents of international public health concern. *Bull World Health Organ* 2005; 83: 928–934.

18. Eckerman I. Chemical Industry and Public Health – Bhopal as an Example. 2001. http://bhopal.bard.edu/resources/research.php (Accessed March 21, 2013).

19. Broughton E. The Bhopal disaster and its aftermath: a review. *Environ Health* 2005; 4(1): 6.

20. Eckerman I. The Bhopal gas leak: Analyses of causes and consequences by three different models. *Journal of Loss Prevention in the Process Industries* 2005; 18: 213–217.

21. Gupta JP. The Bhopal gas tragedy: could it have happened in a developed country? *Journal of Loss Prevention in the Process Industries* 2002; 15(1): 1–4.

22. Sharma DC. Bhopal: 20 years on. *Lancet* 2005; 365(9454): 111–112.

23. Willey RJ, Crowl DA, Lepkowski W. The Bhopal tragedy: its influence on process and community safety as practiced in the United States. *Journal of Loss Prevention in the Process Industries* 2005; 18(4): 365–374.

24. Dunning AE, Oswalt JL. Train Wreck and Chlorine Spill in Graniteville, South Carolina: Transportation Effects and Lessons in Small-Town Capacity for No-Notice Evacuation. *Transportation Research Record* 2007; 2009(1): 130–135.

25. Wenck MA, Van Sickle D, Drociuk D, et al. Rapid assessment of exposure to chlorine released from a train derailment and resulting health impact. *Public Health Reports* 2007; 122(6): 784.

26. Henry C, Belflower A, Drociuk D et al. Public health consequences from hazardous substances acutely released during rail transit–South Carolina, 2005; selected States, 1999–2004. *MMWR* 2005; 54(3): 64–67.

27. United Nations Division for Sustainable Development. Agenda 21. 1992. http://sustainabledevelopment.un.org/content/documents/Agenda21.pdf (Accessed March 21, 2013).

28. United Nations Conference on Sustainable Development. The Future We Want. http://www.uncsd2012.org/thefuturewewant.html (Accessed on March 21, 2013).

29. Strategic Approach to International Chemicals Management (SAICM). International Conference on Chemicals Management on the work of its first session (SAICM/ICCM.1/7), annexes I–III. http://www.chem.unep.ch/ICCM/ICCM.htm (Accessed March 21, 2013).

30. Clifton JC. Mercury exposure and public health. *Pediatric Clinics of North America* 2007; 54(2): 237.e1–237.e45.

31. Ministry of the Environment, Government of Japan. Minamata Disease – The History and Measures. http://www.env.go.jp/en/chemi/hs/minamata2002/ch2.html (Accessed March 21, 2013).

32. Secretariat of the Basel Convention. Basel Convention. www.basel.int (Accessed April 16, 2013).

33. Elliott MR, Wang Y, Lowe RA, Kleindorfer PR. Environmental justice: frequency and severity of US chemical industry accidents and the socioeconomic status of surrounding communities. *Journal of Epidemiology and Community Health* 2004; 58(1): 24–30.

34. U.S. Environmental Protection Agency. Environment Justice. http://www.epa.gov/environmentaljustice (Accessed March 21, 2013).

35. Environmental Protection Agency. Summary of the Emergency Planning and Community Right-to-Know Act (EPCRA). http://www.epa.gov/lawsregs/laws/epcra.html (Accessed March 21, 2013).

36. Levitin HW, Siegelson HJ. Hazardous materials emergencies. In: Hogan DE, Burstein JL, eds. *Disaster Medicine.* 2nd ed. Philadelphia, PA, Lippincott Williams & Wilkins, 2007; 311–325.

37. Chemical Abstracts Service. http://www.cas.org (Accessed September 7, 2015).

38. Walter FG. Hazmat incident response. In: Flomenbaum NE, Goldfrank LR, Hoffman RS, et al., eds. *Goldfrank's Toxicologic Emergencies.* 8th ed. New York, McGraw-Hill, 2006.

39. UNECE. Globally Harmonized System of Classification and Labelling of Chemicals. http://www.unece.org/trans/danger/publi/ghs/ghs_welcome_e.html (Accessed March 27, 2013).

40. UNECE. Globally Harmonized System of Classification and Labelling of Chemicals. 4th revised ed. http://www.unece.org/trans/danger/publi/ghs/ghs_rev04/04files_e.html (Accessed March 27, 2013).

41. National Institute for Occupational Safety and Health (NIOSH). International Chemical Safety Cards (ICSCs): International Programme on Chemical Safety. http://www.cdc.gov/NIOSH/ipcs/icstart.html (Accessed March 27, 2013).

42. OECD. OECD Guiding Principles for Chemical Accident Prevention, Preparedness and Response 2003. http://www.oecd.org/chemicalsafety/risk-management/chemicalaccidents.htm (Accessed March 27, 2013).

43. UNECE. UN Recommendations on the Transport of Dangerous Goods – Model Regulations: 17th revised ed. http://www.unece.org/trans/danger/publi/unrec/rev17/17files_e.html (Accessed March 27, 2013).

44. European Chemical Industry Council (CEFIC). http://www.cefic.be (Accessed March 27, 2013).

45. National Chemical Emergency Centre (NCEC). Hazchem guide. http://the-ncec.com/hazchem (Accessed March 27, 2013).

46. U.S. Department of Transportation (DOT) Pipeline and Hazardous Materials Safety Administration (PHMSA). Emergency Response Guidebook – ERG 2012. http://phmsa.dot.gov/hazmat/library/erg (Accessed March 27, 2013).

47. National Fire Protection Association. NFPA 704, Standard System for the Identification of the Hazards of Materials for Emergency Response. 2012 ed.

48. Environment Directorate, OECD. Guidance concerning health aspects of chemical accidents. 1996. http://www.oecd.org/officialdocuments/publicdisplaydocumentpdf/?cote=OCDE/GD(96)104&docLanguage=En (Accessed September 7, 2015).

49. Garatwa W, Bollin C. Disaster Risk Management – Working Concept. http://www.giz.de/en/html/index.html (Accessed September 7, 2015).

50. Crawford IWF, Mackway-Jones K, Russell DR, Carley SD. Planning for chemical incidents by implementing a Delphi based consensus study. *Emergency Medicine Journal* 2004; 21(1): 20–23.

51. OSHA. Toxic Industrial Chemicals (TICs). http://www.osha.gov/SLTC/emergencypreparedness/guides/chemical.html (Accessed March 21, 2013).

52. Molino LN, Sr. EMS beyond the barricade. In: Ciottone GR, Anderson PD, Auf Der Heide E, et al., eds. *Disaster Medicine.* 3rd ed. Philadelphia, Mosby Elsevier, 2006; 278–282.

53. International Council of Chemical Associations. Responsible Care. http://www.icca-chem.org/en/Home/Responsible-care (Accessed March 21, 2013).

54. International Council of Chemical Associations. Global Product Strategy. http://www.icca-chem.org/Home/ICCA-initiatives/Global-product-strategy (Accessed March 21, 2013).

55. EPA. Emergency Management – Risk Management Plan (RMP) Rule. http://www.epa.gov/emergencies/content/rmp/index.htm (Accessed March 21, 2013).

56. European Commission. Chemical Accidents (Seveso III) – Prevention, Preparedness and Response. http://ec.europa.eu/environment/seveso/index.htm (Accessed March 21, 2013).

57. Gougelet RM. Disaster mitigation. In: Ciottone GR, Anderson PD, Auf der Heide E, et al., eds. *Disaster Medicine.* 3rd ed. Philadelphia, Mosby Elsevier, 2006; 139–144.

58. Scenarios of sustainable hazards mitigation. In: Mileti DS, ed. *Disasters by Design.* Washington, DC, Joseph Henry Press, 1999; 41–64.

59. Department of Energy. Protective Action Criteria (PAC). http://www.atlintl.com/DOE/teels/teel/teeldef.html (Accessed June 19, 2013).

60. National Oceanic and Atmospheric Administration. ALOHA. Http://response.restoration.noaa.gov/oil-and-chemical-spills/chemical-spills/response-tools/aloha.html (Accessed April 30, 2013).

61. Barbisch DFKKL. Understanding surge capacity: essential elements. *Acad Emerg Med* 2006; 13(11): 1098–1102.

62. Keim MEPN, Twum-Danso NA. Lack of hospital preparedness for chemical terrorism in a major US city: 1996–2000. *Prehosp Disaster Med* 2003; 18(3): 193–199.

63. OSHA. http://www.osha.gov (Accessed June 19, 2013).

64. Centers for Medicare and Medicaid Services. EMTALA overview. http://www.cms.hhs.gov/emtala (Accessed February 5, 2013).

65. EPA. Emergency Planning and Community Right-to-Know Act (EPCRA) requirements. http://www.epa.gov/oem/content/epcra/index.htm (Accessed April 1, 2013).

66. The Joint Commission. http://www.jointcommission.org (Accessed February 5, 2013).

67. EPA. Emergency Planning and Community Right-to-Know Act (EPCRA) Local Emergency Planning Requirements. http://www.epa.gov/osweroe1/content/epcra/epcra_plan.htm#plan (Accessed April 1, 2013).

68. Tur-Kaspa ILEI, Hendler I, Siebner R, et al. Preparing hospitals for toxicological mass casualties events. *Crit Care Med* 1999; 27(5): 1004–1008.

69. Northington WEMGM, Hahn ME, Suyama J, Hostler D. Training retention of Level C personal protective equipment use by emergency medical services personnel. *Acad Emerg Med* 2007; 14(10): 846–849.

70. Chan JTYRS, Tang SY. Hospital preparedness for chemical and biological incidents in Hong Kong. *Hong Kong Med J* 2002; 8(6): 440–446.

71. Han KHWR, Kuhri M. An integrated response to chemical incidents–the UK perspective. *Resuscitation* 1999; 42(2): 133–140.

72. Milsten A. Hospital responses to acute-onset disasters: a review. *Prehosp Disaster Med* 2000; 15(1): 32–45.

73. Schwenk MKS, Jaroni H. Toxicological aspects of preparedness and aftercare for chemical-incidents. *Toxicology* 2005; 214(3): 232–248.

74. Barelli ABI, Soave M, Tafani C, Bononi F. The comprehensive medical preparedness in chemical emergencies: 'the chain of chemical survival.' *Eur J Emerg Med* 2008; 15(2): 110–118.

75. Henretig FMCTJ, Eitzen EM, Jr. Biological and chemical terrorism. *J Pediatr* 2002; 141(3): 311–326.

76. Sharp TWBRJ, Keim M, Williams RJ, et al. Medical preparedness for a terrorist incident involving chemical or biological agents during the 1996 Atlanta Olympic Games. *Ann Emerg Med* 1998; 32(2): 214–223.

77. Kreutzer KA. Three-point Hazmat size-up. *Fire Engineering* November 2007: 119–124.

78. Decontamination. In: Briggs SM, Brinsfield KH, eds. *Advanced Disaster Medical Response – Manual for Providers.* Cambridge, MA, Harvard Medical International, Inc., 2003; 35–38.

79. Kenar L, Karayilanoglu T. Prehospital management and medical intervention after a chemical attack. *Emerg Med J* 2004; 21(1): 84–88.

80. United States Department of Labor: Evacuation plans and procedures. http://www.osha.gov/SLTC/etools/evacuation/shelterinplace.html (Accessed April 1, 2013).

81. Byers M, Russell M, Lockey DJ. Clinical care in the "Hot Zone." *Emerg Med J* 2008; 25(2): 108–112.

82. Moles TM, Baker DJ. Clinical analogies for the management of toxic trauma. *Resuscitation* 1999; 42(2): 117–124.

83. Baker D. Medical management of HAZMAT victims in civilian practice. *Current Anesthesia & Critical Care* 1998; 9(2): 52–57.

84. Markel G, Krivoy A, Rotman E, et al. Medical management of toxicological mass casualty events. *Israel Medical Association Journal* 2008; 10(11): 761–766.

85. Garner A, Lee A, Harrison K, Schultz CH. Comparative analysis of multiple-casualty incident triage algorithms. *Ann Emerg Med* 2001; 38(5): 541–548.

86. Hodgetts TJ, Mackway-Jones K. *Major Incident Medical Management and Support: The Practical Approach.* London, BMJ Publishing, 1995.

87. Cone DC, Koenig KL. Mass casualty triage in the chemical, biological, radiological, or nuclear environment. *European Journal of Emergency Medicine* 2005; 12(6): 287.

88. Brennan RJ, Waeckerle JF, Sharp TW, Lillibridge SR. Chemical warfare agents: emergency medical and emergency public health issues. *Ann Emerg Med* 1999; 34(2): 191–204.

89. Holstege CP, Kirk M, Sidell FR. Chemical warfare: nerve agent poisoning. *Critical Care Clinics* 1997; 13(4): 923–942.

90. Nozaki H, Hori S, Shinozawa Y et al. Secondary exposure of medical staff to sarin vapor in the emergency room. *Intensive Care Medicine* 1995; 21(12): 1032–1035.

91. Horton DK, Berkowitz Z, Kaye WE. Secondary contamination of ED personnel from hazardous materials events, 1995–2001. *Am J Emerg Med* 2003; 21(3): 199–204.

92. OSHA. Best practices for hospital-based first receivers of victims from mass casualty incidents involving the release of hazardous substances. 2005. http://www.osha.gov/dts/osta/bestpractices/html/hospital_firstreceivers.html (Accessed June 19, 2013).

93. Geller RJ, Singleton KL, Tarantino ML, et al. Nosocomial poisoning associated with emergency department treatment of organophosphate toxicity-Georgia, 2000. *Clinical Toxicology* 2001; 39(1): 109–111.

94. Leikin JB, Thomas RG, Walter FG, et al. A review of nerve agent exposure for the critical care physician. *Critical Care Medicine* 2002; 30(10): 2346–2354.

95. Advanced Hazmat Life Support. 3rd ed. Tucson, American Academy of Clinical Toxicology and University of Arizona Emergency Research Center, 2003.

96. Agency for Toxic Substances and Disease Registry – ATSDR. Medical Management Guidelines for Phosgene. http://www.atsdr.cdc.gov/mmg/mmg.asp?id=1201&tid=182 (Accessed June 19, 2013).

97. Hazardous Materials Cooperative Research Program. Current Hazardous Materials Transportation Research and Future Needs. April 2012. http://onlinepubs.trb.org/onlinepubs/hmcrp/hmcrp_w001.pdf (Accessed June 19, 2013).

98. National Toxic Substance Incidents Program(NTSIP). http://www.atsdr.cdc.gov/ntsip (Accessed June 19, 2013).

99. UNECE. Convention on the trans-boundary effects of industrial accidents 1992. http://www.unece.org/env/teia/welcome.htm (Accessed June 19, 2013).

SECTION IIIB: Environmental Events

35

FLOODS

Mark E. Keim

Water, water everywhere, and all the boards did shrink;
Water, water everywhere, nor any drop to drink.
Samuel Coleridge, "Rime of the Ancient Mariner"

OVERVIEW

Definition and Classification

The United Nations (UN) defines floods as a "significant rise of water level in a stream, lake, reservoir or a coastal region."[1] Gunn defines floods more specifically as "the overflow of areas that are not normally submerged with water or a stream that has broken its normal confines or has accumulated due to lack of drainage."[2]

Engineers studying past floods use statistics to estimate the chance that floods of various sizes will occur. For example, a flood found to occur on the average of 10 times in 100 years would be called the 10% chance flood or the 10-year flood. A flood that only occurs on the average of once every hundred years would have a 1% chance of occurring in any particular year and would be called the 100-year flood or 1% chance flood.[3]

Floods are classified according to cause (e.g., high rainfall, tidal extremes, structural failure) and nature (e.g., regularity, speed of onset, velocity and depth of water, spatial and temporal scale). This chapter will discuss impacts according to health outcomes. The influence of flood characteristics on health impacts is discussed where appropriate.

Causes of Floods

Floods may be caused by natural processes that are either fluvial (an abundance of rainfall, melting snow) or coastal (a hurricane-related storm surge, coastal inundations, or seismically-induced tsunami) in origin.

Human alterations in the environment may also cause flooding by changes in watershed due to deforestation; overgrazing; the failure of dams, embankments, and levees;[4] channeling of streams, and urbanization of wetlands (which act as a natural flood control by storing water during heavy rains, slowing runoff into streams and reducing flood peaks). Human modifications to the environment affecting global climate change

are also predicted to increase the frequency of flooding hazards worldwide.[5]

Human behaviors can exacerbate flooding severity and impact. Even after prior events, human settlement frequently occurs in flood-prone areas, thereby increasing a community's vulnerability to the effects of flooding. Lack of awareness of the dangers posed by fast-moving floodwaters has led to maladaptive behaviors by people encountering floodwaters. Paradoxically, engineering flood controls such as levee and dam construction may contribute to greater human losses and physical damages after a flood disaster (e.g., levee failure).[6]

Nature of Floods

Fluvial Floods

For the purpose of this discussion, fluvial (or riverine) flooding will be characterized as either a seasonal flood or a flash flood.

Seasonal floods are typified by a gradual rise to flood stage that may extend across large areas over a long duration. Because seasonal floods are usually caused by a relatively gradual accumulation, warning times are generally sufficient to allow safe evacuation of nearby communities. However, seasonal floods also have the propensity to create large and expansive areas of inundation. Two river systems in China (the Yangtze and Huang He) have been associated with seasonal flooding, representing the most catastrophic floods in world history. The Huang He is particularly prone to flooding, having overrun its banks nearly 1,600 times in the past 4,000 years. This is largely due to its course through the flat and densely populated North China plain. The deadliest disaster on record was the 1931 Huang He flood that killed an estimated 3.7 million people.[7]

Flash floods are characterized by a short duration and high volume stream flow, and usually occur within 6 hours of a rain event, after a dam or levy fails, or after the sudden release of water from an ice or debris jam. Once the flash flood has occurred, it is often accompanied by an extremely short warning and response time with potential for great loss of life.[8] The Johnstown, Pennsylvania, flood of 1889 is one example of the capacity for destruction and extreme danger associated with flash floods (as well as the human element of non-sustainable development as a cause of flooding). In the mountains above Johnstown, an old earth dam had been hastily rebuilt to create a lake for an exclusive summer resort patronized by the tycoons of that same industrial prosperity, among them Andrew Carnegie, Henry Clay Frick, and Andrew Mellon.[9]

After torrential rains, a 22-meter high dam located 22.5 km away and 137 meters in elevation above Jamestown collapsed, releasing some 20 million tons of water toward the city. The 18.3-meter high wall of water crashed through 10.36 square kilometers of Johnstown without warning, splintering trees, shattering houses, and killing 2,209 people within 10 minutes. All members of ninety-nine families died, and ninety-eight children were orphaned. It was the first major disaster relief effort managed by the newly formed American Red Cross.[10]

Coastal Floods

Storm surge, produced by the high winds and vacuum effect of low-pressure cyclonic storm systems, can produce dramatically high seas that result in coastal flooding. Storm surge-related drownings account for 90% of worldwide deaths related to cyclonic storms.[4] The 1970 Bhola cyclone that struck East Pakistan (now Bangladesh) is one of the most extreme examples in modern times of mass fatalities caused by drowning due to storm surge. Up to 500,000 people lost their lives in this category 3 tropical cyclone, primarily as a result of the storm surge that flooded much of the low-lying islands of the Ganges Delta.[11–12]

The 1900 Galveston hurricane is one of the deadliest disasters in U.S. history. Coastal flooding caused by the storm surge associated with this category 4 hurricane left over 12,000 dead and 8,000 people homeless, among an original population of only 35,000.[13] Coastal inundations may also occur due to rogue surface waves and cyclonic eddies imparted by weather systems. Seismic events such as earthquakes, landslides, and volcanic eruptions can generate a tsunami pressure wave at sea. Once the tsunami is generated, a series of extremely low frequency, long wavelength ($\sim$300 km) waves are propagated in an expanding radius from the area of displacement. These waves differ importantly from short wavelength surface waves (those caused by wind) or storm surges (those caused by cyclones), in that tsunami waves are propagated throughout the entire depth of the ocean. For this reason, tsunamis represent a tremendous amount of potential energy and can travel at the speed of a jet airliner. As the tsunami enters shallow water near coastlines, the enormous kinetic energy previously spread throughout the large volume of deep ocean water becomes concentrated to a much smaller volume of water, resulting in a tremendous destructive potential as it inundates the land.[14] This remarkable difference in potential energy imparted over a very large distance by a tsunami as compared to other types of floods, is unique in character and public health impact. This discussion will therefore focus on floods other than tsunamis, which are the focus of Chapter 39.

Scope of the Problem

Flooding is the most common type of disaster worldwide, accounting for 49% of all disasters from 1900 to 2013.[15] According to the UN, disasters have affected 2.9 billion people, with over 1.2 million killed from 2001 to 2013.[16] During this same time, floods accounted for 5% of all disaster-related deaths worldwide. In comparison, 6% were caused by epidemics of infectious disease (including HIV and influenza).[15]

From 1900 to 2011, hydrometeorological disasters killed over 19 million people and affected nearly 3.2 billion people world-

Table 35.1. The world's ten deadliest hydrometeorological disasters, 1900–2013, ranked according to number of people killed per nation[15]

Hazard	Country	Year	Number killed (in millions)
Flood	China	1931	3.7
Drought	China	1928	3.0
Flood	China	1959	2.0
Drought	Bangladesh	1943	1.9
Drought	India	1942	1.5
Drought	India	1965	1.5
Drought	India	1900	1.25
Drought	Soviet Union	1921	1.2
Drought	China	1920	0.5
Flood	China	1939	0.5

wide.[15] In particular, meteorological hazards affect a growing number of people and cause increasingly large economic losses, likely related to climate change and increasing vulnerability of the populations affected.[5,15,17] Over the past century, the incidence of extreme weather (hydrometeorological) disasters has increased much more rapidly than that for geological or biological events (Figure 35.1).[15] Floods comprised nearly 34.6% of these disaster-related deaths.

In 2007, the Intergovernmental Panel on Climate Change (IPCC) Fourth Assessment Report (AR4) concluded that these same climate-caused hazards will continue to rise in frequency and severity well into the future.[5]

Floods constituted three of the world's ten deadliest hydrometeorological disasters from 1900–2013, ranked according to number of people killed per nation.[15] Table 35.1 shows the major hydrometeorological disasters that occurred from 1900–2013 and the number of fatalities associated with each event. All of these disasters occurred in developing nations, and all were caused by either floods or droughts.

During 1900–2013, floods also affected the highest percentage of people (43.56%) worldwide among all hydrometeorological disasters (Figure 35.2).[15]

During the past three decades from 1980 to 2011, there have been 7,009 climate-related disaster declarations worldwide, averaging 226 per year (Figure 35.3).[16] Floods have comprised 3,455 (49%) of these disasters.

According to the U.S. National Oceanographic and Atmospheric Administration (NOAA), "In most years, flooding causes more deaths and damage than any other hydrometeorological phenomena. In many years it is common for three-quarters of all federally-declared disasters to be due, at least in part, to flooding."[18]

Parts or all of over 20,000 communities in the United States are subject to a substantial flooding risk. Approximately 7% of the nation's land area, an area almost as big as the state of Texas, is subject to severe flooding.[19] In the United States, floods cause as much as 90% of the damage from disasters (excluding droughts).[20]

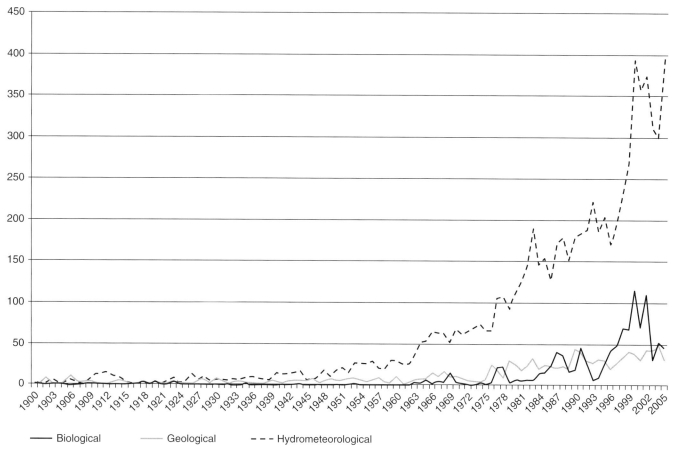

Figure 35.1. Disaster incidence by hazard category, 1900–2005. Adapted from Center for Research on the Epidemiology of Disasters.

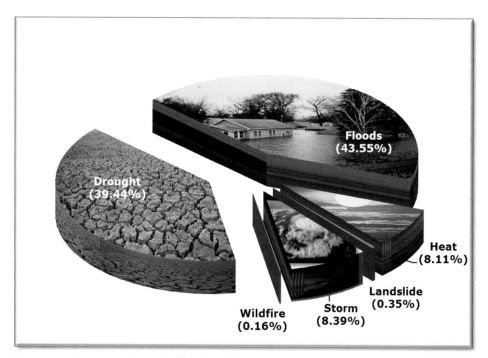

Figure 35.2. Percentage of people affected worldwide according to each category of hydrometeorological hazard, 1900–2013. *Source:* Adapted from EM-DAT: The OFDA/CRED International Database, Belgium 2013.

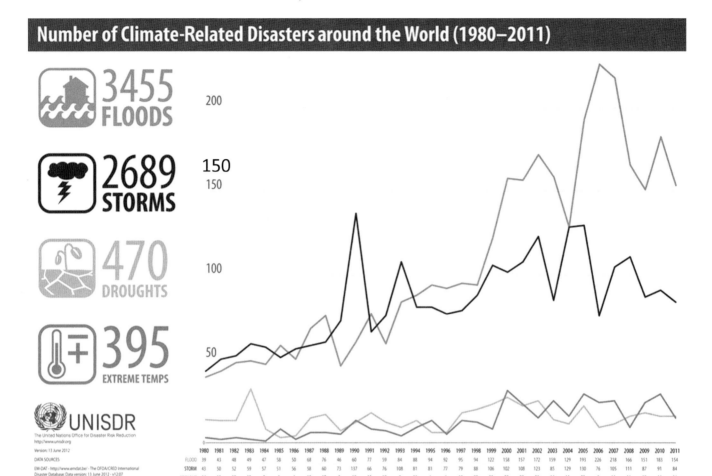

Number of Climate-Related Disasters around the World (1980–2011)

Figure 35.3. Number of climate-related disasters around the world, 1980–2011. *Source:* UN International Strategy for Disaster Reduction, 2013.

Direct economic losses from the 1993 Great Midwestern U.S. floods surpassed $10 billion USD.[21] Estimated flood damage as a result of the 1998 floods in central Texas was approximated at $900 million USD, including damage to 12,000 homes, 700 businesses, and to public property.[22] In the late summer of 2005, flooding after Hurricane Katrina caused more than $200 billion USD in losses, constituting the costliest disaster in U.S. history to that date.[19] Flood-related losses associated with Hurricane Sandy in 2012 are estimated at $25 billion USD.[23] Trends toward increasing population density near coasts and in floodplains suggest a higher probability of future catastrophic flood disasters. The current trend of climate change is projected to have an impact on the frequency and severity of floods worldwide.[5,24] Munich Re, a re-insurance company and member of the UN Environment Programme's (UNEP) Finance Initiative, has been compiling annual records since the 1970s on the cost of disasters. In 2002, Munich Re reported that rain intensities reached unique values worldwide. The report estimated that during 2002, floods caused 42% of worldwide fatalities, 66% of the economic losses, and 64% of insured losses.[24]

Floods are also notable in their capacity to affect extremely large groups of people. The largest single flood during the past century is estimated to have impacted nearly 239 million people.[15] Table 35.2 lists the world's ten largest floods from 1900–2013, ranked according to number of people affected.[15]

Table 35.2. The world's ten largest floods (1900–2013) ranked according to number of people affected[15]

Country	Year	Number affected
China	1998	238,973,000
China	1991	210,232,227
China	1996	154,634,000
China	2003	150,146,000
China	2010	134,000,000
India	1993	128,000,000
China	1995	114,470,249
China	2007	105,004,000
China	1999	101,024,000
China	1989	100,010,000

Public Health Impacts of Flood Disasters

Public health impacts of flooding include damage to homes and consequent displacement of occupants, infectious disease exacerbated by crowded living conditions and compromised personal

Table 35.3. Relative degree of expected public health impact after a flood

Impact	Degree
Drowning mortality	High income nations – Few
	Low income nations – Can exceed 100,000/event
Epidemics	Can occur in low-income nations
Need for trauma care	Rare
Loss of clean water	Can be widespread
Loss of shelter	Can be widespread
Loss of personal and household goods	Can be widespread
Permanent population migration	Rare
Loss of routine hygiene	Can be widespread
Loss of sanitation	Can be widespread
Disruption of solid waste management	Can be widespread
Public concern for safety	High
Increased pests and vectors	Can be widespread
Loss and/or damage of healthcare system	Can be widespread
Worsening of existing chronic illnesses	Can be widespread
Toxic exposures	Possible
Food insecurity	Can occur in low-income nations and remote islands

hygiene, contamination of water sources, disruption of sewage service and solid waste collection, increased vector populations, injuries sustained during clean-up, stress-related mental health and illicit substance use, and death (Table 35.3).[25]

Loss of Safe Water and Adequate Sanitation

During the 1993 Great Midwestern U.S. floods, 9% of the population in the state of Iowa suffered a complete loss of the public water system. Twenty-nine counties in Iowa (representing 37% of the population) reported flood damage to water systems, and thirty-one counties (with 35% of the population) reported flood damage to sewer systems.[26]

Food Insecurity: Crop Losses and Disruption of Food Distribution

Generalized food shortages severe enough to cause nutritional problems usually do not occur after disasters, but may arise among low-income nations in two ways. Food stock destruction within the disaster area may reduce the absolute amount of food available, or disruption of distribution systems may curtail access to food, even if there is no absolute shortage. For example, food security has become a major issue in Southeast Asia, as it has been difficult to deliver food supplies to flood-affected areas.[27] In addition, severe damage to agricultural land and livestock affects those who rely on these forms of food production, with

main food crops severely damaged, along with losses in livestock and poultry.[28] This puts many people out of work, placing a financial strain on the economy and on many businesses and families.[27]

Flooding and sea surges can damage household food stocks and crops, disrupt distribution, and cause major local shortages. Food distribution, at least in the short term, is often a major and urgent need, but large-scale importation/donation of food is usually unnecessary.[29] One notable exception occurs when remote low-lying islands are flooded by seawater to an extent that island aquifer becomes brackish and agricultural land becomes salt-contaminated so that it can no longer support gardens for the next several years. Such an inundation event occurred in the U.S.-associated Pacific island nation of the Federated States of Micronesia during March 2007 and resulted in a loss of food security sufficient enough to warrant a federal disaster declaration.[30,31]

Loss of Shelter and Population Displacement

Floods displace literally millions of people. Displacement is a key risk factor for morbidity and mortality among disaster-affected populations. It creates additional risk for vulnerable populations (see Chapter 10).

The disruption caused by this displacement and the new focus on uncertainties of recovery rather than their previous normal daily routines are a source of high stress. The psychological stress that people suffer after a flood is related to not only reconstruction of their home but also "everything it stood for" in terms of memories and sentiment.[32–34] Flood survivors personally identify with damage and destruction of their homes and personal possessions. Many claim their most devastating losses are the personal possessions that "cannot be replaced."[32]

Misdirected or misguided settlement solutions may increase and prolong the risk of morbidity and mortality among displaced populations by providing shelter below internationally accepted standards for space, nutrition, food, clean water, safety and security, sanitation, hygiene, and access to medical care.[35]

Individual household shelter solutions can be short or long term and subject to the level of assistance provided, land-use rights or ownership, availability of essential services and social infrastructure, and opportunities for upgrading and expanding dwellings. Existing shelter and settlement solutions should be prioritized. If sustainable, involved populations should be allowed to return to the site of the original dwellings. Affected households who cannot return to the site of the original dwellings should be permitted to settle independently within a host community or with host families, whenever possible. Temporary camps and mass shelters should only be used as a last resort, that is, for persons who cannot return to flood-affected areas and cannot settle independently within a host community. Research shows that providing increased social support can significantly lower illness burdens after disasters.[35]

Toxic Chemical Exposures

The mobilization of chemicals either from storage (e.g., underground fuel tanks, pipelines, hazardous landfill sites, and wastewater lagoons) or by remobilization of chemicals already in the environment (e.g., pesticides, dioxin in river/canal sentiment, runoff from roads and bridges, overloaded sewers, and acid mine drainage) has occurred during floods.[36] These chemical hazards are more likely to materialize when industrial and agricultural areas are submerged underwater.[4] One 2004 review identified epidemiological evidence for flood-related adverse health effects following chemical exposures to carbon monoxide, pesticides, agricultural chemicals, dioxin, volatile organic carbons, heavy metals, cyanide, acid waste water, sulfides, and cadmium.[36]

According to local fire department records, 1,200 homes in Grand Forks, North Dakota, affected by the 1997 Red River flood reported problems with fuel oil spills ranging from 190 to 985 liters. Experts from the U.S. Environmental Protection Agency (EPA) conducted a study of thirty-four homes approximately 1 year after the flood occurred. Six homes (17.6%) still had measurable hydrocarbon vapors that were considered a serious health threat. The homeowners were advised to move or undergo major structural work to replace contaminated structures.[37]

Toxic Mold Exposures

In 2004, the U.S. Institute of Medicine (IOM) published a review of the literature regarding health outcomes related to damp indoor spaces. The findings of this report indicate that indoor environmental conditions and personal practices provide mold exposures that may expose residents and remediation workers to risk of negative health effects.[38]

Molds were identified as a potential public health concern arising from the 1993 Midwestern floods.[4] Visible mold growth was found in 46% of homes inspected after flooding caused by Hurricane Katrina.[38] Aspergillus and Penicillum species were the predominant fungi identified, both indoors and outdoors. Although interpreting the significance of measures of airborne mold toxins is complex, indoor air levels were markedly elevated and usual indoor/outdoor ratios for mold were reversed, that is, indoor levels of mold toxin were higher than outdoor.[38,39]

Among the residents interviewed, two-thirds quickly identified particulate respirators as appropriate and necessary respiratory protection for cleaning of mold. Of those who had cleaned up mold, two-thirds did not always use appropriate respirators. Among persons who self-identified as remediation workers, 95% thought mold causes illness and 85% correctly identified particulate filter respirators as the appropriate protection for cleaning up mold. However, 49% of remediation workers had not been fit-tested for respirators and 35% of the same group reported that they did not always use respirators.[38] These findings suggest that a significant proportion of disaster-affected residents and remediation workers may be exposed to potentially hazardous levels of mold. Reasons for this include a lack of understanding of the need for or lack of access to personal protection, or a lack of compliance despite recognition of the need for and availability of protection.[38]

Disruption of Healthcare Services

Flooding may directly damage healthcare entities or it may hinder public access to these facilities by disrupting transportation routes. During the Great Midwestern U.S. floods, five of the ninety-nine counties representing 14% of Iowa's population reported closures of primary care physician offices.[26] In 2008, months of heavy rainfall and rampant flooding in Mozambique, Zambia, Zimbabwe, and Malawi reportedly restricted access to healthcare facilities among patients as well as drug and supply distributors over a very large area of southern Africa.[40]

Floods have a substantial impact on the operation of most emergency medical services systems. The primary effect often results from disruption of usual transport routes due to water. Data concerning air transport in flooding collected during Hurricane Floyd in the United States demonstrated a nearly 650%

increase in helicopter utilization for emergency medical services transports in the affected areas.[6] In most flood-related disasters in the United States approximately 0.02–2% of flood survivors require emergency medical attention.[41]

The Great Midwestern U.S. floods presented multiple challenges to the six metropolitan medical centers in Des Moines, Iowa, when these hospitals lost all public utilities. Healthcare leaders cancelled elective admissions and diverted non-emergency clinical services to alternate facilities. They identified and implemented ancillary resources in order to maintain essential operations. Hospital managers initiated non-routine methods for infection control, sterilization, housekeeping, and food preparation. Planners implemented extraordinary measures in order to maintain adequate amounts of water for laundry, fire protection, cooling, instrument sterilization, renal dialysis, physical therapy, and dietary services.[42]

Disruption of Public Services

During the Great Midwestern U.S. floods, eight counties in Iowa (24% of the state population) reported interruption in public health services (e.g., supplemental food programs and various clinics like those for vaccinations and for treatment of sexually transmitted infections). Ten counties (15% of the population) reported at least one non-operational public sewer system.[26]

Power outages are a common impact of flood disasters. Power outages not related to flooding have been associated with outbreaks of diarrheal illness.[43] The disruption of public access to refrigeration may impact food and also drug safety. For example, life-sustaining medications such as insulin require properly controlled refrigeration in order to remain efficacious.

In addition to flood water disruption of solid waste management services, floods may also generate a large amount of additional solid waste. The degree of extra sold waste generation is proportional to population density and extent of area flooded.[44]

FLOOD MYTHS

Misconceptions regarding the need for large-scale public health interventions related to communicable disease prevention and control are common after flood disasters. Even after learning that there is little scientific basis for implementing such programs, public officials are often tempted to carry through with such plans, sometimes rationalizing that "at least we feel like we're doing something." However, implementing these programs at the time of disasters is often counterproductive and diverts limited personnel and resources from other relief tasks.[6] In addition, these interventions are not without health risk. Officials should therefore carefully weigh the risk versus limited proven benefit (Box 35.1).

Flood-Related Morbidity and Mortality

Flood-Related Mortality

Drowning is the main cause of deaths due to floods. From 1900 to 2011, extreme weather disasters killed over 19 million people and affected nearly 3.2 billion people worldwide.[15] Floods comprised nearly 34.6% of these disaster-related deaths.[15] Floods portended the second highest mortality rate among the top ten disasters for each category of extreme weather hazard worldwide from 1900–2013 (Figure 35.4).[15]

Floods constituted three of the world's ten deadliest hydrometeorological disasters (1900–2013), ranked according to number

Box 35.1. Flood Myths

Mass Vaccination in Absence of an Outbreak

There is often a public demand for typhoid vaccine and tetanus toxoid after floods despite the fact that no epidemics of typhoid or tetanus have occurred after floods in the United States. In some cases, misinformed officials make recommendations for a "flood shot." These recommendations have included immunizations for hepatitis, typhoid, and tetanus.

Mass tetanus vaccination programs are not indicated. Management of flood-associated wounds should include appropriate evaluation of tetanus immunity (and vaccination if clinically indicated) just the same as at any other time.[6]

Some response agencies have recommended typhoid and hepatitis immunization for individuals about to deploy to a flood disaster. This occurs despite the fact that it takes several weeks for antibody to typhoid to develop, and even then vaccination provides only moderate protection.[6] Hepatitis immunization requires a series of vaccinations that are months apart. Thus, in both cases, immunization can create a false sense of security and may contribute to neglect of basic hygiene.

Large-Scale Mosquito Control in Absence of an Outbreak

The public and well-intentioned public officials often expect to implement large-scale mosquito adulticide in the midst of a flood disaster, despite the presumed low risk for mosquito-borne arboviral disease after flood-related disasters in high-income countries.[61] Besides unnecessarily diverting human, fiscal, and logistical resources, the action also increases the possibility of chemical exposures to workers and the public. Vector surveillance is adequate and should be used to guide any consideration of mosquito control.[61]

Fatality Management

The public is often concerned about the danger of disease transmission from decaying corpses. Responsible health authorities should be aware that health hazards such as epidemics associated with unburied bodies are minimal, particularly if death resulted from trauma or drowning (see Chapter 23). It is far more likely that survivors will be a source of disease outbreaks.[29] Mass graves are not necessary when considered solely to prevent the spread of disease caused by mass fatalities. For flood disasters, normal funeral ceremonies and practices should be respected and maintained whenever possible.

---

of people killed per nation (Table 35.2).[15] Seven of these floods occurred in China. All ten occurred in low-resource countries.[15]

Floods are the number one non-terrorist disaster in the United States in terms of lives lost and property damage.[45] Over a 25-year period prior to Hurricane Katrina, floods killed about 140 Americans and cost $6 billion USD in property damage each

year. In the United States, the most common cause of flood-related deaths is drowning.[19]

"The number of deaths associated with flooding is closely related to the life-threatening characteristics of the flood (rapidly rising water, deep flood waters, objects carried by the rapidly flowing water) and by the behavior of the victims."[46] The most

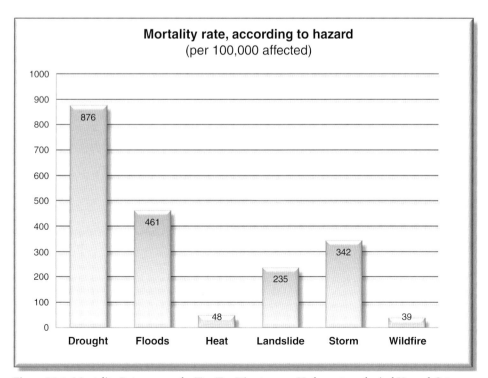

Figure 35.4. Mortality Rate among the Top Ten Disasters per Hydrometeorological Hazard Category, 1900–2013. *Source:* Adapted from EM-DAT: The OFDA/CRED International Database, Belgium, 2013.

readily identifiable flood deaths are those that occur acutely from drowning or trauma, such as can happen after being hit by objects in fast-flowing waters. The number of such deaths is determined by the characteristic of a flood, including its speed of onset, depth, and the extent of flooded area. Information on risk factors for flood-related death remains limited, but men appear more at risk than women. In high-income countries most deaths are due to drowning and, particularly in the United States, are vehicle related.[4,47] The most likely group to drown in their own homes are the elderly.[47]

Flash floods are the number one cause of flooding deaths.[4] Flash flooding is the leading cause of weather-related mortality in United States.[26] In general, higher mortality rates are observed in flash flood incidents, examples of which occurred in Puerto Rico in 1992, Missouri in 1993, Georgia in 1994, and Texas in 2001 when heavy water runoff inundated communities with great immediacy and intensity.[6,25,48] The majority of flood-related drownings occur when a vehicle is driven into hazardous flood waters.[4,22]

The power of water, especially moving water, is astounding. For example, "Two feet [0.6 meters] of water will carry away most automobiles. The lateral force of a foot [0.3 meters] of water moving at 10 mph [16 km/h] is about 500 pounds [227 kg] on the average car. And every foot [0.3 meters] of water displaces about 1,500 pounds [680] of car weight. So two feet of water moving at 10 mph [16 km/h] will float virtually every car."[49]

During the 1998 floods in central Texas, twenty-four of the twenty-nine deaths directly related to the storm were caused by drowning. Of those twenty-four drownings, twenty-two (92%) with known circumstances occurred because the vehicle was driven into high water. These deaths occurred in sixteen separate incidents, some with multiple deaths. Of the sixteen water-crossing incidents, eleven (69%) occurred at locations known to reporting authorities to have a history of flooding; ten (63%) involved trucks and/or sport-utility vehicles.[22]

Prior to the implementation of early warning, evacuation, and shelter systems, drowning from hurricane storm surge accounted for an estimated 90% of cyclone-attributable mortality in both high-income and low-income nations.[4] Approximately 8,000 people died from flooding in 1900 after a large hurricane struck Galveston, Texas. In 1928, 1,836 people died from another hurricane storm surge around Lake Okeechobee in Florida. Large storm surge associated with powerful hurricanes was believed to be the cause of most of these deaths.

Storm surge drowning deaths have markedly decreased in high-income nations due to improvements in population protection measures.[50] One notable exception is that more than 1,300 deaths were attributed to Hurricane Katrina, most of which occurred as a result of flash flooding caused by catastrophic levee failure, making 2005 the third deadliest year in U.S. history for flood deaths to that date.[51]

Flood-Related Morbidity

POVERTY AND FLOOD-RELATED MORBIDITY

Poverty is a key risk factor for human vulnerability to flood disasters. The correlation between poverty and morbidity is seen clearly during flood disasters. Low-income populations within a given society often dwell in locations at higher risk for flooding and have fewer resources available for response and recovery. Rarely, if at all, are any resources available to prepare for or mitigate flood disasters. High-income populations within a society possess a much higher level of resilience and availability of resources that can better afford more cost-effective risk reduction measures. Diseases normally endemic to a given population are typically exacerbated as a result flood disasters. As a result, low-income nations have a higher incidence of flood-related outbreaks of infectious disease, such as leptospirosis, typhoid, malaria, and cholera. High-income nations tend to suffer few flood-related outbreaks, but instead have a higher proportion of flood-related non-communicable diseases, such as injuries, mental illness, cardiovascular disease, and chronic obstructive pulmonary disease.

Causes of flood-related morbidity reported in high-income nations during the first 6 weeks after the disaster are frequently equally divided between injuries and illnesses. Injuries commonly include sprains/strains, lacerations, and abrasions. Many of these injuries occur later during the clean-up phase rather than immediately during the flooding. Communicable and non-communicable diseases cause similar numbers of flood-related illnesses in high-income nations.[26,50]

COMMUNICABLE DISEASES AND FLOOD-RELATED MORBIDITY

The relationship between disasters and communicable diseases is frequently misconstrued. The risk for epidemics is often presumed to be very high in the disaster aftermath. The risk for outbreaks after disasters is often greatly exaggerated by both health officials and the media.[29] The risk of infectious diseases after flood-related disasters is often specific to the event itself, and is dependent on a number of factors. The risk factors for outbreaks after disasters are primarily associated with displacement of highly vulnerable populations. They are related to the proximity of safe drinking water and functioning latrines, the nutritional status of the displaced population, the level of immunity to vaccine-preventable diseases, and the access to healthcare services.[29,43,52] Historically, large-scale, long-term displacement of populations as a result of flood disasters is uncommon. This likely contributes to the low overall risk for outbreaks.[54] In high-income countries with adequate public health infrastructures, post-impact surveillance has only occasionally detected increases in life-threatening infectious diseases after disasters, and these increases have been relatively small.[4,6,52] In comparison, in low-income nations, disaster recovery workers have reported larger outbreaks of endemic infectious diseases including cholera and typhoid, acute respiratory infections, and leptospirosis.[39] Despite frequent public concern to the contrary, non-endemic diseases do not spontaneously emerge after flood disasters. Floods exacerbate diseases that are endemic to the affected populations.

DIARRHEAL ILLNESS

Under flood conditions, there is potential for increased fecal-oral transmission of disease, especially in areas where the population does not have access to clean water and sanitation. Outbreaks of diarrhea occur in both high-income nations and low-income nations and are associated with locally endemic pathogens. The risk of diarrheal illness appears to be less for high-income countries, as compared to low-income countries. Diarrheal illness in high incomes countries most commonly manifests as a self-limiting gastroenteritis without a specifically identified pathogen. Flood-related outbreaks of life-threatening diarrheal diseases (such as paratyphoid and cholera) have been reported in very low-income nations.

Flood-Related Diarrheal Illness in High-Income Nations

In 1983, an outbreak of diarrheal illness was reported in Utah, possibly associated with contaminated water supply that resulted from flooding during the spring snow melt. Five routine bacteriologic samples from the source revealed coliform counts to be elevated above acceptable limits.[35] A similar period of heavy water runoff associated with unseasonably warm weather and ash fall from the Mount Saint Helens volcano eruption in 1980 was also linked to an outbreak of diarrhea due to *Giardia lamblia*.[53]

After flooding caused by Tropical Storm Allison in Houston, Texas, in June 2001, fifty-four (12.9%) surveyed households reported at least one person with illness that occurred after the onset of flooding. Persons living in flooded homes were significantly more likely than those living in non-flooded homes to report illness; the only specific illness significantly associated with residing in a flooded home was diarrhea/stomach conditions.[25] In 2002, in a village near Barcelona, Spain, an outbreak of shigellosis affected over 10% of the population. The outbreak was linked to consumption of drinking water that may have been contaminated after heavy rain caused floods.[54] After Hurricane Katrina in 2006, clusters of diarrheal disease were reported in evacuation centers in four U.S. states; gastroenteritis was the most common acute disease complaint among evacuees in Memphis, Tennessee.[39] Approximately 6,500 of an estimated 24,000 evacuees in Houston shelters visited Reliant Park medical clinic, and 1,169 (18%) persons reported symptoms of acute gastroenteritis. In stool samples from forty-four patients tested, norovirus was confirmed in twenty-two (50%) specimens; no other enteropathogen was identified.[55]

Two cases of toxigenic *Vibrio cholerae* O1 infection were reported in Louisiana after Hurricanes Katrina and Rita.[56-58] However, there was no epidemic and was no evidence to suggest that there was an increased risk of cholera among residents of the Gulf Coast after these hurricanes.[39]

Flood-Related Diarrheal Illness in Low-Income Nations

Surveillance data showed an apparent mortality increase from diarrhea during the 1988 floods in Khartoum, Sudan,[59] but a similar rise was also apparent in the same period of the preceding year.[60] Routine surveillance data and hospital admission records showed diarrhea to be the most frequent cause of death following severe flooding in 1988 in Bangladesh, but again, the effect of the flood was not separately quantified from seasonal influences.[49] Two devastating monsoon-related floods in Bangladesh in 2004 resulted in very large outbreaks of diarrheal disease reaching epidemic proportions throughout the capital city of Dhaka. Healthcare workers evaluated more than 17,000 patients in one hospital during one of these flood periods. Cholera was the most common cause of admission, and enterotoxigenic *E. coli* was also an important cause of acute watery diarrhea, particularly in children less than 2 years of age.[39] In a large study undertaken in Indonesia in 1992 and 1993, flooding was identified as a significant risk factor for diarrheal illnesses caused by paratyphoid fever.[43]

RESPIRATORY INFECTIONS

Whenever there is a lack of clean water among displaced populations, there is often a concomitant difficulty in maintaining adequate hygiene. This lack of hygiene can lead to not only diarrheal illness, but also acute respiratory infections. Reported incidence of acute respiratory infections increased fourfold in Nicaragua in the 30 days after Hurricane Mitch in 1998.[43]

Flooding may also result in episodes of near-drowning and pulmonary aspiration of floodwater. Direct inoculation of the pulmonary system with marine and soil debris may cause serious acute respiratory infections and systemic infections. Flood-related aspiration pneumonia is often polymicrobial.[39]

VECTOR-BORNE DISEASES

The relation between flooding and vector-borne disease is complex. The predicted impact of severe weather or floods on vector-borne illnesses is less certain than that of enteric infections. Severe weather can either increase or decrease the transmission of vector-borne illnesses.[39,49] Such variance probably mirrors the complexity of a given situation, and partly reflects the prevalence of vector-borne diseases in the region before the disaster. Additional factors include: 1) the identity and ecology of the local vectors (some vectors prefer clean water, others prefer organically rich water; some prefer fresh water, others prefer water containing low amounts of salt); and 2) the impact of control programs or other interventions that minimize vector–human contact (for example, the use of larvacidal or insecticidal agents, access of survivors to nets or window screens, and access of survivors to shelters versus sleeping outdoors).[39]

ARTHROPOD-BORNE DISEASES

Flood-Related Arthropod-Borne Disease in High-Income Nations

Floods are often followed by a proliferation of mosquitoes. In the United States, such disasters are rarely followed by outbreaks of arboviral disease, attributable mostly to the relatively low prevalence of vector-borne diseases in the region before the disaster.[39,61]

Heavy rains and flooding have been associated with outbreaks of St. Louis encephalitis in Florida, believed to be associated with the feeding activities of the responsible mosquito vector.[39] In comparison, despite the proliferation of large populations of mosquitoes known to amplify transmission of arboviruses that cause St. Louis encephalitis and Western equine encephalitis after the Great Midwestern U.S. floods, surveillance data indicated minimal risk for arboviral disease above background levels in the disaster area. During the floods, forty-five counties (53% of the population) in Iowa reported vector problems. Mosquito vectors were found to exist in extremely high levels. Serum conversions were not detected in sentinel chicken flocks, nor were there any human cases of illness reported as resulting from mosquito vectors.[26] As a consequence, contingency plans for large-scale mosquito adulticide were not implemented, resulting in an estimated cost saving of over $10 million USD. Despite the presumed low risk for mosquito-borne arboviral disease after flood-related disasters in high-income countries, surveillance programs are useful to assist with determining prevalence of large vector populations and preventing unnecessary expenditures associated with the application of insecticides implemented during prophylactic mosquito control.[61]

Flood-Related Arthropod-Borne Disease in Low-Income Nations

Malaria outbreaks in the wake of flooding have been reported in several very low-income nations with warm climates.[43] Increased numbers of cases of drug-resistant malaria were noted after floods in Sudan[62] and an outbreak of more than 75,000 cases of Plasmodium falciparum malaria occurred in Haiti after Hurricane Flora in 1963.[63] A four- to fivefold increase in malaria incidence also occurred after a flood disaster in 2000 in Mozambique.[61] However, after the 2004 Indian Ocean tsunami, no appreciable increase in the number of malaria cases was reported in Indonesia.[63]

Dengue transmission is influenced by meteorological conditions, however transmission has not been directly attributable to flooding. In Brazil, Indonesia, and Venezuela, rain, temperature, and relative humidity has been associated with patterns of dengue infection.[39] Monsoon rains and floods have been associated with outbreaks of dengue fever in India. In Thailand, dengue was a common cause of fever in children after heavy rain-associated flooding.[39]

RODENT-BORNE DISEASES

Diseases transmitted by rodents may also increase during heavy rainfall and flooding because of altered contact patterns. Humans usually acquire leptospirosis after exposure to fresh water contaminated with the urine of infected animals, such as rats.

There have been reports of flood-associated outbreaks of leptospirosis from a wide range of countries including Argentina, Brazil, Cuba, India, Korea, Mexico, Nicaragua, Philippines, Portugal, Russia, Taiwan, and Hawaii and Puerto Rico in the United States.[23,26,29,64] Investigations in France have documented a significant association between the emergence of leptospirosis and a combination of heavy rainfall and garbage collection strikes. In this case, trash left on the streets led to an increase in the surface rat population.[65]

Chemoprophylaxis with doxycycline is effective as a primary strategy for leptospirosis prevention among people who have high likelihood of occupational exposure or for those in areas of high endemicity. However, study results are inconclusive regarding the efficacy of doxycycline chemoprophylaxis in areas with high endemicity of leptospirosis in the setting of floods.[66]

DERMATOLOGICAL CONDITIONS

Dermatological conditions, usually in the form of nonspecific rashes, are a commonly reported complaint during floods and other disasters.[4,29] Among hurricane evacuees from the New Orleans area, a cluster of infections with methicillin-resistant Staphylococcus aureus (MRSA) was reported in approximately thirty pediatric and adult patients at an evacuee facility in Dallas, Texas. Three of the MRSA infections were confirmed by culture.[58]

WOUND INFECTIONS

Wound infections are common after disasters. The destruction of the regional health infrastructure, the inability to wash wounds with clean water, and a shortage of topical or systemic antimicrobial agents can all lead to severe wound infections, even if the initial trauma was relatively minor. In 2005, after hurricane Katrina, twenty-four cases of Vibrio species bacterial wound infections were identified. Most patients had associated comorbidities that probably increased their risk of Vibrio wound infection, and many had been wading in floodwaters.[39,58]

There is no evidence indicating that the risk of tetanus is increased in flood-related lacerations; therefore standard immunization practices should be an employed, that is, a wound normally classified as "low-risk" remains so even if exposed to floodwaters.[6] In comparison, the incidence of tetanus in the disaster setting has been associated with wounds that are highly contaminated with soil as result of high-energy traumatic inoculation occurring in low-income nations where patients are less likely to have had primary vaccinations and access to post-exposure tetanus prophylaxis. Clusters of tetanus cases were reported after the Indian Ocean tsunami as well as the Pakistan earthquake in 2005. However, these exposures were sustained during the initial trauma on the day of the event and not associated with exposure to floodwater or contaminated water sources. No subsequent cases were reported 2 weeks after the tsunami, indicating an association with the initial traumatic injury on the day of the event and not from wound exposure to floodwaters afterwards.[63]

INJURIES

During a flood disaster, injuries are more likely to occur as people attempt to travel or evacuate through flooded areas and again when they return to dwellings to repair damage and clear debris. Hypothermia, with or without submersion injury, is seen in some flood casualties. Conductive heat loss due to immersion in any water less than 16–21°C may lead to hypothermia. Wet clothing and water immersion tend to conduct away core body heat even when the ambient air temperature is extremely warm, but less than body temperature. Convective heat losses increase in windy conditions.

Electrocutions have occurred as a result of downed power lines, electrical wiring, and improper handling of wet appliances. Injuries from fires and explosions from gas leaks also occur. Musculoskeletal and soft tissue injuries are frequent conditions associated with floods. Lacerations and punctures are common sequelae during post-flood cleanup and recovery activities.[4,6]

Although it is a recurrent public concern that animals such as snakes may be forced to seek refuge from rising floodwaters in areas that may be inhabited by humans, public health surveillance after floods has not indicated that wild animal bites have been a major issue.[4,6] In contrast to wild animals, after Hurricane Floyd there were increases in reports of domesticated dog bites.[50] Epidemiologists reported similar data from Iowa during the same year.[26]

In Missouri after the Great Midwest U.S. floods of 1993, injuries were reported through a routine surveillance system. During a 6-week period, a total of 524 flood-related conditions were reported, and of these 250 (48%) were injuries. These injuries were categorized as sprains/strains (34%), lacerations (24%), abrasions (11%) and other injuries (11%).[8]

MENTAL HEALTH EFFECTS

Multiple studies have reported severe social and health impacts in the setting of flood disasters.[32,35,67–71] Social effects include disruption to people's lives, relationships and communities, and the destruction of people's homes.[32] Long-term effects of flooding on psychological health may be even more significant than those for any other illness or injury.[72,73] For many people, the emotional trauma continues long after the water has receded.

Factors that appear to make people more vulnerable to the development of psychological problems include:

■ Objective and subjective characteristics of the disaster – proximity of the victim to the disaster site; the duration of the disaster; the degree of physical injury; the witnessing of death or injury.[72]

■ Characteristics of the post-disaster response and recovery environment – community cohesion; secondary victimization; disruption of social support systems;[47] lack of home-ownership and duration of displacement from home.[35]

■ Characteristics of the individual or group – history of psychological problems; elderly; unemployed; single parents; children separated from their families.[72]

In one study of the health effects of flooding in thirty locations in the United Kingdom, psychological effects were much more commonly reported after flooding than physical ones. Women also appeared to suffer markedly more frequently than men at the worst time of flooding.[35] A number of psychological effects reported by flood victims have been strongly associated with reporting physical effects, particularly immediate effects.[35]

Increased morbidity and mortality following a flood may also result from heightened psychological stress.[73] Psychiatric examinations of 224 children 2 years after the 1972 flood in Buffalo Creek, West Virginia, showed that 80% of the children were severely emotionally impaired by their experiences during the flood.[74] Five years after the flood caused by Tropical Storm Agnes in Pennsylvania, perceived health problems were reported more commonly by flood-affected respondents than non-affected controls.[74]

Anxiety and Depression

There is considerable evidence for the development of anxiety and depression among flood-affected populations. Most studies are from high- or middle-income countries, including Australia, Poland, the United Kingdom, and the United States, but there is also a study from Bangladesh.[47] A few studies have examined flood-related mental health impacts on children. One 1993 study found post-flood changes in behavior among children 2–9 years old.[47]

Post-Traumatic Stress Disorder

Studies in Europe and North America have revealed post-flood psychiatric disorders among flood-affected populations that meet the criteria for post-traumatic stress disorder (PTSD).[32,47,68,71] One longitudinal study found 15–20% of people affected by a disaster had symptoms of PTSD.[73] Other studies after the 1997 floods in Poland suggested long-term negative effects on the well-being of children aged 11–14 and 11–20 years with increases in PTSD, depression, and dissatisfaction with life. Six months after Hurricane Floyd in the United States, similar findings were described for disaster-affected children aged 9–12 compared with controls.[47]

Studies of flood survivors in India found significantly higher scores for PTSD and depression among people more than 60 years old compared to all other groups.[75] Studies by Huang and colleagues found that a simple risk score model could be used to predict adult PTSD victims after floods in China.[76]

Suicides

Evidence is limited regarding flood-related suicides. One study in a high-income nation indicated that suicide rates increased by 13.8% above pre-disaster rates.[6]

NONCOMMUNICABLE DISEASES

Flood disasters have been reported as a significant cause of both acute and chronic exacerbations of noncommunicable diseases such as cardiovascular and respiratory illnesses. In addition,

Table 35.4. Top ten conditions: from rapid needs assessments performed by cluster sample among persons in Hurricane Katrina evacuation centers between September 10 and 12, 2005

Condition	Incidence per 1,000 residents
Hypertension/cardiovascular	108.2
Diabetes	65.3
New psychiatric condition	59.0
Pre-event psychiatric condition	50.0
Rash	27.6
Asthma/Chronic obstructive pulmonary disease	27.5
Influenza-like illness or pneumonia	26.3
Toxic exposure (including carbon monoxide)	16.0
Other infection	15.6
Diarrhea	12.8

CDC Data. Available at: www.cdc.gov/od/katrina/09-19-05.htm.

flood disasters have also been identified as a contributor to new onset of chronic illnesses.[25,50,80,81]

Short-Term Effects: Acute Exacerbations of Chronic Diseases

Disasters that cause population displacement are often associated with a worsening of chronic diseases.[25,50,80,81] Signs and symptoms of exacerbations involving diabetes and cardiovascular disease (and even cardiac arrests) have been reported from most high-income countries after flooding.[77,78] Increases in chronic respiratory illnesses, especially worsening asthma, are also reported after these events.[77,78] Exacerbations of chronic diseases may represent the majority of medical conditions among flood-affected populations in high-income nations, especially in shelter settings. Table 35.4 illustrates the range of patient conditions after flood displacement in a high-income nation.

This degree of correlation between exacerbations of chronic disease and flood disasters appears to be similar in both rural and urban settings. Results of a rapid needs assessment in rural and urban Iowa following large-scale flooding events in 2008 revealed that 9.0% of urban households and 8.9% of rural households reported the worsening of a chronic condition of someone within their household.[79]

The development of hypertension by male flood victims was reportedly greater than by male non-flood victims in the 5 years after flooding caused by Hurricane Agnes in Pennsylvania.[74] Benin also reported a marked increase in hypertension in Russia after the 1964 flood, and in Moldavia after two successive floods in 1969.[74]

Long-Term Effects: Chronic Exacerbations and New-onset of Chronic Disease

Over the past half century, multiple investigators have studied the long-term health effects from floods. These long-term health effects not only involve worsening of existing chronic diseases among flood-affected populations, but also new onset of chronic disease, mostly related to cardiovascular disease.

Bennett studied 316 flood respondents and 454 non-flood controls for morbidity and mortality in the year after the 1968 Bristol floods in England. He found higher mortality among residents of the flooded sections, especially the elderly. Health status during the year was worse in the flood group as measured by increased hospital admissions for both males and females.[82] Logue studied 407 flood and 155 non-flood female respondents by postal questionnaire to determine their families' mental and physical health status. The development of hypertension by the husbands of flood respondents was significantly greater than by the husbands of non-flood respondents in the 5 years after the flood. Flood-exposed families also reported more respiratory, gastrointestinal, and cardiovascular-related health problems.[83] Logue and Hansen conducted a case-control study of the thirty-one female flood victims who reported the development of hypertension in the 5-year post-disaster survey. Factors such as property loss, financial difficulties, physical work, use of alcohol, and perceived distress were significantly associated with hypertension. Anxiety and difficulty in sleeping also demonstrated significant positive correlations with hypertension.[84]

Benin reported a marked increase in hypertensive disease over the long term in Voroshilovgrad, Russia, after the 1964 flood and in Tiraspol, Moldavia, after two successive floods in 1969. In Tiraspol there was an increase in diabetes as well.[85] Abrahams studied 234 flood families and 163 non-flood families up to 12 months after the Brisbane floods in Australia in 1974. The number of visits to physicians and hospitals by members of the flood group increased after the flood. Psychological problems were more common than physical problems and were more common in females.[86]

Price followed on Abrahams' study, focusing on age-related health effects. He found that women 65 years of age or older experienced significantly more psychiatric symptoms than men.[87]

Floods and Cancer

Numerous researchers report an association between flood disasters and cancer. In 1978, Janench et al. investigated a cluster of lymphoma and leukemia cases in the Canisteo River Valley in New York.[88] Before 1974, the combined rates of leukemia and lymphoma for the river valley towns and the non-river valley towns were similar. In the period from 1974–1977, leukemia and lymphoma rates increased in all three river valley towns, at rates 35% higher than predicted.

Li and colleagues performed a retrospective cohort study in flood-affected areas in Hunan, China, in 1999 and discovered that the standard mortality rates of injuries/poisonings and malignant neoplasms were higher among groups located in the areas of river flood and inadequate soil drainage as compared to those in the non-flood group.[89] The percentage of attributable risk of standard mortality rates was 12.26% and 26.60% in the river flood group and 10.56% among groups located in areas with inadequate soil drainage.

CARBON MONOXIDE POISONING

Carbon monoxide poisonings occur, usually in association with loss of electrical power, when flood-affected populations improperly use carbon monoxide emitting fuel sources within poorly ventilated, enclosed spaces. This happens when people place generators indoors, in garages, or outdoors but near windows. Other carbon-monoxide emitting sources include indoor burning of charcoal for cooking and heating and using leaf

blowers indoors for flood clean up. After the 2004 hurricanes in Florida, 157 persons were treated from fifty-one exposure incidents, with six reported deaths. Of the 167 cases of carbon monoxide poisonings associated with Hurricane Katrina in 2005, 48.5% were treated and released without undergoing hyperbaric oxygen therapy, 43.7% were released after undergoing hyperbaric oxygen therapy, and 7.8% were hospitalized (most for just 1 day). Among these patients, 80% complained of headache, 51.5% nausea, 51% dizziness, 31.5% vomiting, and 16.4% dyspnea; 14.5% experienced loss of consciousness. The mean carboxyhemoglobin level was 19.8%, with a range of 0.2–45.1%.[20]

CURRENT STATE OF THE ART

Sustainable Development and Disaster Risk Management

A widely used international definition of sustainable development is "development which meets the needs of the present without compromising the ability of future generations to meet their own needs."[90] The concept of sustainable development was first codified decades ago during the Declaration of the United Nations Conference on the Human Environment at Stockholm in June 1972. Principle 1 of this declaration stated, "Man has the fundamental right to freedom, equality and adequate conditions of life, in an environment of a quality that permits a life of dignity and well-being, and he bears a solemn responsibility to protect and improve the environment for present and future generations."[90]

Development has the potential to either mitigate or amplify the human health risk posed by flood disasters. Studies of modified aquatic systems in Africa and Asia, involving the damming or impoundment of water sources, have almost universally shown not only a magnification of disease incidence but also changing patterns of occurrence according to time and location.[91-98]

Over time the overall approach to emergencies and disasters among nations has shifted from ad hoc post-impact activities to a more systematic and comprehensive process of risk management that emphasizes the importance of pre-impact risk reduction activities including prevention, mitigation, and preparedness.

Building on these core principles of both sustainable development and disaster risk management, the 2002 World Summit on Sustainable Development plan of implementation stated that, "An integrated, multi-hazard, inclusive approach to address vulnerability, risk assessment and disaster management, including prevention, mitigation, preparedness, response and recovery, is an essential element of a safer world in the twenty-first century."[99] Sustainable disaster risk management is a comprehensive approach to reduce disaster impact to a society over time without transference of additional risk and associated costs to future generations.

Toward Sustainable Flood Risk Management

The risk from disaster occurs when vulnerable populations are exposed to a hazard such as flooding and there are insufficient resources to match the immediate needs. This can lead to excess morbidity and mortality. Risk assessment is used to quantify environmental health risk. For flooding events, the risk equation has been applied to estimations of the likelihood of disaster impact as follows: p(flood hazard) x p(vulnerability or "susceptibility") − p(absorbing capacity or "resilience") = p(disaster impact). The probability of the hazard occurring is based on

Table 35.5. Floodplain Management Strategies and Tools[3]

Strategy	Tools
Modifying Hazard	Dams and Reservoirs
	Dikes, levees, and floodwalls
	Channel alterations
	High flow diversions
	Storm water management
	Shoreline protection
	Land treatment measures
Modifying Vulnerability	Regulations
	Development and redevelopment policies
	Disaster preparedness
	Flood forecasting, warning and evacuation plans
	Flood-proofing and elevation
Modifying Impact	Information and education
	Flood insurance
	Tax adjustments
	Flood emergency measures
	Disaster assistance
	Post-flood recovery
Restoring and Preserving Floodplain Resources	Regulations
	Development and redevelopment policies
	Information and education
	Tax adjustments

models that apply historical data from past floods in the same specific location being analyzed for risk.

The term "floodplain management" embodies the effort to manage the waters and lands subject to flooding to: 1) reduce all losses due to flooding; and 2) protect and enhance the natural values (inherent social, economic, ecological and cultural) of floodplains. It includes actions by all levels of government and the private sector ranging from constructing massive dams to zoning decisions of small communities. It involves concerns with wetlands, water quality, location of new developments, and a host of other considerations. Planning and operationalizing a comprehensive floodplain management program usually requires the cooperative participation of all levels of government and the private sector. The four main strategies of floodplain management relate to: modifying the likelihood of the hazard occurring; the vulnerability (or susceptibility) to the hazard; increasing the resilience or capacity of the society to absorb the impact of the hazard without mismatch of needs and resources; and restoring and preserving natural and cultural resources of the floodplains (Table 35.5).

The prevailing paradigm of sustainable flood management is derived from the concept of sustainable development. A seismic shift has been described as taking place in managing flood risk. Many countries' well-established reliance on structural defenses has been questioned, and cheaper and more sustainable alternatives have been sought.[100]

In the past, due to emphasis on structural defense, alleviation was prioritized above complimentary strategies such as promoting avoidance, raising awareness, and providing assistance. For many decades this paradigm of flood defense has been successful in protecting urban dwellers from riverine inundation and enabling farmers to cultivate or raise livestock right up to the edge of the river or seashore. This strategy, initially questioned because of the threat posed by climate change, is being increasingly abandoned.[100] More cost-effective strategies for disaster risk reduction through flood prevention, preparedness, and mitigation have gained wider application as compared to expensive, non-sustainable cycles of response and recovery.

The Scotland Water Environment and Water Services Act of 2003 states that public officials have a duty "to promote sustainable flood management and act in a way best calculated to contribute to the achievement of sustainable development." In practice this means that officials must balance social, economic, and environmental needs within a framework that incorporates intergenerational equity.[100] Intergenerational equity is a concept based on the fundamental principle of sustainable development that requires meeting current population needs without compromising the ability of future generations to meet their own needs. Present development should not lead to an increased economic burden for future generations in the form of expensive and inefficient response and recovery measures. Each generation is responsible for avoiding public policies and developmental practices that increase the future risk of disasters.

Sustainable flood risk management also seeks to reduce risk at all stages of the disaster cycle, giving preference to more cost-effective disaster risk reduction activities such as prevention, preparedness, and mitigation as compared to more costly and less sustainable response and recovery efforts.

Lessening Public Health Vulnerability to Flood Disasters

In prior times, vulnerability was generally measured in terms of flood damage to infrastructure and commerce. The current state of the art is seeking to further define and measure human vulnerability in terms of indicators for health, socioeconomic status, and quality of life. By focusing on vulnerability and the ability of individuals and communities to recover (resilience), sustainable flood management places individuals at risk at center stage and tasks the responsible authorities with enhancing social equity and promoting community cohesiveness. This is coupled with a heightened sense of individual responsibility.

Vulnerability Reduction

Within the context of disaster risk reduction, vulnerability is defined as the likelihood of suffering an adverse health effect when exposed to a given health hazard. These are characteristics and circumstances that are inherent to the specific person or population. People are not equally susceptible to the same health hazard. Differences among persons are due to such factors as demographics, socioeconomic status, social capital, and health status. The heaviest burden of every disaster most often falls disproportionately on women, children, the frail, the elderly, and those with disabilities. This degree of vulnerability to a given environmental hazard has a direct relationship to the frequency and severity of adverse health outcomes. Persons more susceptible to a disaster hazard have a higher risk for injury and illness as compared with those less susceptible.[102]

In one study of over 25,000 flood victims in Hunan, China, Feng and colleagues found that PTSD in flood victims was significantly associated with social support. Subjective support may play a more important role in mitigating the impact of floods than objective support, such as relief supplies.[101]

Healthy people are less vulnerable to the adverse effects of disaster hazards. Health promotion programs, medical care, social support services, and social integration that result in a reduction of the existing burden of disease and injuries create greater functionality and sustained mobility. They also result in a healthier population that is less susceptible to any given extreme weather hazard. In this sense, equitable and sustainable access to public health, medical, and social services, as well as community cohesion are essential in reducing human susceptibility to extreme weather events.[102]

Fundamental to sustainable flood management is a change in attitude in which a willingness to take on greater personal responsibility for mitigating flood losses replaces undue reliance on government assistance when losses occur.[100] Flood risk assessments commonly focus on protecting property and are the basis for financial decision-making. Environments are often protected irrespective of the cost. The health and social impacts suffered by people affected by floods remain mostly ill considered. In this respect, a better understanding of the social effects of floods is needed. Disruption of people and communities cannot be measured in monetary costs. Floods can cause health impacts that are enduring, including stress and trauma. The psychological effects of flooding can continue for months or even years after the event, and are often more pronounced than the physical health effects.[103] Tapsell et al. proposed a Social Flood Vulnerability Index (SFVI), which measures the impact that floods could have on potentially affected communities. The SFVI is a composite-added index derived from review of the existing literature and hundreds of interviews of disaster victims. It is based on three social characteristics and four financial deprivation indicators. It recognizes that age and financial status of the affected populations are the most important variables, followed by the prior population health status. The seven indicators used for derivation of the SFVI are:

- Unemployment;
- Overcrowding;
- Non-ownership of a car;
- Non-ownership of a home;
- Long-term illness;
- Single-parent family; and
- Elderly.

Strengthening Public Health Resilience to Flood Disasters

After Hurricane Katrina, a 2005 *Lancet* editorial criticized the inadequate support for a resilient public health system that protects human life when disasters occur.[104] Populations that possess a high capacity for access to public health and medical services are more resilient and less vulnerable to flood-related morbidity or mortality. There is growing concern regarding the longer-term impacts of climate change on human health, including flooding.[24,35]

Studies of two villages in Bangladesh found that people in an area with low flooding and with better socioeconomic circumstances are more likely to cope with impacts compared to people in areas with high and sudden flooding. Similarly, households' ability to cope varies depending on people's socioeconomic conditions, such as education, income, and occupation.[105]

The sustainable development of cost-effective public health and medical systems strengthens population resilience to flood disasters. Methods that reduce population vulnerability also increase resilience of the public health against flood-related morbidity and mortality.

Preventing the Public Health Impact of Flood Disasters

The Great Mississippi River flood of 1926–1927 resulted in the Flood Control Act of 1928, which legislated development of the largest levee system in the world. Despite increases in local and federal regulatory requirements and funding for flood hazard mitigation starting in 1926 in both the UK and United States, flood damage has continued to increase.[106] Although flood-related mortality during the past half-century has declined among high-income nations (mostly because of improved warning systems), economic losses have continued to rise due to increased urbanization and coastal development.[107] Many people lack the ability to prevent flood hazards, leaving the public health and medical sectors to play important roles in mitigating and preventing the public health impact of disasters. The most effective means of reducing flood risk in the floodplain is to prohibit development and rebuilding in these areas. For homes allowed in flood risk areas there are measures at the property level that can reduce the damage from future flooding. Homeowners need appropriate risk information as well as expert advice on how to appropriately protect individual properties from flooding.[108]

The majority of disaster-related mortality is directly attributable to drowning. Therefore, population protection measures like evacuation are aimed at preventing drowning by warning populations and moving them away from the flood hazard in a timely fashion. The incidence of flash floods in the United States is increasing; however, the mortality from these floods is decreasing. This decrease in mortality parallels advances in the U.S. National Weather System advanced warning system. Warning has been identified to be a substantial factor in decreasing mortality from flash floods by more than 50%.[4]

Health communication is a valuable tool in educating the public before and after flood impact regarding protective behaviors that help to prevent drowning (i.e., cautions regarding driving vehicles in flooded areas). Other injuries and illnesses can also be prevented through public awareness and education that promote safe and healthy activities during flood response and recovery efforts. Injuries such as electrocutions, burns, and carbon monoxide poisonings are typical examples of flood-related morbidity that are preventable through public awareness and health education campaigns. Chronic psychological and medical illnesses can also be prevented through activities that adequately manage stress in the disaster-affected population.

Governmental and nongovernmental services cannot always be sure that the public has adequate information necessary to avoid dangerous exposures to flood waters. Studies of flash floods in Iran by Adalan et al. revealed that, although local people were aware of their potential exposure to flooding, they were not aware of the existence of a hazard map and their vulnerability. The same study found a local early warning system lacking in its ability to make point predictions of rainfall and a standard warning threshold. There were also shortfalls found in the communications offered by the meteorological office despite the availability of flash flood response plans and guidelines within the provinces' health systems.[109]

Even minor investments to improve risk knowledge, monitoring/warning, dissemination/communication, and response capacity decrease mortality from flash floods. The appropriate use of personal protective equipment (PPE) among disaster-affected populations and recovery workers can help to prevent secondary disaster-related morbidity due to toxic exposures from chemicals or mold. Measures to increase awareness of the appropriate respiratory protection among the public are warranted in order to lessen potential exposures to mold hazards. Public health officials can accomplish this via traditional media announcements and educational sessions for employees of home improvement stores and other commercial entities that sell respirators. In order to decrease the probability of flood-related illness, flood victims and relief workers should practice proper hand hygiene (wash their hands with soap and water) before preparing or eating food, after toilet use, and after participating in flood cleanup or after handling potentially contaminated articles.[110]

Chemical risk assessments are useful to identify and characterize industrial and agricultural hazardous material sites located in flood-prone locations in order to prevent toxic exposures and associated adverse health effects.

Public policy may guide land-use and zoning regulations that prevent population displacement. These efforts subsequently lessen the potential future need for expensive shelter and settlement options that must also include access to basic necessities for space, food, water, sanitation, hygiene, security, and medical care. Lessening population displacement markedly decreases the risk for morbidity and the excessive demand for services as a result of flooding.

Well-established disease surveillance systems are necessary to monitor health effects among the flood-affected population and direct cost-effective public health interventions that may prevent secondary morbidity and mortality. Clinical and laboratory surveillance should be integrated in order to rapidly detect disease and guide therapy.

Early implementation of environmental health capacity related to toxicology, water, sanitation, waste management, and vector control can prevent disease due to toxic, vector-borne, food-borne and water-related illnesses.

Flood disaster risk assessments should be used to guide both local and national decisions regarding location/relocation of critical public health and healthcare facilities outside of floodplains whenever possible, so that secondary disasters (i.e., public health and medical facility evacuations) do not occur at healthcare facilities.

Public health programs that offer primary prevention of chronic disease, as compared with merely managing existing illness, also lessen vulnerability of the disaster-affected population to flood-related morbidity and mortality. In this sense, building and maintaining a baseline robust public health infrastructure also mitigates the public health impact of floods. Population reliance on food sources and distribution systems that are not vulnerable to flooding may prevent any significant public health impact attributable to malnutrition. Reliable and economical access to drugs and medical care also reduces adverse health effects. This is best accomplished through a well-developed and equitable healthcare system.

Mitigating the Public Health Impact of Flood Disasters

The public health impact of floods reflects secondary effects of the disaster such as population displacement and disruption of existing health services. To minimize these secondary effects, public health and healthcare relief efforts must be coordinated within the general emergency management cycle before, during, and after the impact phase and throughout recovery. Strategies should promote early reinstatement of normal routine activities of daily living among disaster-affected populations in order to mitigate ongoing adverse psychological and other health effects.

Mitigation is defined as the reduction of harmful effects of a disaster by limiting its impact on human health and economic infrastructure. In the past, mitigation measures have been used in the traditional fields of engineering and urban planning. Flood-related mitigation activities lessen deaths and injuries by ensuring structural safety through enforcing adequate building codes, promulgating legislation to relocate structures away from flood-prone areas, planning appropriate land-use, and managing coasts and floodplains.[3] Critical public health and medical assets can be identified before flood impact and engineering measures can be taken to mitigate loss of critical health infrastructure and assets during flooding. Key buildings may be designed or strengthened in ways that reduce flood damage risk.

Shelter and settlement solutions for displaced populations must adequately address basic human needs related to space, water, sanitation, hygiene, nutrition, and security in order to mitigate the public health impact of floods. Settlement solutions that do not promote hastening resettlement and minimizing population displacement may contribute to the long-lasting psychological impact of the disaster and its subsequent association with chronic health effects. Therefore, public health workers should be involved in decisions regarding the rapid reinstatement of healthy homes and healthy communities that would have a direct impact on the health of flood-affected populations.

A study in Vietnam confirmed that poor households are more vulnerable to floods than are rich households since their livelihoods tend to depend on natural resources such as agriculture and fisheries that are relatively more affected by floods. Thus a generation of net non-agricultural jobs to achieve livelihood diversification would reduce the physical damage and the vulnerability of poor households.[111]

Preparing for the Public Health Impact of Floods

The public health impact of flood disasters is predictable for both high- and low-income nations. It is therefore possible to prepare emergency response and recovery activities that will lower the risk of flood-related morbidity and mortality. "Public health emergency preparedness is the capability of the public health and health care systems, communities, and individuals, to prevent, protect against, quickly respond to, and recover from health emergencies, particularly those whose scale, timing, or unpredictability threatens to overwhelm routine capabilities."[112]

An emergency management program has the goal to "strengthen the overall capacity and capability of a country to manage all types of emergencies and bring about an orderly transition from relief through recovery and back to sustained development."[113] Keim's Eleven E's of emergency preparedness are:[114]

1. Evaluation and forecasting of hazard
2. Early warning
3. Evacuation
4. Emergency operations planning
5. Education and awareness
6. Exercises and drills
7. e-Health and electronic media
8. Epidemiology
9. Equipment and supplies
10. Enforcement of land-use regulations and zoning codes
11. Economic incentive

In modern times, accurate weather forecasts linked to timely warning systems for hazardous flooding have effectively mitigated the effects of floods on the health and well-being of communities. Emergency operations planning for response and transition planning for recovery are core elements of public health preparedness. Once plans are developed, both the public and response communities must be educated and trained to implement protective behaviors. Exercises test the validity of emergency plans and the effectiveness of education and training. Epidemiological investigations identify the adverse health effects of flood disasters. Surveillance activities monitor health trends, allowing for early warning and intervention. The availability of equipment and supplies (i.e., PPE, boats and helicopters, power generators, water pumps, and water purification units) offers the affected community enhanced absorptive capacity and resilience. Enforcement of land-use regulations and zoning codes also helps to break the response cycle by lessening or eliminating the risk of population exposure to flooding.

Despite the increased level of preparedness, flood-related deaths, diseases, and injuries continue to occur.[4] The development of robust emergency operations plans[29,115,116] and the design of effective messages to prompt desired behavior are key elements for saving lives.

Responding to the Public Health Impact of Floods

Community Needs Assessment

Immediately after the flood impact phase, responder teams conduct rapid needs assessments in order to identify gaps between health and medical needs of a flood-affected community and available resources. A needs assessment typically consists of administering a standardized questionnaire that assesses health, medical, and pharmaceutical needs; the status of public health services; and access to basic services such as water, sanitation and hygiene, food, shelter, sewage, and electricity.

Thorough and accurate documentation of household losses is essential. A study of seasonal flooding in Vietnam revealed that official damage estimates often include public infrastructure; however, these assessments also tend to underestimate damage to households.[117]

Disease Risk Assessment

Responding effectively to the needs of the disaster-affected population requires an accurate disease risk assessment that includes both acute and chronic disease, including injuries as well as illnesses. A systematic and comprehensive post-flood evaluation should identify: 1) diseases that are common and endemic to the affected area; 2) living conditions of the affected population; 3) availability of safe water and adequate sanitation facilities; 4) underlying nutritional status and immunization coverage among the affected population; and 5) degree of access to healthcare and to effective clinical care.[43] Risk assessments can also characterize flood-related toxic exposures.

Clinical Diagnosis and Management of Flood-related Morbidity

Healthcare personnel should anticipate flood-related adverse health effects in order to be prepared to detect and intervene effectively when they occur. Clinicians should maintain a high index of suspicion for illness and injuries commonly associated with floods. Flood-related injuries frequently include soft tissue lacerations, contusions, and abrasions.

Endemic infectious diseases as well as chronic diseases may worsen. Mental illness and toxic exposures (e.g., carbon monoxide and mold) are known to increase after floods but may manifest with nonspecific symptoms such as malaise, anxiety, headaches, and nausea.

Studies of flood disasters have shown that outbreaks of vaccine-preventable diseases rarely result.[53] Despite the fact that these epidemics have not been reported following flood disasters in the United States, public demand for emergency mass immunization, especially against typhoid fever, hepatitis, and tetanus, is common. Assuring the safety of water and food supplies is of paramount importance in preventing enteric disease transmission when water and sewage systems have been compromised. Active surveillance data should be used to justify consideration of an immunization campaign. Basic rules of hygiene and sanitation are far more important than immunizations in preventing infectious disease that floodwaters could potentially spread.[110] Mass immunization in absence of a documented outbreak is usually counterproductive during flood disasters and diverts limited human resources and materials from other more effective and urgent measures.[4,29,53] Mass vaccination would be justified only when the recommended sanitary measures do not have a preventative effect and if there is evidence of the progressive increase in the number of cases of illness with risk of an epidemic.[29]

Disaster Relief Services after a Flood

Overall, regardless of flood exposure, most people do not seek assistance from disaster service agencies. On average, the probability of seeking disaster relief services increases with the number of flood experiences. Racial/ethnic minorities, rural residents, economically challenged individuals, and people with low levels of perceived social support may be more likely than people without these characteristics to request assistance. Public health, along with relief agencies should therefore be aware that vulnerable populations may have a greater need for the services that they provide.[118]

Mass Care and Shelter of Flood-Displaced Populations

Public health officials should be involved in decisions regarding the mass care and settlement of displaced populations in order to assure a safe and healthy environment. Public health workers assist in performing food safety and water quality inspections, and assessment of sanitation and hygiene in mass evacuation and care shelters.

Environmental Health Services for Flood-Affected Populations

The demands for environmental health services and consultation are high during flood disasters. The following are common considerations:[8]

- Purification of drinking and cooking water;
- Disinfection of wells;
- Food safety;
- Sanitation and personal hygiene; and
- Mosquito control.

Flood-Related Morbidity and Mortality Surveillance

Although communicable disease outbreaks worldwide are rare after flooding, some potential exists for disease transmission; therefore, flood-affected communities should be under close surveillance.[110] Mortality surveillance is performed to determine the nature and circumstances surrounding flood-related deaths so that appropriate preventive actions can be initiated to reduce further mortality. Morbidity surveillance is conducted to detect: 1) increases in diseases that are endemic to the area; 2) infectious diseases that must be contained or controlled; and 3) injuries that require public advisories. While important, these drop-in surveillance systems may be difficult to implement during flood emergencies, especially in low-resource countries.

A 2010 flooding event in Pakistan affected approximately 18 million persons. In response to the emergency, Pakistan's Ministry of Health and WHO enhanced an existing disease early warning system (DEWS) for outbreak detection and response. During a 47-day period, approximately 5.6 million new patient visits were reported. Overall, DEWS was useful in detecting outbreaks, but it was limited by inadequate data quality. The challenges of DEWS implementation mirror those of other early warning alert and response network surveillance systems, which have been documented in many emergencies. Alerts for rare diseases should trigger timely investigation and control measures. In practice, however, such systems frequently include monitoring of other infectious diseases of public health importance that occur more frequently, as they did in Pakistan. This is problematic because reporting of these more common diseases can overwhelm resources, negatively affect data quality, and potentially detract from outbreak detection.[119]

Flood-specific surveillance systems are often used to detect increases in vector populations such as mosquitoes. In addition, public health officials should conduct laboratory-based surveillance of drinking water sources such as public and private wells.[4]

Chemical Emergency Response

The role of public health in the investigation of a flooding event that results in a chemical release should include the following activities:[36]

- Hazard identification;
- Risk communication;
- Liaison with other relevant responder agencies;
- Technical advice including aspects of toxicology, decontamination, antidotes, and PPE;
- Registry and follow-up of exposed casualties; and
- Emergency plan development for flooding in other high-risk areas.

The Role of Social Support in Improving Behavioral and Physical Health Outcomes

A complex set of social and other factors defines flood victims' susceptibility to effects on physical and mental health. There is some evidence that effective community and professional agency management of the flooding aftermath can mitigate deleterious mental health outcomes, which in turn are strongly associated with physical health effects.[36] Research from the United States indicates that providing increased social support can significantly lower illness burdens after disasters.[120]

Recovering from the Public Health Impact of Floods

Long-term recovery from the public health impact of flood disasters can take years. Additional financial, health, and emotional costs may continue long after basic utilities and shelters have been reinstated. The public health and medical community must continue to engage in outreach activities long after the flood event itself has occurred.

Stimpson et al. found that after the Great Mississippi River flood only a small proportion of individuals affected by large-scale flooding events actually sought available recovery services.[118] The researchers also found that patients' frequency of exposure to disaster circumstances was positively associated with their willingness to accept assistance.[118]

The disaster recovery phase may also offer a window of opportunity for improving risk reduction strategies, such as improvements in preparedness and mitigation. Recovery strategies that promote future risk reduction should be prioritized. Permanent migrations of populations are rare after disaster floods. Disease surveillance systems are necessary to identify the long-term adverse health effects of flood disasters. Public health and medical services must develop infrastructures sufficiently robust to detect and help patients to manage the long-term risks of flood-associated illness, such as mental illness and cardiovascular disease.

RECOMMENDATIONS FOR FURTHER RESEARCH

Flooding is one of the most devastating disasters, posing multiple risks to human health. Despite this, there has been only limited systematic research on the health outcomes of flooding.[35] There is surprisingly little evidence about the health effects of floods, particularly in relation to morbidity. There are virtually no studies available on the effectiveness of public health measures, other than flood warning systems. A wide range of health risks have been well documented, although there remains scientific uncertainty regarding the strength of association and public health burden for specific health effects.[47] Overall, there are few data on the long-term health impacts of flooding.[73]

Although some studies conducted during and after floods have provided important information on factors contributing to the risk of morbidity and mortality, unresolved inconsistencies remain more than 25 years after being posed as research recommendations.

Research recommendations originally offered by Jean French and Kenneth Holt in 1989 include:[74]

- Factors influencing actions people take in the face of flash flood warning and evacuation notices should be studied further
- Study should be done to assess the circumstances under which there is sufficient time to permit evacuation by car or when it is safer to abandon vehicles and escape to higher ground on foot.
- A cohort of flood victims should be followed over time to determine whether they are at higher risk than a comparable

group of non-flood victims of having adverse physical and mental health effects.

■ Systematic study should be undertaken taken to determine whether an increase in certain biological agents results from disrupted water supplies and sewage systems after floods and whether this is related to geographic location.

■ Systematic studies should be undertaken to examine the release of chemical agents during flooding and the potential for contamination of human pathways from such events.

■ A reporting system should be established to more accurately assess the number of deaths and injuries associated with each flood and the circumstances surrounding each flood death and injury.

There is a need for standardized criteria for estimating flood damage and public health impact. Perception of flood damage is influenced by historical experience. For example, in low-vulnerability U.S. states, floods causing over $1 million USD damage are notable events and are likely to be reported. Conversely, in high-vulnerability states, damage of $5 million USD or more occurs frequently, so smaller damages might seem unremarkable and be underreported.[106]

The effectiveness of detection and warning systems should be evaluated and researchers should make recommendations for appropriate standards for such systems in ensuring greater warning sensitivity.[4] More research into the behavioral outcomes of health risk communication is important. This is especially significant to help prevent the continued cases of drowning related to vehicle use, as well as other preventable morbidity and mortality such as mold-related exposures and carbon monoxide intoxication.

In 2005, Ahern and colleagues identified the following knowledge gaps with respect to managing the public health impact of flood disasters:[47]

■ Mental health impacts of flooding, especially the long-term impacts, and their principal causes.

■ Nature and magnitude of mortality risks in the period after flooding.

■ Quantification of the risks of infectious and vector-borne diseases following floods.

■ Effectiveness of warning systems and public health measures in reducing flood-related health burdens.

■ Defining health-related costs of flooding in terms of how they influence decisions about specific interventions.

■ Quantification of the degree to which land-use and climate change will contribute to flood risk and associated health burdens in different settings.

WHO also recognizes that the mental health consequences of floods "have not been fully addressed by those in the field of disaster preparedness or service delivery," although it is generally accepted that disasters, such as earthquakes, floods, and hurricanes, "take a heavy toll on the mental health of the people involved, most of whom live in developing countries, where capacity to take care of these problems is extremely limited." Areas of particular concern relate to anxiety and depression, PTSD, and suicide.[47] Much work remains to define evidence-based approaches that will decrease morbidity and mortality from floods, a disaster with one the greatest overall public health impacts.

Disclaimer

The material in this chapter reflects solely the views of the author. It does not necessarily reflect the policies or recommendations of the U.S. Centers for Disease Control and Prevention (CDC) or Department of Health and Human Services (HHS).

REFERENCES

1. United Nations Department of Humanitarian Affairs (UNDHA). Internationally Agreed Glossary of Basic Terms related to Disaster Management. DHA 93/36. Geneva, December 1992. http://reliefweb.int/sites/reliefweb.int/files/resources/004DFD3E15B69A67C1256C4C006225C2-dha-glossary-1992.pdf (Accessed August 27, 2013).

2. Gunn SWA. *Multilingual dictionary of disaster medicine and international relief.* Dordrecht, Kluwer Academic Publishers, 1990.

3. Keim M. Flood Disasters. In: Koenig K, Schultz C, eds. *Disaster Medicine.* New York, Cambridge University Press, 2010; 529–542.

4. Malilay J. Floods. In: Noji ER, ed. *The public health consequences of disasters.* New York, Oxford University Press, 1997; 287–300.

5. Intergovernmental Panel on Climate Change (IPCC) Working Group II. Impacts, Adaptation and Vulnerability. United Nations. Geneva, 2007. http://www.ipcc.ch/publications_and_data/ar4/wg2/en/contents.html (Accessed September 28, 2013).

6. Poole J, Hogan D. Floods. In: Hogan D, Burstein J, eds. *Disaster Medicine.* Philadelphia, PA Lippincott, Williams & Wilkins, 2007; 214–214.

7. Life Books. The China Floods. In: *Nature's Fury.* New York, Time Inc., 2008; 61.

8. CDC. Morbidity surveillance following the Midwest flood – Missouri, 1993. *MMWR* 1993; 42(41): 797–798.

9. McCullough D. *The Johnstown Flood.* New York, Simon and Schuster, 1987; 186.

10. Life Books. The Johnstown Flood. In: *Nature's Fury*; 34.

11. Frank N, Husain S. The deadliest tropical cyclone in history? Bulletin of the American Meteorological Society. *American Meteorological Society* 1971; 53(6): 438–444.

12. Life Books. The Bhola Cyclone. In *Nature's Fury*; 76.

13. Life Books. The Galveston Hurricane. In *Nature's Fury*; 37.

14. Keim M. Cyclones, Tsunamis and Human Health. *Oceanography* 2006; 19(2): 40–49.

15. Centre for Research on the Epidemiology of Disasters (CRED). EM-DAT: the international Disaster Database. Brussels, Belgium, Ecole se Sante Publique, Universite Catholique de Louvain. 2009. http://www.emdat.be/disaster-trends (Accessed August 27, 2013).

16. United Nations International Strategy for Disaster Reduction (UNISDR). Disaster Statistics. 2013. http://www.unisdr.org/we/inform/disaster-statistics (Accessed August 27, 2013).

17. Thomalla F. Reducing hazard vulnerability: towards a common approach between disaster risk reduction and climate adaptation. *Disasters* 30(1): 39–48.

18. NOAA. National Weather Service. Natural hazard statistics. http://www.nws.noaa.gov/om/hazstats.shtml (Accessed September 28, 2013).

19. U.S. Department of the Interior, U.S. Geological Survey. Flood Hazards – A National Threat. U.S. Geological Survey Fact Sheet 2006–3026. URL: http://pubs.usgs.gov/fs/2006/3026 (Accessed September 28, 2013).

20. Llewellyn M. Floods and tsunamis. In: *Surg Clin Am* June 2006; 86(3): 557–578.

21. Parret C, Melcher NB, James RW. The discharges in the upper Mississippi River basin. In: *US geological survey circular 1120-a.* Denver, CO, U.S. Government Printing Office, 1993.

22. CDC. Storm-related mortality – Central Texas, October 17–31, 1998. *MMWR* 2000; 49(07): 133–135.

23. Munich Re Group. Natural catastrophe statistics for 2012 dominated by weather extremes. Munich, Germany. Press release. January 3, 2013. http://www.munichre.com/en/media_relations/press_releases/2013/2013_01_03_press_release.aspx (Accessed September 28, 2013).

24. Munich Re Group. Annual Review: Natural Catastrophes 2002. http://www.unep.org/download_file.multilingual .asp?FileID=96 (Accessed August 27, 2015).

25. CDC. Tropical Storm Allison rapid needs assessment Houston, Texas, June 2001. *MMWR* 2002; 51(17): 365–369.

26. CDC. Public health consequences of a flood disaster – Iowa, 1993. *MMWR* 1993; 42: 653–656.

27. ReliefWeb. Cambodia: floods – September 2011. http://reliefweb.int/disaster/fl-2011-000148-khm (Accessed September 26, 2013).

28. Manzanilla DO, Paris TR, Vergara GV, et al. Submergence risks and farmers' preferences: implications for breeding Sub1 rice in Southeast Asia. *Agric Syst* 2011; 104: 335–347.

29. Noji E. Public health issues in disasters. *Crit Care Med* 2005; 33(1): S29–S33.

30. FEMA. Federated States of Micronesia Drought Emergency Declaration. July 31, 2007. http://www.fema.gov/disaster/3276 (Accessed September 28, 2013).

31. Keim ME. Sea-Level-Rise Disaster in Micronesia: Sentinel Event for Climate Change? *Disaster Med Public Health Prep* 2010; 4(1): 81–87.

32. Carroll B, Morbey H, Balogh R, et al. Flooded homes, broken bonds, the meaning of home, psychological processes and their impact on psychological health in a disaster. *Health Place* June 2009; 15(2): 540–547.

33. Guiliani V, Feldman R. Place attachment in a developmental and cultural context. *Journal of Environmental Psychology* 1993; 13: 1–8.

34. Moore J, Placing home in context. *Journal of Environmental Psychology* 2000; 20: 207–217, 540–547.

35. Tunstall S, Tapsell S, Green C, et al. The health effects of flooding: social research results from England and Wales. *J Water and Health* 2006; 3(4): 365–380.

36. Euripidou E, Murray V. Public health impacts of floods and chemical contamination. *J Pub Health* 2004; 26(4): 376–383.

37. Potera C. Fuel damage from flooding: finding a fix. *Env Hlth Persp* 2003; 111(4): A228–231.

38. CDC. Health concerns associated with mold in water damaged homes after hurricanes Katrina and Rita – New Orleans area, Louisiana, October 2005 *MMWR* 2006; 55(2): 41–45.

39. Ivers LC, Ryan ET. Infectious diseases of severe weather-related and flood-related natural disasters. *Current opinions in infectious diseases* October 2006; 19(5): 408–414.

40. Schatz J. Floods hamper health-care delivery in southern Africa. *Lancet* 2008: 371; 799–800.

41. Noji E. Natural Disaster Management. In: Auerbach P, ed. *Wilderness Medicine: Management of Wilderness in Environmental Emergencies.* 4th ed. St. Louis, MO, Mosby, 2001: 1603–1621.

42. Peters M. Hospitals respond to water lost during the Midwest floods in 1993: preparedness and improvisation. *J Emerg Med* 1996; 14(3): 345–350.

43. Watson JT, Gayer M, Connolly MA. Epidemics after natural disasters. *Emerg Infect Dis* January 13, 2007; 1. http://www.cdc .gov/ncidod/EID/13/1/1.htm (Accessed August 31, 2015).

44. Chen JR, Tsai HY, Shen CC. Estimation of waste generation from floods. *Waste Management* 2007; 27: 1717–1724.

45. Kim SH. Flood. In: Ciottone G, ed. *Disaster Medicine.* 3rd ed. Philadelphia, PA, Mosby, 2006: 489–491.

46. WHO Europe fact sheet 05/02. Flooding: health effects and preventive measures. http://www.google.com/url?sa=t&rct=j&q=&esrc=s&frm=1&source=web&cd=1&ved=0CCkQFjAA&url=http%3A%2F%2Fvac.ciifen-int.org%2FdoDownload%3Bjsessionid%3D750444CEFB98416F01D59A889F786C52%3Ffname%3Dfile37749.str%26orname%3Dn-1539-0x.pdf%26mtype%3Dapplication%2Fpdf&ei=72lHUuC9DoTA9gTlk4GwCA&usg=AFQjCNEpfP33mQH1h4kySmGNDlO_RV6Xw&bvm=bv.53217764,d.eWU (Accessed September 28, 2013).

47. Ahern M, Kovats RS, Wilkinson P, et al. Global health impacts of floods: epidemiologic evidence. *Epidemiol Rev* 2005; 27: 36–46.

48. Staes C, Orengo JC, Malilay J, Rullan J, Noji E. Deaths due to flash floods in Puerto Rico, January 1992: implications for prevention. *Int J Epidemiol* 1994; 23: 968–75.

49. American National Red Cross. Flood and flash flood. http://www.redcross.org/services/disaster/keepsafe/flood.html (Accessed September 28, 2013).

50. CDC. Morbidity and mortality associated with Hurricane Floyd–North Carolina, September–October 1999. *MMWR* 2000; 49(17): 369–372.

51. Shultz J. Epidemiology of tropical cyclones: The dynamic of disaster, disease, and development. *Epidemiol Rev* 2005; 27: 21–35.

52. Noji E. The Nature of Disasters. In: Noji ER, ed. *The public health consequences of disasters.* New York, Oxford University Press, 1997; 3–20.

53. CDC. Current trends flood disasters and immunization – California. *MMWR* 1983; 32(13): 171–172, 178.

54. Tuffs A, Bosch X. Health authorities on alert after extensive flooding in Europe. *BMJ* 2002; 325: 405.

55. CDC. Norovirus outbreak among evacuees from hurricane Katrina – Houston, Texas, September 2005. *MMWR* 2005; 54: 1016–1018.

56. CDC. Two cases of toxigenic Vibrio cholerae O1 infection after Hurricanes Katrina and Rita – Louisiana, October 2005. *MMWR* 2006; 55: 31–32.

57. CDC. Vibrio illnesses after hurricane Katrina – multiple states, August–September 2005. *MMWR* 2005; 54(37): 928–931.

58. CDC. Infectious disease and dermatologic conditions in evacuees and rescue workers after Hurricane Katrina – multiple states, August–September, 2005. *MMWR* 2005; 54: 961–964.

59. McCarthy MC, He J, Hyams KC, et al. Acute hepatitis E infection during the 1988 floods in Khartoum, Sudan. Trans R Soc. *Trop Med Hyg* 1994; 88: 177.

60. Woodruff BA, Toole JM, Rodriguez DC, et al. Disease surveillance and control after a flood in Khartoum, Sudan, 1988. *Disasters* 1990; 14: 151–163.

61. CDC. Rapid assessment of vectorborne diseases during the Midwest flood United States, 1993. *MMWR* 1994; 43(26): 481–483.

62. CDC. Report: International notes health assessment of the population affected by flood conditions – Khartoum Sudan. *MMWR* 1989; 37(51 & 52): 785–788.

63. Guha-Sapir D, van Panhuis W. The Andaman Nicobar earthquake and tsunami 2004: impact on diseases in Indonesia. Centre for Research on the Epidemiology of Disasters (CRED). Brussels, Belgium. 2005. http://www.preventionweb.net/english/professional/publications/v.php?id=1916 (Accessed September 28, 2013).

64. CDC. Report: Leptospirosis After Flooding of a University Campus – Hawaii, 2004 *MMWR* 2006: 55(5): 125–127.

65. Socolovschi C, Angelakis E, Renvoisé, A. et al. Strikes, flooding, rats, and leptospirosis in Marseille, France. *Int J Infect Diseases* 2011; 15: 710–715.

66. Bhardwaj P, Kosambiya JK, Vikas KD, et al. Chemoprophylaxis with doxycycline in suspected epidemic of leptospirosis during floods: does this really work? *African Health Sciences* June 2010; 10(2): 199–200.

67. Tapsell SM, Tunstall SM, 2001. The health and social effects of the June 2000 flooding in the NE region. *Report to the environment agency.* Middlesex University, Flood Hazard Research Centre.

68. Tapsell SM, Tunstall SM. I wish I'd never heard of Banbury: the relationship between 'place' and the health impacts of flooding. *Health and Place* 2008; 14(2): 133–154.

69. Auger C, Latour S, Trudel M, Fortin M. Post-traumatic stress disorder after the flood in Sanguenay. *California Academy of Family Physicians* 2000; 46: 2420–2427.

70. Ginexi EM, Weihs K, Simmens SJ, Hoyt DR. Natural disaster and depression: a prospective investigation of reactions to the 1993 Midwest floods. *American Journal of Community Psychology* 2000; 28: 295–518.

71. Verger P, Rotily M, Brenot J, Baruffol E, Bard D. Assessment of exposure to a flood disaster in a mental health study. *Journal of Exposure Analysis and Environmental Epidemiology* 2003; 13: 436–442.

72. Gerrity E, Flynn B. Mental health consequences of disasters. In: Noji ER, ed. *The Public Health Consequences of Disasters.* New York, Oxford University Press, 1997; 101–121.

73. Ohl C, Tapsell S. Flooding and human health: The dangers posed are not always obvious. *BMJ* 2000; 321: 1167–1168 (Editorial).

74. French JG, Holt KW. Floods. In: Gregg MB, ed. *The Public Health Consequences of Disasters.* Atlanta, GA: HHS, Public Health Service, CDC, 1989; 69–78.

75. Telles S, Singh N, Joshi M. Risk of posttraumatic stress disorder and depression in survivors of the floods in Bihar, India. *Indian J Med Sci* August 2009; 63(8): 330–334.

76. Prediction of posttraumatic stress disorder among adults in flood district. *BMC Public Health* 2010; 10: 207.

77. European Commission (NA). Flooding in Europe: health risks. Health and Consumer Protection. 2010. http://ec.europa.eu/health/climate_change/extreme_weather/flooding/index_en.htm (Accessed August 31, 2015).

78. Guha-Sapir D, Thomas Jakubicka T, Vos F, et al. Health impacts of floods in Europe: Data gaps and information needs from a spatial perspective. *Centre for Research on the Epidemiology of Disasters. MICRODIS.* Brussels, Belgium. 2010; 23–25.

79. Quinlisk P, Jones M, Bostick N. Results of Rapid Needs Assessments in Rural and Urban Iowa Following Large-scale Flooding Events in 2008. *Disaster Med Public Health Prep* 2011; 5: 287–292.

80. CDC. Hurricanes and hospital emergency room visits – Mississippi, Rhode Island, Connecticut (Hurricanes Alicia and Gloria). *MMWR* 1986; 34: 765–770.

81. CDC. Needs assessment following Hurricane Georges – Dominican Republic, 1998. *MMWR* 1999; 48: 93–95.

82. Bennett G. Bristol floods 1968 Controlled survey of effects on health of local community disaster. *BMJ* 1970; 3: 454–458.

83. Logue JN. Long term effects of a major natural disaster: The Hurricane Agnes flood in the Wyoming Valley of Pennsylvania, June 1972. DtPH (Dissertation). Columbia University School of Public Health, Division of Epidemiology. New York, 1975.

84. Logue JN, Hansen H. A case control study of hypertensive women in a post-disaster community Wyoming Valley, Pennsylvania. *J Human Stress* June 1980; 2: 28–34.

85. Benin L. *Medical consequences of natural disasters.* New York, Springer-Verlag, 1985; 45–60.

86. Abrahams MJ, Price J, Whitlock FA, William G. The Brisbane floods, January 1974: their impact on health. *Med J Aust* 1976; 2: 936–939.

87. Price J. Some Age Related Effects of the 1974 Brisbane Hoods Australian and New Zealand. *J Psychiatry* 1978; 12(55): 52–58.

88. Janerich UF, Stark AD, Greenwald P, Bryant WS, Jacobson, HI, McCusker, J. Increased leukemia, lymphoma and spontaneous abortion in western New York following a disaster. *Public Health Rep* 1981; 96: 350–356.

89. Li X, Tan H, Li S. Years of potential life lost in residents affected by floods in Hunan, China. *Transactions of the Royal Society of Tropical Medicine and Hygiene* 2007; 101: 299–304.

90. UN Environment Programme. Declaration of the UN Conference on the Human Environment. http://www.unep.org/Documents.Multilingual/Default.asp?DocumentID=97&ArticleID=1503 (Accessed August 27, 2015).

91. Hughes C, Hunter J. Disease and "development" in Africa. *Social Science and Medicine* 1970; 3(4): 443–493.

92. Hunter J. Inherited burden of disease: agricultural dams and the persistence of bloody urine (Schistosomiasishematobium) in the Upper East Region of Ghana, 1959–1997. *Social Science and Medicine* 2003; 56(2): 219–234.

93. Hunter JM, Rey L, Scott D. Man-madelakesandman-made diseases. Towards a policy resolution. *Social Science and Medicine* 1982; 16(11): 1127–1145.

94. Keiser J, De Castro M, Maltese C, et al. Effect of irrigation and large dams on the burden of malaria on a global and regional scale. *American Journal of Tropical Medicine and Hygiene* 2005; 72(4): 392–406.

95. Singh N, Mehra RK, Sharma VP. Malaria and the Narmada – river development in India: a case study of the Bargi Dam. *Annals of Tropical Medicine and Parasitology* 1999; 93(5): 477–488.

96. Sow S, de Vlas SJ, Engels D, Gryseels B. Water-related disease patterns before and after the construction of the Diama Dam in northern Senegal. *Annals of Tropical Medicine and Parasitology* 2002; 96(6): 575–586.

97. Waddy BB. Research into the health problems of manmade lakes, with special reference to Africa. *Transactions of the Royal Society of Tropical Medicine and Hygiene* 1975; 69(1): 39–50.

98. Carrel M, Emch M, Streatfiel P, et al. Spatio-temporal clustering of cholera: the impact of flood control in Matlab, Bangladesh 1983–2003. *Health & Place* 2009; 15: 771–782.

99. World Summit on Sustainable Development. Plan of implementation. Johannesburg, South Africa. http://www.un-documents.net/jburgpln.htm (Accessed September 28, 2013).

100. Werrity A. Sustainable flood management: oxymoron or new paradigm? *Area* 2006; 38(1): 16–23.

101. Feng S, Tan H, Benjamin A, et al. Social Support and Posttraumatic Stress Disorder among Flood Victims in Hunan, China. *Ann Epidemiol* 2007; 17: 827–833.

102. Keim ME. Preventing Disasters: Public Health Vulnerability Reduction as a Sustainable Adaptation to Climate Change. *Disaster Med Public Health Prep* June 2011; 5(2): 140–148.

103. Tapsell S, Penning-Rowsell E, Tunstall S, et al. Vulnerability to flooding: health and social dimensions. *Phil Trans R Soc Lond* 2002; 360: 1511–1525.

104. Anonymous. Katrina reveals fatal weaknesses in US public health. *Lancet* 2005; 366: 867. (Editorial).

105. Paul SK, Routray JK. Flood proneness and coping strategies: the experiences of two villages in Bangladesh. *Disasters* 2010; 34(2): 489–508.

106. Pielke RA, Jr., Downton MW, Miller JZB. *Flood Damage in the United States, 1926–2000: A Reanalysis of National*

Weather Service Estimates. Boulder, CO, UCAR, 2002. http://www.flooddamagedata.org (Accessed September 28, 2013).

107. US Department of Commerce. NOAA. National Weather Service. Floods: the awesome power. www.nws.noaa.gov/om/brochures/Floodsbrochure_9_04_low.pdf (Accessed September 28, 2013).

108. Kovacs P, Sandink D. Best practices for reducing the risk of future damage to homes from riverine and urban flooding. Toronto, Institute for Catastrophic Loss Reduction, 2009; 8.

109. Ardalan A, Naieni H, Kabir MJ, et al. Evaluation of Golestan provinces early warning system for flash floods, Iran, 2006–2007. *Int J Biometerol* 2009; 53: 247–254.

110. CDC. Outbreak of diarrheal illness associated with a natural disaster – Utah. *MMWR* 1983; 32(50): 662–664.

111. Navrud S, Tuan TH, Tinh BD. Estimating the welfare loss to households from natural disasters in developing countries: a contingent valuation study of flooding in Vietnam. *Global Health Action* 2009. 5: 1–11.

112. Nelson C, Lurie N, Wasserman J, et al. Conceptualizing and defining public health emergency preparedness. *Am J Pub Health* 2007; 97(S1): S9–S11.

113. deBoer J, Dubouloz M, ed. *Handbook of Disaster Medicine: Emergency Medicine in Mass Casualty Situations.* 2nd ed. Leiden, International Society of Disaster Medicine, 2000.

114. Keim M. Environmental Disasters. In: Frumkin H, ed. *Environmental Health: from global to local.* San Francisco, CA, John Wiley and Sons, Inc., 2010; 843–875.

115. Keim M. Developing a public health emergency operations plan: a primer. *Pac Health Dialog* 2002; 9: 124–129.

116. Keim ME. O2C3: A unified model for emergency operations planning. *Am J Disaster Med* May–June 2010; 5(3): 169–179.

117. Navrud S, Tuan TH, Tinh BD. Estimating the welfare loss to households from natural disasters in developing countries: a contingent valuation study of flooding in Vietnam. *Global Health Action* 2009; 5: 1–11.

118. Stimpson J, Wilson F, Jeffries S. Seeking Help for Disaster Services After a Flood. *Disaster Med Public Health Prep* 2008; 2: 139–141.

119. CDC. Early Warning Disease Surveillance After a Flood Emergency – Pakistan, 2010 *MMWR* 2012; 61(49): 1002–1007.

120. Lutgendorf SK, Antoni MH, Ironson G, Fletcher MA, Penedo S, Baum A, et al. Physical symptoms of chronic fatigue syndrome are exacerbated by the stress of Hurricane Andrew. *Psychosom Med* 1995; 57: 310–323.

36

CYCLONES, HURRICANES, AND TYPHOONS

Kelly R. Klein and Frank Fuh-Yuan Shih

OVERVIEW

Introduction

In the history of all ancient civilizations, there are tales in which a country or kingdom is saved by divine intervention. For example, when the Mongols sought to conquer Japan and complete their quest for control of all Asia, a divine wind known as the Kamikaze saved the Japanese people from the conquest of Kublai Khan by sinking the invasion fleet. This powerful storm, which saved Japan, is known today as a tropical cyclone.

During the past 100 years on coastlines throughout the world, these storms have caused deaths in the hundreds of thousands and property losses valued in the billions of dollars. The risk seems to be increasing as more people decide to live in vulnerable coastal areas. As discussed in the 1999 Hangzhou Declaration in China, more than half the world's population lives in coastal areas with several of the fastest growing cities (Jakarta, Shanghai, Miami, and New Orleans) projected to have 20–30 million inhabitants by the year 2025. It is estimated that by 2020, the U.S. coastal population will have grown from 123 million to 134 million people.[1] In addition, with the projected increase in number and intensity of tropical cyclones occurring due to climate change, this becomes a significant threat. The focus of this chapter is on the impact of tropical cyclones on human societies. This includes: 1) the consequences for public health; 2) the mortality and morbidity resulting from these events; 3) intervention measures such as evacuation; 4) medical preparedness for the affected population; and 5) mitigation, prevention, and response strategies for the medical community drawn from a global perspective.

Tropical Cyclones

Tropical cyclones, often referred to as hurricanes, cyclones, and typhoons, are given different names depending on their particular geographical locations (Table 36.1). All are capable of producing large-scale devastation.[2] In the northern hemisphere, from the International Date Line to the Greenwich meridian, they are known as hurricanes. In the Pacific, north of the equator and west of the International Date Line, they are

Table 36.1. Classification of Cyclones Based on Geographical Location

Hurricane: the North Atlantic Ocean, the Northeast Pacific Ocean east of the date line, or the South Pacific Ocean east of 160E

Typhoon: the Northwest Pacific Ocean west of the date line

Severe tropical cyclone: the Southwest Pacific Ocean west of 160E or Southeast Indian Ocean east of 90E

Severe cyclonic storm: the North Indian Ocean

Tropical cyclone: the Southwest Indian Ocean

known as typhoons. In the Indian Ocean, they are known as cyclones.

The tropical cyclone, among the most destructive of weather systems, is defined meteorologically as a storm system characterized by a low-pressure center with thunderstorms that produces strong winds and flooding rain.[3] These storms are capable of producing up to 20 billion tons of rainwater per day.[4,5] It is estimated that the strength of a fully developed hurricane contains the equivalent energy of 2 million Hiroshima-sized atomic bombs, although only 3–4% of this potential is ever realized.

These massive storms originate over tropical or subtropical oceans and derive the energy that sustains them from the warm waters. The highly organized storm systems consist of a warm center of low barometric pressure surrounded by a definite cyclonic surface wind circulation. They begin as fragile meteorological entities that require several factors to ensure their formation.

1. Warm oceanic waters that have a temperature of at least 26.5°C.
2. An atmosphere that cools rapidly with moist layers at mid-troposphere elevations to enhance thunderstorm formations.
3. The Coriolis forces to rotate the winds and the near-surface disturbance to create a vortex with minimal vertical wind shear.

Table 36.2. Storm Progression

Storm Type	Top Wind Speeds	Duration	Metrological Features
Tropical/Easterly Wave	variable	24 hours	Low pressure moving westward through the trade wind easterlies. Associated with extensive cloudiness and showers.
Tropical Disturbance	variable	>24 hours	Area of organized convection. Often the first developmental stage of any subsequent tropical depression, storm, or cyclone.
Tropical Depression	<16 m/s (38 mph)		Having 1 or more closed isobars (line drawn on the weather map of equal barometric pressures).
Tropical Storm	>17 m/s (39 mph)		No classical developed eye.
			Rain bands form outward from the center
			Given a name and it is tracked.
Cyclone	>33 m/s (74 mph)		Classic well-developed eye and eyewall. Clear spiral shape with formation of spiral rain bands emanating from eye wall.

Cyclonic systems, which may last over open waters for more than 2 weeks, rotate counterclockwise in the northern hemisphere and clockwise in the southern hemisphere with the general storm movement of east to west. As the storm develops, it progresses through successive meteorological stages: tropical wave, tropical disturbance, tropical depression, tropical storm, and cyclone (Table 36.2). The life cycle of tropical storms may be divided into four distinct stages: formative, deepening, mature, and decay. They strengthen over water by the energy released from differences between water and upper atmospheric temperatures. These cyclones are further defined by degrees of barometric pressure, precipitation counts, and the radius of their cloud mass. Due to reduction of temperature disparity, they weaken on landfall. The moment of landfall is defined as the intersection of the surface center of a cyclone with a coastline. Occasionally two mature-stage tropical cyclones will directly interact with each other in a phenomenon known as the Fujiwhara effect. Under the correct conditions, the Fujiwhara effect occurs when the distance between two cyclones is within 550–1,300 km (300–700 nautical miles) and the two storms begin rotating around each other (Figure 36.1). A recent example was Hurricane Sandy in the United States. This storm, although not considered

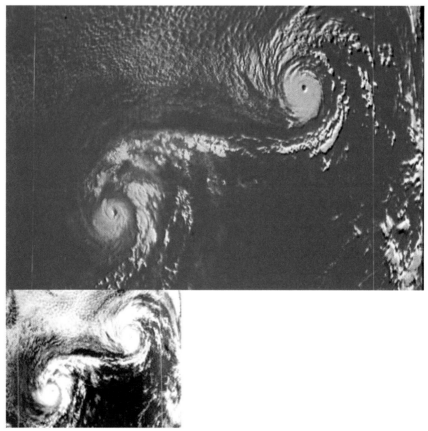

Figure 36.1. Fujiwhara effect, Typhoons Ione and Kirsten, August 24, 1974. Image ID: wea00481, NOAA's National Weather Service (NWS) Collection. *Source:* NOAA Photo Library.

Table 36.3. Saffir-Simpson Hurricane Scale

Category	km/h (mph)	Storm Surge meters (feet)	Damage caused
Tropical Depression	0–62 (0–38)	0 (0)	None
Tropical Storm	63–117 (39–73)	0–0.9 (0–3)	None
1 Minimal	119–153 (74–95)	1.2–1.5 (4–5)	Minimal to buildings and structures; primarily to unanchored mobile homes, shrubbery, and trees; some coastal road flooding and minor pier damage
2 Moderate	154–177 (96–110)	1.8–2.4 (6-8)	Some roofing material, door, and window damage; considerable damage to vegetation, mobile homes, and piers; small craft in unprotected anchorages break moorings
3 Extensive	178–209 (111–130)	2.7–3.7 (9–12)	Structural damage to small residences and utility buildings with a minor amount of curtain wall failures; mobile homes are destroyed; flooding near the coast destroys smaller structures with larger structures damaged by floating debris
4 Extreme	210–249 (131–155)	4–5.5 (13–18)	More extensive curtain wall failures with some complete roof structure failure on small residences; major beach erosions; major damage to lower floors of structures near the shore
5 Catastrophic	>250 (>156)	>5.5 (>18)	Complete roof failure on many residences and industrial buildings; some complete building failures with small utility buildings blown over or away; major damage to lower floors of all structures located less than 3 m (15 ft.) above sea level

powerful if measured by wind speed alone, interacted with a larger extra-tropical storm, imparting more total kinetic energy to the hurricane. Therefore, the destructive impact of Sandy was more consistent with a typical hurricane with higher wind speeds. In addition, the hurricane-storm interaction caused Sandy to move more slowly and unpredictably, making direction and impact area prognostication more difficult.

Tropical cyclones cause loss of life and property damage primarily due to storm surge, strong winds, and floods from the inundating rains. Storm surge is the rising ocean water level driven by wind and the speed of the storm against the coastline along shallow ocean shelves. This results in significant coastal flooding. It is expressed in terms of height above normal tide levels. In 2012, Hurricane Sandy created a catastrophic storm surge due to its tremendous size, causing an estimated 147 direct deaths in the states of New York and New Jersey.[6] In addition, secondary disasters often accompany these cyclones by creating or exacerbating new or existing hazards. Such secondary events induced by a hurricane include tornadoes, landslides, mudslides, and flooding due to levee breaches.

Tropical cyclones are graded based on wind speed using the Saffir-Simpson scale (Table 36.3) or the Australian Tropical Cyclone Intensity scale. Both scales use a 1–5 rating, based on the tropical cyclone's present intensity and peak sustained wind speed. These scales are used to estimate potential property damage and the degree of flooding expected along the coast after the tropical cyclone has made landfall. It is important to remember that although the intensity of the winds is predictive of damage, the speed with which a storm travels through an area also has significant impact. A slow-moving storm can cause more damage by increasing the geographic area exposure time to high winds, rainfall, and flooding.

One of the most devastating meteorological manifestations of the tropical cyclone is its storm surge. The height of the surge can be calculated, and in the United States, the SLOSH (Sea, Lake, and Overland Surges from Hurricanes) computer program is frequently used for this purpose. Depending on the slope of the continental shelf, the storm surge can be quite massive and destructive. Its impact is exacerbated by topographical changes in the local landscape due to deforestation, topsoil erosion, and increased coastal construction. With deforestation and reclaiming of marshlands along coastlines, no natural barriers exist to block the water and wind. Therefore, the cyclone's effects are carried much further inland, increasing the area and population vulnerable to such devastation as landslides and building collapse (Figure 36.2).

As storm surge is the movement of ocean water above high tide, inundation is the height of water on dry land caused by the surge. The severe effects of storm surge are augmented by the phase of the moon, local tide, and the storm's extremely low barometric pressures. Each millibar reduction of air pressure will cause the water surface to rise 1 cm. Therefore, the more intense the storm (lower barometric pressure), the greater the storm surge.[7] In 1899, Tropical Cyclone Mahina produced a surge of 14.6 meters (approximately 48 feet) with fish and dolphins reportedly found on top of 15-meter cliffs.[8] The Galveston, Texas hurricane in the United States that killed 8,000 people in 1900 produced a 5-meter storm surge that flooded the island, which has a maximum height of only 3 meters. In 2005, during Hurricane Katrina, a recorded surge wave averaging 2 meters traveled as far inland as 19 km.

CURRENT STATE OF THE ART

Health Consequences and Public Health

Recent large destructive cyclonic storms such as Hurricanes Katrina and Sandy in the United States, as well as Typhoon Nari in Taiwan reaffirm the complex challenge of providing effective public health planning for such events, especially for those with functional or access needs (special populations). Burkle and Rupp stated that disasters, "keep governments and planners honest by defining public health and exposing its vulnerabilities."[9] Noji noted that a variety of public health emergencies share a

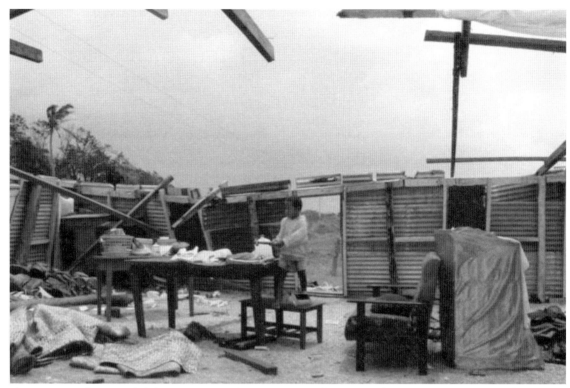

Figure 36.2. Cyclone Evan left devastation over Fiji in 2012. *Source:* http://www.aljazeera.com/news/asia-pacific/2012/12/2012121851221427672.html.

common theme by negatively impacting the public health environment and its protective infrastructure. Specific vulnerabilities include the provision of water, sanitation, shelter, food, and basic health. It is well-known that poverty and social inequality, environmental degradation from inappropriate land use, and a rapid population growth all contribute to the negative public health effects of a tropical cyclone's landfall.[10]

After experiencing a cyclone, levels of resilience to acute and chronic stress and any subsequent catastrophic shock are typically lowered for individuals and groups. An increased risk of susceptibility exists to diseases, both physical and mental. Acutely, the large number of deaths, illnesses, and injuries caused by the cyclone overwhelm the local health services. The destruction of hospitals and clinics by the storm further compromise the immediate medical response and also the provision of long-term care. Depending on the storm's magnitude, the greatest potential for loss of life does not necessarily come from the actual event, but instead from the subsequent everyday health risks such as reduced access to potable water, failure of sanitation systems, lack of care for medical and psychiatric conditions, and exposure to insect vectors.

The public is generally aware that tropical cyclones are capable of causing devastating damage that can severely cripple, if not destroy, a society and its infrastructure. Yet, it is expected by the effected community, both in the United States and internationally, that established public health and healthcare systems will continue to provide services not only in the days leading up to the storm, but during and after the event as well.[11] As a result of these demands, it is imperative that the medical and public healthcare communities are prepared to not only manage injuries caused by the storm, but also to provide continued care for patients with chronic medical conditions and functional or access needs

(see Chapter 10). Typically, these include victims with hypertension, diabetes, renal failure requiring dialysis, mental illness, physical disabilities, and cancer receiving chemotherapy. This is in addition to ensuring safe public drinking water, appropriate sewage disposal, control of disease vectors such as mosquitoes and rats, food distribution, and protection of food supplies from contamination (Table 36.4).

Evacuations

Ideally, no one would be physically present to suffer death or injury during the landfall of a devastating tropical cyclone. In fact, due to their well-defined paths of travel and the use of modern meteorological tracking systems, the movement for 70% of hurricanes will be forecasted 24 hours in advance of their approach to land based on their speed and direction during the previous 24–36 hours.[12] Based on these predictions, people in vulnerable areas are often asked to evacuate voluntarily while local officials assist by changing traffic flow patterns. Often, the contra flow technique is employed, in which both lanes of a roadway are used for outgoing traffic. Researchers have observed that, depending on local and personal experiences, citizens will engage in two opposing types of behavior prior to an evacuation order. They will either spontaneously self-evacuate or, despite storm warnings and subsequent evacuation orders, refuse to comply and remain in their homes, sheltered in the same way they have done in previous years during storms.[13] During Hurricane Sandy, despite strong warnings from emergency management, which included 33,000 telephone calls, use of electronic media and emails, knocking on individual doors, and requesting support from local traditional media sources, thousands of New Yorkers did not evacuate. Data from an official survey conducted by

Table 36.4. Impact of Cyclones and Storm Surges on the Community Components and Indicators of Effects

Categories of Impact	Components Involved	Indicators of Impact
Physical	Inadequate physical protection; poor-quality housing and infrastructure; disruptions of communication, roads, utilities, and public works infrastructure	Trauma-related death tolls; damage/loss of property such as infrastructure, homes, industry, animals, and crops; disruption of normal life; migration to safe places; lack of electricity, potable water, and food; accumulation of waste
Economic	Loss of livelihood and income opportunities; loss of assets and savings; need for recurrent aid; lower socioeconomic stratification	Low income, poverty, unemployment, landlessness, unequal land distribution, lack of relief and rehabilitation, and forced movement of lower-income populations
Agricultural	Land degradation; intrusion of salt water for irrigation increasing seasonal unplanted fields	Low productivity, frequent crop loss, outbreak of migration among the owners of small farms and farm laborers; lack of money for purchasing seed
Social	Disintegration of social organization, increased incidence of female-headed households and resource-poor communities; poor educational services	Social/ethnics crisis; social marginalization, violence, and crime; apathetic attitude; identity crisis; plight of people with decreased options for safety and survival
Environmental	Land and environmental degradation; deforestation, loss of biodiversity and marine resources, increase in salinity, intrusion of salt water, lowering of water table, increase risk to dams	Deforestation; loss of soil fertility; limited biodiversity; increase in refugees, migrants, and the homeless; rising disaster-related deaths
Public Health	Disruptions of healthcare and utility services, inadequate sanitation, lack of qualified physician and clinical services, lack of care for vulnerable groups	Increased mortality and morbidity; poor health and malnutrition; disease epidemics; exacerbation of chronic diseases; increase in PTSD

New York City showed that 22% felt that the storm would not be strong enough to pose a danger, 11% felt that their home was high enough to prevent property flooding, and 8% felt there home was structurally sound enough to withstand the storm.[14]

Evacuation is a very complex undertaking requiring the coordination of multiple unique endeavors, not the least of which is maintaining basic public health services for evacuees. In addition to logistics, cost is an issue. This includes not only the expenses related to the evacuation itself, but also of lost revenue to displaced individuals and to local industry. Therefore, the decision to evacuate an area has significant ramifications.

Hospitals also face the threat of hurricane-induced evacuations. From the years 1971–1999 in the United States, hurricanes prompted more than thirty-eight hospital evacuations.[15] Evidence from hospital evacuations after Hurricane Rita suggest it will take an average of approximately 22 hours (range 6–32 hours) to transfer patients out of a facility.[16]

Many countries other than the United States do not support mass evacuations in the face of a storm. For example, in Taiwan, a community that is frequently subjected to tropical cyclones, most of the buildings are wind-resistant. Only people who live in flood plains, mudslide prone areas, or who are physically disabled or dependent are considered for evacuation.[17]

The decision to evacuate is based on available resources and an estimate of the resulting economic impact as well as the potential loss of life. Because storm landfall predictions can lead to expensive evacuation preparations and subsequent disruptive population movements, individuals involved in making such decisions must consider the potential negative impacts of an evacuation on commercial, healthcare, and other public health activities. Making the decision to evacuate is a challenge for administrators and community leaders, and involves deciding who should be evacuated, when the evacuation should start, and the logistics for the evacuation. Such logistic considerations include mass transportation, traffic patterns, and provision of control and security. There are four major event outcomes for which the evacuation decision will either enhance or damage the credibility of the decision-makers. These are dependent on what happens during the event itself:[18]

■ Evacuation with direct damage to the area or structure evacuated: no lives lost due to the damage nor credibility lost but large economic costs through loss of revenue and expenses incurred.
■ Evacuation with no damage to the area: no lives lost due to the storm but a loss of credibility with large economic costs through loss of revenue and expenses incurred.
■ No evacuation with damage to structures and area: even if no lives lost due to the damage, there is a loss of credibility and a large economic cost due to repair and loss of revenue.
■ No evacuation with no damage to the area in the absence of a direct impact: no lives lost, no credibility lost, and no economic effects.

Research indicates that, once an evacuation decision is made, a considerable amount of time (up to 2 hours using conventional warning practices) may elapse before people in the affected area hear, absorb, and respond to the instructions.[19] The time required to accomplish the evacuation once the physical movement of people is underway depends on the characteristics of the area and on the availability of public transportation and large highways (Table 36.5). It is intuitive to believe that a larger population requires a longer evacuation time, but warning and evacuation times do not necessarily increase with population size and density. This is true, in part, because the infrastructure capacity (for example, street systems and public transportation resources) necessary for moving individuals out of the area is generally more extensive in regions with a greater population.[20]

Table 36.5. Time considerations for phases of evacuation

Evacuation Phase	Time Needed
Reaching an official decision to evacuate	Days
Mobilizing community evacuation resources	Hours
Communicating appropriate protective action instructions to the public	Hours
Individual mobilization of resources to leave the area at risk	Hours to days
Completing the physical evacuation of people occupying the affected area	Days

In areas where a significant reluctance to evacuate exists, the evacuation routes are limited despite the use of contra flow techniques, or population density is high, repeated warnings may be necessary. Characteristics of a good evacuation plan include:

■ Identification of available resources, such as community faith-based organizations and voluntary medical and fire assets.

■ Knowledge of vulnerable populations, which would include those who are elderly, ventilator-dependent, and have language barriers.

■ Awareness of hazardous sites in the area: flood zones, refineries, and hazardous material sites.

■ Knowledge about main transportation assets: highways, trains, buses, and airports.

■ Shelter locations and staging areas for evacuation.

Mortality

In violent tropical cyclones, almost 90% of all primary weather-related deaths are attributed to drowning from the accompanying storm surge. Examples include the cyclones that affected Bangladesh in 1970 and 1991, the Indian coastal states of Andhra Pradesh in 1977 and Orissa in 1999, the Indian state of Gujarat along its coast facing the Arabian Sea in 1998, and the U.S. state of Mississippi in 2005 (Hurricane Katrina). The other 10% result from tornadoes, flying debris, and collapsing structures.[12,21,22] More recently in 2012, Hurricane Sandy on the east coast of the United States caused the direct deaths of more than 147 people, primarily due to storm surge. Almost half of them were more than 65 years of age.[14] In Taiwan and many other Asian/Pacific basin countries, mortality numbers due to storm surge and mudslides remain quite high despite warnings. This has been attributed to deforestation, which allows for mudslides and debris to flow through farming communities during the torrential rainstorms that accompany tropical cyclones. Many countries prone to damage from storm surge have installed early warning systems, which if used in conjunction with timely evacuations and storm-resistant sheltering, can achieve a decrease in mortality rates. Prediction and warning systems have been credited with protecting lives in the Mississippi counties of Mobile and Baldwin. Here, computer models predicted a large storm surge 2 days in advance of the hurricane's arrival, allowing for evacuation and adequate preparation.

In the countries of Bangladesh and Cuba, storm-related mortality rates are lower despite the lack of sophisticated electronic warning systems. This is due to the use of trained volunteers who implement a well-known and easily recognizable flag and siren signal system. When Hurricane Charley struck Cuba, only four deaths occurred despite damages estimated at more than $1 billion USD.[23,24] Conversely, simply having the technology will not guarantee a decrease in mortality. This was seen in Haiti during Tropical Storm Jeanne in 2004. The area had a good electronic warning system, but due to a coup earlier that year, there were no emergency managers available to utilize the system and more than 1,000 people died.[25] In general, the disparity between developing and developed countries remains significant. In developing countries, the majority of cyclone-related deaths result from storm surge in the impact phase, while in developed countries, mortality has declined markedly. The majority of deaths in developed countries that do result from cyclones occur in the post-impact phase.

Morbidity

During a tropical cyclone disaster, there are phase-specific morbidity patterns. Understanding these patterns may help with medical and emergency planning. There are four distinct phases of the disaster that produce morbidity. In the pre-landfall phase, injuries result from storm preparation and evacuation activities. Typical problems include car crashes and falls from ladders. When the tropical cyclone makes landfall, injuries occur from non-reinforced structure collapse, wind-borne debris, falling trees, near-drowning, and downed power lines. In the immediate post-impact phase, traumatic injuries result from electrocution by downed power lines, blunt trauma, or fractures from falling objects and trees, and severe lacerations from chainsaws as people clear debris from houses and roadways. As a result of power outages, burn injuries and carbon monoxide poisoning may occur from devices used improperly for cooking and lighting as well as poorly ventilated gas-powered generators.[21] During the post-impact phase, a surge occurs in the demand for healthcare by citizens with chronic medical conditions. Interventions such as dialysis and medication refills for hypertension, diabetes, psychiatric illnesses, and chronic pain are needed. During the recovery phase of the disaster, acute care needs transition to chronic care. Within weeks, the increased need for generalists, pediatricians, obstetricians, nephrologists, psychiatrists, and cancer specialists replaces the need for surgeons and emergency medicine providers.

The provision of mental health services for victims and rescuers is an important component of any disaster recovery process (see Chapter 9). Therefore, recovery plans should include the involvement of psychiatrists and mental health workers. Patients will require continued treatment of their addictions, depression, schizophrenia, and other psychiatric problems. In addition, services are needed for victims suffering from acute stress syndromes and post-traumatic stress disorder (PTSD).[26]

Many people initially experience fear and distress at the time of tropical cyclone's impact, but the majority of them quickly return to normal. However, some may experience persistent distress that affects functional capability, and a subset of these individuals will progress to PTSD. In the United States, surveillance systems detected increases in rates of psychological disorders after hurricanes. Victims developed new disorders they had not previously experienced and included illnesses such as PTSD, major depression, and anxiety. Risk factors attributable to adverse mental health outcomes include: 1) the severity of an individual's exposure to a family member's injury or death; 2) suffering extensive property loss or displacement; 3) belonging to a vulnerable group such as women, children, the elderly, and the poor; and 4) the presence of existing psychopathology. Social support, high self-esteem, and positive coping strategies can ease the severity of mental health consequences. Early intervention allows mental health professionals to triage those with an increased risk for more severe mental illness.[27]

Infectious and Environmental Disease

The likelihood of infectious disease outbreaks in a community following a tropical cyclone may increase for a multitude of reasons: disruption of public health services and healthcare infrastructure, damage to water and sanitation networks, population displacement, and crowded conditions in temporary shelters. Fecal-oral routes of infection are often the cause and result in outbreaks of diseases such as cholera, hepatitis, Shigella, and other diarrheal illnesses. In crowded shelters, outbreaks of measles and meningitis have been reported, but not in epidemic proportions.

In regions of the globe where infectious disease vectors such as mosquitoes and fleas are already present in the ecosystem, outbreaks of diseases such as typhoid fever, encephalitis, or plague may occur under certain conditions. For example, following flood inundations in tropical areas, ecological conditions are frequently optimal for mosquito reproduction. In 1963, 75,000 cases of *Plasmodium falciparum*, a potentially fatal form of malaria, were recorded in Haiti following Hurricane Flora. This is much higher than the number of infections normally observed.[28] Despite a popular disaster myth, if a disease pathogen is not normally present in the affected area, that particular disease cannot occur in that region despite ideal environmental conditions. [29]

Populations with Functional or Access Needs

Ethics experts have said that the true measure of a society's greatness is how it protects those least able to care for themselves. Recent large cyclonic storms such as Hurricanes Katrina and Rita in the United States and Typhoon Nari in the western Pacific underscore the necessity of meeting the complex challenges of public health planning for individuals with functional or access needs. Disaster coordinators should ensure that emergency management plans address this population (see Chapter 10). Studies in the United States indicate that up to 19% of the general population is disabled. Often, people with functional or access needs have difficulty receiving and understanding public emergency broadcasts due to language barriers or physical limitations. They also have difficulty taking protective actions such as moving to a "special needs" shelter or complying with evacuation orders. In addition to persons with physical disabilities, other individuals that belong to the functional or access needs population include:

- People without access to transportation or who lack financial resources.
- People who do not speak English or who communicate differently (the hearing impaired).
- Migrant workers, homeless persons, visitors, and tourists.
- People who are in congregate facilities (for example, schools, hospitals, nursing homes, and prisons).
- Women and children in countries where they are disenfranchised due to their status in society.

The functional and access needs population is an important but challenging one to include in the disaster planning process. It is clear they will require much in the way of resources during a tropical cyclone disaster. It is essential that emergency managers anticipate the needs of this population and create appropriate plans. These written plans should be practiced and revised through exercises and drills to ensure assistance will be available to this important group.

Hospital Mitigation, Preparedness, Response, and Recovery

Pre-Impact Phase

Pre-event planning for a devastating tropical cyclone is essential for continued hospital operations during and after the disaster, and it starts years before it is needed. As previously stated, the public expects that hospitals and the healthcare system will continue treating current patients and also providing care to those seeking emergent medical attention regardless of what disaster has just occurred.[11] This means that hospitals, clinics, and medical personnel must have planned in advance and now be prepared to deal with the large number of issues associated with a tropical cyclone. These include loss of electricity, absence of fuel or food, emergency generator failure, tainted municipal drinking water supplies, hospital flooding, and personnel shortages. In addition, planning should address feeding the hospital's patients, their families, staff, and the staff's families.

Prior to the tropical cyclone season, it is imperative that emergency management programs are created to address the needs of the hospital and the community it serves. After managers have developed plans to support these comprehensive programs, they must be practiced and modified before the need to use them arises. They should incorporate a list of volunteers that includes medical personnel, environment workers, and social workers along with their current contact information. Plans should also include a current list of hospital assets such as ventilators and autoclaves and possible hospital hazards such as liquid oxygen tanks. Additional plan components should address: 1) morgue capabilities and contingency plans for managing the deceased when the morgue is full or power to cool the area is lost; 2) provision of staff emergency information kits; and 3) memoranda of understanding (MOUs) with other hospitals, vendors, and emergency medical services providers for support. Early evacuation of vulnerable in-patients within hospitals located in the tropical cyclone's path will avoid the danger of evacuation during the time of the storm. Plans should address what pharmaceuticals and the dispensed amounts, if any, to give in-patients when they are discharged (Table 36.6).

An often overlooked point in hospital disaster planning is addressing the needs of vulnerable community members such as the elderly, the infirmed, and those who are ventilator- or oxygen-dependent. These individuals will frequently use the hospital for shelter and basic care when surrounding infrastructure fails and floodwaters rise. In this situation, social workers are incredibly important. They can compile a list of 24-hour pharmacies, oxygen companies that will deliver canisters, and shelters that can accept patients when they are discharged from the hospitals. Social workers often have this information as they manage these issues on a daily basis.

Depending on available resources, preparation should include sandbags, potable water, fuel supply for generators, batteries, functioning backup generators, and communication

Table 36.6. Personal and Institutional Needs

Personal	Institutional Considerations	
A week's supply of prescription medication	Infrastructure	Generators that are biannually tested
An extra pair of glasses or contact lenses plus lens solution		Generators in a location that will not flood
		Fuel tanks for generators in a location that will not flood and taint the fuel
A week's supply of potable water (2.5–3 L/day depending on climate)		Fuel tanks located for easy access to refueling
Full tank of fuel for generators and vehicles		Fuel tanks filled pre-event
Clothing appropriate to weather conditions		Potable water stored
		Morgue on the generator circuit
Flashlight		MOU with fuel vendors to ensure resupply
Family evacuation plan with understood rendezvous points		MOU with emergency generator companies to provide support in case of generator failure
		Sandbags and lumber for windows and doors
		MOU for liquid oxygen supplier
	Operations	Plan for emergency staffing and post-event cleanup staff
		List of essential jobs to include housekeeping, nursing, social work, laboratory technicians, respiratory therapy, cafeteria support staff, and cooks
		Accurate contact list for all personnel
		MOU with food vendors
		MOU with other hospitals in case of evacuation
		MOU with transportation vendors
		MOU with ventilator companies
		Downtime areas for staff and their families
		Pharmacy supplies for staff and families
		Essential medications for discharged patients
		Evacuation plans
		Operating room supplies such as autoclaves, sterile instruments, etc.
		Intensive care operations supplies

alternatives and contacting systems. As an example of such communication alternatives, New York City sent more than 2,000 tweets and gained more than 17,500 social media followers during Hurricane Sandy.[30] Employees should be given information regarding personal preparedness items that they should have for themselves and their family (Table 36.6).

For hospitals not at risk of damage from the tropical cyclone, an adequate number of critical care beds should be available for transfer of patients from other hospitals or in case of mass casualties from the storm. Many hospitals will decide to evacuate at the same time so coordinating these patient movements is ideally done by the regional emergency operations center.[15,30] This was seen during the aftermath of hurricane Katrina, when multiple hospitals in New Orleans evacuated after the levees failed. It was estimated by the New Orleans Times – Picayune on August 31, 2005, that 1,600 hospital patients and 8,600 staff and their families awaited rescue. This number did not include those needing assistance at nursing homes and in assisted living centers. Many of these hospitals had prearranged contracts with ambulance companies, bus companies, and private EMS helicopters. Others did not have such MOUs but were able to secure

verbal agreements when the need arose.[31] After Hurricane Sandy, five hospitals and approximately thirty nursing homes and adult care facilities in New York City had to evacuate due to damage from the storm.[14] Hospital cafeterias should anticipate the need to provide food for all patients, medical staff, their families, and the general public who expect the hospital to remain open.[32] Medical staff should be prepared to remain at the hospital for at least 72 hours or until relief arrives. They should bring with them personal supplies including potable water, non-perishable food, person hygiene items, and personal medications if not provided by the hospital.

Impact Phase and Immediate Aftermath

Typically, hospitals experience a lull in emergency department visits during the time the tropical cyclone makes landfall and in the storm's immediate aftermath. Once the storm has cleared the area, there is a rapid increase in visits to the hospital, mostly for emergency trauma care. In planning for this phase of the disaster, managers should be aware that most patients will not require advanced life support. In fact, medical data from three tropical cyclones affecting Taiwan indicate that only one-fifth of the patients needed an ambulance for transportation to the hospital and that 90% of the patients seen for emergency care did not require hospitalization. The most common injuries recorded were soft tissue trauma followed by head injuries and orthopedic problems such as sprains and fractures.[17]

From a staffing perspective, the hospital will need environmental crews to assist with cleanup and engineers to assess buildings for signs of damage. Other personnel required to support medical care needs include nurses to staff floor beds; operating room staff to care for trauma victims as well as non-disaster related surgical cases such as appendicitis; intensive care unit personnel; and extra emergency department staff to assist with storm-related injuries.

Post-Impact Phase

This phase can last days to years depending on the magnitude of the tropical cyclone and the devastation that it has brought to the area. Hospital effects can vary from minor flooding damage to permanent closure, as was seen in New Orleans after Hurricane Katrina. The functional status of hospitals will influence what actions are necessary to return a community to baseline health and medical status. In many countries, disaster response teams exist that respond quickly and offer assistance provided by medical professionals including surgeons, pediatricians, midwives, and emergency medicine providers. The assignment of such teams to the disaster area is temporary, with deployments lasting a few weeks but generally not months.

If there is widespread devastation, establishing alternate care sites may be an option. This would help hospitals manage the initial onslaught of victims requesting emergency medical care and allow institutions to more effectively distribute the patient load. Surge facilities, staffed by community providers or government assets delivering healthcare to patients with non-acute to moderately acute medical needs, should be available for at least a week after the cyclone makes landfall to meet the transient rapid rise in demand for healthcare.[33] Conversely, if the hospital has sustained only minor damage, then the need for a surge facility would be reduced. Planning for this phase is challenging because it is difficult to anticipate how events will unfold after each tropical cyclone. An example is the impact of Hurricane Katrina on the city of New Orleans. There would not have been the devastation that occurred if the levees had not collapsed and flooded parts of the city.

In the recovery phase, hospitals must be ready to support the community. If there has been a drop in municipal water pressure, water sources must be tested before hospital administrators permit use for drinking and equipment sterilization.[32] In the weeks following a devastating tropical cyclone, trauma and acute care needs gradually evolve to chronic illnesses and psychological needs. Patients with renal failure will need routine dialysis, patients with cancer will require continued chemotherapy or radiation treatments, people will exhaust their supplies of medications and need refills, patients with chronic conditions will suffer acute manifestations, and victims with depression and other debilitating psychological illnesses will present to hospitals requesting assistance. Staffing will be stretched thin and many people might not return to work as their personal life issues will take precedent. Others might move out of the area entirely and seek new employment elsewhere. Within a few weeks to months after the event, the emergency assistance personnel originally dispatched to the disaster zone from outside the area will return to their communities. Those living in the devastated areas must begin rebuilding their community. There are no easy answers or simple templates to support this reconstruction effort. Hard work and communication within the community and with the local and regional governments will facilitate movement toward the goal of return to normalcy.

Pharmaceutical Needs

Part of disaster planning is deciding which medical supplies should be stockpiled for a tropical cyclone and its aftermath. Many of the lists and recommendations available are based on hearsay and personal experiences. There is a paucity of evidence-based literature available for use by hospitals, clinics, or disaster medical teams. Nufer and Wilson-Ramirez examined the medical needs of patients following two hurricanes and found that wounds, musculoskeletal pain, medication refills, upper respiratory infections, rashes, and abdominal complaints were the most common conditions in people seeking emergency care.[34] Following Hurricane Andrew, the U.S. Centers for Disease Control and Prevention conducted a rapid health needs assessment of the impacted population. Analysis of this medical treatment data demonstrated that 16% of households in Florida and Louisiana were unable to obtain prescription drugs to treat acute and chronic medical conditions for 3–10 days after the hurricane.[35] Emergency departments in New York City recorded an increase in patients requesting dialysis and methadone due to unexpectedly prolonged closure of their out-patient treatment facilities after Hurricane Sandy.[30]

Based on this observational literature, an apparent need exists for the following medications in the immediate aftermath of a cyclone: tetanus toxoid, oral and parental antibiotics, insulin and oral hypoglycemics, cardiac medications, respiratory agents, anti-epileptics, analgesics, gastrointestinal drugs, and psychotherapeutics.[36,37] Medications needed after an event can be modeled after an average community hospital's normal emergency department pharmacy usage because chronic diseases will still require treatment.[36] From this information, medications could be easily stockpiled for both emergency treatment and for medication refills until normal pharmacy services are restored or outside assistance is available.

For catastrophic disasters resulting in total collapse of a region's medical infrastructure, World Health Organization, United Nations Children's Fund, High Commissioner for Refugees, Médecins Sans Frontières, International Federation of the Red Cross and Red Crescent Societies, and other groups designed the Interagency Emergency Health Kit in 2011.[38] It was created to meet the primary health needs of a displaced population of 100,000 people for 3 months. The kit includes medicines, disposable items, sterilizable instruments, and basic sterilization equipment. The Basic Unit is intended for use by primary healthcare workers with limited training. The Supplementary Unit is designed for physicians and advanced practitioners and is used to augment the Basic Unit if there are advanced providers available.

RECOMMENDATIONS FOR FURTHER RESEARCH

Tropical cyclones will have a disproportionally greater impact on areas that are socioeconomically depressed. The more extensive the poverty, the more devastating will be the disruption to infrastructure, public health, and ability to provide medical care. In developing countries or poverty-stricken areas of wealthy nations, tropical cyclone mortality continues to be significant, with the majority of deaths occurring from storm surge. In situations where the local and regional infrastructure has been severely damaged, morbidity is more evenly distributed throughout the population, causing devastating and long-term consequences to the affected region. Governments and nongovernmental organizations throughout the world have been working diligently to improve mitigation and preparedness efforts in areas prone to these devastating storms. The frequency and intensity of these events seem to be increasing due to climate change. There have been successes in reducing mortality in many developing and wealthy nations by using early warning systems, improving building codes so structures are better able to withstand tropical cyclone winds, creating storm-safe shelters, and implementing early evacuation in areas at risk from flooding, landslides, and storm surge. These projects work well as long as the government remains stable and provides political and economic support to these mitigation efforts.

Further studies are needed regarding hospital design and construction techniques to minimize flooding of critical areas and generator failures like those seen in the Houston floods in 2001 following Tropical Storm Allison. Hospitals should examine the location of critical patient care areas within their facilities, develop designs that permit expeditious and safe evacuations, and eliminate elements that could make evacuation difficult. Additionally, better studies are needed to create appropriate recommendations for healthcare response teams. Multidisciplinary study groups should investigate alternate methods of population evacuation such as the use of boats, buses, and trains where feasible.

Issues such as evacuation of acute care hospitals and facilities providing long-term care require more in-depth study. Traditionally, most of the papers written about this topic are case reports that do not examine hospital evacuation as a regional process in a systematic manner. The studies by Downey et al. are a major step forward in examining multiple hospital evacuations using a systematic approach and also examining the issue as it integrates with the community response.[16] More such studies are needed to better define how facilities should prepare for and execute an evacuation of large in-patient populations.

The process of mitigation, preparation, response, and recovery from the effects of a tropical cyclone is a very complex and expensive process for public health and hospitals. These entities are expected to remain open and functional regardless of the disaster's intensity. It is important that hospital and public health employees feel secure and that they are adequately prepared. Plans should address infrastructure requirements, staffing, provision of psychological care, and community needs. More intensive investigations in these areas would be useful to ensure healthcare facilities remain functional and can provide appropriate services after a tropical cyclone.

REFERENCES

1. National Coastal Population Report. Population Trends from 1970–2020. http://stateofthecoast.noaa.gov/coastal-population-report.pdf (Accessed August 17, 2013).

2. Holland GJ. Ready Reckoner (see Chapter 9). In: *Global Guide to Tropical Cyclone Forecasting*. WMO/TC-No. 560, Report No. TCP-31. Geneva, World Meteorological Organization, 1993.

3. International Federation of Red Cross and Red Crescent Societies. *World Disasters Report 1993*. Norwell, MS, Kluwer Academic Publishers, 1993.

4. Alvarez R. Tropical Cyclone. In: Ingleton J, ed. *Natural Disaster Management*. Leicester, Tudor Rose, 1999; 34–36.

5. Gray W. General Characteristics of Tropical Cyclones. In: Pielke R, Pielke R, eds. *Storms*. vol 1. London, Routledge, 2000; 145–163.

6. Blake ES, Kimberlain TB, Berg RJ, Cangiolosi JP, Beven JL. Tropical Cyclone Report Hurricane Sandy (AL182012). October 22–29, 2012. National Hurricane Center. 2013.

7. McGuyire B, Mason I, Kilburn C. *Natural Hazards and Environmental Change*. London, Arnold, 2002.

8. NOAA. http://www.aoml.noaa.gov/hrd/tcfaq/E3.html (Accessed May 30, 2013).

9. Burkle FM, Jr., Rupp G. Hurricane Katrina: Disasters keep us honest(Commentary). *Monday Develop*. September 26, 2005; 23(17): 5.

10. Noji EK. The Nature of Disaster: General Characteristics and Public Health Effects. In: Noji EK ed. *The Public Health Consequences of Disasters*. New York, Oxford University Press, 1997; 3–20.

11. PAHO. *Mitigation of disasters in health facilities: Evaluation and reduction of physical and functional vulnerability*. vol. II: *Administrative issues*. Washington, DC, PAHO, 1993.

12. Alexander D. *Natural disasters*. New York, Chapman & Hall, Inc., 1993.

13. Perry RW, Lindel MK. Preparing for Emergency Response: Guidelines for the planning process. *Disasters* 2003; 27: 226–350.

14. Mapping Hurricane Sandy's Deadly Toll. *New York Times*. November 17, 2012. http://www.nytimes.com/interactive/2012/11/17/nyregion/hurricane-sandy-map.html?_r=0 (Accessed May 29, 2013).

15. Sternberg E, Lee GC, Huard D. Counting crises: US hospital evacuations, 1971–1999. *Prehosp Disaster Med* 2004; 1992: 150–157.

16. Downey EL, Andress K, Schultz CH. External Factors Impacting Hospital Evacuations Caused by Hurricane Rita: The Role of Situational Awareness. *Prehosp Disaster Med* 2013; 28(3): 264–271.

17. Shih FY. Risk Analysis of Disasters and Preventive Strategies: Implications for Taiwan. Doctoral dissertation, National Taiwan University, Taipei, 2007.

18. Lindell MK, Prater CS. A Hurricane Evacuation Management Decision Support System (EMDSS). *Nat Hazards* 2007; 40: 627–634.

19. Sorensen JH, Vogt BM, Mileti DS. Evacuation: An Assessment of Planning and Research, Report prepared for FEMA, RR-9, 1987.

20. Vogt BM, Sorensen JH. Evacuation research: a reassessment, ORNL/TM-11908. Oak ridge National Laboratory. Oak Ridge, TN. 1992.

21. Malilay J. Tropical Cyclones. In: Noji E, ed. *The Public Health Consequences of Disasters*. New York, NY, Oxford University Press, 1997.

22. Wisner B, Blaikie P, Cannon T, Davis I. At Risk: Natural hazards, people's vulnerability and disasters. *2nd ed*. New York, Routledge, 2004.

23. Organization of American States (OAS). Disasters, planning, and development: managing natural hazards to reduce loss. Washington, DC, OAS, Department of Regional Development and Environment, Executive Secretariat for Economic and Social Affairs, 1990.

24. Building the Resilience of Nations and Communities to Disasters: Iyogo Framework for Action 2005–2015, UN/ISDR, 2005.

25. Reuters. Talking Point: Why is Haiti so prone to disaster? http://reliefweb.int/report/haiti/talking-point-why-haiti-so-prone-disaster (Accessed September 9, 2015).

26. North CS, King RV, Polatin P, et al. Psychiatric illness among transported hurricane evacuees: acute phase findings in a large receiving shelter site. *Psychiatric Annals* 2008; 38(2): 104–114.

27. Rodriguez SR, Tocco JS, Mallonee S, Smithee L, Cathey T, Bradley K. Rapid Needs Assessment of Hurricane Katrina Evacuees-Oklahoma, September 2005. *Prehosp Disaster Med* 2006; 21(6): 390–395.

28. Toole MJ, Walkman RJ. The public health aspects of complex emergencies and refugee situations. *Ann Rev Public Health* 1997; 18: 283–312.

29. Committee on Research Priorities for Earth Science and Public Health and National Research Council. *Earth Materials and Health: Research Priorities for Earth Science and Public Health.* 1st ed. Washington DC, National Academies Press, 2007.

30. Gibbs LI, Holloway CF. Hurricane Sandy After Action: Report and Recommendations to Mayor Michael R. Bloomberg. May 2013. http://www.nyc.gov/html/recovery/downloads/pdf/sandy_aar_5.2.13.pdf (Accessed May 29, 2013).

31. Moller J. Fuel Shortages, security worry hospitals. *The New Orleans Times-Picayune.* August 31, 2005.

32. Klein KR, Rosenthal MS, Klausner HA. Blackout 2003: preparedness and lessons learned from the perspectives of four hospitals. *Prehosp Disaster Med* September–October 2005; 20(5): 343–349.

33. Meredith JT. Hurricanes. In: Hogan DE, Burstein JL, eds. *Disaster Medicine.* 2nd ed. Philadelphia, PA, Lippincott Williams & Wilkins, 2007.

34. Nufer KE, Wilson-Ramirez G. A comparison of patient needs following two hurricanes. *Prehosp Disast Med* 2004; 19(1): 146–149.

35. Rapid health needs assessment following Hurricane Andrew – Florida and Louisiana, 1992. *MMWR* 1992; 41: 687–688.

36. Rosenthal MS, Klein K, Cowling K, Grzybowski M, Dunne R. Disaster modeling: medication resources required for disaster team response. *Prehosp Disaster Med* 2005; 20: 309–315.

37. Sepehri G, Meimandi MS. The pattern of drug prescription and utilization among Bam residents during the first six months after the 2003 Bam Earthquake. *Prehosp Disaster Med* 2006; 21(6): 396–402.

38. Interagency Emergency Health Kit 2011: Medicines and medical devices for 10,000 people for approximately three months. http://whqlibdoc.who.int/publications/2011/9789241502115_eng.pdf (Accessed August 17, 2013).

37

TORNADOES

Arthur G. Wallace, Jr.

OVERVIEW

A tornado is a narrow, violently rotating column of air extending from the base of a thunderstorm to the surface with variable wind speed that can exceed 482.8 km/h (300 miles per hour) in the strongest of storms. Tornadoes occur in all of the continents with the exception of Antarctica (Figure 37.1).[1] The United States maintains the most detailed records of tornadoes and related data with other countries having lesser or minimal recorded information. The high tornado occurrence countries are the United States, Canada, Bangladesh, Britain, Argentina, and Brazil.[2]

Areas that have a high incidence of these storms share similar geographic and weather-related features that will be reviewed later. Worldwide, tornadoes can occur on any day and at any time. Springtime and the hours between 4:00 PM and 7:00 PM are the most prevalent times, with a peak time of 5:00 PM.[3]

There are a number of variables that determine the extent of physical damage, injury, and death. These include storm strength, population demographics in the storms track, time on the ground, structure design, and advanced warning times. The annual number of tornadoes worldwide is unclear. The United States has the largest number, with averages around 1,000 per year, while Canada comes second with approximately

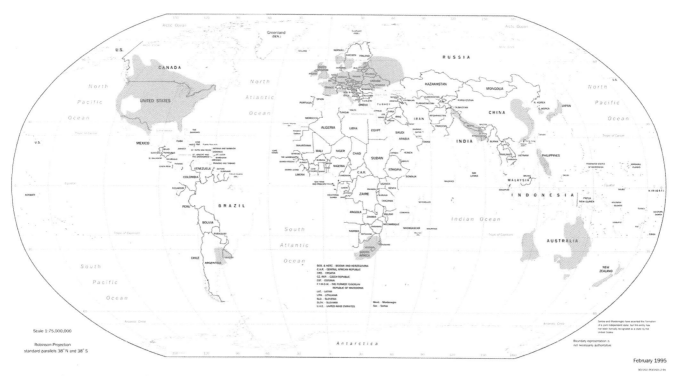

Figure 37.1. Tornadoes Around the World. Courtesy of the National Climatic Data Center of the National Weather Service.

1. 1,300 fatalities in Bangladesh on April 26, 1989
2. 747 fatalities in the United States on March 18, 1925
3. 700 fatalities in Bangladesh on May 13, 1996
4. 681 fatalities in Bangladesh on April 17, 1973
5. 660 fatalities in Bangladesh on April 14, 1969
6. 500 fatalities in Bangladesh on April 4, 1964
7. 500 fatalities in Bangladesh on April 1, 1977
8. 454 fatalities in the United States on April 5–6, 1936
9. 400 fatalities in Russia on June 9, 1984
10. 330 fatalities in the United States on March 21–22, 1932

Figure 37.2. Top Ten Deadliest Tornadoes on Record.

80 annually.[4] Although Bangladesh has fewer storms, it has the highest total mortality. This is due to the high population density, poor quality of construction, and other factors.[4] The most deadly tornadoes by numbers of fatalities and continent are listed in Figure 37.2.[5]

CURRENT STATE OF THE ART

In the framework of disaster management, the subcategories of mitigation, preparedness, response, and recovery will be considered in the context of tornado threats.

Mitigation: Activities that need to be performed before a tornado event include a broad range of categories. In order to reduce injury, death, and adverse health events, advance notification of potential storm risk and warning of imminent threats are paramount. Governmental meteorological agencies typically direct these activities. "Lead time," discussed in more detail later in the chapter, is the time interval from issuing a tornado warning to tornado impact. Some U.S. severe storm experts believe the National Weather Service (NWS) has reached the optimum warning lead time with current technology. They promote the concept that risk will be reduced by public education directed at appropriate protective actions once a warning has been issued, rather than increasing the lead time.[6] Countries with elevated risk for tornadoes have variable degrees of sophistication in detection and warning capabilities.

Building construction practices, which are also inconsistent worldwide, may have an impact on injury and death. Retrofitting homes with safe rooms or shelters has been recommended, as well as maintaining adequate shelters for public gathering places and hospitals.

Preparedness: Routine testing of warning methods (e.g., sirens, public broadcasts, cell phone notifications, other media) should be conducted regularly to check for and address system inadequacies. Testing also provides information to the general population regarding warning methods. Individuals must engage in personal preparedness to understand the protective measures necessary when public health officials issue a warning.

Response: Health systems, public safety, and other response agencies should have action plans in place, practiced and updated as recommended by after-action reviews. In addition, individual behavior can have a major effect on health outcome. The psychological/sociological aspect of an individual's response to warning will be reviewed later in the chapter.

Recovery: Although the impact phase of a tornado has obvious health risks, the post-impact phase has its own set of challenges. During clean-up, the risk of injury from sharp objects, trips and falls, being struck by falling debris, and electrocution from power lines mistakenly thought to be without electricity are potential health risks.

Both event and post-event wound contamination and death from opportunistic infectious agents are concerns that require close monitoring in susceptible populations.[7]

Tornado Science

Tornado Rating Scales

The Enhanced Fujita scale (EF scale) rates the strength of tornadoes in the United States based on the damage they cause. Implemented in place of the Fujita scale introduced in 1971 by Ted Fujita, it became operational in 2007. Canada began using this scale in 2013.[8] Great Britain uses a wind speed scale termed TORRO for tornado rating.[9]

The EF scale is based on U.S.-specific construction practices and its application in other countries may be inexact for rating tornado strength.[10] Figure 37.3 illustrates structural damage as related to wind speed.

Forecasting Thunderstorms

Meteorological science is constantly improving forecasting ability for severe thunderstorms, from which tornadoes are spawned. The Storm Prediction Center (SPC) of the U.S. National Oceanic and Atmospheric Administration (NOAA) produces severe weather outlook forecasts.[11] These incorporate modeling of upcoming atmospheric conditions and compare them to historic weather events. Using probability predictions, the SPC produces data for the current day with projections for the next 8 days.[11]

Worldwide locations with tornado occurrences share similar atmospheric features. Jet stream–driven cold dry air mass travels above a warm moist air mass that creates vertical turbulence and thunderstorm development. In the United States, topography associated with frequent storms is in the Central Midwest and Southeast, as cool dry air mass traveling from the Rocky Mountain range interacts with warm air from the Gulf of Mexico.[4]

In Bangladesh, the cool air mass originates from the Himalayas and the warm air mass from the Bay of Bengal. This results in most storms occurring in a relatively small area of central, south central, and southeast areas regions of the country. March, June, and July are the high-occurrence months.[12]

Southern Ontario and Quebec and the Canadian Prairie Region are the high-occurrence areas in Canada, with June, July, and August being the most likely months of occurrence. In this region of the world, the Rocky Mountain cold front interacts with warm fronts to create thunderstorms.[4]

Forecasting Tornadoes

While predicting thunderstorm probability over the upcoming week is fairly accurate, it is more challenging to predict tornadoes, which are spawned from thunderstorms. Mesocyclone formations within storms are areas of rotation. If the rotating column of air descends and reaches the ground, it is classified as a tornado. Tornadoes can develop within minutes, sometimes leaving a short period of time for detection and warning. Doppler radar, which detects wind circulation within a storm, suggests potential tornado formation. Storm spotters on the ground in contact with the radar operators assist with confirmation by direct visualization.

Figure 37.3. EF0: Winds 65–85 mph, producing light damage. Some damage to chimneys; branches broken off trees; shallow-rooted trees pushed over; signboards damaged. Account for 70% of South Florida tornadoes, yet only result in 5% of tornado casualties (injuries and/or fatalities). EF1: Winds 86–110 mph, producing moderate damage. Peels surface off roofs; mobile homes pushed off foundations or overturned; moving autos blown off roads. Account for 22% of South Florida tornadoes and 20% of tornado casualties (injuries and/or fatalities).
EF2: Winds 113–135 mph, producing considerable damage. Roofs torn off frame houses; mobile homes demolished; boxcars overturned; large trees snapped or uprooted; light-object missiles generated; cars lifted off ground. Account for 8% of South Florida tornadoes and 31% of tornado casualties (injuries and/or fatalities).
EF3: Winds 136–165 mph, producing severe damage. Roofs and some walls torn off well-constructed houses; trains overturned; most trees in forest uprooted; heavy cars lifted off the ground and thrown. Account for 1% of South Florida tornadoes and 44% of tornado casualties (injuries and/or fatalities).
EF4: Winds 166–200 mph, producing devastating damage. Well-constructed houses leveled; structures with weak foundations blown away some distance; cars thrown and large missiles generated. No EF4 tornado has occurred in South Florida.
EF5: Winds >200 mph, producing incredible damage. Strong frame houses leveled off foundations and swept away; automobile-sized missiles fly through the air in excess of 100 meters; trees debarked; incredible phenomena will occur. No EF5 tornado has occurred in Florida.

Scale	Wind speed (Estimated)[4]			Example of damage
	mph	km/h	m/s	
EF0	65–85	105–137	29–37	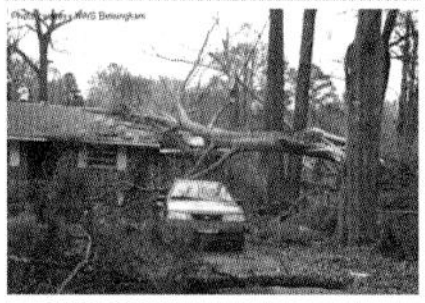
EF1	86–110	138–177	38–49	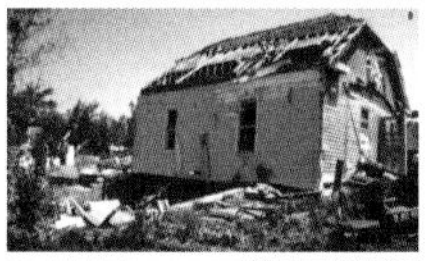
EF2	111–135	178–217	50–60	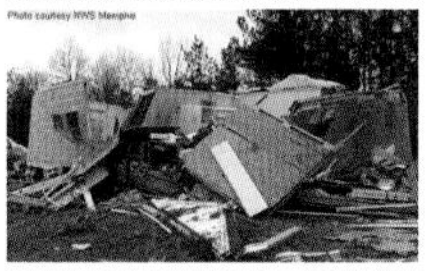
EF3	136–165	218–266	61–73	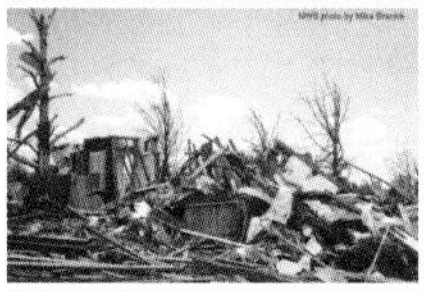
EF4	166–200	267–322	74–90	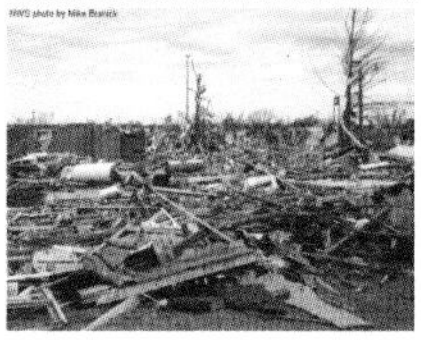
EF5	>200	>322	>90	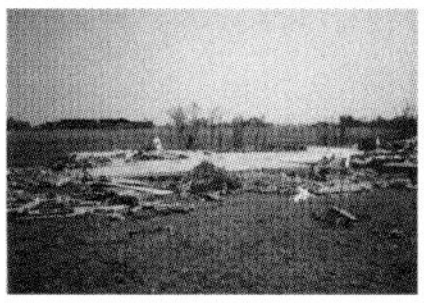

Courtesy of the National Weather Service

Tornado Warning

NWS issues tornado warnings that are disseminated to weather alert radios. NWS partners with various media and communication services that rebroadcast warnings by television, radio, cell phone messaging, and social media. As described previously, the time from issue of warning to tornado impact is termed "lead time." At the time of this writing, NOAA reports an average lead time of 13 minutes in the United States.[13]

American meteorologist Harold Brooks of NOAA and the National Severe Storms Laboratory (NSSL) explains that the lead time has remained unchanged for 25 years and that it has averaged 18.5 minutes. He believes the discrepancies in times

Table 37.1. Bangladesh, Canada, United States: Population, Dispersal, Access to Electronic Devices

	Bangladesh	Canada	United States
Total population	158.5 million	35.7 million	323.1 million
Percentage urban	21%	76%	79%
Percentage with access to television	17%	99%	97%
Percentage with access to landline or mobile phone	7%	100%	80%

Note: Population figures as of January 2015 for each country.

reported are due to the inclusion in more recent reports of "no warning" tornado events (lead time = 0) that skew the data.[14]

Intuitively, longer lead times would allow more time to take protective action and reduce injury and death. However, some weather experts question that premise. They theorize that long lead times indicate that the tornado is large in size and thus was detected sooner and has greater destructive energy. If this were the case, taking refuge inside a structure would increase risk of serious injury or death if that shelter is demolished.[6] A regression model analysis of lead time versus injury and death in more than 18,000 tornado events from 1986–2002 revealed that, when compared to no warning, lead times up to 15 minutes reduced injury and death, while lead times beyond 15 minutes were associated with increased morbidity and mortality.[6,15]

An explanation for this seemingly paradoxical finding is that people erroneously think they have ample time before storm arrival for various activities like getting in a vehicle to outrace the storm. In addition, some people in harm's way have been observed to go outside to watch the storm, mistakenly thinking they would have enough time to get to shelter. Considering that nearly 75% of warnings are false alarms, after 15 minutes, people might assume this is the case and leave the shelter even though they are in a true event.[6]

In Bangladesh, a central government agency, the Bangladesh Meteorological Department (BMD), monitors adverse weather events. BMD uses a sophisticated weather observation and data collection system located centrally and in strategic outlying locations to develop and issue warnings via electronic media.[16] Table 37.1 compares the three countries by population and media capabilities illustrating that Bangladesh's population is mostly rural and without widespread electronic media coverage. Therefore timely advanced warning may be sparse in many areas of the country.[17]

Risk of Injury and Death

Bangladesh

The epidemiology of tornado-related injury and mortality in the developing world is not well documented; however, a retrospective cohort study following a March 20, 2005, tornado in rural Bangladesh provided the following data.[19] Risk factors for mortality:

- Age >60 (adjusted odds ratio [OR] 8.9)
- Being outdoors (adjusted OR 10.4)
- Walls of concrete block or brick compared to thatch or grass (adjusted OR 7.0)

Risk factors for injury:

- Age >60 years (adjusted OR 1.58)
- Female gender (adjusted OR 1.24)
- Being outdoors (adjusted OR 6.6)
- Corrugated tin roofs (adjusted OR 1.3)
- Corrugated tin walls (adjusted OR 1.4)
- Brick or concrete block walls (adjusted OR 2.0)

The higher adjusted odds ratio of death in poorly constructed brick or concrete houses compared to those made of thatch or grass may be due to heavy projectiles causing blunt and penetrating trauma. Figure 37.4 displays the causes of death for this tornado event.

Canada

A case-controlled study following a tornado in Ontario, Canada, on May 31, 1985, yielded the following observations for tornado-related morbidity and mortality.[20] All fatalities were either massive head or trunk injuries.

- Eleven of twelve fatalities died before reaching a hospital.
- Ten of twelve fatalities became airborne, striking the ground or fixed object.
- Two of twelve fatalities were crushed by an object.

Of those with serious injuries resulting in hospitalization, 60% were struck by flying objects, including glass or other debris from both within and outside buildings. Of these, 49% were stuck about the head or neck.

The most common primary diagnosis was fracture, occurring 45% of the time. Concussion or head injury was reported in 26% of the injured. Matched analysis for OR for serious injury or death:

- Previously married (OR 3.0)
- Watching/listening to media 1 hour prior to the storm (OR 2.9)
- Poor building anchorage (OR 3.4)
- Room floor blown away (OR 5.5)
- Location other than basement (OR 9.5)
- Not hiding behind or under objects (OR 9.0)
- Thrown out of vehicle (OR 5.0)
- Vehicle lifted/rolled (OR 2.0)

With unmatched OR for serious injury or death as follows:

- Age >70 years (OR 3.6)
- Hit by objects (OR 2.0).

United States

Risk of injury or death is associated with storm strength, victim age, type of material used for dwelling construction, shelter location, income level, and time of day. The elderly may have reduced physical response ability, impaired sensory function, or reduced access to appropriate shelter. Fabricated and frame houses may not provide protection; a significant number of deaths and injuries occur in individuals sheltering within these structures. Seeking shelter in a basement is associated with injury and death when the house is shifted off the foundation or the basement walls collapse on victims.[21–24] Storms after dark may not be visible or may occur when victims are asleep and unaware

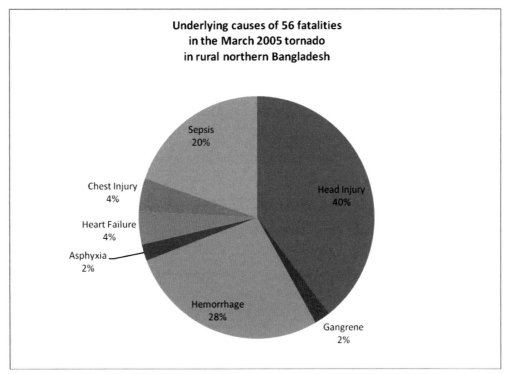

Underlying causes of 56 fatalities in the March 2005 tornado in rural northern Bangladesh

- Sepsis 20%
- Chest Injury 4%
- Heart Failure 4%
- Asphyxia 2%
- Head Injury 40%
- Hemorrhage 28%
- Gangrene 2%

Figure 37.4. Underlying Causes of 56 Fatalities in the March 2005 Tornado in Rural Northern Bangladesh.

or unable to hear a warning siren. Lower-income groups may reside in dwellings that cannot withstand high wind stress or in areas of a community without public warning sirens. Locations where people are at significant risk include schools, churches, and restaurants if they are heavily populated at the time of a direct tornado strike.

The vast majority of tornado deaths occur at the time of impact. The most common mechanisms of death are blunt and penetrating trauma. Victims can be thrown rapidly through the air, accelerated by storm winds, and strike objects. Alternatively, projectiles propelled by the wind can strike people or they can be crushed by collapsing structures. Head, thoracic, and multiple abdominal organ injuries are the frequent causes of mortality.[21–24]

According to National Climatic Data Center, overall mortality rates ranged from 5–10% of all those injured from January 2001 to September 2006 in the United States. NOAA reports the average annual death count from tornadoes in the United States is sixty.[25] However, in 2011 there were 553 tornado deaths, largely due to the April–May multiple storm outbreak in the Southeast that included the deadly May 22 Joplin, Missouri, tornado.[26]

During April 25–28, 2011, the third deadliest tornado disaster occurred in the southeastern United States, despite modern advances in tornado forecasting, advanced warning times, and media coverage. The U.S. Centers for Disease Control and Prevention and Prevention reviewed data from the American Red Cross, death certificates, and NWS to describe fatalities by demographics, shelter used, cause of death, and tornado severity in the affected states of Alabama, Arkansas, Georgia, Mississippi, and Tennessee. Of the 338 deaths, approximately one-third were in older adults; almost half occurred in single-family homes; and a quarter happened in mobile homes. One-half of the twenty-seven tornadoes were rated powerful (EF4 or EF5) and these

were responsible for almost 90% of the deaths.[27] Post-impact causes of death include electrocution, carbon monoxide poisoning from improper generator use, cardiovascular events from stress or physical activity, life support equipment failure from power loss, burns and smoke inhalation from fires while using flammable sources for lighting, and wound infection.[21,22,27]

Injury patterns can be categorized by the time they occur in relation to the storm. This approach informs treatment strategy. Pre-impact injuries can include traffic collisions as people flee ahead of the storm, and falls occurring while running down stairs into basements or storm shelters. Impact phase injuries result from victims being thrown against objects by strong storm winds or being struck by windblown projectiles. The latter phenomenon can lead to wound contamination by organisms that become airborne in high wind events. Wound infection resulting in septicemia, including that from opportunistic organisms in susceptible hosts, is responsible for some in-hospital mortality.[28] Post-impact injury includes puncture wounds and lacerations associated with debris removal, and electrocution while individuals are working around downed power lines erroneously thought to be inactive.

Approximately 50% of injuries seen in hospital emergency care areas are soft tissue wounds, including lacerations, contusions, and punctures. Fractures occur in 30% of victims and are the most common cause for hospital admission. Head injury, including extra and intracranial trauma, accounts for 7% of injuries. Hospital admission rates are typically around 25%.[21–24]

Increased risk for injury and death will likely occur over time due to growing numbers of elderly in the population. Older persons may be more vulnerable to the effects of tornadoes due to decreased sensory perception, reaction times, and sometimes mental acuity. There is a continuing influx of racial and ethnic diversity, which presents language and translation challenges during an emergency.[29] The projected population growth is highest for the West, Southeast, and Gulf states, with the latter two in high tornado risk locations.[29] Finally, the states in the Southeast and Gulf region have between 10–14% occupancy rate of mobile homes, the highest in the country.[30] The death rate is approximately twenty times as high in mobile homes as compared to permanent structures.[31]

Summary

A comparison of three countries with varying demographics shows a close similarity of injury patterns and risk of death from tornadoes. Becoming airborne or being struck by flying debris is a common cause of morbidity and mortality, with head and trunk injuries being the leading causes of mortality. Blunt and penetrating trauma along with soft tissue injuries and fractures make up the majority of injuries. Public education regarding warnings and the proper actions to take and to avoid, along with making proper storm shelters available (especially for occupants of mobile homes) are important public health interventions to mitigate morbidity and mortality.

RECOMMENDATIONS FOR FURTHER RESEARCH

Research on optimal warning systems is required. Harold Brooks and others in NWS are considering using a "warn on forecast" warning instead of the current "warn on detection." This would allow a warning to be issued when forecasting conditions suggest tornado potential rather than waiting for actual tornado formation. The result would be longer lead times and greater opportunities for evacuation of vulnerable patients in hospitals and nursing homes if needed. It would be useful to develop a template for staging movement of patients and necessary supplies and equipment from hospitals to shelters so that efficient and timely transfer can be accomplished with a minimum of patient treatment interruption. In addition to pre-event evacuation, research on strategies for evacuation after a tornado strikes is needed. An example to illustrate this need is the 2011 Joplin tornado during which the St. John Hospital was destroyed by a direct hit and 183 patients were evacuated in 90 minutes.[32]

At NWS, there is interest in studying non-meteorological causes of injury and death in tornadoes. These include morbidity and mortality related to human behavior such as when people do not heed warnings or follow recommendations for protective actions. Should there be required classes in all schools and upper level courses about disaster warnings and appropriate defensive measures? Is there a better way to deliver warnings so the public understands the true nature of the risk and acts accordingly?

Another area of research would be in the development of guidelines for small two to three member paramedic/emergency medical technician/first responder teams to deploy to the impacted area and conduct triage as well as treatment. For example, during the Joplin tornado, the emergency medical services medical director created field treatment stations in an attempt to reduce the influx of minor injuries to the already crowded remaining medical center.[33] This concept has previously been addressed using physicians and nurses at alternate care centers.

Finally, to improve epidemiologic knowledge, development of a standardized classification of injuries from tornadoes, similar to that used for blast injuries, would be useful.

Acknowledgments

I appreciate the professional support and assistance from Dr. Harold E. Brooks, Research Meteorologist NOAA/NSSL; Jim Morgan, DO, emergency department physician and EMS director Joplin, Missouri; and D. Sean Smith, DO, emergency department physician and President Mercy Clinic Joplin and Kansas Division.

REFERENCES

1. http://meteorologicalmusings.blogspot.com/2010/10/map-of-world-tornado-alleys.html. Picture provided by NOAA (Accessed January 15, 2013).
2. www.spc.noaa.gov/faq/tornado/index.html (Accessed January 15, 2013).
3. http://en.wikipedia.org/wiki/Tornado (Accessed March 15, 2013).
4. http://en.wikipedia.org/wiki/Tornado_climatology (Accessed January 15, 2013).
5. http://www.wunderground.com/blog/weatherhistorian/comment.html?entrynum=71 (Accessed March 15, 2013).
6. Dr. Harold E Brooks, Research Meteorologist NOAA/NSSL. Norman, Oklahoma. Personal communication. May 22, 2013.
7. www.cdc.gov/mmwr/preview/mmwrhtml/mm6029a5.htm (Accessed March 28, 2013).
8. http://www.wunderground.com/resources/severe/fujita_scale.asp (Accessed September 1, 2013).
9. http://en.wikipedia.org/wiki/TORRO_scale (Accessed March 30, 2013).
10. www.bama.ua.edu/jcsenkbeil/gy4570/doswell%20et%20al.pdf (Accessed March 30, 2013).
11. www.spc.noaa.gov (Accessed March 1, 2013).
12. http://bangladeshtornadoes.org/bengaltornadoes.html (Accessed January 1, 2013).
13. www.noaa.gov/features/protecting/tornados101.html (Accessed March 1, 2013).
14. www.geography.osu.edu/metclub/Brooks-tornado%20death%20spring%202011.pptx (Accessed March 30, 2013); and personal communication with Harold Brooks, May 22, 2013.
15. Simmons K, Sutter D. Improvements in Tornado Warnings and Tornado Casualties, *Int J Mass Emerg and Disasters* 2006; 24: 351–369.
16. http://www.iawe.org/WRDRR_Bangladesh/Preprints/S4BMD.pdf (Accessed March 30, 2013).
17. www.nationmaster.com (Accessed March 1, 2013).
18. http://www.vanhorne.info/files/vanhorne/F%20Wirasinghe.pdf (Accessed March 30, 2013).
19. www.ncbi.nlm.nih.gov/pubmed/21073669 (Accessed March 30, 2013).
20. http://www.ncbi.nlm.nih.gov/pubmed/2589312 (Accessed March 30, 2013).
21. Centers for Disease Control and Prevention (CDC). Tornado Associated Fatalities – Arkansas 1997. *MMWR* May 16, 1997; 46(19): 412–416.
22. CDC. Texas Disaster – Texas, May 1997. *MMWR* November 14, 1997; 46(45): 1069–1072.

23. Oho Y. Risk Factors for Death in the 8 April 1998 Alabama Tornado *and* Quick Response Report #145. Boulder, CO, Natural Hazards Response Applications Center, 2002. http://www.colorado.edu/hazards/research/qr/qr145/qr145.html (Accessed April 30, 2013).

24. CDC. Tornado Disaster –Illinois 1990 *MMWR* January 18, 1991;40(2): 33–36.

25. http://www.noaa.gov/features/protecting/tornados101.html (Accessed May 1, 2013).

26. http://www.spc.noaa.gov/climo/online/monthly/newm.html (Accessed May 1, 2013).

27. CDC.Tornado-Related Fatalities – Five States, Southeastern United States, April 25–28, 2011. *MMWR* July 20, 2012; 61(28): 529–533.

28. http://www.cdc.gov/mmwr/preview/mmwrhtml/mm6029a5.htm (Accessed May 1, 2013).

29. http://www.fema.gov/pdf/about/programs/oppa/demography_%20paper_051011.pdf (Accessed May 1, 2013).

30. http://www.statemaster.com/graph/hou_per_of_hou_uni_tha_are_mob_hom-housing-percent-units-mobile-homes (Accessed May 2, 2013).

31. http://www.nssl.noaa.gov/users/brooks/public_html/deathtrivia (Accessed May 16, 2013).

32. D. Sean Smith, DO, St. John Hospital. Personal communication, March 28, 2013.

33. http://www.emsworld.com/contact/10645868/jim-morgan (Accessed March 30, 2013).

38

EARTHQUAKES

Carl H. Schultz and Shira A. Schlesinger

OVERVIEW

Earthquakes have posed a significant threat to human lives and property throughout history. During the past 40 years, seismic events have resulted in more than 1.5 million deaths.[1,2,3] Earthquakes are considered one of the most destructive disasters. An average of sixteen earthquakes leading to death occur throughout the world each year with many more leading to injury and property damage.[2] The 2011 Tōhoku Earthquake and Tsunami produced at least $300 billion USD in damage, killed more than 20,000 people, and caused the second worst nuclear disaster in history to that date.[4] This occurred in a nation with sophisticated, modern seismic building codes. Short-term mortality and long-term outcomes are even more severe in less developed countries with greater numbers of population at risk for displacement and public health catastrophes (Table 38.1) The 2010 Haiti Earthquake killed over 300,000 people, and caused an estimated $14 billion USD in direct economic damages.[4,5]

Society's continued vulnerability to the devastating effects of earthquakes is the result of several factors. Earthquakes are sudden-impact disasters that strike quickly and without warning, making mitigation and evacuation efforts difficult. Many of the factors that influence the severity of the earthquake's impact are difficult to control, including the day of the week, time of day, population density, location, and local geological conditions. Yet the quantity of property damage, loss of life, disruption of economic activity, and interference in the provision of important services also varies depending on the degree of preparedness and success of mitigation measures implemented prior to the temblor. Inadequate building materials, structural design deficiencies, and the absence of laws regulating building construction increase susceptibility to seismic damage. Failure to initiate mitigation efforts results in long-term disruption of transportation, communication, and financial infrastructures. Such issues emphasize the importance of adequate education and planning in regions at risk for seismic events.

Worldwide demographics also play a role in mitigating or increasing the impact of seismic events. Many large population concentrations exist along major fault lines. These populations are at higher risk of earthquake-related morbidity and mortality.

Table 38.1. Earthquake Mortality since 2000 (selected examples)

Year	Location	Approximate Deaths
2001	Gujarat, India	20,100
2003	Bam, Iran	31,000
2004	Sumatra, Indonesia (with tsunami)	283,000
2005	Kashmir, Pakistan	80,400
2008	Eastern Sichuan, China	87,600
2010	Port au Prince, Haiti	316,000
2011	Honshu, Japan (with tsunami)	21,000

Despite this high risk, population density continues to increase in many of these regions, exacerbating the potential for future injuries and deaths after a seismic event.

CURRENT STATE OF THE ART

In considering mitigation, preparedness, response, and recovery efforts to address earthquake effects, planners and responders must recognize the interplay of seismic characteristics, the built environment, and human factors.

Earthquake Characteristics

To understand the issues involved with managing the earthquake threat, it is necessary to explore basic concepts related to seismic events. Several theories attempt to explain earthquake behavior. The concept most widely accepted by seismologists is the tectonic plate theory. This theory is based on the structure of the earth's crust, and asserts that in the initial formation of continents, the earth's land mass was aggregated in a single unit. This unit subsequently fragmented, and the sections, known as tectonic

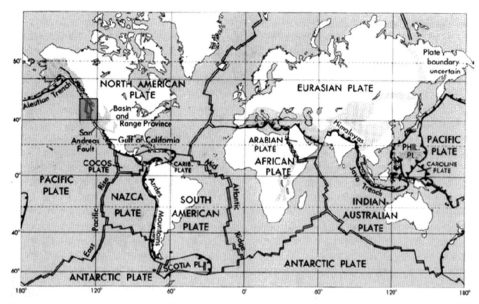

Figure 38.1. Major World Faults. From: http://pubs.usgs.gov/gip/volc/fig 37.gif. Courtesy of United States Geological Survey.

plates, began moving against each other (Figure 38.1).[6] These land sections remain in constant motion. A major fault line is defined where the edges of tectonic plates meet. Surrounding the major faults are minor ones that also give rise to seismic events. A variable degree of deformation associated with increasing stress accumulates along fault lines as land masses move past or against each other. This deformation is eventually released through perceptible seismic motion. Although tectonic plate theory explains most earthquakes, there are seismic events that it cannot adequately clarify, such as activity in the New Madrid zone in the United States, which is located along the Mississippi River Valley approximately 1,600 km (1,000 miles) away from the nearest plate boundary.[7] More information is needed to understand how earthquakes occur in these locations.

Tectonic plates move in relation to one another in three specific patterns described as strike-slip, dip-slip, and oblique-slip (Figure 38.2). Strike-slip faults occur when plates slide horizontally past one another. Dip-slip faults occur when the plates slide over or under each other.[6] These are further characterized as normal faults (where the underlying segment moves upward) and reverse faults (where the underlying segment moves downward). Oblique-slip faults exhibit both types of motion when they rupture. Dip-slip faults are most frequently associated with the development of tsunamis.

The location where the fault rupture begins is known as the hypocenter (or focus) and is located below the earth's surface. The point on the earth's surface directly above the hypocenter is called the epicenter (Figure 38.3). When an earthquake occurs, stress is relieved along the fault lines as the land masses shift and release energy in the form of seismic waves. Temblors produce

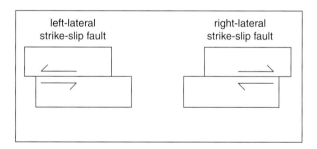

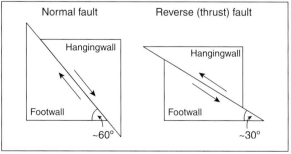

Figure 38.2. Types of Fault Motion Characterizing Strike-Slip and Dip-Slip Faults.

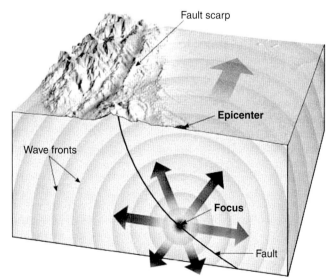

Figure 38.3. Relationship between Hypocenter (Focus) and Epicenter. Modified from http://teampride.yolasite.com/resources/8.1.pdf.

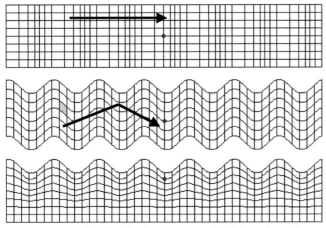

Figure 38.4. Earthquake Shock Waves. Modified from http://home.hiroshima-u.ac.jp/er/Resources/Image195.gif.

three types of seismic waves: primary (P), secondary/shear (S), and surface (L) waves (Figure 38.4). P and S waves are referred to as body waves, meaning that they develop at the hypocenter and radiate in all directions through the earth's interior. L waves are surface waves and can only move through the earth's crust.

P waves are the fastest of the seismic waves, traveling at 4.8 km/s in a longitudinal direction. S waves travel at 3.2 km/s and cause the earth to move at right angles from the direction of the P waves. The difference in velocity between the P and S waves allows determination of the epicenter. Different rates of travel between the P and S waves also produce two separate perceptions by individuals. The P wave generates an acoustic signal that sounds like an approaching train whereas the S wave produces a sharp jolt. The L wave is a slow surface disturbance that causes swaying of tall buildings and large swells in bodies of water. This seismic wave is the major cause of damage and injury from earthquakes.

The frequency and amplitude of the vibrations produced at the surface and the subsequent earthquake severity depend on the amount of mechanical energy released, the distance/depth of the focus, and the structural properties of the soil near the surface.[6,8] Distance from the epicenter is a poorer predictor of severity because the transmission strength of earthquake shock waves is influenced by ground composition, liquefaction, and landslide susceptibility. Soils with high water content transmit energy waves that cause significant mortality, morbidity, and structural damage even at great distances from the epicenter. In contrast, solid rock transmits earthquake energy with a mini-

mum of vibration. This explains why areas in a liquefaction zone situated relatively far from the epicenter can be more severely impacted by seismic intensities than locations nearer the epicenter on bedrock.[6]

Earthquakes are characterized by intensity and magnitude. Magnitude is the total energy generated by the temblor. This energy is measured with a seismograph and then converted using the Richter scale (Table 38.2). The Richter magnitude scale is a logarithmic scale that estimates total energy released by an earthquake. A change of 1 unit in the Richter scale corresponds to a 10-fold change in ground motion and a 32-fold change in radiated energy.[8] Measurements on the Richter scale below 2.0 are not usually felt and measurements on the Richter scale above 5.0 can cause damage. A major earthquake consists of a magnitude 7.0 or greater. A major earthquake may be preceded by preliminary tremors known as foreshocks. There can also be lower magnitude events after the main earthquake known as aftershocks, which can produce significant additional damage and may necessitate additional local or regional evacuations.

The earthquake's intensity is determined by the degree of ground shaking in a particular location. Intensity is calculated using two separate methods: an objective approach using instrumentation and a subjective evaluation based on human observations and perceptions. The first method uses motion detectors to record peak ground velocity (PGV) and peak ground acceleration (PGA). The greater the degree of ground motion, the higher the recorded velocity and acceleration. This information is referred to as the instrumental intensity. PGV and PGA determinations are based on the degree of ground movement measured at localized points obtained by ground sensors placed in earthquake-prone areas. When available, they provide precise estimates of intensity not influenced by the subjective perception of motion or damaged structures. Instrumental intensities recorded during an earthquake are better predictors of injury and lethal outcomes than the rate of building collapse.[9,10,11] However, since sensors are placed in only a few locations, the use of instrumental intensities as a worldwide measure is limited.

The second method of measuring intensity, the Modified Mercalli Intensity (MMI) scale, relies on the extent of observed property damage and the perceived degree of shaking reported by people experiencing the earthquake.[12] Intensity determinations are made using this subjective 12-point scale after an earthquake when U.S. Postal Service employees are interviewed regarding their experiences and the visible structural damage they observe (Table 38.3). Different governmental workers may perform this task in other countries. Using one of the twelve categories on the MMI scale, a value is selected that most accurately represents the

Table 38.2. Richter Scale

Description	Magnitude	Number per year	Approximate energy (J)
Great Earthquake	>8.0	1–2	$>6.3 \times 10^{16}$
Major Earthquake	7.0–7.9	15	$>2 \times 10^{15}$–6.3×10^{16}
Destructive Earthquake	6.0–6.9	134	$>6.3 \times 10^{13}$–2×10^{15}
Damaging Earthquake	5.0–5.9	1319	$>2 \times 10^{12}$–6.3×10^{13}
Minor Earthquake	4.0–4.9	13,000 (estimated)	$>6.3 \times 10^{10}$–2×10^{12}
Smallest Usually Felt	3.0–3.9	130,000 (estimated)	$>2 \times 10^{9}$–6.3×10^{10}
Detected but Not Felt	2.0–2.9	1,300,000 (estimated)	6.3×10^{7}–2×10^{9}

Table 38.3. The Modified Mercalli Intensity Scale

INTENSITY	I	II–III	IV	V	VI	VII	VIII	IX	X+
SHAKING	not felt	weak	light	moderate	strong	very strong	severe	violent	extreme
DAMAGE	none	none	none	very light	light	moderate	moderate/heavy	heavy	very heavy

degree of shaking and damage. This value is then assigned to the pertinent postal code. Recording the MMI values for all postal codes in the earthquake zone yields a representation of the overall intensity. Although MMI scale measurements are subjective, they are generally valid. Researchers have found that MMI values correlate well with structural damage, deaths, and traumatic injuries.[6,10] Electronic resources and social media have increased the potential for data collection in MMI scales. The United States Geological Survey now invites individuals to report their experience of temblors via an online adapted MMI questionnaire (http://earthquake.usgs.gov/earthquakes/dyfi) that contributes to shake maps for seismic events around the globe. Comparisons between the MMI scale, Richter scale, and Instrumental Intensity scale are depicted in Table 38.4.

Table 38.4. Comparison between the Modified Mercalli Scale, the Richter Scale, and the Instrumental Intensity Scale

Modified Mercalli Scale		Richter Scale		Instrumental Intensity Scale				
				Perceived Shaking	Potential Damage	Peak Acceleration (%g)	Peak Velocity (cm/s)	Instrumental Intensity
I	Felt by almost no one		Generally not felt, but recorded on seismometers	Not felt	None	<0.17	<0.1	I
II	Felt by very few people	2.5		Weak	None	0.17–1.4	0.1–1.1	II–III
III	Tremor noticed by many, but they often do not realize it is an earthquake							
IV	Felt indoors by many; feels like a truck has struck the building	3.5	Felt by many people	Light	None	1.4–3.9	1.1–3.4	IV
V	Felt by nearly everyone; many people awakened; swaying trees and poles may be observed			Moderate	Very light	3.9–9.2	3.4–8.1	V
VI	Felt by all; many people run outdoors; furniture moved, slight damage occurs			Strong	Light	9.2–18	8.1–16	VI
VII	Everyone runs outdoors; poorly built structures considerably damaged; slight damage elsewhere	4.5	Some local damage may occur	Very strong	Moderate	18–34	16–34	VII
VIII	Specially designed structures damaged slightly, others collapse			Severe	Moderate/Heavy	34–65	31–60	VIII
IX	All buildings considerably damaged, many shift off foundations; noticeable cracks in ground	6.0	A destructive earthquake	Violent	Heavy	65–124	60–116	IX
X	Many structures destroyed; ground is badly cracked	7.0	A major earthquake	Extreme	Very heavy	>124	>116	X+
XI	Almost all structures fall; very wide cracks in ground							
XII	Total destruction; waves seen on ground surfaces, objects are tumbled and tossed	8.0+	Great earthquake					

Seismology, the study of earthquakes and the propagation of seismic waves, has made progress in estimating the probability of a strong earthquake occurring during any 24-hour period in certain parts of the United States, such as California. These predictions are based on evaluations of previous events and analysis of potential relationships between events. Seismologists cannot currently predict with certainty when or where the next earthquake will occur or its intensity level.[13]

Management Issues

The persistent threat of seismic events and the difficulties involved with mitigating their effects highlight the importance of disaster preparedness for such events. Planning efforts should emphasize the following: 1) protocols outlining predicted modifications of prehospital and hospital medical care during the initial response; 2) efficient use of community resources; 3) awareness of common clinical conditions seen after earthquakes and related treatment options; and 4) recognition that arrival of outside help will not be immediate and likely require more than 48 hours.

Incident Command

In the initial period after an earthquake, a degree of uncertainty arises for individuals in a community and for the local and regional healthcare system. Once it is clear that resource demands in the post-earthquake period exceed what is available under standard operating procedures, establishing a system of command and control, known as an Incident Command System (ICS), becomes essential for effective management. Based on a concept initially used by California firefighters in the 1970s for effective coordination and resource control when battling wildfires, the ICS directs response activities through decisions made by a single individual known as the incident commander and implemented by a formal chain of command. By providing a standardized system of command and control, complex situations can be managed more efficiently during a disaster. In cases in which multiple jurisdictions have a role in management, the ICS becomes a Unified Command System and may include representatives from state and federal levels in addition to local entities.[7,14] A detailed explanation of ICS can be found in Chapter 11.

An incident management system is used at the Emergency Operations Center (EOC) for each responding organization. This center is the location where personnel representing various entities from the public and private sector meet during an emergency event to: 1) coordinate response and recovery actions; 2) conduct strategic decision-making; and 3) manage resource allocation.[7,14]

Prehospital Response

After an earthquake, victims' lives may depend on how rapidly they are extricated from collapsed buildings and how expeditiously they receive medical treatment. In urban areas of developed countries, it is common that paramedics perform initial prehospital care; however, in a large-scale earthquake they may be unavailable for this activity, particularly in systems in which they have primary responsibilities as firefighters (since fires are common after earthquakes). In systems not using paramedics, first responders may be police, firefighters, other ambulance personnel, or even physicians.

Complicating the threat to the population, secondary events that increase the lethality of the initial earthquake can occur after seismic activity. Such events include fires, landslides, floods, and tsunamis, among others.[2,6] The 2004 Indian Ocean (Sumatra-Adanam) Earthquake and Tsunami was one of the most destructive seismic events of the past century. The vast majority of deaths were the result of tsunami activity, rather than the initial earthquake, whose epicenter was over deep water off the coast of Sumatra. During the 1994 Northridge, California, earthquake, fires and burns accounted for 6.1% of the fatalities and 7.3% of the hospitalized injuries respectively, even though nonresidential buildings were the most affected and the fires were quickly controlled.[2]

When fires occur immediately after an earthquake, such as in the 1989 Loma Prieta temblor in northern California and the 1995 Great Hanshin earthquake in Japan, the priority is to minimize the amount of damage resulting from these blazes. Much the same as medical emergencies, fires may quickly outstrip the resources available for conflagration control. Therefore human resources in places where firefighters also share responsibility for medical response or search and rescue will be initially directed to fire suppression.[7,15] This can leave the affected area without paramedic support. Although it was only a moderate-sized earthquake, sections of San Francisco went without paramedic support in the critical early hours following the Loma Prieta temblor because of the prioritization of fire suppression over other aid efforts.

Another problem faced by industrialized populations after an earthquake is exposure to released toxic materials stored in such facilities as power stations and chemical plants. Following the 1989 Loma Prieta earthquake, approximately 20% of the post-earthquake injuries were caused by exposure to toxic chemicals.[12] The 2011 Tōhoku Earthquake and Tsunami resulted in the second worst nuclear accident in history to that date. Under these circumstances, decontamination and evacuation must be addressed to limit the number of exposed victims, and to improve community safety. When managing the threat of toxic exposures, it is reasonable to consider directing human resources to assist with decontamination and evacuation instead of the rescue effort.

Communication between paramedics in the field, base stations providing medical direction for prehospital personnel, and receiving hospitals can be disrupted after a seismic event. Notifying hospitals of victims' impending arrivals becomes difficult, increasing the risk that healthcare resources cannot be effectively managed. Many individuals will not wait for the arrival of paramedics or other prehospital providers. Family and friends will frequently bring victims to the nearest, most familiar, or most accessible hospital, overwhelming the facility's capacity. During the Puerto Limon, Costa Rica, earthquake in 1999 most victims were transported by survivors.[16] Following the 2001 Gujarat, India, earthquake, most of the victims used private transportation to reach hospitals.[17] Major trauma victims will be brought to non-trauma centers and many patients without life-threatening injuries will arrive at trauma centers. This mismatch of medical needs and available resources can potentially overwhelm capacities and result in inefficient utilization, potentially leading to increased morbidity and mortality. While this phenomenon is undesirable, it is difficult to avoid during the first hours after an earthquake.

Breakdown of communication systems makes coordination of field care and disposition difficult, jeopardizing the direction and integration of all prehospital activities. Prehospital provider radios frequently rely on repeaters that can fail, making transmission of radio signals to dispatchers or base station hospitals difficult. Ambulances from different jurisdictions tend to use different radio frequencies, making communication between field units and the central coordinating body problematic even when repeaters function. Complicating the situation is the arrival of unsolicited ambulances from outside regions to areas most impacted by the earthquake. Without functioning communications, individuals responsible for coordinating field activity may remain unaware when this outside assistance arrives. Satellite or cellular (wireless) telephones are also of limited usefulness as circuits quickly become overloaded with a large increase in official and non-official communication. The creation of a globally recognized disaster frequency, or even of nationally recognized disaster frequencies, would make a significant contribution to the improvement of communication under these circumstances.

Many alternate communication systems for response coordination and patient care have been developed to address the challenges arising after disaster events, especially in Europe and in the United States. A wireless transmission system for disaster patient care (WISTA) was developed to assist emergency personnel in treating disaster victims and coordinating medical resources.[18] The Wireless Internet Information System for Medical Response in Disasters (WIISARD) is a project by the University of California, San Diego, designed to support disaster relief operations in the field.[18] The Trauma Patient Tracking System is another initiative that allows integration of information and patient tracking over a wireless network from initial field triage or hospital presentation throughout the disaster event and follow-up. Information is linked to the individual via a barcoded wristband containing a Global Positioning System (GPS) or Radio Frequency Identification (RFID) tracking device.[19] Although these systems show promise, at the time of this writing none has been implemented after an earthquake. Given the additional likelihood of electricity and other infrastructural failures, concern exists that technology-based systems will not be applicable during the initial response period.

Movement into and out of a disaster zone is difficult following an earthquake. Significant damage occurs to transportation infrastructure such as roads, bridges, traffic signals, and road lighting. Following the 2010 Chilean earthquake, nearly 300 roadway bridges in the country were destroyed or damaged, including 20 with collapsed spans.[20] During the 1994 Northridge earthquake, 15% of the fatal injuries were motor vehicle related, primarily as a result of the disruptions in traffic control devices.[10] Forty-three of the sixty-three total deaths following the Loma Prieta event were associated with the collapse of road structures.[10] Individuals involved in earthquake-related motor vehicle crashes are 5.23 times more likely to die at the scene than survive to hospitalization.[2] Landslides, soil settlement, and slope failures, among other events, increase damage to roadways. Ill or injured survivors who require transportation to medical centers will experience delays until safe or passable routes are identified. The early use of law enforcement personnel (including National Guard assets in the United States) to control important transportation areas can improve this situation.[7]

The initial prehospital response should be directed toward the provision of emergency medical assistance, followed by search and rescue activities. Approximately 90% of all earthquake deaths are the result of structural collapse.[6] In some studies, death and

injury rates were 67- and 11-fold higher, respectively, for trapped victims compared to those who did not require extrication.[12,21] Injuries caused by collapsing structures or falling building components were 8.36 times more likely to result in fatalities than in hospitalizations.[2] The consequences of constructing buildings from substandard material and using seismically unsafe designs are clear.

There is a well-documented decrease in survival for victims trapped longer than 24–48 hours after an earthquake, as seen in the Campania-Irpinia earthquake (1980) in Italy and the Tangshan earthquake (1976) in China.[3,8] In Italy, a survey of 3,169 survivors showed that 93% of those who were trapped and survived were extricated within the first 24 hours and 95% of those who died expired before extrication.[21] Estimates of survivability among entrapped victims in Turkey and China indicate that within 2–6 hours, fewer than 50% of those buried were still alive.[3,11,21] In studies of the 1980 Italian and 1988 Armenian earthquakes, investigators concluded that 25–50% of the victims who were injured and died slowly could have been saved if they had received initial life-saving treatment within 6 hours of the event.[3,11,12,21]

Urban Search and Rescue (USAR) teams are among the first types of assistance deployed to earthquake zones. These teams theoretically increase survival by facilitating prompt extrication of trapped victims. In principle, USAR teams can help local leaders with structural assessment, advanced search and rescue techniques, and specialized medical training to limit the period of entrapment and mitigate some of its adverse medical effects.[22] The utility of USAR teams has, however, been questioned. In the United States, for example, it typically requires nearly 24 hours for teams to deploy and begin search and rescue activities in country and even more time to provide international assistance, thereby limiting their usefulness for saving lives after an earthquake.[22] In the Northridge earthquake, 19 hours passed before a USAR team originating in a city only 160 km (100 miles) from the affected area began operations at the collapsed Northridge Meadows Apartments.[7] After the 2011 Tōhoku Earthquake and Tsunami, a major Japanese USAR team had to be called back from its deployment in New Zealand to perform rescue activities in Japan.[23] The first U.S. USAR team sent to Turkey after the 1999 earthquake required 48 hours to begin operations.[7] After the 2010 earthquake in Haiti, airport damage and other access problems delayed arrival of some USAR teams by more than 4 days.[24] Reports show that more than 90% of survivors are rescued by local first responders and civilian volunteers within the first 24 hours after an earthquake event.[21,24]

USAR teams represent an expensive component of the earthquake response, with a heavy equipment team costing an estimated $900,000 USD to deploy for 10 to 14 days (average length of assignment).[24] In addition, the consumption of severely limited resources in the earthquake zone by USAR teams to support the transportation and housing of their equipment and personnel may prevent or delay the deployment of other critically necessary medical aid services to the same area. Increasingly there are questions as to the appropriateness of large funding commitments and diversion of other resources to support USAR teams. Some have suggested that funding mobile field hospitals and other interventions might be more effective.[24] One option is to train local inhabitants and first responders such as law enforcement personnel in basic search and rescue techniques. This would provide survivors who have the desire to assist their families, friends, and neighbors by engaging in search and rescue activity with the appropriate tools and techniques to do so. Reports on previous search and rescue events have noted that civilian participation in these efforts, specifically in providing knowledge of victims' whereabouts to searchers, may greatly enhance opportunities for timely extrication and survival.[25]

After an earthquake, an increased requirement for surgical services is expected during the first 72 hours.[6] Early rapid assessment of the extent of damage and injuries is necessary to direct resources where they are most needed.[10] Rescue workers frequently perform triage, using a system similar to Simple Triage and Rapid Treatment (START). This methodology can theoretically sort patients into groups of increasing acuity; however, controversy exists regarding the efficacy of such systems and data supporting their use are limited. Two studies evaluating START suggest it may be useful.[26,27] A third study evaluating meaningful performance metrics for START in an actual disaster concluded the triage algorithm had an acceptable level of undertriage and was successful in prioritizing transport of the sickest patients to area hospitals.[28] The START system emphasizes basic lifesaving measures such as opening an airway and applying direct pressure for external bleeding control, but rescuers are trained not to provide definitive care procedures at the scene. Chapter 14 contains additional information about the START system.

Hospital and Community Response

Hospitals are the traditional source of medical care after seismic events. However, hospitals can also be impacted by earthquakes, aggravating the initial imbalance between demand for care and response capacity. Healthcare facility closure and evacuation are mandated if management staff identify environmental or structural factors that put patients' safety at risk. An early structural assessment performed by expert engineers or, if not available, by on-site personnel is critical. Institutional disaster plans must include a hospital functional status evaluation.[29] The Applied Technology Council (ATC) provides guidance for structural assessments through documents such as the ATC-20 and ATC-20–2, and via a downloadable smartphone or tablet application ROVER (Rapid Observation of Vulnerability and Estimation of Risk, downloadable at www.atc-rover.org) which were developed with support of the U.S. Federal Emergency Management Agency (FEMA) and other entities.[3] Structure-dependent collapse patterns are documented in the FEMA Structural Engineer Training Manual.[22]

After the 2005 Pakistan earthquake, 65% of hospitals in the affected area were destroyed or badly damaged.[30] All hospitals in the Port au Prince region of Haiti were severely damaged or destroyed in the 2010 earthquake, possibly related to the lack of building codes in the country. Even facilities in areas with strict earthquake building codes may prove vulnerable to earthquake damage and require evacuation. Following the 2011 Tōhoku Earthquake and Tsunami, nearly 80% of hospitals and 30% of clinics in the affected regions were damaged, with many fully destroyed by the tsunami.[31,32] During the Northridge, California, earthquake, eight (9%) of ninety-one acute care hospitals were evacuated. Six of these institutions evacuated patients within the first 24 hours after the temblor, including several constructed under the most updated building codes. Two additional hospitals whose initial inspections revealed no critical damage and therefore continued providing patient care (including elective surgeries) were subsequently evacuated in the following weeks and were eventually demolished.[33] Thus hospitals reported to be secure may later prove vulnerable.

Hospitals that cannot continue providing safe inpatient care need to implement policies and procedures to facilitate the transfer and evacuation of their patients. Additionally, hospitals with patients requiring long-term care may choose to evacuate these patients to more distant facilities or to those without emergency or trauma services, making those beds available for potential disaster victims. Ideally, evacuation should be coordinated by the regional EOC if one exists to ensure effective resource utilization; however, if time is critical, hospitals can successfully evacuate patients independently without assistance from an EOC. Such activity is facilitated if mutual aid agreements with other hospitals are already in place or if the hospital is part of a larger system, such as the Department of Veterans Affairs in the United States. In the 2011 Christchurch, New Zealand, earthquake, a national teleconference was held to coordinate transfer of intensive care unit (ICU) patients from the only hospital with an emergency department in the city to hospitals in other areas of the country.[34] Evacuation transport problems can often be solved by collaboration between military and civilian groups. In the 1999 Marmara earthquake in Turkey, military boats and helicopters were used to transfer patients to remote major cities.[29]

Determining which patients to evacuate first is not always straightforward. Individuals hospitalized in ICUs require extensive resources, which are limited after a seismic event. Evacuating the sickest patients first from hospitals often works best, lessening the burden on healthcare facilities while improving the chances for better care of remaining patients and arriving victims.[7,32] When time is critical and structural collapse is imminent, evacuating the healthiest patients first permits movement of the greatest number of patients in the least amount of time.[7] During the Northridge earthquake, one evacuating institution believed that patients were in immediate danger and chose to evacuate the healthiest patients first, successfully evacuating all patients (334 total) to nearby open areas in 2 hours.[32] Methods to evacuate patients from a hospital may vary. In the Northridge evacuation, supervisors transported patients using available equipment such as backboards, wheelchairs, and blankets.[32] Vertical evacuation of patients (moving patients from one floor of the hospital to another) should use stairwells and not involve elevators until these have been inspected and deemed safe.

Without a thorough understanding of the science, planners might falsely believe that hospitals located near the earthquake epicenter will have a higher probability of structural damage. As such, incident managers may incorrectly assume that hospitals located farther away will remain functional and will preferentially direct patients to these facilities. Although this is true for institutions located at large distances from the epicenter, it does not appear these assumptions are correct for facilities located close to the epicenter. A study examining the association between distance from the epicenter and hospital evacuation found no relationship between these two variables (Figure 38.5).[35] All facilities studied were located within approximately 32 km (20 miles) of the epicenter. In contrast, a strong association existed between PGA and the need for hospital evacuation, regardless of the institution's location. It may be appropriate for incident managers to consult earthquake shake maps before making patient transport decisions during hospital evacuations. In regions with ground motion sensors, computers can generate shake maps identifying the areas of greatest shaking within minutes after a seismic event occurs.

Information about the status of surrounding hospitals is valuable. Some will sustain damage and be unable to accept

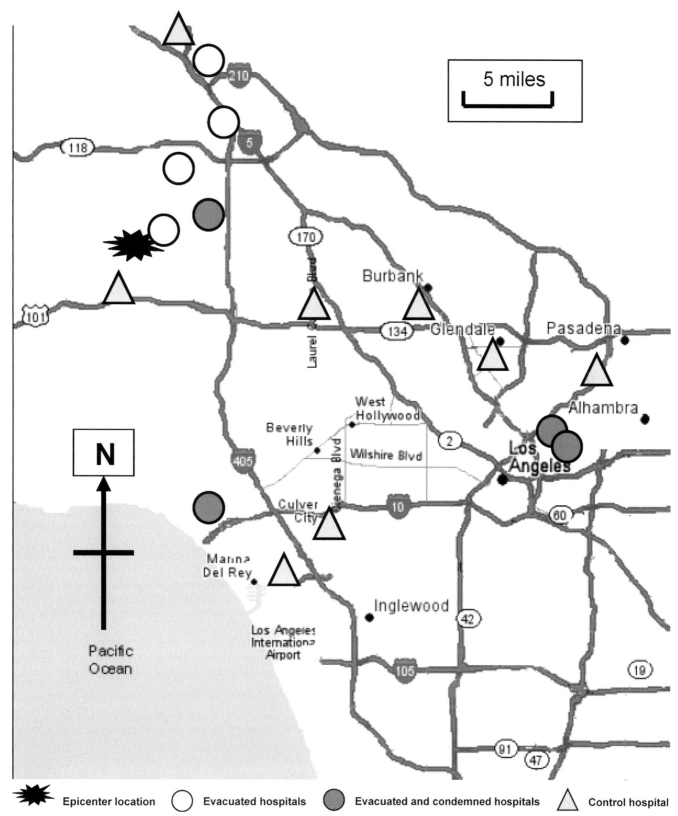

Figure 38.5. Epicenter and hospital locations, Los Angeles County, CA. This map shows the geographic locations of the study and control hospitals, as well as the epicenter of the 1994 Northridge earthquake. From Schultz CH, Koenig KL, Lewis RJ. Decisionmaking in hospital earthquake evacuation: does distance from the epicenter matter? *Ann Emerg Med;* 50(3) 2007: 320–326.

victims from the field. Others will be in the process of evacuation. Remaining functional hospitals can expect an increase in emergency department volume as well as requests to accept patient transfers from damaged institutions. Therefore, it would be extremely useful to establish a hospital communication system that could provide a rapid estimate of status of all regional facilities. Implementation of such a system would permit undamaged hospitals to estimate potential demand for their services in the immediate post-disaster period. Healthcare institutions could then decide whether to cancel elective surgeries, discharge stable patients earlier than planned, or implement other components of their surge plans.[34] Several communications systems currently exist but have not always performed optimally after seismic events.

Functioning hospitals must activate their disaster plans to prepare for the influx of victims. Effective command and control of the facility's response requires implementation of a system that is not dependent on the presence of any specific individual and will function at all time and on all days. A proposed model used by many hospitals is known as the Hospital Incident Command System (HICS) and is based on ICS principles. HICS has been effectively used during previous earthquakes.[7] More information on HICS is available in Chapter 22.

After establishing a command post and implementing an incident management system such as HICS, hospital administration should focus on evaluating personnel availability, communications, and resources. Hospital staff, like the general population, use telephones as a major method of communication. Because standard telephones frequently fail, secondary communication methods should be available. Examples of such methods include: alphanumeric pagers, priority phones, fax machines, Internet/email/instant messaging, cellular phones, wireless systems, ham radio systems, portable two-way radios, satellite telephones, and runners. Use of overhead speakers in patient care areas may be the simplest method of achieving broad communication for updates to in-house staff.

Hospital personnel who are not in the facility after a disaster can be difficult to contact. Therefore, implementation of a disaster callback policy is necessary. Such a policy could state that personnel should report to work in a major disaster unless they are notified to stay at home. Disaster planners can expect that most hospital staff will remain at work and not abandon their responsibilities. After the Northridge earthquake, as in other earthquakes, the majority of staff remained on duty. Communication and transportation disruptions were the main barriers for workers who did not immediately report to the hospital.[7] Notifying suppliers of an abrupt increase in demand for certain products may be difficult.

Patient tracking and the creation of medical records can be problematic after earthquakes. Many patients will not have access to items that document personal information and identity (e.g., medical insurance cards, state-issued identification cards) or will have a health condition that makes gathering information from them impossible (e.g., altered mental status). Therefore, creating a medical record and tracking a patient's movement through the healthcare system can be challenging. Potential solutions include documenting descriptive information such as sex, estimated age, height, color of skin, unique skin marking (mole, tattoo, or scar), eye color, and possibly fingerprints in the medical record.[6] Using records created with generic fictitious names before an event can also solve registration issues. Many trauma centers with electronic tracking systems maintain a large number of these fictitious registration names for quick assignment to unidentified patients. In settings in which patient volume overwhelms hospitals, documenting patient care may not be possible. After the 1991 Costa Rica earthquake, hundreds of patients received medical care even though documentation of these interactions was absent in many instances.[16] No widely accepted solution to the patient-tracking problem has yet been found, although some have suggested using bar codes or RFID devices (see Chapter 28).

In actuality, it is difficult for hospitals to meet the entire demand for medical assistance because they typically operate at a high census with little capacity for accepting additional patients. The solution to providing an effective medical response is optimizing use of all available resources. This requires hospitals to establish plans for maximizing surge capacity after an earthquake, even if hospital structures are damaged or fully occupied.[12] Typical plans include use of additional space not traditionally designated for patient care, such as cafeterias, auditoriums, and parking lots. After a temblor in Puerto Limon, Costa Rica (1999), the only treatment facility was declared structurally unsafe. This resulted in patient evacuations and establishment of treatment areas in the parking lot. After the Northridge and Loma Prieta earthquakes in the United States, treatment areas were established outside several hospitals.[16] Augmenting surge capacity also requires an increase in treatment supplies. To maintain the flow of medical goods, an agreement requiring suppliers to automatically deliver a set amount of material after a seismic event or other disaster should be established as part of a hospital's disaster plan.

In situations in which receiving hospitals become nonfunctional or remain intact but are unable to meet increased service demands, community-based solutions to augmenting surge capacity may be used. One such model is the Medical Disaster Response program. The main advantage of the Medical Disaster Response program is that victims receive rapid advanced medical care even if hospitals are damaged or destroyed. This project, developed by emergency physicians in southern California, trains healthcare personnel in the management of medical problems commonly encountered after earthquakes. It utilizes supplies stored in the community before an earthquake occurs, similar to the concept behind the Strategic National Stockpile, but at the local level. Under austere conditions, the Medical Disaster Response model directs the initial management of casualties by specially trained local personnel who access medical supplies at designated sites within the community.[3] Using this system, local healthcare providers in or near the disaster zone can respond immediately and deliver advanced patient care. Detailed discussion of the Medical Disaster Response project is available in the literature.[3,34,36]

Surge capacity is critical for a health system's disaster preparedness. Deficient capacity limits the ability of healthcare systems to respond to disasters.[37] Surge capacity plans require multidisciplinary collaboration to be successful. With regards to the personnel component of surge capacity, Schultz and Stratton proposed the creation of a database to provide rapid emergency credentialing of volunteers. If implemented, this strategy would offer an accurate, inexpensive, efficient, sustainable, U.S.-based, Joint Commission–compliant tool for rapidly expanding healthcare personnel support for hospital-based patient care. This database is created from a list provided by each hospital of personnel and physicians currently credentialed at their facility with unrestricted privileges. It would be shared with all participating institutions and a county healthcare agency. Volunteers listed in the database could obtain hospital privileges at any hospital within the county for the first 72 hours after a disaster event.[36] Should the database be shared between counties, such individuals could receive emergency privileges in other jurisdictions as well.

The first influx of patients is expected to arrive 30–60 minutes after the temblor, largely by self-transport. These patients will likely present with minor injuries such as uncomplicated lacerations, contusions, or fractures. No consistent relationship between injuries and demographic factors has been reported in the literature; neither age nor sex is considered a risk factor for injury. Because supplies may be limited in a disaster situation, victims with uncomplicated conditions should be quickly evaluated and directed to an observation area, with treatment postponed until more detailed information regarding the overall demand for medical care is available. Many victims suffering from minor injuries never require hospital care. After the 1989 Loma Prieta earthquake, as many as 60% of those with earthquake-related injuries either treated themselves or received treatment in nonhospital settings.[12] When treating uncomplicated lacerations during a disaster, providers should be aware of the risks of infection and missed foreign bodies. To decrease these risks, some experts recommend allowing uncomplicated lacerations to close by second intention or to use delayed primarily closure. There is insufficient evidence to justify any particular treatment recommendation at this time.

The second group of patients to arrive to hospitals is composed of victims with more serious conditions such as crush injuries. In developed nations, these victims are more typically transported via ambulance because they were more difficult to extricate or transport by lay individuals. They may also suffer from other medical conditions, making their initial treatment more challenging. Depending on the scenario, the number and acuity of patients needing acute care at local emergency facilities may overwhelm available resources. Therefore, implementation of a triage process is necessary. Hospital triage decisions must focus on which individuals should be prioritized for medical or surgical treatment. START does not discriminate between those who will consume large amounts of limited resources or whose prognosis will remain poor despite aggressive treatment. To allocate resources more appropriately, a proposed algorithm called the Secondary Assessment of Victim Endpoint (SAVE) was created. The goal of this algorithm is to reduce victim mortality and morbidity by allocating treatment resources only to those who will benefit. This means that not all victims will receive the same degree of care they would under normal circumstances. This treatment approach contradicts the usual medical philosophy of providing potentially unlimited care to each patient.[35]

The SAVE triage algorithm designed for mass casualty events is driven by estimated patient prognosis. It is based on outcomes data from trauma patients and those with other medical conditions who receive standard treatment. It recommends withholding aggressive medical care from those with a less than 50% chance of survival or from those who will essentially deplete all available resources.[35] Implementation of SAVE triage should only occur in situations in which the time for return to standard operations is unknown and rationing of limited resources is necessary. A detailed discussion of SAVE triage is available in the literature.[35]

The need for tools to rapidly prioritize patient care in disasters has received considerable attention. Ultrasonography holds promise as a technology for evaluating mass casualty victims and has many benefits. It is: 1) noninvasive; 2) portable; 3) easily repeatable; and 4) highly sensitive for intraperitoneal blood and many other conditions. Current indications for ultrasound in the evaluation of trauma patients include detection of pleural and pericardial effusions, increased intracranial pressure, pneumothoraces and hemothoraces, and fractures, and for placement of ultrasound-guided nerve blocks for anesthesia. The practical use of sonography has been studied in disaster settings (e.g., following Hurricane Katrina in the United States in 2005) and in the prehospital setting. During the 1988 Armenian earthquake, physicians with two ultrasound machines were able to triage 400 trauma patients over a period of 48 hours in a setting with limited availability of computed tomography.[38] Ultrasound has also been used in Kosovo, Afghanistan, and Iraq by deployed military forces.[39] Concerns regarding use of ultrasound in disaster situations relate to its dependence on functioning electricity and on the operator-dependent nature of its sensitivity. However, newer portable ultrasound devices can be battery-powered over the short-term, and increasing availability of bedside ultrasound in emergency departments, as well as training in their use, will decrease the variability in operator performance and interpretation of scans. It is likely that ultrasound will be increasingly implemented in disaster settings for patient screening and guiding medical care.

Medical Issues

After an earthquake, victims experience various injuries and illnesses that require medical treatment in hospitals or outpatient settings. These injuries can be divided into three major categories: 1) traumatic injuries resulting from the immediate event; 2) injuries and illnesses detected during relief and recovery efforts or resulting from changes in infrastructure or public health frameworks due to the earthquake; and 3) exacerbation of chronic conditions. Typical examples of trauma injuries include fractures, intracranial hemorrhage, spinal cord injuries, and intrathoracic, intra-abdominal, and intrapelvic organ trauma. Medical complications described in previous earthquakes include hypothermia, wound infections, gangrene, sepsis, adult respiratory distress syndrome, exacerbations of chronic pulmonary disease such as asthma, myocardial infarction, and tissue reperfusion syndromes. Although not strictly a complication of seismic activity, many investigators have also noted an increase in childbirths after an event.

Crush and Reperfusion Injuries

Crush injuries and long bone fractures are associated with the development of compartment and crush syndrome, which are commonly found in earthquake victims. Crush syndrome, one of the most common causes of death following a seismic event, results from excessive pressure on areas of significant muscle mass. Damaged muscle tissues leak cell contents into the extracellular space, causing fluid shifts and increased vascular permeability, leading to intravascular depletion.[38] Life-threatening effects of crush syndrome include multisystem organ dysfunction, hypovolemic shock, acidosis, rhabdomyolysis, and electrolyte disturbances (hyperkalemia, hypocalcemia). Untreated, these may produce acute renal failure, respiratory distress syndrome, disseminated intravascular coagulation, and fatal cardiac arrhythmias.[12,40,41]

Mortality rates for patients with crush syndrome who require renal dialysis have been reported to exceed 40%.[42,43] In the 1988

Table 38.5. Critical Ischemic Times by Tissue Type

Tissue Type	Critical Ischemic Time at Normal Temperature
Muscle	4 hours
Fat	13 hours
Bone	4 days

Adapted from: Gillani.[44]

Armenia earthquake, more than 1,000 victims trapped in collapsed buildings demonstrated crush syndrome and 323 developed acute renal failure requiring renal dialysis.[12] During the Kobe earthquake, crush syndrome was observed in 13.8% of hospitalized patients and acute renal failure developed in half of these individuals.[38,40] After the 1991 Costa Rica earthquake, autopsies performed on a sample of victims showed crush injury as the predominant mechanism of injury and cause of death.[16]

The time required before cells become damaged and begin to release their contents, termed the "critical ischemic time," differs between tissues, leading to a variable presentation dependent on the distribution of involved areas and ambient temperature (Table 38.5). Patients with longer extrication times, and/or abdomen or pelvis entrapment may be more likely to demonstrate signs of severe disease during or immediately after extrication.[44] Crush syndrome has been found in patients exposed to compressive forces for as little as 1 hour, but is usually seen in patients subject to high compressive pressures for 6 hours or more. When resources permit, patients with prolonged entrapment should have therapy initiated in the field, and before completion of extrication. Current recommendations of the Renal Disaster Relief Task Force of the International Society of Nephrologists (RDRTF-ISN) include initiation of intravenous fluid resuscitation initially on patient contact, with increased infusion volumes during the extrication process.[45]

Standard therapy for crush syndrome includes large amounts of intravenous fluids (500 to 1,000 ml/hr of isotonic saline), monitoring of cardiac rhythm and urine output, and dialysis if necessary. Due to the high risk for acute renal failure and hyperkalemia, intravenous fluids should be potassium-free. In the 1993 Turkey earthquake, researchers noted that some victims transferred from the field received solutions containing potassium.[39] If possible, isotonic saline with 5% dextrose is preferable as this provides needed glucose in patients with high metabolic demand and may attenuate the hyperkalemia.[44] While previous protocols included alkalinization via addition of bicarbonate to fluids, newer recommendations caution providers regarding complications of excessive alkalinization, including potential for worsening hypocalcemia and volume overload compromising respiratory status. Similarly, given risks of fluid overload and studies on limited efficacy, there is no current consensus on the administration of mannitol to crush victims.[46] Mannitol is contraindicated in anuric patients.[44]

In patients with significant crush injuries or compartment syndrome with potential for acute kidney injury (AKI), urine output should be monitored closely, with an output goal of more than 50 ml/hr. Patients with anuria or oliguria despite adequate rehydration, evidenced by central venous pressure monitoring, ultrasound measurement of the inferior vena cava, leg raise test, or other similar clinical or invasive measurements, should be presumed to have AKI. Further fluid administration should be restricted to avoid hypervolemia and pulmonary compromise. Even patients with mild initial presentations may be at risk for AKI after a crush injury. In the wake of a large disaster, individuals who are clinically stable with lesser pathology on initial evaluation (i.e., well-appearing, no long-bone fractures, no large open wounds) may be discharged to preserve capacity for victims requiring more services. These patients should be instructed to continue aggressive oral hydration, and to return immediately for darkening urine or decreased urine output.[44]

Lower mortality rates are seen when patients with crush injury–associated AKI are treated with adequate dialysis under the supervision of healthcare professionals.[42] Implementing a protocol using intermittent hemodialysis (IHD) during short sessions allows the treatment of several patients per day with a single machine. Continuous renal replacement therapy and peritoneal dialysis are less efficient in removing potassium and urea in comparison to intermittent hemodialysis, although they cause less hemodynamic instability.[38,40,44] There is limited experience with these dialysis therapies in disaster settings.

A major obstacle shared by all dialysis methods is the requirement for relatively large volumes of clean purified water as the dialysate fluid. To address this and related issues, RDRTF-ISN was developed in Europe. This group deploys to disaster locations and provides nephrologic assistance to both AKI patients and to those needing chronic dialysis. In 2010, assessment teams from the RDRTF-ISN deployed to both Haiti and Chile to assist with repairing dialysis equipment and water filtration systems along with designing IHD protocols. Eventually, many patients in Haiti received treatment in the Dominican Republic.[47]

In the austere environment that frequently follows an earthquake, prevention of crush syndrome may be difficult. A victim can deteriorate quickly to the point of death as the crush-injured area is extricated from a collapsed structure.[22,40] During the 1976 Tangshan earthquake in China, many patients died suddenly of cardiac arrest soon after extrication, presumably due to hyperkalemia.[16] When a high degree of suspicion exists that crush syndrome and associated hyperkalemia will develop during or immediately after rescue, it is recommended to delay extrication until personnel can infuse several liters of intravenous isotonic saline.[16,38,39] If large volumes of fluid are not available, amputation of the involved extremity is an option. Another suggested approach to this situation is application of a tourniquet to the compromised limb before extrication. Theoretically, this may avoid sudden death due to the ensuing reperfusion of the crushed extremity.[48] No data currently exist to support this intervention.

When treating crush injuries to an extremity, fasciotomies should be performed only when compartment syndrome is clearly present, such as when intracompartmental pressure measurements exceed 30–35 mmHg or rise to within 30 mmHg of the diastolic blood pressure.[40] Routine fasciotomies to prevent compartment syndrome are contraindicated due to the risk of infection related to the procedure itself. However, if the procedure is performed at a stage when the muscle is still viable, and the wound is kept covered with sterile dressing and allowed to heal by secondary intention, infection is rarely seen. Administration of antibiotics may also improve the prognosis, although this is controversial.[48] Medical management of compartment syndrome using mannitol has been proposed as an alternate to surgical intervention but presents risks of AKI or other complications in hypovolemic patients.[41]

Table 38.6. Mangled Extremity Severity Score (MESS) Score

Shock

Systolic blood pressure maintained above 90 mmHg	0
Transient hypotension	1
Persistent hypotension	2

Age (years)

<30	0
30–50	1
>50	2

Skeletal/soft-tissue injury

Low energy (stab; simple fracture; civilian gunshot wound)	1
Medium energy (open or multiple fractures; dislocation)	2
High energy (shotgun; military gunshot wound; crush injury)	3
Very high energy (as previous, plus gross contamination, soft tissue avulsion)	4

Limb ischemia

Pulse reduced or absent but normal perfusion	1
Pulseless; paresthesia; reduced capillary refill	2
Cool, paralyzed, insensate, numb	3
(Score doubled for ischemia longer than 6 hours)	

Modified table from Robertson.[54]

Amputations play a role in facilitating extrication and in removal of severely mangled extremities. The mangled extremity severity score is a tool that can assist medical providers deciding whether to amputate an injured lower extremity in cases where survival of the limb is questionable (Table 38.6).[49] A total score of 7 or greater indicates a high probability the extremity will be unsalvageable despite aggressive treatment and that amputation should be considered.[35,48,49] This assessment demonstrates specificity between 90% and 100%, making it acceptable for use in disaster settings. When indicated as an emergency procedure, a guillotine amputation performed at the most distal site possible is best technique and has a low incidence of infection, even without antibiotics.[48]

Pain Management

Painful procedures such as amputation, fasciotomy, and fracture reduction require effective anesthesia and analgesia. Available options include regional anesthetics (nerve blocks, Bier blocks) and administration of systemic medications. In the austere setting, it is unlikely that sufficient personnel or equipment will be available for monitoring of many patients simultaneously using general anesthesia. Thus this option should be reserved for those patients requiring major abdominal or thoracic surgery. Following the 2008 Wenchuan earthquake, the arriving anesthesia team effectively used epidural anesthesia or regional plexus blocks on more than 60% of 141 patients requiring emergent surgery.[50] Epidural anesthesia carries a low risk for hypotensive complications or airway compromise. Recent experience in Haiti supports the potential efficacy of ultrasound-guided regional nerve blocks for immediate and continued post-procedural analgesia.[51,52]

With regard to systemic medication, ketamine has emerged as a reliable drug for achieving effective procedural anesthesia and analgesia. Ketamine, a dissociative agent, has been categorized as a rapid-onset, short-acting, safe, and effective drug that preserves airway reflexes and supports the cardiovascular system. In a review of 11,589 patients treated with ketamine, only two healthy patients required intubation. Ketamine has been used safely in unmonitored, austere environments in Afghanistan to facilitate field amputations, and after disasters with minimal adverse events.[3] In the absence of contraindications, ketamine can be administered safely via oral, intravenous, rectal, or intramuscular routes. The recommended dosage to achieve full dissociation with complete amnesia is 2 mg/kg for slow intravenous administration and 4–6 mg/kg for intramuscular injection.[3,48] Although rare, adverse events reported in disaster setting include intra-operative emesis and laryngospasm.[53]

Fluid Resuscitation

Availability of intravenous fluids may be limited in the first 48 hours after a seismic event. Therefore, common practice patterns must be modified regarding the type and amount of fluids used in a disaster setting. Limited data support the use of hypertonic saline for initial resuscitation and normal saline for early maintenance.[3,54] A Cochrane review of studies comparing hypertonic and isotonic fluids for trauma resuscitation found no significant differences in mortality between trauma patients initially resuscitated with isotonic versus hypertonic crystalloids.[55] Doses of 4 ml/kg of hypertonic saline seem to be safe and effective in trauma patients and burn victims, including children.[54,56] If there is improvement with hypertonic saline, patients can be supported with normal saline. Concerns about the development of hypernatremia and a hyperosmolar state limit the amount of hypertonic saline that can be used. The main objective in changing resuscitation fluids is reducing the volume of normal saline that must be kept in inventory for initial patient stabilization. Liter bags of saline are heavy and require significant space for storage. Medical personnel can initially resuscitate two to four times the number of patients with a given volume of hypertonic saline as they can with the same volume of normal saline. Additionally, at least one study using hypertonic solutions in resuscitation of hypovolemic shock from blunt trauma demonstrated a decrease in adult respiratory distress syndrome (ARDS) when hypertonic fluids were used for initial resuscitation.[57] This may be due to decreased third spacing of hypertonic fluids during resuscitation.[58] More information is needed to determine the optimal intravenous solution for resuscitation and stabilization of disaster victims.

Newer data on resuscitation in penetrating torso trauma argues that "permissive hypotension" may increase survival for major trauma patients if a delay in providing definitive care is anticipated. Thus some experts recommend maintaining blood pressure in the moderately hypotensive range, targeting a systolic of 90 mmHg or mean arterial pressure of 60 mmHg. They suggest that normalizing blood pressure may be associated with increased internal hemorrhage and exacerbated morbidity and mortality.[35,54] Definitive evidence for or against this approach is lacking, and the majority of studies with positive findings only addressed penetrating torso trauma, which may not be relevant to many earthquake victims.

After initial resuscitation and stabilization, an assessment of surgical needs and capabilities must be performed, with triage of patients requiring prompt definitive management. Adults who do not respond to fluid resuscitation should be reevaluated with regard to the continuation of aggressive care. Ultrasound can quickly confirm the presence of significant intra-abdominal hemorrhage. If significant or increasing intraperitoneal bleeding is identified, resources are limited, and surgical intervention is unavailable, consideration for the provision of comfort care only is warranted. The opposite is true for children with abdominal trauma; they should be treated aggressively because many will survive even severe intra-abdominal injury without operative intervention.[35]

For those with potential requirements for fasciotomy or other non-abdominal procedures, it may be untenable to deny patients oral intake pending capacity (personnel and equipment) for surgery. In the 2010 Haitian earthquake, oral intake restrictions for trauma patients were liberalized due to the lack of intravenous fluids and the malnutrition status of many patients. Although no clear evidence about the safety of this procedure is reported, groups that used this practice denied any significant adverse events.[52]

Transition from Immediate to Subacute/Ambulatory Care

After a catastrophic earthquake, by the time substantial outside medical resources arrive to the disaster area, most victims have either received initial treatment or are dead. However, the need for maintaining medical care, supporting the damaged healthcare infrastructure, and supplementing limited resources persists. Groups that arrive after the immediate response phase is over are critical to preserving the lives of survivors. Disaster Medical Assistance Teams (DMATs) are available in some countries, including the United States, Japan, and Australia. These teams were created with variable missions and response times. One important function they can provide is to care for ambulatory patients in any location. For example, these teams can decrease the healthcare burden on emergency departments by offering another option for medical care in the days to weeks after the earthquake.

RDRTF can similarly increase dialysis capacity for existing renal patients and for victims suffering AKI from crush syndrome. The positive impact of RDRTF was demonstrated following the Marmara earthquake in Turkey in 1999 and the Yogyakarta earthquake in Indonesia in 2006.[59,60] RDRTF is composed of three divisions: American, European, and Pacific.[38] DMATs and RDRTF are meant to be self-sufficient and to establish patient care capability with limited consumption of local community resources. The time required for these teams to arrive at the disaster zone is often more than 48 hours (sometimes weeks in remote areas), limiting their effectiveness in reducing the burden of acute patient care in many cases.[59] These teams will help in the reconstitution of the basic medical care system because hospitals, clinics, and medical offices may be destroyed or incapacitated for an unknown length of time and sometimes indefinitely.

Overall mortality from earthquake injuries is affected by the availability and efficacy of medical and surgical services within the first week after the event. In the 2010 Haitian earthquake response, many initial hospital capabilities were provided by a mobile field hospital deployed by the Israeli Defense Forces Medical Corps (IDF-MC). This mobile field hospital encompassed a staff of 230 personnel including 44 physicians and 77 additional hospital personnel. They established a 72-bed onsite hospital with laboratory, pharmacy, and surgical capabilities less than 4 days after the event (Figure 38.6).[61] Of note, the 230 individuals arriving with this team included 109 nonmedical personnel (e.g., security, carpenters, plumbers, and information technology personnel). The team provided their own generators, medications, supplies, and electronic equipment, rendering them entirely self-sufficient. Personnel in the IDF-MC field hospital treated 1,111 patients and performed 244 operations by day 14 after the earthquake.[61] Later field hospital arrivals are more likely to provide ongoing care to survivors newly disabled as a result of disaster-related injuries, and to those patients with chronic medical conditions now deprived of regular sources of care. Experiences of other field hospitals differ from that of IDF-MC. Staff and supplies from the University of Chicago arrived nearly 2 weeks after the initial event, but continued their activities for nearly 4 months on-site.[62] During their 4-month deployment, staff in this field hospital provided care to twice the number of patients treated in the 10-day IDF-MC acute care facility. Cost-benefit analyses of field hospital deployments, including their cost-effectiveness and effects on numbers of lives saved and long-term patient outcomes are lacking.

An important area to consider in an ongoing disaster response is public access to information. In the aftermath of an earthquake, locating individuals can be extremely difficult. Many victims will leave the area, die, or be hospitalized. Patient transfers are common and victims will often receive ongoing care in facilities far from where they live. The creation of a public information center will decrease the time and effort people spend looking for relatives and improve family reunification. In recent years, several organizations have used social media and principles of crowd-sourcing to facilitate acquisition and dissemination of information on victim locations, harnessing the increasing penetrance of internet and short message service (SMS) in both high- and low-income nations. Starting with the 2010 Haitian earthquake, the Google Person Finder (https://google.org/personfinder/global/home.html) has invited individuals and organizations to upload and search information via a centralized website. In the United States, the Red Cross Safe & Well program performs a similar function. While initial public and media response has been positive, research is necessary to assess the efficacy of these programs as well as the risks to privacy and the potential for exploitation of disaster victims.

Non-trauma-related Medical Conditions

A review of pertinent literature reveals that more than 20% of patients hospitalized in the first 72 hours after earthquakes suffer from non-traumatic conditions.[11] Many of these indirect health effects from disasters are predictable and preventable.[63] Most manifest as acute exacerbations of chronic conditions such as diabetes, pulmonary diseases, coronary artery disease, chronic kidney disease, hypertension, anxiety, and pregnancy-related complications.[12,60] Beginning on the third day following the 1999 Chi-Chi earthquake in Taiwan, medical diseases became the most common cause for hospitalization.[11] In Haiti, presentations for medical complaints outnumbered those for traumatic complaints within 2 weeks following the temblor.[61] After the 1985 Mexico City earthquake, there was an increase in the number of spontaneous abortions, premature births, and normal deliveries, making those conditions the primary reasons for admission in acute care facilities.[12] Healthcare professionals should be prepared for the increased incidence in these medical conditions following earthquakes. Exposure of displaced populations to extreme weather and crowding in remaining or temporary

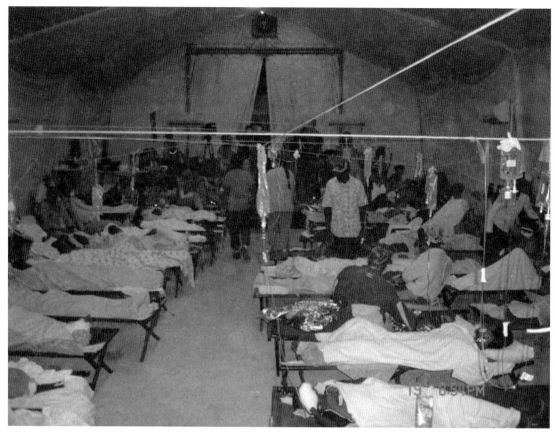

Figure 38.6. Mobile field hospital established by the Israeli Defense Forces Medical Corps in Haiti four days after the 2010 earthquake.

shelters also creates additional potential victims. Variable degrees of hypothermia were documented in patients evacuated from the Armenia earthquake of 1988.[21,22] Increased rates of tuberculosis were reported in both Japan and Haiti after earthquake events.

Myocardial Infarction

Increased numbers of patients presenting with conditions related to cardiovascular disease such as myocardial infraction and cardiac arrest have been reported after earthquakes.[7,63] A 50% increase in cardiac deaths was reported in the first 3 days following the 1981 Athens 6.7-magnitude earthquake.[7,12] Analysis of this phenomenon suggests that it may be caused by psychological stress resulting in an increase in catecholamines promoting vasoconstriction, and not to an increase in physical exertion. The incidence of sudden cardiac death rose dramatically in the first 24 hours after the Northridge earthquake, and then decreased in the following 6 days. This suggests that those who died immediately after the earthquake were already susceptible to cardiac events and may have died in the next several days. It appears the earthquake may have accelerated the process. In most studies, increases in cardiac mortality were reported to occur within a few days following earthquakes; however, after the 7.2-magnitude 1995 Great Hanshin-Awaji earthquake, augmented cardiac mortality was reported over a period of weeks.[63] Earthquakes that cause chronic stress among the population during the recovery and reconstruction stage may result in prolonged cardiac events. In addition, hospital damage and the resultant loss of standard treatment resources increase mortality and worsen prognosis from myocardial infarction.

Acute and Chronic Pulmonary Disease

Respiratory injury is a major cause of death among victims of earthquakes. Early mortality caused by airway obstruction, asphyxiation, and dust-induced fulminant pulmonary edema are possible scenarios. Part of the increased incidence in respiratory diseases after earthquakes is attributable to the inhalation of dust produced by collapsed structures during early search and rescue activities.[12] After the 2011 Tōhoku Earthquake and Tsunami, there was more than a twofold increase over baseline in the number of elderly patients admitted to hospitals in the disaster area for respiratory or pulmonary complaints. The majority of these complaints included pneumonia and exacerbations of chronic obstructive pulmonary disease and asthma. The stress of the event combined with post-disaster conditions combine to impair the ability of fragile groups, particularly the elderly, to perform activities of daily living, increasing their risk for pulmonary injury.[64] However, children and adults are susceptible to these same conditions. In a study of patients treated in a Haiti tent camp during days 15 through 18 after the event, nearly 25% had pulmonary complaints, and fever; respiratory complaints were the major infectious complaint after the Wenchuan earthquake.[65,66]

End-Stage Renal Disease

After a seismic event, there is an increase in the number of patients with chronic end-stage renal disease (ESRD) whose conditions deteriorate. Dialysis-dependent patients may not receive their treatments because the supply of water and electricity required are disrupted. In addition, dialysis centers and materials may be destroyed and personnel may be unavailable. Centers with the capability to perform dialysis can be overwhelmed by new patients with AKI secondary to crush syndrome as well as by patients with ESRD whose usual site of care is not functional. The immediate options for increasing surge capacity for dialysis patients are either to decrease the number of weekly dialysis sessions for each patient or to shorten the duration of each session, as was done after the Marmara earthquake in 1999. In the aftermath of this seismic event, officials not only implemented shortened periods for dialysis but also advised strict dietary and fluid restrictions. Compliance with these recommendations was high. As a result, despite less frequent dialysis, weight gain and blood pressure among these patients did not differ when compared with the pre-disaster period.[60] As new temporary centers for dialysis open or alternate facilities become available, patients can receive their treatments at nearby satellite outpatient units until damaged facilities are restored.[40]

In the first days after a disaster, dialysis-dependent patients should be advised on strict fluid restriction and avoidance of potassium-rich foods. If dialysis treatment centers are inoperative or cannot be reached, potassium exchange resins kept in the home can serve as a temporizing measure to mitigate hyperkalemia.[60] Disaster plans should consider management strategies for ESRD patients because they will consume a large amount of resources needed in the aftermath of a major temblor. In an extreme situation in which the physician needs to prioritize treatment between patients with acute or chronic renal failure, dialysis should be administered first to those with AKI. These individuals, if they survive their critical state, are more likely to live longer and healthier lives.[60]

Management of Psychological Distress

Disasters are associated with a continuum of risk and resilience. They frequently initiate significant new incidences of psychiatric disorders within a population. The psychological impacts of disasters are felt by responders, victims directly impacted by the event, their families, and the surrounding communities. The increase in cardiovascular events after earthquakes is believed to result in part from the increased psychosocial stress from the event. Both the general population and responders may need supportive psychological services.

The first attempt to model population-level disaster mental health impacts was performed for the Southern California "Shakeout Scenario" Exercise. This simulation involved a catastrophic 7.8-magnitude earthquake effecting a population of 21 million over eight counties in Southern California. The exercise used the Psychological Simple Triage and Rapid Treatment (PsySTART) Disaster Mental Health Triage System – a triage system that measures doses of exposure to traumatic loss, disaster-related injury and illness, separation from family members, and severe peri-traumatic stress. Using the PsySTART model in the Shakeout Scenario, and incorporating incident-specific features including deaths, injuries, and home loss, Schreiber and Shoaf estimated the psychological impact of this disaster event. In the 21 million individuals living in the impact area, the number of distressed but resilient individuals was estimated at 8 million, and the point prevalence of new disorders requiring professional assessment and care was 200,000.[67] Disaster preparedness schema should take into account the potential short- and long-term implications of this level of psychological impact. Further detailed discussion of disaster mental health is found in Chapter 9.

Infection and Epidemics

After an earthquake, the effected region is subject to increased rates of infection, and to epidemics of diseases normally endemic in the population. The most important factors contributing to an area's vulnerability to infectious diseases are the loss of adequate drinking water supplies and sanitation systems. Failure of these systems increases the risk for development of water-borne diseases. In addition, earthquakes lead to soft tissue injuries, population displacement, and crowding, all of which have been shown to increase infectious disease exposure and transmission of communicable diseases.[68] In patients with crush injuries and other limb and soft tissue trauma, early initiation of appropriate antimicrobial therapy is important to decrease mortality from wound-related infections. Cultures of infected wounds following two disparate earthquakes – Haiti and China – revealed predominance of Gram-negative bacteria, including *Acinetobacter baumannii*, *Enterobacter cloacae*, *Escherichia coli*, *Klebsiella pneumonia*, and *Pseudomonas aeruginosa*.[69,70] Importantly, in species isolated in Haiti, a majority were resistant to trimethoprim/sulfamethoxazole, and over a third were cephalosporin-resistant. Fluoroquinolones, particularly ciprofloxacin, are currently the recommended first-line agents for empiric therapy of post-earthquake wound infections. Additionally, tetanus vaccination and treatment of at-risk populations is important to prevent infection from tetanus-prone wounds.

Despite the theoretical risks for epidemics in the immediate post-earthquake period, it appears unlikely that they will actually occur, especially for diseases not already endemic to the disaster area.[6,7] Few articles in the literature report outbreaks after an earthquake. A malaria outbreak was reported after the 1999 Costa Rica earthquake. In addition, after the 1994 Northridge earthquake, a coccidiomycosis outbreak was reported.[68] It appears that mass vaccination campaigns, based solely on the fear of possible epidemics, are inappropriate. However, strengthening of public health surveillance systems in the aftermath of earthquakes is important to prevent or control epidemics. Ten months after the 2010 Haitian earthquake a cholera epidemic emerged on the island resulting in more than 400,000 cases and nearly 6,000 deaths. It is believed that the importation of cholera to this non-endemic area was the result of United Nations peacekeeping personnel arriving from an endemic region, Nepal, combined with the poor sanitation facilities for both residents and many aid workers.[71] Residents of camps for Internally Displaced Persons (IDPs) were relatively spared from this epidemic, likely due to their improved sanitation and water facilities as compared with those populations outside of the IDP camps.[72] An epidemiological surveillance system should direct any interventions, including resource investment in vaccination campaigns, based on measured disease activity in the area.

Disposal of Bodies

Decaying corpses represent a concern to the public and to health authorities; however, the belief that an increased risk of disease transmission exists due to decomposing dead bodies in the aftermath of major disasters is a myth. Authorities should be aware that the health hazards related to unburied human remains, principally those of trauma victims, are negligible. Mass burials or cremations are not justified on the basis of public health concerns.[73,74] Such practices require the use of enormous amounts of fuel, destroy any evidence for future identification, and do not respect some religious rituals. One situation in which handling human remains can represent a health risk is during epidemics of transmissible infectious diseases. Even in these situations, there is no reason to deprive families of their wishes to manage their dead relatives according to their customs, as long as they follow certain safety measures (however, this may be difficult in the case of Ebola virus disease).[68] In addition, it is important to identify victims. This has relevance not only to regional governments but also to provide family members a greater degree of stability and closure in reference to their losses. Fingerprints, photographs, dental records, imaging, and DNA analysis can be used to help identify victims (see Chapter 23).[73] Disaster Mortuary Operational Response Teams (DMORTs) consisting of forensic specialists are organized in some nations in parallel with DMATs. These teams assist with victim identification and body disposal.

Prevention

Disaster mitigation and preparedness plans at all levels of government are important factors for reducing earthquake mortality.[16] These plans must provide for early extrication of trapped victims and early treatment of immediate medical conditions with effective use of available resources. Implementation of an incident management system along with previously negotiated mutual aid agreements and transportation networks, including airlifts, can also improve victim prognosis.

Disaster preparedness plans should focus on augmentation of the prehospital response to minimize the lethal impact of earthquakes and maximize lifesaving potential within the first 24 hours after the event. Prehospital providers must be prepared to initiate abbreviated patient assessment protocols designed for disasters rather than continue with everyday responses. Immediate needs assessments associated with an efficient organizational structure are required to optimize disaster response. This must be done with the coordination of local, state, national, and international agencies. It is of great importance to incorporate data obtained from formal training exercises into the disaster planning process and to develop relationships among organizational entities that participate in a disaster response.

The Joint Commission requires hospitals seeking their accreditation to include an evacuation strategy in their emergency management programs. Institutions must periodically test their evacuation plans by using drills that model the disruption of emergency department and hospital activities.[75] Although The Joint Commission requires that disaster drills involve the regional responders needed in an earthquake, hospitals often do so in an ineffective manner, failing to realistically assess overall preparedness.

Education in earthquake risk reduction should be a major focus for healthcare and community members. Preparation programs must include:

- Training of teams for search and rescue operations and needs assessments;
- Identification of safe sites where people can be relocated after the event;
- Education and training of area healthcare professionals regarding common medical conditions in earthquake victims and how to appropriately treat them;
- Maintenance of pharmaceuticals and supplies needed for the most frequent earthquake-related medical presentations;
- Assessing the structural safety of facilities essential to the operation of disaster responses (e.g., hospitals) and requesting upgrades as necessary;

- Arrangement for alternate water supplies;
- Plans for maintenance of viable vehicle transportation corridors;
- Orientation to the operation of emergency communication systems; and
- Training of teams to assess structural and nonstructural damage and determine whether buildings are safe for occupancy.

Critical actions taken before, during, and after a disaster will save lives and minimize property damage. Building damage and structural collapse resulting in loss of life are predictable in settings without seismic construction codes.[21,76] A study of the 1976 Guatemala earthquake concluded that deaths and injury were critically dependent on housing damage and construction materials used.[21] Building codes developed for seismic areas are intended to prevent catastrophic structural failure and reduce mortality with the formation of large void spaces in any structure that does fail.[22] Implementation and enforcement of building codes will help prevent deaths and improve the safety of the population. Yet even stringent building codes are not 100% effective.

Communities at risk for earthquakes must adopt effective response strategies to decrease losses after an event. Substantial numbers of victims are rescued by community members in the first hours after an earthquake. Therefore, planners should train local residents in safe search and rescue activities. To reduce the number of deaths suffered by extricated victims, care should be provided for life-threatening injuries within the first 6 hours.[10] Because insufficient and uncoordinated medical responses are often reported in the aftermath of earthquake events, more attention to a local medical response plan, such as the Medical Disaster Response program, is warranted.

In addition, and particularly in areas where building codes may effectively prevent collapse-related injuries, individuals should be educated on mitigating nonstructural damage by securing loose objects. Bracing bookcases to the wall, securing heavy electronic equipment, and using earthquake hooks to hang glass-containing picture frames are simple prevention activities that can substantially reduce injuries. After the Northridge earthquake, individuals from sixteen hospitals were interviewed and reported that most of the injuries resulting in hospital admission were caused by falls or by being hit by objects.[39] Many tools and devices are currently available for securing both heavy and smaller objects.

RECOMMENDATIONS FOR FURTHER RESEARCH

Although investigators examining the medical and health consequences of seismic events have made significant progress, additional work is necessary to improve the care and outcomes of earthquake victims. These endeavors will require a transdisciplinary approach involving participation from multiple medical, health, and nonmedical professionals. A few projects with the potential for achieving this goal follow.

A rapid and accurate estimate of casualty numbers and the extent of their injuries is necessary to coordinate the size and type of healthcare resources required to provide care to earthquake victims. Delays in obtaining this information will lead to an inappropriate or inadequate medical and health response. Current estimates are based on generalized information gathered from previous seismic events and do not reflect individual variations in building construction or population density.

In addition, current casualty estimation computer programs do not provide estimates in real-time and are not specific for earthquakes. New models are needed that can use population data for individual locations and rapidly generate estimates based on observed building damage. Designing such models is possible using data-mining techniques combining engineering building damage classification data and population injury information.

If a large-magnitude earthquake occurs in a densely populated area, implementing a system for triaging medical casualties will be necessary. There are several triage systems available, but data on their effectiveness are limited. Most research to date has focused on triage tool assessment using drills or models thought to approximate the types of victims caused by seismic activity, such as individual trauma patients. Such investigations produce limited information that does not address how these triage systems will perform in an actual disaster. More investigations are required of mass casualty triage system performance based on meaningful outcomes data in actual earthquakes to clarify which of these tools is most appropriate.

Many countries have made a significant investment in earthquake response by equipping, staffing, and transporting USAR teams to events all over the world. However, the impact of these teams on meaningful outcomes remains unclear. While the rescue of trapped victims days after the earthquake is inspiring, it is possible the resources devoted to sustaining USAR teams might not be cost-effective from a population perspective. Many people die weeks to months after a temblor due to dehydration, exposure, and infectious disease. It is possible many more lives might be saved if the resources invested in USAR teams were instead devoted to public health interventions. Although political forces may create resistance, objective investigations into the value of USAR teams are necessary.[24]

The field management of victims suffering from crush injuries remains controversial. If resources are plentiful, standard treatment protocols apply. Under austere conditions, however, the most appropriate approach to such victims is unknown, especially when supplies of intravenous fluids are limited. The roles for field fasciotomies, amputations, tourniquets applied to crushed extremities before extrication, and the use of hypertonic saline all require additional study. Future possibilities for treatment of AKI in the post-disaster environment may also include regenerative dialysis sorbent systems that require smaller amounts of purified water. These devices are relatively compact and often used in the home. Although the U.S. military has had experience with one of these systems for battlefield treatment of AKI since the 1980s, these particular machines are no longer produced.[77] Development of similar systems is underway.

Developing countries that experience a large seismic event often lack the resources to mount an effective response and require assistance from other countries and the United Nations. However, the coordination of multiple international response assets from governmental and nongovernmental organizations remains a challenge. In addition, the level of skill and professionalism associated with responding medical teams is not currently regulated. No internationally recognized essential standards for responders exist. The events in Haiti have raised the profile of these issues and some efforts are being made to address such concerns. These ongoing efforts must continue until international standards for team professionalization are developed and implemented.

The large number of victims generated by a powerful earthquake requires hospitals to quickly increase surge capacity.

Research has identified the major components of this process and programs exist to support some aspects of surge capacity, including the U.S. National Pharmaceutical Stockpile, community-based programs such as the Medical Disaster Response project, the Emergency System for Advanced Registration of Volunteer Health Professionals, and the creation of Federal Medical Stations. It remains unknown, however, how effective these programs will be. Further investigation is needed to examine what interventions will be successful under actual disaster conditions. If current programs fail to adequately address surge capacity, disaster experts must identify new approaches that can meet the rapidly expanding demand for care.

Identifying the areas most heavily damaged by an earthquake is important. These locations are not evenly distributed near the epicenter, but are scattered over a wide area affected by the temblor. Because most deaths and injuries result from building damage, quickly obtaining such information can provide responders with the locations where most victims will be found. In addition, it can suggest which hospitals remain functional and which are evacuating patients. The current technology using ground motion sensors that measure PGA and PGV can generate shake maps within minutes of a seismic event. These maps depict the intensity of ground motion over a wide area. Although this information suggests areas of higher and lower probability for structural failure, it is insufficient to reliably predict building damage. More sophisticated software that incorporates ground motion along with soil conditions and types of building construction could yield a more accurate prediction of building damage and subsequent injury potential.

Disaster management focuses on needs assessments of the affected population, efficient utilization of resources, prevention of further adverse health effects, and evaluation of relief program effectiveness.[72] Improvements in disaster mitigation and responses for future events will require a carefully organized, multidisciplinary evaluation of their associated consequences. Therefore, a government-sponsored international research center for the multidisciplinary evaluation and study of disasters is needed.

Summary

Earthquakes are spontaneous events associated with increases in morbidity and mortality, and large economic losses, including costly property damage. Understanding the challenges that arise after seismic events can assist with planning, improving strategies for mitigating their effects, and assisting with more effective coordination of local resources. The medical management of earthquake victims remains difficult; however, the amount of data on this subject continues to increase, allowing the development of new recommendations. Implementation of field triage protocols (e.g., START and SAVE) and the use of a unified command system are vitally important in supporting early organizational efforts in the chaotic environment that surrounds catastrophic earthquakes. Acknowledging that hospitals will be overwhelmed during the first 24–48 hours helps responders prepare for that reality, supporting plans to augment surge capacity and thereby decreasing victim mortality and morbidity. Hospital structures remain susceptible to seismic damage and healthcare facilities must prepare and test reliable evacuation plans that incorporate effective strategies used successfully in previous events. Knowledge of common conditions that arise after an earthquake, such as crush syndrome, respiratory symptoms, renal failure, fractures, and lacerations can help healthcare professionals more effectively manage these medical problems. In addition, refining plans for the management of chronic medical conditions, epidemiologic surveillance, and the appropriate disposition of dead bodies are important to improve earthquake response and recovery.

REFERENCES

1. Kazzi AA, Langdorf MI, Handly N, White K, Ellis K. Earthquake epidemiology: the 1994 Los Angeles Earthquake emergency department experience at a community hospital. *Prehosp Disaster Med* 2000; 15(1): 12–19.

2. Peek-Asa C, Kraus JF, Bourque LB, Vimalachandran D, Yu J, Abrams J. Fatal and hospitalized injuries resulting from the 1994 Northridge earthquake. *Int J Epidemiol* 1998; 27(3): 459–465.

3. Schultz CH, Koenig KL, Noji EK. *A medical disaster response to reduce immediate mortality after an earthquake.* N Engl J Med 1996; 334(7):438–444.

4. United States Geologic Survey (USGS). Earthquakes with 1,000 or More Deaths (through the end of 2014). http://earthquake.usgs.gov/earthquakes/world/world_deaths.php (Accessed September 4, 2015).

5. Cavallo EA, Powell A, Becerra O. Estimating the direct economic damage of the earthquake in Haiti. Inter-American Development Bank, 2010. Inter-American Development Paper Working Paper No. 163.

6. Perez E, Thompson P. Natural hazards: causes and effects. Lesson 2 earthquakes. *Prehosp Disaster Med* 1994; 9(4): 260–269.

7. Schultz CH. Earthquakes. In: Hogan DE, Burstein JL, eds. *Disaster Medicine.* 2nd ed. Philadelphia, PA, Lippincott Williams & Wilkins, 2007; 185–193.

8. Adams RD. Earthquake occurrence and effects. *Injury* 1990; 21(1): 17–20.

9. Shoaf KI, Sareen HR, Nguyen LH, Bourque LB. Injuries as a result of California earthquakes in the past decade. *Disasters* 1998; 22(3): 218–235.

10. Ramirez M, Peek-Asa C. Epidemiology of traumatic injuries from earthquakes. *Epidemiol Rev* 2005; 27: 47–55.

11. Chan YF, Alagappan K, Gandhi A, et al. Disaster management following the Chi-Chi earthquake in Taiwan. *Prehosp Disaster Med* 2006; 21(3): 196–202.

12. Naghii MR. Public health impact and medical consequences of earthquakes. *Rev Panam Salud Publica* 2005;18(3): 216–221.

13. Gerstenberger MC, Wiemer S, Jones LM, Reasenberg PA. Real-time forecasts of tomorrow's earthquakes in California. *Nature* 2005; 435: 328–331.

14. Mignone AT, Jr., Davidson R. Public health response actions and the use of emergency operations centers. *Prehosp Disaster Med* 2003; 18(3): 217–219.

15. Sekizawa A, ed. Post-Earthquake Fires and Firefighting Activities in the Early Stage in the 1995 Great Hanshin Earthquake. Nakahara, Mitaka, Tokyo. U.S. Department of Commerce: U.S. Building and Fire Research Laboratory, 1997.

16. Pretto EA, Angus DC, Abrams JI, et al. An analysis of prehospital mortality in an earthquake. Disaster Reanimatology Study Group. *Prehosp Disaster Med* 1994; 9(2): 107–117.

17. Roy N, Shah H, Patel V, Coughlin RR. The Gujarat earthquake (2001) experience in a seismically unprepared area: community hospital medical response. *Prehosp Disaster Med* 2002; 17(4): 186–195.

18. Yuechum C, Xin H, et al. WISTA: A Wireless Transmission System for Disaster Patient Care. 2nd International Conference on Broadband Networks. 2005; 2: 1041–1045.

19. Maltz JS, Ng TSC, Li DJ, Wang J, Wang K, Bergeron W, et al. The Trauma Patient Tracking System: implementing a wireless monitoring infrastructure for emergency response. 2005 27th Annual International Conference of the IEEE Engineering in Medicine and Biology Society, Vols. 1–72005; 2441–2446.

20. Buckle I, Hube M, Chen GD, Yen WH, Arias J. Structural Performance of Bridges in the Offshore Maule Earthquake of 27 February 2010. *Earthquake Spectra* 2012; 28: S533–S552.

21. Noji EK, Kelen GD, Armenian HK, et al. The 1988 earthquake in Soviet Armenia: a case study. *Ann Emerg Med* 1990; 19(8): 891–897.

22. Macintyre AG, Barbera JA, Smith ER. Surviving collapsed structure entrapment after earthquakes: a "time-to-rescue" analysis. *Prehosp Disaster Med* 2006; 21(1): 4–17.

23. *Agence France-Presse.* Japanese search team leaves N.Z. for own crisis. 2011.

24. Peleg K, Kellermann AL. Medical relief after earthquakes: it's time for a new paradigm. *Ann Emerg Med* 2012; 59(3): 188–190.

25. Auf der Heide E. The importance of evidence-based disaster planning. *Ann Emerg Med* 2006; 47(1): 34–49.

26. Garner A, Lee A, Harrison K, Schultz CH. Comparative analysis of multiple-casualty incident triage algorithms. *Ann Emerg Med* 2001; 38: 541–548.

27. Cross KP, Cicero MX. Head-to-head comparison of disaster triage methods in pediatric, adult, and geriatric patients. *Ann Emerg Med* 2013; 61(6): 668–676.

28. Kahn CA, Schultz CH, Miller KT, Anderson CL. Does START Triage Work? An Outcomes Assessment after a Disaster. *Ann Emerg Med* 2009; 54: 424–430.

29. Socna J, Sella T, Shaham D, et al. Facing the new threats of terrorism: Radiologists' perspectives based on experience in Israel. *Radiology* 2005; 237: 28–36.

30. Surviving the Pakistan Earthquake: Perception of the affected one year later. Fritz Institute. 2006. http://www.fritzinstitute.org/prsrmPR-PakistanEarthquakeSurvey.htm (Accessed September 7, 2013).

31. Saito T, Kunimitsu A. Public health response to the combined Great East Japan earthquake, tsunami and nuclear power plant accident: perspective from the Ministry of Health, Labour and Welfare of Japan. *Western Pacific Surveillance and Response Journal* 2011; 2(4): 7–9.

32. Kuroda H. Health care response to the tsunami in Taro District, Miyako City, Iwate Prefecture. *Western Pacific Surveillance and Response Journal* 2011; 2(4): 17–24.

33. Schultz CH, Koenig KL, Lewis RJ. Implications of hospital evacuation after the Northridge, California, earthquake. *N Engl J Med* 2003; 348(14): 1349–1355.

34. Ardagh MW, Richardson SK, Robinson V, Than M, Gee P, Henderson S, et al. The initial health-system response to the earthquake in Christchurch, New Zealand, in February, 2011. *Lancet* 2012; 379(9831): 2109–2115.

35. Schultz CH, Koenig KL. Earthquakes and the practicing physician. *West J Med* 1992; 157(5): 591.

36. Benson M, Koenig KL, Schultz CH. Disaster triage: START, then SAVE – a new method of dynamic triage for victims of a catastrophic earthquake. *Prehosp Disaster Med* 1996; 11(2): 117–124.

37. Schultz CH, Stratton SJ. Improving hospital surge capacity: a new concept for emergency credentialing of volunteers. *Ann Emerg Med* 2007; 49: 602–609.

38. Vanholder R, van der Tol A, De Smet M, et al. Earthquakes and crush syndrome casualties: Lessons learned from the Kashmir disaster. *Kidney Int* 2007; 71(1): 17–23.

39. Brooks AJ, Price V, Simms M. FAST on operational military deployment. *Emerg Med J* 2005; 22(4): 263–265.

40. Vanholder R, Sever MS, Erek E, Lameire N. Acute renal failure related to the crush syndrome: towards an era of seismonephrology? *Nephrol Dial Transplant* 2000; 15(10): 1517–1521.

41. Sever MS, Erek E, Vanholder R, et al. The Marmara earthquake: epidemiological analysis of the victims with nephrological problems. *Kidney Int* 2001; 60(3): 1114–1123.

42. Sever MS, Vanholder R, Lameire N. Management of crush-related injuries after disasters. *N Engl J Med* 2006; 354(10): 1052–1063.

43. Sever MS, Erek E, Vanholder R, et al. Clinical findings in the renal victims of a catastrophic disaster: the Marmara earthquake. *Nephrol Dial Transplant* 2002; 17(11): 1942–1949.

44. Gillani S, Cao J, Suzuki T, Hak DJ. The effect of ischemia reperfusion injury on skeletal muscle. *Injury* 2012; 43(6): 670–675.

45. Sever MS, Vanholder R. Recommendations for the management of crush victims in mass disasters. *Nephrology Dialysis Transplantation* 2012; 27: 1–67.

46. Brown CVR, Rhee P, Chan LK, Evans K, Demetriades D, Velmahos GC. Preventing renal failure in patients with rhabdomyolysis: Do bicarbonate and mannitol make a difference? *Journal of Trauma-Injury Infection and Critical Care* 2004; 56(6): 1191–1196.

47. Vanholder R, Borniche D, Claus S, Correa-Rotter R, Crestani R, Ferir MC, et al. When the earth trembles in the Americas: the experience of Haiti and Chile 2010. *Nephron Clin Practice* 2011; 117(3): c184–c197.

48. Erek E, Sever MS, Serdengecti K, et al. An overview of morbidity and mortality in patients with acute renal failure due to crush syndrome: the Marmara earthquake experience. *Nephrol Dial Transplant* 2002; 17(1): 33–40.

49. Schultz CH, Koenig KL. Preventing Crush Syndrome: Assisting with field amputation and fasciotomy. *JEMS* February 1997: 30–37.

50. Wang Z, Sun Y, Wang Z, Wang Q, Yu W. Anesthetic management of injuries following the 2008 Wenchuan, China earthquake. *European Journal of Trauma and Emergency Surgery* 2011; 37(1): 9–12.

51. Missair A, Gebhard R, Pierre E, Cooper L, Lubarsky D, Frohock J, et al. Surgery under extreme conditions in the aftermath of the 2010 Haiti earthquake: the importance of regional anesthesia. *Prehosp and Disaster Med* 2010; 25(6): 487–493.

52. Jawa RS, Zakrison TL, Richards AT, Young DH, Heir JS. Facilitating safer surgery and anesthesia in a disaster zone. *American Journal of Surgery* 2012; 204(3): 406–409.

53. Mulvey JM, Qadri AA, Maqsood MA. Earthquake injuries and the use of ketamine for surgical procedures: The Kashmir experience. *Anaesthesia and Intensive Care* 2006; 34(4): 489–494.

54. Robertson PA. Prediction of amputation after severe lower limb trauma. *J Bone Joint Surg Br* September 1991; 73(5): 816–818.

55. Bunn F, Roberts IG, Tasker R, Trivedi D. Hypertonic versus near isotonic crystalloid for fluid resuscitation in critically ill patients. *Cochrane Database of Systematic Reviews* 2004; 3.

56. Driessen B, Brainard B. Fluid therapy for the traumatized patient. *J Vet Emerg Crit Care* 2006; 16(4): 1–24.

57. Bulger EM, Jurkovich GJ, Nathens AB, Copass MK, Hanson S, Cooper C, et al. Hypertonic resuscitation of hypovolemic shock after blunt trauma – A randomized controlled trial. *Arch Surg* 2008; 143(2): 139–148.

58. Kobayashi L, Costantini TW, Coimbra R. Hypovolemic Shock Resuscitation. *Surg Clin-North Am* 2012; 92(6): 1403–1423.

59. Klein D, Millo Y, Shuvurum A, Tzur H. The use of alkaline hypertonic saline solution for resuscitation of severe thermally injured patients (our experience). *Ann Medit Burns Club* 1994; 7(4): 194.

60. Sever MS, Erek E, Vanholder R, et al. Features of chronic hemodialysis practice after the Marmara earthquake. *J Am Soc Nephrol* 2004; 15(4): 1071–1076.

61. Kreiss Y, Merin O, Peleg K, Levy G, Vinker S, Sagi R, et al. Early Disaster Response in Haiti: The Israeli Field Hospital Experience. *Annals of Internal Medicine* 2010; 153(1): 45–48.

62. Babcock C, Theodosis C, Bills C, Kim J, Kinet M, Turner M, et al. The Academic Health Center in Complex Humanitarian Emergencies: Lessons Learned From the 2010 Haiti Earthquake. *Acad Med* 2012; 87(11): 1609–1615.

63. Angus DC, Pretto EA, Abrams JI, et al. Epidemiologic assessment of mortality, building collapse pattern, and medical response after the 1992 earthquake in Turkey. Disaster Reanimatology Study Group (DRSG). *Prehosp Disaster Med* 1997; 12(3): 222–231.

64. Yamanda S, Hanagama M, Kobayashi S, Satou H, Tokuda S, Niu KJ, et al. The impact of the 2011 Great East Japan Earthquake on hospitalisation for respiratory disease in a rapidly aging society: a retrospective descriptive and cross-sectional study at the disaster base hospital in Ishinomaki. *BMJ Open* 2013; 3(1): e000865.

65. Broach J, McNamara M, Harrison K. Ambulatory Care by Disaster Responders in the Tent Camps of Port-au-Prince, Haiti, January 2010. *Disaster Med Public Health Prep* 2010; 4(2): 116–121.

66. Zhang L, Liu X, Li Y, Liu Y, Liu Z, Lin J, et al. Emergency medical rescue efforts after a major earthquake: lessons from the 2008 Wenchuan earthquake. *Lancet* 2012; 379(9818): 853–861.

67. Jones LM, Bernknopf R, Cox D, Goltz J, Hudnut K, Mileti D, et al. The ShakeOut Scenario: USGS Open-File Report 2008–1150 and California Geological Survey Preliminary Report. 2008.

68. Floret N, Viel JF, Mauny F, Hoen B, Piarroux R. Negligible risk for epidemics after geophysical disasters. *Emerg Infect Dis* 2006; 12(4): 543–548.

69. Zhang B, Liu Z, Lin Z, Zhang X, Fu W. Microbiologic characteristics of pathogenic bacteria from hospitalized trauma patients who survived Wenchuan earthquake. *European Journal of Clinical Microbiology & Infectious Diseases* 2012; 31(10): 2529–2535.

70. Marra AR, Martino MDV, Ribas MR, Rodriguez-Taveras C, dos Santos OFP. Microbiological findings from the Haiti disaster. *Travel Medicine and Infectious Disease* 2012; 10(3): 157–161.

71. Chin CS, Sorenson J, Harris JB, Robins WP, Charles RC, Jean-Charles RR, et al. The Origin of the Haitian Cholera Outbreak Strain. *N Engl J Med* 2011; 364(1): 33–42.

72. Tappero JW, Tauxe RV. Lessons Learned during Public Health Response to Cholera Epidemic in Haiti and the Dominican Republic. *Emerging Infectious Diseases* 2011; 17(11): 2087–2093.

73. Noji EK. The public health consequences of disasters. *Prehosp Disaster Med* 2000; 15(4): 147–157.

74. Management of Death Bodies after Disaster: A Field Manual for First Responders, Washington, DC: PAHO; 2006. https://www.icrc.org/eng/assets/files/other/icrc-002-0880.pdf (Accessed September 4, 2015).

75. Mattox K. The World Trade Center attack. Disaster preparedness: health care is ready, but is the bureaucracy? *Crit Care* 2001; 5(6): 323–325.

76. Mas Bermejo P. Preparation and response in case of natural disasters: Cuban programs and experience. *J Public Health Policy* 2006; 27(1): 13–21.

77. Chung KK, Perkins RM, Oliver JD. Renal replacement therapy in support of combat operations. *Critical Care Medicine* 2008; 36(7): S365–S369.

39

TSUNAMIS

Samuel J. Stratton

OVERVIEW

A tsunami is a series of waves created when a large volume of ocean water is rapidly displaced. With the current state of the science, tsunami events can be unpredictable. They are best classified as sudden-impact disasters. Commonly, submarine (underwater) earthquakes are associated with tsunamis, but other geophysical events causing mass displacement of water generate tsunami waves. These events may consist of underwater landslides, volcanic eruptions, meteorite impacts, and submarine explosions, including nuclear detonations.[1] Tsunami waves are created as the mass of displaced water radiates relative to gravitational forces across an ocean or sea.

The term tsunami is of Japanese origin from the words "tsu" meaning harbor and "nami" meaning wave.[1] Tsunamis usually occur in a series of nonrhythmic waves as opposed to a single wave. The first tsunami wave to approach a shore is often not the largest in the series. In the open ocean, tsunami waves can have a wavelength of up to 700 km (435 miles) and propagate at speeds of 640 km (400 miles) per hour.[2] In open water, tsunamis may have a wave height (amplitude) of only a few centimeters. Upon reaching shallow beaches and harbors, the waves slow and build to heights with inertial energy well beyond those of wind-generated waves (Figure 39.1).

Tsunamis can cause severe damage to coastal areas as they "run-up" onshore and dissipate wave energy caused by the massive displacement of ocean water. The destructive effect of a tsunami is controlled by the submarine topography in front of the land area that the tsunami approaches. A sloping beach or land positioned on a submarine ridge will sustain damage from the direct impact of high waves, whereas a wide and shallow continental shelf will absorb most of the wave energy and protect a land mass behind it.[2] Tsunamis are different from wind waves and tidal movements because of the large amount of energy they contain and the long, wide character of the waves.

Tsunamis present in two different forms: local and ocean-wide waves. Local tsunami waves arise when earthquakes or undersea disruptions occur near a shore. Local tsunamis can occur after an earthquake or subsurface event has been detected

by residents of the at-risk shoreline. Local tsunami waves runup to shore with little warning other than the preceding event that displaced the large volume of sea water. In the 2004 Indian Ocean tsunami, 130,000 persons in the coastal area of Aceh Province, Indonesia, near the originating earthquake were killed by direct effects of the tsunami and earthquake.[3] The same earthquake generated an ocean-wide tsunami that killed 145,000 persons on distant shores throughout the Indian Ocean in Thailand, the Maldives, India, and Sri Lanka.[3] Ocean-wide tsunamis are generated by distant earthquakes or submarine events that may or may not be felt by affected shoreline residents. A classic example of an ocean-wide tsunami is the 1960 Chilean tsunami that was generated by a devastating magnitude 9.5 earthquake off the coast of southern Chile. The tsunami waves spread across the Pacific, striking Hilo, Hawaii, 14 hours and 48 minutes after the initial quake, killing 61 persons, with the highest wave measuring 10.5 m (35 ft.); it continued on to run-up on the coastal area of Sanriku, Japan, killing 142 persons.[4] This same phenomena occurred with the 2011 Tōhoku Earthquake and Tsunami, with tsunami waves detected in the Hawaiian Islands and throughout the Pacific Rim, including the western United States, Mexico, and South America.[5]

Historically, tsunamis have occurred in all the oceans of the world, with the U.S. coast of Maine struck in 1926 and ancient reports of tsunamis in the Mediterranean Sea.[6] Most tsunamis of consequence strike in the Pacific Ocean. Here they cause significant destruction because ocean topography frequently includes land masses on the edges of ocean canyons rather than on a gently sloping continental shelf.[7] The Pacific Rim is highly active with earthquake activity, raising the risk for tsunamis.[8]

In addition to the immediate destruction that occurs with the run-up of tsunami waves, there is long-lasting environmental damage that occurs in coastal regions. Destruction of natural flora and fauna disrupts ecosystems.[9] Damage to community infrastructure can lead to public health emergencies, including sanitation disruption; interruption of food, water, energy, and transportation systems; and interference with healthcare delivery systems.[9,10] Ecology and infrastructure damage can lead to outbreaks of diseases that are endemic to the disaster region.[11] As demonstrated by the 2011 Tōhoku Earthquake and Tsunami,

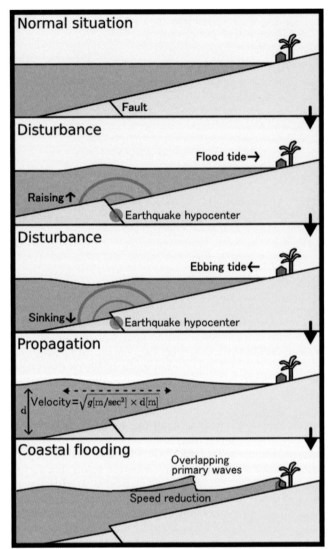

Figure 39.1. Diagram showing the generation of tsunami waves by a submarine earthquake. With disruption of the ocean floor, energy is transferred to the water mass, causing displacement of a large mass of water. The energy of the ocean floor disruption is then dispersed in the form of a water mass or wave. When the tsunami strikes a shoreline, the energy stored in the form of water mass is dissipated on the shoreline.

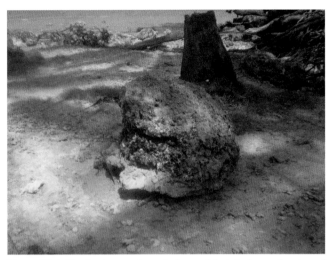

Figure 39.2. During tsunami events, heavy debris is churned onto and off shore, as shown by this large coral rock thrown on shore in the Solomon Islands during the 2007 tsunami. Source: NOAA, by John Beba, Woodlark Mining Limited.

tures. Because tsunamis are high-energy waves, boats and other offshore objects can be torn from moorings. These objects, along with anchors and other fittings, are thrown violently against the shore, causing direct damage to sea walls, buildings, and other objects in the path of the wave. Once tsunami waves run-up on shorelines, it is not uncommon for automobiles, buses, refrigerators, trees, large rocks, and other debris to be thrown against any object in the path of the waves. Many coastal areas have electrical lines close to shore, raising the risk for disruption of these lines and secondary electrical injury to humans and animals. The rolling, crushing nature of tsunami waves can cause release of biological and chemical toxins from storage containers, automobiles, electrical devices, gasoline stations, and other damaged sources.[8]

As tsunami waves recoil, debris and toxins are pulled into the ocean with forces that are close to that of the energy of the oncoming waves (Figures 39.3 and 39.4). Because tsunami waves present in series, debris, chemicals, and suspended material are churned and thrown back and forth to the shoreline and ocean. In addition to damage from heavy objects, toxins, and silt, tsunami

secondary disasters such as radioactive release from a tsunami-damaged nuclear power plant can occur.

CURRENT STATE OF THE ART

On-Shore Tsunami Effects

As tsunami waves run-up onto coastal areas, there is churning of silt, sand, and organic matter that is then thrown onto the shore. Onrushing seawater, sand, and debris cause direct damage to structures and roads (Figure 39.2). In addition, persons in the path of the tsunami waves are swept into onrushing waves. They suffer drowning and aspiration of seawater with suspended material as well as blunt injury from heavy debris captured by the waves. Tsunami waves destroy and damage essential service areas, waste management systems, flood control systems, and struc-

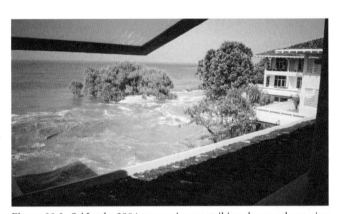

Figure 39.3. Sri Lanka 2004 tsunami wave striking shore, submerging bases of trees and low-lying buildings. Note the forceful churning of water as the wave is striking. Source: NOAA, by Chris Chapman, Cambridge, UK.

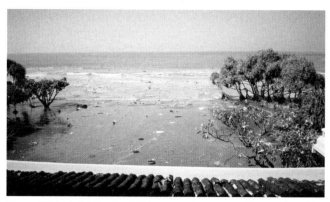

Figure 39.4. A Sri Lanka 2004 tsunami wave receding and pulling debris and objects into the ocean with forces that nearly equal the energy of the incoming wave. Source: NOAA, by Chris Chapman, Cambridge, UK.

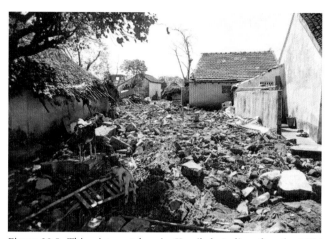

Figure 39.5. This picture taken in Karaikal, India, after the 2004 Indian Ocean tsunami shows the debris field left by the tsunami waves. High-force movement of heavy debris and sharp objects within a tsunami wave cause major injuries to exposed humans and animals. Source: NOAA, by Joseph Trainor, University of Delaware, Disaster Relief Center.

run-ups are associated with on-shore fires as natural gas lines and flammable materials and liquids are exposed.[12]

Tsunami waves have little effect on deep-water structures as they traverse open waters. They dissipate large amounts of energy as they run-up to shore. Shoreline coral reefs and ecosystems can be severely affected by tsunami strikes, causing long-term loss of marine life and habitats, requiring centuries to replace.[12] Loss of coastal marine ecosystems can lead to loss of fishing grounds and affect tourism and other human industries. Tsunami run-ups in industrialized coastal areas can cause release of environmental toxins including paints, oils, gasoline, detergents, and solvents. Release of these toxins can affect both marine and human populations for extended periods. Release of human and animal biological waste can contaminate and damage food and water supplies for extended periods.

Tsunami waves striking industrialized areas often break natural gas and electrical supply lines. As water recedes, the risk of fire is high from ignition of combustible material left in the wake of the waves. Many of the secondary fires are caused by ignition of oil products, including gasoline, diesel fuel, plastics, and solvents. Because water alone will not extinguish these types of fires, and these burning materials are lighter than water, subsequent onrushing tsunami waves can spread fire and burning debris throughout the affected area. Both thermal and chemical burns of survivors are to be expected when tsunami waves strike industrialized shorelines.

Immediate Tsunami Risks for Humans and Animals

Drowning is the obvious risk for humans and animals when a tsunami strikes an inhabited shoreline. Many persons survive the initial effects of an oncoming rolling wave but are swept to sea to drown in open ocean waters that are churning as tsunami waves strike. Because of this phenomenon, children, women, and the disabled are more likely to drown because they may lack the strength to hold onto stationary objects to avoid being swept out to the open ocean.[3] Attempts to survive by clinging to floating debris are often futile because the waves strike and recoil from the shoreline in a churning, mixing motion.

In addition to drowning, death occurs by blunt force injury as heavy objects are thrown against persons and structures as the advancing waves hit the shore. Fatal crush injury and blunt trauma are reported as the second most common cause

of death related to tsunamis.[13] Mortality is also associated with impalement by large pieces of glass and sharp, protruding metal, wood, and vegetable matter formed and exposed by the forces of the tsunami waves (Figure 39.5). Descriptions of persons found impaled through the torso on bamboo shoots, metal rods and pipes, and splintered tree branches and trunks are common. Closed head injury secondary to blunt trauma and blunt force solid organ injury with subsequent hemorrhage are also recognized causes for fatal injury related to tsunami events.[13] Building collapse from tsunami waves undermining structural foundations is another cause for crush injury.[13]

Prolonged serious medical conditions resulting directly from tsunami events are uncommon and most persons either survive to be "ambulatory" or are killed suddenly during the event.[3,14] Table 39.1 lists injuries that can be anticipated in survivors. Lacerations, soft tissue injuries, and orthopedic injuries are most often encountered in the aftermath of a tsunami strike. Because those suffering these injuries are in a contaminated environment, tetanus prophylaxis is a primary concern. In opposition to standard practice in which most soft tissue wounds and lacerations would be immediately sutured or closed, wounds presenting during the acute disaster phase of a tsunami event are often left open to heal by secondary intent or delayed primary closure after thorough irrigation and debridement. Avoiding primary wound closure is necessary because of the contaminated nature of the injuries and concern for retained foreign bodies.

Eye injuries secondary to flying debris and direct injury are common during tsunami events. Frequent episodes of tympanic membrane rupture are also reported and are most likely caused by pressure gradients when victims are submersed in the water of a rolling wave. Facial injuries and dental trauma are also to be expected.

Orthopedic injuries are predominantly long bone fractures but also include pelvic fractures and spinal injuries (including cervical spine injury and compression fractures of the thoracic and lumbar spine regions). Amputation of digits and partial hand and foot amputations are commonly reported and are the result of crushing and severing caused by heavy floating debris churned

Table 39.1. Immediate Tsunami Injury Risks

Submersion

    Drowning

    Aspiration lung injury

    Tympanic membrane rupture

Blunt force injury

    Crush injury

    Closed head injury

    Solid organ blunt force injury

    Spinal injury

        Cervical spine injury

        Compression fracture of thoracic and lumbar spines

    Orthopedic injury

        Long bone fracture and contusion

        Dislocation of shoulder, elbow, knee, digits

        Amputation of digits, hands, feet

        Pelvic fracture

    Eye injury, both blunt and penetrating

    Soft tissue injury

        Laceration

        Contusion/abrasion

Penetrating trauma

    Foot injury from sharp debris

    Penetrating thorax/abdominal injury

Burn

    Thermal

    Chemical

Dental trauma

Table 39.2. Elements of a Rapid Epidemiologic Assessment

1. Determine the overall impact of the event

    Geographical extent

    Number of affected persons

    Estimated duration

2. Assess the impact on health

    Number of casualties

    Number injured

    Number with illness

    Number well and unaffected

3. Determine the integrity of the healthcare system

4. Determine the specific medical and health needs of the survivors

5. Assess the disruption of essential services that contribute to public health

    Water

    Power

    Sanitation

    Communication

    Shelter

    Food

6. Determine the extent of resources needed by local authorities for adequate response and recovery to the disaster

within tsunami waves. Dislocations of the shoulder, elbow, and knee are also to be expected during tsunami events.

Pulmonary injury due to aspiration of contaminated water is frequent in relation to tsunamis.[3] Although pneumothorax due to blunt chest injury and barotrauma would be expected, it has not been reported as a predominate injury. Thermal and chemical burns are reported and expected because caustic toxins can be released from containers and fires occur in the aftermath of a tsunami strike.

Public Health Aspects of Tsunami Events

The immediate public health concerns from tsunami events include loss of shelter, food, water, and clothing. Starvation and hypothermia or sunburn and sun exposure are common public health issues immediately after a tsunami strike.[13] Survivors are often left partially clothed without access to potable water or food. Because debris, including broken glass, splintered trees, and destroyed buildings, are distributed throughout the immediate environment by the waves, mobility is limited and access to food,

water, and shelter is difficult. After tsunami events, initial public health activities generally include environmental health actions to develop safe, protected shelter and ready access to drinking water and clothing.[3] Providing food appropriate to the cultural norms for the area struck by the tsunami is an important public health priority.

When the immediate needs of the surviving population have been addressed and survivors have moved to safe locations, organized assessment of health-related needs should be conducted. Initial assessments include survey of shelters and survivor collection points; random-cluster analysis of the affected community is often preferred as soon as feasible.[15] Knowledge of local health risks and challenges is essential in planning and conducting a rapid health analysis. For example, if it is known that malaria is endemic in an area struck by a tsunami, those doing a health assessment would survey for accessibility to protective mosquito netting for sleeping quarters and access to DEET or other appropriate mosquito repellents. The recovery phase of the 2004 Indian Ocean tsunami provides an interesting illustration of the importance of knowing local health hazards. Outside experts made unnecessary strong recommendations for complicated cholera vaccination programs in areas struck by the tsunami when cholera was not a threat and had not been present in the area for decades.[16]

Information obtained during rapid public health assessments of an affected population is used to plan and implement immediate health responses. Table 39.2 lists the elements most often addressed during a rapid health assessment following a sudden-onset event such as a tsunami. The focus of these health assessments is to make prompt estimates of the health needs of an affected population.[15] Visual inspection, interviews with key personnel, and surveys are the mainstay tools for rapid health assessments.[15]

World Health Organization (WHO) evaluations performed during the December 2004 Indian Ocean tsunami provide examples of the importance of rapid health assessments in tsunami events. Evaluation immediately after the event showed that burial of the dead, sheltering survivors, waste and debris removal, and provision of water and food were crucial first efforts to prevent public health failures within the surviving populations. Later health assessments showed that malnutrition, childhood diarrhea, hazardous waste management, and disposal of rotting animal carcasses were a priority. Importantly, rapid health assessments detected measles cases among children in eastern parts of the affected area, allowing for an intensive vaccination program that prevented a measles outbreak among a generally unvaccinated pediatric population.[17]

Public health providers must know the hazards and risks that exist within a community and anticipate the challenges these may present in a tsunami event. This is illustrated by the 2011 Tōhoku Earthquake and Tsunami with the release of radioactive material when a nuclear power plant was flooded with ocean water. Knowing the risk that the nuclear plant posed allowed for graduated evacuation from radiation zones and permitted public health officials to anticipate the health and welfare needs of those evacuated, including their mental health support requirements.

Tsunami Warning Systems

Although tsunamis can be classified as sudden-onset events, there are often periods of warning before a tsunami wave impact. Local tsunami run-up to a coastal area is frequently preceded by a submarine earthquake or volcanic eruption that can be felt by those occupying hazardous areas of the shoreline. Understanding the association of tsunamis with earthquakes and other underwater disturbances allows for escape to higher ground or inland areas.

As ocean-wide tsunami waves approach a land mass there is often a profound receding of the water along a shoreline as the tsunami rolls in. Appreciating the link between profound receding of shore waters and incoming tsunami waves can allow for initial movement of those at risk away from the shore (Figure 39.6). There have been many anecdotal reports of animals unexplainably rushing to higher ground minutes before the approach of a tsunami as if they are able to sense the incoming wave.

In 1949, the United States created an organized tsunami warning system with headquarters located in Honolulu, Hawaii.[18] In 1960, an earthquake occurring off the southern shore of Chile caused severe local damage and generated an ocean-wide tsunami that impacted Hilo, Hawaii, resulting in significant destruction and killing sixty-one residents. The same tsunami waves proceeded to Japan where they inflicted substantial damage and killed 200 people. After this 1960 tsunami event, a coalition of Pacific nations was formed to develop a warning system to prevent future damage by ocean-crossing tsunami waves. With support of the United Nations, the international Pacific Tsunami Warning Center (PTWC) was developed.[18] Until 1967, PTWC had responsibility for warning Pacific nations of ocean-wide tsunamis. In 1967, following a severe 1964 Alaskan earthquake and tsunami, the West Coast and Alaska Tsunami Warning

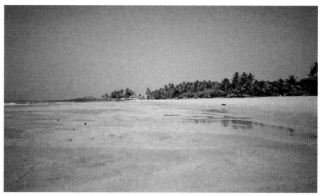

Figure 39.6. The initial receding of water from shore before the run-up of a tsunami wave during the 2004 Indian Ocean tsunami. During this "warning" phase of a tsunami run-up, rocks and sand that are normally submerged along the outer shore become exposed. This receding of the ocean serves as a warning for those along the shore to move to higher ground to avoid a possible incoming tsunami wave. Source: NOAA, by Chris Chapman, Cambridge, UK.

Center (WC/ATWC) was established. WC/ATWC has responsibility for issuing tsunami warnings for Alaska, British Columbia, Washington State, Oregon, and California. PTWC monitors the rest of the Pacific.[19,20]

When the 2004 Indian Ocean tsunami occurred, an organized warning system did not exist for the Indian Ocean area. Subsequently, PTWC added the Indian Ocean, South China Sea, and Caribbean to those areas monitored and warned of tsunami risks.[19]

PTWC currently has twenty-six participating international member states.[20] Officials use multiple tools to determine tsunami risks and events. These technologies include earthquake sensing and information devices, drifting and moored ocean data buoys, satellite observation equipment, Argo floating buoys, integrated on-land observation sites, high-frequency coastal radar, and the Shore Coastal-Marine Automated Network. Equipment supporting this network is located in lighthouses and shore stations that monitor weather and seismic activity.[20,21]

Standard terminology has been developed for tsunami alerts that are released from tsunami warning centers. A "tsunami advisory" indicates that a threat exists but that no tsunami has been detected. A "tsunami watch" indicates that an earthquake or other high-risk tsunami-generating event has been detected and coastal areas are to stand by for further information and alerts. A "tsunami warning" indicates that a tsunami has been generated or that conditions are serious enough for coastal communities to take responsive actions. Information generated with a tsunami warning includes earthquake magnitude, originating location, and arrival times, but not size of waves.[22]

Mitigating the Effects of Tsunamis

Tsunami waves are hazards unique to coastal areas of the world. They are a known hazard because the origins of tsunamis are earthquakes, submarine volcanoes, landslides, and other sources for displacement of large volumes of water. Human-inhabited coastal regions that are in areas of geophysical activity place persons at direct risk for tsunami disaster effects. The coastal region known as the Pacific Rim is a well-recognized tsunami hazard zone.

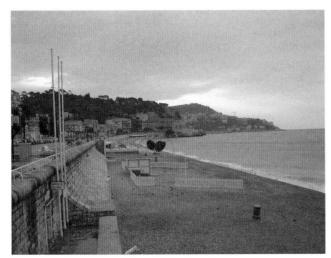

Figure 39.7. A protective sea wall constructed to repel and limit potential tsunami damage along the shoreline of Nice, France. This tsunami sea wall was constructed after Nice was struck by a tsunami triggered by a construction-generated shoreline landslide. *Source:* Samuel J. Stratton.

Human habitation and activity in low-lying coastal lands puts people at direct risk for tsunami injury and loss. Furthermore, recreational use of low-lying coastal lands places visitors to these areas in danger of injury and death from tsunamis. Building structures for human habitation near low-lying shorelines in tsunami hazard areas raises the risk for death and injury as well as economic loss from tsunamis. As with many hazards, ignorance of the threat or ignoring the risks posed by tsunamis leads to inevitable calamity. Such consequences can be avoided by proactive community planning and education.

Japan, a country that has been repeatedly struck by tsunamis, has developed environmental mitigation strategies to protect human populations from the waves' effects by building sea walls along shorelines facing open ocean. Tsunami sea walls range up to 4.5 meters (13.5 ft) in height and provide an initial break for potential incoming tsunami waves (Figure 39.7).[23] Using the same rationale, open low-lying beaches in areas of southern California in the United States use earthen or sand barriers behind open beach to dissipate the energy of incoming storm waves and potential tsunamis. Maintenance of natural wetlands, forest, and vegetation (that often lie immediately adjacent to open beach areas) helps dissipate the energy of incoming tsunami waves and further affords protection for inland structures and habitats. Building standards and laws that limit the use of low-lying coastal lands for construction of houses, factories, schools, airports, energy plants (including nuclear power plants), and other essential human activity is a proactive method for decreasing the risk posed by tsunamis. Despite this, human encroachment into coastal zones has placed much of the world's population at risk for injury and death due to tsunamis.[24–26] Decisions to live in at-risk coastal areas are characterized by the need to satisfy political and short-term economic goals rather than the requirement to implement rational decisions regarding housing and industrial zoning. Individuals responsible for these decisions often lack an understanding of the potential risks.

Community planning for the emergency response to potential tsunami events is important for decreasing risks. As with planning for other disasters, initial community efforts should include a hazards assessment of the affected area. Low-lying coastal lands facing open ocean are at obvious risk for tsunami run-up. In addition, harbors and waterways must also be considered as these entities have the potential to transmit and sometimes funnel the energy of a tsunami inland. Topographical mapping of shorelines is particularly helpful in identifying potential areas at risk. Generally, areas that are less than 10 meters (32.8 ft.) above sea level are at highest risk for tsunami damage.[23]

A key element of tsunami disaster planning is providing a strategy for rapidly evacuating persons in the path of an incoming wave to locations inland and at higher elevation (> 10 m). As noted earlier, tsunamis are sudden-impact events, but usually can be predicted immediately prior to occurrence. A system for warning those at risk of an incoming tsunami after a triggering event (e.g., an offshore earthquake) allows for protective evacuation to higher ground inland. In many areas of the Pacific Rim, warning sirens have been installed to rapidly alert those in an area of immediate risk. Other types of communication warning systems such as social media, email, text messages, and reverse emergency phone trees have not been reported to be effective; thus, sirens continue to be universally used. Warning posters and signs identifying the most efficient route to higher ground are also placed in high-risk areas to facilitate evacuation. Placement of evacuation route direction signs are important interventions. Research shows that many people become directionally disoriented when incoming tsunami waves strike. Total evacuation of a tsunami run-up zone is important as anyone in low-lying areas is at risk for injury or death. This includes emergency first responders and security–law enforcement personnel. More sophisticated plans in developed countries include not only evacuation of emergency first responders and security personnel to higher ground, but also simultaneous movement of essential portable equipment with the personnel.[25,27]

Pre-event education is key to the success of emergency evacuation of those at risk. The resident population must know basic information about tsunamis. Knowledge of the meaning of warning sirens allows persons to respond more quickly when the alarm is sounded. In addition, it is important to educate those visiting, inhabiting, or working in coastal areas that extreme and sudden raising or receding of the ocean shoreline can indicate an incoming tsunami. Persons in tsunami hazard areas should be aware of signage that directs people away from the risk zone. Other important tsunami information includes understanding that the waves come in series and that the first tsunami wave may not be the largest. Furthermore, intervals between waves are not constant and can be markedly asynchronous. After arrival of the initial tsunami wave, further waves in the series can be spread over time and may not strike the shore for more than 2 hours. Because of the predictable delay in arrival of the complete tsunami wave series, rescue personnel and equipment are generally staged away from the shoreline at higher ground for 2 hours after the onset of the first wave to prevent their becoming victims.

Reports show that tsunami warnings sometimes attract sightseers to the coastal area, causing impairment in attempts to evacuate. Control of evacuation perimeters is important. Communication by standard landlines and cellular telephones is often ineffective due to system overload and not available to emergency operations and rescue personnel. Alternate communication methods using radio systems in redundant configurations should be considered for potential responders. Organized amateur radio operators have been valuable in helping communicate and facilitate coordination of response in tsunami events.

Recovery efforts are often prolonged following tsunamis and constitute public health emergencies. Management of the dead and accounting for those lost and probably washed out to sea is an early recovery concern along with providing care to survivors.[28] For the management of survivors, ambulatory care supplies such as tetanus vaccine, sterile irrigation solutions, fracture splinting materials, and dressings are often the first to be depleted.[14] The disaster's impact on the mental health of victims is a particular concern.

Populations that must be considered when planning for tsunamis include visitors and tourists. Many coastal areas are popular vacation locations and those visiting may not be familiar with the risk. This was particularly true with the 2004 Indian Ocean tsunami event. In some areas impacted by this disaster, approximately half of the survivors requiring medical services were tourists and visitors.[3] Basic response information (in multiple languages) for visitors and tourists in tsunami hazard areas is part of comprehensive planning.

RECOMMENDATIONS FOR FURTHER RESEARCH

Although standard plans have been developed for emergency evacuation of areas threatened by incoming tsunamis, there has been little research into the quickest and safest evacuation methods. General recommendations suggest those threatened by tsunamis should seek higher ground, but time taken in moving to higher ground may not be as effective as moving into upper stories of solidly constructed multistory buildings. The development of safe and effective maneuvers for avoiding personal injury from tsunamis represents a significant future research opportunity.

The local and international management of large-scale tsunami events is an area that research can inform. In January 2007, Claude de Ville de Goyet published a comprehensive article describing health lessons from the 2004 Indian Ocean tsunami. His observations are summarized in the following paragraphs.

This tsunami event provides a wealth of information. Between 227,000 and 275,000 persons were lost or died as a result of the tsunami, with 1.7 million displaced.[3,16] The tsunami affected several countries and varying cultures, with Indonesia and Sri Lanka in states of government instability at the time of the tsunami strike.[16] Although thousands of reports and observations of the event are available in journals or on the Internet, few scientifically rigorous studies have been published at the time of this writing. The tsunami-related issues noted by de Ville de Goyet form a basis for a core research agenda for future tsunami disaster research. De Ville de Goyet provides the following observations in his paper on the 2004 Indian Ocean tsunami:

1. Funding was not a primary obstacle to an effective relief response. At a global average, US$7,300 was committed per affected survivor. Yet external responses to the event were ineffective, suggesting that abundant financial resources and technology do not guarantee a successful recovery effort.[16]

2. Few decisions were made based on needs assessments. Accountability of many nongovernmental organizations and United Nations agencies was to their donors rather than to the survivors and local governments. Decisions by outside agencies regarding the types of donations and aid offered were based on political pressures and media influences as opposed to basic epidemiological needs assessments and evaluations.[16]

3. The national public health capacities of the affected countries were minimally impacted by the disaster except for Aceh Province, Indonesia. In Banda Aceh, which was also impacted by earthquake forces, there was loss of healthcare delivery resources. Otherwise, infrastructure damage and human injury and loss occurred in the coastal areas, with inland areas remaining intact. The tsunami did not damage hospitals and public health resources directly. During a tsunami event, people who are in the coastal impact areas drown, die of trauma caused by loose debris, or survive with injuries but remain ambulatory.[14,16] Local, organized responses to tsunami events using inland resources that withstand or are not affected by the tsunami waves have been more successful than medical assistance organized from outside a community.

4. For the Indian Ocean tsunami event, international humanitarian standards were not adapted to local contexts. The Sphere Handbook is an internationally accepted standard for disaster response that uses a needs-based approach to compensate for disaster losses.[29] International standards published in the Sphere Handbook rely on a strong rights-based approach, which was not a predominate norm in many of the countries affected by the tsunami.

The rigid application of lofty international standards to local situations without adapting to local norms during the Indian Ocean tsunami event caused negative consequences. Responding international organizations targeted populations they could easily access, for which the standards could be met, rather than seeking out those populations in locations more difficult to reach. This resulted in a concentration of resources in urban areas, leaving some in rural areas without assistance. Furthermore, tourists and refugees became a primary focus as opposed to those locals trying to survive in rural regions and who experienced a more primitive existence prior to the event. There was also an overextension of the emergency phase and a delay in the recovery phase. The continued influx of donated resources provided an incentive to focus on obtaining more material and volunteer aid rather than transitioning to the more difficult recovery actions required. The international response resulted in a dilemma for local health departments and providers because the medical standards provided could not be sustained after relief efforts ceased. The disaster response medical resources donated and supplied by outside organizations exceeded the local standards available before the event.[16]

The emergency construction of duplicate health centers and medical clinics by international responders resulted in competition between these agencies and was an example of inappropriate international aid.[16] Those providing international aid quickly overwhelmed Aceh and Sri Lanka, causing confusion and frustration for victims of the disaster. Further, the incoming aid workers and equipment added to the stress of managing the event for local emergency operations administrators. This increased demand for logistical support resulted in a second disaster, as local managers struggled to coordinate the invading relief workers and their equipment.[16]

Marginalization of local health authorities by international responders was another challenge. On-site access to foreign assets, such as air transportation, equipment, and communication systems was limited to international responders. Those in the local response groups who were familiar with and culturally aware of the affected populations were provided only pre-event methods and resources. As already noted, local responders not only had to manage the disaster with existing limited resources, but had the added burden of attempting to coordinate and direct incoming responders from the international sector.[16]

An additional factor compounding the difficulties caused by international response groups in the aftermath of this event was the overstating of epidemic risks. The occurrence of major secondary epidemics following sudden-impact disaster events is not the norm.[30] Although there was no evidence for epidemic risks during the tsunami event, humanitarian agencies stimulated fear of epidemics and diverted attention from recovery efforts. Rather than focusing on basic disaster medical science using surveillance techniques and health education, the international effort concentrated on immunizations for cholera, which is logistically and technically complex. This cholera immunization campaign resulted in the loss of scarce operational resources for a nonexistent threat, ignoring more obvious threats such as the large numbers of children who were not immunized for measles. The very real hazard of a measles epidemic was minimized by some international "experts." Nevertheless, the little-publicized but substantial threat from measles was identified and immunization was successfully conducted using standard field surveillance and immunization programs for high-risk populations.[31] As demonstrated here, health priorities should be informed by sound public health hazard and risk assessments based on field work as opposed to theoretical pontification. For the affected population, repairing the environmental (water and sanitation) and economic (fishing and food production) infrastructure proved to be an immediate health priority.[16]

Researchers have described medical and public health challenges encountered following tsunamis in a general sense, but primarily for the acute recovery or response phases. The long-term effects on health have been minimally studied and this area represents an opportunity for further research. In addition, WHO conducted an extensive review and evaluation of the state of knowledge for public health response to tsunami events.[32] Categories for which more evaluation and research are needed are listed in Table 39.3.

Summary

Tsunami waves represent high-energy massive movements of water generated when large volumes of ocean water are displaced by events such as earthquakes and submarine volcanic eruptions. The coastal regions of the Pacific Ocean are the areas of highest risk for tsunamis, but these disasters can strike anywhere that an ocean or sea meets a coastline. Injury and destruction from tsunamis occur as the waves strike the shoreline. The most common cause of death from tsunamis is drowning, followed by blunt injury resulting from loose debris thrown inland by tsunami wave run-up.

The essential elements for prevention of tsunami injury and damage are limiting construction in exposed coastal areas, developing sea walls and coastal protection barriers, and educating those at risk to seek higher ground immediately when the threat of tsunami is high. Recognizable warning systems and planned evacuation routes are keys to tsunami response planning. Tsunami waves come in series, and the first wave to strike shore is not necessarily the largest of the series.

As with other sudden-impact disasters, most of the mortality related to the event occurs immediately with the onset of the event. The majority of survivors requiring medical resources are not critically ill. Most are in need of ambulatory medical care and attention to existing chronic diseases (such as diabetes) that were present prior to the event. Predominate immediate public health needs are for shelter, water, food, clothing, and mental health support. Local health agencies and governments are best at identifying hazards and risks during a tsunami event and at managing the response and should be in the lead. International aid organizations should be in a support role and coordinate their responses with local authorities.

Table 39.3. WHO Recommendation Categories for Development of Evaluation and Research of Tsunami Events[32]

1. Data, information, indicators, and reporting
2. Standardized event magnitude measurement
3. Structural damage correlation
4. Community burdens
5. Assessment methods
6. Evaluation of interventions
7. Public health systems
8. Medical care systems
9. Mental health
10. Coordination and control of relief
11. Communication systems
12. Impact of civil conflict
13. Water and sanitation systems
14. Food and nutrition
15. Transportation and logistics
16. Public works and engineering
17. Energy supply
18. Education
19. Social structures and societal systems
20. Interventions and responses
21. Shelter and clothing
22. Economy
23. Preparedness and planning
24. Military and security

Listed are the major categories identified by WHO for evaluation and research of tsunami events. The listed categories serve as a framework for future tsunami research.

REFERENCES

1.   NOAA. Tsunami Vocabulary and Terminology. http://www .tsunami. noaa.gov/terminology.html (Accessed October 17, 2013).

2. Earth Science Australia. Tsunami...Tidal Waves. http://earthsci.org/education/teacher/basicgeol/tsumami/tsunami.html (Accessed October 23, 2013).

3. WHO. TRIAMS Final Report. http://www.who.int/hac/crises/international/asia_tsunami/triams/triams_report_3.pdf (Accessed October 17, 2013).

4. WHO. Emergency and Disasters Data Base. http://www.em-dat.net (Accessed October 17, 2013).

5. Hunter JC, Crawley AW, Petrie M, Yang JE, Aragon TJ. Local public health system response to the tsunami threat in coastal California following the Tōhoku Earthquake. *PLOS Curr Dis* July 16, 2012. Edition 1. DOI: 10.1371/4f7f57285b804.

6. National Geophysical Data Center/World Data Service (NGDC/WDS). Global Historical Tsunami Database, Boulder, CO. http://www.ngdc.noaa.gov/hazard/tsu_db.shtml (Accessed October 23, 2013).

7. NOAA. Tsunamis. http://www.tsunami.noaa.gov (Accessed October 17, 2013).

8. U.S. Geological Survey. Tsunamis and Earthquakes. http://walrus.wr.usgs.gov/tsunami/CIHH.html (Accessed October 23, 2013).

9. Urabe J, Takao S, Nishita T, Makino W. Immediate ecological impacts of the 2011 Tohoku Earthquake Tsunami on intertidal flat communities. *Plos One* 8(5): e62779.

10. Vaccari M, Collivignarelli C, Tharnpoophasiam P, Vitali F. Wells sanitary inspection and water quality monitoring in Ban Nam Khem (Thailand) 30 months after the 2004 Indian Ocean tsunami. *Environ Monit Assess* 2010; 161: 123–133.

11. Manimunda SP, Sugunan AP, Sha WA, Singh SS, Shriram AN, Vijayachari P. Tsunami, post-tsunami malaria situation in Nancowry group of islands, Nicobar district, Andaman and Nicobar Islands. *Indian J Med Res* 2011; 133: 78–82.

12. NOAA. Potential Ecological Impacts of Indian Ocean Tsunami on Nearshore Marine Ecosystems. http://www.noaanews.noaa.gov/stories2005/s2362.htm (Accessed October 23, 2013).

13. WHO. Injuries and Disability: Priorities and Management for Populations Affected by the Earthquake and Tsunami in Asia. http://www.who.int/violence_injury_prevention/other_injury/tsunami/en/index.html (Accessed October 23, 2013).

14. Stratton SJ, Tyler RD. Characteristics of medical surge capacity demand for sudden-impact disasters. *Acad Emerg Med.* 2006; 13: 1193–1197.

15. Wetterhall SF, Noji EK. Surveillance and epidemiology. In: Noji EK, ed. *The Public Health Consequences of Disasters.* New York, Oxford University Press, 1997: 37–64.

16. de Ville de Goyet C. Health lessons learned from the recent earthquakes and tsunami in Asia. *Prehosp Disaster Med* 2007; 22: 15–21.

17. WHO South Asia Tsunami Situation Reports. http://www.who.int/hac/crises/international/asia_tsunami/sitrep/en (Accessed October 23, 2013).

18. NOAA. PTWC History. http://www.prh.noaa.gov/ptwc/history.php (Accessed October 23, 2013).

19. NOAA. PTWC Responsibilities. http://www.prh.noaa.gov/ptwc/responsibilities.php (Accessed October 23, 2013).

20. NOAA. Tsunami Warning Centers. http://www.nws.noaa.gov/om/brochures/tsunami4.htm (Accessed October 23, 2013).

21. NOAA. Tsunami Warning Systems. http://www.ndbc.noaa.gov (Accessed October 23, 2013).

22. NOAA. How does the Tsunami Warning System Work? http://www.tsunami.noaa.gov/warning_system_works.html (Accessed: October 23, 2013).

23. U.S. National Research Council. *Preventing Earthquake Disasters: The Grand Challenge in Earthquake Engineering a Research Agenda.* Washington, DC, National Academies Press, 2003: 12–25.

24. Dudley WC, Lee M. *Tsunami!* Honolulu, University of Hawaii Press, 1998.

25. National Weather Service. Tsunami Ready. http://www.tsunamiready.noaa.gov (Accessed October 23, 2013).

26. CDC. Tsunamis. http://www.bt.cdc.gov/disasters/tsunamis (Accessed October 23, 2013).

27. American Red Cross. Tsunami. http://www.redcross.org/services/disaster/01082,0_592_,00.html (Accessed October 23, 2013).

28. CDC. Rapid health response, assessment, and surveillance after a tsunami – Thailand, 2004–2005. *MMWR* 2005; 54: 61–64.

29. SPHERE Humanitarian Charter and Minimum Standards in Disaster Response Handbook. Revised 2004 ed. http://www.sphereproject.org (Accessed October 23, 2013).

30. PAHO/WHO. Natural Disasters Myths and Realities. 2001. http://www.paho.org/English/DD/PED/myths.htm (Accessed October 23, 2013).

31. CDC. Assessment of health-related needs after tsunami and earthquake – three districts, Aceh Province Indonesia, July–August 2005. *MMWR* 2006; 55: 93–97.

32. WHO. Conclusions and Recommendations. In: *Tsunami 2004: A Comprehensive Analysis.* New Delhi, World Health Organization, 2013; 247–278.

40

Winter Storms and Hazards

John M. Wightman and William H. Dice

OVERVIEW

Severe winter storms can be life-changing events that isolate and disrupt families; result in closures of schools, businesses, and government; prevent air, ground, and water transportation; and destroy large components of agricultural and service industries. Public safety can be threatened when roads are impassable, power grids are non-functional, and telecommunications are inoperable.

Cold temperatures and wind chill; persistent ice or snow creating slick conditions; avalanches; bodies of water covered by insufficient ice thickness to support objects on their surface; ice-choked waterways; and coastal flooding from higher water levels also create winter hazards temporally unrelated to storms.

Humans can exist in extremely cold environments, but their physiology is best suited for the tropics from which the species originated. Adaptation to cold is most importantly behavioral. Heat loss is slowed or prevented by avoiding contact with cold surfaces and ingestion of cold substances, sheltering from wind and precipitation, wearing protective clothing, and physically moving to a warmer location. Peripheral vasoconstriction and shivering only modestly and temporarily protect humans exposed to very low temperatures. The consequences of many winter storms make it difficult or impossible for unprepared or unassisted humans to achieve the behavioral modifications necessary to mitigate the direct effects of cold, or to obtain the resources needed to maintain health.

This chapter discusses the challenges winter hazards pose for humans with an emphasis on winter storms. The disaster life cycle – mitigation, preparedness, response, and recovery – used here includes a continuous loop of planning and preparedness; warning, if any; the event itself; immediate response, which is almost always local; rapid assessment to identify needed resources; definitive response with ongoing surveillance and repeated assessments; recovery to baseline; and system improvements to increase preparedness for the next event.

Scope of Winter Storms

Winter storms were relatively uncommon causes of disasters in Canada, the United Kingdom (UK), and the United States

until the mid-1990s, after which the number resulting in major federal disaster declarations has been in double digits half of the last twenty winter seasons in the United States alone.[1] Since 1980, ten winter-storm disasters have each cost over $1 billion (normalized to 2011 USD) and a combined total of $29.3 billion USD in economic damages.[2] Four involved catastrophic winter storms in the 1990s with a combined mortality of almost 500 human deaths,[3] but there have been other major storms in the last decade as well.

From January 15–19, 2007, a cyclone over the Netherlands generated a "European windstorm" with high sustained winds and gusts up to 202 km/h. Power was severed to over 50,000 homes in the United Kingdom alone. Several major highways across Europe were forced to close, commuter rail traffic was slowed, and hundreds of commercial flights were cancelled. On navigable waterways, ferries were halted, one freighter ran aground, and another carrying hazardous cargo had to be abandoned. Overall, this storm, named Kyrill, caused widespread damage across the British Isles and Western Europe, and resulted in forty-seven deaths. Falling objects and motor vehicle collisions (MVCs) seemed to dominate as mechanisms of fatal injury.[4]

Three major winter cyclones also made their way across North America the same month: 1) from Texas to southeastern Canada January 11–16; 2) from Texas to the Carolinas January 16–19; and 3) across the U.S.-Canadian border January 19–24. Over 1 million people were without power for days during some portion of the 2-week period. Large portions of several U.S. states, plus the entire state of Oklahoma, were declared disaster areas. MVCs accounted for the majority of the eighty-seven deaths attributed to these storms.[5]

The scope of any individual potential injury/illness-creating event (PICE) in any country does not need to be as great as these to significantly alter baseline societal patterns that – in addition to having a major negative regional or national economic impact – result in patient attempts to access the healthcare system.

Definitions used in this chapter are listed in Table 40.1. Winter precipitation comes in a variety of forms, including rain, freezing rain, sleet, and snow. Colder temperatures and strong

Table 40.1. Winter weather definitions according to the U.S. National Weather Service glossary. This information is in the public domain. It was retrieved from the NWS Glossary at http://www.weather.gov/glossary on October 30, 2007.

Avalanche – A mass of snow, rock, or ice falling down a mountain or incline. In practice, it usually refers to the snow avalanche.

Blizzard – The following conditions are expected to prevail for a period of 3 hours or longer: sustained wind or frequent gusts to 56 km/h (35 mph) or greater; and considerable falling or blowing snow reducing visibility frequently to less than 0.4 km (0.25 mi.).

Blowing Snow – Wind-driven snow that reduces surface visibility. Blowing snow can be falling snow or snow that has already accumulated but is picked up and blown by strong winds. Blowing snow is usually accompanied by drifting snow.

Coastal Flooding – The inundation of land areas adjacent to bodies of salt water connected to the Atlantic Ocean, Pacific Ocean, or Gulf of Mexico, caused by sea waters over and above normal tidal action. This flooding may impact the immediate oceanfront, gulfs, bays, back bays, sounds, and tidal portions of river mouths and inland tidal waterways.

Cyclone – A large-scale circulation of winds around a central region of low atmospheric pressure: counterclockwise in the Northern Hemisphere, clockwise in the Southern Hemisphere.

Drifting Ice – In hydrologic terms, pieces of floating ice moving under the action of wind and/or currents.

Drifting Snow – Drifting snow is an uneven distribution of snowfall/snow depth caused by strong surface winds. Drifting snow may occur during or after a snowfall. Drifting snow is usually associated with blowing snow.

Drizzle – Precipitation consisting of numerous minute droplets of water less than 0.5 mm in diameter.

Flood – Any high flow, overflow, or inundation by water that causes or threatens damage.

Freeze – When the surface air temperature is expected to be 0°C or below over a widespread area for a climatologically significant period of time.

Freezing Rain – Rain that falls as a liquid but freezes into glaze on contact with the ground. Freezing drizzle, fog, and boat/ship spray also occur.

Heavy Snow – Snowfall accumulating to 10.2 cm (4 in.) or more in depth in 12 hours or less; or snowfall accumulating to 15.2 cm (6 inches) or more in depth in 24 hours or less.

Ice Fog – A suspension of numerous minute ice crystals in the air, or water droplets at temperatures below 0°C, based at the earth's surface, which reduces horizontal visibility. Also called freezing fog.

Ice Jam – In hydrologic terms, a stationary accumulation (of ice) that restricts or blocks (water) flow.

Ice Storm – Describes occasions when damaging accumulations of ice are expected during freezing rain situations. Significant accumulations of ice pull down trees and utility lines, resulting in loss of power and communication. These accumulations of ice make walking and driving extremely dangerous. Significant ice accumulations are usually accumulations of 6.4 mm (0.25 in.) or greater.

Lake-Effect Snow – Snow showers that are created when cold, dry air passes over a large warmer lake, such as one of the U.S. Great Lakes, and picks up moisture and heat.

Nor'easter – A strong low-pressure system that affects the U.S. Mid-Atlantic and New England States. It can form over land or over the coastal waters. These winter weather events are notorious for producing heavy snow, rain, and tremendous waves that crash onto Atlantic beaches, often causing beach erosion and structural damage. Wind gusts associated with these storms can exceed hurricane force in intensity. A nor'easter gets its name from the continuously strong northeasterly winds blowing in from the ocean ahead of the storm and over the coastal areas.

Rain – Precipitation that falls to earth in drops more than 0.5 mm in diameter.

Sleet – Pellets of ice composed of frozen or mostly frozen raindrops or refrozen, partially melted snowflakes. These pellets of ice usually bounce after hitting the ground or other hard surfaces. Heavy sleet is a relatively rare event defined as an accumulation of ice pellets covering the ground to a depth of 12.7 mm (0.5 in.) or more.

Snow – Precipitation in the form of ice crystals, mainly of intricately branched, hexagonal form and often agglomerated into snowflakes, formed directly from the freezing (deposition) of water vapor in the air.

Snow Flurries – An intermittent light snowfall of short duration (generally light snow showers) with no measurable accumulation (trace category).

Snow Shower – A short duration of moderate snowfall. Some accumulation is possible.

Snow Squall – An intense, but limited duration, period of moderate to heavy snowfall, accompanied by strong, gusty surface winds and possibly lightning (generally moderate to heavy snow showers). Snow accumulation may be significant.

Wind Chill – A measure of the effects of increased wind speeds that accelerate heat loss from exposed skin.

winds may magnify the ruinous effects of each on the environment. They also have direct individual and combined effects as wind chill on exposed humans and animals. Predominately warm climates may not experience freezing precipitation at all, but heavy winter rains and wind can still put people and property in danger, especially through flooding. In colder climates, flooding may also occur secondary to ice jams or avalanche flow obstructing flowing bodies of water, or as a consequence of melting ice and snow. These events may be unrelated to a storm. Snow avalanches are capable of obliterating or isolating towns.

Winter storms are generally categorized by type of precipitation or by storm type (e.g., blizzards, ice storms, lake-effect storms, nor'easters, European windstorms). Each has unique features, but also common elements that include the following:

■ Cold has direct effects on people, property, and electrical and mechanical systems. Damage can be temporary or permanent. Frostbite and hypothermia are the two medical conditions most commonly associated with cold environments. They can occur indoors when power failure limits heat generation or outdoors when people are stranded in a storm or its aftermath, conducting necessary activities in cold environments, or during winter recreation.

■ Frozen precipitation creates wet conditions that can accelerate heat loss from humans and animals. Unlike liquid water that runs off surfaces, ice and snow accumulate on objects, adding significant weight to structures that may not be designed to withstand the added stress. Ice can pull down power and telecommunication lines (Figure 40.1), crush roofs of buildings, and collapse bridges. Ice flowing on rivers can also damage bridges and watercraft.

■ Dangerous movement results from slick ground conditions, degraded visibility, and icing conditions that affect air and water transportation. These conditions inhibit the ability of people to obtain supplies and resources, as well as make it difficult to obtain assistance when help is needed. They also may indirectly contribute to falls, MVCs, recreational accidents, and other injuries related to snow removal and clean-up operations.

All these features of winter storms create hazardous situations, which slow emergency response and increase the risks for responders during the storm itself and for some time afterward if accumulated frozen precipitation and cold temperatures cause hazards to persist.

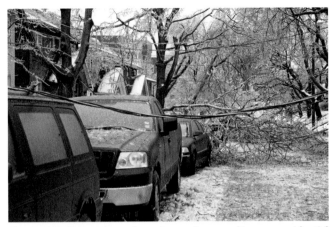

Figure 40.1. Downed tree branches and power lines on residential street in Toronto. Courtesy of istockphoto.

At lower elevations from October to April, populations of American, Asian, and European countries in extra-tropical northern latitudes are at risk from the effects of winter weather. However, regional probabilities for specific types of storms differ. In the United States, winter storms are more frequent in northern states, mountainous regions, and east of the Great Lakes (Figure 40.2). They uncommonly occur in the southern United States, but ice storms are especially treacherous when they do.[6]

As with all PICEs, the impact winter storms have on society is what defines their magnitude. Regions having little experience with winter storms often have the least prepared populations and, therefore, are at even greater risk. These areas may also have

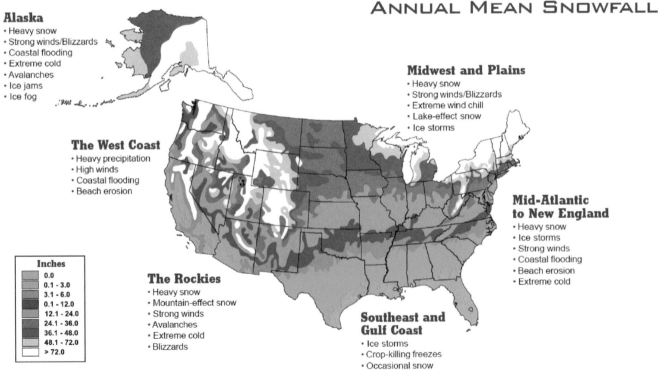

WINTER STORM HAZARDS IN THE U.S.
ANNUAL MEAN SNOWFALL

Alaska
• Heavy snow
• Strong winds/Blizzards
• Coastal flooding
• Extreme cold
• Avalanches
• Ice jams
• Ice fog

Midwest and Plains
• Heavy snow
• Strong winds/Blizzards
• Extreme wind chill
• Lake-effect snow
• Ice storms

The West Coast
• Heavy precipitation
• High winds
• Coastal flooding
• Beach erosion

Mid-Atlantic to New England
• Heavy snow
• Ice storms
• Strong winds
• Coastal flooding
• Beach erosion
• Extreme cold

The Rockies
• Heavy snow
• Mountain-effect snow
• Strong winds
• Avalanches
• Extreme cold
• Blizzards

Southeast and Gulf Coast
• Ice storms
• Crop-killing freezes
• Occasional snow

Inches
0.0
0.1 - 3.0
3.1 - 6.0
0.1 - 12.0
12.1 - 24.0
24.1 - 36.0
36.1 - 48.0
48.1 - 72.0
> 72.0

Figure 40.2. Winter storm hazards in the United States. This graphic is in the public domain. It was reproduced from the National Weather Service's pamphlet entitled *Winter Storms: The Deceptive Killers*.

local and state governments with inadequate capacity to respond rapidly and effectively. Unprepared communities could exponentially increase the human and economic impact of an event. For instance, 1 m (3 ft.) of snow blanketing rural areas of America's Great Plains may minimally disrupt populations and their associated agricultural and ranching industries. In distinction, 1 cm (0.4 in.) of ice from New York City to Washington, DC, could paralyze major commercial, financial, and governmental centers.

Understanding the human impact of catastrophic events, so society can be better prepared for future challenges, is a primary mission for practitioners of emergency management and disaster medicine. With regard to winter storms, the medical literature mostly analyzes events over the last three decades. Health effects of storms that move up the Ohio River Valley from the Texas Gulf Coast and the so-called nor'easters have been the most extensively reported data in the English-language medical literature, likely because of their relative frequency and effects on large population and economic centers in the north-central United States and northeastern seaboard.

A nor'easter that resulted in a major ice storm affecting an area of North America centered over the St. Lawrence River and extending east toward Nova Scotia, January 4–10, 1998, is one of the best described events. The storm resulted in over 4 million people being without electricity – some for up to 33 days – mostly in southern portions of Ontario, Quebec, and Nova Scotia and northern portions of New England.[7] Those who were displaced from their homes in Ontario, and could not move in with a relative or friend, constituted almost 5% of the affected population, placing approximately 140,000 persons in 454 emergency shelters.[8] Some Canadian hospitals were without power for 3 weeks.[9] Estimated total damages for the two countries amounted to as much as 6 billion USD.[7]

Determining a cause of death to be from extreme temperatures is a diagnosis of exclusion, and difficult without awareness of risk factors and circumstances. Databases likely underestimate the numbers as some types of reporting are not required, no precise case definitions exist, and there is little quality control over death certificates. Nonetheless, U.S. data suggest that mortality from excessive cold is less common than from excessive heat.[10] However, this might not be true on a regional basis, or in other countries with different climates.

Deaths from all causes in the United States are more common in January than for any other month. This is especially true for the elderly, and this higher mortality has been specifically linked to colder periods.[11] A study of four consecutive winters in Minnesota showed a slight increase in mortality during cold days, but a greater increase in cardiovascular mortality during periods following snowfall.[12] One report covering 6 consecutive January months in Pennsylvania found that there was a 1.27 times higher relative risk of dying during "extreme climatic conditions" – defined as when the temperature was less than –7°C (19°F) or more than 3 cm (1.2 in.) of snow had fallen.[13] A British study noted a statistically higher risk of dying in winter months from 1986–1996 (1.5% higher for every 1.5°C [2.7°F] decrease in temperature), especially if no central heating was used in the household.[14] The results of both studies demonstrated tight 95% confidence intervals.

The exact risk of storm-related mortality from all causes is not well known. There is no universal requirement to report that any individual's death is or is not directly related to a weather phenomenon. Because of this, any generalized data must be viewed skeptically, unless the data set from which it is derived is specified. Therefore, planners cannot rely on these statistics to predict where resources will be needed to mitigate mortality rates before, during, or after a storm.

A massive blizzard in New England on February 6, 1978, was followed by two public health reports regarding mortality. Twenty-seven storm-related fatalities were identified in Massachusetts, but no overall increase in total mortality was appreciated.[15] In Rhode Island, on the other hand, researchers concluded that there was an increase in total mortality in the first 5 days following the storm,[16] although statistical methods were not used to compare the study group to an unexposed cohort.

Assuming any given healthcare system can maintain its capabilities during and immediately after a winter storm – or rapidly implement its existing plans or ad hoc processes to increase surge capacity – the emergency department (ED) is typically the first functional area affected, because it is the location where ambulances bring patients from the community and where the public is accustomed to seeking unscheduled care.

A Massachusetts study of fifteen hospitals found a significant decrease in ED visits on the day of the blizzard in February 1978, but daily census rapidly returned to baseline.[15] A survey of five major hospitals in northeastern New York State noted a similar trend after a January 1996 blizzard, but this was then followed by a marked increase in ED volume the next day.[17] Only one scientific article could be found that specifically reported the effects of a winter storm on a pediatric ED. The author found that the total daily census increased 35% in the 36 hours before a blizzard hit eastern Pennsylvania and Delaware in January 1996, decreased to very low levels during the storm, then slowly returned to baseline over the next 4 days.[18] A post-event spike frequently reported in adult and combined adult/pediatric EDs was not seen, although there was an increase in the percentages of higher-acuity conditions and a near-tripling of the admission rate.[18]

Following a particularly heavy snow storm in a region of the United States where snow is expected, common storm-related mechanisms of injury (in descending order of frequency) included: slips and falls, MVCs, being struck by falling objects, carbon monoxide (CO) poisoning, and injuries and illnesses related to using clean-up equipment like chainsaws and snowblowers. Morbidity and mortality were also due to deficiencies in access to customary care, lack of home heating due to power loss, and inability to discharge patients to their existing home situations.[17]

Similar findings were reported from a single university medical center in the aftermath of an ice storm that affected much of North Carolina in December 2002, and interrupted power to 1.3 million homes.[19] Ice more commonly downs power lines than does heavy snow. The most common mechanism of injury was from falling objects striking people who were conducting assessments and clean-up outside. An epidemic of CO poisoning was also seen in patients presenting to the same institution. These mechanisms accounted for all the life-threatening injuries, except one elderly patient who likely became hypothermic after a stroke. Slips and falls, injuries associated with darkness, and burns encompassed the other causes of injury. In this study, MVCs could not reliably be determined to be storm-related in many instances, so they were not specifically examined.[19]

One of the first epidemiological reports documenting an increased incidence of fractures associated with a winter storm was published by Ráliš in the aftermath of 5 days of snow and ice over 1 week around the New Year 1978–1979.[20] In a UK ED with a census of over 93,000 patients per year, the number of patients with fractures increased 2.85 times over baseline, peaking at a rate of one in every five patients. In descending order of frequency, the locations of fractures were the wrist and forearm, foot and ankle, hand, hip, leg, chest, spine, and skull.[20]

In the midwestern United States, ice storms have led to numerous orthopedic injuries. Falls on ice, particularly in the elderly, more commonly resulted in extremity fractures than falls during equivalent periods of snow-cover in St. Louis.[21] In the 9 days after a winter storm passed through Indianapolis in February 1994, 327 injuries in 259 individuals who slipped on ice were managed at a single hospital. Most were back injuries of various types, but over a third of patients were diagnosed with fractures of the non-axial skeleton.[22] Following the 13-day ice storm of January 1998, Canadian EDs reported over one-third of the injuries seen were directly storm-related.[23] This was also true in both adult and pediatric populations in Montreal.[9] Physicians at Montreal General Hospital alone performed sixty emergency orthopedic operations for storm-related injuries.[9]

One statewide epidemiological study of 6,047 winter storm–related injuries in Oklahoma revealed that, for every eight injuries, six were due to falls and one was due to an MVC. Additional mechanisms included sledding, CO poisoning, clean-up activities, and "other" categories. Falls were more common in persons ≥40 years, whereas MVCs were more likely in persons <40 years of age. Falls were twice as likely to cause fractures in the older age group.[24]

CO poisoning is generally seen in winter months, and its incidence can be increased by a storm that results in widespread power losses. Sources of CO are usually burning fuel indoors for heat, electricity generation, or cooking with nontraditional fuel sources. Exhaust fumes filling automobiles with snow-obstructed tailpipes is another mechanism of CO poisoning following winter storms.

The rate of CO poisoning cases increased after a winter storm disrupted power to a large portion of the Seattle–Tacoma area of the northwestern United States in 1993.[25,26] Thirty incidents resulted in eighty-one cases at thirteen hospitals through the 3-day storm. Another spike in CO poisoning cases was reported in the same area after two winter storms in late 1996.[26] Following the North American ice storm of January 1998, over 1,000 cases of CO poisoning from at least 700 individual incidents were reported in Quebec alone, and this was likely fewer than actually occurred.[9] Four hospitals in rural Maine reported 42 incidents causing 100 cases with up to 8 patients arriving from a single scene.[27] About half that number was reported for two EDs in just one city in Ontario.[28] After a December 2002 ice storm in North Carolina, a single university hospital saw 200 cases of CO poisoning in 1 week,[29] while another one in a different city saw 48 after the same storm.[19]

Several studies report an increased incidence of fatal and nonfatal acute coronary syndromes (ACS) associated with winter storms.[12,30,31] Specific risk factors could not be identified in a small cohort of patients surviving myocardial infarctions after a January 1979 blizzard in Chicago.[32] Short-term cold exposure was not believed to be the cause of increased ACS when a Canadian study examined 15 years of epidemiological data.[33] On the other hand, a Dutch study concluded that wind chill may have a greater effect on cardiovascular risk than cold air itself.[34]

Heavy snow shoveling has been shown to elicit sustained heart rates near age-calculated maximums with aerobic oxygen demands similar to arm-crank ergometry.[35] Although a Cana-dian study concluded that the incidence of "heart attacks" was independent of snowfall, the ones that did occur were more likely to follow shoveling.[36] In distinction, an American study of ten EDs in one New York county after a January 1996 blizzard affected much of the northeastern United States, found a 6.6 times increased relative risk of ACS events – primarily following snow shoveling, and often in persons without histories of coronary artery disease.[37] Comparing consecutive January months from 1991 to 1996, a Pennsylvania study noted increased risk of cardiac mortality in males – progressively higher in younger age groups: 1.28–2.21 for those > 65 years old; 1.32–2.38 for those 50–64 years old; and 2.35–5.35 for those 35–49 years old.[13] In another study, the rate of non-cardiovascular illnesses was not noted to change.[37]

Scope of Other Winter Hazards

Accidental hypothermia can occur at virtually any ambient temperature, but it is more strongly associated with cold air and cold-water submersion. Death rates in the United States are 0.08–1.99 per 100,000 population in the contiguous 48 states – although, as expected, they are higher in Alaska.[38] Therefore, accidental hypothermia is not a common cause of death, but is a potentially preventable one. Disabled persons, the elderly, and the socially disadvantaged are at particular risk at all times. However, during and after a winter event, these and other groups may have more acute needs due to disruption of power or inability to access assisting services.

Cold-water immersion is a complex phenomenon, which may or may not have coexistent hypothermia. Although epidemiological statistics are readily available regarding drownings in several countries, few are particular to cold-water immersions. One that did specifically address this examined the winter months during the 1991–2000 decade in Canada. Researchers determined that, out of 2007 cold-water immersion deaths, 1,245 (62%) occurred between November and April. Although the human activities just before these incidents were not directly linked to winter months or storms, the relative percentages may be useful for mitigation purposes: 45% occurred during boating or other aquatic activities; 22% while on ice (the majority of these on snowmobiles); 15% during land transportation collisions; and 14% from other falls into water.[39] Epidemiological data regarding nonfatal cold-water immersion injuries were not reported.

Snow avalanche is a natural phenomenon involving snow accumulated over time, but winter storms increase the risks for populations living in avalanche-prone terrain. The financial impact and public health implications of avalanches are often relatively small compared to those from widespread devastating storms. Generally, the consequences of snow avalanche predictably involve human-built structures, transportation systems, and power and telecommunications infrastructure; but people can be injured when caught in their destructive paths.

In North America and Europe, there are about 150 deaths each year attributed to snow avalanches. There were 329 deaths from avalanches in Canada between 1978 and 2007. Outdoor recreation is associated with about nine in ten fatalities. North American avalanche victims most often include snowmobile riders and HeliCat skiers. Snowmobilers are the fastest growing percentage of avalanche victims.

In an autopsy study in Utah, twenty-two avalanche deaths from asphyxiation also had mild to moderate traumatic brain injury, and all six of the cases where trauma was the cause of death had severe brain injury.[40]

In a Canadian autopsy study of 204 avalanche fatalities, the immediate cause of death in 75% of cases was asphyxia. Trauma was the cause of death in 24% and hypothermia in 1% of cases. Of the trauma victims with single-system injuries, 46% were chest-related, followed closely by head injury in 42%, then 8% with neck injury. About half of the trauma casualties were completely buried in snow. Victims of asphyxia were buried in 92% of cases. Trauma victims were buried an average of 90 cm (about 3 ft.), and asphyxia cases were buried an average of 150 cm (about 5 ft.). Burial time averaged 25 minutes for trauma cases and 45 minutes for asphyxia cases.[41]

A study of Austrian avalanche victims from 1994–2005 included 1,745 people. The authors reported 565 cases either partially or completely buried. Records were reviewed on ninety-four victims admitted to Innsbruck Medical Center. There were sixty-seven (71%) survivors to discharge. Cardiopulmonary resuscitation (CPR) was performed on arrival for twenty-three victims, with a mortality rate of 91%. The most frequent diagnosis in this study was hypothermia (56%). Spinal fractures were found in 7%. A protocol that used total-body computed tomography imaging missed only 2.1% of injuries detected later.[42]

The most common nonfatal injuries in avalanche victims are orthopedic, craniofacial, and soft-tissue injuries. In a radiological study of fourteen avalanche victims in Switzerland, 133 imaging studies demonstrated 61% musculoskeletal injuries and 39% extra-skeletal injuries. Fractures of the axial skeleton (26.8%) were more common than the extremities (9.8%). Non-skeletal findings were intrathoracic (39%), intra-abdominal (15%), and intracranial (10%).[43] Chapter 42 contains additional information on avalanches.

CURRENT STATE OF THE ART

Decision-makers must know a situation exists before they can implement preparedness plans and devote resources for a targeted and coordinated response. It is usually easy to detect that a winter storm has dropped precipitation on a given region, but its human impact is much more difficult to assess, especially when aerial over-flights and on-the-ground access to affected areas are limited. Establishing an incident command structure, regardless of size, collects the resources officials need to determine the security and safety of affected areas, identify hazards to responders, and coordinate the support necessary to begin rescue and recovery efforts.

Winter Hazards

Storms and their aftermaths affect both populations and societal systems, the latter of which includes the ability to respond to community emergencies and to deliver healthcare outside and inside hospitals. Public health surveillance and interventions, emergency medical services (EMS) systems, and regional hospital capacity can all be adversely affected by power losses, hazardous driving conditions, and geographic isolation. Snow avalanches can cause similar problems, although generally on more localized scales than widespread storm damage. Cold environments can be treacherous to both the general population and public safety personnel.

Weather Conditions

One of the purposes of government is to protect the public welfare, particularly with resources not available to individuals or private groups. Most developed nations have one or more methods of notifying their populaces of important weather conditions that may adversely impact people or property. In the United States, this responsibility begins with the National Weather Service (NWS).

NWS may issue a "winter storm watch" when there is an increased risk of a hazardous weather or hydrologic event, but its occurrence, location, and/or timing is uncertain. The purpose of a "watch" is intended to alert the population at risk to initiate protective actions. Once its weather predictions are more certain, a "winter storm advisory" or "winter storm warning" may be issued – or the message may be more specific, such as "blizzard warning."

- The term "advisory" highlights special weather conditions that are less serious than a warning. They are for events that may cause significant inconvenience, and if caution is not exercised, could lead to situations that may threaten life or property.
- The term "warning" is issued when a hazardous weather or hydrologic event is occurring, is imminent, or has a very high probability of occurring. A warning is used for conditions posing a threat to life or property.

Although print media is useful for long-range forecasts (i.e., more than 24 hours in the future), broadcast media and the Internet are the most common methods used for more immediate notifications of approaching winter storms. The U.S. National Oceanic and Atmospheric Administration (NOAA) All-Hazards Weather Radio broadcasts important information directly from the nearest NWS office around the clock.

Storm severity categories may help populations at risk, emergency response organizations, and other public and private facilities (e.g., government centers, hospitals) prepare for potential effects. Hurricanes, known as cyclones in some parts of the world, and tornadoes each have a well-known severity index associated with them: 1–5 for the former and 0–5 for the latter. A seven-level categorization scheme, called the Local Winter Storm Scale (LWSS), has also been proposed.[44] It is based on five weighted meteorological factors over any given area: sustained wind speed; speed of wind gusts; snow accumulation; ice accumulation; and visibility. The overall LWSS category may help predict a storm's societal impact. Although it has been correlated to an older Realized Disruption Index, the LWSS has only been retrospectively derived to date, and is not yet in as widespread use as other storm categorization schemes. However, one advantage is that impact predictions can be modified moment-to-moment as constantly updated weather data are received and analyzed.

Responding to emergency scenes is hazardous in any environment. Dangerous winter road conditions and limited visibility caused by winter storms, as well as the increased risk of becoming stranded far from shelter amplify the risk. EMS, fire/rescue, and law enforcement personnel usually receive formal training on emergency driving. However, specific driving instruction for winter weather is often only didactic in nature. Few response organizations provide hands-on training that allows drivers to experience real winter emergency conditions in controlled situations using operational response vehicles, which

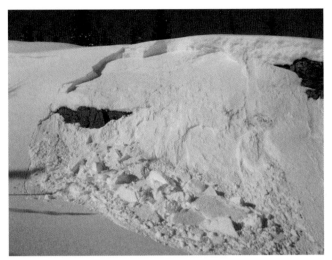

Figure 40.3. Separation of snow from a ridge at the starting zone of an avalanche. Photograph courtesy of William H. Dice, MD.

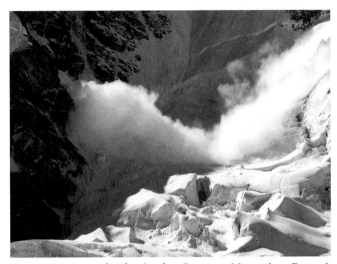

Figure 40.4. An avalanche in the Caucasus Mountains, Bezengi, Kabardino-Balkaria. Courtesy of iStockphoto.

handle much differently than passenger vehicles. Similarly, few private companies or public service organizations – including those delivering healthcare – provide any driver training to those who must respond during or after winter storms. When road conditions exceed driver abilities to navigate them, the number of emergency scenes may increase, and thereby compound the overall demand for rescues and out-of-hospital medical responses.

When driving during or after a winter storm, speed must be reduced to improve traction and decrease distance required to identify hazards and stop safely. Heavy snowfall and wind-swept snow can cause near "white out" conditions with visibility less than 15 meters (50 ft.). Slick conditions on road surfaces increases stopping distances. Negotiating hills and curves may be difficult. Even stepping out of vehicles can be more risky, and slips and falls can injure responders. Parking or exiting a vehicle on a roadway can be very dangerous when other vehicles are moving around it. Distracted by flashing emergency lights, other drivers may lose control of their own vehicles causing impacts with emergency response vehicles and their crews.

"Black ice" is a term referring to a thin layer of ice that cannot be seen when it is adhered to darkly colored road surfaces, yet is just as treacherous as an icy surface several centimeters thick. This invisible ice layer can develop in minutes when a wet roadway at the freezing point suddenly becomes colder due to evaporation via wind or with the loss of the sun's heat (e.g., with clouds, sunset, or shade).

Avalanche Terrain

Avalanches are characterized by three physical zones: a starting zone, where unstable snow layers begin to move (Figure 40.3); a track, where snow flows down a slope below the starting zone; and the runout zone, where snow and debris collect at the bottom. Avalanches containing dry snow usually begin on slope angles greater than 25°, but avalanches on wet snow can begin on shallower slopes. Generally, wind-deposited snow is at greater risk for breaking loose. Places where snow is deposited by wind are near ridge lines, behind trees, and behind high or convex terrain.

Orientation to the sun affects snow stability, and changes with temperature and season. Sunny slopes are more stable in winter, but rapidly become unstable as spring temperatures rise. Shady slopes allow snow to remain cold in winter, with a tendency to form unstable layers from frost. Shady slopes stabilize slowly as spring arrives.

Terrain features also influence the likelihood that snow will begin to slide. Forest cover generally stabilizes the snow. Timber harvesting from steep mountains in Europe was stopped almost 100 years ago to preserve protected forests. Surface obstacles such as tree stumps, boulders, shrubs, and rock formations can anchor snow until it is deep enough to form unstable layers above these features. In rough terrain, more than 1 meter (3 ft.) of snow is required to produce avalanche-favorable conditions.

Avalanche speed and impact pressure determine the destructive power of the slide. Avalanche material can accelerate rapidly near the starting zone and reach over 25 m/s (82 fps) within the first 200 meters (218 yd.). Dry-snow avalanches begin as a slab or as loose snow with a relatively dense core at the bottom of the slide covered by a snow cloud when speeds exceed 10 m/s (33 fps). The overhead cloud can be over 10 meters (33 ft.) high, which can seriously obscure visibility if trying to watch for victims during an observed avalanche (Figure 40.4). The depth of the core is typically 1–2 meters (3–6 ft.), but can be deeper. As the snow slides, friction causes water to form on the surface of snow particles such that, when the moving snow mass comes to rest in the runout zone, it hardens immediately as the water freezes. The hardened snow makes self-extrication nearly impossible, even when persons are only partially buried. Deposit densities from avalanches range from 200 kg/m³ (12.5 lbs./ft.³) for small dry-flow types to over 1,000 kg/m³ (62.4 lbs./ft.³) for large slush-flow types.

Powder-only avalanches lack a dense core, so they tend to cause less physical damage. Dry-flow avalanches are probably the most destructive overall due to their velocities. A dry-flow avalanche at Rogers Pass, British Columbia, generated impact pressures over 600 kPa (87 psi).[45] An impact pressure of 100 kPa (14.5 psi) will uproot a mature tree, and 1,000 kPa (145 psi) will move a reinforced concrete structure. Air blast is a phenomenon where air in front of high-speed avalanche material is compacted into a high-pressure wave. This can cause additional damage in an area wider than the flow itself, but most avalanches are not associated with a significant air blast.

Cold Environments

Other winter hazards are generally less likely to result in disaster situations by themselves, but cold environments can affect indoor living with inadequate heat and complicate many outdoor activities. Recreation can be curtailed if necessary, but emergency responders may have fewer options. They must be prepared for hazardous driving or flying conditions to and from scenes; the effects of cold, wind, and wet conditions on themselves, their patients, and their vehicles; and on potential disruptions to radio, cellular, and satellite service created primarily by atmospheric conditions or secondarily by damage to power and telecommunications systems.

Responders must also ensure that their equipment and supplies are functional in cold environments. Vehicles must be well maintained and prepared for operations in cold weather or slick surface conditions. This is true for all ground-based vehicles, which are subject to maintenance standards at local and national levels in most countries if governmentally owned, but may not be if owned by individuals or businesses (e.g., utility companies). The same applies to aircraft used as ambulances or for other public service applications, the maintenance and operations of which are even more stringently controlled, especially as regards adverse environmental conditions.

Winter temperatures are harsh on vehicles. Engine and transmission oils become more viscous at lower temperatures, requiring longer warm-up times for vehicles kept in unheated locations for any period of time. Water in fuel lines may freeze. Block heaters are used to keep engine fluids warmer to facilitate starting. Windshield wipers become less efficient as rain freezes or turns to sleet or heavy wet snow, hampering visibility. Headlamps can become covered with wet snow, reducing the light output reaching roadways to almost nothing. Snow may also obscure directional signals, parking lights, and emergency flashers, making it difficult for other motorists to see vehicles at sufficient distances to avoid collision on slick roadways.

Crashes and vehicle incapacitation can result in response personnel being stranded while driving in inclement weather, ice, or heavy snow. Radio communications may be degraded and cellular or satellite telephones may be nonfunctional during or immediately after a winter storm. Response personnel must be prepared for the inability to communicate with their own dispatch authority, other emergency response agencies, or an Emergency Operations Center (EOC). Medical control for patient care advice or authorizations beyond an EMS crew's standing orders or scope of practice might be limited. Communications problems may also make it difficult to call for assistance, if stranded.

All emergency response personnel venturing into the winter environment must have operational guidelines for a communications outage or cold-weather vehicle failure. Most authorities recommend that stranded motorists stay with their vehicles, but caution them to guard against cold injury if not heating the interior, and CO poisoning if running the engine or using some other heat source.

Many emergency response vehicles, which operate in areas likely to receive ice and snow, are equipped with chains that can be used either on their tires or in a deployable apparatus under the chassis such that, at the touch of a button, chains are rotated on a horizontal axis near the tires resulting in enhanced traction equivalent to chained tires.

Response personnel must be properly attired, equipped, and trained for work in cold, windy, and wet scenarios. Typical clothing worn by EMS responders on a day-to-day basis may not adequately protect them from the elements, because winter storms may prolong scene times in harsh outdoor environments.

Clothing worn should minimize the risk of injury yet maximize dexterity and function. The overarching goals are to preserve core body heat and to minimize exposure of skin to cold air and surfaces. Knowledge about environmental conditions is essential so that proactive and reactive behaviors will be appropriate to prevent tissue damage. Mental status changes from environmental exposures can lead to deleterious behaviors such as paradoxical undressing. The following are general recommendations for the prevention of cold-induced problems:

- Adequate hydration, nutrition, and rest are essential. Being in excellent physical condition is an advantage. Use of tobacco products is detrimental to good circulation. Clean, healthy skin is better at preventing cold injury, but washing too frequently can dry and damage protective barriers.
- Thermal insulation can be provided by garments themselves and trapped air between fabric layers. The mnemonic for prevention of COLD stands for Clean fabrics; Opening for ventilation during exercise (to avoid wetting perspiration); Loose layers to retain insulating air pockets, and allow for donning and doffing layers as conditions change; and Dry garments, which must be changed if they get wet. The head must be well insulated, because significant body heat can escape from the exposed scalp.
- Avoid tight-fitting clothing and restrictive gloves or boots. Liners improve the insulation of both. When dexterity is not needed, mittens are more effective at retaining heat than are gloves.
- A balance must exist between external water impermeability and the risk of retaining sweat inside protective garments that cannot breathe. Particularly with regard to the feet, wet conditions soften the skin, which can lead to debilitating nonfreezing injuries like trench foot. Extra socks must be available so that damp socks can be exchanged for dry ones.
- Protect exposed skin surfaces from cold and windy air, as well as from cold liquids and surfaces. Avoid damaging skin through ultraviolet radiation directly from the sun or indirectly from reflection off ice, snow, water, windows, or light-colored building surfaces.
- Use the buddy system, especially by trained individuals who consciously and frequently check each other, to decrease the likelihoods of insidious frostbite and hypothermia.

In addition to rescuers, these recommendations apply to all persons living indoors with inadequate heating or outdoors exposed to cold environments.

Local Medical Responders

Winter storms may severely limit the ability of responders to reach callers in a timely manner, or to find victims during a community needs assessment or deliberate search. Once located, care may have to be delivered in relatively austere medical conditions for periods of time that may far exceed those to which first responders and EMS personnel are accustomed. Transportation to a permanent or temporary medical facility, or even to a heated shelter with power and food, may be so treacherous that the risk–benefit ratio is higher than staying in place. Response organizations and systems must consider how to best plan, train, operate, and recover in these environments.

Access

Winter storms may severely limit the ability of responders to access known victims or areas to search for unknown victims. Much has been written in books and journals and posted on the Internet regarding tactics, techniques, and procedures for searching for victims who cannot call for help after a storm with freezing precipitation or after being buried in an avalanche runout zone. However, virtually nothing has been published on best practices for EMS and other public safety personnel who must access persons who have called for help during or after one of these events.

Response efforts need to be coordinated with other community resources when debris or fire, downed power lines, ruptured natural gas or water pipelines, or physical violence threaten the safety of responders. Response should be coordinated through a local or regional EOC functioning under an incident command structure. In advance of a winter storm, a local EOC could prohibit ambulances from traveling off plowed roadways, yet still be responsive to requests for assistance. For instance, response assets could be reorganized into task forces, such that a call for medical help would result in dispatch of a snow plow, a four-wheel-drive vehicle with a command officer and a medic, and a staffed fire engine. These resource groupings could be kept intact between calls. Public health representation could also facilitate data collection for a rapid needs assessment.

Access to avalanche victims is challenging. Survival of those not initially killed from injuries is associated with four parameters: 1) burial depth; 2) the victim's ability to self-extricate; 3) body parts or objects attached to a victim exposed above the snow; and 4) terrain effects on victim access, care, extrication, and evacuation by rescuers.

According to the Colorado Avalanche Information Center, since 1950 about 63% of avalanche survivors were rescued by companions compared to 19% by organized rescue teams. Use of beacons can improve survival. However, in an Austrian study of 109 totally buried victims, only 31.1% of victims had transceivers and none were rescued by companions.[46] It is rare to survive for more than 1 hour when buried. When people are caught in an avalanche, observers should establish a "last-seen point." Rescuers must consider the risk of additional snow slides before entering an area to begin any search. Companions should organize a hasty search beginning from the last-seen point. The hasty search is performed by first looking for visible clues such as equipment or clothing, and listening for voices. If there is no surface clue to locate the victim, a beacon search should be undertaken. If beacons were not attached to individuals or a search for beacon signals fails to locate any victims, a probe search should be initiated. Communication with search-and-rescue teams should occur as soon as possible, but should not delay the hasty search.[47]

Out-of-Hospital Care

Hasty rescue and rapid out-of-hospital care of avalanche victims may be lifesaving. Asphyxiation is the leading cause of death after avalanche burial, mostly from decreasing oxygen and increasing carbon-dioxide fractions within any sealed air pocket. When victims are freed within 15 minutes, the survival rate is over 90%. However, when victims remain buried for 30 minutes, the survival drops to 30%. Survival beyond 30 minutes depends on the size of the air pocket around the victim's face.[48]

Because rescuers may need to remove up to 1.33 metric tons (approximately 3,000 lbs.) of snow to reach a victim buried under just 1 meter (3 ft.) of snow; the priority of rescue efforts should be focused on the victim's head and face. Once cleared of ice and snow, airway management and assisted ventilation, with or without endotracheal intubation, should be completed as soon as access is achievable, before further efforts to free the rest of the body.

With the exception of conditions directly related to heat loss, individual out-of-hospital patient care should be similar to that without winter conditions. Nevertheless, responders must be aware of the risks of cold weather to them and their patients, and must anticipate delays in access and evacuation during storms. Illnesses may be more advanced or complications of injuries may be more manifest when access is delayed. Additionally, the duration of care may be extended for longer than EMS and rescue personnel are otherwise accustomed. Depending on limitations in evacuation options or extensions of transportation times, care may have to be delivered for hours, or perhaps even days in extreme circumstances.

Evacuation delays may necessitate hemorrhage control methods less familiar to civilian EMS responders. Exsanguinating extremity hemorrhage may have to be controlled with a proximal tourniquet, either by inflating a blood-pressure cuff or applying a prefabricated or field-expedient device. Application of dressings or powders containing clot-enhancing agents such as kaolin, mineral zeolite, microporous polysaccharide microsphere, poly-N-acetylglucosamine (chitosan), or fibrin may be useful adjuncts.

Since people routinely postpone seeking medical care when there is no extreme weather, a delayed response under storm conditions may not pose additional challenges for responders. A notable exception is when patients' health conditions require services that are disrupted by the storm, for example, a patient on a home ventilator with failure of back-up power. Injured patients, on the other hand, may be more likely to seek care immediately, yet medically trained providers may not be able to access them rapidly. Delayed complications (e.g., established wound infections, gangrene or tetanus, compartment syndromes) or progressive conditions (e.g., increased intracranial pressure, pulmonary contusions, slow intracavitary hemorrhage) may be less familiar to EMS personnel – and their scope of practice may only allow for supportive care, even when delays in evacuation to definitive care could result in loss of life or limb.

Frostbite and hypothermia are the most common cold-induced conditions. Out-of-hospital management consists of removing the source of the cold insult and supporting the patient during evacuation to a higher level of care. Active rewarming is difficult in the field. In situations of widespread power loss, the only source of added heat may be the interior of an evacuation vehicle. If specialized equipment is available and functional within the response vehicle, this represents an additional rewarming option. In general, though, active rewarming is conducted at a medical facility.

Cold injuries can be divided into nonfreezing and freezing categories. The former includes pernio, trench foot, and immersion foot. Pernio results from the combined effects of wet and cold skin, but may occur in dry nonfreezing conditions. Trench foot may occur in chronically wet feet exposed to near-freezing temperatures and made relatively ischemic by vasospasm and increased tissue pressure induced by standing or tight footwear. Immersion foot results from skin that has become waterlogged after prolonged cold-water immersion. Injuries that actually freeze tissue include frostnip and frostbite.

Pernio, also called chilblains, is a localized inflammatory condition of the skin, which results from an abnormal tissue response that develops over 12–24 hours after cold exposure. There is frequently a history of Raynaud's phenomenon. Pernio most commonly manifests as tender bluish or purplish subcutaneous nodules in exposed areas. These lesions are often associated with edema or blister formation. Treatment consists of local massage to stimulate blood flow and slow rewarming at normal room temperatures. Active rewarming with higher temperatures significantly increases the intense burning and itching associated with resolution.[49] Nifedipine may have a role in hastening clearance of the lesions with less discomfort, and possibly reducing the likelihood of recurrence.[50]

Trench foot and immersion foot are clinically indistinguishable. They both progress insidiously through three phases: pre-hyperemic, hyperemic, and post-hyperemic. Intense vasospasm causes skin blanching and mottling in the pre-hyperemic phase. Peripheral pulses may be diminished. Capillary refill is usually prolonged. Continued exposure results in anesthesia and gait disturbances from damage to sensory and proprioceptive nerves.[49] Rewarming creates a hyperemic condition with erythema, petechiae, swelling, pain, and hypesthesia – yet is still associated with prolonged capillary refill.[51] Epidermal sloughing may occur. Nerves controlling voluntary muscular action and vibratory sensation may be adversely affected. Therefore, the goal of treatment is rewarming core body temperature without directly warming the affected body parts, so as to keep the metabolic demands of the injured tissue low.[49] The post-hyperemic phase is not normally seen in the field, unless evacuation is significantly delayed after rewarming.

Frostnip, which heralds the beginning of tissue ice-crystal formation, is a warning sign that frostbite is imminent. Vasoconstriction leads to pallor, localized pain, and sensory numbness. Clinical manifestations can be readily reversed by preventing additional cooling and by rewarming the affected body parts.[49]

Frostbite represents freezing of extra- and intracellular water with cell injury or destruction leading to tissue damage, which can be compounded by microvascular stasis and ischemia. Typical symptoms progress from feeling local cold to loss of sensation. Pain may occur in a "watershed" area between frostnip and frostbite, typically more proximal to fully involved areas of distal tissue freezing. Frostbitten skin may appear a waxy yellowish white or translucent bluish color. It may be frozen solid.

Prevention of further cooling should be the primary goal prior to in-hospital management of frostbite. Wet, or possibly frozen, clothing should be gently removed. If adhered to the skin, other portions of any garments can be cut away, leaving frozen bits of clothing temporarily attached. Out-of-hospital rewarming of frozen tissue is generally discouraged, unless evacuation to definitive medical care will be significantly delayed.[52] A 10-year Canadian study found that delay to medical care was one factor associated with poor frostbite outcome, so delayed access or prolonged evacuation times may have implications for prognosis.[53] One author suggested 2 hours of field time as a cutoff to begin thawing in the field, but only if no chance of refreezing is possible.[54]

The position of the International Commission for Alpine Rescue provides a useful extrapolation from mountaineering to victims of other winter hazards.[55] Guidelines are divided into whether the victim is out in the open or inside shelter, but commonalities include: removal of wet clothing; orally administered warm fluids; and aspirin up to 1 g or ibuprofen up to 800 mg, if available. In shelter, if active rewarming is performed by immersion into a warm 37°C (99°F) bath, the patient should not be allowed to subsequently use the part, which includes walking if the feet are involved, until after definitive care has been rendered. Because edema will ensue as the part is warmed, the area should be elevated and dry dressings loosely applied.[55]

Prevention of further cooling is also the primary goal for the out-of-hospital treatment of hypothermia. Other field management options are limited. Patients with mild hypothermia (i.e., core body temperature 32–35°C [90–95°F] and still capable of shivering) may warm themselves by being covered with dry, heat-retaining clothing, blankets, or other items. These interventions allow endogenous heat production through metabolism and the shivering reflex, and constitute the passive external rewarming technique. Active external rewarming involves the addition of exogenous heat to the body through a warm environment or radiant heaters. External rewarming interventions can be supplemented by warm oral fluids not containing caffeine or warm intravenous crystalloid fluids, but these field methods of active internal rewarming have only minor temperature-raising effects – although they may have an additional benefit of volume repletion, because many victims of hypothermia are also dehydrated.[52,54,56]

Bradycardia is often observed at core temperatures less than 28°C (82°F). In severe hypothermia, when the temperature is less than 25°C (77°F), more serious cardiac dysrhythmias occur. Development of new atrial fibrillation is ominous, as it may herald progression to ventricular fibrillation. When dysrhythmias complicate hypothermia, the treatment of choice is rewarming. Medications are not likely to be helpful until the heart is warm.[57] Transthoracic pacing is possible, but not required in most cases.[57,58]

The out-of-hospital management of cold-water immersion is much the same as for any drowning, and is primarily supportive. Hypothermia may or may not occur during cold-water immersion, but the field care of hypothermia is the same as delineated previously.[59] However, many successful resuscitations with good neurological outcomes following prolonged submersion in cold water have been reported. Therefore, assuming the resources are available and transportation times reasonable, responders should consider initiating interventions even when immersion times are known to be up to 1 hour or more.

Avalanche victims found in cardiac arrest and buried for less than 1 hour are not likely to have core temperatures below 30°C (86°F), and resuscitation will probably fail because of prolonged asphyxia without hypothermia. An air pocket must be present for a victim to survive long enough to develop hypothermia as a cause of cardiac arrest.[60,61] If the victim is buried for more than 1 hour and uncovered with an intact air pocket, relatively protective hypothermia could exist, and CPR and transport for core rewarming should be considered.

Evacuation

Just as winter weather can affect the ability of first responders to access victims, it can also make it hazardous or difficult to transport them from out-of-hospital scenes to medical facilities. The usual evacuation assets may not be available. Standard ambulances may not be outfitted for driving to or from a victim's initial location. Few have four-wheel drive, so nonmedical vehicles of expediency may have to be used. Moreover, helicopters may not be operational or safe to fly. In a Canadian study, 30% of requested helicopter EMS missions were aborted due to weather, which was the next most common reason behind the 42% combination of the helicopter not being the appropriate vehicle and cancellation by medical control.[62]

Determining the most appropriate destination for patients should be guided by local protocols, but the winter environment may force additional considerations in a disaster setting. Some medical facilities may be directly affected by the winter storm. Impaired ground and air accessibility, power losses, and staff absenteeism are just a few of the reasons a hospital or other facility may not have the capacity to receive new patients from the field. Other facilities may be overwhelmed by high patient volume and higher patient acuity in a storm's aftermath. Routing of transportation assets directly to centers offering specialty services may be required for pediatrics, major trauma, serious burns, and hyperbaric oxygen therapy to name a few; but transportation to these services may not be expedient or safe during hazardous winter conditions.

Finally, the possibility of being stranded during evacuation could be complicated by having to maintain care for one or more patients for much longer durations than medical training, supply quantities, and vehicle power were designed. Telecommunications with medical control, to assist medics in these unfamiliar situations, may or may not be available.

Despite governmental regulations and industry guidelines on operations of emergency vehicles, there are few standards regarding cold-weather storage and use of onboard medical equipment and pharmaceuticals. Ground-based ambulances can often be parked in some kind of a garage while awaiting calls. This is rarely an option for helicopters, especially when they are hospital-based. Two North American[63,64] studies and one European[65] study have examined temperatures inside medication containers on rotary-wing ambulances. Both identified temperatures far outside the range recommended for pharmaceutical storage, although the clinical impact of this is uncertain. An important exception would be cold intravenous fluids, which could be potentially harmful to many patients, if given in any significant quantity.

Local Medical Receivers

A challenge for hospitals is inadequate staffing resources (e.g., inability to surge with off-duty staff due to weather preventing travel from home and on-duty staff overworked due to lack of relief) or capability degradation (e.g., interruption of facility water and power and supply expenditure without replenishment). Nonetheless, patients continue to seek care for a variety of baseline and storm-related problems. As in the field, the care delivered to individual patients is similar to that in other situations, except that cold-induced injury, hypothermia, CO poisoning, and other storm-associated conditions may complicate conventional management. Establishing disaster triage protocols to screen victims for these potentially occult problems is recommended to enhance ED operations following a winter storm.

Primary Triage

Because the ED is the focal point of victim reception, it is also the site of initial triage of persons presenting for care. Patient conditions may or may not be directly attributable to the storm, but all individuals must be screened. In addition to standard triage questions for potentially serious illnesses and injuries, high levels of suspicion for frostbite, hypothermia, and CO poisoning are required when people present to the hospital following a winter storm. Such storm-related conditions can be coexistent with a seemingly unrelated chief complaint. In order to limit the risk of missing these potentially occult conditions, triage personnel should specifically ask about exposure to cold, wet, or windy conditions, as well as the possibility of exposure to burning fuels.

If sufficient resources are available for the volume and acuity of conditions, little or no adjustment to routine operations may be necessary. However, any excessive patient need or limitation in healthcare capacity may require a different approach to triage and activation of facility disaster plans. Protocols should address the probability of various conditions, establish reasonable diagnostic parameters recognizing the potential limitations in laboratory and radiology services, provide management guidelines, and identify admission and discharge criteria that may be different than those under non-disaster circumstances.

Emergency Care

Traumatic injuries directly related to winter storms include those sustained during outdoor movement (e.g., slips and falls, MVCs) clean-up efforts (e.g., snow clearing, tree removal, utility repair) recreational activities (e.g., sledding, snowmobiling), and those due to generally hazardous conditions (e.g., avalanche, ice-covered bodies of water). As most of these mechanisms are familiar to emergency professionals, only those unique to winter weather are discussed in this chapter.

Although often purchased for recreation, snowmobiles can be important transportation sources during and after a winter storm. While able to facilitate transport for both patients and staff, snowmobiles are also associated with increased need for healthcare resources. Snowmobile crashes involve drivers, passengers, pedestrians, and people being pulled on sleds. Most injuries are musculoskeletal, but head, chest, and abdominal injuries occur frequently. Trauma around the knee is common, and fractures of the femur and tibia encompass nearly half of the injuries. In a study of snowmobile collisions in Canada, 74% of victims required emergency surgery with a mean of 1.6 operative procedures per patient.[66]

Complex wounds caused by a variety of mechanisms may present after winter storms (Figure 40.5). Many follow the use of power equipment for clearing debris, fallen trees, and snow. Chainsaw injuries occur throughout the year,[67] but snowblower injuries can be expected following a heavy snowfall.[68] Following a 1997 storm in Rhode Island, seven of eleven patients injured by snowblowers indicated that they placed their hand into a running machine, though three of the remainder said that the machine was off at the time of injury. Amputation was common, as were open fractures and tendon injuries. Ten hand injuries were managed in the ED by hand surgeons and one required inpatient treatment. The majority of cases involved the index, middle, and ring fingers.[69]

Management of open wounds should follow traditional wound care guidelines. Wounds should be thoroughly described with emphasis on size, shape, depth, foreign material, local perfusion, distal circulation, tendon function, neuromuscular strength, and two-point discrimination prior to anesthesia. Plain radiography should be routine. Computed tomography or ultrasound may be used to further evaluate for deep foreign bodies. Bleeding and pain must be controlled prior to imaging studies.

Resuscitation may be required, and significant blood loss might necessitate transfusion. However, administration of blood products in the face of a winter-weather emergency should be

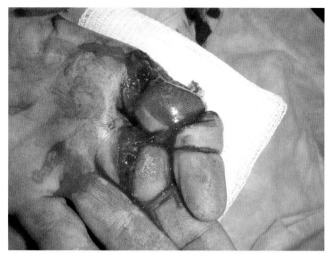

Figure 40.5. Typical snowblower injury. The patient placed his hand into the running auger to remove a chunk of ice with resulting open fractures of index and long fingers. The avascular, denervated index finger was amputated at the metocarpalphalyngeal joint. Photograph courtesy of William H. Dice, MD.

carefully considered, because of the limited ability to replace banked blood. Both regional anesthesia and procedural sedation are useful adjuncts for ED evaluation and management of large complex wounds.

An important prerequisite for complete assessment is a bloodless field. Arterial bleeding can be controlled by ligating small vessels or using a blood-pressure cuff inflated proximally. This tourniquet technique can be applied for up to 2 hours while vascular control is achieved, the wound is explored, and copious irrigation accomplished.

All open injuries from power tools should be considered crushed and contaminated, and thus require thorough cleaning to remove gross debris and reduce bacterial load. Clean tap water is an acceptable alternate to saline for irrigation of wounds. Debridement of devitalized tissue is important.

Every patient with a wound is susceptible to tetanus, even though there are few reported cases in developed nations. Public health authorities recommend a tetanus toxoid booster when there is evidence of a complete initial vaccination series and the last booster was over 5 years prior to any tetanus-prone wound. In the absence of the primary immunizations, tetanus immune globulin plus tetanus toxoid is recommended.

The use of antibiotics by any route in the management of simple wounds offers no clear advantage or disadvantage in preventing infection. In the face of a winter-storm disaster, physicians should consider the potentially limited availability of community pharmacies, and ability of patients to return for any complications when recommending antibiotics or other medications. Use of antibiotics for uninfected simple wounds is a questionable practice, and is generally not supported in the medical literature. However, management guidelines for wounds that involve tendon, bone, nerves, or large vessels generally include antibiotics.

Since a winter storm might delay presentation of patients with complex wounds and availability of consultants may be limited, emergency physicians should consider delayed primary closure, especially for injuries more than 6 hours old. If not prevented from restrictions on travel or limitations in personal resources, the patient could return for daily dressing changes

prior to definitive debridement and closure in 3–5 days. Nonoperative ED management of fingertip amputations is accepted practice, although telephone consultation with a hand specialist is advised prior to repair.

In addition to traumatic injuries, the winter environment is further associated with cold injuries and hypothermia in exposed individuals representing a wide range of demographics.[55,56] Power failures after winter storms lead to use of alternate power and heat sources that are associated with CO poisoning.[27] These three entities can lead to death or permanent disability, but may be clinically occult and missed as a primary or complicating condition, if not actively sought.

Freezing (e.g., frostbite) and nonfreezing (e.g., trench foot and immersion foot) cold injuries should be anticipated following winter storms. The risk for cold injury is markedly higher in both African-American men and women than in whites of either sex. Additional risk factors include alcohol or drug use, psychiatric disease, motor vehicle trauma, and motor vehicle failure. Patients with prior cold injury appear to be more susceptible to recurrence.[56] All of these cold injuries can be permanently debilitating.

Symptoms and signs of cold injury are based on the changes associated with tissue ischemia and the freezing process. Vasoconstriction reduces blood flow when skin temperature falls below 15°C (59°F). Other skin changes occur when extracellular ice crystals form at temperatures below 0°C (32°F). Intravascular sludging occurs, endothelial leakage begins, and edema develops.[55]

Nonfreezing injuries are managed in manners similar to those already discussed for the out-of-hospital setting. Freezing injuries are definitively managed by active rewarming without massage. A practical, four-step approach is required to efficiently care for the frozen tissue: 1) stop ongoing insults by removing any constricting or wet clothing, and gently drying the involved area; 2) examine affected skin areas for signs of ischemia, change in texture (e.g., waxy, inflexible, solid), presence of blisters, and loss of sensation; 3) rapidly rewarm affected parts until all skin out to the most distal portions appears perfused and pliable; and 4) protect the rewarmed tissue from evaporative cooling and direct pressure with loosely applied dry dressings and padding.

Frostbite is treated in the ED with rewarming, hydration, wound care, and pain control. Rapid rewarming is the immediate objective once frostbite is discovered. Dry external heat is not appropriate for frostbite. Rewarming should take place in a water bath at 40–42°C (104–107°F), usually for 15–30 minutes until signs of skin reperfusion are evident (i.e., red or purple color and pliable texture). Systemic fluid resuscitation is usually not required, as it is in thermal burns. Once the part is rewarmed it should be elevated, splinted, and the toes and fingers separated with cotton. Rewarming is painful, so systemic analgesic medications are usually required. Debridement of the blisters that form after rewarming is controversial, and is generally not performed in the ED.

Use of thrombolytic agents showed some promise in reducing tissue loss when given within 24 hours of rewarming.[70] However, later practice excluded the routine use of these medications for frostbite. Other attempts to use agents to enhance blood flow into and through thawed tissue have not been successful in clinical studies. Heparin, dextran, intra-arterial reserpine, hyperbaric oxygen, and surgical sympathectomy have been used in frostbite treatment without dramatic changes in tissue salvage.

Frostbite is categorized as deep or superficial. Some clinicians use a grading system of 1–4. Classification is made after rewarming. Favorable prognostic signs in superficial frostbite include sensation to pinprick, blisters containing clear fluid, and normal skin color. Poor prognostic signs in deep frostbite include non-deforming hard skin, loss of sensation, blisters filled with dark or bloody fluid, and non-blanching cyanotic skin color.[55]

It is difficult to define the full extent of cold injury and provide a prognosis for tissue loss at initial presentation. Best practices usually include a "wait and see" approach to amputation that can be quite prolonged since mummification can take up to 3 months. Researchers have studied the value of magnetic resonance imaging and magnetic resonance angiography in predicting tissue viability with limited success.[71] Technetium (^{99m}Tc) scanning has also been investigated to identify tissue that will require amputation.[72] One study of severely frostbitten hand injuries in France suggested that ^{99m}Tc scanning in the first few days after rewarming predicts the level of amputation for 84% of cases.[73] However, other studies suggest that ^{99m}Tc images do not accurately identify eventual levels of gangrene.[71] Generally, surgeons are reluctant to decide on an amputation level until complete demarcation several months later.

Patients discharged from the ED can experience long-term symptoms from their cold injuries. Nonfreezing trench foot can result in muscle atrophy and contractures. Deep frostbite is associated with cold sensitivity, increased sweating, pain, hypersensitivity, and skin color change. Superficial frostbite can lead to persistent cold sensitivity, numbness, and loss of sensation. Many cold injuries can result in chronic occupational impairment.

The incidence of accidental hypothermia is a public health issue year-round, especially as regards socially disadvantaged persons. These groups are at risk for being disproportionately affected by winter storms or unusually cold environments, while others may be displaced from their residences by power failures or structural damage. Hypothermia can masquerade as other illnesses, especially in people with other risk factors for altered mental status, syncope, and dysrhythmias. Hypothermia can be overlooked in patients who are homeless, use alcohol or drugs, or have chronic conditions like diabetes, hypothyroidism, and psychiatric illness.[74] It can also present in trauma victims, who have more clinically apparent conditions. Triage procedures should include core temperature measurement during cold-weather disasters, which might require use of hypothermia thermometers.

Hypothermia can be a result of infection or a precipitant of infection. In either case, hypothermia associated with infection is associated with higher mortality. Patients with slow rewarming rates (<0.7°C [1.2°F] per hour) and low serum albumin should be carefully assessed for infection and these signs are predictive of outcomes. Hypotension, slow rewarming rates, and bradycardia might be predictors of death during or soon after rewarming.[75] Sepsis should be included in the differential diagnosis for patients with all degrees of hypothermia.

Victims of trauma, particularly vehicle crashes, are at risk for hypothermia as a result of delays in discovery, access, extrication, or evacuation. Trauma patients with a core temperature less than 34°C (90°F) might have increased mortality. Hypothermia is associated with electrolyte abnormalities, acid-base disturbances, coagulopathy, and thrombocytopenia. Hypothermic coagulopathy appears to be similar to disseminated intravascular coagulation, and might require management with plasma, clotting factors, and platelets. Partial thromboplastin and prothrombin times should be measured early in the evaluation of hypothermic trauma patients. Thromboelastography (testing the efficiency of blood coagulation) may also be useful in some patients.

Complete blood count, basic metabolic profile, and arterial blood-gas analysis may be helpful in assessing hypothermic patients. Temperature correction of blood-gas results is not necessary during initial management. Severe hypothermia can be associated with lower cardiac output from loss of plasma volume, which decreases in hypothermic patients. The loss of intravascular fluid can potentially decrease renal blood flow by 50%, which may result in acute renal failure. In the absence of significant electrocardiographic changes, correction of low potassium is generally not required, because warming usually reverses the abnormality.

Endotracheal intubation and mechanical ventilation are necessary for patients with respiratory failure or cardiac arrest. Traditional rapid-sequence induction drugs are acceptable for hypothermic patients. However, care is needed to minimize airway and cardiac stimulation, because of the risk of ventricular fibrillation. Life-threatening arrhythmias associated with hypothermia are notoriously difficult to manage.[57]

Preventing additional heat loss through wet clothing and skin and exposure to ambient air is the first step in the ED management of hypothermia, but core rewarming is the focus of reversing its untoward effects. Passive and active external rewarming techniques are recommended for mild hypothermia, when core temperatures are greater than 32°C (93°F). Covering the patient with blankets accomplishes rewarming by containing and reflecting heat generated by the patient's own metabolism. Active external rewarming can supplement this approach by using radiant warmers or heated air. These techniques can raise body temperature 0.5–0.8°C (0.9–1.8°F) per hour.[52]

Although core temperature "afterdrop" is an anecdotal observation when active external rewarming is used on patients with lower core temperatures, the clinical significance of central temperature, electrolyte, and pH changes – reported when the periphery warms faster than the core – remains elusive. Nonetheless, moderate and severe hypothermia requires more aggressive management using active core-rewarming methods, mostly determined by physician expertise and hospital capabilities.

Active internal rewarming by aerosol inhalation of warm humidified oxygen, gastric lavage, bladder lavage, and warm enemas may be appropriate for moderate hypothermia, but are mostly ineffective for victims with severely depressed core temperatures. Thoracic or peritoneal lavage or both are alternate therapeutic options in the ED. In either technique, two intracavitary tubes are placed into one or both pleural spaces or the peritoneal cavity under aseptic conditions. Sterile water or crystalloid fluid warmed to 40–42°C (104–107°F) is allowed to circulate from one tube to the other and drain by gravity.

Indicators of irreversible hypothermic cardiac arrest include serum concentrations of potassium greater than 10 mmol/L or fibrinogen less than 50 mg/dL.[74] When potentially reversible cardiac arrest complicates hypothermia, cardiopulmonary bypass (CPB) is the treatment of choice when available.[57] The warming rate for CPB is 1–2°C (1.8–3.6°F) every 3–5 minutes. Use of a mechanical chest compression device might be useful when the availability of CPB is delayed.[76] Other indications for CPB are solidly frozen extremities, rhabdomyolysis, or failure of other rewarming techniques.[74] An alternate to CPB is hemodialysis, which achieves similar rewarming rates, and offers some advantage when electrolyte abnormalities, metabolic acidosis, or renal failure complicate hypothermia.[77] However, most hospitals are not equipped to perform emergency CPB or dialysis.

CO poisoning is another hazard that can be confused with nonspecific viral syndromes and other common complaints, as it most commonly presents with headache, nausea, and dizziness.[78] People with other medical conditions such as heart or lung disease might be more susceptible to the effects of CO, and present to the ED for treatment of chest pain or shortness of breath.[79] Severe CO poisoning contributes to ischemic myocardial injury, and can double mortality.[80] Depression, dementia, and psychosis have been reported between 2–28 days after CO poisoning.

Pulse oximetry is unreliable when CO is present, because artificially high saturation readings are associated with carboxyhemoglobin. The standard measurement for the presence or absence of CO is blood carboxyhemoglobin concentration. However, carboxyhemoglobin concentration does not reliably predict delayed neurological sequelae such as an inability to concentrate, learning impairment, memory loss, and abnormal motor function.[81]

The treatment for CO poisoning is removal from the source and administration of a high concentration of inspired oxygen. The half-life of CO breathing room air is about 5–6 hours. The half-life decreases to less than 2 hours by maximizing oxygen inspiration via face mask, positive-pressure mask, or ventilator. Employing hyperbaric oxygen therapy further hastens CO elimination.[78] Hyperbaric chambers traditionally used to treat CO poisoning are located at fixed facilities, but success has also been reported with portable chambers.[82]

Generally, hyperbaric oxygen therapy is indicated for any history or persistence of syncope, altered mental status, neurological impairment, or myocardial ischemia, as well as for most pregnant patients.[78] Hyperbaric treatment might also be indicated in patients found to be at higher risk for long-term cognitive impairment (i.e., patients > 36 years old, exposure >24 hours duration, or "higher" carboxyhemoglobin levels).[83] Hyperbaric facilities may be scarce resources that are difficult to access during the aftermath of a winter storm. How long after exposure hyperbaric oxygen therapy is beneficial remains controversial.

In terms of preparedness for epidemics of CO poisoning, one report of an epidemiological spike during a winter storm found that almost four of every five patients arrived between 6:00 PM and 6:00 AM.[26] In this study, the eighty-one patients were distributed over 3 days and thirteen hospitals,[26] so the impact on individual EDs in that urban area was minimal. However, even at a large university medical center in North Carolina, an epidemic of 200 cases in 1 week resulted in the need for hyperbaric oxygen therapy outstripping available chambers in the area.[29] The chamber at Hôpital du Sacre-Cœur de Montréal was used to treat forty-five patients in the first 9 days after the Ice Storm of 1998.[9]

Secondary Triage

Secondary triage to specialty centers can be interrupted by degraded conditions at sending and receiving facilities in the midst of a weather emergency. Interfacility patient transportation in inclement weather or over dangerous roads can be risky. Regional referral centers have been created for services not available at all hospitals – some of which are for victims of major trauma, serious burns, and conditions requiring hyperbaric therapy. Patients initially presenting to hospitals without these services could require any or all of them. In situations when resource needs exceed availability, referral facilities could be overwhelmed.

Scarce specialty resources may be unavailable, therefore contingency plans must be in place for hospitals to temporarily manage patients normally transferred under less constrained circumstances. Increased needs and evacuation delays may require all healthcare professionals to adjust conventional practices. Tertiary care centers should be prepared to increase capacity for those they can receive, and provide enhanced consultative services by telecommunications to facilities unable to transfer patients.

Changes must be made in ED and hospital discharge planning to accommodate lack of resources. Displaced persons may be unable to return home. Healthcare providers must consider whether a patient has a home; will go to a home without power, heat, or communications; or will go to a shelter environment that may limit the patient's ability to self-manage medical conditions. Patients might need to remain at the hospital for longer periods, potentially restricting the number of additional admissions. Moving patients to less crowded facilities may not be possible due to existing road conditions or weather limiting aeromedical transportation. Even when patients can be discharged, home healthcare services (e.g., oxygen, pharmaceuticals, nursing care) or transportation to return for additional services (e.g., chemotherapy, dialysis) may be unavailable. Follow-up clinics may not be open for days or weeks.

Healthcare Facilities

Hospitals can be adversely impacted by winter storms. The most critical systems for hospital operations are:

- physical plant;
- utilities;
- personnel;
- supplies and equipment;
- internal and external communications;
- transportation; and
- supervisory and managerial support.

Power loss can affect lighting, medical equipment, and safety systems. Frozen pipes can block ready access to clean drinking water, water for personal hygiene, and sewage outflow. Hazardous road conditions make it difficult for surge personnel or the next scheduled shift to report for work. Those already on duty at a facility may have to work extended shifts, or additional days, without relief. Supplies may not be able to be replenished; malfunctioning medical equipment may not be able to be repaired.

Information on the effects of winter storms on healthcare facilities is available in articles on medical care, but healthcare systems studies are more limited. Reports from those that have chosen to share their experiences are typically anecdotal, but may still be illustrative of potential problems others may face in the future.

A November 1996 U.S. ice storm in Washington State interrupted power to up to a third of its population and a number of hospitals. One trauma center required six diesel generators to maintain operations. If it had not had the ability to switch over to a secondary utility feed, it might have been without electricity for 12 days.[84]

In the aftermath of the Ice Storm of 1998, many Canadian hospitals had to operate on generator power for almost 3 weeks.[9] Even in the absence of a disaster situation, one report identified significant facility power losses on the day of a mid-Autumn heavy snow storm. At one hospital, complete power loss resulted in having to hand-ventilate patients in its intensive care unit for 45 minutes.[17] Facilities should know what equipment does not receive power from emergency generators.[84]

During a 2006 October snow storm in western New York State, power failure at a county water treatment plant threatened the potable water supply to the regional trauma center and children's hospital. Hospitals might not be able to use tap water, and delivery of bottled water can be difficult or impossible over icy roads.[85,86]

Telecommunications may be interrupted for a variety of reasons. This may affect telephones and pager systems. One hospital arranged for emergency delivery of numerous cellular telephones just to communicate within the facility itself.[86]

Public and private transportation may be dangerous, difficult, or impossible; thus, staff absenteeism can be a significant concern in the aftermath of winter storms. Emergency vehicles have been used to help personnel get to work and relieve those on duty at the time of the storm.[17]

Transportation can also be problematic in three other situations: moving victims from the community to hospitals or other healthcare facilities; accomplishing interhospital transfers for specialty care; and discharging patients to home or skilled-nursing facilities. After the Ice Storm of 1998, some hospitals opened additional ward beds for discharged patients who could not return home.[85] Providing home healthcare services was a challenge after an ice storm hit southeastern Oklahoma in December 2000.[86]

Sheltering employees and their families often becomes an additional function of a fixed facility. During the prolonged crisis following the Ice Storm of 1998, Montreal General Hospital set up shelters for employees and their families in unused portions of the facility – while providing free food service and child care – in order to ensure it had enough staff to meet patient needs.[9] Ottawa Civic Hospital opened two oncology floors to house staff for up to 3 weeks.[85] Others have reported similar solutions and use of nearby compassionate-care facilities.[84]

Healthcare facilities have also accommodated displaced persons.[86] One psychiatric hospital in Ontario sheltered many of the neediest people in its community, but then found itself having to care for the medical needs of several elderly borders.[87] Serving as a shelter in addition to managing increased ED or inpatient census may require additional security assets.[85]

In addition to fixed facilities, a variety of temporary facilities might be established by governmental and nongovernmental organizations to mitigate the human impact of severe winter storms. Most of these would be for the purposes of providing shelter from the elements and serving as distribution centers for water and food, although limited first aid services might be available at some. In the context of a community's emergency operations plan, the likelihood of limited ground movement in a storm's aftermath would argue for staffing these facilities and notifying the public of their locations in advance of expected severe weather. The media could then use public service announcements to direct persons in need to the shelters that remain functional after the event.

Temporary shelters can house and care for those who are displaced from their homes due to structural damage, lack of power or water, or inability to resupply food or medications. Community centers, schools, churches, and government buildings are commonly used for sheltering. Some of these buildings may remain connected to a functioning power grid or have emergency generators facilitating the provision of heat, water, and amenities such as microwave ovens and televisions. A priority for road access to shelters must be included in plans for winter storm emergencies.

Mental health is a concern for persons requiring shelter. Loud background noise, lack of privacy, and poor sleep cycles in such conditions lead to mental health issues such as anxiety and depression, substance use, psychosis, suicidal ideation or attempts, and possible long-term sequelae such as post-traumatic stress disorder.

Infectious diseases can be difficult to control in shelters. Bacterial and viral respiratory infections, gastrointestinal disturbances, and other maladies can rapidly spread between persons in close-quarter living conditions. A supply of sanitation items such as anti-bacterial hand wipes, alcohol-based hand sanitizers, and surface disinfectants may reduce the risk.

If a potentially contagious disease is identified, measures should be taken to isolate infected and exposed persons. Curtains or hanging sheets and arranging cots to prevent face-to-face relationships can be used to mitigate transmission risk to some degree. To limit cross-contamination, individuals should be restricted from group events (e.g., meals, social activities, gatherings for announcements). In the presence of gastrointestinal infections, strict sanitation must be enforced at toilet facilities.

Water and food availability, storage, preparation, and distribution are a concern in any sheltering situation. In order to mitigate the potential for large-scale food-borne illnesses, care should be taken to ensure that personnel are adhering to health codes. Prepared food must be kept heated or cooled to proper temperatures during preparation, storage, and service. Winter temperatures might allow food storage under ambient outside conditions.

Pots, pans, and utensils used to cook food need to be thoroughly cleaned. If a shelter is without running water, but water can be delivered, a three-bucket system can be used. Hot, soapy water in the first bucket or barrel is used for washing, then subsequent containers are used for a two-stage rinse. Alternatively, dishes and food preparation equipment can be taken to another location for washing. The use of disposable plates, bowls, and utensils can make it feasible to feed hundreds of people and reduce the need for washing of dishes, but this approach comes with additional logistics issues of supply replenishment and waste disposal. The same would apply to use of already packaged meals.

Rapid Needs Assessments

One or more rapid assessments[88] for identifying deficiencies created by a winter storm and determining potential resources required to respond to a storm's impact are necessary to optimize management. The fundamental difficulty is rapidly gathering reliable and useful data in a timely manner sufficient for response decision-making, particularly when ground and air transportation might be difficult and dangerous. Snowmobile drivers and Nordic skiers may be useful in these situations.

Modified cluster sampling is an epidemiological method advocated by the U.S. Centers for Disease Control and Prevention (CDC) to gauge the impact on communities that have sustained severe property damage that make egress and ingress difficult in the initial aftermath of an event.[89,90] The technique involves sampling thirty randomly selected clusters of land in the affected

Table 40.2. Selected survey questions during modified cluster sampling of households in areas affected by a winter storm. This information is in the public domain. It was modified from CDC at http://www.bt.cdc.gov/masscasualties/research/community.asp on July 14, 2013.

- Not enough water or food
- No home (displaced or difficulty returning)
- No running water
- No electricity
- No heat
- No functioning toilet
- No telephone
- No personal vehicle
- No access to commercial or public transportation
- Unable to obtain needed medications or home health services
- Injuries
- Illnesses (acute or chronic)
- Need for medical care
- Need for counseling
- Special needs (e.g., disabilities, extremes of age, mental health issues, pets)

Assessment teams can also inspect homes and shelters for hazardous conditions. Public service information, education, and limited medical care can also be provided.

area, which are then targeted for assessment teams that conduct personal interviews of persons still present. Table 40.2 lists typical questions. Data are then collected and analyzed to estimate rates, which are then extrapolated to total population numbers based on the known pre-event census. The incident commander can then use this information to allocate response resources and start the recovery process.

This sampling method was used in rural Maine following the Ice Storm of 1998, but severe travel limitations delayed the first on-the-ground survey by 10 days.[91] Nonetheless, the assessment was able to determine that 14% of the affected population remained without electricity, 18% were using gasoline-powered generators, and 68% had their utility power restored in that timeframe. Many had no telephone service, but most had access to public service broadcasts through either radio or television.

Needs assessments can also identify victims with injuries and illnesses, either related or unrelated to the storm. Illnesses may be new, or exacerbations of chronic conditions from either the cold environment or inability to access customary care. Healthcare access – in the forms of EMS availability or capabilities of individuals and families to travel to medical offices, clinics, and hospitals – can also be assessed. Of particular note in CDC's assessment after the Ice Storm of 1998, potentially hazardous sources of CO were identified in many homes without electrical power. Furthermore, only 8% of homes had a working CO detector.[91]

External Response

Major disasters can disrupt or overwhelm local response capacity, necessitating outside assistance to help mitigate the human impact of the event. Regional resources can be staged at the county, province, or state levels – the exact terminology differs between countries. As such, specifics are beyond the scope of this chapter, but any response must be coordinated through an inci-

dent management system capable of coordinating all necessary resources.

When local and regional resources do not have the capacity to significantly mitigate the effects of a PICE, national or international resources may be necessary. In the United States, a federal disaster must be declared by the president after formal requests by the governor(s) of the state(s) affected. With regard to winter storm response, local and state governmental and nongovernmental organizations must be prepared for storms of lesser magnitude. Because of an inherent delay in mobilizing any federal governmental or military response – unless deployed in advance of an approaching storm – local jurisdictions must be prepared to be the only response during the first 3–4 days after an event. In the United States, the second edition of the National Response Framework (as revised in 2013) serves as a guide for responding to all types of emergencies.

Disaster Medical Assistance Teams (DMATs) are essential components of the federal response to a public health disaster. DMATs deployed after major winter storms have provided needed medical care when local doctors' offices, clinics, and pharmacies were closed due to lack of power or inability of staff to travel to their places of employment. DMATs have also supported local hospital staffs, which allowed them to rest, tend to their own families, and address damage to their properties. Some DMAT members have also assisted local nursing home staff in caring for residents, while others assisted in shelter clinics on a rotating basis.

Following the Ice Storm of 1998, a mobile mission was devised. A utility vehicle was stocked with equipment, supplies, and medications for a team composed of a physician, nurse, and paramedic. This mobile clinic traveled daily to each shelter in the area. Several house calls were also made to check on families who remained in their homes. Some were treated in place for pneumonia, viral syndromes, strep throat, and other minor illness and injuries. Many people displaced from their homes and staying in shelters had forgotten to bring or had run out of their regular medications. Small supplies of these medicines or close substitutes were provided by DMAT members until local pharmacies were functional and people could safely travel to pick up prescriptions.[6]

Public Information

The ultimate goal of any public educational effort is to prevent problems before they occur. In the United States, CDC has created standardized messages for a variety of events as part of its Public Health Information Network (PHIN).[92] One purpose of this initiative was "to receive, manage and disseminate alerts, protocols, procedures and other information for public health workers, primary care providers, and public health partners in emergency response."[93]

Medically related information disseminated to the public and to healthcare personnel should be based on evidence where it exists. Areas of focus should be on causes of morbidity and mortality that are associated with winter storms: cold exposure; CO poisoning; and injuries such as MVCs, slips and falls, snow removal, and those associated with recreational activities.

Cold Exposure

A number of factors place people at risk for accidental hypothermia. These include extremes of age (particularly <1 year and ≥60 years), male sex (likely behavioral), ethanol ingestion,

Table 40.3. Internet Resources for Public, Individual, and Group Preparedness

Canada	
Public Health Agency	http://www.phac-aspc.gc.ca/cepr-cmiu/index-eng.php
United Kingdom	
Department of Health	https://www.gov.uk/government/uploads/system/uploads/attachment_data/file/213126/KeepWarmKeepWell.pdf
United States	
American Red Cross	http://www.redcross.org/prepare/disaster/winter-storm
Centers for Disease Control and Prevention	http://www.bt.cdc.gov/disasters/winter
DisasterCenter.com	http://www.disastercenter.com/guide/winter.html
Emergency Management	http://www.fema.gov/what-mitigation/plan-prepare
Health and Human Services	http://www.bt.cdc.gov/disasters/winter/staysafe/hypothermia.asp
National Weather Service	http://www.nws.noaa.gov/om/brochures/wntrstm.htm
Occupational Safety & Health	https://www.osha.gov/SLTC/emergencypreparedness/guides/winterstorms.html
Ready.gov	http://www.ready.gov/publications

Many local and state governments, nongovernmental organizations, and universities also have useful information.

treatment with neuroleptic medications, hypothyroidism, and malnutrition. Two populations that are at particular risk are relatively young participants in outdoor sports and recreational activities who sustain overwhelming cold stress, and "vulnerable populations" exposed to moderate indoor cold stress, most specifically the elderly.[11] In a longitudinal study of forty-seven people over 69 years of age in the UK, a progressive decrease in thermoregulatory capacity was noted.[94] Numerous reports have noted greater morbidity and mortality in the elderly following winter storms.[11,21,55] Similarly, ethanol ingestion is a risk factor for frostbite, because shivering is inhibited and skin vasodilatation impairs physiologic thermoregulation.[95] Few data are available regarding the ability of public information campaigns to reduce the incidence of frostbite and hypothermia. The UK has been conducting a campaign called "Keep Warm – Keep Well" for a number of years, but published research regarding its impact on reducing cold-associated morbidity and mortality is unavailable.

Assuming an intact power supply or other Internet access, public information resources can be found online (Table 40.3). As a back-up, documents can be printed prior to need in preparation for possible power loss. Local organizations could also develop similar educational products for their own public awareness programs, tailored to risks and resources specific to a particular jurisdiction.

Carbon Monoxide Poisoning

As is the case at other times of the year, prevention is the key to mitigating the impact of CO poisoning. Because CO is colorless and has no detectable odor or noxious properties, preventive measures involve a combination of public information campaigns and detector/alarm devices.

Efforts to increase public awareness must consider uneven cultural distributions in epidemiology and receptivity to educational programs. Surrounding the 1993 storm affecting the largest urban population center of the U.S. state of Washington, the vast majority of cases related to indoor cooking with charcoal briquettes were represented by Asian minorities, most of whom did not speak English. In contrast, all CO-intoxication cases caused by gasoline-powered electricity generators were seen in non-Hispanic whites.[26] Newspaper, radio, and television were extensively employed – and one fire department distributed 2,000 leaflets door-to-door – but all warnings were communicated only in English.[25] In Rochester, New York, public education may have contributed to the modest reduction in absolute numbers of CO poisoning cases seen during an ice storm in 2003 as compared to a similar storm in 1991. On the other hand, a concomitant decrease in indoor cooking as a source mechanism was also observed.[96] Others have reported difficulty disseminating information when telecommunications were disrupted by a storm.[8]

CO detectors with an audible alarm have the potential to alert exposed individuals, if appropriately installed and maintained. One study concluded that they might prevent up to half of unintentional deaths.[97] However, the same study also found that 42% of those who were likely asleep at the time of fatal poisoning had alcohol in their system. This proportion was similar for victims whose blood alcohol level was either above or below 100 mg/dL.[97] In a report of unintentional non-fire-related CO poisonings following the December 2002 ice storm in North Carolina, the severity of poisonings in households with functioning alarms was much less than in those without them.[98]

Vehicle Incapacitation

The use of any vehicle carries with it the ever-present risk of mechanical breakdown or inability to negotiate winter terrain. When vehicles are incapacitated in non-inclement weather or when help is readily accessible, this usually causes more frustration and aggravation than illness or injury. However, when driving in an inhospitable and dangerous environment, such as the aftermath of a severe winter storm, or when rescue is delayed by environmental conditions or sheer call volume, immobility could rapidly lead to a high risk for morbidity and mortality.

Once stranded, the occupants involved need to make a determination regarding whether to stay with the vehicle or walk to better shelter. History suggests staying with the vehicle is the best course of action in most circumstances. Travel across terrain can be difficult due to snow and ice, especially with no knowledge of the area. Blowing snow can quickly cause disorientation. Land navigation is a learned skill, for which many motorists and emergency responders have no training. A detailed map or portable global positioning system (GPS) device may help, but individuals may still be at risk due to lack of sufficiently protective clothing. Remaining in a vehicle can retain some heat for a short period and will block any wind that can hasten the onset of cold injury and hypothermia. During any overland trek, a fall could be deadly

Table 40.4. Suggested items for a winter storm survival kit to be carried in motor vehicles for the contingency of being stranded. This information is in the public domain. It was modified from CDC at http://www.bt.cdc.gov/disasters/winter/pdf/extreme-cold-guide.pdf on July 14, 2013

- Blankets or sleeping bags
- Flashlight with extra batteries*
- First aid kit
- Knife
- High-calorie, nonperishable food
- Extra clothing, hat, mittens or gloves, boots
- Large empty can and plastic cover with tissues/paper towels for sanitary purposes
- Smaller metal can and waterproof matches to melt snow for drinking water
- Bag of sand or cat litter for tire traction
- Tire chains
- Shovel
- Windshield scraper and brush
- Tool kit
- Emergency tire-repair equipment (canned compressed air and sealant)
- Tow rope
- Booster cables
- Water container
- Road maps and compass or GPS device
- Signal devices (e.g., flares, light-emitting diode [LED[devices, pylons)
- Cellular telephone with charger or citizens band (CB) radio with extra batteries*
- AM/FM and NOAA radios with extra batteries*

* Lithium batteries have longer life and function better in cold temperatures

if an ankle, knee, back, or head injury is sustained in inclement weather. In addition, unwittingly treading on thin ice over a body of water could lead to immersion injury or drowning.

The chances of being seen and rescued are likely much higher when staying with the vehicle, as passing cars may quickly render aid if the road is frequently traveled. If somebody else who is familiar with their travel plans notes that the stranded individuals are overdue, rescue assets will inevitably be dispatched. Attaching a brightly colored object to the antenna, putting up the hood, activating emergency flashers, and deploying road flares all signal distress. In contrast, a dark, unlit car on the edge of the road is much less likely to be recognized.

Fuel tanks should be kept near-full to avoid ice in the tank and fuel lines, and to maintain sufficient fuel to idle the car 10 minutes each hour for heat if stranded. Care should be taken to prevent the buildup of snow against the exhaust system of a running vehicle, which could cause CO poisoning without warning. NOAA and CDC suggest being prepared by carrying a storm-survival kit when driving during the winter season (Table 40.4). Motorists should not travel alone whenever possible.

Other Injuries

While MVCs are a common cause of injury and death following a winter storm,[4,5,17,21] there are other hazards associated with winter driving. CDC has stated that "officials should consider the following recommendations during blizzards: 1) early

in the storm, warn against non-essential driving; 2) announce publicly that persons who must drive should have extra clothes and food with them and remain in their vehicles if stranded; and 3) advise extreme caution if the heating system is used while the vehicle is stopped (even for short periods) because exhaust systems may become blocked with snow and ventilation adequacy is hard to determine."[99]

Heavy snow can collapse the roofs of buildings not designed for the added weight. Family, friends, and the media often advise homeowners to clean snow from their roofs, but this can be a hazardous undertaking for people who do not have the agility and balance, strength and dexterity, or safety equipment to undertake the task. Official broadcasts should warn the public about the potential dangers of clearing rooftop snow, and offer alternate resources for those who do not feel safe or capable of doing it. Media announcements regarding the cardiovascular risks of shoveling and the safe use of snowblowers and other power equipment might also be considered, but their potential impact on the epidemiology of injuries is unclear. The same is true for warnings about injuries related to winter recreational activities.

Fall prevention is a long-standing part of the research agenda for geriatric medicine. With regard to slippery conditions caused by a winter storm, the elderly are the population at highest risk.[21] Some prevention strategies may have application to other populations as well. Others may need to be developed, but none can be expected to have significant impact on incidences and outcomes without ongoing surveillance programs to better elucidate the epidemiology of winter slips and falls.

Avalanche Mitigation

Reducing the risk of avalanche damage and injury are based on three principle questions. First, what is the frequency of prior avalanches in a particular location? Second, what would be the likely track of an avalanche if the snowpack releases? Finally, are people, buildings, critical infrastructure, and response assets exposed to the avalanche path?

There are four categories of avalanche protective measures available to emergency planners: temporary or permanent control of the likelihood of snowpack release; and temporary or permanent control of human vulnerability to impact.

Avalanche-control activities are familiar to snow skiers, who may have to wait for an area to open while explosives are used to safely trigger avalanches that threaten a resort. Another example of temporary avalanche control is compacting snow at avalanche starting zones. Permanent solutions to control the impact of avalanches involve constructing devices that prevent the snow from releasing at the starting zone, deflecting the snow as it runs down the slope, or slowing the snow as it reaches the runout zone. Protective forests can slow and deflect avalanches, reducing the risk to areas below.

Protecting people from high-risk avalanche paths might require emergency managers to temporarily close roads, evacuate buildings, and provide safe travel routes to responders. In avalanche-prone areas, permanent solutions include relocating buildings, rerouting roads and power lines, and constructing protective shelters. Avalanche detection systems are used primarily by railroads to reduce derailments caused by debris on the tracks. These systems use sensors that include wires that stretch or break, radar, vibration, sound, or photoelectric triggers. When triggered, the sensor sends a signal to activate a siren, warning light, or message sign.[100,101]

RECOMMENDATIONS FOR FURTHER RESEARCH

As with many research questions in public health, it is difficult to measure what is prevented. Particularly in the field of disaster medicine, comparisons can often only be made to baseline rates of morbidity and mortality before a PICE. Evaluating any data between different events, even those caused by the same insult type such as a winter storm, is made extremely difficult by the heterogeneity of multiple characteristics of the incident itself and the region affected. Determining the effectiveness of any change in medical interventions or response tactics, techniques, or procedures often lacks any valid cohort to which new data can be compared. Numbers are often small, especially when trying to identify subsets of populations that might derive the most benefit from any change in standard practices.

Although numerous disaster medicine centers have evolved since the early 1990s, no nationally or internationally coordinated research agenda has been disseminated. The U.S. National EMS Research Agenda[102] made no specific call for outcomes research in disaster medicine, and it has not been updated since its release in 2001. With specific regard to winter storms, no recommendation was made to study the potential occupational safety and health effects of driving in hazardous winter conditions or working in cold environments, better methods for managing cold-induced conditions in the field, or out-of-hospital management of patients for prolonged periods of time.

Most disaster research needs to be multidisciplinary and collaborative, with relationships made and responsibilities delineated before an event. Until more consistent data are collected for more events over a greater period of time, winter storm research will need to focus primarily on population effects, with the goal being to develop better methods of rapidly identifying populations at risk for adverse health impacts caused by difficult outdoor movement, widespread power losses, and limited healthcare access. Specific areas of research should include risk mitigation; system preparedness; out-of-hospital access, care, and evacuation; rapid needs assessments; preventive medicine; and infrastructure recovery.

Risk Mitigation

No known force can stop a winter storm. However, the risks to potentially vulnerable populations can be mitigated. Research should focus on making society less susceptible to disruption. Developing solutions requires a cost-benefit analysis based on sound evidence. For instance, one method for potentially decreasing the incidence of accidental hypothermia and CO poisoning might be to equip every building determined to be at risk with a safe gasoline-powered generator and ample fuel. However, it might be too expensive to supply millions of homes with this emergency capacity in order to save at most a few hundred lives every year. A pre-disaster public education campaign might be more cost-effective. Neither option, nor any of a myriad of other programs in the spectrum of cost versus benefit, should be implemented without quality population-based research in one or more representative geographical regions or vulnerable populations.

One key feature to any pre-event risk-mitigation policy is having quantitative and qualitative data on vulnerable populations updated as often as practicable. Census data are useful, but much more is necessary during a PICE. Are there buildings at higher risk for power loss than others? Which of those have

safe alternate sources? Which households have infants, elderly, or disabled persons? Which have persons requiring home health services like oxygen, antibiotics, chemotherapy, or dialysis that could not be delivered due to hazardous road conditions?

System Preparedness

Protection of the public safety and healthcare infrastructure against physical hazards (e.g., power loss, inaccessibility) and system breakdown (e.g., victims' needs overwhelming resources) should also be researched. How can rescue capacity, EMS response, and hospital capabilities be preserved during and after a major winter storm? How fast can roads be cleared? How well can response vehicles traverse the affected area? Should EMS personnel be more dispersed throughout the community prior to storm arrival? Should hospital staffing be bolstered before some storms to decrease absenteeism and allow for those on duty to maintain more normal work–rest cycles? Emergency management tactics, techniques, and procedures for planning, operations, safety, and overall effectiveness should also be scrutinized through research. It is unclear whether these or any other interventions will improve medical or mental health outcomes after an event. Only proactive research will be able to answer these questions.

Emergency Services

True research into evidence-based best practices for locating, rescuing, and providing out-of-hospital medical response to victims of a winter storm is virtually nonexistent. As such, there are many questions that need to be answered to prevent significant funds from being invested in unproven equipment and technologies.

What balance of weather conditions and population needs make it unsafe to attempt or continue access efforts? What are the best search techniques for victims who cannot call for help? What types of vehicles or vehicle equipment should be used to access victims who request assistance? Which agencies are needed to facilitate access to neighborhoods with ice or snow cover, felled trees, and downed power lines? How can rescue and EMS personnel be best protected when working in cold environments? What are the caloric and fluid requirements of response personnel? Should work–rest cycles be different under cold stress?

In a mass casualty situation, what triage methodologies result in the best outcomes for populations affected by a winter storm? Preventing additional heat loss is most likely beneficial; but should active-external, or even active-internal rewarming be undertaken in the field or in an ambulance? If so, what are the best methods of accomplishing it? What degree of rewarming prior to hospital arrival would improve outcomes? Is the care of a victim of cold-water immersion any different than of one suffering "dry" hypothermia? How does frostbite or hypothermia complicate other medical conditions for which EMS may have been primarily called? Should medic training include the diagnosis and treatment of advanced complications that occur when healthcare access is significantly delayed? Should medics be trained and authorized to manage patients for longer periods of time than usual when evacuation times are limited by weather or road conditions? What balance of conditions and patient medical requirements make it unsafe to attempt evacuation? Which patients should receive care but not be evacuated? Can protocols be used for these decisions or must medical control be consulted by radio or telephone in order to achieve safe dispositions for patients?

What types of vehicles or vehicle equipment should be used to evacuate victims? Is there any benefit to air versus ground versus water evacuation? Are field-expedient nonmedical vehicles safe for some patients? If so, which ones, and who makes the decision what vehicle to use? What is the best destination for a severely hypothermic or frostbitten patient? If it is a tertiary referral center, is there degradation of benefit over time? Should an intervening stop at a less-capable ED be made for immediate care, before secondary triage and transfer to the referral center?

Rapid Needs Assessments

The U.S. CDC has recommendations for community studies in the early aftermath of any event that causes widespread property damage.[90] The first step is to identify neighborhoods or other specific areas that are the most severely affected. This could be accomplished by satellite data, aerial over-flights, or by reports from reliable observers within the distressed area. Once ground access is possible, surveyors collect data (Table 40.2) from members of households, occupants of business and public buildings, and emergency responders to determine the demographics of affected persons and families, their general and mental health plus their medical needs, and their living conditions plus additional resources required. Local and external organizations can then use this information as analyzed by the modified cluster-sampling technique to target subsequent relief efforts. While currently in use, these methods of data collection and analysis need further study to assess their accuracy and utility.

Repeated assessments throughout the response and recovery phases should be used to verify the effectiveness of measures taken. This is frequently neglected, resulting in estimating the impact of the event but not the impact of various aspects of emergency management. Comparing prior community assessments within the same event would have more validity than comparing them to a different historical event. If relief efforts or other interventions are deemed unsuccessful, this could focus inter-event research on new methods or technologies that may be more useful in similar circumstances following a future PICE.

Preventive Medicine

Preventive medicine measures to control injuries and illnesses in the wake of a disaster differ in some respects after a winter storm than they do following other events affecting a wide geographical region and its societal services. Some experts suggest that the best public awareness campaigns are extensions of existing community injury prevention and control measures. However, continuous research efforts in injury epidemiology and clinical management are needed to determine best practices for incidence reduction and improved outcomes. Information on subpopulations with medical and health issues related to winter storms could be collected within larger population-based databases.

Infrastructure Recovery

Although recovery should begin at the same time as the initial response, the latter will dominate early and the former will dominate late in the continuum of the disaster life cycle. Systematic and targeted data collection must be conducted throughout all four phases of emergency management. What worked and what did not, costs and benefits of different approaches, and proposed plans for the next event must be shared with other communities facing similar challenges. As yet, except in limited regional contexts, there is no single, readily-available repository for best practices in response and recovery.

Analysis of recovery data from the last event in a given region, or a critical review of past events in other regions, should produce better preparedness for the next event. Not all PICEs are the same, but similar events cause similar problems from which information can be analyzed, and solutions proposed and tested before they are needed to save lives and protect property and systems.

REFERENCES

1. FEMA. Major disaster declarations, emergency declarations, and fire management assistance declarations. http://www.fema.gov/news/disasters.fema (Accessed June 2, 2013).
2. Smith AB, Katz RW. US billion-dollar weather and climate disasters: data sources, trends, accuracy, and biases. *Natural Hazards* 2013; 67: 387–410.
3. National Climactic Data Center. Billion-dollar weather/climate disasters. NOAA. at http://www.ncdc.noaa.gov/billions/events (Accessed June 2, 2013).
4. Kyrill. Wikipedia. http://en.wikipedia.org/wiki/Kyrill_(storm) (Accessed September 4, 2015).
5. January 2007 North American ice storm. Wikipedia. http://en.wikipedia.org/wiki/North_American_ice_storm_of_2007 (Accessed November 10, 2007).
6. Wightman JM, Fenno JA, Dice WH. Winter storms. In: Koenig KA, Schultz CH, eds. *Koenig & Schultz's Disaster Medicine: Comprehensive Principles and Practices.* 1st ed. Cambridge, Cambridge University Press, 2010; 586–608.
7. North American ice storm of 1998. Wikipedia. http://en.wikipedia.org/wiki/North_American_ice_storm_of_1998 (Accessed November 10, 2007).
8. Riddex L, Dellgar U. The ice storm in eastern Canada 1998: KAMEDO-Report No 74. *Prehosp Disaster Med* 2001; 16: 50–52.
9. Hamilton J. Quebec's Ice Strom '98: "all cards wild, all rules broken" in Quebec's shell-shocked hospitals. *CMAJ* 1998; 158: 520–524.
10. Dixon PG, Brommer DM, Hedquist BC, et al. Heat mortality versus cold mortality: a study of conflicting databases in the United States. *Bull Am Meteorol Soc* 2005; 86: 937–943.
11. Kilbourne EM. Cold environments. In: Gregg MB, ed. *The Public Health Consequences of Disasters.* Atlanta, GA: CDC, 1989; 63–68.
12. Baker-Blocker A. Winter weather and cardiovascular mortality in Minneapolis–St Paul. *Am J Public Health* 1982; 72: 261–265.
13. Gorjanc ML, Flanders WD, VanDerslice J, Malilay J. Effects of temperature and snowfall on mortality in Pennsylvania. *Am J Epidemiol* 1999; 149: 1152–1160.
14. Aylin P, Morris S, Wakefield J, Grossinho A, Jarup L, Elliott P. Temperature, housing, deprivation and their relationship to excess winter mortality in Great Britain, 1986–1996. *Int J Epidemiol* 2001; 30: 1100–1108.
15. Glass RI, O'Hare P, Conrad JL. Health consequences of the snow disaster in Massachusetts, February 6, 1978. *Am J Public Health* 1979; 69: 1047–1049.
16. Faich G, Rose R. Blizzard morbidity and mortality: Rhode Island, 1978. *Am J Public Health* 1979; 69: 1050–1052.

17. Geehr EC, Salluzzo R, Bosco S, Braaten J, Wahl T, Wallenkampf V. Emergency health impact of a severe storm. *Am J Emerg Med* 1989; 7: 598–604.

18. Attia MW. The blizzard of 1996: a pediatric emergency department. *Prehosp Emerg Care* 1998; 2: 285–288.

19. Broder JA, Mehrotra A, Tintinalli J. Injuries from the 2002 North Carolina ice storm, and strategies for prevention. *Injury* 2005; 36: 21–26.

20. Ráliš ZA. Epidemic of fractures during periods of snow and ice. *BMJ* 1981; 282: 603–605.

21. Lewis LM, Lasater LC. Frequency, distribution, and management of injuries due to an ice storm in a large metropolitan area. *South Med J* 1994; 87: 174–178.

22. Smith RW, Nelson DR. Fractures and other injuries from falls after an ice storm. *Am J Emerg Med* 1998; 16: 52–55.

23. Hartling L, Pickett W, Brison RJ. The injury experience observed in two emergency departments in Kingston, Ontario during "Ice Strom '98". *Can J Public Health* 1999; 90: 95–98.

24. Piercefield E, Wendling T, Archer P, Mallonnee S. Winter storm-related injuries in Oklahoma, January 2007. *J Safety Res* 2011; 42: 27–32.

25. CDC. Unintentional carbon monoxide poisoning following a winter storm – Washington, January 1993. *MMWR* 1993; 42: 109–111.

26. Houck PM, Hampson NB. Epidemic carbon monoxide poisoning following a winter storm. *J Emerg Med* 1997; 15: 469–473.

27. Daley WR, Smith A, Paz-Argandona E, Malilay J, McGeehin M. An outbreak of carbon monoxide poisoning after a major ice storm in Maine. *J Emerg Med* 2000; 18: 87–93.

28. Hartling L, Brison RJ, Pickett W. Cluster of unintentional carbon monoxide poisonings presenting to the emergency departments in Kingston, Ontario during "Ice Strom '98." *Can J Public Health* 1998; 89: 388–390.

29. Ghim M, Severance HW. Ice storm-related carbon monoxide poisonings in North Carolina: a reminder. *South Med J* 2004; 97: 1060–1065.

30. Glass RI, Zack MM. Increase in deaths from ischaemic heart disease after blizzards. *Lancet* 1979; 1: 485–487.

31. Spitalnic SJ, Jagminas L, Cox J. An association between snowfall and ED presentation of cardiac arrest. *Am J Emerg Med* 1996; 14: 572–573.

32. Glass RI, Wiesenthal AM, Zack MM, Preston M. Risk factors for myocardial infarction associated with the Chicago snow storm of Jan 13–15, 1979. *JAMA* 1981; 245: 164–165.

33. Anderson TW, Richard C. Cold snaps, snowfall and sudden death from ischemic heart disease. *CMAJ* 1979; 121: 1580–1583.

34. Kunst AE, Groenhof F, Mackenbach JP. The association between two windchill indices and daily mortality variation in the Netherlands. *Am J Public Health* 1994; 84: 1738–1742.

35. Franklin BA, Hogan P, Bonzheim K, Bakalyar D, Terrien E, Gordon S, Timmis GC. Cardiac demands of heavy snow shoveling. *JAMA* 1995; 273: 880–882.

36. Persinger MA, Ballannce SE. Snow fall and heart attacks. *J Psychol* 1993; 127: 243–252.

37. Blindauer KM, Rubin C, Morse DL, McGeehin M. The 1996 New York blizzard: impact on noninjury emergency visits. *Am J Emerg Med* 1999; 17: 23–27.

38. CDC. Hypothermia-related deaths – United States 1999–2002 and 2005. *MMWR* 2006; 55: 282–284.

39. Canadian Red Cross Society. Drownings and Other Water-Related Injuries in Canada: 10 Years of Research. 2006.

40. McIntosh SE, Grissom CK, Olivares CR, Kim HS, Tremper B. Cause of death in avalanche fatalities. *Wilderness Environ Med* 2007; 18: 293–297.

41. Boyd J, Haeheli P, Abu-Laban RB. Patterns of death among avalanche fatalities: a 21 year review. *CMAJ* 2009; 180: 507–512.

42. Wick M, Weiss R, Hohlrieder M, et al. Radiological aspects of injuries of avalanche victims. *Injury* 2009; 40: 93–98.

43. Grosse A, Grosse C, Steinbach L. Imaging findings of avalanche victims. *Skeletal Radiol* 2007; 36: 515–521.

44. Cerruti BJ, Decker SG. The local winter storm scale: a measure of the intrinsic ability of winter storms to disrupt society. *Bull Am Meteorol Soc* 2011; 92: 721–737.

45. McClung DM, Schaerer PA. Characteristics of flowing snow and avalanche impact pressures. *Ann Glaciology* 1985; 6: 9–14.

46. Hohlrieder M, Thaler S, Wuertl W, et al. Rescue missions for totally buried avalanche victims: conclusions from 12 years of experience. *High Alt Med Biol* 2008; 9: 229–233.

47. Radwin MI, Grissom CK. Technological advances in avalanche survival. *Wilderness Environ Med* 2002; 13: 143–152.

48. Boyd J, Brugger H, Shuster M. Prognostic factors in avalanche resuscitation: a systematic review. *Resuscitation* 2010; 81: 645–652.

49. Jurkovich GJ. Environmental cold-induced injury. *Surg Clin North Am* 2007; 87: 247–267.

50. Rustin MH, Newton JA, Smith NP, et al. The treatment of chilblains with nifedipine: the results of a pilot study. *Br J Dermatol* 1989; 120: 267–275.

51. White JC, Scoville WB. Trench foot and immersion foot. *N Engl J Med* 1945; 232: 415–422.

52. Biem J, Classen D, Koehncke N, Dosman J. Out of the cold: management of hypothermia and frostbite. *CMAJ* 2003; 168: 305–311.

53. Urschel JD. Frostbite: predisposing factors and predictors of poor outcome. *J Trauma* 1990; 30: 340–342.

54. Bracker MD. Environmental and thermal injury. *Clin Sports Med* 1992; 11: 419–436.

55. Syme D, ICAR Medical Commission. Position paper: on-site treatment of frostbite for mountaineers. *High Alt Med Biol* 2002; 3: 297–298.

56. Giesbrecht GG. Prehospital treatment of hypothermia. *Wilderness Environ Med* 2001; 12: 24–31.

57. Vanden Hoek TL, Morrison LJ, Schuster M, et al. *Circulation* 2010; 122: S829–S861.

58. Ho JD, Heegaard WG, Brunette DD. Successful transcutaneous pacing in 2 severely hypothermic patients. *Ann Emerg Med* 2007; 49: 678–681.

59. Ducharme M, Steinman A, Giesbrecht G. Pre-hospital management of immersion hypothermia. In: Bierens JJLM, ed. *Handbook on Drowning: Prevention, Rescue, Treatment.* Berlin, Springer-Verlag, 2006; 497–501.

60. Brugger H, Sumann G, Meister R, et al. Hypoxia and hypercapnia during respiration into an artificial air pocket in snow: implications for avalanche survival. *Resuscitation* 2003; 58: 81–88.

61. Brugger H, Durrer B, Elsensohn F, et al. Resuscitation of avalanche victims: evidence-based guidelines of the International Commission for Mountain Emergency Medicine (ICAR MEDCOM) intended for physicians and other advanced life support personnel. *Resuscitation* 2013; 84: 539–546.

62. Lawless J. Aborted air medical missions: a 4-year quality review of a Canadian province-wide air medical program. *Air Med J* 2005; 24: 79–82.

63. Madden JF, O'Conner RE, Evans J. The range of medication storage temperatures in aeromedical emergency medical services. *Prehosp Emerg Care* 1999; 3: 27–30.

64. DuBois WC. Drug storage temperatures in rescue vehicles. *J Emerg Med* 2000; 18: 345–348.

65. Helm M, Castner T, Lampl L. Environmental temperature stress on drugs in prehospital emergency medical service. *Acta Anaesthsiol Scand* 2003; 47: 425–429.

66. Stewart RL, Black GB. Snowmobile trauma: 10 years' experience at Manitoba's tertiary trauma centre. *Can J Surg* 2004; 47: 90–94.

67. Haynes CD, Webb WA, Fenno CR. Chain saw injuries: review of 330 cases. *J Trauma* 1980; 20: 772–776.

68. Istre GR, Tinnell C, Ouimette D, Gunn RA, Shillam P, Smith GS, Hopkins R. Surveillance for injuries: cluster of finger amputations from snowblowers. *Public Health Rep* 1989; 104: 155–157.

69. Proano L, Partridge R. Descriptive epidemiology of a cluster of hand injuries from snowblowers. *J Emerg Med* 2002; 22: 341–344.

70. Bruen KJ, Ballard JR, Morris SE, Cochran A, Edelman LS, Saffle, JR. Reduction of the incidence of amputation in frostbite injury with thrombolytic therapy. *Arch Surg* 2007; 142: 546–551, discussion 551–553.

71. Barker JR, Haws MJ, Brown RE, Kucan JO, Moore WD. Magnetic resonance imaging of severe frostbite injuries. *Ann Plast Surg* 1997; 38: 275–279.

72. Cauchy E, Chetaille E, Lefevre M, Kerelou E, Marsigny B. The role of bone scanning in severe frostbite of the extremities: a retrospective study of 88 cases. *Eur J Nucl Med* 2000; 27: 497–502.

73. Cauchy E, Marsigny B, Allamel G, Verhellen R, Chetaille E. The value of Technetium 99 scintigraphy in the prognosis of amputation in severe frostbite injuries of the extremities: a retrospective study of 92 severe frostbite injuries. *J Hand Surg [Am]* 2000; 25: 969–978.

74. Ulrich AS, Rathlev NK. Hypothermia and localized cold injuries. *Emerg Med Clin N Am* 2004; 22: 281–298.

75. Delaney KA, Vassallo SU, Larkin GL, Goldfrank LR. Rewarming rates in urban patients with hypothermia: prediction of underlying infection. *Acad Emerg Med* 2006; 13: 913–921.

76. Wik L, Kiil S. Use of an automatic mechanical chest compression device (LUCAS) as a bridge to establishing cardiopulmonary bypass for a patient with hypothermic cardiac arrest. *Resuscitation* 2005; 66: 391–394.

77. Hernandez E, Praga M, Alcazar JM, Morales JM, Montejo JC, Jimenez MJ, Rodicio JL. Hemodialysis for treatment of accidental hypothermia. *Nephron* 1993; 63: 214–216.

78. Weaver LK. Carbon monoxide. In: Dart RC, Caravati EM, McGuigan MA, et al., eds. *Medical Toxicology*. 3rd ed. Philadelphia, PA, Lippincott Williams & Wilkins, 2004; 1146–1154.

79. Henry CR, Satran D, Lindgren B, Adkinson C, Nicholson CI, Henry TD. Myocardial injury and long-term mortality following moderate to severe carbon monoxide poisoning. *JAMA* 2006; 295: 398–402.

80. Satran D, Henry CR, Adkinson C, Nicholson CI, Bracha Y, Henry TD. Cardiovascular manifestations of moderate to severe carbon monoxide poisoning. *J Am Coll Cardiol* 2005; 45: 1513–1516.

81. Raub JA, Benignus VA. Carbon monoxide and the nervous system. *Neurosci Biobehav Rev* 2002; 26: 925–940.

82. Lueken RJ, Heffner AC, Parks PD. Treatment of severe carbon monoxide poisoning using a portable hyperbaric oxygen chamber. *Ann Emerg Med* 2006; 48: 319–322.

83. Weaver LK, Valentine KJ, Hopkins RO. Carbon monoxide poisoning: risk factors for cognitive sequelae and the role of hyperbaric oxygen. *Am J Respir Crit Care Med* 2007; 176: 491–497.

84. Dealing with power failure: how Spokane hospitals survived the ice storm. *Hosp Secur Saf Manage* 1997; 17: 3–4.

85. The ice storm of the century: how affected hospitals and communities dealt with the challenges of a unique, prolonged emergency. *Hosp Secur Saf Manage* 1998; 18: 5–9.

86. The Oklahoma ice storm: a Y2K disaster that arrived one year later – how two rural hospitals coped and what they learned. *Hosp Secur Saf Manage* 2001; 22: 5–8.

87. Hunter DG, MacDonald D, Peever L. Ice storm: a crisis management diary. *Hosp Q* 1998; 1: 69–73.

88. Malilay J. Public health assessments in disaster settings: recommendations for a multidisciplinary approach. *Prehosp Disaster Med* 2000; 15: 167–172.

89. Malilay J, Flanders WD, Brogan D. A modified cluster-sampling method for post-disaster rapid assessment of needs. *Bull World Health Organ* 1996; 74: 399–405.

90. CDC. Rapid community needs assessment using modified cluster sampling methods. Centers for Disease Control and Prevention. http://www.bt.cdc.gov/masscasualties/research/community.asp (Accessed June 23, 2013).

91. CDC. Community needs assessment and morbidity surveillance following an ice storm – Maine, January 1998. *MMWR* 1998; 47(17): 351–354.

92. Public Health Information Network. CDC. Last updated June 10, 2007. http://www.cdc.gov/phin (Accessed June 23, 2013).

93. CDC. IT Functions and Specifications (also known as the Public Health Information Network Functions and Specifications). Version 1.2. December 18, 2002. http://www.bt.cdc.gov/planning/continuationguidance/docs/appendix-4.doc (Accessed November 10, 2007).

94. Collins KJ, Dore C, Exton-Smith AN, Fox RH, Macdonald IC, Woodward PM. Accidental hypothermia and impaired temperature homoeostasis in the elderly. *BMJ* 1977; 1(6057): 353–356.

95. Freund BJ. Alcohol ingestion and temperature regulation during cold exposure. *J Wilderness Med* 1994; 5: 88–98.

96. Lin G, Conners GP. Does public education reduce ice storm-related carbon monoxide exposure? *J Emerg Med* 2005; 29: 417–420.

97. Yoon SS, Macdonald SC, Parrish RG. Deaths from unintentional carbon monoxide poisoning and potential for prevention with carbon monoxide detectors. *JAMA* 1998; 279: 685–687.

98. CDC. Use of carbon monoxide alarms to prevent poisonings during a power outage – North Carolina, December 2002. *MMWR* 2004; 53: 189–192.

99. CDC. Public health impact of a snow disaster. *MMWR* 1982; 31: 695–696.

100. Fuches S, Brundl M. Damage potential and losses resulting from snow avalanches in settlements of the Canton of Grisons, Switzerland. *Natural Hazards* 2005; 34: 53–69.

101. McClung D, Schaefer P. *The Avalanche Handbook*. 3rd ed. Seattle, WA, The Mountaineers, Inc., 2006.

102. National Highway Traffic Safety Administration et al. *National EMS Research Agenda*. Washington, DC, DOT and HHS, 2001.

41

EXTREME HEAT EVENTS

Carl Adrianopoli and Irving Jacoby

OVERVIEW

This chapter addresses the medical and public health implications of extreme heat events (EHEs) and the associated mortality and morbidity. EHE conditions can be defined by summertime weather that is substantially hotter and/or more humid than average for a location during a comparable time period. History is filled with the failures of great civilizations caused by significant climate changes reacting with human adaptations. Examples include the collapse of the north African "Bread basket" for ancient Rome, the wind-swept droughts in Oklahoma's "Dust bowl" during the 1930s, the vast European droughts in the Middle Ages, and the severe 1921 drought in extensive areas of the former Soviet Union that resulted in millions of deaths.[1] Even the genocide in the Darfur region of west Sudan has a weather-related component. The ongoing drought has pit herders against farmers, with the added elements of race and religion exacerbating the situation.

There have been more than twenty EHEs that have killed hundreds or even thousands of people across the world since 1901, including the deadly 2003 EHE in Europe that killed more than 35,000 people, with 15,000 dead in France alone.[2,3] In the United States, up to 800 died of EHEs in Chicago and Milwaukee in 1995. Additional thousands have died in Philadelphia, St. Louis, Kansas City, and other major U.S. cities since the early 1990s. In New York City during the period from 2000 to 2011, an annual average of 447 residents were treated and released from an emergency department (ED) for heat illness, another 152 were hospitalized, and another 13 died. Seventy of the 154 total deaths in that period were as a result of two severe heat waves in 2006 and 2011.[4] EHEs in U.S. mid-Atlantic and midwest cities can be accompanied by glaring sun with no cloud cover, temperatures in the 35–40°C range, and heat indexes (temperature and humidity) from 43–51°C or more. This results in crowded hospital EDs on diversion and media stories of the elderly found dead in tightly shut, overheated urban apartments.

EHEs are not determined by the absolute temperature alone, but are dependent on other conditions specific to each location. An EHE in sub-Saharan Africa in June, for example, will be much hotter in absolute temperature than an EHE in Minneapolis-St. Paul in a comparable period. In addition to overall temperatures, other environmental factors such as humidity, air circulation, building type, and nighttime temperatures can intensify the health effects of EHEs.

Health personnel are concerned with EHEs because rising temperatures result in increasing heat-related mortality and morbidity. Global warming and climate change will intensify this phenomenon. Thermal trends between 1901 and 2010 show an upward movement in both land and ocean temperatures (Figure 41.1). Unless scientists determine a way to alter the weather, the best approach for protecting people around the globe will be to improve weather prediction and strengthen public health and medical system management of EHEs. Most serious health effects of EHEs can be effectively prevented or addressed by providing timely warning to vulnerable populations, access to air conditioning, adequate potable water (in the developing world), and shelter from the sun. As will be discussed, these simple solutions can be hindered by complex physiological, environmental, medical system, and even political and sociocultural restrictions.

Increasing global warming, urbanization, and population numbers require improvement in effective EHE management. This is true not only across the developed world, but more significantly in the sprawling cites and barren rural areas of the developing world. The fact that there are more than 1 billion people living without access to potable water complicates other EHE-related effects.[5] There is little likelihood of technological and engineering solutions to global warming in the near future. The political will to address global warming by strong and effective restrictions and planning programs (e.g., fuel-efficient automobiles, less burning of high-carbon fuels such as coal and wood, carbon taxes/exchange programs, and strong land-use regulations) has been variable. Until better mitigation strategies are in place to prevent EHEs, local and national governments need to address growing heat-related morbidity and mortality with effective mitigation, preparedness, response, and recovery measures.

Annual deaths from EHEs typically exceed those from hurricanes, lightning, tornadoes, floods, and earthquakes combined.

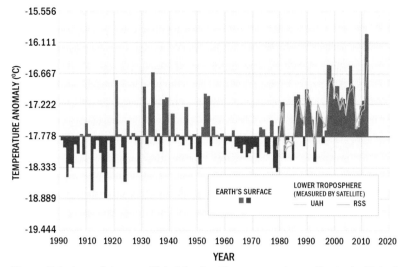

Figure 41.1. Annual Average Global Surface Temperature Anomalies in the United States, 1901–2010. *Source:* Environmental Protection Agency, http://www.epa.gov/climatechange/science/recenttc.html. Reviewed/modified by Tom Javorcic, 2013.

During the period from 1979 to 1999, there were 8,015 heat-related deaths recorded.[6] Despite the fact that EHE deaths often exceed those from all other weather-related sources,[7] EHEs have rarely been addressed as serious weather events with high mortality.[8] More recently, EHEs affecting vast parts of the world for weeks at a time appear to be altering this longstanding misperception. Figure 41.2 compares fatalities from EHEs documented by death certificates to fatalities from other weather-related disasters over a 29-year period.

Mortality documented by death certificates frequently underestimates actual heat-related deaths occurring during an EHE.

Accurate calculation of the number of individuals who have died of temperature-related causes during an EHE is difficult. A traditional method has been to estimate "excess mortality," defined as the difference between the number of deaths observed and the number expected, based on the crude death rates for the same geographical area, during the same period when no heat wave or other unusual circumstances were present.[9] Substantial inconsistencies often exist between the "excess deaths" that are calculated for the period of an EHE and the exact number of deaths that have been certified as heat-related by a medical examiner or a coroner. In U.S. and European examples, the average annual

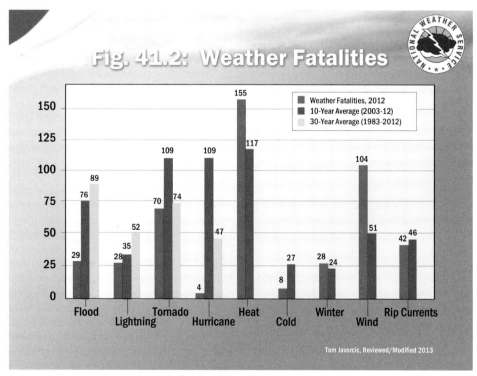

Figure 41.2. Weather Fatalities. *Source:* NOAA, Summer 2010.

rate of heat-related deaths increased during EHEs in each age group, except for children aged 14 years and younger. This was particularly true for persons 75 years and older. Because other causes of death (e.g., cardiovascular and respiratory diseases) also increase during heat waves, heat-related deaths due directly to weather conditions represent only a portion of heat-related mortality.[10–12]

In 1980, when U.S. summer temperatures reached all-time high levels until that date, there were 5,000 deaths above the expected number, with more than the 1,700 cases documented as having been caused by heat.[9] In contrast to violent weather events, an EHE is a "silent killer" that is dramatically less apparent than other hazards, especially at the outset.[7] There are credible estimates as high as 160,000 deaths annually across the world from EHEs and other weather disasters, with most of these deaths occurring in developing nations.[12,13]

Even advanced nations are not immune to what might otherwise appear to be a problem of teeming urban areas in poorer countries that lack adequate supplies of potable water, decent shelter for their populations, and a clear recognition of the dangers posed by EHEs. Kalkstein, using data from his study of forty-four large American cities, estimates that 1,840 excess deaths occur annually due to the presence of high-risk air masses during a "present-day typical summer."[14] This estimate is consistent with studies demonstrating that only a portion of the increase in mortality during EHEs is documented on death certificates.[9,15,16] Previous studies have estimated that the combined EHE-attributable summertime mortality (excess deaths) for several vulnerable U.S. metropolitan areas is well above 1,000 deaths per year.[17,18,19] The U.S. Centers for Disease Control and Prevention (CDC) found that heat-related deaths have been underestimated by 22–100%.[9,10,20] Similar research on EHE-attributable mortality confirmed this finding in rural areas.[21] The fact that many victims of heat stroke die later from organ failure may result in incomplete detection of the true health burden of an EHE.

Public awareness of potentially deadly EHEs has generally lagged behind reality. In Europe, for example, despite cataclysmic, heat-related death tolls in recent years, the Europeans have had a difficult time in changing their basically benign, "friendly to people" view of the summer's heat.[22] Global warming/climate change data may modify these perceptions.

Global warming/climate change is likely to result in progressively more serious and frequent EHEs across the developed and developing world.[23] Urban populations in non-industrialized countries continue to be particularly vulnerable to the direct effects of climate change.[24] The world political community has generally accepted the human involvement paradigm that the burning of carbon-based fossil fuels to a great degree causes global warming.[25] At the 2005 United Nations (UN) Summit on Global Warming, Janez Drnovšek in a succinct and prescient statement called for integrated worldwide planning, a search for solutions, and the raising of politicians' and the public's consciousness.[26] Worldwide efforts to mitigate the effects of EHEs in developing nations generally have been neither extensive nor successful. The 2013 International Climate Change Panel reported, "Warming of the climate system is unequivocal, and since the 1950s, many of the observed changes are unprecedented over decades to millennia. The atmosphere and ocean have warmed, the amounts of snow and ice have diminished, seal levels have risen, and the concentrations of greenhouse gases have increased."

CURRENT STATE OF THE ART

Health Risk Factors from Extreme Heat Events

Physics, Physiological, and Meteorological Effects of Heat Exposure

Increasing heat and humidity affect the body's ability to maintain its homeostatic balance, but similar heat indexes (temperatures and humidity) will affect individuals differently based on personal, geographical, sheltering, and other aspects of the mini-climates in which they live. The temperature of the air, its humidity and motion, and the amount of radiant heat energy to which an individual is exposed are the most important factors in human heat stress. Of these, air temperature can have the greatest impact.[27] Although there may be intense temperature fluctuations on the outer surfaces and extremities of the human body, thermal homeostatic mechanisms attempt to maintain a relatively stable core temperature. There are four aspects to this homeostatic process: 1) metabolic heat gain; 2) heat loss from perspiration/evaporation; 3) conductive and invective heat loss or gain; and 4) the effects of radiant energy.[9] When air temperature is low, heat generated metabolically is more easily lost from the body to the air. As air temperature increases, convective heat loss is no longer possible, and heat can be gained from the air. High humidity limits the cooling effects of perspiration evaporation.[9]

The interpretation of any heat index value will be affected by differences in an individual's age, medications, clothing, and body habitus. In addition, these numbers will fluctuate significantly when compared with other values obtained if one could measure the various microclimates to which individuals are exposed.[9] For example, those older than age 52 tend to produce significantly less perspiration than those who are younger.[28] Differences in hydration patterns can complicate the application of general heat indices to individuals or groups. Elderly populations with little shelter from the sun's direct rays, or those shuttered tightly within steaming, unventilated brick buildings in inner-cities will experience drastically different reactions to the heat than middle-class, middle-aged suburban dwellers with air-conditioned homes.

Increasing temperatures, humidity, and direct exposure to the sun can increase the heat stress that individuals experience during EHEs. Heat index tables often assume that temperatures are taken in a shaded area, with little wind. In addition, most heat index tables note that direct sunlight can increase heat index figures by up to approximately 8°C and that exposure to dry winds can further increase health risks by promoting rapid dehydration (Figure 41.3).[29] Ultimately, any meteorological conditions that increase heat indexes will increase heat stress and health risk. All else being equal, the shock effect of the increased heat is greater the earlier in the summer the EHE occurs.[30,31] In a similar fashion, health risks increase with the duration of the EHE, the amount of time spent above minimum temperature thresholds, and the rapidity of the rise in the heat index.[17,32–36] Residents become increasingly acclimated to the heat as the season progresses. It is not absolute temperature, but rather the extent of upward deviation from usual local summer temperatures that seems to be the key variable affecting mortality.[35] As Table 41.1 demonstrates, there is striking similarity across the continents (with the exception of Antarctica) in the array of the highest-ever recorded temperatures.

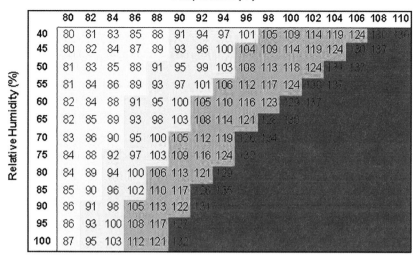

Figure 41.3. Likelihood of Heat Disorders with Prolonged Exposure or Strenuous Activity. *Source:* NOAA, http://www.srh.noaa.gov/ssd/html/heatwv.htm. Reviewed/modified by Tom Javorcic, 2013.

Diagnosis and Treatment of Heat Stress Illnesses

There are several clinical syndromes that comprise heat stress illnesses or conditions: 1) heat cramps; 2) heat edema; 3) heat syncope; 4) heat exhaustion; and 5) heat stroke. They represent variations and overlap in a continuum of heat illness, from minor complaints to overwhelming heat stress that can lead to death.[36]

Heat cramps present as pain and spasm in heavily exercised muscles. Their presentation can vary, from the parade marcher who complains of abdominal pain, to the athlete with cramping in the calves. The mechanism is thought to result from an imbalance in water and sodium intake, leading to hyponatremia, either measurably or locally at the cellular level. Clinically the body temperature is normal, with little evidence of frank dehydration. Measurement of electrolytes may reveal hypokalemia, hyponatremia, respiratory alkalosis, hypomagnesemia, and hypophosphatemia. On the scale of severity, this is usually a benign condi-

tion, treatable with rest, removal from the heat source, and oral or parenteral fluid and electrolyte replacement. Pitfalls that may occur include the attribution of abdominal cramping to heat cramps, when in fact the patient has an alternate diagnosis, such as infectious peritonitis or internal bleeding from a ruptured viscus or hemorrhagic ovarian cyst. Additionally, rhabdomyolysis can occur in the setting of severe exertion or repetitive muscular contraction, leading to myoglobinuric renal failure and life-threatening hyperkalemia with its attendant effects on cardiac conduction. Thus, evaluation in the setting of significant muscle pain should include laboratory studies that can detect these conditions.

Heat edema is a mild condition resulting in swelling of the hands or feet, related to prolonged peripheral vasodilation followed by orthostatic pooling of blood in the extremities. It is usually responsive to elevation of the affected limbs. It must

Table 41.1. Highest Temperature Extremes

Locator #	Continent	Highest Temp (°C)	Place	Elevation(m)	Date
1	Africa	58	El Azizia, Libya	112	13 Sept. 1922
2	North America	57	Death Valley, CA (Greenland Ranch)	−54	10 July 1913
3	Asia	54	Tirat Tsvi, Israel	−220	22 June 1942
4	Australia	53*	Cloncurry, Queensland	190	16 Jan. 1889
5	Europe	50	Seville, Spain	8	4 Aug. 1881
6	South America	49	Rivadavia, Argentina	206	11 Dec. 1905
7	Oceania	42	Tuguegarao, Philippines	22	29 Apr. 1912
8	Antarctica	15	Vanda Station, Scott Coast	15	5 Jan. 1974

* This temperature was measured using the techniques available at the time of recording, which are different from the standard techniques currently used in Australia. The most likely Australian high-temperature record using standard equipment is an observation of 50.7°C recorded at Oodnadatta in 1960.

be differentiated from renal failure, deep vein thrombosis, and congestive heart failure in susceptible populations.

Heat syncope is characterized by sudden loss of consciousness and is also related to peripheral venous blood pooling with subsequent orthostatic hypotension. It occurs with prolonged standing, or rising quickly from a sitting position. Such persons should not be "held up" or supported, but rather gradually lowered to the ground. First aid treatment consists of laying the patient on the ground and lifting the legs up slightly to restore blood flow to the head. Maintaining the patient in an upright position may prolong the period of poor cerebral perfusion. Rehydration should ensue, and an electrocardiogram should be obtained to ensure no heart blocks or other cardiac conduction abnormalities are occurring.

Heat exhaustion occurs in the setting of excess diaphoresis in a hot, humid environment, leading to volume depletion. Core body temperature will be elevated above normal, but typically remains less than 40.5°C, which usually defines the level for heat stroke. Symptoms are profuse sweating, malaise, fatigue, headache, dizziness, nausea, and vomiting. If left untreated, the condition will likely progress to classic heat stroke. Tachycardia and hypotension may be present, but major neurological dysfunction does not occur. Treatment consists of cooling, oral rehydration, or intravenous rehydration in someone who is hypotensive or fails to respond to oral fluid replacement within a few hours.

Heat stroke is the most life-threatening condition related to heat stress. It is defined as an elevated core body temperature usually equal to or greater than 40.5°C in association with significant acute mental status or behavioral changes. Mental status changes can consist of confusion, bizarre behavior, hallucinations, delirium, unresponsiveness, seizures, posturing, or coma. Loss of sweating as a mechanism for body cooling is a late finding. The observation that sweating ceases is found in only 50% of cases, and those patients with exertion-related hyperthermia are more likely to be sweating. Heat stroke is a medical emergency and occurs when heat production exceeds physiological cooling capacity such that heat dissipation no longer occurs. Hyperthermia is characteristically differentiated from fever, in that fever occurs due to an upward adjustment of the temperature set point in the hypothalamus. In hyperthermia, the hypothalamus set point is normal, but the body is unable to eliminate acquired or self-generated heat, leading to excessive body temperature.

With the onset of heat stroke, widespread cellular and organ damage ensues, characterized initially by tachycardia, increased cardiac index, and central venous dilation. Critical deterioration continues, progressing to hypotension, acute renal and hepatic failure, gut ischemia, rhabdomyolysis and cardiovascular collapse. Manifestations include coagulopathy in association with hepatic, renal, and cardiac failure. Hemostatic disturbances are marked by drops in platelet counts and fibrinogen and consumption of clotting factors. Although usually attributed to direct cellular injury by heat, a contribution from inflammation has been proposed in the last decade. Specifically, a role of the systemic inflammatory response syndrome (SIRS) in the development of multi-organ system dysfunction is theorized.[37] Thermal injury to the vascular endothelium[38] activates platelet aggregation, which is irreversible, even following cooling. Excess deposition of fibrin ensues in arterioles and capillaries, which may lead to vascular thrombosis causing occlusion of blood supply in various organ beds. Coagulation often persists until

platelets and coagulation proteins are consumed at a faster rate than they are produced, even after normalization of fibrinolysis following cooling. As coagulation proceeds, platelets and coagulation proteins are consumed, resulting in blood loss from multiple tissue sites, such as gums and venipuncture wounds. High circulating levels of cytokines correlate with morbidity and mortality in heat stroke. Few controlled studies have been performed examining the efficacy of anti-cytokine, anti-endotoxin or anti-coagulation drugs on patient outcome with heat stroke.[37]

Classic heat stroke is described during EHEs, particularly in the elderly. Exertional heat stroke may also occur in young, fit populations such as athletes and military recruits undergoing training. Several high-profile deaths in professional athletes have been reported by the media, demonstrating the importance of prevention when weather conditions increase the risk of such heat stress. In that setting, marked rhabdomyolysis and myoglobinuric renal failure are often observed along with acute hepatic failure and disseminated intravascular coagulation. Mortality ranges from 10–70% in series of heat stroke patients, with higher mortality rates found when treatment is delayed more than 2 hours.[39] Predictors of multi-organ dysfunction include respiratory failure, metabolic acidosis, elevated creatinine phosphokinase, and liver function test elevations greater than twice normal.[40]

Treatment requires rapid cooling to avoid further cellular and organ damage by extreme hyperpyrexia. In the field or on arrival to the ED, ice or cold liquids should be placed in contact with the patient (especially in the axillae and groin), and additional cooling measures instituted as available, while airway, breathing, and circulation are assessed and managed. Airway management may include endotracheal intubation. If severe hyperpyrexia is suspected, use a rapid sequence paralytic agent that does not induce hyperkalemia, i.e., avoid using succinylcholine. Due to altered mental status, an immediate glucose determination is needed to allow rapid diagnosis and treatment of hypoglycemia. Breathing assessment should include oxygen saturation monitoring. Circulatory support includes cardiac monitoring and fluid resuscitation when indicated to support blood pressure, perfusion, and urine output. Caution is necessary when managing the geriatric population that may have antecedent cardiac, pulmonary, and/or renal disease. In addition to ice packing, when fans are available, cooling can be accomplished by spraying the undressed patient with tepid (not cold) water while blowing air from large fans across the body surface to maximize evaporative heat loss. More invasive methods such as ice water lavage of the stomach through a nasogastric tube or the peritoneum through a peritoneal lavage catheter, and even cardiopulmonary bypass have had reported anecdotal success. These aggressive treatments have limited evidence of benefit, however, and may actually be harmful and are therefore not recommended by some experts.[41,42] A newer modality of using intravenous catheters containing cooling coils offers an additional treatment option.[43] Frequent monitoring of the core body temperature is essential to avoid overshooting and creation of further problems due to hypothermia. It is not necessary to reduce body temperature to normal, but only to the level thought not to produce cellular injury; a goal of 38.9°C is reasonable. Risks and benefits of each of these techniques have been reviewed.[44]

Recreational drug use may also contribute to heat-related mortality. The number of fatal cocaine overdoses appears to correlate with higher ambient temperatures. In a New York

City study, the mean daily number of cocaine overdose deaths increased by 33% on days with a maximum temperature of 31.1°C or higher, in comparison to days when the mean temperature was below this point.[45] This appears to be related to the fact that both cocaine and heat stress cause significant thermoregulatory instability. Other risk factors for developing heat stroke found in the New York City EHEs were neighborhood poverty, lack of access to working air conditioning, chronic medical and psychiatric conditions, and obesity.[4]

Emergency Medical Services, the ED, and Extreme Heat Events

In nations with well-developed emergency services, prehospital emergency medical services (EMS) and the ED play significant roles during EHEs. The EMS system is the triage and transportation system that initiates patient contact when dispatched, often initiates treatment in the field, and transports patients to EDs. During EHEs, just as the number of patients increases, so too do the requests for ambulances. The average number of ambulance calls increased by 10% on those days considered oppressively hot over the 4-year period from 1999 to 2002 in a study in Toronto, Canada.[46] Data from two EHEs in Adelaide, Australia, in 2008 and 2009 demonstrated a 10% increase in ambulance calls in the first event, and 16% in the second.[47] In the Sydney, NSW, Australia study of the 8-day EHE in 2011, a 10% increase in ambulance calls was noted in the age group <75 years old, while it increased 17% in the age group >75 years old.[48] Augmentation of EMS capabilities may be a reasonable intervention during an EHE.

EDs are the major hospital point of entry for most victims suffering heat-related illnesses and therefore have a large role in preventing escalating morbidity and mortality. EDs should be prepared to manage surges of EHE patients with adequate cooling equipment. Thus, ED managers must ensure sufficient supplies of water spray bottles, cooling packs, fans, cooling catheters, and ice during EHEs. Informational handouts can be printed as part of discharge instructions in advance of such emergencies as well as during the events. This should become part of the general community educational program, much as is done for other types of safety issues. Increased visits to the EDs in affected areas should be expected.

Using a wide variety of measures to predict EHEs is a complex process that can involve a national weather service, local health departments and emergency management agencies, first response EMS agencies, hospitals, medical examiners/coroners' offices, and many other local agencies and community organizations. No matter how effective the ED may be as a heat mortality sentinel, it cannot provide sufficient warning to reduce the impact of these emergencies. Systems designed to predict EHEs in a timely manner should augment rather than substitute for the longer-range prediction times that air mass monitoring systems allow. The EHE has already started by the time patients begin presenting to EDs. Earlier real-time identification of presenting symptoms of patients to the EMS system may identify the onset of an EHE sooner. A study of atmospheric circulation phenomena identified a five-wave pattern of anomalous planetary waves that tended to precede the onset of heat waves by 15 to 20 days. This was not necessarily linked to tropical heating, suggesting that EHEs are predictable beyond the typical weather forecast range of 7 to 10 days.[49] EHEs tend to quickly generate many patients so that, in systems where it is permitted, many EDs implement diversion status. As three Institute of Medicine (IOM) reports delineate, the U.S. emergency medical care system "is woefully inadequate and unprepared for a pandemic, bioterrorist attack, natural disaster or other national crisis."[50] IOM found the U.S. emergency care system to be underfunded, too fragmented to communicate and cooperate effectively across levels and geographical areas, and possessing little surge capacity to manage a disaster. The IOM also found that emergency care staff members are often inadequately trained to respond to large-scale disasters or to care for pediatric patients. While this analysis focused on the United States, findings are likely similar in other countries.

During Chicago's July 1995 EHE, there were 1,072 more hospital admissions than average for comparative weeks, with 838 (35%) more patients aged 65 years and older being admitted than expected. There was also strong anecdotal evidence of increased ED visits. An analysis of excess hospital admissions during the heat wave defines who was admitted and why. The primary reasons for a hospital visit were dehydration, heat stroke, or heat exhaustion. The susceptible population at risk for admission had comorbid cardiovascular illnesses, endocrine disorders, liver and kidney diseases, or nervous system disorders. Within this population, the elderly were disproportionately represented, in large part due to their altered thirst perception and related conditions.[51] On the second day of the EHE, only a few Chicago EDs were on diversion and directing ambulances to other hospitals. By the fourth day, however, eighteen city EDs were diverting patients to other facilities.[7] A study of the 1993 heat wave in Philadelphia found a 26% increase in total mortality and a 98% increase in cardiovascular mortality associated with the EHE. In adjacent counties, the risk for dying of cardiovascular disease rose significantly for people older than 65 years, for both sexes and all races.[52]

During the European heat wave of 2003, heat-related deaths in a Parisian hospital occurred mostly in elderly patients (mean age 84), and 69% were women. Patients who died differed from those who survived.[53] The former were characterized by greater levels of dependency and by a more abnormal initial clinical presentation (such as elevated temperature, lower blood pressure, and altered mental states). They were also more likely to have existing ischemic cardiomyopathies and to be taking psychotropic medications.[53] In London during the same period, 2,091 deaths occurred (17% more than for the same period in earlier years); 23% of the deaths were among those 75 years of age or older.[54] Investigators report similar findings in Australia, where high environmental temperatures are common, although it is rare that these exceptional conditions produce elevated levels of heat-related morbidity and mortality. In four major teaching hospitals in Adelaide, most patients presenting with heat-related conditions (85%) were aged 60 years or older, with 20% from institutional care, and 30% with poor mobility. Peak presentation followed high daily temperatures for 4 consecutive days. Severity was related to existing cognitive impairment, diuretic use, presenting temperature, heart rate, blood pressure, serum sodium, and serum creatinine. The mortality rate was 12%, and 17% required a more dependent level of residential care on discharge.[55] There were comparable findings in a 1999 study in Wisconsin where heat-related illnesses led to twenty-one deaths. Death rates were highest among the elderly; particularly those aged 65–84 years (2.2/100,000). Heat was attributed as the underlying cause of death for twelve of the twenty-one victims. Cardiovascular conditions resulted in another eight deaths and were a contributing cause for an additional seven.[56]

Hospital/ED Surge Capacity and Extreme Heat Events

For years, emergency managers have considered "surge capacity" in their catastrophic planning (see Chapter 3). Although an EHE would likely stress existing healthcare facility resources, it is unlikely that most EHEs would last long enough and generate enough patients to necessitate the use of external surge facilities. A review of surge capacity, however, is helpful to the extent that the strategies similar to those used for external expansion can be used to support and extend services within existing fixed facilities.

U.S. hurricanes in 2004 and 2005 provide an example of the devastating health and medical effects of weather disasters. Hurricanes Katrina and Rita and subsequent flooding caused the same types of damage to many local healthcare facilities as they did to other types of buildings. Many hospitals and federal and state medical support agencies were forced to establish operations in temporary locations such as shuttered retail stores and veterinary hospitals.[57] Freestanding or support/augmentation facilities were also constructed at airports, sports complexes, and adjacent to existing institutions. These surge hospitals addressed the increase in demand for medical care and contained triage, treatment, and sometimes surgical capacities.[57]

Using the United States as an example, federal disaster support to hospitals is only a small part of the national emergency management system. This system is a complex network of public, private, and nonprofit organizations (ranging from the American Red Cross to professional organizations such as the American Hospital Association, local hospital councils, and community groups in the vicinity of hospitals) as well as individual benefactors. It also includes federal, state, and local government agencies, special districts and quasigovernmental bodies, nonprofit service and charitable organizations, ad hoc volunteer groups and individuals, and private sector firms that provide governmental services by contract.[58] Collaboration with this huge array of emergency preparedness agencies and entities in a coordinated and effective manner requires hospital preparedness staff whose perspectives are broader than just the individual hospital's concerns. Planners must also be knowledgeable about the complex and rapidly growing scientific evidence base related to disasters.

Surge planning in U.S. hospitals includes consideration of The Joint Commission requirements for: 1) establishing hospital incident command systems as the chain of command for disasters; 2) all-hazard emergency management plans; 3) mutual aid agreements and processes with other hospitals, systems, and local, state, and federal agencies; 4) coordination with local emergency management agencies; and 5) the requirement to maintain comprehensive documentation on decision making, victim destinations, patient tracking, and reimbursement.[59] Existing rules and waivers under the federal Medicare program can also significantly influence a hospital's ability to manage surge requirements. Other recommendations that address surge planning appear in the publication *Medical Surge Capacity and Capability: A Management System for Integrating Medical and Health Resources during Large-Scale Emergencies.*[60] Those that have the most relevance to EHEs include:

■ Redundancy. Developing redundancy in hospital operations systems to ensure backup capability during an emergency. Backup systems should be evaluated for their vulnerability to hazards, particularly those most likely to affect primary systems.

Table 41.2. External Support for Hospital EDs before/during EHEs (U.S. examples)

■ Longer shifts, intra- and interhospital agreements
■ Mutual aid, provided by state/local agencies, groups, or through the Emergency Medical Assistance Compact (EMAC), administered by the National Emergency Management Association (NEMA)
■ State/local Departments of Public Health assets, such as the Illinois Mobile Emergency Response Team (IMERT), or the Special Operations Response Team (SORT) in North Carolina
■ The National Disaster Medical System
■ The Medical Reserve Corps

■ Testing of backup and support systems. Establishing programs for testing, inspection, and preventive maintenance of backup systems and facility safety features.

The U.S. National Foundation for Trauma Care has made several key recommendations for improving the capacity of trauma centers to provide care to victims of a terrorist event.[61] Those relevant to EHE surge planning include:

■ Fund disaster medical care at cost and develop sustainable funding because existing federal programs (pre- and post-disaster) do not provide sufficient fiscal support.
■ Sustainment (e.g., staff and supplies) for more than 3 days is required.
■ Fund statewide (and multistate) resource monitoring systems.
■ Provide adequate funding to train staff, based on the proximity and the threat of the hazard.
■ Provide aftercare for the chronically ill and displaced persons.
■ Mutual aid agreements and memoranda of understanding (MOUs) must be developed.

Auf der Heide published response strategies for hospitals during disasters. Those that are directly applicable to EHEs are:

■ Establish EMS/hospital radio networks to rapidly collect hospital status information and direct the flow of those casualties who are transported by ambulance. Since a truly interoperable system that is effective, affordable, and easy to use does not currently exist, overall communications redundancy is desirable.
■ Ensure that hospitals/EMS radio systems are established to facilitate early warning to hospitals from responders in the field. A number of sophisticated systems exist that report hospital bed status availability (as a marker of patient care capacity), hospitals on diversion, and other key information.[62]

The Joint Commission found that legal and reimbursement issues are among the most critical, non-patient, care-related challenges that hospitals face when developing surge capacity.[57] During surge conditions, state and federal waivers can protect emergency medical workers. During Hurricane Katrina, for example, the governor of Louisiana waived state licensure restrictions for those practitioners licensed out of state. The Department of Health and Human Services (HHS) afforded liability protection to healthcare workers who volunteered, and waived the Emergency Medical Treatment and Active Labor Act. A number of U.S. laws and agreements (e.g., the Emergency System for Advanced Registration of Volunteer Health Professionals) as well as a proposed hospital-based credentialing system have made it potentially easier to accommodate volunteers who respond to a disaster.

Other U.S. federal and state programs that can provide healthcare staff resources during surge conditions include the National Disaster Medical System, the U.S. Public Health Service Commissioned Corps, and the Medical Reserve Corps. The Emergency Management Assistance Compact, administered by NEMA, can also provide volunteers (Table 41.3). Individuals recruited by this program (31,000 for Hurricanes Katrina and Rita alone) played important roles in the responses to the four hurricanes in 2004 and to Katrina and Rita the following year.[57,63]

Mortality and Morbidity from Heat Exposure

There is a relatively consistent correlation between mortality and increases in heat measured by temperatures, heat index (a measure of temperature and humidity), or by air-mass conditions.[12,14,64-66] Using sophisticated air-mass models, researchers demonstrated a clear relationship between heat-related mortality and EHEs in forty-four major U.S. metropolitan areas.[14] In a study of twenty-eight metropolitan areas within the United States, heat-related deaths during EHEs significantly exceeded the expected totals for time of year and were in substantial agreement with the previous findings.[19] Overall, however, heat-related mortality trends declined between 1964 and 1998, as temperatures and heat stress conditions have risen. This suggests that a relative "desensitization" of the U.S. metropolitan population to weather-related heat stress has occurred. Such desensitization can be attributed to a variety of factors, including improved medical care, increased air conditioning use, better public awareness programs, and both human physiological and urban medical/emergency response systems adaptations. The irony is clear: traditionally hotter metropolitan areas have lower heat-related mortality.

EHEs also increase morbidity. The majority of studies emphasize the most serious incidents that result in ED visits and hospital admissions.[67] Semenza studied 1,072 hospital admissions during the 1995 Chicago EHE and found the majority of excess admissions were due to dehydration, heat stroke, and heat exhaustion among people with existing conditions.[51] Rydman also studied intense heat-related morbidity from the same event through an analysis of ED visits and found that heat-related morbidity was an antecedent of mortality.[68] Knowlton et al.[69] collected data from the 2006 California heat wave showing a substantial rise in morbidity, with dramatic increases across a wide range of morbidities statewide. ED visits far exceeded excess hospitalizations. Heat-related illnesses, electrolyte imbalances, acute renal failure, nephritis and nephrotic syndrome, diabetes and cardiovascular diseases were the main reasons for the increase in ED visits. Heat-related ED visits increased 6-fold statewide, and more than a 10-fold increase was seen in heat-related hospitalizations. Kilbourne searched for the most effective responses to heat-related illnesses and determined that universal access to air conditioning may be the most effective intervention, even with the relatively high costs of providing this service to the poor.[35] More recent studies found that basic behavioral changes and adaptations (e.g., use of air conditioning, adequate hydration, heat emergency plans, warning systems, and illness management

plans) could significantly mitigate heat-related morbidity and mortality.[70]

The most precise definition of mortality related to heat waves is that given by a medical examiner or a coroner in the formal determination of death. After serious EHEs in Philadelphia in 1993, and in Chicago in 1995, the National Association of Medical Examiners recommended the following definition of heat-related death: "a death in which exposure to high ambient temperature either caused the death or significantly contributed to it."[71] The committee also recommended that the diagnosis of heat-related death be based on a history of exposure to high ambient temperature and the reasonable exclusion of other causes of hyperthermia. The diagnosis may be established from the circumstances surrounding the death, investigative reports concerning environmental temperature, or measured antemortem body temperatures at the time of collapse being at least 40.6°C. Under those conditions, the cause of death should be certified as heatstroke or hyperthermia. In cases in which the antemortem body temperature cannot be established, but the environmental temperature at the time of collapse was high, appropriate heat-related diagnosis should be listed as the cause of death or as a significant contributing factor.[71]

Heat stroke survivors have been shown to have significant elevations in their 30-year mortality rates when compared with individuals that never experienced heat stroke. Many heat stroke victims in Europe succumbed to multi-organ failure during the weeks, months, and years following the heat event, despite acute hospital treatment.[72,73]

Demographic and Individual Factors in Heat Exposure

Individuals at highest risk of becoming ill or dying during EHEs are the very young, the elderly (socially isolated, without access to air conditioning, bedridden, and with ischemic heart disease or other chronic conditions), the poor, minorities, and those taking certain medications such as neuroleptics or antiparkinson agents.[9,28,55,66,68,74-79] Behaviors that can result in heat stroke from dehydration and impaired judgment include strenuous exercise or work in hot or humid weather (even by the young and physically fit), alcohol consumption, and the use of some nonprescription drugs (e.g., antihistamines and sleeping pills).[9,80] Cocaine overdose, which is associated with hypertension, tachycardia, coronary vasospasm, arrhythmias, and increased core temperature, was linked with a significant increase in mortality in Marzuk's 1998 study of New York City.[45,78]

Use of cooling centers by individuals was not shown to be significantly protective, probably because so few visited them.[74] Walking down flights of stairs, with the mobility limitations often accompanying older age, and crossing potentially unsafe streets to attend cooling centers are unlikely options for many of the at-risk elderly.[74] European mortality patterns in the August 2003 heat wave mirrored those seen in the United States, with 70% of those dying from heat-related causes being 75 years or older.[81] Accurate demographic estimates and projections of those sickened or dying from heat-related causes are complicated because susceptible groups often remain in the city, creating a bias in predicted excess deaths.[82] Most often, there are more females affected by adverse heat-related conditions than males. This probably reflects the higher proportion of women in the elderly population, their possible higher susceptibility, and their higher rates of living alone (Figure 41.4).[82]

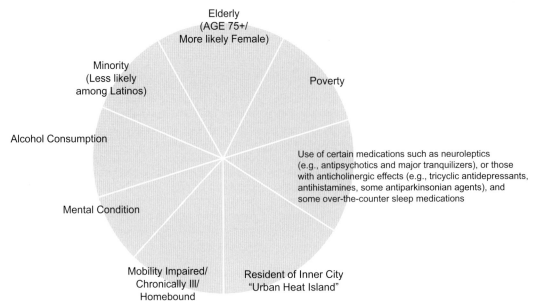

Figure 41.4. The Demographic and Individual Risk Factors of Heat-Related Mortality.

During Chicago's 1995 heat wave, hospital admissions were up 11% for the week of the heat event, with a 35% increase for patients 65 years of age and older. The majority of the excess admissions (59%) represented patients requiring treatments for dehydration, heat stroke, and heat exhaustion. With the exception of acute renal failure, no other primary discharge diagnoses were significantly elevated. In contrast, analysis of comorbid conditions revealed 23% excess admissions for underlying cardiovascular diseases, 30% for diabetes, 52% for renal diseases, and 20% excess admissions related to nervous system disorders. Patient admissions for emphysema and epilepsy were also significantly elevated during the heat event.[51] Other risk factors for developing heat stroke found in the New York City EHEs were neighborhood poverty, lack of access to working air conditioning, chronic medical and psychiatric conditions, and obesity.[4]

Geographical Factors in Heat Exposure

Average summer temperatures appear to have no effect on heat deaths. Kilbourne observed that it is not the absolute temperature value, but rather the extent of upward deviation from the usual summer temperature that seems to influence mortality.[35] For example, in the United States, southwestern cities such as Phoenix, Arizona, have fewer heat-related deaths but have higher average temperatures than midwestern cities such as St. Louis, Missouri, or Chicago, Illinois, which have experienced high mortality from heat waves. Neither excess mortality nor prominent heat-related health effects were noted in Phoenix in July 1980 despite temperatures that averaged 2.4°C above baseline and a highest monthly temperature of 46°C. As expected, based on reports in the international literature, cities that normally have a cool climate (those located in the north) reported the highest excess mortality.[83] Reasons for these differences have not been studied extensively. Possible explanations include differences in population age/acclimatization, architectural style/building materials, and air conditioning use. In 2002, researchers at the University of Delaware reported a list of temperature levels that raise mortality and morbidity in select, large American cities whose populations have been subjected to various degrees of heat stress. These are listed in the emergency response plan of the City of New York (Table 41.3).[85]

There is evidence of a geographical and physiological basis for the lower death rates in urban areas that have higher average temperatures. Kilbourne observed that heat seems to cause fewer health problems in characteristically warm areas than in

Table 41.3. Threshold Heat Temperatures That Result in an Increased Local Mortality Rate

Location	Threshold Temperature (°C)
Atlanta, Georgia	34
Chicago, Illinois	33
Cincinnati, Ohio	33
Dallas, Texas	39
Denver, Colorado	32
Detroit, Michigan	32
Kansas City, Kansas	37
Los Angeles, California	27
Memphis, Tennessee	37
Miami, Florida	32
Minneapolis, Minnesota	34
New York City, New York	33
Philadelphia, Pennsylvania	33
St. Louis, Missouri	36
Salt Lake City, Utah	35
San Francisco, California	29
Seattle, Washington	31

those that are more variable in climate; the temperature level required to increase mortality is actually higher in hotter climates.[14,35,85] DiMaio reported that when individuals live in a temperate zone, many of their nascent sweat glands become permanently inactive during childhood.[86] If, however, the individual lives in the tropics, the glands remain functional throughout life. Other adaptations include reduction in sodium loss from sweat to 3–5 g/day, after 4–6 weeks of acclimatization. A person who sweats profusely may lose as much as 15–30 g/day of sodium chloride until becoming acclimated.

Chestnut demonstrated geographical patterns in heat-related mortality.[87] The highest hot weather–related mortality rates are in northern metropolitan areas of the United States, even though average summer temperatures are higher in southern metropolitan areas. This suggests that biological/behavioral adaptations occur in areas that are consistently hot, but not where minimum daily temperature variability is great. The availability of air conditioning, standards of living, and housing quality contribute to differences in mortality, but these explain a much smaller share of the fatalities than does variability in minimum daily temperatures.[87] Kalkstein found that consecutive days of hot, oppressive weather caused a continued rise in mortality.[88] Chestnut also reported that areas with higher average temperatures and more frequent hot weather episodes do not necessarily experience more hot weather–related mortality during summer months.[87] Several southern metropolitan areas with very hot, humid summer weather experience much lower or no statistically significant hot weather–related mortality. It remains unclear whether these data apply to the degree of mortality or morbidity from increases in the temperature, duration, and frequency of hot weather episodes in the tropics.[1]

Death rates related to EHEs do not occur on the days with the highest average temperatures. In a study of heat-related mortality from the September 1970 heat wave in New York and other eastern seaboard cities, the highest mortality levels occurred on the third day, when the temperatures were less than those on the first 2 days (Figure 41.5).[9,89,90] In Chicago's 1995 EHE, a slightly different pattern manifested, with the number of deaths peaking 2 days after the maximum heat-index recording.[91] This is consistent with previous studies demonstrating that during EHEs, the maximum number of heat deaths tends to lag behind the days with the highest temperatures.[92,93] It has also been suggested that EHE-related mortality may reflect the tendency of heat stress to precipitate death in persons who are already ill from a wide variety of chronic diseases and would die in the near future.[9] Evidence of this potential effect has been sought but not found. For example, no significant decrease in the number of deaths was reported following the EHE in New York in 1972.[9,89,90]

Urban Heat Islands as Risk Factors

Urban Heat Island and Bioclimates

The long-established concept of the "urban heat island" is pervasive in the American and European literature on EHEs, and applies, to a lesser extent, to urban areas in developing countries.[94,95] This phenomenon describes urban and suburban temperatures that are 1°C–6°C hotter than in nearby rural areas. Elevated temperatures can affect communities by increasing peak energy demand, air conditioning costs, air pollution levels, and heat-related illness and mortality.[96] A typical urban heat island profile is shown in Figure 41.6. Important aspects of the

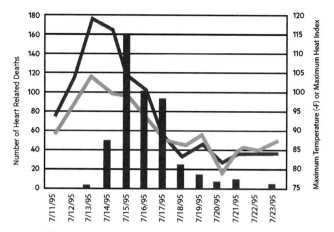

Heat Related Deaths - Chicago
Maximum Temperature and Heat Index

This graph tracks maximum temperature, heat index, and heat-related deaths in Chicago each day from July 11 to 23, 1995. The gray line shows maximum daily temperature, the blue line shows the heat index, and the bars indicate number of deaths for the day.

Figure 41.5. Heat-Related Deaths, Chicago, July 1995.
Source: National Synthesis Team, U.S. Global Change Research Program, published in 2000.

urban heat island literature include themes regarding poverty, social isolation, social class, race/minority status, crime, poor housing, inadequate healthcare, and mobility limitations. Ultimately, most of these factors are related to poverty and unemployment. Studies of heat islands do not generally indicate bioclimatic aspects (effects of weather and climate on life forms, including humans) and are therefore of limited use for urban planners.[97]

Urban areas tend to be warmer because of their "masses of stone, brick, concrete, asphalt, and cement."[27] These darker surfaces, which absorb more solar heat during the day, radiate that energy into the environment at night.[84] All of these factors, including diminished wind and cooling air currents create the heat storing and absorbing urban heat island. The Atlanta Metropolitan Area Heat Profile appears in Figure 41.7 with red, and dark and light orange and yellow denoting hotter and colder areas. Heat wave response planning is of interest in intensely developed urban areas that are large enough, dense enough, and often old enough to have potentially damaging urban heat islands. U.S. studies analyzing data from the last 100 years confirm this finding and recognize associations among: 1) large masses of cityscape (e.g., cement, asphalt, and high percentages of multiple unit dwellings); 2) a relative lack of trees and other vegetation; and 3) poor wind and air circulation patterns. These areas have experienced relatively high EHE-related morbidity and mortality.[9,34,84,87] Klinenberg termed urban heat islands "Urban Loneliness Islands," referring to the physical and social isolation of many elderly heat victims.[98]

After the deadly Chicago heat wave of 1995, the National Oceanic and Atmospheric Administration (NOAA) observed, "There is sufficient circumstantial evidence to conclude that the urban heat island was at least partially responsible for . . . conditions in Chicago's south side. . . . [T]he elderly and infirm . . . in urban areas are in the greatest danger during heat

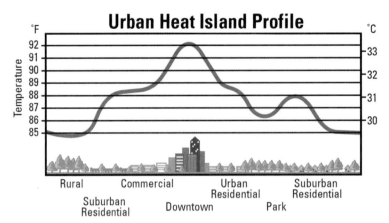

Urban Heat Island Profile

Heat islands are often largest over dense development but may be broken up by vegetated sections within an urban area.

Figure 41.6. Urban Heat Island Profile. *Source:* Environmental Protection Agency, http://www.epa.gov/heatisland/about. Reviewed/modified by Tom Javorcic, 2013.

waves."[7] During EHEs, health risks are magnified by increasing exposure time and maximum temperature.[2]

Urban populations in non-industrialized countries are likely to be particularly vulnerable to such effects when compounded by climate change.[99] Worsening economic conditions exacerbate this impact. A statement by Lord May, President of the British Royal Society, makes clear that climate change and its related and unexpected costs could ruin efforts to elevate Africa out of poverty.[4] Vulnerable populations can, however, be spared many of the effects of EHEs through relatively uncomplicated human interventions, including the use of advanced early warning systems and providing access to potable water, shelter, emergency medical care, and air conditioning.[17]

Concentrations of asphalt, concrete, stone, and brick are relatively new, and make up relatively smaller parts of urban areas in developing nations. Poor immigrants to the city, and even the emerging middle class, usually live in a different environment. These areas are characterized by quasi-traditional, owner-constructed, single- or extended-family housing, frequently densely packed, and usually with dirt rather than asphalt or cement roads. These typically large barrios, favelas, kam-

pungs, or townships are not really heat islands, due to their lack of a genuine urban infrastructure. Yet these communities are where almost all deaths and illnesses from EHE events occur.

Heat in the Indoor Environment

Kovats and Jendritzky found that there are three main factors associated with indoor heat exposure.[100]

1. Thermal capacity of the building – A heavy building will warm up more slowly in a heat wave, particularly if it is well insulated.
2. Position of apartment – The upper floors of a building will generally be hotter than the lower floors because the roof provides inadequate insulation and warmer air tends to rise.
3. Behavior and ventilation – Occupants will adapt as best they can to hot environments using fans (which can actually cause harm at higher temperatures) and opening windows to let in cool evening air. The fact that many people tend to wear the same clothing regardless of season or temperature demonstrates the complexity of decision processes and determinants of behavior.

Givoni categorized the variables that influence the inner bioclimate:[97,101,102]

- The geometrical configuration of the building;
- The orientation of the building;
- The size and location of the windows;
- The properties of the building materials;
- The colors of the external surfaces.

Givoni also described aspects of external design that influence urban climate.

- Size and density of the built up area:
  - The microclimate in the immediate vicinity of green spaces differs from that prevalent in unplanted areas.
  - Vegetation has lower heat capacity than building materials.

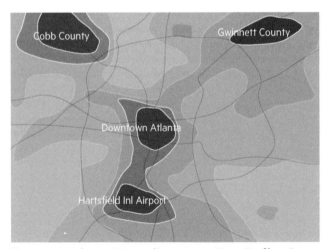

Figure 41.7. Atlanta Metropolitan Area Heat Profile. *Source:* Environmental Protection Agency, http://www.epa.gov/heatisland/about/measurement.html. Reviewed/modified by Tom Javorcic, 2013.

■ Solar radiation is absorbed so that reflected radiation is very small (low albedo).

■ Green spaces have higher evapotranspiration rates than unplanted areas.

■ Plant leaves can filter dust out of the air.

■ Layout and width of streets and their orientation to prevailing winds.

■ The height, shape, and relative location of buildings.

■ Shading conditions along streets and parking areas.

■ Ensuring short distances for walking.

There is a need for further health research on the relationship between housing types and heat effects. In addition, there is little information about how people behave in their homes. When do they use their air conditioners? What is the effect of electrical costs? When do they open their windows for cooling or when do they close them to keep out pollution or noise?

Air Conditioning

Air conditioning is a "special case" in Europe, which relies much less on air conditioning than the United States, even in many healthcare institutions. The European research on air conditioning is not definitive, but supports the use of unit-wide, central air conditioning as opposed to single room air conditioning. The latter has been found to be minimally, if at all protective, unless the housing unit has enough window air conditioners to approximate the coverage of central air conditioning.[103] Although Europeans recognize the protective nature of air conditioning in EHEs, they stress that air conditioning requires sealed buildings that create stagnant, polluted air issues, and that air conditioning itself uses energy that contributes to global warming. When power grids fail, people are often left in relatively airtight buildings.[97] In Europe, air conditioning is advised only in cases in which ill health is present.[100]

Planning for Extreme Heat Events

The Extreme Heat Event Planning Process

Despite the many examples of deadly EHEs, a 2004 review of plans from 18 U.S. cities at risk for heat-related mortality found that many had inadequate plans or no plans at all.[104] Another study of 120 of the largest U.S. cities found that only 29 had developed single-purpose response plans and these were of varying quality and scope. In a 2010 review, 31 cities were found to have adopted plans.[105,106,107] Although there is no mechanism for coordinated U.S. EHE response planning, there has been significant activity at the federal level. These efforts include the development and mass circulation of a comprehensive, interagency extreme heat event guide (2006), the federally sponsored Heat Wave Workshop in 1996, the National Weather Service's (NWS) growing use of sophisticated air mass prediction systems, CDC's coverage of EHEs in its *Morbidity and Mortality Weekly Reports*, and study results published on multiple Web pages by EPA, CDC, and NOAA.

Urban EHE response planning has developed into a unique policy area with its own literature that is scattered among larger disciplines. It is supported by a growing public awareness and constantly reinforced by heat wave alerts. During recent decades, a modestly growing number of urban governments in Europe, Canada, and the United States, have reacted to EHEs by developing EHE response plans. These include alert/watch/warning systems based on an analysis of deadly air masses that provide more "early warning time" than previous systems. In addition to such strategies, existing urban EHE response plans have included the following: 1) public utility bill forgiveness or modified bill payment; 2) free air conditioner distributions; 3) public cooling centers; 4) public information hotlines; 5) public education and information systems; 6) registries for the elderly and other at-risk populations; and 7) aggressive outreach programs. Such policies could be adopted in developing countries, although international donors may need to supply the necessary resources. The most plausible cooling sites are usually government offices and elite hotels, places often reluctant to admit poor people. Khogali and Rosenfeld divide response strategies into primary, secondary, and tertiary levels. Their recommendations are specific and proactive with the goal to reduce heat-related disease in the workplace and at sports venues.[107]

Primary prevention addresses adequate and effective building design to maximize comfortable cooling and ventilation, and to reduce radiant and convective heat using mechanical aids.

Secondary prevention includes a wide variety of workplace and sports-related preventative measures that are placed in two groups. The first is referred to as selection and acclimation. These interventions can include pre-event deployment and placement of medical examination resources/equipment in occupational settings and pre-event medical examinations of those participating in sports activities. The second measure is appropriate administrative personnel behavior. This emphasizes modification of the work–rest cycle or the exercise–rest cycle and provision of cool rest areas with fluids.

Tertiary prevention strategies aim at diagnosing heat illness syndromes as early as possible. Khogali and Rosenfeld stress workplace and organized athletic participation.

Certain characteristics are associated with individual municipalities that have developed an EHE response plan. A logistic regression analysis of the twenty-nine U.S. cities with such documents showed that cities with larger populations, higher percentages of multiple unit dwellings, fewer residents age 25 or older with bachelor's degrees, higher violent crime rates, and a member of a heat wave advocacy coalition working or living within the jurisdiction were more likely to have developed a plan. Violent crime was a significant predictor. If such correlations are not spurious, they offer further evidence of widespread perceptions that heat waves are law-and-order problems to the extent that dangerous neighborhoods will tend to minimize people traveling to cooling centers, opening windows to let in cooler night air (when that is available), or have the social cohesion of safer neighborhoods. Cities with a political rather than a professional administration are more likely to have a plan, suggesting "political" solutions as more plausible than purely "technocratic" ones.

Well-designed EHE plans can be cost-effective. Semenza, for example, concluded that those at greatest risk of dying during Chicago's 1995 heat wave were people with medical illnesses, socially isolated, and without air conditioning. Such groups could benefit from simple interventions.[66]

In both Chicago and Milwaukee during the 1995 events, NWS issued warnings of the developing heat wave several days in advance and these were quickly broadcast by the local media. Given this advance warning, many of the heat-related deaths associated with this event were preventable.[108] Despite these timely warnings and effective media coverage, this information either failed to reach or was not used effectively by the people who succumbed to heat-related deaths. This included the victims themselves as well as members of the healthcare community who did not always understand the scope of the impending calamity.[7] Much more than effective media announcements are needed to avoid serious heat wave mortality and morbidity.[66,68,109–112] The development of pre-event plans that integrate public and private assets is necessary to coordinate and effectively deploy lifesaving resources.

It is difficult to use scientific evidence to judge the post facto efficiency of EHE response plans because no two heat waves are the same, and because of the large number of interrelated variables. Researchers analyzed the 1995 EHEs in St. Louis and Chicago and compared them to the 1999 EHEs in those same cities. Although noting differences, they saw more effective and faster responses in 1999 that appeared to save lives that would have been lost in 1995. These cities learned from prior experiences and improved their EHE response plans.

The only intervention that was not widely reflected in the content of existing plans was equipment grant subsidies (e.g., for air conditioners) for poor residents. Not surprisingly, bill forgiveness, bill postponement, and related programs involve real losses for utility companies. Such programs reflect a confluence of creativity, resources, cooperation, and public spirit. In developing countries, air conditioners would rank low among priorities for the poor as compared with receiving advanced notice of the impending increase in temperature, better education, potable water, adequate shelter, and healthcare. In addition, a large number of air conditioners would likely cause local circuits to fail or create a demand that electricity-generating facilities could not fulfill.

Community Prevention and Mitigation Plans for EHEs

The U.S. National Center for Environmental Health within CDC conducted a nationwide survey of local heat wave preparedness plans in an effort to develop guidelines for cities.[8,113] CDC's National Center for Environmental Health reviewed EHE preparedness plans from twelve U.S. cities at risk for heat wave–related morbidity. Cities were selected based on location and population. Examination of their respective plans focused on assessing key elements. These included: 1) inclusion of community organizations; 2) plans for early information dissemination; 3) targeting of high-risk populations; 4) heat monitoring methods and plan activation; 5) interventions; and 6) evaluation. The important elements of these plans are discussed.

Community Participation

Effective heat wave response plans require collaboration between a wide variety of government agencies including departments of public health, emergency management agencies, urban and regional planning departments, agencies for the elderly, and community and volunteer organizations. Community organizations can lend and donate equipment or supplies, provide air-conditioned cooling sites, and assist with identification of high-risk populations for outreach. The previously referenced survey reported that, although the departments of health and community organizations were generally included in plans, incorporation of the police, media, hospitals, utility companies, and local businesses varied. Communications systems between organizations appeared in all plans, but only six provided complete and updated contact information.

Early Information Dissemination

Heat-related illnesses can be prevented by the dissemination of early public information, and such educational endeavors are essential to successful prevention efforts. These should include recognition of health threats posed by high heat and humidity, appropriate precautionary and response measures, and encouragement to check on family members and neighbors in high-risk groups. Eight of twelve plans included early educational messages to city residents.

High-Risk Populations

Although eight of the twelve surveyed plans targeted educational messages and interventions toward the elderly populations, only four developed specific methods to reach socially isolated individuals. Furthermore, only one plan addressed individuals with chronic illnesses, and two addressed those on medications affecting thermoregulation. Three focused on the disabled and two on the homeless. While clinics, pharmacies, physicians, visiting nurses, and home health workers can help with public education, they were not included in many plans.

Heat Monitoring Methods and Plan Activation

Each plan involved methods for monitoring heat. Typically, monitoring was performed by the local office of NWS. Six plans included the medical examiner's office and EDs for evaluating heat-related mortality and morbidity. Ten plans used a three-level public warning system for advisory, watch, and warning levels. Only three described criteria for deactivation.

Interventions

All twelve cities surveyed had plans to provide air-conditioned shelters. Ten municipalities used hotlines, and six provided transportation to the shelters. Two provided air conditioners and "check-in" services for the elderly, and two could procure emergency funds for cooling packs, beverages, and transportation services. Four provided water, suspension of utility disconnection, and extension of community swimming pool hours. Two cities provided translation services and four provided telecommunication devices for the deaf.

Evaluation

Only one proposal outlined a method of evaluating the plan following its implementation. After the EHE and the response conclude, the lead organization should conduct an evaluation of the city's efforts and document the results in an after-action report. This evaluation should include data/input from participating organizations and from the public. This will help improve future responses to heat wave emergencies.

Elements of Effective Extreme Heat Event Plans

Effective EHE preparedness and response plans vary, based on different local circumstances. The EHE experts who developed the *Excessive Heat Events Guidebook* reviewed multiple information sources, including the preparedness and response literature, views of other experts in the field, and best examples of existing plans.[17] They selected a number of elements key to the development of effective EHE preparedness and response plans (Table 41.4).

Extreme Heat Event Prediction: Ensure Prediction of Extreme Heat Event Conditions 1–5 Days in Advance

Adequate advanced warning is the most important factor in preventing EHE related morbidity and mortality. EDs need time to augment staffing and hospitals must adjust to

Table 41.4. Elements of Effective EHE Plans

■ Ensuring prediction of EHE conditions 1–5 days in advance
■ Quantitative links between temperature and health effects
■ EHE notification and effective governmental responses: hotlines, public information, at-risk registries, direct action
■ Mitigation by urban builders and urban governmental regulators

Table 41.5. Urban Strategies to Reduce Heat Island Effects

■ Cities foster urban gardens/roof gardens
■ Builders use light colors (especially on roofs or any reflective surfaces)
■ Cities support tree and shrub intensity
■ Cities integrate cooling airways into urban design, creating or taking advantage of existing wind patterns

summer vacations, staff rotations, and the suspension of elective procedures. Ambulance services require similar preparation and coordination. If importing medical support from other jurisdictions is necessary, pre-event planning is critical. Since the pool of paramedics and emergency medical technicians is a relatively inelastic group, the practice of assigning individuals to serve in a variety of capacities will likely be ineffective and lead to highlighting of existing shortages and limited staff availability.

Forecasting the development and characteristics of an EHE is critical to both EHE risk assessment and implementation of notification and response systems. NWS provides this information across the United States and has begun using more sophisticated air-mass models that provide improved notification. The system was originally developed by Kalkstein at the Center for Climatic Research at the University of Delaware. Toronto and a growing number of U.S. cities, as well as a number of cities around the world, use this sophisticated air mass–based prediction system that incorporates local factors. Air mass occurrences can be predicted up to 48 hours in advance with the use of model output statistics guidance forecast systems.[114]

Extreme Heat Event Risk Assessment of Potential Health Impacts from Rising Temperatures

Whichever agency coordinates the response to EHEs, it must develop quantitative estimates of potential health effects from the rising temperatures. Planners must consider increased demands on EDs and hospitals as well as requirements for populations whose special needs and circumstances make them more vulnerable. Emergency managers can access records of facilities and locations with significant concentrations of high-risk individuals to use as the basis for health needs projections. Estimating resource needs based on the risk assessment should lead to outreach activities to those most likely to be affected.

Extreme Heat Event Notification and Effective Response Actions

Coordinating public broadcasts of information about the anticipated timing, severity, and direction of EHE conditions as well as information regarding implementation of various protective measures is important. Emergency facilities, healthcare providers, and hospitals require notification regarding the timing of EHEs so that emergency staffing plans can be invoked. Emergency phone lines must be created as soon as early weather warnings are issued.

Mutual aid plans are necessary so that staff and facility shortages can be managed effectively. In addition to mutual aid assistance, in the United States, a variety of state and federal programs provide staffing during EHEs. These include the National Disaster Medical System (NDMS), the Emergency Management Assistance Compact (EMAC), and the Medical Reserve Corps.

Local hospital councils and hospital networks may also provide mutual aid support.

Outreach activities for high-risk groups including the elderly and homeless must be initiated as soon as possible after early weather warnings are issued. Utility shutoffs should be suspended during the period of the EHE and the recovery phase. Cooling shelters must be staffed and operational, with transportation and security measures taken. Rescheduling of some public events may be required.

Extreme Heat Event Mitigation

Strategies currently exist that can reduce the effects of urban heat islands and general EHE conditions. City managers can develop and publicize urban garden and vegetation programs. Contractors can construct buildings using lighter colors (particularly on roofs) and use the reflective quality of certain building materials, particularly in public structures, to reduce EHE effects.

The Philadelphia Extreme Heat Event Response Plan

In response to a deadly EHE in 1993, a multiagency task force developed an integrated EHE preparedness and response plan. As the *Excessive Heat Events Guidebook* observes, the Philadelphia plan is often described as the "Benchmark" Plan. The Philadelphia Plan includes:[17]

■ Public announcements associated with intense education and preparation of the media;
■ Buddy system advocacy for checking on local high-risk residents throughout the event (includes block captains);
■ Public hotline activation;
■ Home visits by health department staff;
■ Halt to service shutoff during high heat warning periods;
■ Increased emergency medical service staffing;
■ Increased outreach for the homeless;
■ Cooling shelter/senior refuge;
■ Outreach by public posting of key numbers and other public messaging on local landmark buildings.

Basic strategies for reducing heat-related mortality based on a review of the EHE response literature and several model city plans are presented in Table 41.5.[17]

The Chicago Heat Wave of 1995

The Chicago heat wave of 1995 was a relatively short but extreme event that resulted in deaths within vulnerable populations and damaged the reputation of the political system that was slow in recognizing and coping with its consequences. The effects of heat-related emergencies extend beyond morbidity and mortality and include intensely emotional and political components. During the Chicago heat wave, a brief but intense confrontation between the medical examiner and the city's mayor ensued regarding the definition of heat-related deaths. By varying accounts, Chicago experienced approximately 500–700 excess deaths, most of which were classified as heat-related during the roughly 5-day heat wave period.[66] The African-American community had the highest rate of heat-related mortality of all minority groups.[115] In Chicago's case, there was an existing heat wave emergency plan, but it was not as detailed or as extensive as the one that was developed after the event. The plan in effect during the heat wave was very brief and not comprehensive. It was the focus of an intense media debate regarding its value, the lack of urgency of the city's initial response, and the definition and numbers of "excess" heat-related deaths. In the midst of a growing controversy, two reporters for the *Chicago Sun Times* wrote, "Chicago's 1½ page heat plan is thin on details about getting relief to the people who need it most. And during last week's heat emergency, they failed to follow that plan until the death toll started rising."[116]

During the first days of the heat wave, the mayor was under attack for his response to the deadly event, and, like most Chicagoans, he did not anticipate the problem. The Cook County medical examiner reported more than 370 heat-related deaths, and accurately predicted that the final count would be more than 400. The newspapers reported that when confronted with such numbers, the mayor responded to the medical examiner by saying, "Every day people die of natural causes.... You can't put everything as heat-related."[117] The nightly news aired images of crowded funeral homes and refrigerated trucks outside the county morgue.[118] The medical examiner's figures and methods were supported by later research.[77] Once the magnitude of the crisis became clear, an improved plan was quickly developed. In the interim, community groups called for the resignation of top cabinet members involved in the heat crisis.[119]

Extreme Heat Events in the Developing World

A scientific consensus has developed regarding the belief that global temperatures are warming and that there is an association with humankind's growing use of carbon-based fuels. In 1988, under the guidance and auspices of the UN, scientists and government officials from around the world inaugurated the Intergovernmental Panel on Climate Change (IPCC). This body produced massive world assessment reports in 1990, 1995, 2001, 2007, and 2013, further refining and corroborating the global warming paradigm as both anecdotal and scientifically validated evidence continued to grow.[120] A meta-analysis was reported in the journal *Science* in 2004, stating that of 928 papers presented, "none of the papers" disagreed with the thesis that global warming exists and that human activity is a cause.[25] A significant amount of planning and analysis has emerged from the United States and Europe in response to deadly heat waves. Given that 2007 had the highest January temperatures on record to that date, planning for EHEs across the world will likely intensify (Figure 41.8).[9,17,121,122,123] Planning related to global warming has its limitations. Robert J. Samuelson said, "we don't know enough to relieve global warming, and – barring major technological breakthroughs – we can't do much about it." He cites projections from the International Energy Agency demonstrating that "unless we condemn the world's poor to their present poverty – and freeze everyone else's living standards, greenhouse gases will double by 2050. No government will adopt the draconian restrictions on economic growth and personal freedom

Table 41.6. Interlocking EHE Problems in Urban Megacities of the Developing World

- Shortages of potable water
- Weak government services
- Lack of access to air-conditioned structures
- Crowded shelters
- Unplanned, tightly packed neighborhoods with casual structures

that might curb global warming."[124] World population growth and development will likely proceed as expected, exemplified by China's construction of one new coal-fired power plant each week.[124] The urban megacities of the developing world are subject to the interlocking problems of shortages of potable water, weak government services, lack of access to air-conditioned structures, and crowded shelters (Table 41.6).

Despite the history of EHEs, there is consensus that many adverse outcomes are preventable.[17,125] Reducing future undesirable outcomes requires improving the awareness of public health officials and the general public regarding the associated health risks while continuing to develop and implement effective EHE notification and response programs.[124] EHEs are public health threats because they often increase the number of daily deaths and other nonfatal adverse health outcomes in affected populations. The most vulnerable groups can be found living in urban heat islands.[124,126,127] Future unfavorable health impacts could be reduced through early forecasting of EHEs and subsequent implementation of low-cost and effective responses.

The effects of global warming are intensified by two crucial issues: population growth and the shift to living in cities. For those residing in developing countries, the cities often provide only rudimentary infrastructure and poverty significantly impacts quality of life.[128] At the end of 2008, the world's population reached more than 6.87 billion and it is expected to reach 7.4 billion by 2016. Two-thirds of these individuals will live in cities by 2020 with estimates of up to 1 billion now living as squatters in informal housing, mainly across the developing world.[129,130] As of 2015, there were 35 "megacities" (cities with >10 million inhabitants each) in existence, with the majority of these in the developing world. This does not imply, however, that urban density is necessarily negative. London's stylish Kensington and Chelsea have densities three times those of poorer boroughs.[127]

The available support from international organizations is insufficient to ameliorate EHE disasters in meaningful ways, so a search for solutions to these growing public health problems is a pressing global need. Industrialized nations can play a significant role as informed leaders of public opinion, selecting the best domestic and international policies. The situation in several cities will be highlighted to illustrate the problems.

The following discussion focuses on two cities from South America (Caracas, Venezuela, and Rio de Janeiro, Brazil); Africa (Cairo, Egypt, and Nairobi, Kenya); and southeast Asia (Jakarta, Indonesia, and Kuala Lumpur, Malaysia). There are many interesting differences among these cities, but the cities' surprising similarities will be discussed. Because political and economic constraints on adequate preparations for EHEs are significant, these will be addressed for developing nations.

Each of these cities has the following characteristics: 1) a high-rise commercial center representing a heat island that is smaller in relation to the city's total surface area than in the west;

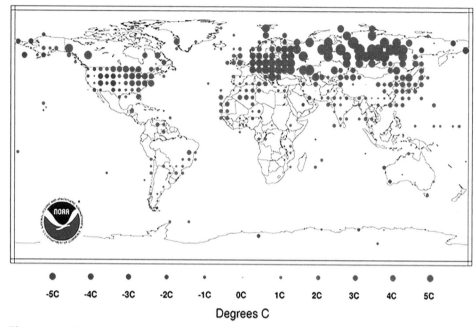

Figure 41.8. Temperature Anomalies, January 2007 (with respect to a 1961–1990 base period). *Source:* NOAA, http://www.noaa.gov. Reviewed/Modified by Tom Javorcic, 2013.

2) spacious elite residential areas occupied by foreigners and ethnic minorities whose success can evoke resentment among the poor; 3) huge residential areas occupied by lower socioeconomic status individuals in search of employment (often recent migrants from rural areas); and 4) a better-educated, emerging middle class that cannot afford elite residences. The areas where the poor reside are called barrios, favelas, alleys, townships, or kampungs. There, the physical infrastructure, roads, electricity, sewage facilities, potable water, communication networks, schools, clinics, and hospitals range from grossly overstretched to virtually nonexistent. For example, in some regions, extreme, monsoon-like rains cause sewage-laden flooding that does not drain because the open ditches built by local residents do not connect to each other.[131] Social safety nets and bureaucratic competence are also lacking. Individuals have few net benefits from citizenship. This exacerbates problems with any response to EHEs. While military and security institutions exist, these powerful resources are not generally available to manage EHEs.

Each vulnerability exacerbates the others and compounds the impact of disasters, ensuring persistent malnutrition, insecure residential status, and deteriorating public safety.[132] Traditional coping techniques are ineffective in these urban areas. Personal savings do not exist so people cannot afford to replace their homes when destroyed by disasters.[127] The poor are essentially segregated from mainstream markets and the economic opportunities these markets offer, as well as from basic education and healthcare. Even under conservative assumptions about population growth, land use, and industrial production in developing countries, computer models predict serious health consequences from a warmer world.[133]

High levels of air and water pollution in these cities will exacerbate the deleterious effects of EHEs for the majority who cannot afford any mitigating interventions, even bottled drinking water. Breathing the air of Jakarta (daytime population 12 million) has the estimated health effect of smoking two packs of cigarettes a day. This impact is magnified because many Jakartans do smoke

two or more packs of cigarettes a day as well. Carbon dioxide concentrations and diesel exhaust contribute to a high incidence of asthma and other respiratory problems. The absence of any interconnected sewer drains means a greatly increased risk of hepatitis, gastroenteritis, cholera, meningitis, typhoid, and even polio – especially for children.[134]

It is extremely difficult for the poor to help themselves, or compel the authorities to provide assistance. There are few if any realistically available "cooling centers" in these six cities. The main venues – government offices and elite hotels – do not welcome temporary occupation by the poor. It might be thought that tax incentives would prompt corporations to occasionally open their cooled offices to those living in poverty, but some corporations have already made arrangements to avoid paying taxes, and others do not provide such shelter for practical or security-related reasons. Some of the poor can attempt to seek shelter in the badly polluted underground car parks or similar structures, but will likely be deterred by inhospitable police. The prevalence of rice paddies in the suburbs of Asian cities offers some cooling, as does the prevalence of Australian eucalyptus trees, but their deep roots lower the water table.

Elitism, or rule by a small and powerful politically insulated group, is more frequent, even in ostensibly democratic countries in the developing world. The six cities and countries discussed have varying degrees and types of democracy. Elitism is far from absent in western politics, but there are countervailing powers and pressures on elitism in the west, so it does not always determine political outcomes. Analogous powers and pressures have yet to emerge in most developing countries. In the cities/countries under discussion, elitism simply correlates with increasing inequality and a resistance to reform.[135] In these cities, one of the only recourses for the poor is to engage in political demonstrations or civil unrest. These tactics usually do not improve their situation to any great degree. This is a major reason why elites, and the police and military forces they support, treat EHEs primarily as law-and-order problems.

The state of administration in most developing countries is also problematic. In the west, disaster planning and implementation is the province of trained and motivated professionals. In contrast, there is little bureaucratic altruism in most developing countries and little evidence of professionally trained management. Elite interests are typically far removed from EHEs. Attempts to plan and implement EHE policies are thwarted by low levels of administrative competence, especially at the municipal level, and public mistrust, because few benefits are conferred by this bureaucracy. It is impractical for a bureaucrat to specialize in healthcare planning, because these administrators are regularly transferred for reasons unrelated to their expertise or the public's needs. Low bureaucratic salaries and sometimes a culture of corruption often mean that actual management decisions run contrary to any reasoned elaborations of the public interest. Persons imbued with an ethos of professionalism will be less likely to exhibit such behavior.[136,137]

All problems cannot be attributed to political and administrative underdevelopment. Even the best of intentions are stymied by an acute shortage of resources. The western mix of clinics, hospitals, and specialty service providers is in short supply. The few services that exist are mostly dedicated to elite use. Emergency responses are usually directed toward regime stability, and often involve the military and police rather than public health. Because overall elite fortunes are also tied to issues such as severe acute respiratory syndrome and avian influenza, there can be public health responses in these areas. Ideally, UN agencies, western governments, and nongovernmental organizations (NGOs) such as Oxfam could, and no doubt will, coordinate efforts in future events.

Egypt (Cairo), Kenya (Nairobi), and Indonesia (Jakarta) are acutely dependent on aid from multilateral donors. Organizations such as the International Monetary Fund, WHO, the World Bank, and the U.S. Agency for International Development provide EHE resources and expertise. They could demand implementation of effective policies as conditions for providing assistance; however, this is unlikely to occur. Many of the best intentioned NGOs and international aid organizations are not sensitive enough to EHE-related needs at their highest administrative levels. At present, donors are unlikely to consider extreme weather before other types of development projects, although growing worldwide awareness of global warming/climate change may alter this.[131]

Could international organizations improve on extreme-weather preparedness for developing countries? Will they develop a regional or global warning system for EHEs and a strategy for more effective city planning before an extreme-weather equivalent of the 2004 tsunami occurs? This is what Anna Tibaijuka, the head of UN Habitat, calls "the biggest problem confronting humanity in the 21st Century."[129] The background paper for the 3rd World Urban Forum recommends that cities form new partnership networks with multilateral institutions and donors, national and provincial governments, the private sector, and the urban poor to create resource commitments for planning, implementation, and upgrading of slums.[137] As the Hyogo Framework for Action, 2005–2015 notes,

> Disaster loss is on the rise with grave consequences for the survival, dignity and livelihood of individuals, particularly the poor... [since this loss interacts with] changing demographic and socio-economic conditions, unplanned urbanization... environmental degradation, climate variability and change [including El Niño/La Niña],... competition for scarce resources, and the impact of epidemics such as HIV/AIDS.

> Events of hydrometeorological origin [i.e., floods, droughts, landslides, tropical cyclones, hurricanes and typhoons] constitute the large majority of disasters.

> The Yokohama Strategy... [of 1994 addressed] disaster risks in the context of sustainable development [and identified gaps and challenges that still remain unfilled and unmet] in five main areas. (a) Governance: organizational, legal and policy frameworks; (b) Risk identification, assessment, monitoring and early warning; (c) knowledge management and education; (d) Reducing underlying risk factors; (e) Preparedness for effective response and recovery.[138]

WHO seems ideally placed to undertake these actions, especially because it already collaborates effectively with similar organizations such as the UN Habitat and the UN Environmental Program on other issues. Additional plausible coordinators are the World Bank (with its augmented mission to take account of global warming), or the International Monetary Fund. Regardless of what organization takes the lead, the same stumbling blocks are likely to remain: a scarcity of resources and political/bureaucratic entanglements.

International leadership is just one issue. The question also arises as to which level of government is most appropriate for managing EHEs in developing countries? In Europe, citizens look toward national ministries or even the national chief executive. Responsibility in the United States lies almost exclusively on the municipal level by default. In developing countries, mayors or regional governors are frequently unskilled and lack leadership training. Instead, they are usually people who have performed well in elite patron–client networks and are given their positions as a reward by prominent national politicians. It is these latter politicians that the public will hold responsible. Therefore, one solution is to assign formal authority for EHE response planning to these individuals.

Ideally, such a plan would be technocratic in its creation and supported by sufficient political power and legitimacy to enhance implementation. Matters are frequently complicated, however, as the concept of elitism and the lack of a technologic ability in developing countries illustrate. One potential innovation that can partially circumvent uncooperative administrations and supply needed technocracy is use of an advocacy coalition. These entities are groups of respected politically independent professionals who work together to identify a problem and to develop solutions. Often these groups are composed of weather professionals, government officials, public health personnel, and medical and emergency management experts who advocate for EHE planning.[139] Such groups exist in the United States and in Europe. With a legitimacy based on their nonprofit volunteerism, such advocates could collaborate directly with interested municipalities and national NGOs.

Factors that correlate highly with injury and death from EHEs in the United States are also associated with death from these events in the developing world. These factors include poverty and social isolation, race, age older than 75 years, the percentage of people living in multiunit dwellings, population density, and high rates of violent crime. Many of these are often combined into the single variable identified as the urban heat island, described previously. Other than poverty, however, many of these factors are absent from the cities under discussion. For example, although general levels of violent crime have historically been low in Cairo, Jakarta, and Kuala Lumpur, the Arab Spring, other bouts of political instability, and similar conditions have increased violence rates significantly. The additional factors relevant to developing countries remain unclear. Ideal research projects designed to answer such questions will encompass large populations. The relative scarcity of resources and the wider scope of competing needs in developing countries suggest that smaller, less sophisticated evaluations are more relevant.

In contrast, Europeans demonstrate a broader, more integrated approach that better links building codes, wetlands/shoreline protections, land-use regulations, control over rates of urbanization and deforestation, and management of industry locations. Some extreme-weather events are so new to Europe that the tailoring of responses to a specific event remains insufficient, as illustrated by the lack of sufficient numbers of air-conditioned hospitals and cooling centers. Developing countries can select between adaptable U.S. and European approaches to create a strategy that meets local needs.

The generally modest external support available to developing nations for solving EHE-related health problems is less problematic than it appears. Developing nations, generally with sophisticated external support, have implemented cost-effective interventions and accomplished major public health successes even under conditions of extreme poverty, weak or nonexistent healthcare infrastructure, and civil war or unrest. For example, as recently as 1988, 125 countries were endemic for polio; however, by mid-2013, just three countries had endemic polio concerns. Efforts were launched in 1974 to kill the black fly that spreads disease and blindness. By 2002, these interventions prevented up to 600,000 cases of blindness.[140] Nevertheless, the challenges associated with EHEs requires a much more rapid response (a matter of days) than that for traditional public health conditions resulting from infectious diseases.

RECOMMENDATIONS FOR FURTHER RESEARCH

Hospitals/EDs/EMS in the United States

EDs Can and Should Be Used to Predict the Healthcare Burden and Epidemiological Consequences of Environmental Disasters

Computerized networks of ED databases should be developed and incorporated into existing reporting mechanisms.[68] These networks would report the prevalence of heat-related conditions treated in the ED in real time. Although ED data create an accurate picture of the EHEs current impact, they will not provide the 1–5 day lead time for area-wide EHE preparations and response. Air mass monitoring systems are the major strategy to supply this advanced warning.[141]

Individual Hospitals and Medical Systems Should Arrange for Extra Medical Staffing in Support of ED Services

The rising demand for medical care associated with EHEs will place additional burdens on the EMS system, individual hospitals, and medical systems to increase emergency services capacity.[17] Increased staffing of EDs, individual hospitals, and hospital systems in response to a forecasted EHE can prevent the EMS from becoming overwhelmed. This enhances the opportunity to avert negative outcomes or at least address them at an earlier and less severe stage.[17] EDs must be aware that many of the additional support staff needed in emergency situations have multiple commitments. They are often members of local, state, and federal emergency teams, as well as the National Guard and other organizations.

Local Emergency Medical Systems Need Fiscal and Institutional Support at the Regional, State, and Federal Levels

It is likely that the onset of EHE conditions will result in significant increases in demand for emergency care in the form of EMS calls and visits to EDs. Existing local and state resources supported by mutual aid agreements, state emergency management assistance compacts, as well as the resources of federal governments may provide the necessary additional medical support that individual hospitals or hospital systems require. Evaluation of the applicability and availability of these resources must occur before the onset of EHE conditions.[17]

Studies published by IOM emphasize that although demands on emergency and trauma care have grown dramatically, the capacity of the system has not kept pace.[142] Meeting the need for medical care in the face of increasing patient volume and limited resources remains challenging. Balancing existing system utilization with the huge demands that EHEs could place on EDs requires extensive area-wide planning coupled with effective integration of existing response assets and systems.

Local and Regional Governments

Urban Areas at Substantial Risk for EHEs Should Develop Listings of Vulnerable Individuals, Especially Those Older than 75 Years of Age

Detailed registries are difficult to develop and maintain and can be costly. In their absence, however, the municipal government's ability to conduct effective outreach to those vulnerable to EHEs is extremely limited. Information for compiling such lists can be obtained from religious and social organizations. Another option is to require owners of dwellings in which the elderly reside to report critical data to local health and welfare agencies. City departments of urban and regional planning and Administration on Aging offices can also be very helpful in supporting the development of registries.

Research Exploring the Effectiveness of EHE Preparedness and Response Strategies as well as the Association between EHEs and Morbidity Is Necessary to Aid in the Development of Evidenced-Based Plans

McGeehin and Mirabelli discussed the need for broad-based research into EHEs, including further investigations of critical weather parameters as they relate to EHEs and urban design.[70]

International Initiatives

An International Institute Is Needed to Coordinate the Various Aspects of EHE Preparedness and Response, Focusing on Emergency Management and Planning Efforts Related to Weather, Public Health, Medical, Structural, Environmental, and Urban and Regional Planning Issues

A number of federal, state, and municipal organizations as well as universities have served as focal points for research and development activities for EHEs. To continue and intensify the growing interest in EHE response planning and the related areas of medical, weather, and emergency management research, a single-purpose institute dedicated to the study of EHEs should be developed.

Proposed Solutions to the Challenges of EHEs in Cities of the Developing World

What should response organizations, administrators, and politicians do to mitigate the effects of EHEs in developing countries? The U.S. and, to some extent, European experiences provide potential EHE preparedness and response activities for developing countries to consider. In practical terms, these are more likely to be addressed by international NGOs and be coordinated by entities such as WHO.

Weather Prediction Based on Air Mass Modeling from Entities Such as NOAA and the European Union Should be Used as the Basis for Alert/Watch/Warning Systems

Air mass monitoring systems can provide an additional 1–5 days of early warning regarding EHEs. They are already in place in a growing number of urban areas across the world and are being instituted in the U.S. by the NOAA's NWS.

Education and Communication with Residents of Urban Areas Is Necessary. These Efforts Must Anticipate Cultural and Religious Diversity and Be Externally Funded

EHE preparedness and response efforts must be extremely sensitive to local religious and cultural practices. As in most proposals discussed in this section, external funding from NGOs and international aid coordinated by organizations such as WHO are required. These efforts may be complicated by local practices and a general lack of governmental and political support.

Targeted Funding for Specific Public Health Measures Is a Necessity

The underfunded status of emergency medical and public health systems in most developing nations is likely to continue, as is the lack of governmental resources and political determination to address EHEs. Therefore, financial support for specific public health measures is required. Otherwise, assistance will continue to come from international NGOs and other external sources of international aid.

Effective Urban and Regional Planning Is Needed in Cities That Feature Extensive Areas of Slum Housing

Unless EHE infrastructure issues are considered along with other medical and public health systems needs, there is little chance of addressing existing resource shortfalls.

Distribution of Bottled Water and Potable Water Systems Can Be Effective Short-Term Solutions to EHEs

Although initially effective, water distribution does not address the long-term needs of developing nations regarding adequate supplies of potable water. It highlights the traditional approach of meeting short-term disaster needs as opposed to addressing the much larger, long-term resource and political/governmental problems that are the root cause of most medical and public health problems.

Future Research Directions

The following examples illustrate research that could improve the effectiveness of EHE management. These areas of research have been generally under-investigated by public health and medical

planners. The research selections that appear reflect significant aspects of the urban reality from which EHEs have developed. Unlike most public health and medical research, it is not primarily empirically derived. Rather, it is process-driven, and recognizes that good plans will not automatically result in good outcomes unless time and thought are spent on the implementation aspects. In fact, a whole research literature in political science and public administration has been dedicated to how laws, plans, and concepts are implemented.[143]

Experts in the field of urban and regional planning have spent decades studying how plans are implemented into effective methods of solving specific problems. Implicit in this research is how the public, the urban governance leadership (public and private), and other groups are brought together to operationalize plans. The types of responses that various U.S. or European cities crafted cannot be directly transferred to cities in the developing world without some modification. There are, however, important elements of these strategies that can be adopted. Although it will not be possible to implement some systems that depend on effective and relatively well-equipped bureaucracies, potentially useful technologies can be applied successfully if the particular political, ethnic, sociocultural, and other urban-based realities are understood. The projects can be grouped in nine categories.

1. **Remote sensing**. Such techniques could have an important role in refining and quantifying the widely accepted effects of urban heat islands. These procedures are not referenced in any of the plans reviewed in this chapter, although the weather prediction and heat island literatures are becoming more incorporated into related areas of investigation. For example, NASA Landsat space imaging shows a clear correlation between demographic changes and physical landscape changes. Future international coordination efforts, taken in conjunction with such prediction innovations as air mass modeling, can be expected to predict localized risks for heat-related morbidity and mortality.[144]

2. **The effects of information on participants in the problem-solving process.** Urban and regional planning research recognizes the value of information as part of the problem-solving process. A good example is the widespread and effective public information campaign that educated citizens about the buddy system in Philadelphia. This plan had a positive and lifesaving impact as people evaluated each other's states of health during EHEs.[145]

3. **Rational arguments and irrational audiences.** When policymakers address technological issues such as power plant locations, they often confront hostile and apparently irrational audiences. Sometimes frustrated technocrats will turn to behavioral science for solutions. Whether or not the audience is really "irrational" depends on understanding their perceptions of the problem. In the developing world, belief systems and social and class orientations may dissuade people from what appears to be the most prudent technological solutions. An example would be resistance to the brief use of large, air-conditioned spaces in tourist hotels to prevent heat-related deaths.[146]

4. **Consensus building: mistaken interests in the discourse model of planning.** Researchers have demonstrated that mistaken judgments about individual and group self-interest could be addressed by structured rational discourse; however, more work is needed. In the complicated ethnic and political milieus of modern urban areas, mistaken motives still lead to failure. For example, many urban EHE plans include cooling

centers that require individuals to use public transportation, travel through dangerous areas, and overcome personal mobility issues. In this case, the planners either need to modify their consensus to ensure the public can easily access the sites or abandon the concept.[147]

5. **Planning through consensus building.** In an investigation of eight case studies, research proved that those whose interests are directly impacted will actively participate if they are approached. Borrowed from the urban development experience, the author followed eight projects and found that arriving at a consensus involving the major stakeholders is normally required if a plan is to be effectively implemented. In U.S. cities, this means that EHE interventions such as cooling centers must be tested among urban elderly poor, as well as with the utility companies and major government agencies. In developing nations, it means arriving at consensus will require participation by NGOs, local and/or world advocacy groups, impoverished citizens, and the local elite, whose support is required.[148]

6. **Discussion and rationality.** Researchers found some indication that discussion enhanced rationality among the participants; however, increased rationality among the participants may not be sufficient to foster the outcomes that are desired by planners.[149]

7. **Confronting a fractured public interest.** The researcher reviewed models addressing urban ethnic conflict in Johannesburg, Belfast, and Jerusalem. In Johannesburg, government planners confronted racism, poverty, and vast cultural gaps as they improved services to the squatter-shack areas in Alexandria Township. They concentrated their efforts on addressing the poor quality of water, sanitation, housing, and public health services. The planners balanced the need to reduce apartheid patterns and provide access to the more affluent white areas for blacks while serving as mediators for the interest of all groups. Addressing urban and regional planning problems required that political, social, and racial problems also be resolved. This type of organizational research on the political and ethnic environments in the developing world also applies to the increasingly diverse urban and rural populations in the United States.[150]

8. **Planning and chaos theory.** Some of the ideas about randomness or chaos emerging in various fields of the natural, social, and applied sciences have major implications for EHE planning. Research suggests that the world may be both easier and more difficult to understand than previously believed and that untidy cities may not be as dysfunctional as is assumed. This is another way of saying that just because order is not perceived, does not mean there is none. This knowledge is very important in the cultures of urban areas in developing nations as emergency management professionals work with supportive local networks to advocate for implementation of EHE plans.[151]

9. **Judging the relative effectiveness of various EHE plan components in reducing EHE-related mortality and morbidity.** As global climate change intensifies, the effects of EHEs and research into the cost effectiveness of the various plan components will become more prevalent and more complex.[152]

In summary, the technologic aspects of EHE management are far less complicated than are the influences of political, sociocultural, and ethnic issues. Only through the application of coordinated transdisciplinary approaches to research will the morbidity and mortality of EHEs be reduced.

Acknowledgment

The editors and authors acknowledge the contributions to this chapter of Paul H. Brietzke and Jerome H. Libby, sadly now both deceased, as well as Laurie Adrianopoli and Tom Javorcic for their help with the figures.

REFERENCES

1. Menne B, with contributions from Wolf T. In: Kirch W, Menne B, Bertollini R, eds. *Extreme Weather Events and Public Health Responses.* Berlin/Heidelberg, Springer-Verlag, 2005; xxviii.
2. Kobasa P, ed. *Heat Waves: Library of Natural Disasters.* Chicago, World Books, Inc., 2008; 10.
3. The National Weather Service. http://www.wrh.noaa.gov/sto/heatwave.php (Accessed December 11, 2008).
4. Heat Illness and Deaths – New York City, 2000–2011. *MMWR* 2013; 62(31): 617–621.
5. Kinver M. Water Policy "Fails world's poor." *BBC One Minute World News.* Updated March 9, 2006. Based on the UN World Water Development Report, outlined at the World Water Forum in Mexico, 2006. http://news.bbc.co.uk/2/science/nature/4787758.stm (Accessed March 24, 2007).
6. U.S. Centers for Disease Control and Prevention (CDC). Heat Illnesses and Death, CDC Media Relations: *MMWR* July 4, 2003. www.cdc.gov/od/oc/media/mmwrnews/n030704.htm (Accessed December 11, 2008).
7. National Oceanic and Atmospheric Administration (NOAA). *July 1995 Heat Wave: National Disaster Survey Report.* Washington, DC, U.S. Department of Commerce, National Weather Service; 1995; viii: 17–52.
8. CDC. *Heat Wave Emergency Response: A Review by the National Center for Environmental Health.* Atlanta, The National Center for Environmental Health, Division of Environmental Hazards and Health Effects, 1999.
9. Kilbourne EM. Heat waves and hot environments. In: Noji EJ, ed. *The Public Health Consequences of Disasters.* New York, Oxford University Press, 1997; 249.
10. Ellis FP, Prince HP, Lovan G, Whitington RM. Mortality and morbidity in Birmingham during the 1976 heatwave. *Q J Med* 1980; 49: 1–8.
11. Heat-related mortality – United States, 1997. *MMWR* 1998; 47: 3–5.
12. Bhattacharya S. European heatwave caused 35000 deaths. http://www.newscientist.com/article/dn4259-european-heatwave-caused-35000-deaths.html (Accessed December 11, 2008).
13. Doyle A. 160000 said dying yearly from global warming. Planet Ark. http://www.planetark.org/dailynewsstory.cfm/newsid/22420/story.htm (Accessed December 11, 2008).
14. Kalkstein LS, Greene JS. An evaluation of climate/mortality relationships in large U.S. cities and the possible impacts of climate change. *Environ Health Perspect* 1997; 105(1): 84–93.
15. Ellis FP. Mortality from heat illness and heat-aggregated illness in the United States. *Environ Res* 1972; 5: 1–58.
16. National Center for Health Statistics. Mortality Public Use Computer Data Tapes for the Years 1979–1991. Hyattsville, MD, National Center of Health Statistics, 1994.
17. U.S. Environmental Protection Agency (EPA). *Excessive Heat Events Guidebook. EPA contract 430-B-06–005.* Washington, DC, Environmental Protection Agency, June 2006.

18. Kalkstein LS. Climate and human mortality: relationship and mitigating measures. *Adv Bioclimatol* 1997; 5: 161–177.

19. Davis RE, Knappenberger PC, Michaels PJ, Novicoff WM. Changing heat-related mortality in the United States. *Environ Health Perspect* 2003; 11: 12–18.

20. Henschel A, Burton LL, Margolies L, Smith JE. An analysis of the heat deaths in St. Louis during July 1966. *Am J Public Health* 1969; 59: 2232–2242.

21. Sheridan SC, Dolney TJ. Heat, mortality, and level of urbanization: measuring vulnerability across Ohio, USA. *Clim Res* 2003; 24: 255–266.

22. Cohen JC, Veysseire JM, Bessemoulin P. Bio-climatological aspects of summer over France. In: Kirch W, Menne B, Bertollini R, eds. *Extreme Weather Events and Public Health Responses.* Berlin/Heidelberg, Springer-Verlag, 2005; 34.

23. Meehl GA, Tebaldi C. More intense, more frequent, and longer lasting heat waves in the 21st Century. *Science* 2004; 305: 994–997.

24. Kovats S, Haines A. The potential health impacts of climate change: an overview. *Med War* 1995; 11: 168–178.

25. Oreskes N. Beyond the ivory tower: the scientific consensus on climate change. *Science* 2004; 306: 1686.

26. UN News Centre. National leaders at UN Summit call for stepped-up action to fight climate change. http://www.un.org/apps/news/story.asp?NewsID=15833#.VevRfRFVhBc (Accessed September 5, 2015).

27. Kilbourne EM. Heat waves. In: Gregg MB, ed. *The Public Health Consequences of Disasters.* Washington, DC, HHS, Public Health Service, CDC, 1989; 51

28. Kilbourne EM, Choi K, Jones TS, Thacker SB. Risk factors for heat stroke. A case-control study. *JAMA* 1982; 247: 3332–3336.

29. *Excessive Heat Events Guidebook, 2006.* Washington, DC, EPA. http://www.epa.gov/heatisland/about/pdf/EHEguide_final.pdf (Accessed December 11, 2008).

30. Kalkstein LS, Davis RE. Weather and human mortality: an evolution of demographic and interregional responses in the United States. *Ann Assoc Am Geograph* 1989; 79: 44–64.

31. Sheridan SC, Kalkstein LS. Progress in heat watch-warning system technology. *Bulle Am Meteorolog Soc* 1989; 85: 1931–1941.

32. Greene JS, Kalkstein LS. Quantitative analysis of summer air masses in the eastern United States and an application to human mortality. *Clim Res* 1996; 7(1): 43–53.

33. Stein J, Kaplan S. Scientists Probe Why Heat Wave Became A Killer. *Chicago Tribune.* July 26, 1995; 1, 13, sec. 1.

34. Kunkel KE, Chagnon SA, Reinke BC, Arritt RW. The July 1995 heat wave in the midwest: a climatic perspective and critical weather factors. *Bull Am Meteorolog Soc* 1996; 7: 1507–1517.

35. Kilbourne EM. Heat-related illness: current status of prevention efforts. *Am J Prevent Med* 2002; 22: 328–329.

36. Vlum LN, Bresolin LB, Williams MA for the council on Scientific Affairs. Heat-related illness during extreme weather emergencies. *JAMA* 1998; 279: 1514.

37. Leon LR, Helwig BG. Heat stroke: Role of the systemic inflammatory response. *J Appl Physiol* 2010; 109(6): 1980–1988.

38. Bouchama A, Hammami MM, Haq A, Jackson J, Al-Sedairy S. Evidence for endothelial cell activation/injury in heatstroke. *Critical Care Med* 1996; 24(7): 1173–1178.

39. Hoppe J, Sinert R, Kunihiro A, Foster J. Heat exhaustion and heat stroke. The continually updated medical site. http://www.emedicine.com/emerg/topic236.htm (Accessed December 11, 2008).

40. Varghese GM, John G, Thomas K, et al. Predictors of organ dysfunction in heatstroke. *Emerg Med J* 2005; 22: 185–187.

41. http://emedicine.medscape.com/article/770413-treatment (Accessed December 20, 2008).

42. http://usariem.army.mil/heatill/histroke.htm (Accessed December 20, 2008).

43. Hoedemaekers CW, Ezzahti M, Gerritsen A, van der Hoeven JG. Comparison of cooling methods to induce and maintain normo- and hypothermia in intensive care unit patients: a prospective intervention study. *Critical Care* 2007; 11: R91. http://ccforum.com/content/11/4/R91 (Accessed November 4, 2013).

44. Bouchama A, Knochel JP. Heat stroke. *N Engl J Med* 2002; 346: 1978–1988.

45. Marzuk P, Tardiff K, Leon A, et al. Ambient temperature and mortality from unintentional cocaine Overdoses. *JAMA* 1998; 279: 1795–1800.

46. Dolney TJ, Sheridan SC. The relationship between extreme heat and ambulance response calls for the city of Toronto, Ontario, Canada. *Environ Research* 2006; 101: 94–96.

47. Nitschke M, Tucker GR, Hansen AL, Williams S, Zhang Y, Bi P. Impact of two recent extreme heat episodes on morbidity and mortality in Adelaide, South Australia: a case-series analysis. *Environ Health* 2011; 10: 42.

48. Schaffer A, Muscatello D, Broome R, Corbett S, Smith W. Emergency department visits, ambulance calls and mortality associated with an exceptional heat wave in Sydney, Australia, 2011: a time-series analysis. *Environ Health* 2012; 11: 3.

49. Teng H, Branstator G, Wang H, Meehl GA, Washington WM. Probability of US heat waves affected by a subseasonal planetary wave pattern. *Nature Geoscience* October 27, 2013. http://www.natre.com/ngeo/journal/vaop/ncurrent/full/ngeo1988.html (Accessed November 3, 2013).

50. Institute of Medicine (IOM). Emergency health system unprepared for disasters. News Release by the Center for Infectious Disease Research and Policy. Academic Health Center, University of Minnesota. *CIDRAP News* June 20, 2012; 1.

51. Semenza JC, McCullough JE, Flanders WD, et al. Excess hospital admissions during the July 1995 heat wave in Chicago. *Am J Prevent Med* 1999; 16: 269–277.

52. Wainwright SH, Buchanan SD, Mainzer HM, et al. Cardiovascular mortality – the hidden peril of heat waves. *Prehosp Disaster Med* 1999; 14: 222–231.

53. Davido A, Patzak A, Dart T, et al. Risk factors for heat-related death during the August 2003 heat wave in Paris, France, in patients evaluated at the emergency department of the Hospital European 'Georges Pompidou.' *EMJ* 2006; 23: 515–518.

54. Johnson H, Kovats R, McGregor G, et al. The impact of the 2003 heat wave mortality and hospital admissions in England. *Health Stat Q* 2005; 25: 6.

55. Faunt JD, Wilkinson TJ, Henschke P, et al. The effete in the heat: heat-related hospital presentations during a ten day heatwave. *Aust NZ J Med* 1995; 25: 117.

56. Rajpal RC, Weisskopf MG, Rumm PD, et al. Wisconsin, July 1999 heat wave: an epidemiologic assessment. *WJM* 2000; 99: 41–44.

57. The Joint Commission on Accreditation of Healthcare Organizations and Joint Commission Resources. Surge Hospitals: Providing Safe Care in Emergencies. 2006. http://www.jointcommission.org/assets/1/18/surge_hospital.pdf (Accessed September 5, 2015).

58. Waugh WL. *Living with Hazards, Dealing with Disasters: An Introduction to Emergency Management.* Armonk, NY, M. E. Sharpe, 2000; 3, 4.

59. Landesman LY. *Public Health Management of Disasters: The Practical Guide.* Washington, DC, American Public Health Association, 2001; 35, 6.

60. CNA Medical Surge Capacity and Capability: A Management System for Integrating Medical and Health Resources During Large-Scale Emergencies. This document was prepared under

Contract Number 233–03–0028 for HHS. CAN Corp., 2004; 2–8.

61. The National Foundation for Trauma Care. *United States Trauma Care Proposals for a Terrorist Attack in the Community: The Study of the Impact of a Terrorist Attack on Individual Trauma Centers.* Atlanta, GA, CDC, 2006; 3–5.

62. Auf der Heide E. The importance of evidence-based disaster planning. *Ann Emerg Med* 2006; 47: 34–46.

63. Delinger RF, Gonzenbach K. The two-hat syndrome: determining response capabilities and mutual aid limitations. In: Kayyem JN, Pangi RL, eds. *First to Arrive: State and Local Responses to Terrorism.* Cambridge, MA, MIT Press, 2003; 193–205.

64. Patz J, McGeehin M, Bernard S, et al. The potential health impacts of climate variability and change for the United States: executive summary of the report of the health sector of the U.S. National Assessment. *Environ Health Perspect* 2000; 108: 367–376.

65. Patz J, Engleberg D, Last JJ. The effects of changing weather on public health. *Ann Rev Public Health* 2000; 21: 271.

66. Semenza JC, Rubin K, Selanikio J, et al. Heat-related deaths during the July 1995 heat wave in Chicago. *N Engl J Med* 1996; 335: 84–90.

67. Environmentl Protection Agency. *Excessive Heat Events Guidebook, 2006.* Citing the American Medical Association Council on Scientific Affairs, 1997. Heat-Related Illness During Extreme Weather Emergencies. Report 10 of the Council on Scientific Affairs (A-97).

68. Rydman RJ, Rumoro DP, Silva JC, et al. The rate and risk of heat-related illness in hospital emergency departments during the 1995 Chicago heat disaster. *J Med Syst* 1999; 23: 41, 53–54.

69. Knowlton K, Rotkin-Ellman M, King G, et al. The 2006 California heat wave: impacts on hospitalizations and emergency department visits. *Environ Health Perspectives* 2009; 117(1): 61–67.

70. McGeehin M, Mirabelli M. The potential impacts of climate variability and change on temperature-related morbidity and mortality in the United States. *Environ Health Perspect* 2001; 109(Suppl. 2): 185–189.

71. Donoghue ER, Graham MA, Jentzen JM, et. al. Criteria for the diagnosis of heat-related deaths: National Association of Medical Examiners. Position paper. National Association of Medical Examiners Ad Hoc Committee on the Definition of Heat-Related Fatalities. *Am J Forensic Med Pathol.* March 1997; 18(1): 11–14.

72. Argaud L, Ferry T, Le QH, Marfisi A, Ciorba D, Achache P, Ducluzeau R, Robert D. Short- and long-term outcomes of heatstroke following the 2003 heat wave in Lyon, France. *Arch Int Med* 2007; 167: 2177–2183.

73. Wallace RF, Kriebel D, Punnett L, Wegman DH, Amoroso PJ. Prior heat illness hospitalization and risk of early death. *Environ Research* 2007; 104: 290–295.

74. Naughton MP, Henderson A, Mirabelli MC, et al. Heat-related mortality during 1999 heat wave in Chicago. *Am J Prevent Med* 2002; 22: 221–227.

75. Adams BE, Manoguerra AS, Lilja GP, Long RS, Ruiz RW. Heatstroke associated with medications having anticholinergic effects. *Minnesota Med* 1977; 60: 103–106.

76. Heat-wave-related mortality – Milwaukee, Wisconsin, July 1995 *JAMA*1996; 276: 275.

77. Whitman S, Good G, Donoghue ER, et al. Mortality in Chicago attributed to the July 1995 heat wave. *Am J Public Health, Public Health Briefs* 1997; 9: 87.

78. Heat-related illnesses, deaths, and risk factors – Cincinnati and Dayton, Ohio, 1999, and the United States 1979–1999. *MMWR* 2000; 49(21): 470–473.

79. Lee DH. Seventy-five years of searching for a heat index. *Environ Res* 1980; 22(2): 331–356.

80. Poulton TJ, Walker RA. Helicopter cooling of heatstroke victims. *Aviation Space Environ Med* 1987; 58(4): 358–361.

81. Vendentorren S, Empereur-Bissonnet P. Health impacts of the 2003 heat-wave in France. In: Kirch W, Menne B, Bertollini R, eds. *Extreme Weather Events and Public Health Responses.* Berlin/Heidelberg, Springer-Verlag, 2005; 82.

82. Michelozzi P, de'Donato F, Bisanti L, et al. Heat waves in Italy: cause specific mortality and the role of educational level and socio-economic conditions. In: Kirch W, Menne B, Bertollini R, eds. *Extreme Weather Events and Public Health Responses.* Berlin/Heidelberg, Springer-Verlag, 2005; 126.

83. Conti S, Meli P, Minelli G, et. al. Epidemiological study of mortality during summer 2003 in Italian regional capitals: results of a rapid survey. In: Kirch W, Menne B, Bertollini R, eds. *Extreme Weather Events and Public Health Responses.* Berlin/Heidelberg, Springer-Verlag, 2005; 119.

84. *Heat Emergency Preparedness Guide.* New York, Department of Emergency Management. 2002.

85. Keating WR, Donaldson CG, Cordioli E, et al. Heat related mortality in warm and cold regions of Europe: observational study. *BMJ* 2000; 321: 670–673.

86. Di Maio DJ, Di Maio VJM. *Forensic Pathology.* London, CRC Press, 1992; 379.

87. Chestnut LG, Breffle WS, Smith JB, Kalkstein LS. Analysis of differences in hot-weather-related mortality across U.S. metropolitan areas. *Environ Sci Pol* 1998; 1: 59.

88. Kalkstein LS. A new approach to evaluate the impact of climate on human mortality. *Environ Health Perspect* 1991; 96: 145.

89. Ellis FP. Mortality from heat illness and heat-aggravated illness in the United States. *Environ Res* 1978; 5: 1–58.

90. Ellis EP, Nelson F, Pincus L. Mortality in the elderly in the heat wave in New York City July 1972 and August and September, 1973. *Environ Res* 1975; 10: 1–13.

91. CDC. Heat-related mortality – Chicago, July 1995. *MMWR* 1995; 44: 577–579.

92. Lyster WR. Deaths in summer. *Lancet* 1976; 2: 469 (Letter).

93. Oeschli FW, Buechley WB. Excess mortality associated with three Los Angeles September hot spells. *Environ Res* 1970; 3: 277–284.

94. Okle TR. City size and the urban heat island. *Atmosphere Environ* 1972; 7: 769–779.

95. Akbari H, Rosenfeld A. *Cooling our Communities: A Guidebook on Tree Planting and Light-Colored Surfaces,* Washington, DC, EPA, 2003.

96. EPA. Climate Change – Health and Environmental Effects. http://www.epa.gov/climatechange/effects/health.html (Accessed December 12, 2008).

97. Koppe C, Kovats S, Jendritzky G Menne B. *Heat-Waves: Risks and Responses.* Geneva, WHO, 2004.

98. Klinenberg E. *Heat Wave: A Social Autopsy of Disaster in Chicago.* Chicago, University of Chicago Press, 2002.

99. Kovats S, Haines A. The potential health impacts of climate change: An overview. *Med War* 1995; 11: 168–178.

100. Kovats RS, Jendritzky G. Heat-waves and human health. In: Menne B, Ebi KL, eds. *Climate Change and Adaptation Strategies in Human Health.* Darmstadt, Steinkopf Verlag, 2004: 79–82.

101. Givoni B. Design for climate in hot, dry, cities. In: Oke TR, ed. *Urban Climatology and its Applications with Special Regard to Tropical Areas.* Proceedings of the Technical Conference, Mexico D.E. November 26–30, 1984. Geneva, World Meteorological Organization (WMO No. 652), 1986; 87–513.

102. Givoni B, et al. Outdoor comfort research issues. *Energy Buildings* 35; 2003: 77–86.

103. Rogot E, Sorlie P, Backlund E. Air-conditioning and mortality in hot weather. *Am J Epidemiol* 136; 1992: 106.

104. Bernard SMJ, McGeehin MA. Municipal heat wave response plans in practice. *Am J Public Health* 94; 2004: 1520–1522.

105. McGowan KJ, ed. *Terrorism and Disaster Management: Preparing Healthcare Leaders for the New Reality*. ACHE Management Series. Chicago, Health Administration Press, 2004; 129–130.

106. Adrianopoli C, Culhane P. Heat Waves and Heat Response Planning in American Cities. Presented at the Annual Meeting of the Midwest Political Science Association, Chicago, The Palmer House, April 7, 2005.

107. Adrianopoli C, Culhane P. Responding to Deadly Extreme Heat Events. *PA Times*. July/August/September, in the Smart EM Response Issue. 2013; 36: 3.

108. Palecki MA, Chagnon SA, Kunkel KE. The nature and impacts of the July 1999 heat wave in the Midwestern United States. *Bull Am Meteorolog Soc* 2001; 82: 1353–1367.

109. NOAA 96–21. Many of the 1995 Heat Wave Deaths Were Preventable According to NOAA Report. http://www.publicaffairs.noaa.gov/pr96/apr96/noaa96-21.html (Accessed September 5, 2015).

110. CDC. Heat-related illnesses and deaths – United States, 1994–1995. *MMWR* 1995; 44(25): 465–468.

111. CDC. Heat-wave related mortality – Milwaukee, Wisconsin, July1995. *MMWR* 1996; 45: 505–507.

112. Kellerman AL, Todd KH. Killing heat. *N Engl J Med* 1996; 335: 126–127 (Letter).

113. Dematte JE, O'Mara K, Buescher RW, et al. Morbidity and mortality associated with the July 1980 heat wave in St. Louis and Kansas City, MO. *JAMA* 1982; 247: 327–331.

114. CDC Extreme Heat Bibliography. Extreme Heat website. http://emergency.cdc.gov/disasters/extremeheat/bibliography.asps (Accessed March 15, 2008). See also, *The Excessive Heat Events Guidebook*, EPA 430-B-06–005. A project supported by EPA, NOAA, CDC, and the National Disaster Medical System, then a component of FEMA/U.S. Department of Homeland Security. Washington, DC, EPA, Office of Atmospheric Programs (6207J), June 2006; 20460.

115. Kalkstein L, Jamason PF, Greene JS, et al. The Philadelphia hot weather-health watch. Warning system: development and application. *Bull Am Meteorolog Soc* 1996; 7: 1519–1528.

116. Kaiser R, Le Terte A, Schwartz J, CA, et al. The effect of the 1995 heat wave in Chicago on all-cause and cause-specific mortality. *Am J Public Health* 2007; 97: 158–162.

117. Nelson S. Hundreds Die In Chicago Heat Wave. *The Militant* August 1995; 59(29). http://www.themilitant.com/1995/5929/5929_9.html (Accessed September 6, 2015).

118. Neal S. Daley's leadership wilted in heat crises. *Chicago Sun Times* July 25, 1995: 25.

119. Mitchell MA. Daley details heat emergency plan: call for alerts, outreach to elderly. *Chicago Sun Times* July 21, 1995: 3.

120. Mooney C. Some like it hot. *Mother Jones* May/June 2005: 42.

121. WHO. *Working Paper of the Fourth Ministerial Conference on Environment and Health, Budapest, Hungary, 23–35 June 2004*. Geneva, WHO Europe, 2004.

122. Kirch W, Menne B, Bertolini R, eds. *Extreme Weather Events and Public Health Responses*. Berlin/Heidelberg, Springer-Verlag, 2005.

123. Menne B, Ebi KL, eds. *Climate Change and Adaption Strategies for Human Health*. Berlin/Heidelberg, Springer-Verlag, 2006.

124. Samuelson RJ. Global Warming's Real Inconvenient Truth. *The Washington Post*, Blog July 5, 2006. http://www.washingtonpost.com/wp-dyn/content/article/2006/07/04/AR2006070400789.html (Accessed September 6, 2015).

125. CDC. Extreme Heat: A Prevention Guide to Promote Your Personal Health and Safety. http://www.bt.cdc.gov/disasters/extremeheat/heat_guide.asp (Accessed December 13, 2008).

126. Khogali M. Heat illness alert program. Practical implications for management and prevention. *Ann NY Acad Sci* 1997; 813: 530–532.

127. American Medical Association Council on Scientific Affairs. Heat-Related Illness During Extreme Weather Emergencies. Report 10 of the Council on Scientific Affairs (A-97). Presented at the 1997 AMA Annual Meeting.

128. Madon S, Sahay S. ICTs and cities in the developing world: A network of flows. *Inform Technol People* 2001; 14(3): 273–286.

129. Ajayi J. Development: From Slums to Sustainability. (June 16, 2003) From the IPS (Inter Press Service) for Journalism and Communications for Global Change. http://ipsnews.net/news.asp?idnews/33650 (Accessed January 13, 2007).

130. Neuwirth R. *Shadow Cities: A Billion Squatters. A New Urban World*. New York/London, Routledge, 2006; 9.

131. World Bank. Poverty and climate change: Reducing the Vulnerability of the Poor Through Adaption. http://siteresources.worldbank.org/INTCC/817372–1115381292846/20480614/PovertyAndClimateChangePresentation2003.pdf (Accessed December 13, 2008).

132. *World Urban Forum III. Our Future: Sustainable Cities*. UN Habitat. Background Paper. 2006.

133. Perkins S. Dead heat: the health consequences of global warming could be many. *Science News* 2004; 166(1): 10. http://www.phschool.com/science/science_news/articles/dead_heat.html (Accessed December 13, 2008).

134. Valente M. 2006. Open Sewers a Health and Environmental Risk. From the IPS (Inter Press Service) for Journalism and Communications for Global Change. http://ipsnews.net/news.asp?idnews/33012 (Accessed January 13, 2007).

135. Brietzke P. The politics of legal reform. Washington University. *Global Studies Law Rev* 2004; 3(1): 1–47, at 4–12. Id. at 4–5, 6–9, 11.

136. Brietzke P. Democratization and . . . administrative law. *Oklahoma Law Rev* 1999; 52: 1–47, at 43–47, passim.

137. Brietzke P, Adrianopoli C. Climate change in cities of the developing world. *Journal of Environmental Law and Litigation*. 2010; 25: 85–121.

138. UN International Strategy for Disaster Reduction. *Hyogo Framework for Action. 2005–2015: Building the Resilience of Nations and Communities to Disasters*. Extract from the final report of the World Conference on Disaster Reduction (A/CONF.206/6). http://www.unisdr.org/files/1037_hyogoframeworkforactionenglish.pdf (Accessed September 6, 2015).

139. The Hyogo Framework for Action 2005–2015: Building the Resilience of Nations and Communities to Disasters. Hyogo, International Strategy for Disaster Reduction. www.unisdr.org/wcdr/intergover/official-doc/L-docs/Hyogo-framework-for-action-english.pdf (Accessed December 13, 2008).

140. Sabatier PA, Jenkins-Smith HC. The advocacy coalition framework: an assessment. In: Sabatier PA, ed. *Theories of the Policy Process*. Davis, CA, Westview Press, 1999; 117–166.

141. Jamison D, Breman J, Measham A, et al. *Priorities in Health: The Disease Control Priorities Project*. Washington, DC, The World Bank, 2006; 27–31.

142. Sheridan SC, Kalkstein LS. Progress in heat watch-warning system technology. *Bull Am Meteorolog Soc* 2004; 85: 1931–1941.

143. Committee on the Future of Emergency Care in the United States Health System, IOM of the National Academies. *Hospital-Based Emergency Care: At the Breaking Point.* Washington, DC, National Academies Press, 2006; 1.

144. Hill M, Hupe P. *Implementing Public Policy: Governance in Theory and in Practice.* London, Sage Publications, 2002; 1–40.

145. Wagner R. Using Remotely Senses Imagery to Detect Urban Change: Viewing Detroit from Space. *JAPA* 2001; 76: 327.

146. Hanna KS. The paradox of participation and the hidden role of information. *JAPA* 2000; 66: 398.

147. Kartz JD. Rational arguments and irrational audiences. *JAPA* 1989; 55: 445.

148. Taylor NT. Mistaken interests and the discourse model of planning. *JAPA* 1998; 64: 64–75.

149. Innes JE. Planning through consensus building: a new view of the comprehensive planning ideal. *JAPA* 1996; 62: 460–472.

150. Wilson RW, Payne M, Smith E. Does discussion enhance rationality? A report from transportation planning practice. *JAPA* 2003; 69: 354–367.

151. Bollens SA. Urban planning and intergroup conflict: confronting a fractured public interest. *JAPA* 2002; 68: 22–42.

152. Cartwright TJ. Planning theory and chaos. *JAPA* 1991; 57: 44–56.

42

LANDSLIDES

Iain T. R. Kennedy, David N. Petley, and Virginia Murray

OVERVIEW

Mass movements of dry materials, commonly referred to as landslides, occur frequently, and are increasing around the globe. While technical and geological aspects of landslides are well documented, details of the health and social impacts, and the challenges of rescue and recovery from these disasters are less well researched.

After defining landslides, including classification types and common features, this chapter describes their epidemiologic features. Found everywhere there are slopes, landslides are particularly common around the Himalayan belt, Central America, Caribbean, and in the Pacific, especially the Philippines and Indonesia. Data suggest there were over 80,000 deaths attributable to landslides in one 7-year period.[1]

Direct causes of mortality are typically related to suffocation or asphyxiation from becoming entrapped in the landmass; however other landslide effects are less clearly explained. Mental health consequences are the best described, with high rates of post-traumatic stress disorder (PTSD) and major depressive disorder.[2,3,4] The evidence suggests that landslide survivors may have worse mental health outcomes than the survivors of other disasters, notably floods.[3,5] Physical health outcomes include direct injuries, which can result in crush syndrome, and indirect effects, including increases in infectious diseases, notably malaria.

The keys to reducing the medical and health effects of landslides are disaster risk reduction and mitigation strategies. This chapter describes projects of different scales in variable locations – from the comprehensive system in Hong Kong, to low-cost local projects in the Caribbean. These case study descriptions demonstrate that disaster risk reduction measures are possible in any setting.

Finally this chapter calls for further research into the impacts of landslides and the policies and procedures for immediate response and recovery. Compared to other disaster types, these areas have been relatively neglected, and would benefit from better documentation and analysis. Findings from such studies would help improve the preparation for and response to landslides.

CURRENT STATE OF THE ART

Definition

Landslides are defined as the "downhill and outward movement of slope-forming materials under the influence of gravity."[6] They include a wide variety of phenomena, including rockfalls, debris flows, rock avalanches and soil slides, but exclude avalanches primarily consisting of snow and/or ice. Landslides are commonly triggered by intense or prolonged rainfall; earthquakes; snowmelt and human activity, although a small proportion result from forces acting within the slope and have no external trigger. Research into the mechanisms and impacts of landslides is extensive and detailed; Clague and Stead provide a 2012 state-of-the-art review.[7] However, investigations of the health and social consequences of landslides remain scarce. Research in these areas is urgently needed given the incidence of landslides is increasing with time.[8] This trend is likely to continue due to a combination of population increases (especially in Asia), migration to poorly planned communities on steep slopes on the margins of urban areas, increases in rainfall intensity, and the conversion of forest land to agriculture.

Landslides are important both for their ubiquity – instances have been recorded in every global environment in which slopes are present – and for the role they play in increasing the impact of other hazards. During the 2008 Wenchuan (Sichuan) earthquake in China, nearly 200,000 landslides were triggered,[9] directly killing more than 20,000 people.[10] In the aftermath of the earthquake, rescue and recovery operations were severely hampered by the blockage of roads by landslides.[11] Given the short time window for rescuing victims trapped in buildings, landslides effectively increase the mortality rate from the primary hazards. Finally, considerable resources had to be diverted from rescue operations toward mitigating landslides that had blocked river channels, which created unstable lakes that threatened over 1 million people in the event of a catastrophic collapse of the barrier.[12]

Types of Landslides and Their Characteristics

The nature of the impacts caused by landslides is closely related to their mechanisms of movement. Landslides are commonly

Table 42.1. The simple landslide classification based on movement mechanism and material type.

Mechanism of movement			Type of material		
			Bedrock	Engineering soils	
				Predominantly fine	Predominantly coarse
Falls			Rockfall	Earth fall	Debris fall
Topples			Rock topple	Earth topple	Debris topple
Slides	Rotational		Rock slump	Earth slump	Debris slump
	Translational	Few units	Rock block slide	Earth block slide	Debris block slide
		Many units	Rock slide	Earth slide	Debris slide
Lateral spreads			Rock spread	Earth spread	Debris spread
Flows			Rock flow	Earth flow	Debris flow
			Rock avalanche		Debris avalanche
			Deep creep	Soil creep	
Complex and compound			Combination in time and/or space of two or more principal types of movement		

From Varnes D. Figure 2.1 in Chapter 2: Slope Movement Types and Processes. In: Special Report 176: Landslides: Analysis and Control. Copyright, National Academy of Sciences, Washington, DC, 1978. Reproduced with permission of the Transportation Research Board.

classified according to the materials from which they are formed (generally subdivided into rock, debris, and soil) and the dominant nature of the movement (typically falling, sliding, or flowing) (Table 42.1).[13] In the context of landslide impacts it is also useful to consider rates of movement. Some very large landslides (often with masses in excess of 1 billion metric tons) travel at rates in the order of millimeters per year, and pose no direct threat to life, while a single, free-falling 1-kg block can be fatal. However, in general, larger landslides cause greater levels of fatalities, especially when rates of movement are high. For example, 80% of deaths caused by landslides in Italy resulted from rapid events, such as debris flows and mudflows. However, when slower-moving landslides do cause fatalities, the number of lives lost in each event tends to be higher than for the more rapid events. This is likely due to unanticipated building collapses.[14]

As landslides often contain dense materials like rock, soil, or debris mixed with water and travel at high speeds, human bodies are extremely vulnerable to their impacts. Survival usually requires either protection from a hard structure, such as a building or vehicle, or that the victim remains on the surface of the landslide. When unprotected victims become incorporated into the landslide, mortality is very high, such as in the Beichuan Middle School event where there were over 800 victims and no reported survivors (Figure 42.1).

While landslides are ubiquitous in areas with slopes, their highest rates of occurrence are in areas with high relief, steep gradients, weak materials, and energetic triggering events. Highest rates of landsliding are recorded in mountains through the Alpine–Himalayan belt; in tropical volcanic areas such as the Indonesian archipelago and the Philippines; and in steep areas (even if the total elevation is low) affected by tropical cyclones, such as Taiwan, Hong Kong and southwestern China. Finally, human activities are important in determining patterns of occurrence of landslides. In many cases, people increase landslide

occurrences. For example, landslides are common on reservoir banks created by large dams.[15] Furthermore, in Nepal, landslide occurrence has been greatly increased by the construction of poorly designed and engineered rural roads.[16] On the other hand, in Hong Kong a major program of slope management and engineering over a 30-year period has probably reduced landslide occurrence to significantly lower than its natural background rate.

Landslide Epidemiology

Data on the impact of landslides in terms of global loss of life over a 7-year period (2004–2010) are available in the Durham Fatal Landslide Database, compiled by Petley.[1] Investigators collected information on a daily basis through disaster management agency data sets, newspaper reports, scientific papers, and local correspondents. The researchers report a total of 80,058 deaths (estimated error –5/+20%).[16] Of these, 47,736 were attributable to landslides triggered by earthquakes, with the majority of the remainder being associated with intense rainfall events. This analysis excluded morbidity data, although numbers of injured persons associated with each landslide were recorded for rainfall-induced landslides. Fatality data are collected for earthquake-induced landslides (for example, hundreds of the 8,900 fatalities resulting from the 25 April 2015 Nepal earthquake resulted from landslides),[17] but numbers of injuries are not known as this information is not recorded by agencies responding to such events. As the physics of seismically induced and other landslides are the same, and the vulnerable populations are also similar, the ratio of deaths to injuries may be broadly similar.

To date, no systematic quantitative analysis has been undertaken of injury versus fatality rates for landslides. Researchers performed an analysis of the Durham Fatal Landslide Database for rainfall-induced landslides. Globally, the data indicate there

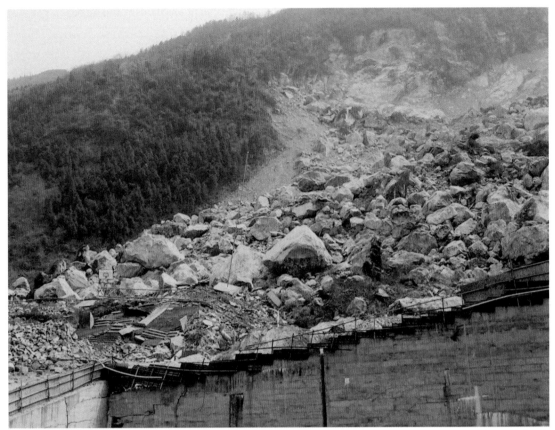

Figure 42.1. Beichuan Middle School landslide, China, 2008. Unprotected victims were incorporated into the landslide, resulting in over 800 victims with no survivors. © David Petley http://blogs.agu.org/landslideblog/2009/03/25/beichuan-photos-of-the-aftermath-of-a-natural-catastrophe.

were 32,322 fatalities and 9,408 reported physical injuries for the 2,620 landslide events in the database, a 77.5% mortality rate. This rate, which is unusually high when compared with other hazards, is a consequence of the extremely violent physical processes associated with landslide events.

Haiti has the highest mortality rate (99.8%) and Norway the lowest (32.6%), suggesting that availability of well-equipped rescue teams and high-quality medical care both at the landslide sites and in the prehospital and hospital environments might be a critical factor in determining this ratio. It is likely that, if similar resources were available in poor countries as are available in the more developed world, then the mortality rate from landslides would be reduced. This pattern is reproduced on a continental basis (Figure 42.2). The highest mortality ratio is recorded in the Caribbean; in this case the data are dominated by the ratio in Haiti. High ratios are also recorded in Central and South America, and Africa. The lowest ratio is recorded in Europe, reflecting the availability of high-quality medical care and rapid emergency response. The low ratio in central Asia may signify the continued existence of disaster management agencies begun in the Soviet era. The low ratio in Southeast Asia could be explained by the influence of the Philippines and Indonesia, both of which have comparatively strong disaster management agencies, providing a rapid response to landslide accidents.

The spatial distribution of the landslide impacts is heterogeneous, with hotspots located along the Alpine–Himalayan belt (especially in the mountainous areas of India, Pakistan, Nepal, Bhutan, and Bangladesh), Central America, the Caribbean, the Andes (especially in Colombia), the Philippines, and Indonesia (Figure 42.3). This reflects a combination of causal factors for landslides and vulnerable populations.

Data regarding the economic costs of landslides are lacking, but would likely show a reverse pattern to mortality ratios, with the highest monetary losses occurring in mountainous areas of developed countries with significant financial assets. For example, the Bingham Canyon copper mine landslide in April 2013 in the U.S. state of Utah was predicted to inflict net economic

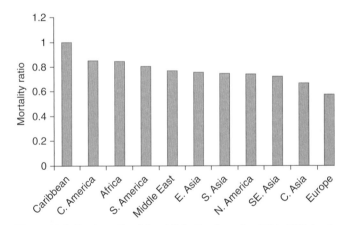

Figure 42.2. Durham Fatal Landslide Database for 2004–2010 landslide mortality ratios by continent (Petley, personal communication, 2013).

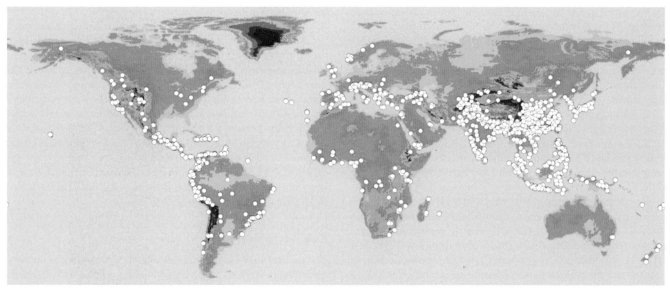

Figure 42.3. In 2004–2010, fatal landslides (white dots) were concentrated in southwestern India, eastern Asia, Central America and the Caribbean. (Petley, personal communication, 2013).

losses in excess of $500 million USD, primarily through lost production in the mine and the costs of excavating the 160 million ton landslide mass.

Health Impacts

As described earlier, a large proportion of direct physical health impacts of landslides are deaths. The most detailed study of a single event[17] examined risk factors for forty-three fatalities during debris flows in Chuuk, Micronesia, in 2002. The predominant cause of death was suffocation caused by being buried in the landslide (39/43), with one victim suffering blunt trauma including severe head injury. Three people died later of traumatic injuries, one of which was complicated by sepsis. On the day of the event, forty-eight survivors were treated in the emergency department with minor injuries, consisting mainly of lacerations and contusions, with concussions and fractures seen less commonly. A further forty-three survivors were admitted to the hospital due to their injuries.[17]

In this event, being younger than 15 years of age was a statistically significant risk factor for increased mortality. Awareness that landslides had recently occurred in the vicinity, and being aware of hazard warning signs, such as "rumbling water," lowered mortality risk. However, no association between the size of the landslide or the slope angle and its impact on health was found.

Even when the victim is not buried by the landslide, injury can be sustained from being struck by rocks or other debris.[18] Landslides also cause indirect health impacts by destroying road and rail links; for example, there are reports of fatalities caused by vehicles striking landslide debris.[19]

Because of the significant weight of debris, landslide survivors are susceptible to crush syndrome, which is characterized by rhabdomyolysis, renal failure, and hyperkalaemia.[20] In severe cases, crush syndrome leads to development of multiorgan pathologies and ultimately death. Although crush syndrome is a common cause of death after disasters, it is treatable, particularly if detected early. Fluid resuscitation and dialysis are mainstays of treatment (see Chapter 38).[21]

Post-Disaster Infectious Diseases

As with other disasters, landslides are associated with outbreaks of infectious diseases. As landslides tend to destroy infrastructure such as housing and community facilities, temporary facilities are used. These facilities can promote infectious disease. For example, a study of a post-landslide camp in Eastern Uganda found there was insufficient access to clean water or latrines, which was exacerbated by many residents using a river water source, despite it being contaminated. There was significant burden of infectious disease, with 8.8% of respondents reporting a household member having diarrhea. However, respiratory infections (58.3% of respondents) and malaria (47.7% of respondents) were more common.[22]

Increase in malaria incidence has been reported elsewhere, including during landslides after the 1991 Costa Rica earthquake. Depending on the region of the country, peak monthly reported rates were between 1,600% and 4,700% higher than the pre-earthquake rates. Landslides were a key factor in this, as they induced deforestation and changes in river flow patterns, which in turn increased mosquito breeding.[23]

Landslides can also directly pollute water supplies through disruption of normal waste management systems and the transportation of soil and other materials into water courses. For example, after a landslide in the Karnaphuli Estuary, Bangladesh, in May 2007, there was a rise in bacterial growth, including a 10-fold increase in fecal coliforms. There was also an upsurge of *Vibrio cholerae* populations, though this was smaller than after the preceding typhoon.[24]

Psychosocial Effects and Impacts on Mental Health

Landslides can significantly impact psychosocial and mental health. Mental health, particularly PTSD, is the most-studied health impact from landslides. Although some of the literature is old, and the diagnostic criteria have changed several times since their publication, they demonstrate that PTSD and major depressive disorder (MDD) are common among landslide survivors in settings as diverse as Italy, Mexico, Puerto Rico, and Taiwan.

A controlled prevalence study after the 1998 landslide disaster in Sarno, Italy, demonstrated that survivors were twenty times more likely than members of a control group to suffer from PTSD (27.6% vs. 1.4%). One year after the disaster, PTSD symptoms were nearly universal in the population of Sarno, with 90% of the study sample displaying PTSD symptoms relating to intrusive experiences.[2]

In 2010, Typhoon Morokot triggered landslides across much of southern Taiwan, killing 650 people. Diagnostic interviews with 277 adolescents displaced by landslides found 25.8% of the adolescents had PTSD 3 months after the disaster. Female gender, being injured during the landslide, and bereavement as a result of the disaster were all associated with increased PTSD risk.[3]

Researchers also studied the effects of a variety of factors on suicide risk in this population. Factors associated with a direct effect on increased suicide risk were female gender, higher frequencies of experiences of being exposed to disasters, PTSD, and MDD. High perceived levels of family support were found to have a protective effect. These data, however, may not be applicable to other populations as they describe a small group of adolescents who survived some of the worst effects of the disaster.[4]

Landslides have been reported to have more severe psychosocial impacts than other disaster types. The authors of the Taiwan study contrasted the prevalence of PTSD in their cohort of 25.8% with a prevalence of 4.5% in a similar cohort after a 1999 earthquake in Greece. Similarly, after an extreme rainfall event in Mexico in 1999, a longitudinal study of people from a locality affected primarily by landslides was compared with people from an area affected by flooding. The landslide survivors had a higher prevalence of PTSD (46%), as measured by diagnostic interviews 6 months post-disaster, compared to the group exposed to flooding (14%). Although the prevalence dropped faster in the landslide survivors, the rate remained higher than for the flooding group (19% vs. 8% at the end of a 2-year follow-up period).[5] While both studies have confounding factors, the type of disaster may account for some of these differences.

Separate from psychological, social impacts were also measured for the Mexico event.[25] Subjects who experienced landslides were more likely: to have been bereaved (60.0% vs. 12.8%); to have lost larger amounts of property (58.5% vs. 44.2%); to have new interpersonal conflicts (29.8% vs. 19.4%); or to have had changes in social networks (social withdrawal) (71.2% vs. 60.9%) than those from flood-affected areas. These factors reduce community resilience. Women generally perceived they had received less social support than did men.

The role of social support in families was also studied after landslides in Puerto Rico in 1985. Alcohol use, depression and total psychiatric symptomatology were found to be higher when there was a lower level of emotional support. Examining the role of family support, contrary to the authors' hypothesis, single and married parenthood did not affect level of symptoms, whereas those without spouses or children had the highest levels of alcohol use.[26]

The 1985 Puerto Rico landslide event was compared to that of survivors of a flood and resultant chemical release in the U.S. city of St. Louis in 1982–1983, where there was a different pattern of psychosocial response. In St. Louis, married parents not directly exposed to the disaster fared best, while married parents who were exposed to the disaster, and single parents regardless of their exposure status, had similar levels of psychological symptomology. The variable exposures of the two groups, methodological differences, and unknown confounders may account for

the disparity in psychosocial response; however, the distinctive cultural responses of the two groups may also have contributed.[26]

A further study of the 1985 Puerto Rico disaster highlighted the importance of the role of cultural norms in disaster response. Investigators used modified diagnostic interviews to assess the prevalence of "*ataques de nervios*" (literally "attack of nerves"). While described in the paper as a "Puerto Rican popular category of distress," and considered to be culturally "normal" in that community, some of the accounts of survivors' *ataques de nervios* symptoms appear sufficiently serious to suggest they would meet diagnostic criteria for acute stress reactions or other psychological disorders.[27] In fact, survivors who described *ataques de nervios* were more likely to have a mental disorder such as PTSD or major depressive disorder.[28]

Risk Perception

The perception of disasters is mediated by a number of factors, including the type of disaster, previous experience with disasters, gender (e.g., men consider hazards less risky than women), and length of education (in years).[29] Researchers describe that survivors of landslides report higher negative perceptions of control and impact from these events than survivors of floods.

The complexity of risk perception is demonstrated in the high landslide risk area of La Paz, Brazil. Known risk, a lack of trust in city officials, a "culture of silence," vested interests, and political implications of alternate strategies resulted in the building of housing, much of it illegal, on high-risk slopes around La Paz. Nathan showed that the occupation of dangerous slopes can be explained as a rational attempt by local people to build resilience to political and social threats, which they perceive as being greater risks than landslides.[30]

In their 2001 study of a landslide in a U.S. National Park, De Chano and Butler demonstrated that the risk perception of those not caught in a landslide does not change after the event, even with respect to the locations where landslides might occur.[31] However, perceptions of the authorities' response to the disaster can change. After a landslide in Stoze, Slovenia, in 2000, public distrust of later interventions from national agencies was compounded by poor communications, conflicting advice, and lack of enforcement (e.g., by ordering evacuation but not enforcing it).[32]

Mental models, which vary in complexity and accuracy, help individuals perceive risks of activities that have not yet occurred. The mental models for flash floods are more developed than those for landslides;[33] possibly because the physical processes for landslides are less well understood by the public. As personal experience, use of multiple sources of information, and higher levels of fear about the hazard lead to better mental models, educational materials on landslide risk should draw on this personal experience and be visually impactful, including the use of pictures of previous local disasters.

Risk Mitigation/Reduction Measures

Landslide risk management is challenging. In more developed countries, large amounts of resources are spent engineering slopes against failure along transportation lines. For example, railway corridors usually consist of a combination of embankments, which can fail, undercutting the line, and cuttings, which can generate landslides that cover the track. Therefore, sophisticated techniques have been developed to investigate, design, manage, and monitor slopes. These techniques are also widely used along highways in urban areas and to protect mountain communities. Failure rates of engineered slopes are low where these techniques are used, and high levels of safety result.

This is best illustrated by Hong Kong, which has the world's most successful slope management program. In response to a series of landslides in the early to mid-1970s, claiming almost 200 lives, the Hong Kong administration established the Geotechnical Control Office (now the Geotechnical Engineering Office), to manage slopes. A variety of techniques have been used to manage the risk, including:

- relocation of the most exposed communities;
- upgrading of manufactured slopes;
- enforcement of strict design codes;
- accreditation of engineering and geological specialists;
- development of a landslide warning system;
- management of natural catchments likely to generate debris flows; and
- public awareness and information campaigns.

As a result of these techniques, summarized by Hencher and Malone in 2012,[34] there has been a dramatic reduction in loss of lives from landslides in Hong Kong, with only three fatalities having occurred in the last decade.

Similar risk mitigation measures for landslides have been identified by communities in other settings. Researchers studying the response to the Stoze, Slovenia, landslide disaster proposed simple legislation. This required clarifying agency responsibilities, sharing best practices, using local hazard assessment experts in area response teams, development of early warning systems, preparation of effective evacuation plans, and inclusion of disaster risk and response reduction into school curricula as a means of improving local and national interventions.

In Thailand, the installation of community early warning systems, first aid training, evacuation drills, and health education programs helped improve psychological well-being and adaptation (as a human coping mechanism) of the local population.[35] These risk mitigation measures therefore improve the resilience of communities to landslide disasters.

Comprehensive landslide management programs are extremely expensive, even for areas as small as Hong Kong, so are usually not practicable at the national scale. High mountain areas face additional challenges since the slopes are often too large or too remote to allow management in this way. For example, the 2010 Attabad landslide in Northern Pakistan had a volume of about 60 million cubic meters. In this case, management is best achieved through a combination of monitoring coupled with relocation of the most threatened communities and infrastructure when necessary. Landslide hazard mapping can help planners to prevent inappropriate development, although this assumes planning authorities are capable of enforcing the resultant regulations.

Work since 2004 in the East Caribbean covering communities containing unplanned housing, predominantly St. Lucia and Dominica, has demonstrated local implementation of affordable risk reduction strategies. Where implemented, slopes which had previously failed under lower rainfall levels were stable against a 1-in-4-year 24-hour storm and a 1-in-50-year 15-day rainfall. There were additional benefits in economic improvements, government relationships, and community resilience. This pro-gram included an organizational framework which provided engagement with vulnerable communities that allowed them to take ownership, gave project guidance, provided employment by engaging contractors from within the community, and built self-esteem.[36]

Disaster Response and Recovery

The emergency response to landslide disasters is usually led by fire and rescue teams. However, there is little guidance available as to the most appropriate ways to search for trapped victims. The location of a victim within a landslide depends on the nature of the movement. Fall events tend to engulf a victim in situ, whereas slides tend to push victims ahead of the main body of the landslide. Landslides undergoing flow-type movement tend to incorporate victims into the mobile mass, rendering locating them much more difficult.

Without a structure to protect a victim, survival time for an individual who is engulfed by the mass is likely to be short, so response must be rapid. A depth of only 30 cm of beach sand can be sufficient to prevent lung inflation.[37] Hence, with a mass of about 2.5 tons per square meter, wet soil or rock may be fatal at shallow depths. After movement ceases, water within the landslide tends to percolate to the base of the slide, which becomes saturated, potentially drowning victims. The same process can lead to drying out of the upper surface of the landslide, making excavation more difficult. Rescues are often delayed by the need to safeguard the rescue team. Landslide events are frequently followed by subsequent failures; it is not unusual for these to be larger than the original collapse. These secondary collapses are caused by over-steepening of the slope by the initial failure, or because the failed block has split into two or more sections that fail sequentially. In the case of debris flows, twenty or more repeat events may occur during a single rainfall.[38]

Almost all landslides leave scars that initially spall rocks or cause small failures. It is extremely difficult to identify whether these indicate another large failure is imminent, even for experienced landslide practitioners. Fire and rescue teams need to seek specialist advice and use unique monitoring equipment to ensure safety is maintained.[39] Nonetheless, people are successfully rescued from within landslides, especially when protected within a well-constructed building. Extraction of victims is very challenging. The weight of landslide material can make it difficult to move by hand; mechanical excavators are better suited for this task, but their use is complicated when the location of buried victims is unknown. Rescue teams must balance speed against the risk of injuring a victim and their own safety. It is difficult to ensure this balance is achieved.

Delay in use of specialist search and rescue teams, with advanced search technology such as acoustic listening and sonar devices, costs lives. In 2006, there was a 5-day delay in obtaining technical support for search and rescue to a large landslide in the Philippines. Buildings, including a school, were displaced about 500 meters down slope before engulfing victims, such that initial search efforts were focused in the wrong area. In this period, the water table rose and drowned people who might have been saved if technical support had been available at the start of the response.[40]

The expectations after landslides of residents of affected areas and those of response and recovery personnel can be very different. A study from Taiwan showed rescuers and survivors agreed that finance and reimbursement of loss should be the highest priority, and public information the lowest. However, residents felt patient care and supportive activities were the second and third priorities, while rescuers believed command and control was the second priority followed by patient care, with supportive activities being the second-lowest priority. Residents were more likely to prioritize housing, food, and sanitation.

These findings suggest responders are more focused on the immediate rescue phase, and may be less concerned with post-disaster recovery, whereas survivors concentrate on recovering losses. Responders should be sensitive to these motivations when assessing needs of the affected community.[41]

Early integration of recovery in the response phase has been shown to lead to better outcomes. A case study examines the impact of a series of landsides in Guatemala that buried a town, including directly impacting the local hospital.[42] The hospital was operational within 16 days of the disaster at a temporary site. Factors that promoted successful movement from disaster response to recovery included an early shared vision of the recovery process. Local control of funds, good links with external aid agencies, and key personnel being invested in the project also improved the transition to recovery.

In addition to victims of the event, the psychosocial well-being and mental health of rescue workers and their families is at risk during and after disasters. Rescue work is labor-intensive and hazardous, and can be complicated by stressors, including fatigue, frustration, fear for personal safety, personal knowledge of the victims, and media exposure. Programs of psychological support that include on-scene and longer-term follow-up for individuals and families are beneficial.[43] However, there is no evidence that single session individual psychological debriefing is beneficial and it may even increase rates of PTSD (see Chapter 9).[44]

RECOMMENDATIONS FOR FURTHER RESEARCH

Geological and engineering aspects of landslides are well understood. Further research is needed on the health impacts of landslides, and how to minimize them. The most effective means of search and rescue and strategies for disaster risk reduction for landslides are additional areas where data from scientific studies may help improve response.

Routine collection of information on nonfatal medical and health effects of landslides would allow a better assessment of health burden, allowing investigation of injuries and mental health impacts. Basic studies, such as that reporting on the 2002 event in Micronesia,[18] can be performed to gain a much greater insight into the human impact of landslides. Examination of the cause of death could also be carried out through retrospective review of post-mortem data.

Further research into health impacts will help inform rescue and recovery operations, and ensure providers have the necessary tools to maximize survival rates. More research on how best to integrate response and recovery phases, while concurrently meeting the needs and expectations of local populations, would also be valuable. As described in this chapter, there has already been exemplary landslide risk reduction and mitigation work, including community education and leadership, carried out in a number of different settings, with variable risk and resource levels. Further detailed reporting of these programs would allow the trialing of good practice in other areas to demonstrate portability of disaster risk reduction measures for landslides. Additionally,

results of studies of disaster risk reduction and mitigation from other disasters could be better leveraged to identify best practices for landslide events.

Acknowledgments

The authors would like to thank Professor Richard Williams, OBE, TD, FRCPsych, DMCC, Professor of Mental Health Strategy, Welsh Institute for Health and Social Care University of Glamorgan, Cardiff, and Pontypridd, and Honorary Consultant Disaster Psychiatrist, Public Health England, for his advice and guidance.

REFERENCES

1. Petley DN. Global patterns of loss of life from landslides. *Geology* 2012; 40(10); 927–930.

2. Catapano F, Malafronte R, Lepre F, et al. *Psychological consequences of the 1998 landslide in Sarno*, Italy: A community study. *Acta Psychiatrica Scandinavica* 2001; 104(6): 438–442.

3. Yang P, Yen C-F, Tang T-C, et al. Post-traumatic stress disorder in adolescents after Typhoon Morakot-associated mudslides. *Journal of Anxiety Disorders* 2011; 25(3): 362–368.

4. Tang TC, Yen CF, Cheng CP, et al. Suicide risk and its correlate in adolescents who experienced typhoon-induced mudslides: a structural equation model. *Depression & Anxiety* 2010; 27(12): 1143–1148.

5. Norris FH, Murphy AD, Baker CK, Perilla JL, Post-disaster PTSD over four waves of a panel study of Mexico's 1999 flood. *Journal of Traumatic Stress* 2004; 17(4): 283–292.

6. Cruden DM, Varnes DJ. Landslide Types and Processes. In: Turner AK, Schuster RL, eds. *Landslides: Investigation and Mitigation*. Washington, DC, Transport Research Board Special Report 1996; 247: 26–75.

7. Clague JJ, Stead D, eds. *Landslides Types, Mechanisms and Modeling*. Cambridge, Cambridge University Press, 2012.

8. Clague JJ, Roberts NJ. Landslide hazard and risk. In: Clague JJ, Stead D, eds. *Landslides Types, Mechanisms and Modeling*. Cambridge, Cambridge University Press, 2012.

9. Xu C, Xu X, Yao X, Dai F. Three (nearly) complete inventories of landslides triggered by the May 12, 2008 Wenchuan Mw 7.9 earthquake of China and their spatial distribution statistical analysis. *Landslides* June 2014; 11(3): 441–461.

10. Yin Y, Wang F, Sun P. Landslide hazards triggered by the 2008 Wenchuan earthquake, Sichuan, China. *Landslides* 2009; 6(2): 139–152.

11. Marui H, Nadim F. Landslides and multi-hazards. In: Sassa K, Canuti P, eds. *Landslides – Disaster Risk Reduction*. Berlin, Springer-Verlag, 200: 435–449.

12. Cui P, Dang C, Zhuang J, et al. Landslide-dammed lake at Tangjiashan, Sichuan province, China (triggered by the Wenchuan Earthquake, May 12, 2008): risk assessment, mitigation strategy, and lessons learned. *Enviro Earth Sci* 2012; 65(4): 1055–1065.

13. Varnes. D. Slope Movement Types and Processes. In: Schuster RL, Krizek RJ, eds. *Landslides, analysis and control*. Transportation Research Board Sp. Rep. No. 176, Nat. Acad. of Sciences, 1978; 11–33.

14. Guzzetti F, Stark CP, Salvati P. Evaluation of flood and landslide risk to the population of Italy. *Environmental Management* 2005; 36(1): 15–36

15. Petley DN. Large landslides and dams; International conference, Vajont. Thoughts and analyses after 50 years since

the catastrophic landslide; October 2013. http://blogs.agu.org/landslideblog/2013/11/20/landslides-and-large-dams/ (Accessed September 5, 2015).

16. Petley DN, Hearn GJ, Hart A, Rosser NJ, Dunning SA, Oven K, Mitchell WA. Trends in landslide occurrence in Nepal. *Natural Hazards* 2007; 43(1): 23–44.

17. Sanchez C, Lee T-S, Young S, et al. Risk factors for mortality during the 2002 landslides in Chuuk, Federated States of Micronesia. *Disasters* 2009; 33(4): 705–720.

18. Kariya Y, Sato G, Mokudai K, et al. Rockfall hazard in the Daisekkei Valley, northern Japanese Alps, on 11 August 2005. *Landslides* 2007; 4: 91–94.

19. Guzzetti F, Reichenbach P, Cardinali M, et al. The impact of landslides in the Umbria region, central Italy. *Natural Hazards and Earth System Science* 2003; 3: 469–486.

20. Redmond AD. ABC of conflict and disaster: natural disasters. *BMJ* 2005; 330(7502): 1259–1261.

21. Sever MS, Vanholder R, Lameire N. Management of crush-related injuries following disasters. *N Engl J Med* 2006; 354: 1052–1063.

22. Atuyambe LM, Ediau M, Orach CG, et al. Landslide disaster in eastern Uganda: rapid assessment of water, sanitation and hygiene situation in Bulucheke camp, Bududa district. *Environmental Health* 2011; 10: 38.

23. Saenz R, Bissell RA, Paniagua F. Post-disaster malaria in Costa Rica. *Prehosp and Disaster Med* 1995; 10(3): 154–160.

24. Lara RJ, Neogi SB, Islam MS, et al. Influence of catastrophic climatic events and human waste on Vibrio distribution in the Karnaphuli estuary, Bangladesh. *EcoHealth* 2009; 6(2): 279–286.

25. Norris FH, Baker CK, Murphy AD, Kaniasty K. Social support mobilization and deterioration after Mexico's 1999 flood: Effects of context, gender, and time. *American Journal of Community Psychology* 2005; 36(1–2): 15–28.

26. Solomon SD, Bravo M, Rubio-Stipec M, Canino G. Effect of family role on response to disaster. *Journal of Traumatic Stress* 1993; 6(2): 255–269.

27. *Diagnostic and Statistical Manual of Mental Disorders.* 5th ed. Washington, DC, American Psychiatric Association, 2013.

28. Saenz R, Bissell RA, Paniagua F. Post-disaster malaria in Costa Rica. *Prehosp and Disaster Med* 1995; 10(3): 154–160.

29. Ho M-C, Shaw D, Lin S, Chiu Y-C. How Do Disaster Characteristics Influence risk perception? *Risk Analysis* 2008; 28: 3.

30. Nathan F. *Risk perception, risk management and vulnerability to landslides in the hill slopes in the city of La Paz,* Bolivia. A preliminary statement. *Disasters* 2008; 32: 3.

31. DeChano LM, Butler DR. Analysis of public perception of debris flow hazard. *Disaster Prevention and Management* 2001; 10(4): 261–269.

32. Mikos M. Public perceptions and stakeholder involvement in the crisis management of sediment related disasters and their mitigation: The case of the Stože debris flow in NW Slovenia. *Integrated Environmental Assessment and Management* 2011; 7(2): 216–277.

33. Wagner K. Mental Models of Flash Floods and Landslides. *Risk Analysis* 2007; 27(3): 671–682.

34. Hencher SR, Malone AW. Hong Kong Landslides. In: Stead D, Clague J, eds. *Landslides types, mechanisms and monitoring.* Cambridge, Cambridge University Press, 2012; 373–382.

35. Oba N, Suntayakorn C, Sangkaewsri R, et al. The enhancement of adaptation and psychological well-being among victims of flooding and landslide in Thailand. *J Med Assoc Thai* 2010; 93(3): 351–357.

36. Anderson MG, Holcombe E, Esquivel M, Toro J. The efficacy of a programme of Landslide Risk Reduction in areas of unplanned housing in Eastern Caribbean, Ghesquiere. *Environmental Management* 2010; 45: 807–821.

37. Zarroug AE, Stavlo PL, Kays GA, et al. Accidental burials in sand: A potentially fatal summertime hazard. *Mayo Clinic Proceedings* 2004; 79: 774–776.

38. Jakob M, Hingr O. *Debris flow hazards and related phenomena.* Berlin, Spring-Praxis, 2005; 739.

39. Hervas J. *Lessons learnt from landslide disasters in Europe.* Ispra, Nedies Project Report EUR 20558 N, JRC, 2003; 91 pp.

40. Lagmay AMA, Tengonciang AMP, Rodolfo RS, et al. Science guides search and rescue after the 2006 Philippine landslide. *Disasters* 2008; 32: 416–433.

41. Lam C, Lin M-R, Tsai S-H, et al. Comparison of expectations of residents and rescue providers of community emergency response after mudslide disasters. *Disasters* 2007; 31(4): 405–416.

42. Peltan ID. Disaster relief and recovery after a landslide at a small, rural hospital in Guatemala. *Prehosp and Disaster Med* 2009; 24(6): 542–548.

43. Clifford B. The New South Wales Fire Brigades' critical incident stress management response to the Thredbo Landslide. *International Journal of Emergency Mental Health* 1999; 1/2: 127–133.

44. Rose SC, Bisson J, Churchill R, Wessely S. Psychological debriefing for preventing post traumatic stress disorder (PTSD). *Cochrane Database of Systematic Reviews* 2002, 2; Art. No. CD000560.

43

VOLCANOES

Peter J. Baxter

OVERVIEW

Introduction

An understanding of how people are killed and injured in volcanic eruptions is essential for advancing disaster mitigation, as well as for managing casualties in actual events (Table 43.1).[1] The main aims of mitigation, one of the four phases of comprehensive emergency management, are the prevention of direct human deaths and injury and reduction of economic losses that can adversely affect health through poverty and social inequalities.[1] A surprisingly large number of lethal phenomena are associated with eruptions, and health hazards can arise even when volcanoes lie dormant. Compared with floods, windstorms and earthquakes, volcanic eruptions occur much less frequently. In recent decades there were on average only two to four events worldwide per year that involved fatalities and most people living in active volcanic regions have only a low statistical risk of a serious event happening in their lifetimes. However, the inexorable growth of populations around volcanoes is increasing the likelihood that eruptions will have much more dramatic impacts in the twenty-first century, as presaged at the last eruption of Merapi, the most active volcano in Indonesia. The population on its slopes has surpassed 1 million. While the populace has been living harmoniously with its small eruptions every 4–6 years and the attendant small loss of life, in October–November 2010 an unexpected and sudden escalation of explosive activity led to the emergency evacuation of 400,000 people to official shelters, the destruction of thousands of homes, and over 200 people being killed before they could escape from its extensive pyroclastic flows.[2]

The resurgence of a dormant volcano in a densely populated area should trigger a state of emergency, like a warning for an approaching hurricane or storm surge. Forecasting an eruption in a state of unrest requires a team of experienced volcanologists equipped with the latest monitoring technology to make a rapid appraisal based on what is known about the particular volcano and by drawing on analogies from similar volcanoes and how they behave. Although most of these potential crises do not lead to a major eruption, and states of unrest can remain in place for years, the scientific uncertainty surrounding eruption fore-

Table 43.1. Main Injury Agents in Volcanic Eruptions

Hazard	Injury Agent	Impact
Flow Processes		
Pyroclastic flows & surges	Heat	Skin & inhalation burns
	Dynamic pressure	Body displacement
	Hot particles	Asphyxia
	Missiles	Multiple Trauma
Lahars	Lateral loading & crushing	Multiple Trauma
		Traumatic asphyxia
	Slurry	Asphyxia, infected wounds
Lava	Radiant heat	Skin burns
Fall Processes		
Tephra	Collapsed roofs	Multiple trauma
	Roofs with ash infill	Asphyxia
	Respirable particles	Exacerbation of existing lung conditions
	Crystalline silica	Silicosis (chronic effect)
	Ballistic projectiles	Multiple trauma
	Pumice/lava fragments	Multiple trauma
Other		
Gases	Irritant acid gases & aerosols	Exacerbation of asthma, bronchitis (sulfur dioxide)
Earthquakes	Collapsing houses	Multiple trauma

casting and the possibility that a serious eruption can happen with little or no warning means that evacuation decisions may have to be made very quickly.[3] As the development of emergency planning at most volcanoes is still in its infancy, a state of unrest at a volcano usually arises in a community with a poor state of

Table 43.2. Best Estimates of the Human Impacts of Twentieth Century Volcanic Events[4]

Human Consequence	Number of Events	Number of People
Killed	260	91,724
Injured	133	16,013
Homeless	81	291,457
Evacuated/affected	248	5,281,906

disaster preparedness. These and other issues surrounding unfamiliarity with volcanic phenomena increase the probability of mass casualties and emphasize the need for health professionals to participate in planning for eruptions. This chapter outlines potential eruption hazards and the key elements of volcanic disaster planning for health sector workers.

Recent Historical Record of Volcanic Eruptions

The most comprehensive database for global volcanic disasters and incidents in the twentieth century (Tables 43.2 and 43.3) shows how the numbers of dead, injured, homeless, and evacuated or otherwise affected persons are attributable to a relatively small number of large events.[4]

The historical record is a poor predictor of present-day volcanic risk. By the end of the twentieth century, about 10% of the world's population was living in areas of active volcanism. No fewer than sixty-seven metropolitan areas with populations of more than 100,000 people are in range of volcanic hazards[5] and there is scant evidence that this knowledge is being used to guide their future development.

Vulnerability to Volcanic Disasters

Volcanic hazards gained worldwide attention in the 1980s after two major eruptions. The cataclysmic explosive eruption of Mount St. Helens in the Cascade Range of the western United States on 18 May 1980, transformed modern volcanology by providing a rare glimpse into the earth's most violent forces. Despite scientists' close monitoring of the volcano for 2 months after a state of unrest began, a giant landslide occurred without any immediate warning, unleashing from the interior of the volcano a directed lateral blast in the form of a pyroclastic surge that destroyed trees in a 180° sector extending as far north as 28 km. Only fifty-seven lives were lost because the volcano was situated in a wilderness, but what if, in the place of the 10 million downed trees, there had been buildings and people?[6] The eruption continued for hours with an ash plume that spread across several states and left central Washington State with near zero visibility for 6 days as the fine ash hung suspended in the air, halting all forms of transport and raising fears about its respiratory health effects.

In 1984 the world was shocked by horrific scenes at Nevado del Ruiz volcano in Colombia, where 23,000 people died mangled and buried in massive volcanic mudflows, known as lahars, which had been triggered by a sudden summit eruption that partially melted the summit glacier, sending torrents of meltwater and pyroclastic debris toward the town of Armero. A warning system was in place, but it was inadequate, and there was no evacuation plan.[7] The blindness of the responsible authorities to the hazard led to this entirely foreseeable and avoidable disaster, and the scale of the tragedy became an important stimulus for the United Nations declaration of the 1990s as the International Decade for Natural Disaster Reduction, the main goal of which was to transfer technology and know-how to developing countries to enable them to improve their mitigation and preparedness for reducing disaster risks. The importance of disaster risk reduction has since become widely accepted and there has been considerable progress in understanding the vulnerability of human beings and their settlements to volcanic eruptions.

Other notable volcanic crises have left their marks, either because of devastating eruptions or, paradoxically, because the

Table 43.3. Top 10 Volcanic Events in the Twentieth Century by Impact[4]

	Killed		*Injured*		*Homeless*		*Evacuated/Affected*	
Rank	Event	Number of People	Event	Number of People	Event	Number of People	Event	Number of People
1.	Pelée, 1902	29,000	Nevado del Ruiz, 1985	4,470	Pinatubo, 1991	53,000	Guagua Pichincha, 1999	1,200,400
2.	Nevado del Ruiz, 1985	23,080	Awu, 1966	2,000	Kelut, 1919	45,000	Pinatubo, 1991	967,443
3.	Santa Maria, 1902	8,750	Ambrym, 1979	1,000	Galunggung, 1982	22,000	Pinatubo, 1992	787,042
4.	Kelut, 1919	5,110	Dieng, 1979	1,000	Pinatubo, 1992	15,700	Agung, 1963	332,234
5.	Santa Maria, 1929	5,000	Lake Nyos, 1986	845	Tokachi, 1926	15,000	Vesuvius, 1906	100,000
6.	Lamington, 1951	2,942	Taal, 1965	785	El Chichón, 1982	15,000	Popocatépetl, 1994	75,000
7.	El Chichón, 1982	2,000	El Chichón, 1982	500	Merapi, 1930	13,000	Soufrière Guadeloupe, 1976	73,500
8.	Lake Nyos, 1986	1,746	Merapi, 1994	500	Merapi, 1961	8,000	Mayon, 1984	73,000
9.	Soufrière St. Vincent, 1902	1,565	Merapi, 1998	314	Soufrière Hills, 1995	7,500	Arenal, 1976	70,000
10.	Merapi, 1930	1,369	Vesuvius, 1906	300	Colo (Una Una), 1983	7,101	Galunggung, 1982	62,755
Total		80,562		11,714		201,301		3,741,374

Table 43.4. Volcanic Crises and Cities since 1980

Campi Flegrei, Italy	1982–1984	Naples
Galeras, Colombia	1989, ongoing	Pasto
Popocatapetl, Mexico	1994	Mexico City, Puebla
Colima, Mexico	1994	Colima
Guagua Pichincha, Ecuador	1998–2001	Quito
Tungurahua, Ecuador	1999, ongoing	Banõs
Reventador, Ecuador	2002	Quito
Nyiragongo, Dem. Rep. Congo	2002, ongoing	Goma
Merapi, Java	2010	Yogyakarta

threat of an eruption failed to materialize (Table 43.4). The former have included El Chichon, Mexico, in 1984 when more than 2,000 people died in pyroclastic flows, and Mt. Pinatubo, Philippines, in 1991, in which more than 300 people died in the ash fallout that collapsed roofs.[8] However, more than 50,000 people were evacuated in time from the paths of lethal pyroclastic flows and surges.[2]

A typical type of "failed eruption" occurred at Guagua Pichincha volcano, which lies close to Quito, the capital city of Ecuador, and the densely populated Inter-Andean valley. Its resumption of activity in 1998 raised widespread concerns of a repeat of its last major eruption in 1660, when heavy ash falls impacted on Quito's city center and lahars (mudflows) triggered by heavy rain on the ash deposits devastated the slopes of the volcano complex, which today are an integral part of the city. In the event, this "worst case" eruption failed to materialize and evacuation and other mitigation measures were unnecessary, but the uncertainty affected the city population of more than 1 million and its economy for several years until the activity finally ceased. Some crises have continued to be unresolved for years, including Galeras, Colombia, near the city of Pasto (200,000 people), and Tungarahua, Ecuador, close to the city of Banõs (25,000 people), with most people having decided to remain in their homes and carry on their lives in the shadows of the restless, unpredictable volcanoes, despite earlier warnings from volcanologists that the populations should move. Galeras began its activity in 1989 and has had several small summit eruptions over the years. Tungurahua volcano in Ecuador had renewed activity on September 14, 1999, and the president of Ecuador ordered a hurried evacuation of the city 3 days later. There were no preparations in place for the relocation of the 25,000 people and by the end of December many had forced their way back into their homes despite the risk of dying in pyroclastic flows. At the time of writing, the threatening state of the volcano remains for the 17,000 people who returned.

These examples show how major volcanic crises and eruptions can continue for years, leading to substantial disruption and impact on local economies as businesses lose confidence and move elsewhere, or wide exclusion zones are established leaving thousands evacuated until the activity eventually declines. These chronic situations are often accompanied by a high level of uncertainty where the people may start to develop a dangerous level of risk fatigue and become less responsive to warnings from scientists monitoring the volcano. Crisis management can therefore be very different from the so-called sudden-onset events like

floods and earthquakes, with which volcanoes are often misleadingly linked. Much of the apparent apathy of government and academia toward volcanic risk mitigation lies in a profound lack of understanding by both of the unique hazards and the complexity of the risks volcanoes can create in densely populated regions, including volcanic islands.

CURRENT STATE OF THE ART

Types of Volcanoes and Their Eruptions

A simplified approach to volcanoes and their hazards is to recognize whether they are mainly explosive or effusive (a non-explosive outpouring of fluid lava) in behavior.[9,10] An essential guide to this is the stratigraphic (geological) record which provides the evidence from past eruptions. Explosive eruptions involve rapid energy changes whereby magma, or molten rock, is so violently expelled from a deeper environment that it fragments into pyroclastic fragments. The silica-rich composition of the magma lends it a high viscosity and these volcanoes are found in subduction zones, an example of which is the Ring of Fire around the Pacific Ocean. Mount St. Helens belongs to this category. The most hazardous and least predictable phenomena of explosive eruptions are pyroclastic density currents (PDCs), also known as pyroclastic flows and surges. These are burning hot clouds of gases and ash that can travel at hurricane speeds for many kilometers and flow over topographic obstacles. Their destructive impacts are due to their velocity and density (dynamic pressure) and high temperatures. Material ejected in eruptions is known as tephra, which includes ash clouds and rapidly cooling rocks with a wide range of sizes (lapilli, clasts, and blocks). Volcanic ash is defined by its diameter (particles less than 2 mm.). Fragmentation of magma may also be produced by steam explosions and the thermal shock when magma comes into contact with water below the earth's surface or when it erupts into surface water, ice or wet sediments. Explosive eruptions are often accompanied by small, viscous lava flows.

At the other end of the spectrum, volcanoes with silica-poor rocks are found mainly at mid-ocean ridges, and most have fluid lava eruptions. The best-known volcanoes with effusive eruptions are on the Big Island of Hawaii. Volcanoes of intermediate magmas can have features of both types. Mount Etna, Italy, is an example of a mainly effusive volcano whose hazard is mostly lava flows, but spectacular eruptions in 2001 and 2002 reminded people that it also has explosive potential. Lava flows are comprised of hot molten rock that ignites or overwhelms objects in its path. Heroic engineering efforts to divert them into less hazardous directions are rarely attempted and have occasionally been met with limited success.

Explosiveness is also governed by the percentage of volatile components (dissolved gases) in the magma. Viscous magmas are more resistant to deformation from the action of forces and mechanical stress, and so the gases do not so readily escape. This leads to increased gas pressure and risk of a sudden, explosive release. Typically, only low levels of pressure develop in eruptions involving more fluid magmas. The main volatiles are water, carbon dioxide, and sulfur dioxide. A small percentage of emissions consist of other gases. These include hydrogen chloride (hydrochloric acid), hydrogen sulfide, and traces of hydrogen, carbon monoxide, and methane.[9] Volcanic gas emissions and gas bursts are human hazards in populated areas.

Locations of Volcanoes

Volcanoes are not found everywhere on earth. Volcanoes and their gas emissions were responsible for the formation of the earth's atmosphere. In modern times, plate tectonics and the volcanism arising from this are likely essential for maintaining the atmosphere in a state that enables life to continue on earth. Eruptions and earthquakes are the deleterious events that maintain this planetary homeostasis. Eighty percent of volcanoes are in subduction zones at convergent plate boundaries, which include the Ring of Fire around the Pacific Ocean (including the Cascades and Mount St. Helens in the United States), and island arcs, such as Indonesia and the islands of the Caribbean; these are explosive. In contrast, about 10% of volcanoes occur at mid-ocean ridges and are effusive.[9] There are about 700 sub-aerial volcanoes in the world, of which 170 are currently active.

Scale of Eruptions

The most devastating eruptions are explosive in nature, but as a general rule large eruptions are uncommon in comparison to small events. Volcanoes that erupt most frequently are likely to be the best studied, for obvious reasons; funding usually exists for scientists to regularly monitor these, especially if they are in densely inhabited areas. The most frequently active volcanoes in Italy and Japan are closely monitored, whereas a lack of resources makes it impossible to focus attention on more than a handful of the 100 known active volcanoes close to large populations in the Indonesian archipelago. When a volcano near a populated area that has been dormant for many years shows signs of activity, scientists will need to install monitoring devices or intensify current monitoring efforts to keep the volcano under close surveillance. If scientists determine that a volcano is beginning to move toward an eruption, they will advise authorities to declare a state of unrest.

The size of an eruption relates to its magnitude (mass of material discharged, or tephra volume) and the intensity or rate of discharge (mass flow rate). A volcanic explosive index (VEI) is a measure of both of these parameters.[9] The largest eruptions are in the super-volcano league, such as Yellowstone, whose eruptions are at average intervals of a hundred thousand years. Yellowstone would impact most of the United States with its ash fall and produce a global catastrophe through persistent atmospheric effects lasting several years after the event. None of these tremendous eruptions has been witnessed in historic times.[11] Eruptions on the scale of Tambora, Indonesia, in 1815, which temporarily lowered global temperatures and triggered crop failures in parts of the world, occur once every several hundred years on average, and an eruption today would have major consequences for global food supplies. A Krakatau-type (Java, 1883) volcano has a frequency in the geological record of about twice every 100 years, and one the size of Mount St. Helens (1980) once every 10 years somewhere in the world. Types of explosive eruptions include the largest and most energetic and destructive – the plinian and sub-plinian, which erupt with heavy ash falls over wide areas and pyroclastic flow activity – to the smaller strombolian and vulcanian, which do not. Plinian eruptions produce high ash and gas-laden atmospheric columns that penetrate into the stratosphere and can interfere with climate and weather on a global scale.[10] Interest in the rarer but high-consequence type of eruption is increasing as the world becomes more aware of the fragility of its ecosystems and climate, and the global interconnections of its economy.[11]

Evaluating Hazards and Risks in Volcanic Eruptions

The main eruptive hazards can be divided into fall and flow processes. Air falls of tephra – airborne fragments of rock and lava of any size or shape expelled during explosive eruptions – are the commonest and most hazardous fall process.

Pyroclastic flows and surges, lahars and debris flows, and lava flows can, for emergency planning purposes, be envisaged by "thinking visually," or intuitively, but their behavior belongs to the world of flow, or fluid dynamics, on which the understanding of the blood circulation, meteorology, and aeronautics is based. The concepts that describe the motions of fluids – viscosity, vorticity, waves, instability, and turbulence – apply to the complexity and behavior of pyroclastic flows and surges, which move along the ground and over obstacles with features of both gases and liquids. This latter feature makes them unpredictable to at least some degree, but advances in computer simulation modeling are enabling scientists to capture some of the main features of their behavior to assist in emergency planning.

Pyroclastic Density Currents

Pyroclastic flows and surges (also called pyroclastic density currents; Box 43.1) are the most hazardous eruptive phenomena. As hot mixtures of particles and gases, they may initially be propelled by volcanic explosions and then move along slopes under gravity, being denser than air despite their high temperature. As well as heat, their hazard is related to lateral loading on structures due to high lateral overpressures which, as pyroclastic flows, can

---

BOX 43.1 Pyroclastic Flows and Surges (Pyroclastic Density Currents)

Pyroclastic surges form more dilute, turbulent suspension clouds than pyroclastic flows and settle when they stop moving into a thin layer of well-sorted and fine-grained deposits. Pyroclastic flows, in contrast, are much denser, having high particle concentrations and are more topographically controlled in that they readily follow valley bottoms and settle as a massive, poorly sorted deposit.[9,10] Many pyroclastic density currents have characteristics of either flows or surges during their run-out, which is why the term has become more widely used for these phenomena.

Another important aspect is the propensity of flows to produce dilute surges that decouple or detach from them and extend beyond where the pyroclastic flow would be expected to travel. Their formation is hard to forecast, but their high temperatures can be lethal and trigger fires (Figure 43.1). All pyroclastic density currents move as gravity (density) currents, being denser than air, and some have extra impetus from explosions at their source in the volcano. Most hazard maps produced for emergency planning for the delineating of evacuation or exclusion zones are governed by the foreseen limits of the pyroclastic density current run-outs, as estimated by volcanologists.

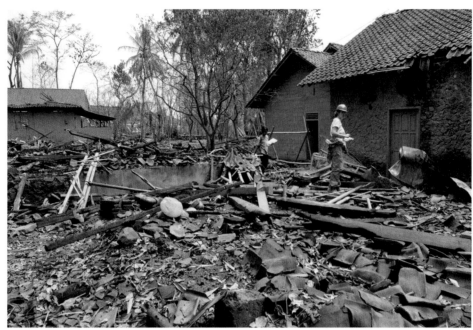

Figure 43.1. Merapi volcano eruption, Indonesia, 2010: Bronggang village. Damage caused by a surge detaching from a pyroclastic flow moving down the nearby Gendol river valley. Destruction of traditional wooden houses by fire, due to firebrands entrained in the surge cloud igniting flammables in lean-tos outside kitchens and then spreading to the interiors of the buildings. Villagers who had failed to evacuate were also killed by the intense heat of the surge (see text).

flatten and bury most things in their paths. This chapter focuses on the human impacts of very violent, dilute surges of moderate volume as they have been responsible for most recent volcanic disasters.[12]

To be caught in a fast-moving dilute surge in the open is almost invariably fatal for human beings. The effects of instantaneous burning heat (temperatures over 200°C), dense and irrespirable concentrations of ash, and lateral loading (dynamic pressure) form a lethal combined impact. At ordinary temperatures, the minimum concentration of inhalable dust (<100μ diameter) capable of causing asphyxia is reported to be 0.1kg/m^3, but this figure is not well founded.[13] Autopsies performed on victims whose bodies could be retrieved from the surge deposits at Mount St. Helens in 1980 showed ash occluding the tracheas or lining the airways.[14]

Exposure to dry, motionless air at 200–230°C can reportedly be survived by a lightly clad person for 2–5 minutes, but in the open, the convective heat transfer from a fast-moving pyroclastic density current at this temperature quickly causes severe thermal injury and rapid death in the absence of protective clothing. Inhaling dry air free from hot particles at this temperature is also tolerable for only a few minutes, but the presence of steam, or water vapor, or inhalable amounts of hot, fine ash reduces the temperature that can be tolerated to below 100°C, because of the risk of thermal injury to the airways in the absence of respiratory protection.[13]

The dose of heat in some dilute pyroclastic density currents may be low enough for a victim to escape severe body burns, especially if the individual is well-protected by clothing, and the duration of exposure is short enough for the hot surge cloud to be replaced by cool air. Pyroclastic density currents push away the air ahead of them and also entrain some air as they flow, but the atmosphere may become intolerable to breathe as well as being low in oxygen. Some survivors talk about gasping for air, or

breathing as if in a vacuum. Some surges may be saturated with water vapor that will increase the amount of heat delivered to the respiratory tract and skin. Humans cannot survive for long breathing saturated air hotter than about 60°C, since at 50°C the heat transfer to the deep lung could be comparable with that of dry air at 200°C, while at 80°C the oxygen concentration of saturated air would be 10–11%, a critically low level not even allowing for the presence of ash particles.[13] Thus, inhalation of saturated air that also contains an abundance of inhalable ash particles at temperatures between 50–100°C could be very hazardous, giving rise to acute bronchoconstriction, pulmonary injury, and hypoxia. A base surge from a steam explosion due to magma–water interaction could also present this hazard. Irritant volcanic gases such as sulfur dioxide might also be present in the surge cloud mixed with the entrained air.

In the outdoors, ordinary clothing may offer little protection and become combusted in the heat of the surge, or be torn off the body by the violence of the surge impact (dynamic pressure). But indoors, or outside under shelter and with brief exposure to the hot current in the periphery of a surge, the heat transfer would be much less so that even light clothing could limit the total body surface area (TBSA) affected. Thus a person wearing a suit might receive a minimum of 20% TBSA burns if the hot ash was in uniform contact with the unprotected exposed skin, whereas for someone with a t-shirt and shorts about 40% TBSA would be affected. These patterns have been observed, for example, in casualties at the eruptions of Unzen, Japan, in 1991 and Merapi, Indonesia, in 2010.

Explosion Hazards to Scientists and Tourists

Although certain eruptions and volcanoes are referred to as explosive, the release of energy is much slower and in a different form than with nuclear weapons or conventional explosives.[12] The "blast wave" of a typical pyroclastic surge has dynamic pressure resulting solely from the lateral loading of the gravity current; there is no peak overpressure as produced in a supersonic wave. Minor explosions from volcanoes can be steam-driven (phreatic) with rocks being hurled without warning from fumaroles or craters that are capable of killing people within range. Six scientists and three tourists were killed in an explosion in the crater at Galeras, Columbia, in 1993 from injuries due to multiple trauma caused by flying rocks blasted from the lava dome.[15]

In most explosive eruptions, shock or blast waves do not usually present hazards far from the eruptive vent. Instead, it is the dynamic pressure and heat of a pyroclastic surge or flow, together with the kinetic energy of entrained loose materials and projectiles that cause the injurious impacts. Velocity measurements of projectiles have been estimated for explosions at the craters in the 1968 eruption at Arenal Volcano (300–400 meters per second) and at Ngauruhoe in 1975 (220–260 meters per second).[16] Although loud sound waves can rattle or even break windows, supersonic blast waves are uncommon and their direct effects are limited mainly to the vicinity of the crater.

Lava Flows

Lava flows from most volcanoes are slow moving. Thus, in contrast to pyroclastic flows and surges, they usually cause few deaths and injuries as people are able to move out of their path in time. The main hazards are from their high temperature (800–900°C) which can cause combustion of buildings by their direct contact or just by radiant heat. Lava flows are notable for engulfing and collapsing buildings in their paths. It is for this destruction of property that they are most feared, although some success has been achieved with diverting lavas, the best example being the intervention of the Italian Civil Protection in the flow from the eruption of Mount Etna in 2003. Sixty-eight lateral vent eruptions have occurred at Mount Etna from 1600 to 2011, but these have been of minimal threat to human life. However, volcanogenic earthquakes arise when fissures open and these can weaken and cause buildings to collapse and occasionally kill people from their cumulative shaking effect.

Secondary hazards from lava flows can arise in several different ways. Lava flows entering the sea generate clouds of steam and hydrogen chloride gas. Occasionally people getting close to still-hot lava flows can be asphyxiated or badly burned in heavy rain because of trapped rainwater suddenly flashing to form a jet of steam. Lava flowing over densely vegetated areas can trap pockets of methane and organics which can then explode and scatter lethal projectiles of lava.[17] More rarely, a lava flow moving down a slope can disintegrate on meeting a sudden incline and form a small but potentially lethal pyroclastic flow.

A few volcanoes in the world can erupt very fluid and fast-moving lava and their lava flows can be highly hazardous. The most important example of this type of volcano is Nyiragongo, located near the city of Goma in the Eastern Democratic Republic of Congo and in the midst of one of the world's worst humanitarian crises. Over 4 million lives have been lost there as a result of conflicts involving local militia groups and their consequences since 1998.[18] In 1977, 500 people living high up on the flanks of the volcano died in a sudden rifting eruption that drained the crater lava lake. The volcano then remained dormant until January 18–19, 2002, when new rifting suddenly extended farther down the flank towards Goma, trapping 170 villagers in flows moving at over 60 km/h. Two main flows reached Goma, by which time they were moving much more slowly, the largest

arriving at about 6:00 PM on the first day. More than 300,000 people escaped from the advancing lava as it drove a path through the city center, destroying the main commercial areas and more than 120,000 homes before the end of the day.[19,20]

The chaotic self-evacuation of the people of Goma and then their rapid return within 2 days before the main lava flow had even ceased flowing raised many concerns about the health hazards they would face. The most important was the risk of outbreaks of endemic cholera and dysentery from the consumption of untreated (chlorinated) water from nearby Lake Kivu, the main source of drinking water. International aid agencies flew workers in to erect emergency chlorination stations and provide water tankers along the side of the lake. The loss of food supplies and charcoal for cooking would have led to hunger very quickly in a population with an already high prevalence of acute malnutrition, but aid workers averted a food crisis. Crowding increased the risk of other infectious disease outbreaks and responders rapidly initiated an immunization campaign (e.g., for measles and meningitis). Most people had to escape from the lava flows with relatively little warning, leaving all their possessions behind. The psychological stress of losing all their property and livelihoods to the lava flows was one of the most significant factors for the population. Only about 13,000 people had to be accommodated in relief camps, the remainder being taken in by relatives or others from the same ethnic group.[19]

The absence of governmental organizations due to the existing complex humanitarian emergency meant that the population was entirely dependent on a swift and effective response by the international agencies and without this, the loss of life from epidemics and other secondary consequences of the eruption would have been much greater.

Lahars

Lahars, or volcanic mudflows, are slurries of water and sediment (60% or more by volume), which can flow at speeds of a few tens of kilometers per hour to more than 100 km per hour on the steep slopes of a volcano. They can flow and set like concrete. In the disaster at Nevado del Ruiz volcano in 1984, in which 23,000 people died, as much as 85% of the town of Armero was left covered in 3–4 meters of hardened mud. In the rescue operation over the following 5 days, 1,244 survivors, mainly from Armero, were admitted to hospitals and 138 of these subsequently died. The lahar struck the town at around 11:30 PM local time and was preceded by a river of water that flowed along the streets and which was fast and deep enough in places to overturn cars and sweep away people.[7] When the lahar arrived it was traveling at an estimated velocity of 12 meters per second and flowed for 10–20 minutes, during which time most of the town was devastated as buildings collapsed under the load of the moving flow. Survivors clung to moving pieces of debris or were swept along on top of the mud. Overall, the several inundations of mud lasted about 2 hours, with two slower-moving major pulses being accompanied by several smaller pulses over this time period.

The head of the lahar was turbulent and contained all manner of debris, including large boulders. The slurry mass buried victims or hurled them against stationary objects, and they were contorted and crushed by debris such as trees and collapsed parts of buildings. Stones and other sharp objects caused deep lacerations. The slurry forced its way into the mouth, eyes, ears and open wounds. Pressure against the chest inhibited breathing in those buried up to the neck as they were swept along in the flow, resulting in death by traumatic asphyxia.

The main injuries sustained by the hospitalized patients were severe crush injuries with open fractures, hemorrhagic, hypovolemic or traumatic shock, chest trauma (flail chest, pneumothorax), mud aspiration, and wound sepsis. More than two-thirds of the in-hospital deaths were ascribed to overwhelming infection, such as gas gangrene, ischemic gangrene, tetanus, and generalized sepsis or septic shock. Some patients had limbs amputated for the treatment of wound infections.[21]

An important cause of wound sepsis was primary suturing of infected or deep and extensive wounds without performing adequate debridement, instead of leaving them open for 5 days before closing (delayed primary closure) according to surgical best practice.

A small number of victims who were rescued after being immersed in the slurry for at least 3 days developed life-threatening necrotizing fasciitis caused by anaerobic and aerobic organisms in synergistic combinations. Zygomycetic organisms were identified in patients with more severe and rapidly progressing lesions. This dreaded complication was due to normally non-pathogenic soil organisms replicating in wounds in the absence of oxygen, and is notoriously resistant to medical treatment.[22]

The reason for so many people surviving when trapped in the lahar was due to its granular or sandy consistency. Lahars diluted by water in this way are called non-cohesive, because they contain relatively little clay, in contrast to the significantly denser cohesive types, which contain much clay derived from chemically altered rocks. However, the sandy consistency made access to the injured difficult and many had to be air-lifted from the slurry by helicopters. The lahar was originally hot enough to scald some victims, and so would have retained heat over several days; otherwise many trapped victims would have died from hypothermia before they could be rescued.

Mount Rainier in the U.S. state of Washington is the most hazardous volcano in the Cascade Range because of its potential for forming massive lahars that can travel long distances into areas that have become heavily populated.[23] Mount Rainier – at 4,393 meters (14,410 feet) above sea level – is the highest peak in the Cascade Range and its load of glacier ice exceeds that of any mountain in the contiguous United States.

Emergency planning and land utilization in the volcano's shadow are based on the footprint of the lahar hazard, which volcanologists say dominates the risk scenario above all other eruptive phenomena according to its past history and range of potential hazards. More fluid, non-cohesive lahars can form in future volcanic activity if huge quantities of meltwater are produced from glacier meltwater (as occurred at the Nevado del Ruiz tragedy in Colombia), but cohesive lahars can also form with little, if any warning, as in the early stages of activity when magma is forcing its way to the surface. This can occur because the flanks are formed by substantial volumes of unstable, water-rich, hydrothermally altered rock that can readily collapse to become either a dry debris flow or a dense lahar.[23]

In Ecuador, a vast, fast-moving lahar developed at Cotopaxi (5,897 meters high) from the melting of the summit ice in its last eruption in 1877. At the time of writing, the worst expected volcanic disaster in this country would be a repeat of the 1877 event in the Chillos valley, which has become much more populated since the nineteenth century, with the town of Lattacunga (population 80,000) only 50–70 minutes travel time for the lahar along its path. The damage to property and infras-

tructure, as well as the potential for extreme loss of life, would dwarf the losses suffered in the Nevado del Ruiz disaster given the greater economic development that has occurred in this high-risk zone.

Even small, non-cohesive lahars can be very dangerous. They commonly arise when thick ash deposits produced by eruptive activity become mobilized by heavy rains almost anywhere on a volcano. A serious complication in an eruption is the triggering of lahar formation when heavy rainfall is produced as large quantities of fine ash particles mix with rain clouds. Lahars can present lethal hazards for several years after large eruptions. This leaves thick ash deposits on flanks, as was seen following the Mount Pinatubo eruption in 1991, with resultant deaths and other very disruptive consequences for thousands of people living along the far end of the slopes of the volcano.

Ash Fall

Tephra is the ash and larger solid material emitted in the atmosphere during a volcanic eruption. The temperature of the erupted material and the mass eruption rate determine the height of the eruption column. These factors, along with wind strength and direction, are the principal controls on the long-distance transport and fallout of the tephra. Ash is defined by geologists as tephra less than 2 mm in diameter, but in explosive eruptions is typically fine-grained and forms thinner deposits with increasing distance downwind from the eruptive vent.[9,10]

Ash falls can affect very wide areas downwind of an erupting volcano, as far as hundreds of kilometers away and can have many different impacts on health and human activity over these long distances. The mixture of ash, gases, and aerosols that are injected into the atmosphere can circle the earth and have temporary effects on global weather and climate.[9,10] The most important aspects for disaster medicine are the immediate health and safety hazards that arise in a typical heavy ash fall, including those created by damage to infrastructure. A large conurbation would be most vulnerable to many of these, such as disruption to transport (including air travel), breakdown of utilities, and the injuries and loss of life from weaker structures collapsing under the accumulated weight of ash. The experiences of people present at the eruption of Mount St. Helens in 1980 provided important information for disaster planning for ash falls at most explosive volcanoes that have moved into a state of unrest.[24]

The first experience downwind of an eruption of this size is the cloud passing overhead and darkness growing as ash starts to fall. In some instances, pumice and other clast material in the fallout can be large enough to smash windshields and cause head injuries, so people should rapidly seek shelter. When fine ash settles on windshields it soon leaves smears if the windshield wipers are turned on; when wiper fluid is depleted, the driver can no longer see out of the windshield. If the ash fall is heavy, visibility can become zero. After dry ash has settled, moving motor vehicles resuspend it in the air and visibility may become severely limited. Rain accompanying an ash fall can make roads very slippery, resulting in collisions. Even without rain, steep inclines can become hazardous as vehicle wheels lose their grip on the road. Ash soon clogs engine air filters and can bring vehicles to a halt. All transport, including planes and trains, will grind to a halt if visibility becomes bad, a situation that lasted for 6 days in central Washington State after the eruption of Mount St. Helens on May 18, 1980, until an unseasonal rainfall in a normally arid area cleared the air of ash that was being constantly resuspended by winds. Volcanic ash severely damages jet engines and airplanes' superstructure, so airports will close after even a light deposit of ash on the runway. During the 6-week eruption of the Eyjafjallajökull volcano in Iceland in 2010, the ash plume persistently blew for 6 days over Europe. Although very little ash fell on the ground, the plume halted commercial air traffic during this period through fear it might damage the jet engines of aircraft in flight.

Ash settling on unprotected electrical insulators at substations can lead to outages from short circuits as it is a good conductor of electricity when it is wet. These outages in turn can stop water supplies, which depend on pumping. Drains and sewage systems can become blocked with the mass of ash when it is washed away by rain. Electronic equipment and computers are readily penetrated by fine ash (laptops depend on a small inside fan for drawing in air for cooling) and can be rendered useless. Hospital systems and equipment can fail. Falling ash and lightning strikes (frequent in some eruptions) can lead to serious communications disruptions, including the unavailability of wireless phones, television, radio, and any other technology requiring transmitters or repeaters.

Rates of accumulation of ash on horizontal surfaces can be as high as 10–20 cm/hour and weak roofs begin to collapse with an accumulated depth of wet ash of only 10 cm. The type of roof and its condition will determine the extent of damage. A collapsing roof can kill or injure the building's occupants by striking them with roof members and by burial in the inrushing ash leading to asphyxia.[25]

The respiratory health effects of ash from volcanoes may need specialized investigation and advice given to the populations affected, especially if an eruption continues intermittently over years, as there will be concern over potential long-term as well as acute effects to the lungs and airways.[26] Ash particles in explosive eruptions can comprise a high mass-proportion of respirable size (<4 μm), which can reach the alveoli, and thoracic size (<10 μm), which can enter the upper airways through the mouth and nose. The raised concentrations in ambient air of particles less than 10 μm in aerodynamic diameter (PM_{10}) can irritate the airways and provoke symptoms in people suffering from asthma and asthmatic bronchitis, as well as exacerbate the conditions of others with chronic cardiopulmonary diseases. The fine ash from silica-rich lava dome eruptions can contain very elevated levels of crystalline silica (cristobalite, quartz), and long-term exposure to repeated ash falls over many years has the potential to cause silicosis. This risk is apparent on Montserrat; long-term health checks and chest X-ray surveys are needed to confirm the effectiveness of the measures for preventing the disease in the general and working populations.[26]

Ballistic projectiles do not usually travel farther than 5 km from the crater. They are an important reason for evacuating a population living close to a volcano, even though other more critical hazards may dominate the eruption scenario. Hot ballistics, even of small size, can smash through corrugated metal roofs leaving small holes of entry but then shatter into fragments over furniture and trigger fires. Blocks a meter or more in size can leave large impact craters. A shower of ballistics is a very frightening experience and can leave an area with damaged or burned-out houses, roads and infrastructure (e.g., downed power lines).[27]

Volcanic Gases

A few volcanoes emit substantial amounts of gases in the plumes from their craters for years without showing any other activity. The summits of most volcanoes are so elevated that the plume does not result in hazardous concentrations in the ambient air. However, at a few low-lying volcanoes (e.g., Masaya, Nicaragua; Poas, Costa Rica), gas plume emissions can present health hazards for kilometers downwind of a volcano's vent. This is due to the irritant effects of sulfur dioxide on the airways, while soluble acid gases damage vegetation by direct fumigation or by making rain water intensely acid. Volcanologists entering crater areas to collect samples are at risk of being overcome by carbon dioxide and hydrogen sulfide.[28]

Soil gases can permeate into the atmosphere from the slopes of dormant volcanoes and their concentrations can accumulate in the indoor air of buildings with gas-permeable foundations.[29,30] Carbon dioxide is the main hazard, and the gas can also act as a carrier of the radioactive gas radon which is known to be a causal factor for lung cancer and can accrue inside poorly ventilated houses.[29,30]

A change in the composition of plume or soil gas and an increase in emission rate from a volcano can be the first sign of magma on the move, so these gases are routinely monitored for evidence of a renewal of volcanic activity.

A rare but important hazard in volcanic areas is an accumulation of carbon dioxide in solution in a pressurized hydrothermal system of a volcano or the buildup of huge amounts of carbon dioxide dissolved under the hydrostatic pressure of deep lakes. An event that triggers the sudden release of the carbon dioxide can lead to the formation of a lethal, denser than air cloud of asphyxiating gas. In the Dieng Plateau in Java, Indonesia in 1979, carbon dioxide was suddenly released from a vent in the ground, flowed down a slope, and killed 149 villagers fleeing from an incipient minor eruption.[31] Two thousand people died when a cloud of carbon dioxide was released late at night from Lake Nyos in Cameroon in 1986, with victims lying unconscious on the ground for hours before dying or regaining consciousness when the gas dispersed in the early morning.[32] Many deep lakes in volcanic areas around the world have been studied for carbon dioxide accumulation since that time, but only Lake Kivu in the Eastern Democratic Republic of Congo and Lake Albano near Rome have been identified so far as potential candidates for such releases. In a future eruption of Nyiragongo, the fissuring could extend into Goma and Lake Kivu, which is a highly stratified and deep lake (maximum depth 485 m) containing a huge quantity of carbon dioxide and methane dissolved in its deeper waters. These gases, derived from volcanic sources under the lake and from biodegradation of organic matter, have accumulated over the centuries and would be highly dangerous if suddenly released in a cloud that was blown over the populated shore (e.g., if a lava eruption occurred in the floor of the lake and its heat drove upwards gas-filled layers of water from depth). While the technology for degassing lakes before they become saturated with gas and highly hazardous (as occurred at Lake Nyos) is available, it is lacking for identifying hydrothermal systems below ground that might be waiting to explode when disturbed by the onset of volcanic activity.

Emergency Planning for Cities and Islands

At least half a million out of a megacity of 4 million people in the Bay of Naples area are at risk from pyroclastic flows and surges in a future eruption of Vesuvius, the volcano for which most emergency planning for a future eruption is being undertaken.[33] The event that leads the eruption risk and hence the planning scenario is its largest eruption in the last millennium, which occurred in 1631. A working maxim in volcanology is that the past behavior of the volcano is an important starting point in planning for a future eruption. In the 1631 event, pyroclastic density currents invaded a relatively sparsely inhabited area around the volcano which today is occupied by half a million people. Computer simulation modeling assists in defining their future run-outs, dynamic pressures, and temperature profiles, which can also be reconstructed in part from study of the deposits laid down in the 1631 eruption.[9] Civil protection has produced plans to evacuate the area of greatest hazard as defined by the scientists in a future emergency. Other, less extreme scenarios from previous eruptions exist, but as the size and type of eruption cannot be forecast with certainty, a hazard-based approach[34] acting on the basis of the worst expected event has been adopted at the time of writing. When the eruption will occur is unknown, but the hazard is potentially so serious that planning (and monitoring of the volcano) is performed on a continuing basis.

Populated volcanic islands present special challenges. On Montserrat in 1997 (over 2 years after the eruption had begun), the volcano's activity had gradually escalated to a level that a large pyroclastic density current-forming eruption could happen and destroy the remainder of the inhabited parts of the island, but such an event could not be forecast with certainty.[35] To provide the needed support for any decision, a group of scientists undertook an evidence-based risk assessment, the first ever of its kind in a volcanic crisis. It confirmed the volcanologists' judgment that beyond the prevailing high-risk areas and exclusion zone, the immediate risk to life from the volcano in its then eruptive state was similar to the background risks from other island hazards, namely earthquakes and hurricanes. Thus, a decision to evacuate the whole island was not needed. The methodological approach proved to be an important precedent for future volcanic crises.[33]

Lava flows have not entered a modern city, but the invasion of Goma by two lava flows in 2002 described previously shows how the destruction can be severe. In a complex emergency, such an eruption could lead to high mortality from ethnic conflict and expose thousands to infectious disease epidemics and the risk of starvation. At Mount Rainier, the horrors of Armero in 1984 could be visited on the large population in the Puget Sound lowland area, but monitoring and warning systems and emergency planning are in place to help prevent such a disaster.[23] While actual experience is limited in terms of the direct and indirect impacts of ash on the health and safety of an urban population (and what mitigation measures will be feasible to offset the immediate risks), a large ash fall with a depth of 0.5–1 meter on a city would most likely lead to complete paralysis of the city's functioning. Massive and costly clearance operations to remove the vast quantities of ash would be required to restore the city's infrastructure.

Ideally, the response of emergency planners and decision-makers should be proportionate to the potential hazards and risks of the volcano, as foreseen by volcanologists and based on available evidence about the volcano itself and its past eruptions, as well as the data from previous eruptions at other similar volcanoes. As mentioned earlier, the response of the public may be very variable, depending on whether they understand the nature of the hazards they may encounter; whether they trust the officials, the scientists, and the media; and whether they can come to terms with the options they may face for

the future of their homes, families, and livelihoods. This is complicated by the inevitable uncertainty over the volcano's behavior and scientists' limitations in precise forecasting of the type, size, and duration of the eruption. Consequently, an eruption of an explosive volcano in a densely populated region or small island places onerous challenges on emergency responders.

The Need for Medical Planning

The largest volcanic catastrophe in the twentieth century was the obliteration of the city of St. Pierre in Martinique in 1902 when it was struck by a violent surge from the volcano Mont Pelée after it had been threatening catastrophe for weeks beforehand. The population of at least 28,000 had been living in fear while officials were unable, on the limited understanding of volcanoes at the time, to take decisive action and move them away from the danger. They died within minutes from a fireball that was ignited by the hot ash as the pyroclastic density current swept through the entire city, leaving only two survivors. This eruption led to a fatalism amongst volcanologists that remained in place for decades. The thought was that such eruptions cannot be survived, which has influenced planners to this day, who may see little point in preparing for mass casualties and instead focus on evacuation measures and rely on volcanologists to provide adequate warning.

Uncertainly surrounding eruption forecasting coupled with unpredictable behaviors of sometimes hundreds of thousands of people under threat makes management of a crisis that results in a major explosive eruption without loss of life extraordinarily challenging, even by the most competent officials and volcanologists.

An example of the need for medical preparedness was the eruption of Merapi in 2010 when the volcanic activity increased faster than expected and people had little time to evacuate. The volcano is situated 25–30 km north of the metropolitan area of Yogyakarta, Indonesia, and in October–November 2010, decades of small to moderate eruptions were overturned with little warning. Over a period of 11 days, swathes of the volcano's slopes were swept by pyroclastic density currents in the most explosive eruption for 100 years. About 10,000 to 20,000 lives were saved by three rapid-phased evacuations called by a group of international volcanologists closely monitoring the volcano.[36] The scientists initially raised the alert level to indicate that there was increased activity on September 20, but the volcano did not become threatening until October 25, when they gave the first call to evacuate, which included everyone within 10 km of the summit. This was followed by a blast-driven pyroclastic density current only 35 hours later; twenty-five of thirty-nine people who refused to leave the area were killed outright and four of the eleven who were treated for their severe burns in hospital survived. The second call to extend the evacuation zone to 15 km on November 3 increased the number of displaced people to 100,000 and was followed 1.5 hours later by pyroclastic density currents travelling to 12 km, but without casualties. Then, only 2 days later, the activity rose rapidly to a climax and a rushed call to extend the evacuation area was followed by another major explosive event within a few hours (just after midnight); at least 200 people who had not left the danger area in time were killed as a pyroclastic density current ran 15.5 km down a main valley and over-spilled into the still-occupied houses along the banks, causing fires and fatal burns.

In contrast, volcanic crises that continue for months and years without major eruptions can induce risk fatigue, leading to evacuees returning against official advice and being killed by a sudden, dangerous turn in the volcano's state. On Montserrat, nineteen people died instantly in a pyroclastic density current in such a tragic event.[37] An emergency medical plan had been in place from early on in the crisis for medical assistance to be sent when needed from the nearby island of Guadeloupe; five casualties were air-lifted there by helicopter for treatment of burns in this incident.

Triage and Treatment of Burns in Surge Eruptions

Due to the rarity of eruptions in densely populated regions, the evidence base to guide management and treatment of mass casualties in dilute pyroclastic density current eruptions is sparse. Early reports were discouraging. At a surge eruption at Mount Unzen in Japan in 1991, forty-one onlookers, including three volcanologists, were engulfed in a surge and thirteen people who survived with severe burns were transported to a nearby hospital that had conducted a mass casualty exercise for such an eventuality only 5 days before. They arrived in 20 to 40 minutes; endotracheal intubation was performed in six patients and tracheostomy was necessary in seven who had the most severe airway injuries. Their ages were 16–43 years. Only one patient, who had 40% TBSA and did not have inhalation injury, recovered. Six of the victims died in the first 2 days: their burns were 90–100% TBSA. The remainder comprised four patients with >80% TBSA and two patients with 40% TBSA who had severe inhalation injury. The former group were in the periphery of the surge and although badly burned were able to walk out of the impacted area; they eventually died in the hospital from acute renal failure. The latter group of patients was standing farther inside the surge. Although their bodies were somehow more protected, the hot ash was driven into their mouths and lungs and was found as far as the alveoli; they died from their lung injuries.[38] Three fit loggers were rescued at the Mount St. Helens eruption in 1980; they had been working together when struck by the surge and had similar burn severity (33–46% TBSA), but only the one who had not suffered inhalation injury recovered after hospital treatment.[39]

The largest series of volcano burn casualties in the world is derived from two eruptions that included surges of Merapi volcano in 1994 and 2010, which briefly enveloped victims, exposing them to hot ash clouds at temperatures at 200–300°C. The first was a dome collapse eruption in which a pyroclastic density current ran down a valley and two dilute surges detached and ran into a small village and a wedding party; the second was the large-scale eruption in 2010. In the 1994 event, twenty-four died at the scene, eighty-one were admitted to the main hospital in Yogyakarta, and twenty-three of these patients survived. In 2010, in two separate surge events (October 26 and November 5), seventy-nine died at the two scenes or on the way to the Yogyakarta hospital; twenty-nine lived to be treated in hospital, of which nine survived. The mortality rate was highest in the first 2–3 days of admission, mainly in the patients with severe burns who also had severe inhalation injury from breathing in the hot ash.

The management of mass burn casualties represents a challenges as it requires substantial resources. Even well-resourced countries have limited burn unit capacity with specialist surgical and nursing care and would be ill-prepared for management of a large number of severely burned patients. Treatment should be prioritized according to age and percent TBSA, with elderly (>60 years) suffering over 40% TBSA being lowest priority, as they are least likely to benefit from intensive treatment. Children under 2 years require highest priority.

An example of a provisional matrix scale of burn severity in volcanic eruptions as a guide for casualty management is suggested for a pyroclastic surge striking an urban area. Many victims would be killed instantly by exposure to intense heat in an irrespirable ash cloud, including most of those caught outdoors, as already explained. However, in locations sheltered by topography or other buildings, burns to the skin, airways, and lung would be the main cause of life-threatening injury:

Level 1. Minor effects of heat (e.g., singed hair, superficial burns to uncovered skin). Low mortality.
Level 2. Burns to 20–40% TBSA; moderate inhalational lung injury. Mortality dependent on treatment resources, patient age, and existing illnesses. Without early treatment in a large-scale disaster, many may die.
Level 3. Burns >40% TBSA; severe inhalation injury. Mortality risk high in first few days because of inhalation injury.
Level 4. Burns >40% and advanced age, existing chronic cardiopulmonary or other systemic diseases raising vulnerability. Probably poor response to treatment. Mortality nearing 100%.

Other injuries can be expected, such as lacerations from broken glass when windows are imploded by the pressure impact of the surge, and smoke inhalation from fires ignited by the hot ash in contact with combustible materials in streets and inside dwellings.

More than a small number of casualties with 20–40% TBSA burns would exceed the national burn unit capacity of most countries, yet this group could comprise a large number of the volcano victims. Survival would be largely dependent on the speed of search and rescue operations and time taken until they received definitive treatment. National and international burns centers would need to be available to receive patients in transfer when local facilities were overwhelmed.

At the time of writing, few large events involving mass burn casualties have occurred; the most notable were the Los Alfaques camping ground explosion in Spain in 1978,[40] and the Ufa gas explosion in the Soviet Union in 1989.[41] However, the scenario in a volcanic eruption would be altogether different. Rescue attempts would be hampered by the continuing eruption, with previous ash falls and resuspended ash preventing access. A thick deposit of hot ash on the ground would prevent immediate entry to the disaster area by road (tires can catch fire and shoes ignite on contact with thick pyroclastic deposits before they have cooled). Concern that the eruption was not yet over, and the threat of a further pyroclastic surge, would keep rescuers away for hours until it seemed likely that the activity had subsided. Helicopters would be needed for rapid movement of rescuers and patients, but these might not fly if too much ash were in the air as this could interfere with the engines.

RECOMMENDATIONS FOR FURTHER RESEARCH

A risk-based (probabilistic) approach in planning for volcanic crises has gained wide acceptance. Experts begin by setting out

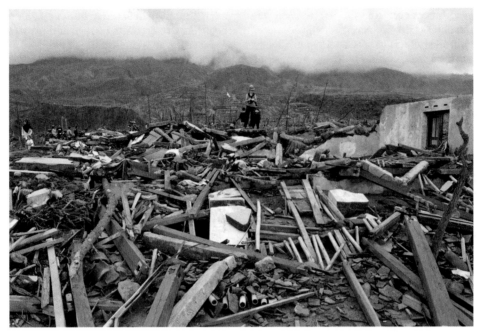

Figure 43.2. Merapi volcano eruption, Indonesia, 2010: buildings in Kinarhejo village flattened by a directed blast surge from volcano in background and hidden by cloud. High temperature of ash deposit not intense enough to burn or char wood. The timbers lie orientated in the direction of the blast. Area evacuated in advance.

the reasonably foreseeable eruptive events in a logic (or event) tree. The full range of eruption scenarios can be developed from this and the tree branches can be populated with conditional probabilities derived through a formal elicitation and expert judgment process. This approach was first applied to a volcanic crisis in Montserrat in 1997[35] and is analogous to the evidence-based methods and decision trees that are used in medicine in diagnosis or treatment in the face of clinicians' uncertainty.[33] This methodology seems especially applicable to the complex (chaotic) behavior of volcanoes and is beginning to be more widely used as a powerful way to quantify risk and to identify the most important eruptive scenarios for emergency planning purposes.

Rapid advances in computer simulation modeling of flow hazards and ash fallout, combined with studies of building and road vulnerability, are being applied in hazard and risk formulation through the involvement of supercomputers. They are also beginning to be used to support decision making in crises. The MESIMEX exercise in the fall of 2006 in Naples was the first "real-time" exercise to test emergency plans during a state of unrest lasting 5 days and escalating toward an eruption. The exercise incorporated computer modeling for forecasting the direction of the wind and the building damage footprint under the ash plume, so as to inform decisions "in real-time" on the safest routes for evacuation of the population around Vesuvius.

Models to estimate casualties from tephra fallout[42,43,44] and pyroclastic surges[45,46,47] based on the vulnerability of buildings and their occupants to impacts quantified by numerical simulation are beginning to be applied in civil protection planning at Vesuvius and Campi Flegrei. For the first time, three-dimensional numerical simulation modeling of pyroclastic surges using supercomputer technology[48] opens up new opportunities for disaster planning in cities and greater scope for interaction between volcanologists and decision-makers.

Conclusion

Volcanic activity is infrequent compared with other hazards. There is less public awareness than for events like earthquakes, floods, and windstorms, until a dangerous volcano moves out of a state of repose and threatens a nearby populated area. Planners need to be prepared for a wide range of volcanic hazards and the possibility that a state of unrest or an actual eruption could last for months or even years. This compounds the complexity of the level of emergency management needed.

Timely evacuation is the main goal in emergency management of major volcanic threats, but disaster planners must also recognize the scientific uncertainties in making relocation decisions and managing public risk perception. Complete or partial relocations may last months and measures to support displaced persons are essential, or people may soon prefer to accept a high risk and demand to return to their homes against the advice of scientists and governmental authorities. In a prolonged crisis in which a forecasted major eruption fails to occur, public perceptions can quickly become highly distorted as a disillusioned population becomes habituated to risk taking and starts to ignore official warnings. Despite the striking developments in technologies for monitoring volcanoes with field and satellite equipment and the benefit these have provided in some crises and with certain types of volcanoes, substantial limitations on forecasting eruption scenarios remain.[49] The potential for events with mass casualties from the unforeseen may remain throughout the duration of most volcanic crises, not just when an eruption begins.[50]

Pyroclastic density currents can be formed in several different ways. Among the most dangerous are lateral blasts, as occurred at Mount St. Helens, when the side of the volcano suddenly gave way after two months of unrest during which the volcano was inflating and weakening under internal pressure.[6] The Soufrière Hills volcano on Montserrat has been erupting since 1995, with its most significant events being caused by the growth and collapse of large domes of heaped-up, viscous lava, extruded slowly over weeks and months like toothpaste from its conduit in the crater and cooling to form dome rock. This then breaks up in each major collapse to fragment into pyroclastic density currents that flow into low lying areas.[35] At other volcano types, large explosive eruptions often begin with vertical eruption columns, which can last several hours and sometimes days. At any stage, parts of the column of ash and gases may lose their buoyancy and descend as pyroclastic density currents down the flank of the volcano, as occurred in the famous eruption of Vesuvius in AD 79 that destroyed Pompeii and killed the remnants of the population who had not left the city.[42] As these eruptions lose more of their energy, pyroclastic density currents may also form by a process known as "boiling over" the crater rim. Pyroclastic density current impacts depend mainly on their temperature, density and velocity, all of which can vary widely according to how they are generated and other factors like the topography of the volcano. Most fast moving surges have devastating potential (Figure 43.2).

REFERENCES

1. Baxter PJ. Medical effects of volcanoes. 1. Main causes of death and injury. *Bull Volcanol* 1990; 52: 532–544.
2. Jenkins S, Komorowski J-C, Baxter PJ, et al. The Merapi 2010 eruption: an interdisciplinary impact assessment methodology for studying pyroclastic density current dynamics. *J Volcanol Geotherm Res* 2013; 261: 316–329.
3. Newhall CG, Punongbayan RS. The narrow margin of successful volcanic risk mitigation. Scarpa R, Tilling RI, eds. *Monitoring and mitigation of volcano hazards*. Berlin, Springer, 1996; 809–838.
4. Witham CS. Volcanic disasters and incidents: a new database. *J Volcanol Geotherm Res* 2005; 148: 191–233.
5. Heiken G. *Dangerous Neighbors: Volcanoes and Cities*. Cambridge, Cambridge University Press, 2013.
6. Newhall CG. Mount St Helens, master teacher. *Science* 2000; 288: 1181–1183.
7. Voight B. The management of volcanic emergencies: Nevado del Ruiz. Scarpa R, Tilling RI, eds. *Monitoring and mitigation of volcano hazards*. Berlin, Springer, 1996; 719–769.
8. Spence RJS, Pomonis A, Baxter PJ, et al. Building damage caused by the Mount Pinatubo eruption of June 15, 1991. In: Newhall CG, Punongbayan RS, eds. *Fire and Mud: eruptions and lahars at Mount Pinatubo, Philippines*. Seattle, University of Washington Press, 1996; 1055–1061.
9. Schmincke H-U. *Volcanism*. Berlin, Springer, 2004.
10. Oppenheimer C, Francis P. *Volcanoes*. 2nd ed. Cambridge, Cambridge University Press, 2004.
11. Oppenheimer C. *Eruptions that Shook the World*. Cambridge, Cambridge University Press, 2011.
12. Baxter PJ, Boyle R, Cole P, et al. The impacts of pyroclastic surges on buildings at the eruption of the Soufrière Hills volcano, Montserrat. *Bull Volcanol* 2005; 67: 292–313.
13. Baxter PJ, Neri A, Todesco M. Physical modeling and human survival in pyroclastic flows. *Natural Hazards* 1998; 17: 163–176.
14. Eisele JW, O'Halloran RL, Reay DT, et al. Deaths during the May 18, 1980, eruption of Mount St Helens. *N Engl J Med* 1981; 305, 931–936.
15. Baxter PJ, Gresham A. Deaths and injuries in the eruption of Galeras volcano, Colombia, 14 January 1993. *J Volcanol Geotherm Res* 1997; 77: 325–338.
16. Morrisey MM, Mastin LG. Vulcanian eruptions. In: Sigurdsson H, Houghton BF, McNutt, SR, Rymer H, Stix J, eds. *Encyclopedia of Volcanoes*. San Diego, CA, Academic Press, 2000; 463–475.
17. Tilling RI, Peterson DW. Field observation of active lava in Hawaii: some practical considerations. In: Kilburn CRJ, Luongo G, eds. *Active Lavas: monitoring and modeling*. London, UCL Press, 1993; 147–174.
18. Salama P, Spiegel P, Talley L, Waldman R. Lessons learned from complex emergencies over past decade. *Lancet* 2004; 364: 1801–1813.
19. Baxter P, Allard P, Halbwachs M, et al. Human health and vulnerability in the Nyiragongo volcano eruption and humanitarian crisis at Goma, Democratic Republic of Congo. *Acta Vulcanologica* 2002–2003; 14–15: 109–114.
20. Komorowski J-C, Tedesco D, Kasareka M, et al. The January 2002 flank eruption of Nyiragongo volcano (Democratic Republic of Congo): chronology, evidence for a tectonic rift trigger, and impact of lava flows on the city of Goma. *Acta Vulcanologica* 2002–2003; 14–15: 27–62.
21. Organización Panamericana de la Salud. Cronicas de Desastres. Erupción Volcánica en Colombia. November 13, 1985.
22. Patiño JF, Castro D, Valencia A, Morales P. Necrotizing soft tissue lesions after a volcanic cataclysm. *World J Surg* 1991; 15: 240–247.
23. Hoblitt RP, Walder JS, Driedger CL, et al. *Volcano hazards from Mount Rainier, Washington. Open file report 98–428*. Denver, U.S. Geological Survey, 1998.
24. Buist AS, Bernstein RS, eds. Health effects of volcanoes: an approach to evaluating the health effects of an environmental hazard. *American Journal of Public Health Medicine* 1986; 76(Suppl.): 1–90.
25. Pomonis A, Spence R, Baxter P. Risk assessment of residential buildings for an eruption of Furnas volcano, São Miguel, the Azores. *J Volcanol Geotherm Res* 1999; 92: 107–131.
26. Horwell CJ, Baxter PJ. The respiratory health hazards of volcanic ash: a review for volcanic risk mitigation. *Bull Volcanol* 2006; 69: 1–24.
27. Blong RJ. *Volcanic hazards: a sourcebook on the effects of eruptions*. Sydney, Academic Press, 1984.
28. Allen AG, Baxter PJ, Uttley CJ. Gas and particle emissions from Soufrière Hills Volcano, Montserrat. *Bull Volcanol* 2000; 62: 8–19.
29. Baxter PJ, Baubron J-C, Coutinho R. Health hazards and disaster potential of ground gas emissions at Furnas volcano, Sao Miguel, Azores. *J Volcanol Geotherm Res* 1999; 92: 95–106.
30. Carapezza ML, Badalamenti B, Cavarra L, Scalzo A. Gas hazard assessment in a densely inhabited area of Colli Albani Volcano (Cava dei Selci, Roma). *J Volcanol Geotherm Res* 2003; 123: 81–94.
31. Le Guern F, Tazieff H, Faivre Pierret RX. An example of health hazard: people killed by gas during a phreatic eruption Dieng Plateau (Java), Indonesia, February 20th 1979. *Bull Volcanol* 1982; 45(2): 153–156.
32. Baxter PJ, Kapila M, Mfonfu D. Lake Nyos disaster, Cameroon, 1986: the medical effects of large scale emission of carbon dioxide? *BMJ* 1989; 298: 1437–1441.
33. Baxter PJ, Aspinall WP, Neri A, et al. Emergency planning and mitigation at Vesuvius: a new evidence-based approach. *J Volcanol Geotherm Res* 2008; 454–473.
34. Rosi M. Quantitative reconstruction of recent volcanic activity: a contribution to forecasting of future eruptions. In: Scarpa R,

Tilling RI, eds. *Monitoring and mitigation of volcano hazards.* Berlin, Springer, 1996; 631–674.

35. Druitt TH, Kokelaar BP, eds. *The eruption of Soufrière volcano, Montserrat, from 1995 to 1999.* London, Geological Society, Memoirs, 21, 2002.

36. Surono, Jousset P, Pallister J, et al. The 2010 explosive eruption of Java's Merapi volcano – a "100-year" event. *J Volcanol Geotherm Res* 2012; 241–242: 121–135.

37. Loughlin SC, Baxter PJ, Aspinall WP, et al. Eyewitness accounts of the 25 June 1997 pyroclastic flows and surges at Soufrière Hills volcano, Montserrat, and implications for disaster mitigation. In: Druitt TH, Kokelaar BP, eds. *The eruption of Soufrière Hills volcano, Montserrat, from 1995 to 1999.* London, Geological Society, Memoirs, 21, 2002; 211–230.

38. Kobayashi K, Hirano A, Murakami R, et al. Pyroclastic flow injury: Mount Unzen-Fugen, June 3, 1991. *Journal of the Japanese Society for Burns Injury* 1993; 19: 226–235.

39. Parshley PF, Kiessling PJ, Antonius JA, et al. Pyroclastic flow injury. Mount St. Helens May 18, 1980. *Am J Surg* 1982; 143: 565–568.

40. Arturson G,. The Los Alfaques disaster: a boiling-liquid, expanding vapour explosion. *Burns* 1981; 7: 233–251.

41. Kulyapin AV, Sakhautdinov VG, Temerbutalov VM, et al. Bashkiria train-gas pipeline disaster: a history of the joint ASSR/USA collaboration. *Burns* 1990; 16: 339–342.

42. Dobran F, Neri A, Todesco M. Assessing the pyroclastic flow hazard at Vesuvius. *Nature* 1994; 367: 551–554.

43. Barberi F, Macedonio G, Pareschi MT, Santacroce R. Mapping the tephra fallout risk: an example from Vesuvius, Italy. *Nature* 1990; 344: 142–144.

44. Spence RJS, Kelman I, Calogero E, et al. Modeling expected physical impacts and human casualties from explosive eruptions. *Natural Hazards and Earth System Sciences* 2005; 5: 1003–1015.

45. Spence RJS, Kelman I, Baxter PJ, et al. Residential building and occupant vulnerability to tephra fall. *Nat Hazards Earth Syst Sci* 2005; 5: 1–18.

46. Spence RJS, Zuccaro G, Petrazzuoli S, Baxter PJ. Resistance of buildings to pyroclastic flows: analytical and experimental studies and their application to Vesuvius. *Natural Hazards Review*, 2004(b); 5: 48-59.

47. Spence R, Kelman I, Brown A, et al. Residential building and occupant vulnerability to pyroclastic density currents in explosive eruptions. *Nat Hazards Earth Syst Sci* 2007; 7: 219–230.

48. Neri A, Ongaro TE, Menconi G, et al. 4D simulation of explosive eruption dynamics at Vesuvius. *Geophys Res Lett* 2007; 34: L04309.

49. Sparks RSJ, Aspinall WP. Volcanic activity: frontiers and challenges in forecasting, prediction and risk assessment. In: *The State of the Planet: Frontiers and Challenges in Geophysics.* Geophysical Monograph 150, IUGG 2004; 19: 359–373.

50. Simkin T, Siebert S, Blong R. Volcano fatalities – lessons from the historical record. *Science* 2001; 291: 255.

INDEX